INTRODUCTION TO
Critical Care Nursing

INTRODUCTION TO

Critical Care
Nursing

FIFTH EDITION

Mary Lou Sole, PhD, RN, CCNS, CNL, FAAN
Professor
College of Nursing
University of Central Florida;
Clinical Nurse Research Scientist
Orlando Regional Medical Center
Orlando, Florida

Deborah G. Klein, MSN, RN, CCRN, CS
Clinical Nurse Specialist
Cardiac ICU and Heart Failure Special Care Unit
Cleveland Clinic;
Clinical Instructor
Frances Payne Bolton School of Nursing
Case Western Reserve University
Cleveland, Ohio;
Adjunct Clinical Associate
School of Nursing
Kent State University
Kent, Ohio

Marthe J. Moseley, PhD, RN, CCRN, CCNS, CNL
Clinical Nurse Specialist, Critical Care
South Texas Veterans Health Care System;
Adjunct Associate Professor
University of Texas Health Science Center School of Nursing
San Antonio, Texas;
Professor
Rocky Mountain University of Health Professions
Provo, Utah

SAUNDERS

ELSEVIER

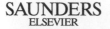

SAUNDERS
ELSEVIER

11830 Westline Industrial Drive
St. Louis, Missouri 63146

Introduction to Critical Care Nursing   ISBN: 978-1-4160-5656-0

Notice

Knowledge and best practice in this field are constantly changing. As new research and experience broaden our knowledge, changes in practice, treatment and drug therapy may become necessary or appropriate. Readers are advised to check the most current information provided (i) on procedures featured or (ii) by the manufacturer of each product to be administered, to verify the recommended dose or formula, the method and duration of administration, and contraindications. It is the responsibility of the practitioner, relying on their own experience and knowledge of the patient, to make diagnoses, to determine dosages and the best treatment for each individual patient, and to take all appropriate safety precautions. To the fullest extent of the law, neither the Publisher nor the Authors assumes any liability for any injury and/or damage to persons or property arising out of or related to any use of the material contained in this book.

The Publisher

Previous editions copyrighted 2005, 2001, 1997, 1993

Library of Congress Cataloging-in-Publication Data
Introduction to critical care nursing / [edited by] Mary Lou Sole, Deborah G. Klein, Marthe J. Moseley.—5th ed.
        p. ; cm.
    Includes bibliographical references and index. ISBN 978-1-4160-5656-0 (hardcover : alk. paper)   1. Intensive care nursing.   I. Sole, Mary Lou.   II. Klein, Deborah G.   III. Moseley, Marthe J.   IV. Title: Critical care nursing.
[DNLM: 1. Critical Care.   2. Nursing Care. WY 154 I618 2009] RT120.I5.I58 2009
616.02′8—dc22

                                                                        2008032381

Managing Editor: Maureen Iannuzzi
Senior Developmental Editor: Jennifer Ehlers
Publishing Services Manager: Deborah Vogel
Project Manager: Brandilyn Tidwell
Designer: Paula Catalano

Printed in the United States of America

Last digit is the print number: 9   8   7   6   5   4   3   2   1

To my daughter, Erin, and husband, Bob, who continue to "allow" mom time to "work on the book" while asking, "When will you be done with it?" To the many students learning critical care concepts, and their teachers, who provide ongoing feedback to make this textbook better and better.

MLS

To the critical care nurses, patients, and their families, who are always teaching me. To my husband, Ron, and my sons, David and Seth, for their support in all that I do. To my parents, Rena Goldenberg, RN, BSN, and Ira Goldenberg, MD, for their guidance and inspiration.

DGK

To my colleagues, especially Dean Harden, Rick Barfield, Kelly Echevarria, Dr. Antonio Hernandez, and Dr. Marcos Restrepo; graduate students, Dave Allen and Max Martell, who care about critical care and caring for patients, families, and teams; most especially to my son, Nicholas. To Marjory Olson, MSN, RN, and Sandra Berrigan, RN, MSN, MHA, who support all that I do.

MJM

About The Authors

MARY LOU SOLE

Mary Lou Sole, PhD, RN, CCNS, CNL, FAAN, has extensive experience in critical care practice, education, consultation, and research. She is a Professor at the University of Central Florida College of Nursing in Orlando, Florida. She also has a per diem appointment as a Clinical Nurse Research Scientist at Orlando Regional Medical Center. As part of her teaching assignment, Dr. Sole often teaches the undergraduate critical care elective course and teaches the acute care clinical nurse specialist courses. She began her career as a diploma graduate from the Ohio Valley General Hospital School of Nursing in Wheeling, West Virginia. She received a BSN from Ohio University, a master's degree in nursing from the Ohio State University, and a PhD in nursing from the University of Texas at Austin. Dr. Sole has published over 50 articles in peer-reviewed journals, the majority of articles focusing on critical care nursing and nursing education. She has received grant funding from the National Institutes of Health to study airway management in critically ill patients. Dr. Sole has been active locally and nationally in many professional organizations, including the American Association of Critical-Care Nurses. She has received numerous local, state, and national awards for clinical practice, teaching, and research. In 1997, she was inducted as a Fellow of the American Academy of Nursing. In 2008, she received the University of Central Florida's top honor, the Pegasus Professor.

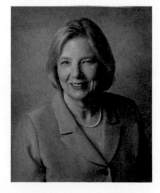

DEBORAH G. KLEIN

Deborah G. Klein, MSN, RN, CCRN, CS, has more than 30 years of experience in critical care practice, education, consultation, and research. She is currently Clinical Nurse Specialist for the Cardiac ICU and Heart Failure Special Care Unit at the Cleveland Clinic in Cleveland, Ohio. She is a Clinical Instructor at Frances Payne Bolton School of Nursing, Case Western Reserve University; and Adjunct Clinical Associate at Kent State University School of Nursing. She received her BSN and MSN from Frances Payne Bolton School of Nursing, Case Western Reserve University, in Cleveland, Ohio. She is active both locally and nationally in professional organizations, including the American Association of Critical-Care Nurses. She has served on editorial boards of several critical care nursing journals and has published over 35 book chapters and articles on critical care topics in peer-reviewed journals. Mrs. Klein has received local and national awards for clinical practice and teaching.

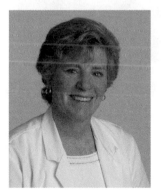

MARTHE J. MOSELEY

Marthe J. Moseley, PhD, RN, CCRN, CCNS, CNL, has more than 20 years of experience in critical care practice, education, consultation, and research. She is currently a Clinical Nurse Specialist for Critical Care at the South Texas Veterans Health Care System in San Antonio, Texas. She also has a Professor position at Rocky Mountain University of Health Professions in Provo, Utah, and has an Adjunct Associate Professor position at the University of Texas Health Science Center School of Nursing at San Antonio, Texas. As a role component of the Clinical Nurse Specialist, Dr. Moseley regularly facilitates orientation to critical care. She received a bachelor of arts degree in nursing from Jamestown College in Jamestown, North Dakota, following the completion of a BA degree in health, physical education, and biology from Concordia College in Moorhead, Minnesota. She completed her MSN and PhD at the University of Texas Health Science Center in San Antonio, Texas. She has been active locally and nationally in professional organizations, specifically the American Association of Critical-Care Nurses, as well as within the VA system. She is on the editorial board for several critical care journals and has published in peer-reviewed journals on critical care topics. Dr. Moseley has received local and national awards for clinical practice and teaching.

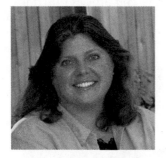

Contributors

Karla S. Ahrns-Klas, BSN, RN, CCRP
Trauma Burn Services Coordinator
Trauma Burn Center
University of Michigan
Ann Arbor, Michigan
Burns

Christina Amidei, MSN, RN, CNRN, CCRN, CS
Instructor
College of Nursing
University of Central Florida
Orlando, Florida
Nervous System Alterations

Mamoona Arif, MSN, RN, CCRN
MRICU Nurse Clinician
Virginia Commonwealth University Hospital
Richmond, Virginia
Comfort and Sedation

Zara R. Brenner, MS, ACNS, BC
Assistant Professor of Nursing
State University of New York at Brockport
Brockport, New York;
Clinical Nurse Specialist and Care Manager
Rochester General Hospital
Rochester, New York
Endocrine Alterations

Robin Donohoe Dennison, DNP, RN, CCNS
Assistant Professor of Clinical Nursing
College of Nursing
University of Cincinnati
Cincinnati, Ohio;
Critical Care Nursing Consultant
Robin Dennison Presents, Inc.
Winchester, Kentucky
Shock, Sepsis, and Multiple Organ Dysfunction Syndrome

Janet Goshorn, MSN, ARNP, BC
Nurse Practitioner
Florida Hospital Medical Center
Orlando, Florida
Acute Renal Failure

Mary Jo Grap, PhD, RN, ACNP, FAAN
Professor, Adult Health Nursing
School of Nursing
Virginia Commonwealth University
Richmond, Virginia
Comfort and Sedation

Joseph Haymore, MS, RN, CNRN, CCRN, ACNP
Neurosurgery and Neurocritical Nurse
    Practitioner
NeuroCare Associates
Kensington, Maryland
Nervous System Alterations

Carolyn D. Hix, DNP, RN, CNAA
Assistant Professor
Middle Tennessee State University
Murfreesboro, Tennessee
Acute Respiratory Failure

Max Hosmanek, MSN, RN, CCRN
Staff Nurse
Surgical Intensive Care Unit
South Texas Veterans Health Care System
San Antonio, Texas
The Critical Care Experience

Douglas Houghton, MSN, ARNP, CCRN
Nurse Practitioner
Trauma Intensive Care Unit
Ryder Trauma Center
Jackson Health System
Miami, Florida
End-of-Life Care in the Critical Care Unit

Melissa L. Hutchinson, MN, RN, CCRN, CWCN
Clinical Nurse Specialist, MICU/CCU
VA Puget Sound Healthcare System
Seattle, Washington
Nutritional Support

Deborah G. Klein, MSN, RN, CCRN, CS
Clinical Nurse Specialist
Cardiac ICU and Heart Failure Special Care
    Unit
Cleveland Clinic;
Clinical Instructor
Frances Payne Bolton School of Nursing
Case Western Reserve University
Cleveland, Ohio;
Adjunct Clinical Associate
School of Nursing
Kent State University
Kent, Ohio
*Code Management; Nervous System Alterations;
    Transplantation features*

Carl Laffoon, MSN, ARNP, CEN, EMT-P, FACHE
Doctor of Nursing Practice Candidate
Rocky Mountain University of Health Professions
Provo, Utah
Gastrointestinal Alterations

Susan Loyola, MSN, RN
Regional Education
Baptist Health System
San Antonio, Texas
Dysrhythmia Interpretation and Management

Mary Beth Flynn Makic, RN, PhD, CNS, CCNS, CCRN
Clinical Nurse Specialist/Educator
Burn Trauma ICU and Neuroscience ICU
University of Colorado Hospital
Denver, Colorado;
Senior Instructor
University of Colorado Health Sciences Center
School of Nursing
Arvada, Colorado
Trauma and Surgical Management

Marthe J. Moseley, PhD, RN, CCRN, CCNS, CNL
Clinical Nurse Specialist, Critical Care
South Texas Veterans Health Care System
Adjunct Associate Professor
University of Texas Health Science Center School
   of Nursing
San Antonio, Texas;
Professor
Rocky Mountain University of Health Professions
Provo, Utah
*Hemodynamic Monitoring; Cardiovascular Alterations;
   Gastrointestinal Alterations*

Jana L. Nohrenberg, MSN, APRN-BC, CCNS
Major, United States Army Nurse Corps
William Beaumont Army Medical Center
Intensive Care Unit
El Paso, Texas
Hemodynamic Monitoring

Lynelle N. B. Pierce, MSN, RN, CCRN
Clinical Assistant Professor
University of Kansas School of Nursing;
Critical Care Clinical Nurse Specialist
University of Kansas Hospital
Kansas City, Kansas
Ventilatory Assistance

Jeanne Powers, MS, RN, CCRN
Clinical Nurse Specialist
Medical Intensive Care Unit
Rochester General Hospital
Rochester, New York
Endocrine Alterations

Maryjane N. Randels, JD, BSN, RN
Orlando, Florida
Ethical and Legal Issues in Critical Care Nursing

Mary Lou Sole, PhD, RN, CCNS, CNL, FAAN
Professor
College of Nursing
University of Central Florida;
Clinical Nurse Research Scientist
Orlando Regional Medical Center
Orlando, Florida
*Overview of Critical Care Nursing; The Critical Care
   Experience; Hemodynamic Monitoring; Ventilatory
   Assistance*

Linda M. Tamburri, MSN, RN, CCRN, CS
Clinical Nurse Specialist
Critical Care Medicine
Robert Wood Johnson University Hospital
New Brunswick, New Jersey
Acute Respiratory Failure

Jayne M. Willis, MSN, RN
Patient Care Administrator
Orlando Regional Medical Center
Orlando, Florida
Ethical and Legal Issues in Critical Care Nursing

Chris Winkelman, PhD, RN, ACNP, CCRN
Assistant Professor
Frances Payne Bolton School of Nursing
Case Western Reserve University
University Heights, Ohio
Genetics features

Patricia B. Wolff, MSN, APRN, BC, AOCNS
South Texas Veterans Health Care System
Medical Oncology
San Antonio, Texas
Hematological and Immune Disorders

Reviewers

Cynthia Gurdak Berry, MSN, RN
Assistant Professor
Ida V. Moffett School of Nursing
Samford University
Birmingham, Alabama

Marylee Bressie, MSN, RN, CCRN, CEN
Instructor
Department of Nursing
Spring Hill College
Mobile, Alabama

Janet E. Burton, MSN, RN, CMSRN
Nursing Instructor
Division of Health Sciences–ASN Nursing Program
Ivy Tech Community College
Columbus, Indiana

Marilyn Caldwell, MS, RN
Assistant Professor of Nursing
Morrisville State College
Morrisville, New York

Jane B. Haertlein, RN
Faculty
Division of Nursing
Bob Jones University
Greenville, South Carolina

Sandra Hale, MS, RN
Associate Professor of Nursing
Lander University
Greenwood, South Carolina

Rebecca Hickey, RN
University of Cincinnati–Raymond Walters College
Liberty Urgent Care
Cincinnati, Ohio

Linda A. Howe, PhD, CNS, CNE
Associate Professor
Clemson University
School of Nursing
Clemson, South Carolina

Roni DeLao Kerns, PhD, RN
Nursing Instructor
Eastern Arizona College
Thatcher, Arizona

RuthAnne Kuiper, PhD, CCRN, CNE
University of North Carolina–Wilmington
School of Nursing
Wilmington, North Carolina

Jacqueline LaManna, MSN, ARNP-BC, ADM, CDE
Instructor/Nursing Lab
University of Central Florida School of Nursing–
Brevard Campus
Cocoa, Florida

Janice Garrison Lanham, MSN, RN
Nursing Faculty/Critical Care Clinical Nurse
Specialty
Clemson University
Department of Nursing
Clemson, South Carolina

Kristine L'Ecuyer, MSN, RN
Associate Professor
School of Nursing
Saint Louis University
St. Louis, Missouri

Carmen Long, MSN, RN
Clinical Instructor and Lecturer
Department of Nursing
Columbus State Community College
Columbus, Ohio

Jo Voss, PhD, RN, CNS
Assistant Professor
College of Nursing
South Dakota State University
Rapid City, South Dakota

Preface

Critical care nursing deals with human responses to life-threatening health problems. Critically ill patients continue to have high levels of acuity and complex care needs. These patients are cared for in critical care units, step-down units, outpatient settings, and at home. The critical care nurse is challenged to provide comprehensive care for these patients and their family members. The demand for critical care nurses who can work across the continuum of care continues to increase.

A solid knowledge foundation in concepts of critical care nursing is essential for practice. Nurses must also learn the assessment and technical skills associated with management of the critically ill patient.

The goal of this fifth edition of *Introduction to Critical Care Nursing* is to facilitate attainment of this foundation for critical care nursing practice. The book continues to provide essential information in an easy-to-learn format for nurses who are new to critical care; it is not intended to be a complete reference on critical care nursing. Information common to all of critical care nursing, regardless of setting, is presented. The textbook is targeted to both undergraduate nursing students and experienced nurses who are new to critical care. Both groups have found past editions of the book beneficial.

ORGANIZATION

Introduction to Critical Care Nursing is organized into three sections. Part I, Fundamental Concepts, introduces the reader to critical care nursing; psychosocial concepts related to patients, families, and nurses; and legal, ethical, and end-of-life issues related to critical care nursing practice. Part II, Tools for the Critical Care Nurse, remains a unique feature of this text. Chapters in this section provide vital information concerning comfort and sedation, nutrition, recognition of dysrhythmias, hemodynamic monitoring, airway management and mechanical ventilation, and management of life-threatening emergencies.

The final 10 chapters of the book complete Part III, Nursing Care during Critical Illness. The nursing process is used as an organizing framework for each chapter. Nursing care plans continue to be included so that nurses new to critical care become familiar with nursing diagnoses and interventions common to many critically ill patients. A summary of anatomy and physiology is provided, as are pathophysiology

diagrams for common problems seen in critical care. Features of each chapter include pharmacology tables, evidence-based practice boxes, clinical and laboratory alerts, geriatric considerations, critical thinking questions, case studies, and new features on genetics and transplantation. Additions and revisions have been made based on reader feedback and current trends.

SPECIAL FEATURES

This edition features a new full-color design with updated full-color figures to enhance reader understanding. Many new and revised learning aids appear in the fifth edition to highlight chapter content:

- **Evidence-Based Practice** boxes identify problems in patient care, ask pertinent questions related to the problems, supply evidence addressing the questions, and offer implications for nursing practice. Most boxes provide references to systematic reviews and meta-analyses that provide a greater synthesis of the research evidence related to a problem.
- **Genetics** features discuss disorders with a genetic component, including diabetes, Marfan's syndrome, and cystic fibrosis.
- **Transplantation** features address cardiac, renal, liver, and lung transplantation within the relevant chapters.
- **Clinical Alerts** highlight particular concerns, significance, and procedures in a variety of clinical settings to help students understand the potential problems encountered in that setting.
- **Laboratory Alerts** detail both common and cutting-edge tests and procedures to alert students to the importance of laboratory results.
- **Geriatric Considerations** alert the user to the special needs of the older patient in the critical care environment.
- Client-specific **Case Studies** with accompanying questions help students apply the chapter's content to real-life situations while also testing their critical-thinking abilities. Discussions for these questions, along with the **Critical Thinking Questions,** found at the end of each chapter, are included on the Evolve site for this title, which is free to instructors upon adoption.

- **Nursing Care Plans** have been redesigned and updated to describe patient diagnoses, outcomes, nursing interventions, and rationales.
- **Pathophysiology Flow Charts** expand analysis of the course and outcomes of particular injuries and disorders.
- **Pharmacology Tables** reflect the most current and most commonly used critical care medications.

New Chapter

In addition to the new and updated special features, a new chapter on end-of-life care is found in this edition. End-of-life concerns are increasingly encountered in critical care nursing practice, and this chapter addresses some of the most crucial issues, including the withholding, limiting, and withdrawing therapy; the effects on the health care team; palliative care; and legal and ethical concerns.

EVOLVE RESOURCES

We are pleased to offer additional content and learning aids to both instructors and students on our Evolve Resources companion Web site, which has been customized for the new edition and is available at http://evolve.elsevier.com/Sole/.

For Students

This edition comes with a new companion Evolve site for students that includes the following resources:

- **Open-Book Quizzes,** consisting of fill-in-the-blank, matching, and multiple-choice questions for each chapter.
- **Animations, Images, Video Clips,** and **Audio Clips,** which feature innovative content from supplemental materials.
- More than 250 **Audio Pronunciations** from Dorland's Dictionary.
- **Crossword Puzzles** for each chapter.
- **Online Concept Map Creator,** a one-of-a-kind program that allows students to create customized concept maps. Students are prompted to enter the following client data: medical diagnosis, pathophysiology, risk factors, clinical manifestations, nursing diagnoses, collaborative problems, expected outcomes, and nursing interventions. The program then generates a concept in two formats: (1) a graphic

"map" that clearly illustrates the relationships among various client data and components of the nursing process, and (2) a tabular word processing file that students may print and use to record client response/evaluation data, thereby completing the nursing process.

For Instructors

The Instructor's Resource is available on the Evolve site and includes the following additional content:

- An **Instructor's Manual,** which provides objectives for each chapter, suggested teaching and learning activities related to the chapter content outline, and answers to the Critical Thinking Challenges from the PowerPoint Presentations.
- Answers to the Critical Thinking Questions and Case Study Questions presented in the textbook.
- A **PowerPoint Presentation** collection of more than 1000 slides, offering a presentation for every chapter.
- An electronic **Test Bank** of more than 500 questions.
- An **Image Collection** including all of the images from the text.

Instructors have access to the student resources as well. Evolve can also be used to do the following:

- Publish your class syllabus, outline, and lecture notes.
- Set up "virtual office hours" and e-mail communication.
- Share important dates and information through the online class calendar.
- Encourage student participation through chat rooms and discussion boards.
- Also available for WebCT and Blackboard systems.

Critical care nursing is an exciting and challenging field. Health care organizations need critical care nurses who are knowledgeable about basic concepts as well as research-based practice, are technologically competent, and are caring toward patients and families. Our hope is that this edition of *Introduction to Critical Care Nursing* will provide the foundation for critical care nursing practice.

MLS
DGK
MJM

In Memory

Dr. Marilyn Lamborn

1946-2007

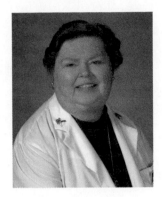

Around 1990 Dr. Jeannette Hartshorn casually mentioned an idea for a critical care nursing textbook to Dr. Marilyn Lamborn and me during lunch. At the time, we were faculty colleagues at the University of Texas Health Science Center in San Antonio School of Nursing, and we all had a passion for critical care nursing. That conversation led to a partnership, hard work, and the publication of *Introduction to Critical Care Nursing*. We collaborated on the first three editions of this textbook and our teamwork and collaboration made the textbook what it is today.

Unfortunately, Dr. Marilyn Lamborn died December 12, 2007, after a lengthy illness. At the time of her death, Dr. Lamborn was Professor Emeritus at the University of West Florida, where she had served as Associate Professor and Chair of the Department of Nursing. Dr. Lamborn had many accomplishments during her career. During her tenure at the University of West Florida, Dr. Lamborn established a basic baccalaureate degree program to complement the existing RN to BSN program, and she provided leadership for the chartering of Upsilon Kappa Chapter, Sigma Theta Tau International. One accomplishment that she was most proud of was being an editor of this textbook, and the fact that the second edition was translated into Chinese! She taught critical care and cardiovascular nursing to many undergraduate nursing students and beamed when she was able to use or recommend this textbook. Dr. Lamborn was from the Atlanta area, where she received her diploma from Georgia Baptist Hospital. Her additional nursing degrees were awarded at the Medical College of Georgia (BSN, MSN) and the University of Texas at Austin (PhD).

This fifth edition of the textbook is dedicated to Dr. Lamborn, her never-ending spirit, and her passion for critical care nursing education.

Mary Lou Sole

Contents

PART I

Fundamental Concepts

CHAPTER 1

Overview of Critical Care Nursing

Mary Lou Sole, PhD, RN, CCNS, CNL, FAAN

DEFINITION OF CRITICAL CARE NURSING

Critical care nursing is concerned with human responses to life-threatening problems, such as trauma, major surgery, or complications of illness. The human response can be a physiological or psychological phenomenon. The focus of the critical care nurse includes both the patient's and family's responses to illness and involves prevention as well as cure.

The critical care nurse is considered to be the patient's advocate. Expected roles of the nurse as advocate are described in Box 1-1.[5] Competencies for critical care nursing practice are listed in Box 1-2.

EVOLUTION OF CRITICAL CARE

The specialty of critical care has its roots in the 1950s, when patients with polio were cared for in specialized units. In the 1960s, recovery rooms were established for the care of patients who had undergone surgery, and coronary care units were instituted for the care of patients with cardiac problems. The patients who received care in these units had improved outcomes. Critical care nursing evolved as a specialty in the 1970s with the development of general intensive care units. Since that time, critical care nursing has become increasingly specialized. Examples of specialized critical care units are cardiovascular, surgical, neurological, trauma, transplantation, burn, pediatric, and neonatal units.

Critical care nursing has expanded beyond the walls of traditional critical care units. For example, critically ill patients are cared for in emergency departments; postanesthesia units; step-down, intermediate care, and progressive care units; and interventional radiology and cardiology units. Acutely ill patients

with high-technology requirements, complex problems, or both, such as patients who are ventilator dependent, may be cared for in medical-surgical units, in long-term acute care hospitals, or at home.

Critical care nurses practice in varied settings to manage and coordinate care for patients who require in-depth assessment, high-intensity therapies and interventions, and continuous nursing vigilance. Critical care nurses also function in various roles and levels, such as staff nurse, educator, and advanced practice nurse.

PROFESSIONAL ORGANIZATIONS

Several professional organizations specifically support critical care practice. These include the American Association of Critical-Care Nurses (AACN) and the Society of Critical Care Medicine (SCCM).

American Association of Critical-Care Nurses

The AACN is a professional organization that was established in 1969 to represent critical care nurses. The AACN is the largest nursing specialty organization in the world. In addition to the national organization, more than 240 chapters are in existence to support critical care nurses at the local level.[3] The mission of the organization is to provide leadership to establish work and patient care environments that are respectful, healing, and humane. The vision of the organization supports creating a health care system driven by the needs of patients and families in which critical care nurses make their optimal contributions.[4]

The association promotes the health and welfare of critically ill patients by advancing the art and science of critical care nursing, and supporting work

---

BOX 1-1   Role of the Critical Care Nurse as Patient Advocate

- Support the right of the patient or surrogate to autonomous, informed decision making.
- Intervene to support the best interests of the patient.
- Help the patient to obtain necessary care.
- Respect the patient's values, beliefs, and rights.
- Provide education and support to help the patient or surrogate make decisions.
- Represent the patient based on his/her choices.
- Support the decisions of the patient or surrogate.
- Intercede for patients who cannot speak for themselves.
- Monitor and safeguard the quality of care.
- Act as liaison between the patient, family, and health care providers.

Data from American Association of Critical-Care Nurses. (2007). *Key statements, beliefs and philosophies behind the American Association of Critical-Care Nurses (AACN)*. Retrieved August 25, 2007, from www.aacn.org.

BOX 1-2   Desired Competencies of Nurses Caring for the Critically Ill

- Clinical judgment and clinical reasoning skills
- Advocacy and moral agency in identifying and resolving ethical issues
- Caring practices that are tailored to the uniqueness of the patient and family
- Collaboration with patients, family members, and health care team members
- Systems thinking that promotes holistic nursing care
- Response to diversity
- Clinical inquiry and innovation to promote the best patient outcomes
- Role as patient/family educator to facilitate learning

Data from Curley, M. A. (1996). The synergy model of certified practice: Creating safe passage for patients. *Critical Care Nurse, 16*(4), 94-99; Curley, M. A. (1998). Patient-nurse synergy: Optimizing patients' outcomes. *American Journal of Critical Care, 7*(1), 64-72.

environments that promote professional nursing practice. Values of the organization include accountability, advocacy, integrity, collaboration, leadership, stewardship, lifelong learning, quality, innovation, and commitment. These values are supported through education, research, and collaborative practice.[4]

The benefits of AACN membership include continuing education offerings, educational advancement scholarships, research grants, and the following official publications: *Critical Care Nurse, American Journal of Critical Care*, and *AACN Advanced Critical Care*. The organization also publishes *Practice Alerts*, which present succinct, evidence-based practices that are to be applied at the bedside. Membership information and other general information are available by contacting the AACN at 1-800-899-AACN or online at www.aacn.org.

Society of Critical Care Medicine

The SCCM is a multidisciplinary scientific and educational organization. The SCCM was founded in 1970 by a group of physicians, and it has grown to more than 13,000 members. The mission of the organization is to secure the highest-quality care for critically ill patients through a multidisciplinary, multispecialty approach. The vision of the SCCM is to have a health care system in which all critically ill and injured persons receive care from a multiprofessional health care team under the direction of a physician specializing in intensive care. These teams use knowledge, technology, and compassion to provide patient care timely, safely, effectively, and efficiently.[35]

The SCCM is dedicated to ensuring excellence and consistency in critical care practice through education, research, and advocacy.[35] Membership in the SCCM is open to physicians and other health care providers who support critical care, including nurses, respiratory therapists, and pharmacists. The SCCM publishes *Critical Care Medicine, New Horizons: The Science and Practice of Acute Medicine*, and *Pediatric Critical Care Medicine*. Membership and other information are available online at www.sccm.org.

Other Professional Organizations

Other professional organizations also focus on improving care of critically ill patients. Examples include the American College of Chest Physicians (www.chestnet.org), the American Thoracic Society (www.thoracic.org), and the professional scientific councils of the American Heart Association (www.americanheart.org). Nurses can apply for membership in these and other related professional organizations.

CERTIFICATION

Critical care nurses are eligible for certification. Certification validates knowledge of critical care nursing, promotes professional excellence, and helps nurses to maintain a current knowledge base.[6] The AACN Certification Corporation oversees the critical care certification process.

The certification for nurses in bedside practice is known as CCRN or PCCN. The CCRN certification is available for nurses who provide care of critically ill adult, pediatric, or neonatal populations. The PCCN is for nurses who provide acute care in progressive care, step-down, telemetry, and similar units. Each certification has minimum clinical eligibility requirements that must be met to take the examination. After passing the written examination, nurses may use the CCRN or PCCN credential after their name. Continuing education and ongoing care for acute or critically ill patients are required for recertification. Once nurses achieve the CCRN or PCCN credential, they may be eligible to sit for additional subspecialty certification in cardiac medicine (CMC) or cardiac surgery (CSC).[2]

Advanced practice certification for critical care nurses is also available. Acute and critical care clinical nurse specialists can seek the CCNS credential. Acute care nurse practitioners can become certified as ACNPC™. A master's degree in the specialty and clinical practice in the field are required for advanced certification.[2]

The AACN certification credentials are based on a synergy model of practice. The synergy model of certified practice states that the needs of patients and families influence and drive competencies of nurses (see Box 1-2). Each patient and family is unique, with a varying capacity for health and vulnerability to illness. Patients who are more severely compromised have more complex needs, and nursing practice is based on meeting these needs.[14,15]

STANDARDS

Standards serve as guidelines for clinical practice. They establish goals for patient care and provide mechanisms for nurses to assess the achievement of patient goals, regardless of the setting for practice.

The *AACN Standards for Acute and Critical Care Nursing Practice* describe practice for nurses who care for critically ill patients.[28] The standards of care delineate the nursing process: collect data, determine diagnoses, identify expected outcomes, develop a plan of care, implement interventions, and evaluate the outcomes of interventions.[28] The standards of professional practice (Box 1-3) describe expectations of the critical care nurse.

BOX 1-3   Standards of Critical Care Professional Practice

The Nurse Caring for Acute and Critically Ill Patients:
- Systematically evaluates the quality and effectiveness of nursing practice
- Reflects knowledge of professional practice standards, laws, and regulations
- Acquires and maintains current knowledge and competency in patient care
- Contributes to the professional development of peers and other health care providers
- Acts ethically on behalf of patients and family members
- Collaborates with the health care team to provide care in a healing, humane, and caring environment
- Uses clinical inquiry in practice
- Considers factors related to safety, effectiveness, and cost in patient care delivery

Data from Medina, J. (2000). *Standards for acute and critical care nursing practice* (3rd ed.). Aliso Viejo, CA: American Association of Critical-Care Nurses.

TRENDS AND ISSUES

As changes in health care delivery evolve, critical care nursing continues to expand and develop to meet patients' needs. Critical care nurses must be aware of current and emerging trends that impact their practice and patient care.

Critical illnesses have increased complexity, and critically ill patients are sicker than ever before. The critical care nurse is challenged to provide care for patients who have multisystem organ dysfunction and complex needs. Contributing to this trend is the increasingly aging population. The elderly have more chronic illnesses that contribute to the complexity of their care than do younger patients. They also tend to develop multisystem organ failure, which requires longer hospital stays, increases cost, and increases the need for intensive nursing care.

Costs for critical care services account for a large portion of an institution's budget and a high percentage of total health care costs. Critical care nurses are challenged to provide comprehensive services while reducing costs and lengths of stay. Changing nurse-to-patient ratios and employing unlicensed assistive personnel are strategies being implemented to reduce costs. However, outcomes associated with changes in staffing need to be monitored and evaluated to ensure that outcomes and patient safety are not compromised.

Quality and safety are essential components of patient care. Nurses and other health care professionals have been challenged to reduce medical errors and promote an environment that facilitates safe practices. For example, the Joint Commission has identified *National Patient Safety Goals* to be addressed in hospitals, long-term care facilities, and other agencies that it accredits.[22] Examples are shown in Box 1-4. Staff nurses are responsible for assisting in implementation of the goals.

Effective communication has been identified as an essential strategy to reduce patient errors and resolve issues related to patient care delivery. The "SBAR" approach is one strategy to improve communication. SBAR stands for Situation, Background, Assessment, and Recommendation. It provides an easy-to-use framework to guide effective communication among health care providers. The SBAR technique is being widely implemented across health care settings.[16,31]

Another strategy to improve patient safety is the implementation of rapid response teams or medical emergency teams to address changes in patients' conditions. These teams bring critical care expertise to the bedside to assess and manage patients whose conditions are deteriorating. The goal of a rapid response team is to identify and manage unstable patients, and those at high risk for cardiopulmonary arrest, to prevent unnecessary deaths. Critical care nurses are often the leaders on such teams.[17,29,36]

The Institute for Healthcare Improvement has introduced several strategies for improving outcomes in the critical care setting. Through its *100,000 Lives* and *Protecting 5 Million Lives from Harm* campaigns, it has challenged hospitals to adopt changes in care to

---

BOX 1-4   Examples of Patient Safety Goals

Improve Accuracy of Patient Identification
- Use at least two methods of patient identification
- Conduct a final verification ("time-out") before any invasive procedure

Improve Communication among Health Care Providers
- Verify verbal and telephone orders for accuracy with a "read-back" procedure
- Standardize abbreviations; create a list of abbreviations that are not to be used (those that contribute to errors)
- Improve reporting of critical test results
- Implement a standardized method for "handoff" communication, including question and answer opportunities

Improve Medication Safety
- Prevent errors involving look-alike and sound-alike medications
- Label all medications and containers
- Reduce harm associated with administration of anticoagulants

Reduce Risk of Health Care–Associated Infection
- Comply with guidelines for hand hygiene
- Treat unanticipated death or major loss of function as a sentinel event

Reconcile Medications across the Continuum of Care
- Compare patient's current (home) medications with those ordered during hospitalization
- Communicate a complete list of medications to the next provider when patients are transferred within an organization or to another setting
- Provide patient with a complete list of medications upon discharge

Reduce Risks Associated with Patient Falls
- Implement programs to reduce patient falls and evaluate effectiveness

Reduce Risk of Influenza and Pneumococcal Disease in Older Adults
- Develop protocols for administration and documentation of vaccination
- Develop protocols for identifying and managing outbreaks of influenza

Encourage Patients and Family Members to Be Actively Involved in Care
- Develop mechanisms for patients and family members to report concerns

Prevent Pressure Ulcers
- Assess risk and address identified risks

Recognize and Respond to Changes in Patient's Condition
- Develop method for staff to request assistance from specialty-trained individuals

Data from The Joint Commission. (2007). *National Patient Safety Goals*. Retrieved August 25, 2007, from www.jointcommission.org/PatientSafety/NationalPatientSafetyGoals.

BOX 1-5 Interventions to Reduce Harm and Prevent Injury

- Activate rapid response team at the first sign of patient deterioration
- Deliver evidence-based care for acute myocardial infarction and heart failure
- Implement "bundles of care" to prevent:
  - Central line infection
  - Acute myocardial infarction
  - Ventilator-associated pneumonia
  - Surgical site infection
  - Sepsis
- Implement procedures for medication reconciliation
- Prevent harm:
  - High-alert medications such as anticoagulants, sedatives, narcotics, and insulin
  - Complications of surgery
  - Pressure ulcers
  - Methicillin-resistant *Staphylococcus aureus*

Data from Institute for Healthcare Improvement. (2007). *Protecting 5 million lives from harm campaign.* Retrieved August 26, 2007, from www.ihi.org.

BOX 1-6 Items to Consider in Daily Multidisciplinary Rounds

- Discharge needs
- Greatest safety risk
- Implementation of ventilator "bundle"
  - Head-of-bed elevation
  - Titration of sedation for assessing readiness to extubate
  - Prophylaxis for peptic ulcer disease
  - Prophylaxis for venous thromboembolism
- Assessment and recommended follow-up
  - Cardiac and hemodynamic status
  - Volume status
  - Neurological status
  - Pain management
  - Sedation needs
  - Gastrointestinal status, including bowel management
  - Nutrition
  - Skin issues
  - Activity
  - Infection status (culture results/therapeutic levels of antibiotics)
  - Laboratory results
  - Radiological test results
- Assess need for all ordered medications
- Identify whether central lines and invasive catheters/tubes can be removed
- Issues that need to be addressed
  - Family needs—educational, psychosocial, spiritual
  - Code status
  - Advanced directives
  - Parameters for calling the physician

save lives and prevent patient injuries.[21] Examples of practices are described in Box 1-5. Many of the focuses of the *5 Million Lives* campaign assist in implementation of the Joint Commission's *National Patient Safety Goals.* A component of many of the Institute for Healthcare Improvement interventions is the concept of *bundles of care.* Bundles are described as evidence-based best practices that are done as a whole to improve outcomes.[7,25,27]

Clinical practice guidelines are being implemented to ensure that care is appropriate and based on research. Examples of guidelines include management of sedation, and nutritional support of critically ill patients. The National Guideline Clearinghouse provides a compendium of guidelines published by various professional organizations and health care agencies (www.guideline.gov). Nurses are encouraged to implement care that is evidence based and to challenge practices that have "always been done" but are not supported by clinical evidence. Advance practice nurses can assist the staff in developing practice guidelines based on research findings.[10,11,18]

Today's environment emphasizes collaborative practice teams for the care of patients. The goal of these teams is to provide comprehensive patient care in a cost-effective manner while recognizing and using each others' talents and expertise. Intensivist-led rounds and daily goal setting are recommended to address patient care issues and adherence to rec-

ommended guidelines and "bundles."[32] Examples of daily goals to be addressed are noted in Box 1-6.

Technology that assists in patient care is growing at a rapid pace. Invasive and noninvasive monitoring systems are used to facilitate patient assessment and to evaluate responses to treatment. Many technological interventions have been introduced to improve patient safety.[8,30] Point-of-care laboratory testing is done at the bedside to provide immediate values to expedite treatment. Computerized physician order entry and nursing documentation are becoming commonplace. In many institutions, data from monitoring equipment are automatically downloaded into the computerized medical record. Nurses must become increasingly comfortable with the application of technology, troubleshooting equipment, and evaluating the accuracy of values. The use of technology must be balanced with delivering compassionate care.

As more technological advances become available to sustain and support life, ethical issues have skyrocketed. Termination of life support, organ and cell transplantation, and quality of life are just a few issues that nurses must address in everyday practice. Nurses must be comfortable addressing ethical issues as they arise in the critical care setting. Increased attention to end-of-life care in the critical care unit is also needed (see Chapters 3 and 4). Palliative care for all patients is an important intervention that must be embraced by those working in critical care units.

The use of telemedicine in the management of critically ill patients is another emerging trend. Technology allows experts to provide consultation and evaluation of patients who may be a great distance from a tertiary critical care center. Data from monitors are transferred for evaluation, and the expert conducts an assessment from a distant location.[9,13] These virtual critical care consultations have resulted in improved patient outcomes. Nurses consult with those providing the telemedicine service based on established protocols and parameters, and when they identify changes in patients' conditions that need to be addressed. These telemedicine strategies will not replace the high-touch, hands-on care delivered by nurses in the critical care unit, but they will assist health care workers at remote sites in decision making.

The critical care environment itself is changing. Units are being redesigned with the interests of both patients and nurses in mind. Equipment is becoming more portable, thus making the transfer of patients for diagnostic testing or to other units easier and safer. Some institutions have adopted a universal care model of patient care, or *acuity-adaptable* rooms. In this setting, patients remain in one unit throughout their hospitalization. The level of nursing care is adjusted to meet the needs of the patient. The universal care model eliminates the need to transfer patients to other units and promotes continuity of care.[19]

Patients are being transferred from critical care units much earlier than before and are discharged from the hospital often while they are still acutely ill. Nurses must ensure that patients and their family members are able to provide care in the home setting, which may be challenging given the reduced length of hospital stays.

Last, and most important, the United States is facing a shortage of critical care nurses. Many factors contribute to the shortage: decreased supply and higher demand for critical care nursing services, increased number of acute and critical care beds in hospitals, issues related to retention in the workplace, and greater availability of other career choices. Priorities for recruiting, educating, and retaining more nurses to work in critical care settings are essential. A related issue is hiring new graduates to work in critical care settings. Before the nursing shortage, many believed that every nurse should have at least one year of medical-surgical experience before working in critical care. That belief has been challenged by many who recognize the need to increase the critical care workforce. In addition, many new graduates want to specialize in critical care. New graduates can be successful in the critical care setting with adequate supervision, orientation, and mentorship.[12,20,23,33] A critical care course, which often includes simulation, is an important strategy to ensure successful orientation.[1,24,26,34] Adequate time in orientation, under the guidance of a supportive preceptor to develop and learn the critical care nursing role, is also essential.

These and other trends will continue to shape the future of critical care practice. Each nurse must continue to monitor trends. One of the best ways to influence practice in an ever-changing environment is through participation in nursing organizations. Reading print and online journals on a regular basis is also important.

SUMMARY

Because the boundaries of critical care have expanded, all nurses will be providing care for critically ill patients. Knowledge of professional organizations and of the scope and standards of practice is important for the nurse entering critical care practice. The purpose of this textbook is to provide fundamental information essential to the care of critically ill patients. The reader is challenged to apply the concepts discussed throughout this book to daily practice.

CRITICAL THINKING QUESTIONS   *evolve*

1. Discuss critical care nursing practice and what it means to you.
2. Compare perceptions of critical care from the viewpoints of student, nurse, patient, and family.
3. Give examples of various environments of critical care nursing practice.
4. Discuss the contributions of professional organizations to critical care nursing practice.
5. Debate the pros and cons of hiring new graduates to work in a critical care unit.
6. Envision the critical care unit of the future. Describe the environment and how care could be delivered.

evolve Be sure to check out the bonus material, including free self-assessment exercises, on the Evolve Web site at http://evolve.elsevier.com/Sole.

REFERENCES

1. Ackermann, A. D., Kenny, G., & Walker, C. (2007). Simulator programs for new nurses' orientation: A retention strategy. *Journal for Nurses. Staff Development, 23*(3), 136-139.
2. American Association of Critical-Care Nurses (AACN). (2006). *Role of the critical care nurse* [position statement]. Aliso Viejo, CA: AACN.
3. American Association of Critical-Care Nurses. (2007). *AACN Certification Corporation home page.* Retrieved August 25, 2007, from www.aacn.org/CERTCORP/certcorp.nsf/home.
4. American Association of Critical-Care Nurses. (2007). *Chapters.* Retrieved August 25, 2007, from www.aacn.org.
5. American Association of Critical-Care Nurses. (2007). *Key statements, beliefs and philosophies behind the American Association of Critical-Care Nurses (AACN).* Retrieved August 25, 2007, from www.aacn.org.
6. American Association of Critical-Care Nurses. (2007). *Value of certification.* Retrieved August 25, 2007, from www.aacn.org/certcorp/certcorp.nsf/vwdoc/BenefitsofCert.
7. Aragon, D., & Sole, M. L. (2006). Implementing best practice strategies to prevent infection in the ICU. *Critical Care Nursing Clinics of North America, 18*(4), 441-452.
8. Bakken, S. (2006). Informatics for patient safety: A nursing research perspective. *Annual Review of Nursing Research, 24,* 219-254.
9. Ceron, M. I. (2007). Bringing virtual technology to the ICU. Constant, expert care of critically ill patients. *Healthcare Executive, 22*(2), 40, 42.
10. Chester, L. R. (2007). Many critical care nurses are unaware of evidence-based practice. *American Journal of Critical Care, 16*(2), 106.
11. Chulay, M., & Hall, J. (2007). The American Association of Critical-Care Nurses (AACN) publishes several evidence-based documents, including *Practice Alerts, Procedure Manuals,* and *Protocols for Practice.* What are the differences among these 3 publications and when should each one be used? *Critical Care Nurse, 27*(2), 82-83.
12. Coombs, M., Chaboyer, W., & Sole, M. L. (2007). Advanced nursing roles in critical care—A natural or forced evolution? *Journal of Professional Nursing, 23*(2), 83-90.
13. Cummings, J., Krsek, C., Vermoch, K., & Matuszewski, K. (2007). Intensive care unit telemedicine: Review and consensus recommendations. *American Journal of Medical Quality, 22*(4), 239-250.
14. Curley, M. A. (1996). The synergy model of certified practice: Creating safe passage for patients. *Critical Care Nurse, 16*(4), 94-99.
15. Curley, M. A. (1998). Patient-nurse synergy: Optimizing patients' outcomes. *American Journal of Critical Care, 7*(1), 64-72.
16. Haig, K. M., Sutton, S., & Whittington, J. (2006). SBAR: A shared mental model for improving communication between clinicians. *Joint Commission Journal on Quality and Patient Safety, 32*(3), 167-175.
17. Halvorsen, L., Garolis, S., Wallace-Scroggs, A., Stenstrom, J., & Maunder, R. (2007). Building a rapid response team. *AACN Advanced Critical Care, 18*(2), 129-140.
18. Hedges, C. (2007). Show me the guidelines! *AACN Advanced Critical Care, 18*(1), 88-90.
19. Hendrich, A. L., & Lee, N. (2005). Intra-unit patient transports: Time, motion, and cost impact on hospital efficiency. *Nursing Economic$, 23*(4), 147, 157-164.
20. Ihlenfeld, J. T. (2005). Hiring and mentoring graduate nurses in the intensive care unit. *Dimensions of Critical Care Nursing, 24*(4), 175-178.
21. Institute for Healthcare Improvement. (2007). *Protecting 5 million lives from harm campaign.* Retrieved August 26, 2007, from www.ihi.org.
22. Joint Commission. (2007). *National patient safety goals.* Retrieved August 25, 2007, from www.jointcommission.org/PatientSafety/NationalPatientSafetyGoals.
23. Kelly, S., & Courts, N. (2007). The professional self-concept of new graduate nurses. *Nurse Education in Practice, 7*(5), 332-337.
24. Lindsey, G., & Kleiner, B. (2005). Nurse residency program: An effective tool for recruitment and retention. *Journal of Health Care Finance, 31*(3), 25-32.
25. Litch, B. (2007). How the use of bundles improves reliability, quality and safety. *Healthcare Executive, 22*(2), 12-14, 16, 18.
26. Marcum, E. H., & West, R. D. (2004). Structured orientation for new graduates: A retention strategy. *Journal for Nurses in Staff Development, 20*(3), 118-124; quiz 125-126.
27. McMillan, T. R., & Hyzy, R. C. (2007). Bringing quality improvement into the intensive care unit. *Critical Care Medicine, 35*(Suppl. 2), S59-S65.
28. Medina, J. (2000). *Standards for acute and critical care nursing practice* (3rd ed.). Aliso Viejo, CA: American Association of Critical-Care Nurses.
29. Offner, P. J., Heit, J., & Roberts, R. (2007). Implementation of a rapid response team decreases cardiac arrest outside of the intensive care unit. *Journal of Trauma, 62*(5), 1223-1227; discussion 1227-1228.
30. O'Neill, A. E., & Miranda, D. (2006). The right tools can help critical care nurses save more lives. *Critical Care Nursing Quarterly, 29*(4), 275-281.
31. Powell, S. K. (2007). SBAR—It's not just another communication tool. *Professional Case Management, 12*(4), 195-196.
32. Pronovost, P., Berenholtz, S., Dorman, T., Lipsett, P. A., Simmonds, T., & Haraden, C. (2003). Improving communication in the ICU using daily goals. *Journal of Critical Care, 18*(2), 71-75.

33. Reddish, M. V., & Kaplan, L. J. (2007). When are new graduate nurses competent in the intensive care unit? *Critical Care Nursing Quarterly, 30*(3), 199-205.

34. Seago, J. A., & Barr, S. J. (2003). New graduates in critical care. The success of one hospital. *Journal for Nurses in Staff Development, 19*(6), 297-304.

35. Society of Critical Care Medicine. (2007). *About SCCM*. Retrieved August 25, 2007, from www.sccm.org/SCCM/About+SCCM/.

36. Thomas, K., VanOyen Force, M., Rasmussen, D., Dodd, D., & Whildin, S. (2007). Rapid response team: Challenges, solutions, benefits. *Critical Care Nurse, 27*(1), 20-27.

CHAPTER 2

The Critical Care Experience

Max Hosmanek, MSN, RN, CCRN
Mary Lou Sole, PhD, RN, CCNS, FAAN

INTRODUCTION

Care of the critically ill patient is no longer restricted to the critical care unit. The American Association of Critical-Care Nurses (AACN) defines critically ill patients as those who are at high risk for actual or potential life-threatening health problems.[4] Patients meeting this definition are cared for in a variety of settings including critical care units, emergency departments, telemetry units, step-down units, and throughout acute care facilities.

Ongoing research into the experiences of critically ill patients and their families consistently supports the premise that care of the patient and the patient's family must be considered holistically. Advances in life-sustaining procedures and treatments present complicated ethical considerations in caring for the most seriously ill, and it is often family members who weigh the efficacy and ethics of extending life versus the potential loss of quality of life (see Chapter 3). In addition, social and demographic changes such as an aging population, and changes in family structure, have altered the traditional definition of what constitutes *family*. Critical care nurses assume an advocacy role in caring for patients and their family members who have life-threatening illnesses and problems. The purpose of this chapter is to describe the critical illness experience and its effects on patients, their families, critical care nurses, and the critical care environment.

THE CRITICAL CARE ENVIRONMENT

The *built environment*, or physical layout, of a critical care unit has a subtle but profound effect on patients, families, and the critical care team. Amid an apparent confusion of wires, tubes, and machinery, a critical care unit is designed for efficient and expeditious life-sustaining interventions. Patients and their family members are cared for in this environment with little or no advance preparation, often causing stress and anxiety. The resultant high stress levels are compounded by the often unrelenting sensory stimulation of light and noise, loss of privacy, and lack of nonclinical physical contact, as well as emotional and physical pain resulting from medical and nursing procedures and the illness itself. Maintaining the safety, dignity, and confidentiality of patients under such circumstances presents an ongoing challenge. Issues related to the environment include sensory overload, noise, and sensory deprivation.

Many studies have documented the detrimental effects of the sensory overload found in a typical critical care unit.[38] Noise is a major factor contributing to sensory overload. The World Health Organization established guidelines for hospital noise levels that recommend daytime levels no greater than 35 dB, and nighttime levels of 30 dB.[39] High levels of noise are associated with many deleterious effects—sleep disruption, decreased oxygen saturation, elevated blood pressure, delayed wound healing, and a potentially greater incidence of rehospitalization. Yet noise levels in hospitals routinely exceed those recommended (Table 2-1). Noise affects not only patients but the critical care team as well, often leading to increased stress, emotional exhaustion and burnout, and increased fatigue.[41] Excessive noise can lead to difficult communication, distractions, or both, and may contribute to medical errors.[39] In addition, loud conversations may compromise patient confidentiality if communication with patients and family members, or between health care providers, is heard throughout the unit.

Several strategies have been identified to reduce noise within the acute care environment: private rooms, installation of sound-absorbing acoustical ceiling tiles, modifying overhead paging systems, and initiating programs to raise awareness among staff

11

about their role in reducing noise.[39] Providing "sedative" music is another strategy to reduce anxiety and discomfort associated with increased noise levels. Such music has no accented beats, no percussion, a slow tempo, and a smooth melody.[15,16] Confidentiality can be improved by designating a private place for communication with family members and closing the door during conversations that may be overheard by others.

Lighting is another issue in the critical care environment. Adequate and appropriate exposure to light is a therapeutic modality for the health of both patients and staff.[37] Inadequate or poorly placed lighting makes transcription of orders more difficult, affects the legibility of reading medication labels, and complicates adequate physical assessment of patients. In addition, the constant artificial lighting present in most critical care units tends to override patients' natural circadian rhythms, resulting in increased disorientation and agitation.[37] Simple measures, such as

designing rooms to take advantage of natural light, can have a number of positive effects including decreased episodes of depression, improved sleep quality, and more effective pain management.[37,38]

A study of physical design identified several critical care units as meeting *best practices* for design. Positive aspects of these units' designs included private rooms that promoted safety, privacy, and comfort; easy access to patients from all sides of the bed; accessible sinks and waste disposal; and natural lighting. Environmental factors that resulted in limited or restricted access of family members to the critical care unit were considered negative aspects of design.[53]

Many hospitals are currently being built in the United States. Demographic factors such as an aging and geographically shifting population have created the need for more hospitals. The boom in hospital building presents an opportunity to design hospitals to best meet the needs of patients, families, and staff members.[60] When planning construction of new health care facilities, cost constraints must be weighed against the evidence of the design effects of on the health and safety of patients and staff.[38] It is important for members of the health care team to work with architects and others planning these hospitals and critical care units to design a safe and healing environment.[35,61] Factors such as adequate ventilation, lighting, and noise abatement must be considered. Design considerations include easy access to the patient and physiologic monitoring devices, ergonomic and safety features, and adequate hygiene (e.g., sinks, disposals, storage) to reduce the risk of infection.

Critical Care Culture

The culture of a critical care unit includes its shared values, attitudes and beliefs, which in turn reflect behavioral norms that guide the functional dynamics of staff interaction. As the dominant professions in critical care, medicine and nursing have distinct cultures shaped by education, training, and their unique approaches to illness and wellness. Although medicine and nursing both value the well-being of patients, they differ as to their beliefs regarding the definition of well-being and how it is achieved. These divergent approaches can enhance patient care by offering different perspectives, and generally are regarded as strengths within the overall context of the patients' plan of care. However, they can be an impediment if they foster a condescending attitude towards other viewpoints.[7] One strategy to improve collaboration is joint education of physicians and nurses to foster shared cultural values, expose each profession to the others' worldview, and focus on skilled communication.[44]

TABLE 2-1 Noise Levels Associated with Patient Care Devices and Activities

Activity	Sound Level [dB(A)]
Toilet flushing	44-76*
Cardiac monitor alarm	44-78*
Scraping of chairs/stools across floor	46-86*
Call-bell lights	48-63*
Oxygen/chest tube bubbling, ventilator	49-70*
Adding medication to/adjusting intravenous line	58-60*
Conversations (staff, patients, and family)	59-90*
Voice over intercom	60-70*
Telephone ringing	60-75*
Television (normal volume at 12 feet)	65†
Raising/lowering head of bed	68-78*
Pneumatic tube arrival	88*
Raising/lowering side rails on bed	90*
Shouts among staff	90†
Addressograph machine	100†
Dropping a stainless steel bowl	108*

*Data from Sommargren, C. (1995). Environmental hazards in the technological age. *Critical Care Nursing Clinics of North America, 7*(2), 287-295.
†Data from Grumet, G. (1994). Noise hampers healing and curbs productivity. *Health Facilities Management, 7*(1), 22-25.

Interactions among providers, especially nurses and physicians, affect patient safety, clinical outcomes, and the recruitment and retention of nurses. Landmark studies conducted by the Institute of Medicine examined the risks inherent in the health care system in the United States, and the estimated death toll that resulted. Deficiencies in care delivery—including a hierarchical, failure-prone system—have been identified as factors related to errors and poor outcomes. In response to these findings, the AACN initiated its Healthy Work Environment campaign. The campaign goal is to create work environments that are safe, healing, and humane. Essential components of healthy work environments include respect, responsibility, and acknowledgment of the unique contributions of patients, families, nurses, and health care team members (Box 2-1).[2] Communication and collaboration warrant additional discussion as they provide the foundation for achieving a healthy work environment (Figure 2-1).[39]

Communication

Effective communication is essential to delivering safe patient care. According to the Joint Commission, a majority of adverse events in accredited institutions are directly attributable to faulty communication.[36]

Adapted from American Association of Critical-Care Nurses. (2005). AACN standards for establishing and sustaining healthy work environments: A journey to excellence. *American Journal of Critical Care, 14*(3), 187-197.

At least half of all communication breakdowns occur during so-called handoff situations, when patient information is being transferred or exchanged.[57] Common handoff situations include nursing shift reports, transcription of verbal orders, and interfacility patient transfers. Barriers to effective handoffs are noted in Box 2-2.

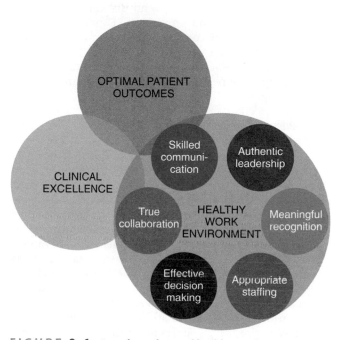

FIGURE 2-1. Interdependence of healthy work environment, clinical excellence, and optimal patient outcomes. *(From AACN. [2005]. AACN standards for establishing and sustaining healthy work environments: A journey to excellence. American Journal of Critical Care 14[3], 189.)*

Data from Adamski, P. (2007). Implement a handoff communications approach. *Nursing Management, 38,* 10; Arora, V., & Johnson, J. (2006). A model for building a standardized hand-off protocol. *Joint Commission Journal on Quality and Patient Safety, 32,* 646.

In recognition of these potential dangers, the Joint Commission has mandated that facilities implement a standardized approach to handoff communications.[36] One technique to improve information exchange uses the acronym SBAR—Situation, Background, Assessment, Recommendation (Box 2-3).[30,51] With this technique, information is delivered in a way that is brief and action oriented. These characteristics are especially useful in communications between nurses and physicians.[5] Other strategies to improve handoff communication include standardized processes for the handoff situation, checklists to prompt and document essential information, and training of all personnel in effective communication techniques.[1,6]

Communication Techniques from Industry: Crew Resource Management

Communication techniques and protocols from other high-risk industries are being implemented in health care settings to improve patient safety.[26,49,52,58] One technique comes from the aviation industry—crew resource management (CRM). Flight crews depend on precise communication to ensure passenger safety. Data analysis of aviation accidents demonstrates a pattern of communication failures among crew members as a principal cause.[24,36] CRM was developed to promote communication and accountability among team members. In a CRM environment, everyone from the captain of the aircraft to the baggage handlers on the ground shares responsibility for safe flight operations. Differences in training are acknowledged and respected, but each member of the team is empowered and has the autonomy to address problems without fear of retaliation or ridicule.

Several components that underpin the effectiveness of CRM are pertinent to critical care nursing.

BOX 2-3   Situation, Background, Assessment, Recommendation (SBAR)

S— Situation: State what is happening at the present time that has warranted the SBAR communication.

B— Background: Explain circumstances leading up to this situation. Put the situation into context for the reader/listener.

A— State what you think is the problem.

R— State your recommendation to correct the problem.

From Haig, K. M., Sutton, S., & Whittington, J. (2006). SBAR: A shared mental model for improving communication between clinicians. *Joint Commission Journal on Quality and Patient Safety, 32,* 167.

During high-risk procedures such as takeoffs and landings, crew members cross-monitor each others' actions by double-checking, verifying, and when necessary, correcting inaccurate or ambiguous information.[24] A comparable situation in nursing is administration of blood products, where an additional verifier is required. Administration of high-risk medications, such as insulin or heparin, also falls into this category.

Situational awareness is a second component of CRM, and means being aware of one's surroundings. The expectation is that if something seems wrong, individuals should trust their "gut instinct" and speak up to correct the situation.[24] A related tool, referred to by the acronym CUS—short for "I'm Concerned, I'm Uncomfortable, this isn't Safe"—is used as a shorthand method to convey concern about a situation. An example of the CUS system is as follows. A central line was to be inserted into a critically ill patient. Supplies were obtained, and the physician asked the nurse to open the insertion kit because the physician had already donned sterile gloves. The nurse states, "I'm concerned, I'm uncomfortable, this isn't safe. Everyone in the patient's room is required to have full barrier precautions on—gown, gloves, mask, hat, and protective eye wear. In addition, the patient needs 'a full body drape' placed appropriately before we start the procedure. You will need to take off your sterile gloves and get everything ready before we start." This method of communication quickly conveys the concern of safety for the patient before the start of the procedure for line insertion.

Collaboration

Collaboration implies teamwork in its most basic sense. In the critical care setting, this primarily involves the interactions between nurses and physicians. The ultimate goal of true collaboration in critical care is to create a *culture of safety,* defined as a nonhierarchical culture where all members have the opportunity, as well as duty, to ensure safe and effective care.[56] As with effective communication, collaboration is founded on mutual respect and the recognition that each discipline involved in patient care brings distinct skills and perspectives to the table.

Many problems associated with the current system of health care delivery can be traced to its hierarchical nature, which is rapidly becoming obsolete. A health care system that is medicine driven and nurse implemented predisposes to noninterdisciplinary, isolationist decision-making behavior.[44] Instead, a culture of quality and safety is important, where collegial nurse-physician relationships are valued as indispensable to delivering superior patient care.[36,56] The unique contributions of each discipline, as well as the importance of support personnel, must be recognized. In high-performance organizations, the most important team member at any given time is the one with the most valuable information.[12]

One strategy for collaboration is the implementation of interdisciplinary bedside rounds one to two times per shift. Here, all disciplines offer collaborative interventions to best meet the needs of the critically ill patient and family members. In addition, patients and families are continually kept up to date about the patient's condition with this increased frequency of communication.

Conducting morning briefings before interdisciplinary rounds is another strategy to improve communication, collaboration, and patient safety. Suggested content of the morning briefings include answers to three questions: (1) What happened during the night that the team needs to know (e.g., adverse events, admissions)? (2) Where should rounds begin (e.g., the sickest patient who needs the most attention)? and (3) What potential problems have been identified for the day (e.g., staffing, procedures)?[59]

THE CRITICALLY ILL PATIENT

Individual response to critical illness is influenced by many factors. These may include age and developmental stage, experiences with illness and hospitalization, family relationships and social support, other stressful experiences and coping mechanisms, and personal philosophies about life, death, and spirituality.

Many stressors related to treatment and the critical care environment affect patients. For example, the experience of mechanical ventilation, along with difficulty communicating, pain, dyspnea, fatigue, and the need for endotracheal suctioning, creates a common stressful scenario for the critically ill patient. Additional major stressors that have been identified by patients when recalling their critical care experience are listed in Box 2-4. The cumulative effect of these stressors can promote anxiety and agitation, and in some cases lead to the development of post-traumatic stress disorder and delirium. Nursing interventions to reduce stress are to ensure safety, reduce sleep deprivation, and minimize noxious sensory overload. One effective intervention is to group nursing activities and medical procedures together to maximize patients' resting periods. Chapter 5 further discusses interventions to promote comfort and reduce anxiety.

Receiving information and feeling safe are predominant, complementary needs of critically ill patients and their family members. Of all the members of the critical care team, nurses spend the most

BOX 2-4 Patients' Recollection of the Critical Care Experience

- Difficulty communicating
- Pain
- Thirst
- Difficulty swallowing
- Anxiety
- Lack of control
- Depression
- Fear
- Lack of family or friends
- Physical restraint
- Feelings of dread
- Inability to get comfortable
- Difficulty sleeping
- Loneliness
- Thoughts of death and dying

time at the bedside with patients and as such are usually the first to hear about any perceived unmet needs.[25] Frequent updates on the patient's condition, anticipated therapies or procedures, and goals of the critical care team are an easy and effective way to allay anxiety while building a relationship of mutual trust.

Even if patients are sedated or unconscious, it is important to remember that many patients can still hear, understand, and respond emotionally to what is being said. Thus, nurses as well as family members should make every effort to simply talk to patients, regardless of the patients' ability to interact. Conversation topics might include reorienting patients to time and place, updates on their progress, and reminders that they are safe and have family and people nearby who care about their well-being.

It is important to increase pleasant sensory input, such as encouraging familiar voices of the family and family touch, and to reestablish day-night cycles by positioning the patient by a sunny window during the day and reducing light levels in the patient's room at night. Reorienting the patient every 2 to 4 hours and addressing the patient directly helps to minimize confusion. Instead of repeatedly questioning the patient (e.g., "Do you know what day it is? Do you know where you are?"), a less demeaning and less frustrating way to reorient the patient is to incorporate this content into normal conversation (e.g., "It's 8 o'clock in the morning on the fifth of September. You are still in the critical care unit. Your family will be here to see you in about 10 minutes"). Conversations about other patients and personal issues are conducted outside the patient's hearing range because such information can increase confusion on the part of the patient and can contribute to sensory overload. It is also very helpful to have objects that facilitate orientation, such as a clock, a calendar, and windows, within the patient's visual field. Personal and meaningful items brought from home by the family may also help to reorient the patient.

Cultural Considerations

The diversity of society in general is mirrored in the patient population of the typical critical care unit. Different cultural orientations require increased sensitivity to the responses and beliefs of patients and their families to illness and hospitalization. Especially important in the critical care environment are beliefs about health and healing, personal space and touch preferences, social organization, and the role of family. Cultural background influences patients' approaches to health care and responses to health care information. Many hospitals have programs to teach cultural sensitivity and competence. Rather than an end in itself, however, such training might better be approached as an ongoing learning process. Table 2-2 lists considerations for some of the cultural groups that may be cared for in critical care areas. These are general concepts that must be assessed in each patient.

Another consideration is the communications challenge posed when treating nonnative speakers, or those with limited English proficiency. It may be especially difficult to explain treatment options, obtain relevant medical information and history, and to reassess such patients after medical interventions. Hospitalized patients with limited English proficiency have a higher incidence and a greater

TABLE 2-2	Cultural Considerations		
Culture of Origin	**Health and Healing Beliefs**	**Space and Touch Preferences**	**Families and Social Organization**
Asian	Traditional health and illness beliefs May rely on traditional practitioners, such as herbalists	Prefer minimal physical contact	Strong family ties Particularly loyal to elders Devoted to family traditions
Anglo-Americans	Rely on modern health care systems, particularly for illnesses perceived as critical or life threatening	Prefer minimal physical contact	Nuclear families most common
Black/African American	Belief in traditional folk medicines and healers	Close personal space	Large, extended families, often female head of household Strong church affiliation
Native American	Belief in traditional folk medicine and healers (e.g., medicine man)	Minimal spatial boundaries Strive to be at one with the universe and surrounding beings	Strong, extended family ties Highly respectful of elders and family traditions
Latino/Mexican American	Belief in traditional folk medicine and healers (e.g., curandero)	Comfortable with tactile relationships, touching, and embracing	Nuclear and extended families Godparents play important role

Modified from Arnault, D. (2006). Framework for culturally relevant psychiatric nursing. In E. Varcarolis (Ed.), *Foundations of psychiatric mental health nursing* (5th ed.). Philadelphia: Saunders; and Bushy, A. (1999). The need for cultural linguistic competent care for families with special health problems. In J. Sebastian & A. Bushy (Eds.), *Special populations in the community: Advances in reducing health disparities.* Gaithersburg, MD: Aspen.

severity of adverse events resulting in harm than do English-speaking patients.[23] One solution to reducing harm is increased use of interpreters, who may also serve as cultural guides in directing care.[5,64]

Discharge from Critical Care and Quality of Life after Critical Care

A growing percentage of critically ill patients survive critical illnesses and injuries. Although discharge from a critical care area represents progress toward recovery, many patients are discharged "quicker and sicker" either to units that care for patients with lesser acuity or to home. Survival to discharge is a goal of critical care nursing, but it is only one aspect of the overall patient and family experience.

Transfer or discharge from the critical care unit can result in stress for both patients and families.[14] Patients may experience physiological or psychological disturbances, or both, referred to as *relocation stress* as a result of transfer from one environment to another. They may also feel a sense of abandonment, and fear losing the security of the higher level of care afforded in the critical care unit.[13,19,45,47,54] Poorly managed transfers from the critical care unit can result in readmission to the hospital and to the critical care unit.[63]

A variety of patient complaints including fatigue, muscle weakness, sleep disturbance, pain, poor concentration, memory impairment, and poor appetite have been reported by survivors of critical illness.[28] Despite these complaints, former critically ill patients and their family members would still be willing to undergo critical care and mechanical ventilation again in most cases to prolong survival.[46]

Additional data show evidence of an increased risk of patients and family members developing post-traumatic stress disorder after a critical care experience.[8] Once home, the demands of follow-up care can place an enormous burden on family members, who may be ill-prepared or unwilling to shoulder such a burden. The time investment and attendant financial costs may be overwhelming.

Discharge planning and patient teaching are essential nursing interventions to improve patient and family outcomes. One technique used by some hospitals is a so-called teach-back method, in which patients are asked to repeat the information and instructions they have been given.[38] Patient-family teaching is an integral part of nursing care. Ongoing family involvement and teaching, beginning at admission and continuing throughout the hospital stay, are crucial interventions to ensure optimal patient outcomes.

Geriatric Concerns

Each individual patient's response to critical illness is influenced by various factors, including age and developmental stage, prior experiences with illness and hospitalization, family relationships and social support, prior stressful experiences and coping mechanisms, and personal philosophies about life, death, and spirituality. Some elderly patients have a diminished ability to adapt and cope with the major physical and psychosocial stressors of critical illness. This is often the result of multiple losses over the years, including loss of physical function, loss of family members, and loss of resources, such as homes and income. Yet some elderly patients with chronic illnesses who have endured multiple critical illnesses demonstrate amazing resilience. Patients who have survived a prior critical illness generally have less anxiety during subsequent admissions. For other patients, their only prior experience with critical illness may have ended with the death of a family member. This scenario can add considerably to the patient's fears and anxiety.

Although the fears and concerns of the geriatric patient are similar to the concerns of younger critically ill patients, the elderly patient may be at greater risk of negative outcomes. An extensive review of the literature related to health-related quality of life (HRQOL) and functional outcomes in elderly survivors of critical illness reported mixed results. Some studies found that elderly patients (defined as age 65 or older) had no changes in HRQOL and were satisfied with their experiences. Increased mortality, functional decline, and a decrease in HRQOL were noted in other studies, especially after a prolonged length of stay in critical care and in the very elderly ($\geq$85 years).[32]

FAMILY MEMBERS OF THE CRITICALLY ILL PATIENT

Family-centered care is the concept of treating the patient and family as an inseparable entity, recognizing that illness or injury of one family member invariably affects all other family members (see Evidence-Based Practice feature).[33] A holistic approach to critical care nursing requires that the family be included in the plan of care.

For many families, both hospitals and the critical care unit are "alien" environments. The media portrayal of hospitals may lead to preconceptions about the hospital and critical care environment. In addition, ready access to medical information—whether reliable or not—regarding the patient's illness may also foster unrealistic expectations. Health literacy is

EVIDENCE-BASED PRACTICE

PROBLEM

Family-centered care has been advocated in critical care units. Yet many practices and traditions result in care that does not focus on the family.

QUESTION

What critical care practices support family-centered care in critical care units?

REFERENCE

Davidson, J. E., Powers, K., Hedayat, K. M., et al. (2007). Clinical practice guidelines for support of the family in the patient-centered intensive care unit: American College of Critical Care Medicine Task Force 2004-2005. *Critical Care Medicine, 35*, 605-622.

EVIDENCE

Members of a multidisciplinary task force sponsored by the American College of Critical Care Medicine reviewed more than 300 articles related to several topics, including decision making, coping, staff member stress, cultural and spiritual support, visitation, family presence, and palliative care. The majority of the studies were case studies or expert opinion articles, indicating many opportunities for critical care nursing research. The group made 43 recommendations based upon the best available evidence on these many topics. Recommendations were to be given a grade of A, based on the highest level of evidence, to D, based on expert opinion. Interestingly, no recommendations were given an "A." Twenty-five recommendations for the multiprofessional health care team that received a grade of C (based on some evidence) or better are as follows:

DECISION MAKING

- Make decisions based on a partnership between the patient, family, and the health care team.
- Communicate the patient's status and prognosis to family members and explain options for treatment.
- Hold family meetings with the health care team within 24 to 48 hours after intensive care unit (ICU) admission and repeat as often as needed.
- Train ICU staff in communication, conflict management, and facilitation skills.

FAMILY COPING

- Train ICU staff in assessment of family needs, stress, and anxiety levels.
- Assign consistent nursing and physician staff to each patient if possible. Update family members in language they can understand. Keep the number of staff members who provide information to a minimum.
- Provide information to family members in a variety of formats.
- Provide family support using a team effort, including social workers, clergy, nursing, medicine, and support groups.

STAFF STRESS

- Keep all health care team members informed of treatment goals to ensure that messages given to the family are consistent.
- Develop a mechanism for staff members to request a debriefing to voice concerns with the treatment plan, decompress, share feelings, or grieve.

CULTURAL SUPPORT OF FAMILY

- If possible, match the provider's culture to that of the patient.
- Educate staff on culturally competent care.

SPIRITUAL AND RELIGIOUS SUPPORT

- Assess spiritual needs and incorporate into the plan of care.
- Educate staff in spiritual and religious issues that facilitate patient assessment.

FAMILY VISITATION

- Facilitate open visitation in the adult intensive care environment if possible.
- Determine visitation schedules in collaboration with the patient, family, and nurse; consider the best interest of the patient.
- Provide open visitation in the pediatric ICU and neonatal ICU 24 hours a day.
- Allow siblings to visit in the pediatric ICU and neonatal ICU (with parental approval) after participation in a previsit education program.
- Do not restrict pets that are clean and properly immunized from visiting the ICU. Develop guidelines for animal-assisted therapy.

FAMILY ENVIRONMENT OF CARE

- Build new ICUs with single-bed rooms to improve patient confidentiality, privacy, and social support.
- Develop signage (e.g., easy-to-follow directions) to reduce stress on visitors.

FAMILY PRESENCE DURING ROUNDS

- Allow parents or guardians of children in the ICU to participate in rounds.

EVIDENCE-BASED PRACTICE—cont'd

- Allow adult patients and family members to participate in rounds.

FAMILY PRESENCE DURING RESUSCITATION

- Develop a process to allow the presence of family members during cardiopulmonary resuscitation.

PALLIATIVE CARE

- Educate staff in palliative care during formal critical care education.

IMPLICATIONS FOR NURSING

Nurses must be aware of research-based strategies to support patients and family members. Nurses can include these recommendations into the plan of care for patients. Nurses should also participate in education to enhance their skills in patient and family-focused care, such as cultural competence and palliative care strategies. Nurses can conduct additional research to test interventions to improve family-centered care in the ICU.

---

the ability to obtain and understand health information to make decisions regarding health care. Lack of health literacy skills may also limit the ability of some families to grasp explanations of a loved one's diagnosis and prognosis. This is true among English-speaking and non–English-speaking families alike.[64]

Family Assessment

Once the patient has been admitted to the critical care unit, an assessment of the family provides valuable information for preparation of the nursing care plan. Essential information is gathered during the admission assessment, and additional information is obtained as available, often during visitation.

Several models are available to guide family assessment, including the Calgary Family Assessment Model. This model consists of three major categories: structural, developmental, and functional.[62] Each nurse determines which categories are appropriate to explore with each family at a given point in the critical illness trajectory. The *structural assessment* includes the internal structure (who is in the family), the external structure (examining extended family and larger systems), and family context (including ethnicity, race, social class, religion and spirituality, and the environment).[62] Assessment of the family structure is the first step and is essential before specific interventions can be designed. The *developmental* assessment includes information related to the family's developmental stages, tasks, and attachments. The *functional* family assessment is concerned with how family members function and behave in relation to one another, and includes instrumental and expressive aspects.[62] The instrumental aspect of family functioning refers to activities of daily living, such as eating, sleeping, and cooking. For family members experiencing the critical illness trajectory, this can be a particularly important area because many of the family's routines

and habits are disrupted. The expressive aspect of family functioning refers to communication patterns, problem-solving abilities, beliefs, roles, and alliances within the family. These aspects are extremely important for the critical care nurse to assess because communication patterns within the family are often altered by the stress of critical illness. Thus, communication has been shown to be a vital component of quality family care.[7]

An early, proactive approach is advised when assessing a patient's family. The family assessment may reveal whether the family members are angry, feeling guilty, or have unaddressed concerns regarding the patient's condition and care. An illness within the family may also uncover underlying conflicts among family members, especially when family members are estranged or have other unresolved issues.

Although assessment data can be challenging to gather for complex family units, recording the collected data in a concise manner can be even more daunting. It is important to identify key information related to family assessment that is shared among all nurses caring for the patient.

Family Needs

Many researchers have identified a predictable set of needs of family members of critically ill patients: receiving assurance, remaining near the patient, receiving information, being comfortable, and having support available.[42,43] Meeting these needs increases family satisfaction and may reduce the development of posttraumatic stress disorder in family members.[7,8]

Lack of communication is a principal complaint when families are dissatisfied with care.[22,25] Nurses can facilitate better communication by providing a simple, honest report of the patient's condition, free of medical jargon. A follow-up assessment to gauge the family's level of understanding helps to tailor the care plan accordingly.

Some family members may be demanding or disruptive, or may insist on constant vigilance from the nursing staff. Such behavior may reflect a sense of loss of control or possibly memories of an adverse outcome during a previous hospitalization. In such cases, it is important to reassure the family member that everything is being done for the patient, and communicate that standards of critical care practice are being followed.

Some nurses have difficulty interacting with family members who want confirmation that everything is being done for the patient. It is important for the nurse to establish a partnership with the family built on mutual respect as well as credibility, competence, and compassion. One strategy is to encourage family members to assist in patient assessment (e.g., identify changes) and participate in selected aspects of the patient's care. Depending on institutional policy, it may be possible to enlist family members to help with tasks such as oral care, hygiene, range-of-motion exercises, or repositioning the patient. These activities give family members a sense of purpose and control, as well as potentially provide an additional layer of safety when the nurse is unavailable.[9] One of the Joint Commission's *National Patient Safety Goals* is to encourage active involvement by both patients and families in reporting safety concerns.[36] Simple acts of helping can also facilitate patient-family bonding and togetherness; promote patient healing and comfort; decrease a family member's sense of helplessness and anxiety; and assist family members in grasping their loved one's condition.[10]

Visitation

Visitation is among the most contentious and widely researched issues in nursing. In the past, critical care units have operated under their own set of rules regarding visitation, often enacting strict controls on both the timing and the length of visits. Proposals to liberalize visitation rules have frequently met resistance from critical care staff. Reasons cited for opposition to liberal visitation include the presumed increased physiological stress for the patient, family interference with the provision of care, and physical and mental exhaustion of family and friends.[11] An additional concern is that family members will be intrusive or overly critical of the nurse's performance. However, visitation in critical care units has been studied extensively. Study findings on family visitation have found no adverse effects on patient stability and infection, or negative consequences on the patient or family.[55] Contrary to traditional thinking, family presence more often has a positive effect on the patient's condition.[27]

A recent national study on visitation practices in critical care units found that 44% of critical care units still have restricted visitation policies. However, 45% of units had policies that were open at all times, or restricted only during rounds and change of shift.[40] Most acute care institutions prohibit visitation by children; however, research to support this policy is limited. Decisions regarding allowing children in critical care units should be based on factors such as developmental stage of the child and adequate preparation of the child for the visit.[34,48] One study showed that allowing children to visit family members in the critical care unit reduced negative behavioral and emotional outcomes of the patient.[48]

Animal-assisted therapy may be beneficial to a patient's recovery. Some critical care units have extended visitation to include pet therapy. These institutions have policies that permit the family pet or designated therapy animals to visit the patient.[17,18,20,29]

Nurses can assist in promoting policy changes to affect open visitation policies.[11] A significant benefit of a liberal visitation policy is its positive impact on the opinions of both patients and families regarding the quality of nursing care. Information is a crucial component in family coping and satisfaction in critical care settings. Visitation promotes information exchange. When combined with family support, as demonstrated by the nurses' caring behaviors and interactions, liberal visitation is influential in shaping the critical care experience for both patients and families.

Family Presence during Procedures and Resuscitation

In conjunction with more liberal visitation policies, many institutions have implemented policies to allow families to be present during invasive procedures and cardiopulmonary resuscitation (CPR). (See Chapter 10 for an in-depth discussion of family presence during CPR.) Factors cited for limiting family members' presence include limited space at the bedside, violations of patient confidentiality, not enough staff members available to assist family members, increased stress on health care staff members (e.g., performance anxiety and risk for litigation), and increased stress and anxiety for family members.[31] However, these factors have not been substantiated by research. Research studies have found that allowing family members to observe invasive procedures and resuscitation efforts promotes increased knowledge of the patient's condition, and allows a witnessing that everything was done, reduces

---

BOX 2-5   Benefits of Family Presence

Being Present Helps Family Members to:
- Remove doubt about the patient's condition
- Witness that everything possible was done
- Decrease their anxiety and fear about what was happening to their loved one

Being Present Facilitates Family Members':
- Need to be together with their loved one
- Need to help and support their loved one
- Sense of closure and grieving should death occur

---

fear and anxiety, and promotes adaptation.[31] Box 2-5 presents the benefits of family presence.

The AACN published a practice alert titled *Family Presence During CPR and Invasive Procedures*. Two recommendations are specified in the document: (1) provide family members of all patients undergoing CPR and invasive procedures the option of being present at the bedside, and (2) develop a written policy for presenting the option of family presence during CPR and bedside invasive procedures.[3] The policy includes education for the staff members on the benefits of family presence; strategies that facilitate family presence, such as the use of trained facilitators; and support for family members who do not want to be present during procedures or CPR.

THE CRITICAL CARE NURSE

As the demand for critical care beds increases, critical care nurses face increasing challenges in balancing expanding work responsibilities with limited resources. Well-educated and highly motivated critical care nurses may bring to the job perfectionist tendencies and unrealistic expectations of self, further contributing to high stress levels. In addition, critical care nurses encounter occupational hazards on a daily basis. For example, the increase in the number of obese patients poses health and safety risks for the nurse when these patients are turned or moved. There is also the constant risk of exposure to communicable diseases.

Like the population in general, practicing nurses are growing older. The reality of an aging population being cared for by an aging nursing workforce is likely to continue. To accommodate this workforce, hospitals are focusing attention on the ergonomics of nursing stations and patient care equipment. Innovative staffing solutions will also be required to continue to tap into the wealth of clinical knowledge and expertise of older nurses who may no longer want or be able to work full-time or 12-hour shifts. As nurses retire or otherwise leave the profession, pressure grows to educate and hire enough qualified replacements. Any decrease in the number of practicing nurses disproportionately affects critical care because of the additional education and training required to achieve competency. For those nurses who remain in critical care, or who are new entrants to the field, the environment in which they practice will become a central issue. Nurse-to-patient ratios, clinical performance and outcomes, nurse burnout, and job satisfaction are related issues that are important to recruitment and retention of critical care nurses.

As the need for critical care nurses continues to grow, support to ensure that critical care nurses focus their care efforts on critical care nursing interventions is a priority. Many tasks that critical care nurses often perform can be delegated to paraprofessional personnel who are educated and trained. Such tasks include cleaning the environment, patient hygiene, and selected treatments such as drawing blood. These activities often can be delegated and cannot be delayed, but are secondary domains of direct nursing care.[50] The primary domain of the critical care professional practice cannot be delegated and often is delayed or deferred while the nurse completes nonnursing tasks. Essential nursing practices include monitoring and assessment; reassessment, interpreting information, and problem solving; evaluation of progress to outcomes; development of sustainable evidence-based practice; coordination of team activities and the plan of care; patient and family education; and team skill development.[50] These professional practice interventions need to be reprioritized for critical care nurses.

AACN SYNERGY MODEL FOR PATIENT CARE

Needs of patients and their family members are important aspects of critical care nursing practice. The AACN Synergy Model for Patient Care was developed to link clinical practice with patient outcomes. Synergy is described as a result of the efforts of two or more parties working together that is greater than that which each could produce if working separately. In other words, the resultant whole is greater than the sum of the parts. The synergy model posits that optimal patient outcomes result when patients' and nurses' characteristics are matched.[21] The unique needs or characteristics of patients and their families influence and drive the competencies of the nurses who care for them. Nursing care reflects an integration of knowledge, skills, experience, and attitudes needed to meet the needs of patients and families.[21]

Eight patient characteristics that span the continuum of health and illness (Box 2-6) and eight nursing competencies (Table 2-3) comprise the synergy model. Patients move among different points along the seven continua. Thus, to create synergy, nurses use various competencies to best meet patient needs. Although all eight nursing competencies are essential for nursing practice, each assumes more or less importance based on the patient's unique characteristics.[21] Several assumptions regarding patients, families, and nurses guide the synergy model. First, all patient and nurse characteristics are viewed in context. Second, patients are biological, psychological, social, and spiritual entities who present at a particular developmental stage. The needs of the whole patient (body, mind, and spirit) are considered. Third, the patient, family, and community all contribute to providing a context for the nurse-patient relationship. Finally, patients and nurses can be described by certain characteristics. All

---

BOX 2-6 American Association of Critical-Care Nurses Synergy Model Patient Characteristics

- Resiliency: the capacity to return to a restorative level of functioning using compensatory/coping mechanisms; the ability to bounce back quickly after an insult
- Vulnerability: susceptibility to actual or potential stressors that may adversely affect patient outcomes
- Stability: the ability to maintain a steady-state equilibrium
- Complexity: the intricate entanglement of two or more systems (e.g., body, family, therapies)
- Resource Availability: extent of resources (e.g., technical, fiscal, personal, psychological, and social) that the patient/family/community bring to the situation
- Participation in Care: extent to which patient/family engages in aspects of care
- Participation in Decision Making: extent to which patient/family engages in decision making
- Predictability: a characteristic that allows one to expect a certain course of events or course of illness

From Kaplow, R. (2007). Synergy model: guiding the practice of the CNS in acute and critical care. In M. G. McKinley (ed.). *Acute and critical care clinical nurse specialists: synergy for best practices* [p. 30]. St. Louis: Elsevier.

TABLE 2-3 American Association of Critical-Care Nurses Synergy Model Nurse Competencies

- Clinical Judgment—clinical reasoning, which includes clinical decision-making, critical thinking, and a global grasp of the situation, coupled with nursing skills acquired through a process of integrating formal and informal experiential knowledge and evidence-based guidelines.
- Advocacy and Moral Agency—working on another's behalf and representing the concerns of the patient/family and nursing staff; serving as a moral agent in identifying and helping to resolve ethical and clinical concerns within and outside the clinical setting.
- Caring Practices—nursing activities that create a compassionate, supportive, and therapeutic environment for patients and staff, with the aim of promoting comfort and healing and preventing unnecessary suffering. Includes, but is not limited to, vigilance, engagement, and responsiveness of caregivers, including family and health care personnel.
- Collaboration—working with others (e.g., patients, families, health care providers) in a way that promote/encourage each person's contributions toward achieving optimal/realistic patient/family goals. Involves intra- and interdisciplinary work with colleagues and community.
- Systems Thinking—body of knowledge and tools that allow the nurse to manage whatever environmental and system resources exist for the patient/family and staff, within or across health care and non–health care systems.
- Response to Diversity—the sensitivity to recognize, appreciate and incorporate differences into the provision of care. Differences may include, but are not limited to, cultural differences, spiritual beliefs, gender, race, ethnicity, lifestyle, socioeconomic status, age, and values.
- Facilitation of Learning—the ability to facilitate learning for patients/families, nursing staff, other members of the health care team, and community. Includes both formal and informal facilitation of learning.
- Clinical Inquiry (Innovator/Evaluator)—the ongoing process of questioning and evaluating practice and providing informed practice. Creating practice changes through research utilization and experiential learning.

Adapted from Kaplow, R. (2007). Synergy model: guiding the practice of the CNS in acute and critical care. In M. G. McKinley (ed.). *Acute and critical care clinical nurse specialists: synergy for best practices* [p. 34]. St. Louis: Elsevier.

characteristics and competencies contribute to each other and cannot be understood in isolation. The interrelated dimensions paint the profile of the patient and nurse.

SUMMARY

This chapter has provided an overview of the critical care environment and the experience of critical illness from the perspective of the patient, family, and nurse. As key players among equals on the critical care team, nurses are ideally positioned to shape the future of critical care by ensuring that the patient remains the focus of that care. By understanding the critical care experience from a variety of perspectives, critical care nurses are better able to tailor their responses and interventions to meet what is both desired and required by critically ill patients and their family members. The resulting synergy is essential to achieving optimal patient, family, and critical care nurse outcomes.

CRITICAL THINKING QUESTIONS · evolve

1. What are some of the potential pitfalls in using cultural categorizations when caring for critical care patients from other cultures?
2. You are leading a work group charged with revising the ICU visitation policy, specifically with regard to open visitation. The majority of the staff is skeptical. What are some of the objections you might encounter, and how would you address them?
3. You are caring for a patient whose family members include other medical professionals (e.g., RN, nurse practitioner, MD). The family is frequently critical of the patient's management and is constantly making suggestions regarding nursing care. How do you respond?
4. The family members of a critically ill patient are trying to decide whether to terminate life-support measures and have asked for your opinion.

evolve Be sure to check out the bonus material, including free self-assessment exercises, on the Evolve Web site at http://evolve.elsevier.com/Sole.

REFERENCES

1. Adamski, P. (2007). Implement a handoff communications approach. *Nursing Management, 38*(1), 10, 12.
2. American Association of Critical-Care Nurses. (2005). AACN standards for establishing and sustaining healthy work environments: A journey to excellence. *American Journal of Critical Care, 14,* 187-197.
3. American Association of Critical-Care Nurses. (2004). *Family presence during CPR and invasive procedures.* Aliso Viejo, CA: AACN.
4. American Association of Critical-Care Nurses. (2006). *Role of the critical care nurse* [position statement]. Aliso Viejo, CA: AACN.
5. Arford, P. (2005). Nurse-physician communication: An organizational accountability. *Nursing Economic$, 23*(2), 72-77.
6. Arora, V., & Johnson, J. (2006). A model for building a standardized hand-off protocol. *Joint Commission Journal on Quality and Patient Safety, 32,* 646-655.
7. Azoulay, E., Pochard, F., Chevret, S., et al. (2003). Family participation in care to the critically ill: Opinions of families and staff. *Intensive Care Medicine, 29,* 1498-1504.
8. Azoulay, E., Pochard, F., Kentish-Barnes, N., et al. (2005). Risk of post-traumatic stress symptoms in family members of intensive care unit patients. *American Journal of Respiratory and Critical Care Medicine, 171,* 987-994.
9. Benner, P. (2001). Creating a culture of safety and improvement: A key to reducing medical error. *American Journal of Critical Care, 10,* 281-284.
10. Benner, P., Hooper-Kyriakidis, P., & Stannard, D. (1999). *Clinical wisdom and interventions in critical care: A thinking-in-action approach.* Philadelphia: Saunders.
11. Berwick, D. M., & Kotagal, M. (2004). Restricted visiting hours in ICUs: Time to change. *Journal of the American Medical Association, 292,* 736-737.
12. Blue Ridge Academic Health Group. (2005). *Report 9: Getting the physician right: Exceptional professionalism for a new era.* Atlanta, GA: Emory University Woodruff Health Sciences Center.
13. Chaboyer, W. (2006). Intensive care and beyond: Improving the transitional experiences for critically ill patients and their families. *Intensive and Critical Care Nursing, 22,* 187-193.
14. Chaboyer, W., Kendall, E., Kendall, M., et al. (2005). Transfer out of intensive care: An exploration of patient and family perceptions. *Australian Critical Care, 18,* 138-145.
15. Chlan, L., Evans, D., Greenleaf, M., et al. (2000). Effects of a single music therapy intervention on anxiety, discomfort, satisfaction, and compliance with screening guidelines in outpatients undergoing flexible sigmoidoscopy. *Gastroenterology Nursing, 23,* 148-156.

16. Chlan, L. L. (2000). Music therapy as a nursing intervention for patients supported by mechanical ventilation. *AACN Clinical Issues, 11,* 128-138.

17. Connor, K., & Miller, J. (2000). Animal-assisted therapy: An in-depth look. *Dimensions of Critical Care Nursing, 19*(3), 20-26.

18. Connor, K., & Miller, J. (2000). Help from our animal friends. *Nursing Management, 31*(7), 42-46.

19. Coyle, M. A. (2001). Transfer anxiety: Preparing to leave intensive care. *Intensive and Critical Care Nursing, 17,* 138-143.

20. Cullen, L., Titler, M., & Drahozal, R. (1999). Family and pet visitation in the critical care unit. *Critical Care Nurse, 19*(3), 84-87.

21. Curley, M. A. (1998). Patient-nurse synergy: Optimizing patients' outcomes. *American Journal of Critical Care, 7,* 64-72.

22. Davidson, J. E., Powers, K., Hedayat, K. M., et al. (2007). Clinical practice guidelines for support of the family in the patient-centered intensive care unit: American College of Critical Care Medicine Task Force 2004-2005. *Critical Care Medicine, 35,* 605-622.

23. Divi, C., Koss, R. G., Schmaltz, S. P., et al. (2007). Language proficiency and adverse events in US hospitals: A pilot study. *International Journal for Quality in Health Care, 19*(2), 60-67.

24. Doucette, J. N. (2006). View from the cockpit: What the airline industry can teach us about patient safety. *Nursing, 36*(11), 50-53.

25. Downey, L., Engelberg, R. A., Shannon, S. E., et al. (2006). Measuring intensive care nurses' perspectives on family-centered end-of-life care: Evaluation of 3 questionnaires. *American Journal of Critical Care, 15,* 568-569.

26. Dunn, E. J., Mills, P. D., Neily, J., et al. (2007). Medical team training: Applying crew resource management in the Veterans Health Administration. *Joint Commission Journal on Quality and Patient Safety, 33,* 317-325.

27. Duran, C. R., Oman, K. S., Abel, J. J., et al. (2007). Attitudes toward and beliefs about family presence: A survey of healthcare providers, patients' families, and patients. *American Journal of Critical Care, 16,* 270-279.

28. Fletcher, S. N., Kennedy, D. D., Ghosh, I. R., et al. (2003). Persistent neuromuscular and neurophysiologic abnormalities in long-term survivors of prolonged critical illness. *Critical Care Medicine, 31,* 1012-1016.

29. Giuliano, K. K., Bloniasz, E., & Bell, J. (1999). Implementation of a pet visitation program in critical care. *Critical Care Nurse, 19*(3), 43-50.

30. Haig, K. M., Sutton, S., & Whittington, J. (2006). SBAR: A shared mental model for improving communication between clinicians. *Joint Commission Journal on Quality and Patient Safety, 32*(3), 167-175.

31. Halm, M. A. (2005). Family presence during resuscitation: A critical review of the literature. *American Journal of Critical Care, 14*(6), 494-511.

32. Henneman, E. A., & Cardin, S. (2002). Family-centered critical care: A practical approach to making it happen. *Critical Care Nurse, 22*(6), 12-19.

33. Hennessy, D., Juzwishin, K., Yergens, D., et al. (2005). Outcomes of elderly survivors of intensive care: A review of the literature. *Chest, 127,* 1764-1774.

34. Ihlenfeld, J. T. (2006). Should we allow children to visit ill parents in intensive care units? *Dimensions of Critical Care Nursing, 25,* 269-271.

35. Jastremski, C. A. (2000). ICU bedside environment. A nursing perspective. *Critical Care Clinics, 16,* 723-734.

36. Joint Commission. (2007). *National patient safety goals.* Retrieved August 25, 2007, from www.jointcommission.org/PatientSafety/NationalPatientSafetyGoals.

37. Joseph, A. (2006). *The impact of light on outcomes in healthcare settings* (Issue Paper No. 2). Concord, CA: The Center for Health Design.

38. Joseph, A. (2006). *The role of the physical environment in promoting health, safety, and effectiveness in the healthcare workplace* (Issue Paper No. 3). Concord, CA: The Center for Health Design.

39. Joseph, A., & Ulrich, R. (2007). *Sound control for improved outcomes in healthcare settings* (Issue Paper No. 4). Concord, CA: The Center for Health Design and the Robert Wood Johnson Foundation.

40. Kirchhoff, K. T., & Dahl, N. (2006). American Association of Critical-Care Nurses' national survey of facilities and units providing critical care. *American Journal of Critical Care, 15,* 13-27.

41. Kohn, L. T., Corrigan, J. M., & Donaldson, M. (2000). *To err is human: Building a safer health system.* Washington, DC: National Academies Press.

42. Leske, J. S. (1991). Overview of family needs after critical illness: From assessment to intervention. *AACN Clinical Issues in Critical Care Nursing, 2,* 220-229.

43. Leske, J. S. (1992). Needs of adult family members after critical illness: Prescriptions for interventions. *Critical Care Nursing Clinics of North America, 4,* 587-596.

44. McCauley, K., & Irwin, R. S. (2006). Changing the work environment in intensive care units to achieve patient-focused care: The time has come. *American Journal of Critical Care, 15,* 541-548.

45. McKinney, A. A., & Melby, V. (2002). Relocation stress in critical care: A review of the literature. *Journal of Clinical Nursing, 11,* 149-157.

46. Mendelsohn, A. B., Belle, S. H., Fischhoff, B., et al. (2002). How patients feel about prolonged mechanical ventilation 1 year later. *Critical Care Medicine, 30,* 1439-1445.

47. Mitchell, M. L., Courtney, M., & Coyer, F. (2003). Understanding uncertainty and minimizing families' anxiety at the time of transfer from intensive care. *Nursing & Health Sciences, 5,* 207-217.

48. Nicholson, A. C., Titler, M., Montgomery, L. A., et al. (1993). Effects of child visitation in adult critical care units: A pilot study. *Heart and Lung, 22,* 36-45.

49. Oriol, M. D. (2006). Crew resource management: Applications in healthcare organizations. *Journal of Nursing Administration, 36,* 402-406.

50. Ott, K. (2005). Differentiation of practice: Complimentary and effective roles. Presented at Clinical Nurse Leader Core Competencies Training, Nashville, TN.

51. Powell, S. K. (2007). SBAR: It's not just another communication tool. *Professional Case Management, 12,* 195-196.

52. Powell, S. M., & Hill, R. K. (2006). My copilot is a nurse: Using crew resource management in the OR. *AORN Journal, 83,* 179-180, 183-190, 193-198.

53. Rashid, M. (2006). A decade of adult intensive care unit design: A study of the physical design features of the best-practice examples. *Critical Care Nursing Quarterly, 29,* 282-311.

54. Roberts, B. L., Rickard, C. M., Rajbhandari, D., et al. (2007). Factual memories of ICU: recall at two years post-discharge and comparison with delirium status during ICU admission: A multicentre cohort study. *Journal of Clinical Nursing, 16,* 1669-1677.

55. Roland, P., Russell, J., Richards, K. C., et al. (2001). Visitation in critical care: Processes and outcomes of a performance improvement initiative. *Journal of Nursing Care Quality, 15*(2), 18-26.

56. Smith, A. P. (2004). Partners at the bedside: The importance of nurse-physician relationships. *Nursing Economic$, 22,* 161-164.

57. Solet, D. J., Norvell, J. M., Rutan, G. H., et al. (2005). Lost in translation: Challenges and opportunities in physician-to-physician communication during patient handoffs. *Academic Medicine, 80,* 1094-1099.

58. Sundar, E., Sundar, S., Pawlowski, J., et al. (2007). Crew resource management and team training. *Anesthesiology Clinics, 25,* 283-300.

59. Thompson, D., Holzmueller, C., Hunt, D., et al. (2005). A morning briefing: Setting the stage for a clinically and operationally good day. *Joint Commission Journal on Quality and Patient Safety, 31,* 476-479.

60. Ulrich, R., Quan, X., Zimring, C., et al. (2004). *The role of the physical environment in the hospital of the 21st century: A once-in-a-lifetime opportunity.* Concord, CA: The Center for Health Design.

61. Williams, M. (2001). Critical care unit design: A nursing perspective. *Critical Care Nursing Quarterly, 24,* 35-42.

62. Wright, L. M., & Leahey, M. (2005). *Nurses and families: A guide to family assessment and intervention* (4th ed.). Philadelphia: F. A. Davis.

63. Wu, C. J., Coyer, F. (2007). Reconsidering the transfer of patients from the intensive care unit to the ward: A case study approach. *Nursing & Health Sciences, 9,* 48-53.

64. Wynia, M., & Matiasek, J. (2006). *Promising practices for patient-centered communication with vulnerable populations: Examples from eight hospitals.* New York: The Commonwealth Fund.

CHAPTER 3

Ethical and Legal Issues in Critical Care Nursing

Jayne M. Willis, MSN, RN
Maryjane N. Randels, JD, BSN, RN

INTRODUCTION

Critical care nurses are often confronted with ethical and legal dilemmas related to informed consent, withholding or withdrawal of life-sustaining treatment, organ and tissue transplantation, confidentiality, and increasingly, justice in the distribution of health care resources. Many dilemmas are byproducts of advanced medical technologies and therapies developed over the past several decades. Although technology provides substantial benefits to critically ill patients, extensive public and professional debate occurs over the appropriate use of these technologies, especially those that are life sustaining. One of the primary concerns in critical care is whether patients' values and beliefs about treatment can be overridden by the technological imperative, or the strong tendency to use technology because it is available.

Although many ethical dilemmas are not unique to critical care, they occur with greater frequency in critical care settings. Therefore, it is crucial that nurses examine the nature and scope of their ethical and legal obligations to patients.

The ethical and legal issues that frequently arise in the nursing care of critical care patients are examined in this chapter. The discussion includes problems that surround patients' rights and nurses' obligations, professional negligence, informed consent, withholding and withdrawal of treatment, and organ and tissue transplantation. The elements of ethical decision making and the involvement of the nurse are discussed.

ETHICAL OBLIGATIONS AND NURSE ADVOCACY

Critical care nurses' ethical and legal responsibilities for patient care have increased dramatically since the early 1990s. Evolving case law and current concepts of nurse advocacy and accountability indicate that nurses have substantial ethical and legal obligations to promote and protect the welfare of their patients.

The duty to practice ethically and to serve as an ethical agent on behalf of patients is an integral part of nurses' professional practice. The nurse's duty is stated in the *Code of Ethics for Nurses with Interpretive Statements*, which was adopted by the American Nurses Association (ANA) in 1976 and was revised in 2001.[5] The code for nurses delineates the moral principles that guide professional nursing practice, and serves the following purposes: (1) it delineates the ethical obligations and duties of every individual who enters the profession; (2) it is the profession's nonnegotiable ethical standard; and (3) it is the expression of nursing's own understanding of its commitment to society.[5] The 2001 *code of ethics for nurses* consists of nine provision statements. The first three describe fundamental values and commitments of the nurse, the next three describe the boundaries of duty and loyalty, and the last three describe duties beyond individual patient encounters. Nurses in all practice arenas, including critical care, must be knowledgeable about the provisions of the code and must incorporate its basic tenets into their clinical practice. The code is a powerful tool that shapes and evaluates individual practice, as well as the nursing profession. However, situations may arise in which the code provides only limited direction. Critical care nurses must remain knowledgable and abreast of ethical issues and changes in the literature so they may make appropriate decisions when difficult situations arise in practice. Additional ANA position statements related to human rights and ethics are available from the ANA Web site (www.nursingworld.org).

Nurses' ethical obligation to serve as advocates for their patients is derived from the unique nature of the nurse-patient relationship. Critical care nurses assume a significant caregiving role that is characterized by intimate, extended contact with persons who are often the most physiologically and psychologically vulnerable, and with their families. Critical care nurses have a moral and professional responsibility to act as advocates on their patients' behalf because of their unique relationship with their patients and their specialized nursing knowledge. The American Association of Critical-Care Nurses (AACN) published *An Ethic of Care*,[1] which illustrates the ethical foundations for critical care practice. Ethics involves the interrelatedness and interdependence of individuals, systems, and society. When ethical care is practiced, individual uniqueness, personal relationships, and the dynamic nature of life are respected. Compassion, collaboration, accountability, and trust are essential characteristics of ethical nursing practice.[1] The AACN ethic of care statement is available from the organization's Web site (www.aacn.org).

ETHICAL DECISION MAKING

As reflected in the ANA code of ethics, one of the primary ethical obligations of professional nurses is protection of their patients' basic rights. This obligation requires nurses to recognize ethical dilemmas that actually or potentially threaten patients' rights and to participate in the resolution of those dilemmas.[5]

An ethical dilemma is a difficult problem or situation in which conflicts exist about the making of morally justifiable decisions. In identifying a situation as an ethical dilemma, certain criteria must be met. More than one solution must exist, and there is no clear "right" or "wrong." Each solution must carry equal weight and must be ethically defensible. Whether to give the one available critical care bed to a patient with cancer who is experiencing hypotension after chemotherapy, or to a patient in the emergency department who has an acute myocardial infarction, is an example of an ethical dilemma. The conflicting issue in this example is which patient should be given the bed, based on the moral allocation of limited resources.

Several warning signs can assist the critical care nurse in recognizing that an ethical dilemma may exist:[11]

- Is the situation emotionally charged?
- Has the patient's condition changed significantly?
- Is there confusion or conflict about the facts?
- Is there increased hesitancy about the right course of action?
- Is the proposed action a deviation from customary practice?
- Is there a perceived need for secrecy around the proposed action?

If these warning signs occur, the critical care nurse must reassess the situation and determine whether an ethical dilemma exists and what additional actions are needed.

Arriving at a morally justifiable decision when an ethical dilemma exists can be difficult for patients, families, and health professionals. Critical care nurses must be careful not to impose their own value system on that of the patient. Each patient and family has a set of personal values that are influenced by their environment and culture.

One helpful way to approach ethical decision making is to use a systematic, structured process, such as the one depicted in Figure 3-1. This model provides a framework for evaluation of the related ethical principles and the potential outcomes, as well as relevant facts concerning the contextual factors and the patient's physiological and personal factors. Using this approach, the patient, family, and health care team members evaluate choices and identify the option that promotes the patient's best interests.

Ethical decision making includes implementing the decision and evaluating the short-term and long-term outcomes. Evaluation provides meaningful feedback about decisions and actions in specific instances, as well as the effectiveness of the decision-making process. The final stage in the decision-making process is assessing whether the decision in a specific case can be applied to other dilemmas in similar circumstances. In other words, is this decision useful in similar cases? A systematic approach to decision making does not guarantee that morally justifiable decisions are reached or that the outcome is beneficial to the patient. However, it ensures that all applicable information is considered in the decision.

ETHICAL PRINCIPLES

As reflected in the decision-making model, relevant ethical principles should be considered when a moral dilemma exists. Principles facilitate moral decisions

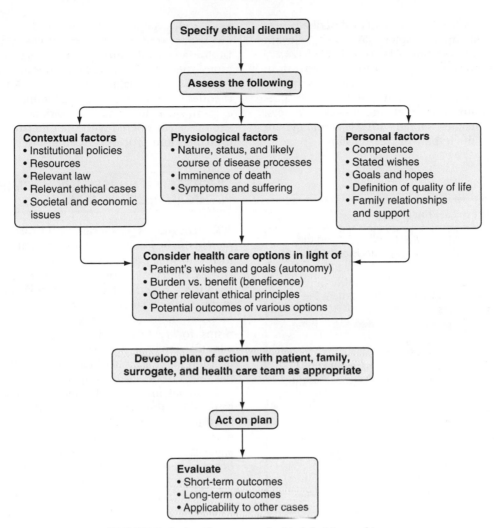

FIGURE 3-1. The process of ethical decision making.

by guiding the decision-making process, but they may conflict with each other and may force a choice among the competing principles based on their relative weight in the situation. Several ethical principles are pertinent in the critical care setting. These principles are intended to provide respect and dignity for all persons (Box 3-1).

Principlism is a widely applied ethical approach based on four fundamental moral principles to contemporary ethical dilemmas: respect for autonomy, beneficence, nonmaleficence, and justice.[6] The principle of *autonomy* states that all persons should be free to govern their lives to the greatest degree possible. The autonomy principle implies a strong sense of self-determination and an acceptance of responsibility for one's own choices and actions. To respect autonomy of others means to respect their freedom

of choice and to allow them to make their own decisions.

The principle of *beneficence* is the duty to provide benefits to others when in a position to do so, and to help balance harms and benefits. In other words, the benefits of an action should outweigh the burdens. A related concept is *futility*. Care should not be given if it is futile in terms of improving comfort or the medical outcome. The principle of *nonmaleficence* is the explicit duty not to inflict harm on others intentionally.

The principle of *justice* requires that health care resources be distributed fairly and equitably among groups of people. The principle of justice is particularly relevant to critical care because most health care resources, including technology and pharmaceuticals, are expended in this practice setting.

In addition to the four principles described previously, the following principles may also be relevant in the critical care setting. The principle of *veracity* states that persons are obligated to tell the truth in their communication with others. The principle of *fidelity* requires that one has a moral duty to be faithful to the commitments that one makes to others. These two principles, along with *confidentiality*, are the key to the nurse-patient relationship.

BOX 3-1   Ethical Principles

- Autonomy: Respect for the individual and the ability of individuals to make decisions with regard to their own health and future (the basis for the practice of informed consent).
- Beneficence: Actions intended to benefit the patients or others.
- Nonmaleficence: Actions intended not to harm or bring harm to others.
- Justice: Being fair or just to the wider community in terms of the consequences of an action. In health care, justice is described as the fair allocation or distribution of health care resources.
- Veracity: The obligation to tell the truth.
- Fidelity: The moral duty to be faithful to the commitments that one makes to others.
- Confidentiality: Respect for an individual's autonomy and the right of individuals to control the information relating to their own health.

Moral Theories

Utilitarianism, deontology, and casuistry are three moral theories that may be used when approaching ethical decision making (Table 3-1).[6] Although these theories do not solve ethical dilemmas, they provide a framework for making decisions. Such theories should be considered with the other relevant ethical principles and processes of ethical decision making.

INCREASING NURSES' INVOLVEMENT IN ETHICAL DECISION MAKING

Although nurses play a significant role in the care of patients, they often report limited involvement in the formal processes of ethical decision making. Nurses' perception of limited involvement in the resolution of ethical dilemmas may be related to many factors, such as lack of formal educational preparation in ethics, lack of institutional mechanisms for review of dilemmas, perceived lack of administrative or peer support for involvement in decision making, concern about reprisals, and lack of perceived decision-making authority.

If nurses are to fulfill their advocacy obligations to patients, they must become active in the process of ethical decision making at all levels. Ethical dilemmas are among the many issues that can lead to *moral distress* for critical care nurses. Moral distress occurs when the nurse knows the ethically appropriate action to take but is unable to act upon it, or when the nurse acts in a manner contrary to personal and professional values. Moral distress is one

---

TABLE 3-1   Moral Theories

Theory	Definition	Decision Making
Deontology: obligation-based theory	Deontological ethics is the theory of duty or moral obligation.	In deontology, ethical decisions are made according to ethical principles, which are interpreted to fulfill a set of duties or values for the care of the individual patient.
Utilitarianism: consequence-based theory	Utilitarians believe that it is the consequences that count, not the intentions.	In utilitarianism, ethical decisions are made considering the greatest good for the greatest number including the patient, family, and society.
Casuistry: case-based reasoning	Casuistry is the school of ethical thought that argues that specific cases inform moral principles.	Casuists advocate that the best starting point for ethical decision making is examining particular cases and the respective decisions made about those cases.

Data from Beauchamp, T. & Childress, J. (2001). *Principles of biomedical ethics* (5th ed.). Oxford, England: Oxford University Press.

of the key issues affecting the workplace environment.[3] Moral distress contributes to the loss of nurses from the workforce and threatens the quality of patient care. Ways for nurses to address moral distress and increase their participation in ethical decision making starts with open communication with the health care team, the patient, and the family regarding the patient's wishes and ethical concerns. A critical element for true collaboration is that health care organizations ensure unrestricted access to structured forums such as ethics committees, and make available the time to resolve disputes among critical participants, including patients, families, and the health care team.[2] Actively addressing ethical dilemmas and avoiding moral distress are crucial factors to creating a healthy workplace where critical care nurses can make optimal contributions to patients and their families.

The Joint Commission requires that a formal mechanism be in place to address patients' ethical concerns. Bioethics committees are one way to address this need. A multidisciplinary committee of health professionals serves as an education and policy-making body and, in some cases, provides ethics consultation on a case-by-case basis. Typical membership of bioethics committees includes physicians, nurses, chaplains, social workers, and, if available, bioethicists. The purpose of ethics consultation is to improve the process and outcomes of patient care by helping to identify, analyze, and resolve ethical problems. This service should be used when the issues cannot be resolved among the health care team, patient, and family. Box 3-2 lists examples of situations where an ethics consultation may be considered.

Nurses can become more involved with ethical decision making through participation in institutional ethics committees, multidisciplinary ethics forums and ethics roundtables, peer review and quality assurance committees, and institutional research review boards. Nurses can also improve and update their knowledge through formal and continuing education courses on bioethics, as well as through telephone and computerized electronic consultation and reference services. Educational programs and ethics consultation services are available through several ethics and law centers in the United States. A few key programs and services are listed in Box 3-3. Additional Internet educational resources are available (Box 3-4).

BOX 3-2 Situations Where Ethics Consultation May Be Considered

- Disagreement or conflict exists on whether to pursue aggressive life-sustaining treatment in a seriously ill patient, such as attempted cardiopulmonary resuscitation, or emphasize comfort/palliative care.
- Family demands to provide life-sustaining treatment such as mechanical ventilation or tube feeding that the physician and nurses consider futile.
- Competing family members are present wanting to make critical decisions on behalf of the patient.
- A seriously ill patient is incapacitated and does not have a surrogated decision maker or an advance directive.

BOX 3-3 Ethics Consultation Services

AMERICAN NURSES ASSOCIATION CENTER FOR ETHICS AND HUMAN RIGHTS
8515 Georgia Avenue
Suite 400
Silver Springs, MD 20910
Telephone: (301) 628-5000
E-mail: ethics@ana.org
http://nursingworld.org/ethics/
CENTER FOR NURSING ETHICS, LAW AND POLICY
University of Texas Medical Branch at Galveston
School of Nursing
301 University Boulevard
Galveston, TX 77555-1132
Telephone: (409) 772-1181
www.son.utmb.edu/nursing/ethicslp/
KENNEDY INSTITUTE OF ETHICS
Georgetown University
P.O. Box 571212
Washington, DC 20057-1212
Telephone: (202) 687-8089
www.georgetown.edu/research/kie

BOX 3-4 Internet Resources for Bioethics

American Journal of Bioethics
http://bioethics.net
American Society for Bioethics and Humanities
www.asbh.org
University of Pennsylvania Center for Bioethics
http://bioethics.upenn.edu
National Institutes of Health Bioethics Resources on the Web
http://bioethics.od.nih.gov/

LEGAL ACCOUNTABILITY IN NURSING

In addition to ethical obligations, nurses in the critical care setting have legal responsibilities to patients. Legal responsibilities have expanded dramatically since the early 1990s as nursing standards of care have been developed and used as a benchmark for defining professional responsibilities.

Lawsuits can be brought against nurses for a variety of reasons: criminal charges or medical malpractice. Most nurses are unaware of the criminal aspect, while more are aware of the medical malpractice lawsuits. Preventing situations that compromise patients is far preferred to defending one's actions in court, but prevention is possible only if nurses have a clear, current knowledge of their legal obligations to patients. This section of the chapter briefly explores legal concepts relevant to critical care practice.

Licensure and Mandatory Education

Nursing is a profession, and as professionals, nurses are required to keep a valid license. A variety of things can affect licensure, such as not meeting state-mandated continuing education unit (CEU) requirements or being named in a criminal lawsuit.

Completion of CEU requirements is one way nurses can document that they meet a certain standard of competence. Many critical care nurses work at large facilities, which offer ample opportunities to acquire CEUs. It is important for nurses to maintain adequate records of CEUs and to submit reports as requested by the state board of nursing.

Hospitals often require additional education and training requirements for those working in critical care. This additional training and certification are required to ensure that nurses are practicing according to the established standards and have the education and training needed for competent care of critically ill patients. For example, critical care nurses are expected to have current expertise in advanced life support. Demonstration of competence in advanced and specialized skills related to the patient population, such as the intraaortic balloon pump and continuous renal replacement, may also be required. Hospitals may also mandate certification in the specialty, such as certification in critical care (CCRN).

Criminal Lawsuits

Criminal lawsuits can arise out of what a nurse does to a client. For instance, a nurse who touches a patient against the patient's will commits the crime of battery in some states. Other examples of criminal lawsuits include assault (threatening to batter a patient), aggravated battery on a person 65 years or older (simple battery on an older adult), and false imprisonment (preventing an alert and oriented patient from leaving against the patient's will), as well as many others.

A criminal charge can arise out of simple situations, and a lawyer can bring both a criminal and a civil suit. Criminal suits have a much higher standard for proof, but just being charged with a criminal suit can cause a nurse's license to get suspended. For example, one nurse was charged with a battery. A year and a half later, the nurse was cleared of all charges. Meanwhile, she could not work as a nurse because her license had been suspended by the Board of Nursing.

It is important for nurses as professionals to protect themselves from criminal charges. Since charges can arise from various clinical situations, it is essential that nurses perform their jobs right the first time, and each and every time. Accidents or incidents are less likely to happen with consistent job performance. Another way to prevent a lawsuit is for nurses to be nice to their patients and family members! Patients and family members who are satisfied with the nursing care are less likely to initiate a lawsuit.

Medical Malpractice

According to Black's Law Dictionary, malpractice is defined as "negligence or incompetence on the part of a professional. Medical malpractice is also defined as a tort that arises when a doctor violates the standard of care owed to a patient and the patient is injured as a result."[8] Malpractice is not limited to physicians; the charge of medical malpractice can be levied against other medical professionals.

Negligence is defined by Black's Law Dictionary as (1) "the failure to exercise the standard of care that a reasonably prudent person would have exercised in the same situation," and (2) "a tort grounded in this failure, usually expressed in terms of the following elements: duty, breach of duty, causation, and damages."[8] As health care professionals, nurses have a duty to provide a certain standard of care to their clients. Failure to practice according to the standard of care frequently results in injury to patients, resulting in nurses being sued under tort law. Torts are civil lawsuits brought against people for monetary damages.

From a legal perspective, a standard is defined as the general recognition of, and conformity to, established practice. A plaintiff who is able to establish that the nurse's failure to perform to an accepted standard of care caused an injury may win a judgment against the nurse. Standards of care are derived from external sources, including expert nurse testimony, state nurse practice acts, the ANA standards of practice, accreditation standards and regulations, authoritative publications, and internal institutional policies and protocols. In addition, courts may review nursing job descriptions and nursing documentation. An acceptable standard of care is the minimum a professional nurse should do in a specific situation. Because baseline standards of care are continuously evolving, the critical care nurse has a responsibility to maintain current knowledge in the field.

Each state has established a statute of limitations for bringing about medical malpractice claims. Lawsuits for medical malpractice often occur months or years after the event that caused the damage to the client. In medical professional negligence cases, the plaintiff (the person bringing the suit) has the burden of proving that the defendant (the person being sued) is liable, or responsible for, an injury. For a professional negligence claim against a nurse to be successful, the plaintiff must establish proof of the following elements:

- The nurse had a specific professional duty to the patient.
- The nurse did not carry out the duty (i.e., breached a duty).
- The nurse caused injury to the patient.
- The patient suffered an injury as a result of the nurse's negligent action.

For example, an unconscious patient develops a corneal ulcer. The nurse caring for the patient has a duty to assess and protect an unconscious patient's eyes from injury. If the nurse failed to assess and protect the patient's eyes, he or she breached the standard of care. If the patient and the patient's legal team prove the nurse's failure to meet the standard of care resulted in the patient's corneal ulcer (the injury), professional negligence exists.

Because lawsuits may be filed long after a nurse has cared for a patient, it is important for critical care nurses to follow some simple strategies. Thorough and accurate documentation is of prime importance. It is difficult for a nurse to prove that an action was performed unless it is documented. In a medical malpractice lawsuit, the case is easier to win for the plaintiff, and the damages go up if there is no or little documentation of actions. Documentation must also be legible. Lawsuits have been won because of an inability of medical professionals to read their handwriting.

Duty to Treat and Abandonment

Nurses have a duty to treat regardless of personal feelings about the patient or the patient's illness. From a legal perspective, a nurse's duty to provide care is derived from a contract or relationship with the employing agency. Abandonment is defined as the unilateral severance of a professional relationship while a patient is still in need of health care.[8] A general rule of thumb: if a patient is accepted by a nurse, the nurse cannot leave that patient without arranging for another nurse to oversee the patient's care. This includes breaks and lunchtime. Nurses who believe they cannot care for a patient because of personal or religious reasons should request a reassignment of the patient to another qualified nurse and ensure the transfer of care. However, the patient must be cared for until another nurse is available and has assumed the responsibilities for patient care.

A nurse should discuss potential moral conflicts with a potential supervisor before employment, to determine whether the employer has policies regarding situations in which moral conflict may arise. This approach allows both the nurse and the employer to be aware of potential issues and to make informed choices about employment at the agency as well as assignments.

SELECTED ETHICAL AND LEGAL ISSUES

Informed Consent

Many complex dilemmas in critical care nursing concern informed consent. Consent problems arise because patients are experiencing acute, life-threatening illnesses that interfere with their ability to make decisions about treatment or participation in a clinical research study. The doctrine of informed consent is based on the principle of autonomy; competent adults have the right to self-determination or to make decisions regarding their acceptance or rejection of treatment.

Elements of Informed Consent

Three primary elements must be present for a person's consent or decline of medical treatment or research participation to be considered valid: competence, voluntariness, and disclosure of information. Competence (or capacity) refers to a person's ability to understand information regarding a proposed medical or nursing treatment. Competence is a legal term and is determined in court. Health care providers evaluate mental capacity. The ability of patients to understand relevant information is an essential prerequisite to their participation in the decision-making process and should be carefully evaluated as part of the informed consent process. Patients providing informed consent should be free from severe pain and depression. Critically ill patients usually do not have the mental capacity to provide informed consent because of the severe nature of their illness or their treatment (e.g., sedation). If the patient is not mentally capable to provide consent, informed consent is obtained from the designated health care surrogate or legal next of kin. State law governs consent issues, and legal counsel should be consulted for specific questions.

Consent must be given voluntarily, without coercion or fraud, for the consent to be legally binding. This includes freedom from pressure from family members, health care providers, and payers. Persons who consent should base their decision on sufficient knowledge. Basic information considered necessary for decision making includes the following:

- A diagnosis of the patient's specific health problem and condition
- The nature, duration, and purpose of the proposed treatment or procedures
- The probable outcome of any medical or nursing intervention
- The benefits of medical or nursing interventions
- The potential risks that are generally considered common or hazardous
- Alternative treatments and their feasibility
- Short-term and long-term prognoses if the proposed treatment or treatments are not provided

The nurse's job is not to provide a patient with the information to obtain informed consent—this is the role of the physician. The nurse's responsibility is to witness signatures on the informed consent. In addition, if the patient asks questions of the nurse and the nurse believes the patient does not understand the procedure enough to give informed consent, it is the nurse's duty to have the physician or assigned medical professional explain the procedure again to the patient. Even though it sometimes is not pleasant for the nurse, especially if the physician gets angry, it is much better to listen to an angry physician than to be cited in a medical malpractice suit.

Informed Consent of Adolescents

Adolescents are a special case when it comes to consent. Unless a procedure is needed emergently, a parent or legal guardian is required to provide consent for a minor (a person younger than 18 years). Depending on statute and case law, which vary from state to state, minors may provide consent for treatment if they are emancipated (legally considered independent persons, not under the control of a parent or legal guardian). Emancipated minors include those who are (1) self-supporting, not living at home, or both; (2) married; (3) pregnant or a parent; (4) in the military; or (5) declared to be emancipated by a court. Some states also give decision-making authority to minors who are considered to be mature or who are seeking treatment for certain conditions, such as sexually transmitted diseases or pregnancy. Information on state laws related to emancipated minors can be found on the Juvenile Law Center Web site (www.jlc.org/index.php/factsheets/emancipationus).

Decisions Regarding Life-Sustaining Treatment

Care of persons who are terminally ill or in a persistent vegetative state raises profound questions about the constitutional rights of persons or surrogates to make decisions related to death or life-sustaining care, as well as the rights of the state to intervene in treatment decisions. Table 3-2 reviews three landmark legal cases—Quinlan, Cruzan, and Schiavo—that have influenced legal and ethical precedents in the right-to-die debate. Box 3-5 lists definitions for some terms pertinent to these issues.

The issue of treatment for persons whose quality of life is severely compromised, as in irreversible coma or brain death, is often a result of advanced biomedical technology. Technology frequently sustains life in persons who would have previously died of their illnesses. The widespread use of advanced life-support systems and cardiopulmonary resuscitation (CPR) has changed the nature and context of dying. A "natural death" in the traditional sense is rare; most patients who die in health care facilities undergo resuscitation efforts.

The benefits derived from aggressive technological management often outweigh the negative effects, but the use of life-sustaining technologies for persons with severely impaired quality of life or for those who are terminally ill has stimulated intensive debate and litigation. Two key issues in this debate are the appropriate use of technology and the ability of the seriously ill person to retain decision-making rights. These issues are based on the ethical principles of beneficence and autonomy.

At the heart of the technology controversy are conflicting beliefs about the morality and legality of allowing persons who are terminally ill or severely debilitated to request withdrawal or withholding of medical treatment. In these situations, two levels of treatment must be considered: ordinary care and extraordinary care. These levels of care are at two ends of a continuum of potential treatment options. Although, based on one's beliefs, some therapies could be put in either category, this distinction is still helpful from a legal and ethical perspective. However, ethicists believe that any treatment can become extraordinary whenever the patient decides that the burdens outweigh the benefits.

TABLE 3-2   Landmark Legal Cases in the Right-to-Die Debate

Case	Events	Impact
Karen Quinlan	Karen Ann Quinlan was the first modern Icon of the right-to-die debate. The 21-year-old Quinlan collapsed at a party after swallowing alcohol and the tranquilizer Valium on April 14, 1975. Doctors saved her life, but she suffered brain damage and lapsed into a "persistent vegetative state." Her family waged a much-publicized legal battle for the right to remove her life-support machinery. They succeeded, but in a final twist, Quinlan kept breathing after the respirator was unplugged. She remained in a coma for almost 10 years in a New Jersey nursing home until her 1985 death.	In finding for the Quinlan family, the courts identified a right to decline lifesaving medical treatment under the general right of privacy. According to the court, her right to privacy outweighed the state's interest in preserving her life, and her father, as her surrogate, could exercise that right for her.
Nancy Cruzan	Nancy Cruzan became a public figure after a 1983 auto accident left her permanently unconscious and without any higher brain function. She was kept alive only by a feeding tube and steady medical care. Cruzan's family waged a legal battle to have her feeding tube removed. The case went all the way to the U.S. Supreme Court, which ruled that the Cruzans had not provided "clear and convincing evidence" that Nancy Cruzan did not wish to have her life artificially preserved. The Cruzans later presented such evidence to the Missouri courts, which ruled in their favor in late 1990. The Cruzans stopped feeding Nancy in December of 1990, and she died later the same month.	The Cruzan case had a significant impact on end-of-life decision making across the country. After the Cruzan decision, the Patient Self-Determination Act was passed by Congress to allow patients to make their own decisions about end-of-life care and/or routine care, should they be unable to make decisions for themselves. The case prompted the development of hospital ethics councils and increased the number of advance directives.
Theresa Schiavo	Theresa Marie "Terri" Schiavo was a Florida woman who sustained brain damage and became dependent on a feeding tube. She collapsed in her home in 1990, experienced respiratory and cardiac arrest, leading to 15 years of institutionalization and a diagnosis of persistent vegetative state. In 1998, her husband, who was her guardian, petitioned the court to remove her feeding tube. Terri Schiavo's parents opposed the removal, arguing that Terri was conscious. The court determined that Terri would not wish to continue life-prolonging measures. Subsequently a 7-year battle occurred that included involvement by politicians and advocacy groups. Before the court's decision was carried out on March 18, 2005, the Florida legislature and the United States Congress had passed laws to prevent removal of Schiavo's feeding tube. These laws were later overturned by the Supreme Courts of Florida and the United States. On March 31, 2005, after a complex legal history in the courts, Terri Schiavo died at a Florida hospice at the age of 41.	This recent case received national and international media attention with very public debate regarding the moral consequences of withdrawing life support. The movement to challenge the decisions made for Terri Schiavo threatened to destabilize end-of-life law that had developed principally through the cases of Quinlan and Cruzan. Although the Schiavo case had little effect on right-to-die jurisprudence, it illustrated the range of difficulties that can complicate decision making concerning the termination of treatment in incapacitated persons.

Traditionally, extraordinary care includes complex, invasive, and experimental treatments such as resuscitation efforts by CPR or emergency cardiac care, maintenance of life support through invasive means, or renal dialysis. Experimental treatments such as gene therapy also are extraordinary therapies.

Ordinary care usually involves common, noninvasive, and tested treatments such as providing nutrition, hydration, or antibiotic therapy. In the critical care setting the noninvasive criterion does not apply; ordinary care is defined as usual and customary for the patient's condition. Maintenance of hydration and nutrition through a tube feeding is an example of a treatment that falls somewhere between ordinary and extraordinary care, and is a highly debatable issue. Therefore, it is important for individuals to document their wishes rather than relying on the members of the health care team to assist in

BOX 3-5   Definitions in Critical Care Decision Making

Concept	Definition
Advance directive	Witnessed written document or oral statement in which instructions are given by a person to express desires related to health care decisions. The directive may include, but is not limited to, the designation of a health care surrogate, a living will, or an anatomical gift.
Living will	A witnessed written document or oral statement voluntarily executed by a person that expresses the person's instructions concerning life-prolonging procedures.
Health care decision	Informed consent, refusal of consent, or withdrawal of consent for health care, unless stated in the advance directive.
Incapacity or incompetent	Patient is physically or mentally unable to communicate a willful and knowing health care decision.
Informed consent	Consent voluntarily given after a sufficient explanation and disclosure of information.
Proxy	A competent adult who has not been expressly designated to make health care decisions for an incapacitated person, but is authorized by state statute to make health care decisions for the person.
Surrogate	A competent adult designated by a person to make health care decisions should that person become incapacitated.
Terminal condition	A condition in which there is no reasonable medical probability of recovery and can be expected to cause death without treatment.
Persistent vegetative state	A permanent, irreversible unconsciousness condition that demonstrates an absence of voluntary action or cognitive behavior, or an inability to communicate or interact purposefully with the environment.
Brain death	Complete and irreversible cessation of brain function.
Clinical death or cardiac death	Irreversible cessation of spontaneous ventilation and circulation.
Life-prolonging procedure	Any medical procedure or treatment, including sustenance and hydration, that sustains, restores, or supplants a spontaneous vital function. Does not include the administration of medication or treatments deemed necessary to provide comfort care or to alleviate pain.
Resuscitation	Intervention with the intent of preserving life, restoring health, or reversing clinical death.
Do not resuscitate (DNR) order	A medical order that prohibits the use of cardiopulmonary resuscitation and emergency cardiac care to reverse signs of clinical death. The DNR order may or may not be specified in patients' advance directives.
Allow natural death	An alternate term with less negative connotations, but essentially meaning DNR.

Adapted from Florida Statutes Chapter 765.101 definitions. Retrieved July 31, 2007, from www.flsenate.gov/statutes.

the decision-making process related to nutrition and hydration.

Cardiopulmonary Resuscitation Decisions

The goals of emergency cardiovascular care are to preserve life, restore health, relieve suffering, limit disability, and reverse clinical death.[4] Frequently, ethical questions arise about the use of CPR and emergency cardiac care, as such treatment may conflict with a patient's desires or best interests. The critical care nurse should be guided by scientifically proven data, patient preferences, and ethical and cultural norms.

The American Heart Association provides guidelines for providers for making the difficult decision to provide or withhold emergency cardiovascular care.[4] The generally accepted position is that resuscitation should cease if the physician determines the efforts to be futile or hopeless. Futility constitutes sufficient reason for either withholding or ceasing extraordinary treatments.

Withholding or stopping extraordinary resuscitation efforts is ethically and legally appropriate if patients or surrogates have previously made their preferences known through advance directives. It is also acceptable if the physician determines the resuscitation to be futile, or has discussed the situation with the patient, family, and/or surrogate as appropriate, and there is mutual agreement not to resuscitate in the event of cardiopulmonary arrest. For the nurse not to initiate the resuscitation, a *do not resuscitate* (DNR) order must be written. Most physicians also write supporting documentation regarding the order in the progress notes, such as conversations held with the patient and family members.

Withholding or Withdrawal of Life Support
Withholding of life support, withdrawal of life support, or both, can range from not initiating hemodialysis (withholding) to terminal weaning from mechanical ventilation (withdrawal). Decisions are made based on consideration of all factors in the ethical decision-making model. In all instances of withholding and withdrawing of life support, comfort measures are maintained, including management of pain, management of pulmonary secretions, and other symptom management as needed (see Chapter 4).

Most decisions regarding withdrawing and withholding of life support are not made in the courts. They are made based on open communication with the patient, family, and surrogate, as appropriate. An ethical decision-making approach is used to decide on the best actions to take or not take in the situation. If ethical or legal questions arise, ethics consultation services, ethics committees, and risk managers can provide assistance. The value of clearly stating in writing one's end-of-life issues before becoming critically ill (advance directive) is key to avoiding having treatment given or not given against one's wishes.

End-of-Life Issues

Patient Self-Determination Act
In response to public concern about end-of-life decisions and the overall lack of consistent hospital policies, the United States Congress enacted the Patient Self-Determination Act.[10] This act requires that all health care facilities that receive Medicare and Medicaid funding inform their patients about their right to initiate an advance directive, and the right to consent to or refuse medical treatment.

Discussions regarding advance directives and end-of-life wishes should be made as early as possible, preferably before death is imminent. The ideal time to discuss advance directives is when a person is relatively healthy, not in the critical care or hospital setting. This allows more time for discussion, processing, and decision making. Nurses in every practice setting should assess patients regarding their perceptions of quality of life and end-of-life wishes in a caring and culturally sensitive way and should document the patient's wishes. Patients should be strongly encouraged to complete advance directives, including living wills and durable power of attorney, to ensure that their wishes will be fol-

lowed if they are terminally ill or in a persistent vegetative state.

Advance Directives
An *advance directive* is a communication that specifies a person's preference about medical treatment should that person become incapacitated. Several types of advance directives exist, including DNR orders, allow-a-natural-death orders, living wills, health care proxies, and other types of legal documents (Box 3-5). It is important for nurses to know whether a patient has an advance directive and that the directive be followed. Failure to follow an advance directive may result in a lawsuit.

The *living will* provides a mechanism by which individuals can authorize which specific treatments can be withheld in the event they become incapacitated. Although living wills provide direction to caregivers, in some states, living wills are not legally binding and are seen as advisory. When completing a living will, individuals can add special instructions about end-of-life wishes. Individuals can change their directive at any time.

The *durable power of attorney for health care* is more protective of patients' interests regarding medical treatment than is the living will. With a durable power of attorney for health care, patients legally designate an agent whom they trust, such as a family member or friend, to make decisions on their behalf should they become incapacitated. This person is called the *health care surrogate* or proxy. A durable power of attorney for health care allows the health care surrogate to make decisions whenever the patient is incapacitated, not just at the time of terminal illness. Some legal commentators recommend the joint use of a living will and a durable power of attorney to give added protection to a person's preferences about medical treatment.

Ultimately, if self-determination and informed consent are to have real value, patients or their surrogates must be given an opportunity to consider options and to shape decisions that affect their life or death. Communication and shared decision making among the patient, family, and health care team regarding end-of-life issues are key.[9] Unfortunately, this frequently does not happen before admission to a critical care unit. The critical care nurse must be part of the team that educates the patient and family, so they can determine and communicate end-of-life wishes.

The critical care nurse is legally responsible for providing care according to the advance directives. Some situations may result in moral distress for the nurse. A nurse who is unable to follow these legal documents because of personal or religious beliefs must ask to have the client reassigned to another nurse. For instance, some advance directives may call for withdrawing life support when certain conditions are met, and this may conflict with the nurse's personal or religious beliefs. Nurses who frequently ask to be reassigned to another client may need to think about another nursing specialty where they do not come into conflict with advance directives.

The nurse must also be cognizant of the facility's policies regarding advance directives. For example, if a DNR order is on the chart, does it meet all the requirements for a legal document per facility policy? Is it signed by the physician? Is the chart notated properly? Is there a health care proxy? Are the forms proper? Is there a living will? It is very important for the nurse to know the answers to all of these questions because if an advance directive is not per policy, then a lawsuit will likely follow. Consider the case of a patient with a DNR order in which this information is not passed on in report or notated in the medical record properly. The patient requires CPR. CPR may be implemented, and the family may sue based on the rescue efforts, even if the client lives.

Organ and Tissue Transplantation

Improved surgical methods and increasingly effective immunosuppressive drug therapy have improved the number and the type of successfully transplanted organs and tissues. Table 3-3 lists tissues and organs that are transplanted and the medical indication.

Despite the successes in transplantation, there is a severe shortage of organs to meet the growing demand. The United States Congress enacted the National Organ Procurement and Transplantation Network to facilitate fair allocation of organs and tissues for transplantation. This system is administered by the United Network for Organ Sharing, a group that maintains a list of patients who are awaiting organ and tissue transplantation and helps to coordinate the procurement of organs. In 2007, more than 97,000 people were on the organ transplantation waiting list for the United States.[13] This shortage has motivated multiple efforts to increase the organ supply. These efforts include creating registries for donors and including organ donor designation on driver's licenses. There are legal mandates for *required request* and mandatory organ procurement organization notification when a patient's death is imminent. In some situations, removal of the organ to be transplanted is not life threatening and can be accomplished without causing significant harm to a living donor (e.g., kidneys and bone marrow). Other types of organ and tissue removal (e.g., heart) are performed only in donors who meet the legal definition for brain death. A controversial effort to increase the donor pool has resulted in expanded criteria for non–

TABLE 3-3	Organ and Tissue Transplantation
Material Transplanted	**Necessitating Condition**
Bone	Conditions requiring facial/bone reconstruction
Bone marrow	Leukemias
Brain tissue	Parkinson disease
Cartilage	Conditions requiring facial/bone reconstruction
Corneas	Corneal damage, agenesis
Fascia	Conditions requiring repair of tendons, ligaments
Heart	End-stage cardiomyopathy
Heart valves	Diseased valves
Kidneys	End-stage renal disease
Liver	End-stage liver disease
Lungs	End-stage lung disease
Pancreas	Diabetes mellitus
Skin	Burns (temporary cover)
Veins	Diseased veins/arteries

heart-beating organ donation. This involves donation after cardiac death from older or sicker donors.

Since the 1968 Harvard Medical School Ad Hoc Committee's brain death definition, organs have primarily been removed from patients with cardiac function who have been pronounced dead on the basis of neurological criteria but continue to receive mechanical ventilation. The concept of brain death is distinct from the concept of persistent vegetative state or irreversible coma. In brain death, complete and irreversible cessation of brain function occurs, whereas in irreversible coma or persistent vegetative state, some brain function remains intact. Tests to determine brain death are outlined in Box 3-6. If a patient is a designated organ donor and brain death is determined, the patient is pronounced to be dead; however, perfusion and oxygenation of organs are maintained until the organs can be removed in the operating room. Even with optimal artificial perfusion and oxygenation, organs intended for transplantation must be removed and transplanted quickly.

The most rapid increase in the rate of organ recovery from deceased persons has occurred in the category of donation after cardiac death—that is, a death declared on the basis of cardiopulmonary criteria (irreversible cessation of circulatory and respiratory function) rather than brain death.[12] Most commonly,

BOX 3-6   Criteria Used to Determine Brain Death*

- Absence of spontaneous respiration
- Absence of spontaneous movement
- Cessation of brain function, including absence of all function of the brainstem and cerebral hemispheres, and verified by:
  - No response on neurological examination
  - Isoelectric electroencephalogram
  - Bilateral absence of cortical response to median somatosensory-evoked potentials
  - Absence of cerebral blood flow in the absence of hypothermia or drug-induced states

*These tests are formalized into criteria for brain death by different institutions or groups, such as the Harvard Medical School Ad Hoc Committee or the National Institute of Health Collaborative Study of Cerebral Survival. No absolute standardization exists for "brain death criteria."

the kidneys, liver, and pancreas are recovered after cardiac death because of the length of time in which these organs can be deprived of oxygen and still be transplanted successfully. In 2005, a conference on donation after cardiac death concluded that it is an ethically acceptable practice to retrieve organs after cardiac death to increase the number of organs available for transplantation.[7] Nonetheless, the practice remains controversial because of the complexities required during the transition from end-of-life care to organ donation.

Critical care professionals must ensure that the decision to withdraw care is made separately from the decision to donate organs. In addition, donation after cardiac death is often performed in the operat-ing room. Critical care personnel need to create a plan of care should the patient not die as expected. Donors must be dead according to specified hospital policy before organ procurement. The process of organ procurement cannot be the proximate cause of death.

Everyone in the United States has the legal right to donate organs. To uphold that right, family members or significant others must be given the opportunity to donate organs or tissues on behalf of their loved ones if there is no advance directive. Local organ procurement organizations have designated requestors whose role is to seek consent for organ donation. The role of the critical care nurse is to refer potential organ donors to the organ procurement organization. Because the consent rate for organ donation is only about 50%, it is important to approach potential donors sensitively and with awareness of cultural and religious implications. The designated requestors are trained to address donation with regard to such issues.

Ethical Concerns Surrounding Transplantation

Organ and tissue transplantation involve numerous and complex ethical issues. The first consideration is given to the rights and privileges of all moral agents involved: the donor, the recipient, the family or surrogate, and all other recipients and donors. Important ethical principles that are useful in ethical decision making regarding transplantation include respect for persons and their autonomous choices, beneficence and nonmaleficence, justice, and fidelity. Three of the most controversial issues in transplantation are the moral value that should be placed on the human body part, the just distribution of a human body part, and the complex problems inherent in applying the concept of brain death to clinical situations.

CASE STUDY   evolve

Mr. W. is a 67-year-old patient in the coronary care unit who has severe heart failure and chronic obstructive pulmonary disease. Mr. W. has been in and out of the hospital for 3 years and requires oxygen therapy at night. He has severe, chronic chest pain and dyspnea. He had a respiratory arrest and was put on the ventilator last night. He awakens after the resuscitation and communicates that the breathing tube be removed and that he be allowed to die. He is tired of the pain and dyspnea. He asks for medication to make him comfortable after the tube is removed. His family agrees with the plan of care.

Mr. W.'s wishes are followed. He is extubated and is given morphine for sedation and comfort. Mr. W.'s family members all remain at the bedside, taking turns holding his hand and talking to him.

QUESTIONS

1. Apply the ethical decision-making model discussed in this chapter to this case. What are the relevant ethical principles? Are there other areas that must be assessed before proceeding?
2. As the critical care nurse caring for Mr. W., what are your priorities at this point? On what ethical principles are these priorities based?
3. Suppose that you have strong religious beliefs about withdrawal of life support. If you were assigned to Mr. W., what actions should you take?

SUMMARY

The ethical and legal responsibilities of nurses who work in acute care settings have increased dramatically since the early 1990s. Based on evolving case law, state statutes, and state nurse practice acts, nurses are held to a high standard of care and are also held directly accountable for their individual nursing actions. Nurses must maintain and continually update their knowledge base and clinical competencies. Failure to do so could not only cause harm to patients but could also put nurses and their employers at risk for allegations of professional negligence.

Nurses who care for critically ill patients are challenged by legal and ethical dilemmas on a daily basis. In their role of patient advocate, ethical decision making and open communication must be facilitated. Numerous resources are available to assist with developing the knowledge and skill to do this well. There are no easy answers to ethical dilemmas. A formal decision-making model assists the nurse, but some situations may still remain very ambiguous. Appropriate ethical nursing responses are based on wanting to do the right thing for the patients and families that you care for and initiating the steps to advocate for the patient.

CRITICAL THINKING QUESTIONS   *evolve*

1. You are taking care of Mrs. H., a 90-year-old patient with gastrointestinal bleeding. She has developed numerous complications and requires mechanical ventilation. She is unresponsive to nurses and family members. She has been in the hospital for 2 weeks and requires a transfusion nearly every day to sustain adequate hemoglobin and hematocrit levels. Her prognosis is poor. Before this hospitalization, she lived independently at her own home. Her children tell you they are tired of seeing their mother suffer. How do you respond to the family, and what follow-up do you perform?

2. You are taking care of Mr. J., a 23-year-old man with a closed head injury. During the night shift, you note a change in the level of consciousness at 3:00 AM. You call the physician, who tells you to watch Mr. J. until the physician attends rounds the next morning. He tells you not to call him back. Mr. J.'s neurological status continues to deteriorate. What actions do you take? What is the rationale for your actions?

3. It is 2 days later, and Mr. J., as described earlier, now has a herniated brainstem and is declared brain dead but remains on life support. His wife is at the bedside and is fully aware of the situation. You do not know whether Mr. J. signed an organ donor card. What are your ethical and legal obligations regarding organ donation at this point? How would you approach the situation?

4. You are caring for Mrs. M., a 68-year-old woman with an acute myocardial infarction. She is in the coronary care unit after a successful angioplasty. Her husband brought in her living will, which states that Mrs. M. does not desire resuscitation. Mrs. M. is pain free and alert. As you start your beginning-of-shift assessment, Mrs. M. says, "You know, now that I've made it through the angioplasty, I realize that tubes and machines may not be so bad after all. I haven't made it this far to give up now. If I go into cardiac arrest, I want you to do all that you can for me." What ethical principle is Mrs. M. using? As her nurse, what actions should you take and why?

5. You are the charge nurse of a nine-bed critical care unit. You have one open bed. The house supervisor calls and tells you that there are two patients who need a critical care bed. The first is a 23-year-old female patient currently in the operating room after multiple trauma. The second patient is a 78-year-old man who is in the emergency department with severe septic shock. According to the supervisor, both patients are going to need mechanical ventilation and inotropic therapy. What are your decisions and actions at this point? What ethical principles are your actions based on?

evolve Be sure to check out the bonus material, including free self-assessment exercises, on the Evolve Web site at http://evolve.elsevier.com/Sole.

REFERENCES

1. American Association of Critical-Care Nurses. (2002). *An ethic of care.* Retrieved June 29, 2007, from www.aacn.org/AACN/Memship.nsf/.
2. American Association of Critical-Care Nurses. (2005). *AACN standards for establishing and sustaining healthy work environments.* Retrieved June 29, 2007, from www.aacn.org/hwe.

3. American Association of Critical-Care Nurses. (2006). *Position statement, moral distress*. Retrieved June 29, 2007, from www.aacn.org/AACN/pubpolcy.nsf/Files/MDPS.

4. American Heart Association. (2005). *American Heart Association 2005 guidelines for cardiopulmonary resuscitation and emergency cardiopulmonary care*. Retrieved July 1, 2007, from www.americanheart.org.

5. American Nurses Association. (2001). *Code of ethics for nurses with interpretive statements*. Silver Springs, MD: Author.

6. Beauchamp, T., & Childress, J. (2001). *Principles of biomedical ethics* (5th ed.). Oxford, England: Oxford University Press.

7. Bernat, J. L., D'Alessandro, A. M., Port, F. K., et al. (2006). Report of a national conference on donation after cardiac death. *American Journal of Transplantation, 6*, 281-291.

8. Garner, B. (2006). *Black's law dictionary* (3rd pocket ed.). Rochester, NY: Thompson-West Publishing.

9. Heyland, D. K., Tranmer, J., & Feldman-Steward, D. (2000). End-of-life decision making in the seriously ill hospitalized patient: An organizing framework and results of a preliminary study. *Journal of Palliative Care, 16*, S31-S39.

10. Public Law No. 101-508, 4206, 104 Stat. 291. (1990). The Self-Determination Act amends the Social Security Act's provisions on Medicare and Medicaid. Social Security Act 1927, 42 U.S.C. 1396.

11. Rushton, C. H., & Scanlon, C. (1998). A road map for negotiating end-of-life care. *MedSurg Nursing, 6*(1), 59-62.

12. Steinbrook, R. (2007). Organ donation after cardiac death. *New England Journal of Medicine, 357*(3), 209-213.

13. United Network for Organ Sharing. (2007). *Data*. Retrieved July 1, 2007, from www.unos.org/.

CHAPTER 4

End-of-Life Care in the Critical Care Unit

Douglas Houghton, MSN, ARNP, CCRN

INTRODUCTION

Advances in technology during the past several decades have vastly improved the ability of health care providers to care for the sickest patients and have led to increasingly successful outcomes. However, the appropriate use of these often invasive and frequently expensive resources is still a matter of debate, leading to ethical issues in the care of persons with a critical illness. A recent epidemiological study found that approximately 38% of all deaths in the United States occur in an acute care setting, with 22% of the deaths occurring after admission to an intensive care unit.[4] This finding is disturbing, since research evidence has shown that the vast majority of Americans would like to die in the comfort of their home environment.[20] However, most critical care units remain a relatively hostile, often uncomfortable and impersonal place for dying patients and their families.[17] The landmark Study to Understand Prognoses and Preferences for Outcomes and Risks of Treatment (SUPPORT) revealed many disparities between patients' care preferences and the care they received. The most significant findings from the study included a lack of clear communication between patients and health care providers, a high frequency of aggressive care, and widespread pain and suffering among inpatients.[45] Subsequently, increasing national attention to the issue has stimulated the growth of funding for research and development of medical and nursing care guidelines for the care of the dying person in the critical care unit.

Multiple factors have been identified as influencing the continuation of aggressive care in the face of a poor or futile prognosis.[37,38] The failure of clinicians, family members, and patients to openly and honestly discuss prognoses, end-of-life issues, and preferences is one of the most significant factors preventing early identification. Changes in management of those persons are not likely to benefit from further aggressive critical care measures.[10,37,57] The fact that no valid assessment tools exist to accurately predict when care is medically futile is another major contributing factor to many conflicts at the end of life[14,26] (Box 4-1). The identification of the dying patient is often subjective, based on the individual health care providers' opinions and interpretations of patient response/results.

Societal values and those of health care providers also play a significant role in how end-of-life care in the United States is provided. These values include a commonly held belief that patients die of distinct illnesses, which implies that such illnesses are potentially curable.[13] Dying is often viewed as failure on the part of the system or providers. The purpose of the health care system in the United States is to treat illness, disease, and injury, and this "lifesaving" culture continues to drive aggressive care even when it becomes obvious that the ultimate outcome will be the death of the individual.[17,23]

ETHICAL AND LEGAL CONCERNS

Real-life drama and ethical dilemmas present themselves on a regular basis to critical care clinicians, who are often poorly prepared educationally to deal with such situations. The issues described above lead to conflict among health care team members, as well

BOX 4-1   Definition of Medical Futility

> *Medical futility:* Situation in which therapy or interventions will not provide a foreseeable possibility of improvement in the patient's health condition. Legal and organizational definitions may vary, and much controversy exists.[8]

as conflict between the team, patients and families, and even within families themselves. (See Chapter 3 for additional discussion.) For example, the legal battle in Florida concerning the withdrawal of enteral nutrition for Terri Schiavo demonstrated how divisive a situation can become when family members express disagreement about the patient's wishes.[9,16] This case brought national attention and debate to what otherwise might have been a routine and peaceful withdrawal of care. The key legal issues revolved around the use of surrogate decision making.[9,16] This legal precedent is based on the constitutional principle of self-determination. Should an individual become incapacitated due to illness, injury, or heavy sedation, decisions about health care are made by either the patient's designated health care surrogate or a legally designated proxy who is appointed to make decisions for the person. This is a common scenario in the critical care setting.[46,47] Ideally, the surrogate or proxy should be familiar with how the incapacitated person would make health care decisions in a situation if the person were capable.[21] Health care surrogates may need to be reminded that they should act as they believe the patient would act in a similar situation, not as their personal values dictate. Evidence has shown that surrogates frequently do not correctly identify patients' preferred wishes, which raises concerns especially when dealing with withdrawal-of-care issues near the end of life.[30,42] End-of-life decision making can be best facilitated through open and frequent communication between the health care team and the family, in which the family is provided ample opportunity to speak. This process will successfully resolve most end-of-life conflicts, with less stress on the part of both the health care team and the family.[9,27,28,53]

Advance directives describe a patient's preferences for treatment in a terminal or vegetative state and are a legally recognized means of clarifying end-of-life treatment preferences.[27] However, many patients have not executed advance directives. In-depth discussions between the family and the health care team are essential in arriving at mutually agreed upon and clearly understood treatment choices that reflect perceived patient preferences in the situation.

To further complicate the issues, many patients in critical care units lack both an advance directive and a surrogate decision maker.[24] Providing end-of-life care in these situations is ethically and legally challenging, and research has suggested that physicians often substitute their own judgment in these cases.[40,56] Recommendations for managing these situations are found in published guidelines.[2,3]

Effects on Nurses and the Health Care Team

Many clinicians experience personal ethical conflicts when providing painful interventions and aggressive care to patients when they believe the situation is futile, causing significant moral distress that can lead to burnout.[5,18,33,41] Care choices made by patients, surrogates, or both, may also differ from those that clinicians might personally make, causing further strain in remaining nonjudgmental in such a situation.

Patients' dignity may be impaired during a critical care unit stay, and their preferences and wishes may be ignored, dictated for them by providers, or unknown. Such situations contradict basic nursing ethical principles, causing further moral distress.[18,58] At times, health care providers do not clearly communicate a futile prognosis to patients or the family members, denying them the ability to make informed choices.[53,56] When care is withdrawn and patients die, caregivers often experience a sense of loss or grief, especially if the patient's stay was lengthy. Attendance at funerals or unit debriefing sessions after a death may help to resolve emotional strain, but finding a balance between maintaining a professional, healthy distance and being authentic and humane in our care is a difficult task.

DIMENSIONS OF END-OF-LIFE CARE

Nursing care in the critical care setting at the end of life is focused on five dimensions. These dimensions of nursing care consist of alleviation of distressing symptoms (palliation); communication and conflict resolution; withdrawal, limiting, or withholding of therapy; emotional/psychological care of the patient and family; and caregiver organizational support.

Palliative Care

Palliation is the provision of care interventions that are designed to relieve symptoms of illness or injury that negatively impact the quality of life of the patient and/or family.[12,32] Common distressing symptoms that may occur with multiple disease states include pain, anxiety, hunger/thirst, dyspnea, diarrhea, nausea, confusion/agitation, and disturbance in sleep patterns.[32,45] Palliative care should be viewed as an integral part of every ill or injured patient's care and should not be reserved only for the dying patient. Relief of distressing symptoms should always be provided whenever possible, even when the primary focus of care is lifesaving or aggressive treatment. An important part of palliative care consists of "simple" nursing interventions, such as frequent repositioning, good hygiene and skin care, and creation of a peaceful environment to the extent possible in the critical care setting.

For those patients with recognized life-limiting illness or injury, palliative care consultations with experts in symptom management can provide significant benefits to critically ill persons and their families. The use of palliative care experts to assist in managing patients' care decreases hospital lengths of stay and resource utilization. Improved patient/family communication and better management of pain and other symptoms are additional benefits noted.[12,15,32,48]

Earlier identification of patients who are unlikely to benefit from further aggressive care, and improved management of pain and other symptoms, are effective strategies to improve end-of-life care.[6,7] Frequent nursing assessment for symptoms of pain should be considered the "fifth vital sign," and nurses should be cognizant of the fact that people express pain in different ways, which may vary between cultural groups and individuals.[32] Medications to control pain and relieve anxiety in the critically ill patient are described in Chapter 5.

Communication and Conflict Resolution

Clear, ongoing, and honest communication between the members of the health care team and the patient/family is a key factor in improving the quality of care for the dying patient in the critical care unit.[28,34,37] Interventions testing various communication strategies when dealing with end-of-life issues have had positive results. Guidelines for effective communication are described in Box 4-2.

Withholding, Limiting, or Withdrawing Therapy

The majority of deaths in the critical care unit are preceded by some manner of withholding, withdrawal, or limiting of medical therapy.[32,57] Such a decision should be made with input and agreement in a shared decision-making model.[55] Appropriate

---

BOX 4-2 Guidelines for Effective Communication to Facilitate End-of-Life Care

- Present a clear and consistent message to the family. Mixed messages confuse families and patients, as do unfamiliar medical terms. The multidisciplinary team needs to communicate and strive to reach agreement on goals of care and prognosis.[6,7]
- Allow ample time for family members to express themselves during family conferences.[28,31] This increases their level of satisfaction and decreases dysfunctional bereavement patterns after the patient's death.
- Aim for all (health care providers, patients, and families) to agree on the plan of treatment. The plan should be based on the known or perceived preferences of the patient.[9,53] Arriving at such a plan through communication minimizes legal actions against providers, relieves patient/family anxiety, and provides an environment in which the patient is the focus of concern.
- Emphasize that the patient will not be abandoned if the goals of care shift from aggressive therapy to "comfort" care (palliation) only.[54] Let the patient/family know who is responsible for their care, and that they can rely on those individuals to be present and available when needed.
- Facilitate continuity of care.[32,35] If a transfer to an alternate level of care, such as a hospice unit or ventilator unit, is required, ensure that all pertinent information is conveyed to the new providers. Details of the history, prognosis, care requirements, palliative interventions, and psychosocial needs should be part of the information transfer.

---

withdrawal, limiting, or withholding of therapy does not constitute euthanasia or assisted suicide, both of which are illegal in the United States (with the exception of Oregon, where assisted suicide is permitted in select instances). Minimal moral distress on the part of the health care team, patients, and families should result if generally accepted ethical and legal principles are followed during this process (Box 4-3).[21]

Preparing patients (if conscious) and families for what will likely occur during the withdrawal process is key to alleviating anxiety and undue distress.[32] A nursing care priority should be anticipating patient symptoms, such as dyspnea during ventilator withdrawal, and medicating to alleviate such symptoms, even if high doses of medications are required. Assessment of patient response (e.g., comfort) is

---

BOX 4-3   Ethical Principles for Withholding and Withdrawing Life-Sustaining Treatment

1. Death occurs as a consequence of the underlying disease. The goals of care are to relieve suffering and not to hasten death.
2. Withholding life-sustaining treatment is morally and legally equivalent to withdrawing treatment. Both actions require the same degree of active physician/nurse participation as any other procedure.
3. Any treatment can be withdrawn or withheld, including nutrition, fluids, antibiotics, or blood products.
4. Any dose of analgesic or anxiolytic medication may reasonably be used to relieve suffering, even if the medication has the potential to hasten death. Signs of suffering include dyspnea, tachypnea, diaphoresis, grimacing, accessory muscle use, nasal flaring, and restlessness.
5. Life-sustaining treatment should not be withdrawn while a patient is receiving paralytic agents. After discontinuation of such drugs, the patient must demonstrate sufficient motor activity to allow thorough clinical assessment before withdrawal of support.
6. Cultural and religious views influence the perspectives of patients and family members regarding life-sustaining treatment. These issues should be openly discussed and an effort made to accommodate various perspectives. Pastoral or spiritual care providers may assist in this process.

Adapted from University of Washington/Harborview Medical Center physician orders. Retrieved July 21, 2007, from http://depts.washington.edu/eolcare/instruments/wls-orders2.pdf.

the sole means of deciding how much medication is appropriate in a given situation, and therapy should be titrated to relieve emotional and physical distress even if such dosing hastens the death of the patient as a secondary effect.[11] Commonly used medication regimens include morphine sulfate and intravenous benzodiazepines for anxiolysis (Figure 4-1). Recent data have supported the perception that most patients die in comfort during the withdrawal process.[39]

Ventilator Withdrawal

The most commonly withheld or withdrawn medical intervention in the critical care setting is mechanical ventilation. Some debate and regional practice variations exist, but excellent practice guidelines for ventilator withdrawal are available from the American Association of Critical-Care Nurses Web site (Box 4-4).[49,56] This process is known as "terminal weaning" (see Clinical Alert) and can consist of titration of ventilator support to minimal levels, removal of the ventilator but not the artificial airway, or complete extubation.[11] Nurses should consult their institution's policy and procedure manual for specific requirements or variation.

CLINICAL ALERT
Ventilator Withdrawal

During terminal weaning of ventilatory support, patients may exhibit symptoms of respiratory distress, such as tachypnea, dyspnea, or use of accessory muscles. Pain medication and sedation should be titrated as needed to relieve such symptoms.

Other Commonly Withheld Therapies

Vasopressors, antibiotics, dialysis, and nutritional support are other common therapies that may be ethically withheld when goals of treatment shift to palliation instead of cure. Again, the primary nursing responsibility is to assess and ensure patient comfort during the withdrawal or withholding process.

Emotional and Psychological Care of the Patient/Family

One of the most challenging aspects of end-of-life care is addressing the emotional and psychological needs of the patient and family. Needs are as variable as family situations, and it is important for the nurse to carefully assess what the patient's and family's needs *are* instead of making assumptions about what they *ought* to be. Nonjudgmental assessment, in which the nurse is keenly aware of the patient's and family's personal feelings or values about the situation, is essential in determining priorities in this dimension of care (see Evidence-Based Practice feature). Keep in mind that "family" can consist of many different persons in an individual's life, and may include unmarried life partners (same or opposite sex), close friends, and "aunts," "uncles," or "cousins" who may actually have no legal relationship to the patient.

For some families, spiritual counseling from a religious figure might be a priority. For others, the

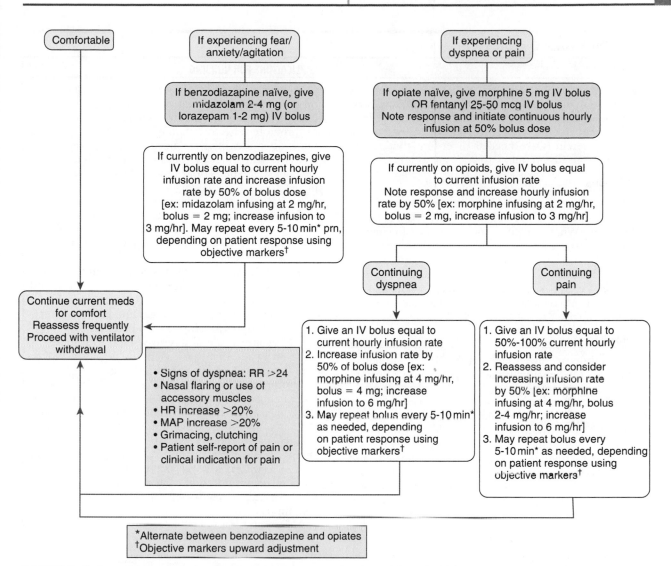

FIGURE 4-1. Guidelines for pharmacological interventions during withdrawal of life support. *(From Virginia Commonwealth University Hospital, Richmond, VA.)*

need may be for statistics documenting their loved one's chances of survival with a particular diagnosis.[52] One common need is the need for clear, consistent, and accurate information about the patient's condition, what to expect during the withdrawal and dying process (if applicable), and reassurance that the patient will not suffer during the dying process.[13,29] Coordinating the communication process between the patient/family and the health care team is a key nursing action in end-of-life care.

Many institutions have bereavement counselors with extended training in assisting patients/families through the dying process and its aftermath. Social workers, spiritual care providers, or licensed mental health professionals can frequently be of assistance in meeting the needs of families. Cultural sensitivity is essential to accurately determine situational priorities, meanings, and perceptions, which may vary widely across cultures.

Maintaining the patient's dignity during the dying process is of the utmost importance. The nurse should make time to listen to family accounts of the patient's life before the illness/injury and acknowledge the patient's individuality and humanity. A calm manner and voice, a quiet and private environment, and allowing unrestricted family access to the bedside as much as possible are key nursing interventions before, during, and after the patient's death.[6]

EVIDENCE-BASED PRACTICE

PROBLEM

Supporting family members of critically ill patients who are dying is an important part of nursing care. Holding end-of-life family conferences may be a strategy to provide this support. Guidelines for organizing such conferences are needed to ensure that family members' needs are met.

QUESTIONS

What are the outcomes associated with end-of-life family conferences for family members of the critically ill patient. What guidelines should be used to conduct such conferences?

REFERENCE

Lautrette, A., Ciroldi, M., Ksibi, H., Azoulay, E. (2006). End-of-life family conferences: Rooted in the evidence. *Critical Care Medicine, 34*(Suppl.), S364-S372.

EVIDENCE

The authors reviewed eight observational studies of families of patients who died in the critical care unit and 13 interventional studies designed to improve communication during end-of-life care. Poor communication, lack of communication, and an increased incidence of posttraumatic stress were reported in the observational studies. Increased satisfaction was associated with frequent and clear communication, and compassion. Withdrawal of life support that was explained clearly, occurred as expected, and was comfortable for the patient was also associated with increased satisfaction. A variety of interventions were studied, such as ethics consultations, intensive communication strategies, and active participation of nurses, physicians, and social workers. Collectively, interventions that improved satisfaction and also resulted in reduced lengths of stay focused on early, ongoing, and intensive communication between family members and health care providers.

IMPLICATIONS FOR NURSING

Communication that is proactive is essential for family members who are making decisions at the end of life. Participation in family conferences is one way to promote effective family communication. The nurse often identifies the need for such a conference and is instrumental in coordinating the conferences. Several suggestions for end-of-life conferences are made:

- Organize the conference at a time that family members and health care providers can all be present. Schedule in a quiet place with all participants seated at the same level, such as a conference table.
- Identify what the team knows about the family before the conference (family assessment), and resolve any issues and conflicts among the health care providers regarding proposed treatment options before the conference.
- Encourage the family to write down questions or issues that they want to be answered or addressed during the conference.

During the conference, make the family comfortable talking about death and dying issues, discuss what the family understands, and allow them to talk about the family member's life and medical history. Provide honest information about the patient's prognosis. Discuss goals for palliative care, emphasizing that patient comfort will be maintained. Use skills of effective communication such as reflection, empathy, and silence. Conclude with a plan and follow-up communication.

It is important to provide items for family comfort, such as tissues, a refreshment, or a chair. When no words seem appropriate, maintaining a respectful conscious presence can speak volumes. The patient's death may be a relatively routine part of the nurse's day, but it is important to keep in mind that family members will likely remember the situation and the actions of the nurse and health care team, for many years. Nursing interventions are summarized in Box 4-4.

Caregiver Organizational Support

Providing end-of-life care requires much time, and staffing patterns have been identified as a barrier to provision of optimal care.[6,7,36] Nursing administrators should keep this in mind when staffing to allow nurses time to adequately care for the dying patient. Should staffing ratios be less than adequate, assistance from colleagues can help relieve the nurse caring for a dying patient of other responsibilities.

BOX 4-4   Nursing Interventions to Support Care at the End of Life

- Assess patient's and family members' understanding of the condition and prognosis to address educational needs.
- Educate family members about what will happen when life support is withdrawn to decrease their fear of the unknown.
- Assure family members that the patient will not suffer.
- Assure family members that the patient will not be abandoned.
- Provide for emotional support and/or spiritual care resources, such as grief counselors and spiritual care providers.
- Facilitate physician communication with the family.
- Provide for visitation/presence of family and extended family. Most family members do not want the patient to die alone.

BOX 4-5   End-of-Life Online Resources

- http://depts.washington.edu/eolcare/aboutus/index.html (University of Washington/Harborview Medical Center)
- www.aacn.nche.edu/elnec (American Association of Colleges of Nursing)
- www.aacn.org/AACN/PalCare.nsf/vwdoc/RWJ (American Association of Critical-Care Nurses)
- www.apa.org/pi/eol/homepage.html (American Psychological Association)
- www.nlm.nih.gov/medlineplus/endoflifeissues.html (National Library of Medicine)
- www.eperc.mcw.edu (Medical College of Wisconsin)
- www.dyingwell.org (Dr. Ira Byock)
- www.endoflife.northwestern.edu (Northwestern University)

In addition to providing adequate staffing resources, helpful organizational behaviors include bereavement programs for families, and assistance or guidance in making funeral arrangements. Debriefing or support sessions for staff members often ease the stress of caring for dying patients.[32]

Critical care nurses have expressed the need for provider and public education concerning end-of-life issues.[6] Efforts to educate the public on a variety of end-of-life issues are vital to improving care, through promotion of advance directives and conversations with loved ones concerning life support options.

Nurses have also identified the need for professional end-of-life education.[6,58] The American Association of Colleges of Nursing first developed the *End-of-Life Competency Statements for a Peaceful Death*, which has spurred the improvement of end-of-life education in undergraduate nursing curricula.[1] Training is also available to prepare nurse educators to educate nurses in bedside practice to deliver competent and compassionate care to the dying patient.[32] Additional online resources can be found in Box 4-5.

CULTURALLY COMPETENT END-OF-LIFE CARE

Many clinicians believe that they lack the skills and preparation to tackle difficult end-of-life issues with patients and families of critically ill patients.[10,37]

This discomfort may be magnified when clinicians deal with patients and families from a different cultural or ethnic background than that of their own.[25,44,51] Cultural influences on care at the end of life are highly variable, even by region.[19]

The United States is well recognized as a nation of people from increasingly diverse cultural backgrounds and ethnicities.[50] Therefore, it is necessary to understand how cultural and ethnic differences affect crucial end-of-life decision-making processes and communication preferences in diverse groups, and how these may vary during stressful situations.[41] Better understanding of these cultural differences in end-of-life care preferences will lead to more effective and satisfying care and communication with patients and families.

Religious doctrine and beliefs profoundly influence patients' and families' choices for end-of-life care. Significant differences in perspective may exist between and within many major religious groups, and these values are often deeply and subtly ingrained in belief systems underpinning care choices, including those of health care providers.[25,37]

Research on end-of-life care preferences in various cultural/ethnic/religious groups remains poorly developed. In general, Caucasians prefer less invasive and aggressive options near the end of life, while African Americans tend to choose more aggressive treatment.[25,44,51] Nurses are encouraged to become familiar with the values and beliefs of common cultural groups in their practice setting, as well as to recognize the influence of personal religious/cultural context.

CASE STUDY

evolve

M.O. is a 26-year-old Hispanic man who sustained severe injuries in a high-speed motorcycle accident, requiring admission to the critical care unit. He had previously been in perfect health other than having mild asthma as a child, according to his mother. His most significant injuries are a cervical spine fracture and quadriplegia at the C2 level, and a devastating traumatic brain injury consisting of a subarachnoid hemorrhage and diffuse axonal injury. He has subsequently developed acute respiratory distress syndrome (ARDS), requiring high levels of mechanical ventilation during the first 3 days of his hospitalization. His prognosis for functional recovery from his brain injury is deemed to be "poor" by the neurosurgeon, and because of his high quadriplegia, he will remain ventilator dependent for life. M.O.'s family is Cuban, very close-knit, and religious (Catholic), and consists of two sisters, his father and mother, and a grandmother who lives with them. Many of them do not speak English well, including his mother who is his designated legal surrogate. All are very

tearful and devastated by his injuries but remain hopeful that "God will help him recover and move again." His 20-year-old sister, in a private conversation with the nurse, states that her brother had told her before that he would prefer to die if he was ever paralyzed "like Christopher Reeve." She is afraid to verbalize these feelings with the rest of the family, because she thinks her mother will accuse her of not loving her brother or of wanting to kill him.

QUESTIONS

1. What should the nurse say to M.O.'s sister? What course of action could the nurse recommend?
2. What resources in the institution would be most helpful to this family at this time? Why?
3. How does the family's cultural/religious background influence its perspective on this situation?
4. What learning needs does this family have? How could these be most appropriately met?

SUMMARY

End-of-life care is challenging, but many nurses find it to be an extremely rewarding element of their practice. Making a positive difference in a person's life at this critical time requires skill, compassion, education, and self-awareness. Key dimensions of end-of-life care include alleviation of distressing symptoms (palliation); communication and conflict resolution; withdrawal, limiting, or withholding of therapy; emotional and psychological care of the patient and family; and caregiver organizational support.

CRITICAL THINKING QUESTIONS

evolve

1. When communicating with families concerning the process of withdrawal of life support such as mechanical ventilation, what concepts are important to convey to the family?
2. What is palliative care, and does it apply only to patients with a terminal illness?
3. The nurse assesses that significant disagreement exists among family members with regard to what course of treatment is best for the patient. What action would be most effective in improving the situation?

evolve Be sure to check out the bonus material, including free self-assessment exercises, on the Evolve Web site at http://evolve.elsevier.com/Sole.

REFERENCES

1. American Association of Colleges of Nursing. (2002). *End-of-life competency statements for a peaceful death.* Washington, DC: Author.

2. American Geriatrics Society. (2002). *AGS position statement: Making treatment decisions for incapacitated elderly patients without advance directives.* Retrieved March 29, 2007, from www.americangeriatrics.org/products/positionpapers/treatdec.shtml.

3. American Medical Association, Council on Ethical and Judicial Affairs. (2004). *Code of medical ethics: Current opinions with annotations.* Chicago: Author.

4. Angus, D. C., Barnato, A. E., Linde-Zwirble, W. T., Weissfeld, L. A., Watson, S., Rickert, T., et al., on behalf of the Robert Wood Johnson Foundation ICU End-of-Life Peer Group. (2004). Use of intensive care at the end of life in the United States: An epidemiologic study. *Critical Care Medicine, 32,* 638-643.

5. Badger, J. M. (2005). Factors that enable or complicate end-of-life transitions in critical care. *American Journal of Critical Care, 14,* 513-522.

6. Beckstrand, R. L., Callister, L. C., & Kirchhoff, K. T. (2006). Providing a "good death:" Critical care nurses' suggestions for improving end-of-life care. *American Journal of Critical Care, 15*(1), 38-46.

7. Beckstrand, R. L., & Kirchhoff, K. T. (2005). Providing end-of-life care to patients: Critical care nurses' perceived obstacles and supportive behaviors. *American Journal of Critical Care, 14*(5), 395-403.

8. Bernat, J. L. (2005). Medical futility: Definition, determination, and disputes in critical care. *Neurocritical Care, 2*(2), 198-205.

9. Bloche, M. G. (2005). Managing conflict at the end of life. *New England Journal of Medicine, 352*(23), 2371-2373.

10. Boyle, D. K., Miller, P. A., & Forbes-Thompson, S. A. (2005). Communication and end-of-life care in the intensive care unit. *Critical Care Nursing Quarterly, 28*(4), 302-316.

11. Campbell, M. L. (2004). Terminal dyspnea and respiratory distress. *Critical Care Clinics, 20*(3), 403-417.

12. Campbell, M. L. (2006). Palliative care consultation in the intensive care unit. *Critical Care Medicine, 34*(Suppl. 11), S355-S358.

13. Cook, D., Rocker, G., Giacomini, M., Sinuff, T., & Heyland, D. (2006). Understanding and changing attitudes toward withdrawal and withholding of life support in the intensive care unit. *Critical Care Medicine, 34*(Suppl. 11), S317-S323.

14. Council on Ethical and Judicial Affairs, American Medical Association. (1999). Medical futility in end-of-life care. *Journal of the American Medical Association, 281*(10), 937-941.

15. Curtis, J. R. (2005). Interventions to improve care during withdrawal of life-sustaining treatments. *Journal of Palliative Medicine, 8*(Suppl. 1), S116-S131.

16. Ditto, P. H. (2006). What would Terri want? On the psychological challenges of surrogate decision making. *Death Studies, 30,* 135-148.

17. Dracup, K., & Bryan-Brown, C. W. (2006). Dying in the intensive care unit. *American Journal of Critical Care, 14,* 456-458.

18. Elpern, E. H., Covert, B., & Kleinpell, R. (2005). Moral distress of staff nurses in a medical intensive care unit. *American Journal of Critical Care, 149,* 523-530.

19. Fassier, T., Lautrette, A., Ciroldi, M., & Azoulay, E. (2005). Care at the end of life in critically ill patients: The European perspective. *Current Opinion in Critical Care, 11*(6), 616-623.

20. Field, M. J., & Cassel, C. K. (Eds.). (1997). *Approaching death: Improving care at the end of life.* Washington, DC: National Academy Press (Institute of Medicine).

21. Gavrin, J. R. (2007). Ethical considerations at the end of life in the intensive care unit. *Critical Care Medicine, 35*(Suppl. 2), S85-S94.

22. Reference deleted in proofs.

23. Kaufman, S. R. (2005). *And a time to die: How American hospitals shape the end of life.* New York: Simon and Schuster.

24. Kirchhoff, K. T., Anumandla, P. R., Foth, K. T., Lues, S. N., & Gilbertson-White, S. H. (2004). Documentation on withdrawal of life support in adult patients in the intensive care unit. *American Journal of Critical Care, 13*(4), 328-334.

25. Kwak, J., & Haley, W. E. (2005). Current research findings on end-of-life decision making among racially or ethnically diverse groups. *The Gerontologist, 45*(5), 634-641.

26. Lamont, E. B. (2005). A demographic and prognostic approach to defining the end of life. *Journal of Palliative Medicine, 8*(Suppl. 1), S12-S21.

27. Lang, F., & Quill, T. (2004). Making decisions with families at the end of life. *American Family Physician, 70*(4), 719-723, 725-726.

28. Lautrette, A., Darmon, M., Megarbane, B., Joly, L. M., Chevret, S., Adrie, C., et al. (2007). A communication strategy and brochure for relatives of patients dying in the ICU. *New England Journal of Medicine, 365*(5), 469-478.

29. Levy, M. L., & McBride, D. L. (2006). End-of-life care in the intensive care unit: State of the art in 2006. *Critical Care Medicine, 34*(Suppl. 11), S306-S308.

30. Lewis, C. L., Hanson, L. C., Golin, C., Garrett, J. M., Cox, C. E., Jackman, A., et al. (2006). Surrogates' perceptions about feeding tube placement decisions. *Patient Education and Counseling, 61,* 246-252.

31. McDonagh, J. R., Elliott, T. B., Engleberg, R. A., Treece, P. D., Shannon, S. E., Rubenfeld, G. D., et al. (2004). Family satisfaction with family conferences about end-of-life care in the intensive care unit: Increased proportion of family speech is associated with increased satisfaction. *Critical Care Medicine, 32*(7), 1484-1488.

32. Medina, J., & Puntillo, K. (Eds.). (2006). *AACN protocols for practice: Palliative care and end-of-life issues in critical care.* Sudbury, MA: Jones and Bartlett.

33. Meltzer, L. S., & Huckabay, L. M. (2004). Critical care nurses' perceptions of futile care and its effect on burnout. *American Journal of Critical Care, 13*(3), 202-208.

34. Mosenthal, A. C., & Murphy, P. A. (2006). Interdisciplinary model for palliative care in the trauma and surgical intensive care unit: Robert Wood Johnson Foundation demonstration project for improving palliative care in the intensive care unit. *Critical Care Medicine, 34*(Suppl. 11), S399-S403.

35. Mularski, R. A., Curtis, J. R., Billings, J. A., Burt, R., Byock, I., Fuhrman, C., et al. (2006). Proposed quality measures for palliative care in the critically ill: A consensus from the Robert Wood Johnson Foundation Critical Care Workgroup. *Critical Care Medicine, 34*(Suppl. 11), S404-S411.

36. Nelson, J. E. (2006). Identifying and overcoming the barriers to high-quality palliative care in the intensive care unit. *Critical Care Medicine, 34*(Suppl. 11), S324-S331.

37. Nelson, J. E., Angus, D. C., Weissfeld, L. A., Puntillo, K. A., Danis, M., Deal, D., et al. (2006). End-of-life care for the critically ill: A national intensive care unit survey. *Critical Care Medicine, 34,* 2547-2553.

38. Robichaux, C. M., & Clark, A. P. (2006). Practice of expert critical care nurses in situations of prognostic conflict at the end of life. *American Journal of Critical Care, 15*(5), 480-489.

39. Rocker, G. M., Heyland, D. K., Cook, D. J., Dodek, P. M., Kutsogiannis, D. J., & O'Callaghan, C. J. (2004). Most critically ill patients are perceived to die in comfort during withdrawal of life support: A Canadian multicentre study. *Canadian Journal of Anaesthesia, 51,* 623-630.

40. Rubenfeld, G. D., & Elliott, M. (2005). Evidence-based ethics? *Current Opinion in Critical Care, 11,* 598-599.

41. Rushton, C. H. (2006). Defining and addressing moral distress. *AACN Advanced Critical Care, 17*(2), 161-168.

42. Shalowitz, D. I., Garrett-Mayer, E., & Wendler, D. (2006). The accuracy of surrogate decision makers. *Archives of Internal Medicine, 166,* 493-497.

43. Shrank, W. H., Kutner, J. S., Richardson, T., Mularski, R. A., Fischer, S., & Kagawa-Singer, M. (2005). Focus group findings about the influence of culture on communication preferences in end-of-life care. *Journal of General Internal Medicine, 20,* 703-709.

44. Siriwardena, A. N., & Clark, D. H. (2004). End-of-life care for ethnic minority groups. *Clinical Cornerstone, 6*(1), 43-48.

45. SUPPORT Principal Investigators. (1995). A controlled trial to improve care for seriously ill hospitalized patients: The Study to Understand Prognoses and Preferences for Outcomes and Risks of Treatments (SUPPORT). *Journal of the American Medical Association, 274*(20), 1591-1598.

46. Thompson, D. R. (2007). Principles of ethics: In managing a critical care unit. *Critical Care Medicine, 35*(Suppl. 2), S2-S10.

47. Tonelli, M. R. (2005). Waking the dying: Must we always attempt to involve critically ill patients in end-of-life decisions? *Chest, 127*(2), 637-642.

48. Treece, P. D., Engleberg, R. A., Shannon, S. E., Nielsen, E. L., Braungardt, T., Rubenfeld, G. R., et al. (2006). Integrating palliative and critical care: Description of an intervention. *Critical Care Medicine, 34*(Suppl. 11), S380-S387.

49. Truog, R. D., Meyer, E. C., & Burns, J. P. (2006). Toward interventions to improve end-of-life care in the pediatric intensive care unit. *Critical Care Medicine, 34*(Suppl. 11), S373-S379.

50. U.S. Census Bureau. (2002). *Race and Hispanic or Latino origin by age and sex for the United States: 2000.* Retrieved March 24, 2007, from www.census.gov/population/cen2000/phc-t08/phc-t-08.pdf.

51. Valente, S. M. (2004). End of life and ethnicity. *Journal for Nurses in Staff Development, 20*(6), 285-293.

52. Wall, R. J., Engelberg, R. A., Gries, C. J., Glavan, B., & Curtis, J. R. (2007). Spiritual care of families in the intensive care unit. *Critical Care Medicine, 35*(4), 1084-1090.

53. Weissman, D. E. (2004). Decision making at a time of crisis: Near the end of life. *Journal of the American Medical Association, 292*(14), 1738-1743.

54. West, H. R., Engleberg, R. A., Wenrich, M. D., & Curtis, J. R. (2005). Expressions of nonabandonment during the intensive care unit family conference. *Journal of Palliative Medicine, 8*(4), 797-807.

55. White, D. B., & Curtis, J. R. (2006). Establishing an evidence base for physician-family communication and shared decision making in the intensive care unit. *Critical Care Medicine, 34*(9), 2500-2501.

56. White, D. B., Curtis, J. R., Lo, B., & Luce, J. M. (2006). Decisions to limit life-sustaining treatment for critically ill patients who lack both decision-making capacity and surrogate decision-makers. *Critical Care Medicine, 34*(8), 2053-2059.

57. White, D. B., Engleberg, R. A., Wenrich, M. D., Lo, B., & Curtis, J. R. (2007). Prognostication during physician-family discussions about limiting life support in intensive care units. *Critical Care Medicine, 35*(2), 442-448.

58. Wlody, G. S. (2007). Nursing management and organizational ethics in the intensive care unit. *Critical Care Medicine, 35*(Suppl. 2), S29-S35.

PART II

Tools for the Critical Care Nurse

CHAPTER 5

Comfort and Sedation

Mamoona Arif, MS, RN, CCRN

Mary Jo Grap, PhD, RN, ACNP, FAAN

INTRODUCTION

Maintaining an optimal level of comfort for the critically ill patient is a universal goal for physicians and nurses.[40] Patients in the critical care unit experience pain from preexisting diseases, invasive procedures, or trauma. Pain can also be caused by monitoring devices (catheters, drains), noninvasive ventilating devices, endotracheal tubes, routine nursing care (airway suctioning, dressing changes, and patient positioning), and prolonged immobility. It has been reported that 64% of patients recall having pain as a stressful experience during their critical care unit stay.[33]

Unrelieved pain may contribute to inadequate sleep, which may lead to exhaustion, anxiety, disorientation, and agitation. A recent study reported that 26% of critically ill patients experienced delusional memories such as dreams, hallucinations, nightmares, and the illusion that people were trying to hurt them.[86] These delusional memories have been linked to the development of posttraumatic stress disorder (PTSD).[43]

The patient's perception, expression, and tolerance of pain and anxiety may vary because of different psychological and social influences.[69] Evidence of ethnic differences in pain perception has also been reported.[64,83] Therefore, it is important for health care providers to assess and manage pain and anxiety appropriately. Hospitals and health care accrediting agencies have recognized that pain and anxiety are major contributors to patient morbidity and length of stay. According to a National Patient Safety Goals Survey, pain assessment remains one of the top standards of noncompliance among hospitals (19%).[41] The Joint Commission requires that pain be assessed in "all patients" and that it be considered the "fifth vital sign." The Joint Commission also recommends that tools to evaluate pain should be specific to the age and disease state of the patient and to the site of pain.[41] Promoting rest, comfort, and frequent reorientation are important nursing interventions to reduce pain and anxiety for a critically ill patient. The treatment of pain and anxiety should be individualized to the patient's needs for analgesia and sedation. Many critically ill patients have underlying chronic pain, thus making assessment and management more challenging. This chapter focuses on the assessment and management strategies for the critically ill patient experiencing acute pain, anxiety, or both.

DEFINITIONS OF PAIN AND ANXIETY

The International Association for the Study of Pain defines pain as an unpleasant sensory and emotional experience associated with actual or potential tissue damage.[68] This explanation of pain alludes to the global nature of pain. McCaffery[59] defines pain as "whatever the experiencing person says it is, existing whenever he says it does." With the use of this definition, the patient becomes the true authority on the pain that is being experienced, and the patient's pain should be managed based on this description. Many theoretical bases for the development of pain have been proposed. The gate control theory is the most widely used in research and therapy (Box 5-1).[39]

Anxiety is a state marked by apprehension, agitation, autonomic arousal, and/or fearful withdrawal.[60] It is a prolonged state of apprehension in response to a real or perceived fear. Anxiety must be assessed in the same way used to assess pain: the patient's level of anxiety is whatever the patient reports.

Pain and anxiety are often interrelated and may be difficult to differentiate because the physiological and behavioral findings are similar for each. The relation between pain and anxiety is cyclical (Figure 5-1), with each exacerbating the other.[17] Inadequately treated pain leads to greater anxiety, and anxiety is associated with higher pain intensity.

BOX 5-1   Gate Control Theory of Pain

Innocuous (nonpainful) stimuli transmitted by large afferent nerve fibers may prevent the transmission of painful stimuli. Stimulation of larger nerve fibers causes synapses in the dorsal horn of the spinal cord to cease firing, thus creating a "closed gate." A closed gate decreases the stimulation of trigger cells, decreases transmission of impulses, and diminishes pain perception. Persistent stimulation of the large fibers may allow for adaptation, allowing pain signals to reach the spinal cord and brain.

Modified from Heuther, S., & DeFriez, C. B. (2006). Pain, temperature regulation, sleep, and sensory function. In K. L. McCance & S. E. Heuther (Eds.), *Pathophysiology: The pathologic basis for disease in adults & children* (5th ed., pp. 447-489). St. Louis: Mosby.

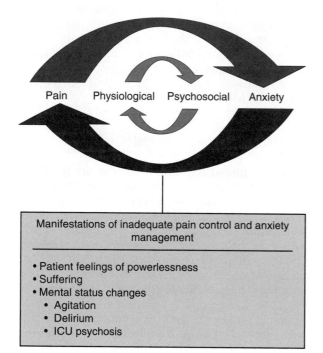

FIGURE 5-1. The anxiety-pain cycle. *(From Cullen, L., Greiner, J., & Titler, M. G. [2001]. Pain management in the culture of critical care. Critical Care Nursing Clinics of North America, 13[2], 151-166.)*

Anxiety may contribute to pain perception by activating pain pathways, altering the cognitive evaluation of pain, increasing aversion to pain, and increasing the report of pain.[17] If pain and anxiety are unresolved and escalate, the patient may experience feelings of powerlessness, suffering, and psychological changes such as agitation and delirium. Anxiety is not a benign state, and unrelieved anxiety may lead to greater morbidity and mortality, especially in patients with cardiovascular disease. PTSD may occur after intensive care unit (ICU) discharge.[18,42]

Because interventions to manage pain may differ from those used to manage anxiety, the nurse must be astute to the patient's precipitating problem. If pain is being treated in a patient who is experiencing anxiety only, the anxiety may worsen as potentially ineffective management strategies are used. For example, the pharmacological agents used to treat pain have very different properties compared with those agents used to treat anxiety. Pain management involves antiinflammatory and analgesic medications, whereas sedative medications are used to treat anxiety.

PREDISPOSING FACTORS TO PAIN AND ANXIETY

Many factors inherent to the critical care environment place patients at risk of developing pain and anxiety. Pain perception may occur as a result of preexisting diseases, invasive procedures, monitoring devices, nursing care, or trauma. The perception of pain is also influenced by the expectation of pain, prior pain experiences, a patient's emotional state, and the cognitive processes of the patient.[12] Although pain perception involves conscious experience, new evidence shows a higher prevalence of pain in adult patients with impaired cortical function, or cortical immaturity during early development in children.[11,67] Yet, these vulnerable populations receive fewer analgesics as compared with patients with intact cognitive function.[15,47]

Anxiety is likely to result from the inability to communicate; the continuous noise of alarms, equipment, and personnel; bright ambient lighting; and excessive stimulation from inadequate analgesia, frequent assessments, repositioning, lack of mobility, and uncomfortable room temperature. Sleep deprivation and the circumstances that resulted in an admission to the critical care unit may also increase patient anxiety. Recent research has found that intubated patients receiving mechanical ventilation experience moderate levels of anxiety.[14]

PHYSIOLOGY OF PAIN AND ANXIETY

Pain

All pain results from a signal cascade within the body's neurological network. Pain is initiated by signals that travel through the peripheral nervous

TABLE 5-1	Physiological Responses to Pain and/or Anxiety
Tachycardia	Diaphoresis
Tachypnea	Increased glucose production (gluconeogenesis)
Hypertension	
Increased cardiac output	Nausea
Pallor and/or flushing	Urinary retention
Cool extremities	Constipation
Mydriasis (pupillary dilation)	Sleep disturbance

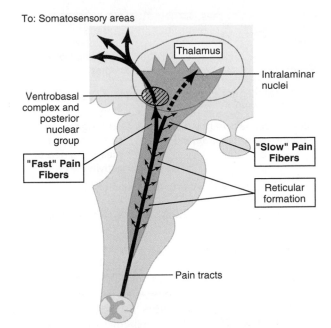

To: Somatosensory areas

FIGURE 5-2. Transmission of pain signals into the brainstem, thalamus, and cerebral cortex by way of the "fast" pain pathway and "slow" pain pathway. *(From Guyton, A., & Hall, J. (2006). Textbook of Medical Physiology (11th ed.). Philadelphia: Saunders.)*

system to the central nervous system for processing.[19] Pain can be classified as acute or chronic, malignant or nonmalignant, and nociceptive or neuropathic. In all forms of acute pain, the sympathetic nervous system (SNS) is usually activated quickly, and several physiological responses typically occur (Table 5-1). In contrast, some forms of chronic pain may result in less activation of the SNS and a different clinical presentation.

The sensation of pain is carried to the central nervous system by activation of two separate pathways (Figure 5-2). The fast (sharp) pain signals are transmitted to the spinal cord by slowly conducting, thinly myelinated A-delta afferent fibers. A-delta fibers are activated by high-intensity physical (hot and cold) stimuli that are important in initiating rapid reactions. Conversely, slow (burning; chronic) pain is transmitted by the unmyelinated, polymodal C fibers, which are activated by a variety of high-intensity mechanical, chemical, hot and cold stimuli.[45]

The most abundant receptors in the nervous system for pain recognition are nociceptors whose cell bodies are located in the dorsal root ganglia.[45] The sensation of pain received by peripheral endings of sensory neurons is called nociception. The nociceptive pain is divided into somatic and visceral. Nociceptive pain is detected by specialized transducers attached to A-delta and C fibers. Somatic pain results from irritation or damage to the nervous system. Visceral pain is diffuse, poorly localized, and often referred.[45]

Mechanical, chemical, and thermal stimuli activate nociceptors to produce a painful sensation. Examples of mechanical stimuli include a crushing injury or a surgical wound. A chemical stimulus is any substance that produces skin irritation, and burn injury is a thermal stimulus for pain. Identifying the correct pain-inducing stimulus is important in the effective management of pain. Removal of the stimulus should always precede other treatment measures in managing pain.[35]

Nociceptors differ from other nerve receptors in the body in that they adapt very little to the pain response. If the stimulus for pain is not removed, the body continues to experience pain until the stimulus is discontinued or other interventions (e.g., analgesic agents) are initiated. This is a protective mechanism so the body tissues being damaged will be removed from harm.

Nociceptors usually lie near capillary beds and mast cells. When tissue injury occurs, the nociceptor initiates an inflammatory response near the injured capillary.[28,62,70] The mast cells in the damaged tissues degranulate, releasing histamine and chemotactic agents that promote infiltration of injured tissues with neutrophils and eosinophils. As neutrophils move into the site of injury, more neurotransmitter-like substances (acetylcholine, bradykinins, substance P, and enkephalins) are released from the neutrophils into the surrounding tissue. These substances act as mediators and may induce or suppress pain. Endogenous cytokines that suppress pain induction are commonly referred to as the endorphins.

Current advances in neuroimaging studies have identified a more complex level of processing of pain

TABLE 5-2   Neuroimaging Studies

Method	Application in Pain Studies
Functional magnetic resonance imaging (fMRI)	Localizing brain activity
Electroencephalography (EEG); Magnetoencephalography (MEG)	Detecting temporal sequences and measuring neuronal activity.
Single photon emission computed tomography (SPECT); Positron emission tomography (PET)	Identifying neurotransmitter systems and drug uptake
MR spectroscopy	Detecting long-term changes in brain chemistry

Data from Apkarian, A. V., Bushnell, M. C., Treede, R. D., & Zubieta, J. K. (2005). Human brain mechanisms of pain perception and regulation in health and disease. *European Journal of Pain, 9*, 463-484.

in the human cerebral cortex. The neuroimaging studies have identified multiple nociceptive pathways that deliver parallel imputs to somatosensory, limbic, and associative structures.[3,50] These techniques (Table 5-2) allow noninvasive examination of brain mechanisms involved in acute and chronic pain processing.

Anxiety

The physiology of anxiety is less clearly understood in comparison with pain and is a more complex process because no actual tissue injury is thought to occur. Anxiety stimulates the SNS response.

Anxiety has been linked to the reward and punishment centers within the limbic system of the brain. Stimulation in the punishment centers frequently inhibits the reward centers completely.[35] The punishment center is also responsible for helping a person escape from potentially harmful situations. The punishment center has dominance over the reward center for the person to escape harm.

POSITIVE EFFECTS OF PAIN AND ANXIETY

In the healthy person, pain and anxiety are adaptive mechanisms used to increase mental and physical performance levels to allow a person to move away from potential harm. When the SNS is activated, the person usually becomes more vigilant of the environment, especially to potential dangers. Once dangers are recognized, the person makes a choice whether to flee the situation or combat the possible threat. For this reason, SNS activation has become known as the "fight-or-flight" response.

NEGATIVE EFFECTS OF PAIN AND ANXIETY

Physical Effects

Both pain and anxiety activate the SNS. Catecholamine levels increase, which may place a significant burden on the cardiovascular system, especially in a critically ill patient. Activation of the SNS results in tachycardia and hypertension, which leads to increased myocardial oxygen demand. Patients with silent myocardial infarction do not experience chest pain and therefore do not seek immediate medical treatment.[34] These patients are at high risk for increased morbidity and mortality. Anxiety is also associated with recurrent cardiac events and mortality for cardiac patients.

The physiological response to stress also interferes with the healing process and impairs perfusion and oxygen delivery to tissue.[9] Hemodynamic instability, immunosuppression, and tissue catabolism may also occur.[93] Any large organ that experiences an increase in oxygen consumption places the critically ill patient at risk of increased rates of complications related to end organ ischemia.[56]

Hyperventilation (tachypnea) can be stressful to the patient because rapid breathing requires a significant amount of effort with the use of accessory muscles. Hyperventilation may cause respiratory alkalosis. Respiratory alkalosis may result in impaired tissue perfusion, and many vasoactive medications become less effective.

If the patient is mechanically ventilated, an increased respiratory rate leads to feelings of breathlessness. As the patient "fights" the mechanical ventilator, further alveolar damage ensues, and the endotracheal or tracheostomy tube creates a "choking" sensation and increased anxiety. Anxiety may also result in increased dyspnea and delayed ventilator weaning.

Psychological Effects

Many patients in the critical care unit report feelings of panic and fear. Pain and anxiety exacerbate reports of lack of sleep, nightmares, and feelings of bewilderment, isolation, and loneliness. The effects of a critical care unit stay may persist long after discharge, and many patients develop PTSD as a result of their critical care unit experience.[42]

Extreme anxiety, pain, and adverse effects of medications can also lead to agitation, which is commonly seen in the critically ill patient. Agitation is associated with inappropriate verbal behavior, physical aggression, and increased movement that may lead to harm to the patient or caregiver.[26,91]

ASSESSMENT

Quality pain management begins with a thorough assessment, reassessment, and documentation to facilitate treatment and communication among health care providers.[32] The 2005 American Pain Society guidelines recommend a five-step hierarchy approach to pain assessment:[32]

- Pain should be assessed and treated promptly in all patients. Pain assessment and documentation should be clearly communicated with other health care providers.
- The patient should be actively engaged in the pain management plan.
- Health care providers need to provide preemptive treatment with analgesics to provide safe, effective, and equitable pain management.
- Pain should be reassessed and treatment adjusted to meet the patient's needs.
- Health care facilities need to establish a comprehensive quality improvement program that monitors both health care provider practice and patient outcomes.

Pain assessment is challenging in patients who cannot communicate; these patients represent the majority of critically ill patients. Factors that alter verbal communication in critically ill patients include endotracheal intubation, altered level of consciousness, restraints, sedation, and therapeutic paralysis.[30,40,90]

The American Pain Society guidelines mandate evaluation of both physiological and behavioral response to pain in patients who are unable to communicate.[38] At present, no universally accepted pain scale for use in the noncommunicative (cognitively impaired, sedated, paralyzed, or mechanically ventilated) patient exists.[40] Optimal pain assessment in adult critical care settings is essential since it has been reported that nurses underrate the patient's pain.[36,79,80] Nurses often undermedicate the critically ill patient as well. One study reported that more than 60% of critically ill patients did not receive any medications before and/or during painful procedures such as central line insertions, wound dressing changes, and suctioning.[82] Inaccurate pain assessments and resulting inadequate treatment of pain in critically ill adults can lead to significant physiological consequences.

Assessment involves the collection of the patient's self-report of the pain experience as well as behavioral markers. Nurses can ask the patient to describe the pain or anxiety being experienced, or to provide a numerical score to indicate the level of pain or anxiety. In addition, behavioral or physiological findings of pain are phenomena that are observed. For example, increased blood pressure or a facial grimace or frown may indicate pain or anxiety. Typical physiological responses related to pain are detailed in Table 5-1. In the healthy person, these responses are adaptive mechanisms and result from activation of the SNS in an attempt to ready the individual for the fight-or-flight response. In the critically ill patient, these changes may induce further stress on an already compromised individual.

As part of the assessment of pain and anxiety, the nurse must be aware of what procedures may cause pain, and the effectiveness of interventions.[81] When patients exhibit signs of anxiety or agitation, the assessment also includes identification and treatment of the potential cause, such as hypoxemia, hypoglycemia, hypotension, pain, and withdrawal from alcohol and drugs. When possible, patients should be asked about any herbal remedies used as complementary and alternative medical therapies and whether they take them along with prescription or over-the-counter medications.[89] These products may lead to adverse herb-drug interactions, especially in the elderly who are more likely to be taking multiple drugs.

Pain Measurement Tools

In the assessment of pain, the nurse asks the patient to identify several characteristics associated with the pain. These characteristics include the precipitating cause, severity, location (including radiation to other sites), duration, and any alleviating or aggravating factors. Any pain assessment should address these pain characteristics or the assessment is not complete. Patients with chronic pain conditions, such as arthritis, may be able to provide a detailed list of effective pain remedies that may be useful during the present hospitalization.

Several tools are available to ensure that the appropriate pain assessment questions are asked. One tool used in assessing the patient with chest pain is the PQRST method. The PQRST method allows the nurse to remember a mnemonic so all chest pain characteristics are documented.

P—*Provocation or position.* What precipitated the chest pain symptoms, and where in the chest area is the pain located?

Q—*Quality.* Is the pain sharp, dull, crushing?

R—*Radiation.* Does the pain travel to other parts of the body?

S —*Severity or symptoms associated with the pain.* The patient is asked to rate the pain on a numerical scale and to describe what other symptoms are present.

T—*Timing or triggers* for the pain. Is the pain constant or intermittent, and does it occur with certain activities?

One of the most common methods to determine pain severity is to ask for a pain score. Patients are asked to rate their pain on a numbered scale such as 0 to 10. A score of 0 indicates no pain, and a score of 10 indicates the worst pain the patient could possibly imagine. The pain score is reassessed after medications or other pain-relieving measures have been provided. Institutional policy provides guidelines for the method and frequency of pain assessment. Some institutions require nurses to intervene for a pain score greater than a predesignated number. The pain score method should be used only with patients who are cognitively aware of their surroundings and are able to follow simple commands. It is possible for patients with mild to moderate dementia to self-report pain, but this ability decreases with progression of the disease.[38] Numeric rating is not an appropriate method to assess pain in patients who are disoriented or have severe cognitive impairment.

A second tool is known as the FACES Pain Scale. Patients are asked to describe how they feel by pointing to a series of faces ranging from happy to distressed faces (Figure 5-3). The FACES method involves a higher level of emotional intellect because the patient must be able to process different yet similar visual stimuli accurately.[51] The most common versions of the FACES scale use between five and seven different images.

Another widely used subjective pain measurement tool is the Visual Analog Scale (VAS). The VAS is a 10-cm line that looks similar to a timeline. The scale may be drawn horizontally or vertically, and it may or may not be numbered. If numbered, 0 indicates no pain, whereas 10 indicates the most pain

(Figure 5-4). When using the VAS, the nurse holds up the scale, and the patient points to the level of pain on the line. If the patient is able to communicate in writing, the patient can place an "X" on the VAS with a pencil. The VAS can also be used to evaluate a patient's level of anxiety, with 0 representing no anxiety and 10 the most anxiety. The VAS must be used for patients who are alert and able to follow directions. It is effective for awake nonverbal patients, such as those who are being supported by mechanical ventilation.

Pain Measurement Tools for Nonverbal Patients

Identification of the optimal pain scales for noncommunicative patients has been the focus of several studies. To date, no one tool is universally accepted for use in this patient population.[37,40] Assessment of pain intensity may be quantified by using the behavioral-physiological scales.

Adult Behavioral Pain Tools

Several behavioral pain tools are available to assess critically ill adult patients. Widely used and validated, the Behavioral Pain Scale was developed to assess pain in the critically ill adult who is nonverbal and unable to communicate (Table 5-3).[77] The Behavioral Pain Scale provides critical care nurses with an objective and reliable pain measurement tool.[77,78] It has been researched only in the mechanically ventilated patient and therefore may not be appropriate in other patients.

Another recently developed behavioral pain tool is the Critical-Care Pain Observation Tool (Table 5-4). It was initially validated in cardiac surgery patients and most recently in patients in other ICUs.[29,31] The Critical-Care Pain Observation Tool is appropriate for the assessment of patients with or without an endotracheal tube.[29]

The Checklist of Nonverbal Pain Indicators[25] provides a good indicator of the patient's distress by being attentive to pain-related behaviors. The tool was initially developed because of concerns that

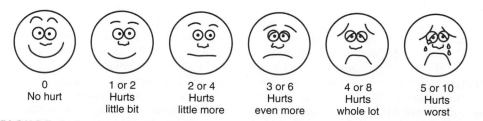

FIGURE 5-3. A version of the FACES scale. *(From Hockenberry:* Wong's Essentials of Pediatric Nursing *[7th ed., p. 663]. St. Louis: Mosby.)*

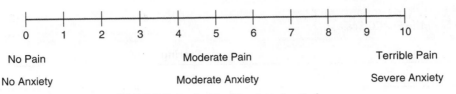

FIGURE 5-4. The Visual Analog Scale.

TABLE 5-3	The Behavioral Pain Scale*	
Item	**Description**	**Score**
Facial expression	Relaxed	1
	Partially tightened (e.g., brow lowering)	2
	Fully tightened (e.g., eyelid closing)	3
	Grimacing	4
Upper limbs	No movement	1
	Partially bent	2
	Fully bent with finger flexion	3
	Permanently retracted	4
Compliance with ventilation	Tolerating movement	1
	Coughing but tolerating ventilation most of the time	2
	Fighting ventilator	3
	Unable to control ventilation	4

*Each of the categories—facial expression, upper limbs, and compliance with ventilation—is scored from 1 to 4. The values are added together for a total score between 3 and 12.
From Payen, J.-F., Bru, O., Bosson, J. L., Lagrasta, A., Novel, E., Deschaux, I., et al. (2001). Assessing pain in critically ill sedated patients by using a behavioral pain scale. *Critical Care Medicine, 29*(12), 2258-2263.

TABLE 5-4	Critical-Care Pain Observation Tool	
Indicator		**Score**
Facial Expression		
• Relaxed, no muscle tension		0
• Tense facial muscles (brow lowering, orbit tightening, and levator contraction)		1
• Grimacing with tense facial muscles		2
Body Movements		
• Absence of movements		0
• Protection		1
• Restlessness		2
Muscle Tension in Upper Extremities		
• Relaxed		0
• Tense, rigid		1
• Very tense or rigid		2
Compliance with the Ventilator		
• Tolerating ventilator or movement		0
• Coughing but tolerating ventilator		1
• Fighting ventilator		2
Non-Ventilator, Vocalization		
• No sound		0
• Sighing, moaning		1
• Crying out, sobbing		2
Total Score		—

Data from Gelinas, C., Fillion, L., Puntillo, K. A., Viens, C., & Fortier, M. (2006). Validation of the critical-care pain observation tool in adult patients. *American Journal of Critical Care, 15*, 420-427.

some of the cognitively impaired patients are not able to respond reliably to the yes/no questions about pain. This tool showed no significant differences in observed pain behaviors between the cognitively impaired group and the cognitively intact group. The Checklist of Nonverbal Pain Indicators has been tested in acute and long-term care settings to assess acute and chronic pain in elderly patients.[25,74]

Pediatric Pain Tools

Similar to noncommunicative critically ill adults, newborns, infants, and preverbal toddlers are unable to report and describe pain. In the pediatric population, the FLACC (Table 5-5) tool is used to assess pain in children who lack the verbal and cognitive skills to provide pain intensity reports. The acronym FLACC (face, legs, activity, cry, and consol-ability) was developed to remind users of the five different categories of the scale.[66] Scores greater than 4 to 5 necessitate intervention. The FLACC tool has been used in critically ill adults, but the tool has yet to be researched in this patient population.

The COMFORT Scale is widely used in pediatric critical care unit settings and has been recently used in adult critical care units. It contains behavioral and physiological factors to evaluate pain and to assess distress.[2] The scale has not been extensively validated in adult critically ill patients.

TABLE 5-5　The FLACC Scale

Categories*	Scoring		
	0	**1**	**2**
Face	No particular expression or smile	Occasional grimace or frown, withdrawn, disinterested	Frequent to constant quivering chin, clenched jaw
Legs	Normal position or relaxed	Uneasy, restless, tense	Kicking, or legs drawn up
Activity	Lying quietly, normal position, moves easily	Squirming, shifting back and forth, tense	Arched, rigid, or jerking
Cry	No cry (awake or asleep)	Moans or whimpers, occasional complaint	Crying steadily, screams or sobs, frequent complaints
Consolability	Content, relaxed	Reassured by occasional touching, hugging, or being talked to; distractible	Difficult to console or comfort

*Each of the five categories (F) Face; (L) Legs; (A) Activity; (C) Cry; (C) Consolability is scored from 0 to 2. The values are added together for a total score between 0 and 10.

From Merkel, S. I., Voepel-Lewis, T., Shayevitz, J. R., Malviya, S. (1997). The FLACC: A behavioral scale for scoring post-operative pain in young children. *Pediatric Nursing, 23*(3), 293-297. Reprinted with permission of the publisher, Jannetti Publications, Inc., East Holly Avenue, Box 56, Pitman, NJ 08071-0056; Phone (856) 256-2300; Fax: (856) 589-7463. For a sample copy of the journal, please contact the publisher.

Anxiety and Sedation Measurement Tools

Sedation Scales

No objective tool is considered the gold standard for determining a patient's level of anxiety. Anxiety typically produces hyperactive psychomotor functions including tachycardia, hypertension, and movement. Patients are typically sedated to limit this hyperactivity. The level of sedation can be measured by using objective tools or scales. An ideal sedation scale provides data that are simple to compute and record; accurately describes the degree of sedation or agitation within well-defined categories; guides the titration of therapy; and has validity and reliability in critically ill patients.[40]

When administering medications to sedate a patient, the goal is to achieve a level of sedation with the lowest dose. By using lower doses of medications, the patient is less likely to experience drug accumulation or adverse effects. These adverse effects include increased hospital stay, delayed ventilator weaning, immobility, and increased rates of ventilator-associated pneumonia. Conversely, not enough sedation may lead to agitation, inappropriate use of paralytics, increased metabolic demand, and an increased risk of myocardial ischemia.[61] Sedation scales assist in the accurate identification and communication of sedation level. The most frequently used sedation scales are the Richmond Agitation-Sedation Scale (RASS), the Ramsay Sedation Scale, and the Sedation-Agitation Scale.

The RASS is a 10-point scale, from +4 (combative) through 0 (calm, alert) to −5 (unarousable). The patient is assessed in three steps using discreet criteria, over 30 to 60 seconds (Table 5-6).[88] Raters using the RASS have consistent agreement in their assessment of the patient. The RASS is useful in detecting changes in sedation status over consecutive days of critical care unit care, and correlates with the administered dose of sedative and analgesic medications.[22]

The Ramsay Sedation Scale was developed for postoperative evaluation of patients emerging from general anesthesia.[84] The scale includes three levels of wakefulness and three levels of sedation (Table 5-7). The nurse makes a visual and cognitive assessment of the patient. Scores range from 1 (awake) to 6 (asleep/unarousable).

The Sedation-Agitation Scale (Table 5-8) describes patient behaviors seen in the continuum of sedation to agitation.[85] Scores range from 1 (unarousable) to 7 (dangerously agitated).

The appropriate target level of sedation depends on the patient's disease process and therapeutic or support interventions required. A common target level of sedation is a calm patient who is easily aroused; however, deeper levels of sedation may be needed to facilitate mechanical ventilation.

Continuous Monitoring of Sedation

No technological device provides the bedside nurse with an absolute measurement of the patient's pain or anxiety. Technological devices are being used in

TABLE 5-6   Richmond Agitation-Sedation Scale

Term	Score
Combative	+4
Very agitated	+3
Agitated	+2
Restless	+1
Alert and calm	0
Drowsy—sustains (>10 sec) awakening, with eye contact to voice*	−1
Light sedation—sustains (<10 sec) awakening with eye contact to voice*	−2
Moderate sedation—any movement (but no eye contact) to voice*	−3
Deep sedation—no response to voice, but any movement to physical stimulation*	−4
Unarousable	−5
Score	

*In a loud voice, state patient's name and direct patient to open eyes and look at speaker.

From Sessler, C. N., Gosnell, M. S., Grap, M. J., Brophy, G. M., O'Neal, P. V., Keane, K. A., et al. (2002). The Richmond Agitation-Sedation Scale: Validity and reliability in adult intensive care unit patients. *American Journal of Respiratory and Critical Care Medicine, 166,* 1338-1344.

the operating room and the critical care unit to measure a patient's level of consciousness to verify anesthesia and sedative dosing. Since pain and anxiety activate the SNS, a heightened level of consciousness may result. Technological devices attempt to measure these physiological changes by assessing the patient's brain activity.

The electroencephalogram (EEG) records spontaneous brain activity that originates from the cortical pyramidal cells on the surface of the brain. Any

TABLE 5-7   The Ramsay Sedation Scale

Level	Scale
1	Patient awake, anxious and agitated or restless, or both
2	Patient awake, cooperative, oriented, and tranquil
3	Patient awake; response to commands only
4	Patient asleep; brisk response to light glabellar tap or loud auditory stimulus
5	Patient asleep; sluggish response to light glabellar tap or loud auditory stimulus
6	Patient asleep; no response to light glabellar tap or loud auditory stimulus

From Ramsay, M. A., Savege, T. M., Simpson, B. R., Goodwin R. (1974). Controlled sedation with alphaxalone-alphadolone. *British Medical Journal, 2*(90), 656-659.

TABLE 5-8   Sedation-Agitation Scale

Score	Characteristic	Examples of Patient's Behavior
7	Dangerously agitated	Pulls at endotracheal tube, tries to remove catheters, climbs over bed rail, strikes at staff, thrashes from side to side
6	Very agitated	Does not calm despite frequent verbal reminding of limits, requires physical restraints, bites endotracheal tube
5	Agitated	Anxious or mildly agitated, attempts to sit up, calms down in response to verbal instructions
4	Calm and cooperative	Calm, awakens easily, follows commands
3	Sedated	Difficult to arouse, awakens to verbal stimuli or gentle shaking but drifts off again, follows simple commands
2	Very sedated	Arouses to physical stimuli but does not communicate or follow commands, may move spontaneously
1	Unarousable	Minimal or no response to noxious stimuli, does not communicate or follow commands

From Riker, R. R., Fraser, G. L., Simmons, L. E., & Wilkins, M. L. (2001). Validating the Sedation-Agitation Scale with the bispectral index and Visual Analog Scale in adult ICU patients after cardiac surgery. *Intensive Care Medicine, 27*(5), 853-858.

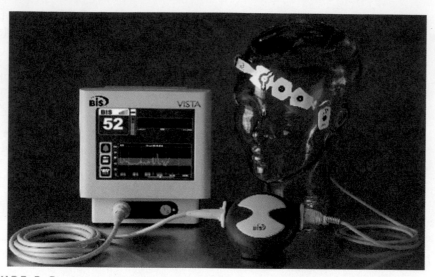

FIGURE 5-5. The Bispectral Index (BIS) monitor and electrode. *(Courtesy of Aspect Medical Systems, Newton, MA.)*

major brain activity produces a resultant peak in activity on the EEG monitor. The EEG monitor receives data from 21 electrodes that are placed in key positions on the patient's head. The number of electrodes may be decreased depending on the patient's head size and the purpose for the EEG procedure.[58] In the critical care unit, the EEG is used infrequently to assess levels of sedation because it takes significant time (up to 60 minutes) to acquire proper electrode placement and a high level of skill to interpret the EEG recording.

The EEG generally changes from a low-amplitude, high-frequency signal while the patient is awake to a large-amplitude, low-frequency signal when the patient is deeply anesthetized.[6] Devices that monitor continuous EEG signals without using the traditional 21-electrode system are frequently used to assess levels of sedation in the critically ill patient. These newer devices digitize the raw EEG signal and apply a complex algorithm that results in a numeric score ranging from 0 (isoelectric EEG) to 100 (fully awake).[27] Examples of such devices are the Bispectral Index Score (BIS) monitor (Aspect Medical Systems, Newton, MA) and the Patient State Index (PSI) Analyzer (Physiometrix, North Billerica, MA). The resulting score provides an objective analysis of the level of wakefulness.[48] To obtain a signal, an electrode is placed across the patient's forehead and is attached to a monitor. The monitor displays the raw EEG and the BIS or PSI value. The BIS monitor and electrode are shown in Figure 5-5.

A value greater than 90 typically indicates full consciousness, and a score of 40 to 60 represents deep sedation. A BIS value of >60 is associated with patient awareness and recollection. Therefore, a BIS value of less than 60 should be the goal in critically ill patients who require sedation.[27]

A score is usually documented with each set of vital signs. When using BIS or PSI monitoring, results must be correlated with the patient's clinical assessment and correct electrode placement. All muscle activity may not be completely filtered, which may affect the value. These devices are especially useful for critically ill patients who are treated with medications that produce deep sedation or neuromuscular blockade. They provide a continuous evaluation of sedation that may also be less affected by rater bias. However, studies comparing these values to sedation scales have shown only moderate agreement, indicating that neither is ideal as a single method of sedation assessment in the critically ill.[27]

PAIN AND ANXIETY ASSESSMENT CHALLENGES

Many situations may lead to an incomplete assessment and/or management of pain or anxiety. These include delirium and the administration of neuromuscular blocking (NMB) agents.

Delirium

A relationship exists among acute delirium, pain, and anxiety. Delirium is characterized by an acutely changing or fluctuating mental status, inattention, disorganized thinking, and altered levels of consciousness. Acute delirium is common in critically ill patients; more than 80% of patients develop some form of delirium during their stay.[95]

Delirium is categorized according to the level of alertness and level of psychomotor activity. It is divided into three clinical subtypes: hyperactive, hypoactive, and mixed (Table 5-9). Patients with hyperactive delirium are agitated, combative, and disoriented.[95] These patients place themselves or others at risk for injury because of their altered thought processes and resultant behaviors.[4] Psychotic features such as hallucinations, delusions, and paranoia may be seen. Patients may believe that members of the nursing or medical staff are attempting to harm them.

Hypoactive delirium is often referred to as quiet delirium. The mixed subtype describes the fluctuating nature of delirium. Some agitated patients with hyperactive delirium may receive sedatives to calm them, and then may emerge from sedation in a hypoactive state.

The exact pathophysiological mechanisms involved with the development and progression of delirium are unknown. However, they may be related to imbalances in the neurotransmitters that modulate the control of cognitive function, behavior, and mood.[95] Risk factors for the development of delirium include hypoxemia, metabolic disturbances, electrolyte imbalances, head trauma, the presence of catheters and drains, and certain medications. Neurotransmitter levels are affected by medications with anticholinergic properties. Benzodiazepines, opioids, and other psychotropic medications are associated with an increased risk of developing delirium (Table 5-10).

Since delirium occurs in many patients receiving mechanical ventilation and is independently associated with more deaths, longer hospital stays, and higher costs, all critically ill patients should be monitored for delirium.[21,40,94] Older patients are especially at risk for delirium.[7] The first delirium assessment method for the critical care unit (CAM-ICU) is an adaptation of the Confusion Assessment Method (Box 5-2)[20] and is designed to be a serial assessment tool for use by bedside nurses and physicians. It is easy to use, takes only 2 minutes to complete, and requires minimal training.[95]

Management of delirium focuses on keeping the patient safe. The least restrictive measures are used because unnecessary use of restraints or medication may precipitate or exacerbate delirium. Splints or binders may be needed to restrict movement if the patient is pulling at catheters, drains, or dressings. Any type of tubing should be removed as soon as possible, particularly nasogastric tubes, which are irritating to agitated patients.[44] If these measures are not successful, medication may be necessary to improve cognition, not to sedate the patient. Haloperidol, a neuroleptic agent, is the recommended medication for delirium because it has few anticholinergic and hypotensive effects. In the critically ill patient, the intermittent intravenous route of

TABLE 5-9	Clinical Subtypes of Delirium
Subtype	**Characteristics**
Hyperactive	Agitation
	Restlessness
	Attempts to remove catheters or tubes
	Hitting
	Biting
	Emotional lability
Hypoactive	Withdrawal
	Flat affect
	Apathy
	Lethargy
	Decreased responsiveness
Mixed	Concurrent or sequential appearance of some features of both hyperactive and hypoactive delirium

Truman, B., & Ely, E. W. (2003). Monitoring delirium in critically ill patients: Using the Confusion Assessment Method for the intensive care unit. *Critical Care Nurse*, 23(2), 25-36.

TABLE 5-10	Risk Factors for Delirium
Older than 70 years	
Transfer from a nursing home	
History of depression, dementia, stroke	
Alcohol or substance abuse	
Electrolyte imbalance	
Hypothermia or fever	
Renal failure	
Liver disease	
Cardiogenic or septic shock	
Human immunodeficiency virus infection	
Rectal or bladder catheters	
Tube feedings	
Central venous catheters	
Malnutrition	
Presence of physical restraints	
Visual or hearing impairment	

Modified from Truman, B., & Ely, E. W. (2003). Monitoring delirium in critically ill patients: Using the Confusion Assessment Method for the intensive care unit. *Critical Care Nurse*, 23(2), 25-36.

BOX 5-2   The Confusion Assessment Method for the Critical Care Unit

Delirium is diagnosed when both Features 1 and 2 are positive, along with either Feature 3 or Feature 4.

Feature 1. Acute Onset of Mental Status Changes or Fluctuating Course
- Is there evidence of an acute change in mental status from the baseline?
- Did the (abnormal) behavior fluctuate during the past 24 hours, that is, tend to come and go or increase and decrease in severity?
  Sources of information: Serial Glasgow Coma Scale or sedation score ratings over 24 hours as well as readily available input from the patient's nurse or family.

Feature 2. Inattention
- Did the patient have difficulty focusing attention?
- Is there a reduced ability to maintain and shift attention?
  Sources of information: Attention screening examinations by using either simple picture recognition or random letter test. These tests don't require verbal response, and thus they are ideally suited for mechanically ventilated patients.

Feature 3. Disorganized Thinking
- Was the patient's thinking disorganized or incoherent, such as rambling or irrelevant conversation, unclear or illogical flow of ideas, or unpredictable switching from subject to subject?

- Was the patient able to follow questions and commands throughout the assessment?
  1. "Are you having any unclear thinking?"
  2. "Hold up this many fingers."
  3. "Now, do the same thing with the other hand." (not repeating the number of fingers)

Feature 4. Altered Level of Consciousness: Any Level of Consciousness Other Than "Alert"
- **Alert:** normal, spontaneously fully aware of environment and interacts appropriately
- **Vigilant:** hyperalert
- **Lethargic:** drowsy but easily aroused, unaware of some elements in the environment, or not spontaneously interacting appropriately with the interviewer; becomes fully aware and appropriately interactive when prodded minimally
- **Stupor:** difficult to arouse, unaware of some or all elements in the environment, or not spontaneously interacting with the interviewer; becomes incompletely aware and inappropriately interactive when prodded strongly
- **Coma:** unarousable, unaware of all elements in the environment, with no spontaneous interaction or awareness of the interviewer, so that the interview is difficult or impossible even with maximal prodding

---

delivery is preferred because it results in better absorption and fewer side effects than the oral or intramuscular formulations. Haloperidol produces mild sedation without analgesia or amnesia. Prolongation of the QT interval on the ECG may be seen and can result in torsades de pointes. Patients with cardiac disease are at higher risk for this dysrhythmia. Other side effects include neuroleptic syndrome, as evidenced by extreme anxiety, tachycardia, tachypnea, diaphoresis, fever, muscle rigidity, increased creatine phosphokinase levels, and hyperglycemia.

Neuromuscular Blockade

NMB agents, historically used in the operating room, are being used more in critically ill to facilitate endotracheal intubation and mechanical ventilation, to control increases in intracranial pressure (ICP), and to facilitate procedures at the bedside (e.g., bronchoscopy, tracheostomy). The goal of neuromuscular blockade is complete chemical paralysis.

During a difficult endotracheal intubation, the use of a rapid-acting NMB agent allows the airway to be secured quickly and without trauma. Some patients are unable to tolerate mechanical ventilation despite adequate sedation. Long-acting NMB agents may improve chest wall compliance, reduce peak airway pressures, and prevent the patient from "fighting" the ventilator (ventilator dyssynchrony). Neuromuscular blockade promotes tolerance of newer modes of mechanical ventilation, including inverse ratio and pressure control.[57] The result is improved gas exchange with increased oxygen delivery and decreased oxygen consumption. In patients with elevated ICP, suctioning, coughing, and agitation can provoke dangerous elevations in ICP. NMB agents diminish ICP elevations during these activities. In some patients, complete immobility may be required for a short period for minor surgical and diagnostic procedures performed at the bedside.

NMB agents do not possess any sedative or analgesic properties. Any patient who receives effective neuromuscular blockade is not able to communicate or to produce any voluntary muscle movement, including breathing. Therefore, any patient receiving these agents must also be sedated. Many institutions start continuous infusions of sedative medications, before they initiate an NMB agent.

EVIDENCE-BASED PRACTICE

PROBLEM

Patients who require mechanical ventilation commonly require sedation and analgesia. Neuromuscular blockade is also needed for some patients. Although pharmacological support is an important intervention, administration of analgesics, sedatives, and neuromuscular blockade often results in prolonged mechanical ventilation and related consequences such as ventilator-associated pneumonia.

QUESTIONS

Which medications are preferred for sedation of the critically ill patient? Should protocols be used to wean patients from sedation?

REFERENCE

Vender, J. S., Szokol, J. W., Murphy, G. S., & Nitsun, M. (2004). Sedation, analgesia, and neuromuscular blockade in sepsis: An evidence-based review. *Critical Care Medicine*, *32*(Suppl.), S554-S561.

EVIDENCE

The authors worked within a committee structure and expert panel to review research related to sedation, analgesia, and neuromuscular blockade in patients with sepsis. After reviewing the body of research, they graded recommendations for practice. Research related to administration of diazepam, lorazepam, midazolam, and propofol was inconclusive regarding the best agent to administer. Lorazepam has been noted to provide easier management of sedation at a lower cost than other agents. Propofol has the benefit of more rapid awakening for assessment; it may be more useful

in some patients, such as those who need frequent neurological assessment. For pain management, opioids are recommended; however, no specific agent is preferred over another. Fentanyl has a more rapid onset of action and may be useful if rapid onset of analgesia is required. Morphine has a longer duration of action but is associated with hypotension. Research is strong related to administration of sedation using protocols and sedation scales. Sedation protocols reduce duration of mechanical ventilation and lengths of stay. Protocols include sedation goals and standardized methods for assessing sedation.

IMPLICATIONS FOR NURSING

Although the systematic review focused on the septic patient, findings apply to all critically ill patients. Different medications are available for administration; the nurse must assess the effects of medications on achieving goals for sedation and pain management, while monitoring for side effects. Different medications may be required based on assessment findings. Administration of sedation via protocols using standardized assessment tools is important in achieving target goals. Nurses must be knowledgeable of the sedation protocols at their facility and must be competent in using standardized sedation assessment tools. Assessment with standardized tools, such as those described in this chapter, allows for the patient to be monitored and treated using the same criteria, regardless of who is completing the assessment. Target sedation goals can easily be established, and effectiveness of meeting these goals can be evaluated.

Patients receiving NMB therapy are closely monitored for respiratory problems, skin breakdown, corneal abrasions, and the development of venous thrombi. If a patient experiences pain or anxiety while receiving an NMB agent, an increase in heart rate or blood pressure may be noted. Nursing care for patients receiving NMB therapy is presented in Box 5-3.

One important nursing intervention is assessing the level or degree of paralysis by using a peripheral nerve stimulator to assess a train-of-four (TOF) response. The TOF evaluates the level of neuromuscular blockade to ensure that the greatest amount of neuromuscular blockade is achieved with the lowest dose of NMB medication. The peripheral nerve stimulator delivers four low-energy impulses, and the number of muscular twitches is assessed. The ulnar nerve and the facial nerve are the most frequently

used sites for peripheral nerve stimulation. Four twitches of the thumb or facial muscle indicate incomplete neuromuscular blockade. The absence of twitches indicates complete neuromuscular blockade. The TOF goal is two out of four twitches. An example of a peripheral nerve stimulator is shown in Figure 5-6.

No tools or devices can adequately assess pain and sedation in patients receiving NMB agents. The patient is monitored for physiological changes (Table 5-1), and if changes do occur, the nurse must determine whether pain or anxiety is the potential cause. These patients may be the best candidates for assessment by nontraditional means such as the BIS or PSI monitoring system.

Although several NMB agents are available, the most frequently used are outlined in Table 5-11. Succinylcholine (paralytic), when administered with

BOX 5-3   Nursing Care of the Patient Receiving Neuromuscular Blockade

- Perform train-of-four testing before initiation, 15 minutes after dosage change, then every 4 hours, to monitor the degree of paralysis.
- Ensure appropriate sedation.
- Lubricate to eyes to prevent corneal abrasions.
- Ensure prophylaxis for deep vein thrombosis.
- Reposition the patient every 2 hours as tolerated.
- Monitor skin integrity.
- Provide oral hygiene.
- Maintain mechanical ventilation.
- Monitor breath sounds; suction airway as needed.
- Provide passive range of motion.
- Monitor heart rate, respiratory rate, blood pressure, and oxygen saturation.
- Place indwelling urinary catheter to monitor urine output.
- Monitor bowel sounds; monitor for abdominal distention.

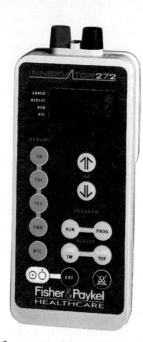

FIGURE 5-6. A train-of-four peripheral nerve stimulator. (Courtesy of Fisher & Paykel Healthcare, Auckland, New Zealand.)

etomidate (sedative), is frequently used for rapid sequence intubation because of its short half-life. However, succinylcholine should not be used in the presence of hyperkalemia because ventricular dysrhythmias and cardiac arrest may occur. Pan-

curonium is a long-acting NMB agent. When it is given in bolus doses, tachycardia and hypertension may result. The effects of pancuronium are prolonged in patients with liver disease and renal failure. Newer NMB agents such as atracurium are given in the critically ill because they are associated with fewer side effects and can be used safely in patients with liver or renal failure. Atracurium was succeeded by cisatracurium, whose pharmacodynamic and adverse effect profile proved to be superior to that of atracurium. Cisatracurium does not cause histamine release, provides better hemodynamic stability, and elimination of the drug is independent of the hepatic and renal function.[65]

MANAGEMENT OF PAIN AND ANXIETY

Nonpharmacological Management

Nonpharmacological approaches to manage pain and anxiety are early strategies because many medications used for analgesia or sedation have potentially negative hemodynamic effects. Efforts to reduce anxiety include frequent reorientation, providing patient comfort, and optimizing the environment. For example, a nurse's explanation to the patient and family of the different types of alarms heard in the critical care unit may lessen anxiety levels. Many of these nonpharmacological approaches are clustered under the heading complementary or alternative therapies. These therapies are rapidly being integrated into the critical care environment. The three most commonly used complementary therapies in the critical care unit are environmental manipulation, guided imagery, and music therapy.

Environmental Manipulation

The nurse may decrease patient anxiety and pain by changing the environment so it appears less hostile. Explanations of the monitoring equipment, alarms, and nursing care will help to decrease anxiety. The presence of calendars and clocks is helpful. For a patient experiencing delirium, continual reorientation and repetition of explanations and information is helpful. Family members often benefit from role modeling, as nursing staff members offer support and reassurance to patients while avoiding arguments with patients who have irrational ideas or misperceptions.

Another effective strategy is altering the patient's room. Patients and families should be encouraged to bring in personal items from home. Pictures of family members and other small keepsakes provide diversions from the stressful critical care environment. In

Text continued on p. 72

PHARMACOLOGY

TABLE 5-11   Drugs Frequently Used in the Treatment of Anxiety, Pain, or for Neuromuscular Blockade*

Drug	Action/Uses	Dosage/Route	Side Effects	Nursing Implications
Treatment of Anxiety				
Midazolam (Versed)	Benzodiazepine; anxiety/sedation	IV loading dose: 0.5-4 mg; may repeat in 10-15 min Infusion: 1-7 mg/hour	CNS depression Hypotension Respiratory depression Paradoxical agitation	Titrate infusion slowly in increments. Monitor blood pressure and respiratory status. Administer fluids as indicated. Slowly wean drug after prolonged therapy.
Diazepam (Valium)	Benzodiazepine; anxiety/sedation	PO: 2-10 mg bid-qid IM/IV: 2-20 mg, depending on assessment; may repeat in 1 hr *Elderly* 2-2.5 mg 1-2 times/day; increase gradually PRN	Hypotension Respiratory depression Paradoxical agitation	Monitor blood pressure and respiratory status. Inject slowly over 1 min (5 mg/mL). Unstable in plastic (PVC) infusion bags; possibility of precipitation.
Lorazepam (Ativan)	Benzodiazepine; anxiety/sedation	PO: 2-6 mg/day given bid-tid IV 2 mg initially; may repeat 1-2 mg in 10 min Mild anxiety: 0.5-1 mg Moderate-severe anxiety: 2-4 mg *Elderly* 1-2 mg/day, PRN	Hypotension (less than midazolam) Respiratory depression Paradoxical agitation Hyperosmolar metabolic acidosis (IV prolonged infusion)	Monitor blood pressure and respiratory status. Assess acid-base status with prolonged infusion.
Propofol (Diprivan)	Nonbenzodiazepine; sedative/anesthetic	Initial infusion: 5 mcg/kg/min for 5 min; increase dose in 5-10 mcg/kg/min increments over 5- to 10-min until sedation target achieved Maintenance: infusion rate of 5-50 mcg/kg/min (or higher)	Hypotension Fever, sepsis Hyperlipidemia Respiratory depression CNS depression	Patient should be intubated and mechanically ventilated. Monitor blood pressure and hemodynamic status. Change infusion set every 12 hours. Monitor plasma lipid levels.

Continued

*All dosages are for adult patients; this table does not account for typical dose adjustments used with the geriatric population.
bid, Two times per day; *CNS*, central nervous system; *g*, gram; *IM*, intramuscular; *IV*, intravenous; *PO*, by mouth; *PR*, per rectum; *PRN*, as needed; *qid*, four times per day; *SC*, subcutaneous; *tid*, three times per day; *TD*, transdermal.
Data from Reilly, C., et al. (2007). *Drugs facts and comparison* (61st ed.). Philadelphia: Lippincott Williams Wilkins. McKenry, L., Tessier, E., & Hogan, M. (2006). *Mosby's pharmacology in nursing*. St. Louis: Mosby; Lehne, R. (2007). *Pharmacology for nursing* (6th ed.). Philadelphia: Saunders.

PHARMACOLOGY

TABLE 5-11   Drugs Frequently Used in the Treatment of Anxiety, Pain, or for Neuromuscular Blockade—cont'd

Drug	Action/Uses	Dosage/Route	Side Effects	Nursing Implications
Dexmedetomidine (Precedex)	Selective alpha$_2$-adrenoreceptor agonist; anesthetic; sedative	IV: loading dose: 1 mcg/kg over 10 min (must dilute) Infusion: 0.2-0.7 mcg/kg/hr	Hypotension Nausea Bradycardia	Give only by continuous infusion, not to exceed 24 hours. Evaluate hepatic and renal function.
Management of Pain				
Fentanyl (Sublimaze [IV]/ Duragesic [patch])	Opioid; treat pain	Infusion: 1-3 mcg/kg/hr TD: 25 mcg/hr, titrate as needed	Hypotension Muscle rigidity Decreased gastric motility Respiratory depression Bradycardia Itching	Titrate infusion slowly in increments. Monitor blood pressure, heart rate, and respiratory status. Administer fluids as indicated. Give as an infusion for extended therapy. Patch: avoid direct heat (e.g., heating blanket), which accelerates fentanyl release. Change patch every 72 hours.
Hydromorphone (Dilaudid)	Opioid; treat pain	PO: 2-4 mg every 4 to 6 hours SC/IM: 1-2 mg every 4 to 6 hours PRN IV: 1-2 mg every 4 to 6 hours slowly over 2-3 min	Hypotension Decreased gastric motility Respiratory depression	Titrate infusion slowly in increments. Monitor blood pressure, heart rate, and respiratory status. Administer fluids as indicated.
Morphine (Duramorph/MS Contin/Roxanol)	Opioid; treat pain	SC/IM: 5-10 mg every 4 hours PRN PO: 5-30 mg every 4 hours PRN Extended release: 15-60 mg every 8 to 12 hours IV: 4-10 mg every 2 to 4 hours PRN Epidural: 5 mg	Hypotension Decreased gastric motility Urinary retention Respiratory depression Nausea and vomiting Itching or rash	Titrate infusion slowly in increments. Monitor blood pressure, heart rate, and respiratory status. Administer fluids as indicated.
Aspirin (Ecotrin/Bayer)	Nonsteroidal antiinflammatory drug (NSAID)	PO/PR: 325-650 mg every 4 hours PRN, not to exceed 4 g/day (analgesic)	Bleeding Gastrointestinal ulcers Tinnitus Thrombocytopenia	Administer with food if taking PO. Do not exceed recommended doses. Monitor complete blood count and renal function.

Drug	Classification/Use	Dosage	Adverse Effects	Nursing Considerations
Ketorolac (Toradol)	Nonsteroidal antiinflammatory drug (NSAID)	IV/IM: 30 mg every 6 hours (max 120 mg); duration should not exceed 5 days	Headache Dyspepsia Nausea Acute renal failure	Monitor complete blood count. Monitor renal and liver function.
Acetaminophen (Tylenol)	Nonnarcotic analgesic	PO/PR: 325-1000 mg every 4 to 6 hours PRN, not to exceed 4 g/day	Renal failure with chronic overdosage Blood dyscrasias Hepatic toxicity	Monitor renal and liver function. Assess other drugs for acetaminophen content (e.g., Percocet).
Delirium				
Haloperidol (Haldol)	Neuroleptic; used to treat delirium and alcohol withdrawal	PO: 0.5-5 mg bid or tid; maximum 30 mg/day IM: 2-5 mg every 1 to 8 hours PRN IV: 2-5 mg every to 8 hours Mild agitation: 0.5-2 mg Moderate agitation: 5 mg Severe agitation: 10 mg; may require dosing every 30 min (maximum single dose, 40 mg)	Drowsiness Prolonged QT interval Extrapyramidal symptoms Euphoria/agitation Paradoxical agitation Neuroleptic malignant syndrome Tachycardia	Measure QT interval at start of therapy and periodically. Monitor blood pressure with initial treatment or change in the dose. Use with caution when patient is receiving other proarrhythmic agents. Administer anticholinergic for extrapyramidal symptoms.
Therapeutic Paralysis				
Atracurium (Tracrium)	Neuromuscular blockade	IV: loading dose: 0.4-0.5 mg/kg Maintenance infusion: 5-10 mcg/kg/min to a maximum of 17.5 mcg/kg/min	Hypotension Tachycardia Rash	Ensure adequate airway. Safer than other paralytic agents in patients with hepatic or renal failure.
Succinylcholine	Neuromuscular blockade; short-term use	IV: loading dose: 1-1.5 mg/kg; maximum 2 mg/kg	Hyperkalemia	Secure airway. Avoid in patients with elevated serum potassium.

some critical care units, it may be possible to move the patient's bed so it faces a window. Some patients may benefit from being moved to a different room. Physically moving the patient to a different location prevents the patient from becoming tired of the surroundings, and it may provide some sense of clinical improvement for the patient and family. There are also critical care units in which the monitoring equipment are concealed behind cabinetry to provide a homelike atmosphere.

Family involvement is one of the most important strategies to decrease the patient's anxiety or pain. The patient's family is often able to interpret patient behaviors to the nursing staff, especially those associated with pain or anxiety. Families should be asked to participate in the care whenever the patient's condition allows it. Examples of family participation include coaching during breathing exercises, assisting with passive range of motion, and providing hygiene measures.

Guided Imagery

Guided imagery is a mind-body intervention intended to relieve stress and to promote a sense of peace and tranquility.[96] It involves a form of directed daydreaming. It is a way of purposefully diverting and focusing thoughts. Guided imagery is a very powerful technique in controlling pain and anxiety. Critically ill patients may be instructed in the use of guided imagery during painful procedures or weaning from mechanical ventilation. For example, when performing a needlestick puncture, the nurse may tell patients to think about their children or imagine walking on a beach.

In a randomized study, relaxation and guided imagery were used to reduce anxiety and depression in gynecological and breast cancer patients undergoing brachytherapy. The experiment group showed statistically significant reductions in anxiety, depression, and body discomfort compared with the control group.[55] Guided imagery with gentle touch or light massage has also been shown to decrease pain and tension in preoperative and postoperative cardiac surgery patients.[49] Benefits of the guided imagery program included reduced stress and anxiety, decreased pain and narcotic consumption, decreased surgical side effects, decreased length of stay, reduced hospital costs, enhanced patient's sleep, and increased patient satisfaction.[8,96] Guided imagery is a very simple and inexpensive strategy that all nurses can easily incorporate into their daily practice during most procedures and interventions.

Music Therapy

Similar to guided imagery, a music therapy program offers patients a diversionary technique for pain and anxiety relief. Some medical institutions have staff members dedicated solely to music therapy. When appropriate, a music therapist comes to the patient's bedside in the critical care unit and offers one-on-one therapy.[87]

Music therapy may be effective in reducing pain and anxiety if patients are able to participate. Patients who are heavily sedated, chemically paralyzed, or physically restrained may not benefit from this type of therapy. Music therapy is an ideal intervention for patients with low energy states who fatigue easily, such as those who require ventilatory support, because it does not require the focused concentration necessary for guided imagery.

Musical selections without lyrics that contain slow, flowing rhythms that duplicate pulses of 60 to 80 beats per minute decrease anxiety in the listener.[13] Music can also provide an alternative focus on a pleasant, comforting stimulus, rather than on stressful environmental stimuli or thoughts. Music therapy can reduce anxiety, and some studies show, duration of intubation.[53,97] Careful scrutiny of musical selections and of personal preferences of what is considered relaxing is important for success.

Pharmacological Management

Even with the most aggressive nonpharmacological therapies, many critically ill patients require medications to relieve pain, anxiety, or both. The appropriate management of pain may result in improved pulmonary function, earlier ambulation and mobilization, decreased stress response with lower catecholamine concentrations, and lower oxygen consumption, leading to improved postoperative outcomes.[10,16,93] Table 5-11 summarizes pharmacological therapies used in managing pain and anxiety.

Opioids

Medications for managing pain include opioids and nonsteroidal antiinflammatory drugs (NSAIDs) (see Clinical Alert). The most commonly used opioids in the critically ill are fentanyl, morphine, and hydromorphone. The selection of an opioid is based on its pharmacology and potential for adverse effects. The benefits of opioids include rapid onset, ease of titration, lack of accumulation, and low cost. Fentanyl has the fastest onset and the shortest duration, but repeated dosing may cause accumulation and prolonged effects. Morphine has a longer duration of action, and intermittent dosing may be given. However, hypotension may result from vasodilation, and its active metabolite may cause prolonged sedation in patients with renal insufficiency. Hydromorphone is similar to morphine in its duration of action.

There is a rapidly growing demand for safe and
effective pain management. Management of mild
to moderate pain has traditionally been based upon
the use of NSAIDs (aspirin, ibuprofen) and acetaminophen (Tylenol). Both the NSAIDs and acetaminophen are effective for mild to moderate pain
and are widely administered. However, NSAIDs
may not be tolerated because of gastrointestinal
symptoms and can cause potentially fatal peptic
ulceration and bleeding. Selective COX-2 inhibitors
(Celebrex) were developed to reduce the gastrointestinal side effects and complications. They are
used mostly in people with arthritis and various
pain conditions. COX-2 inhibitors have caused cardiovascular events. The Food and Drug Administration issued advice to apply cautions and restrictions
when prescribing COX-2 inhibitors, particularly for
patients at increased cardiovascular risk and for
long-term use. They have recommended using the
lowest effective dose for the shortest duration.

Reference Article: Langford, R. M. (2006). Pain management today: What have we learned? *Clinical Rheumatology,
25*(Suppl. 1), S2-S8.

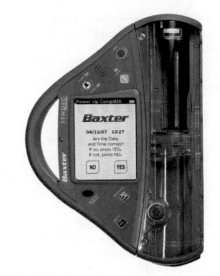

FIGURE 5-7. A patient-controlled analgesia infusion
pump. *(Courtesy of Baxter Healthcare, Deerfield, IL.)*

Adverse effects of opioids are common in critically
ill patients. Respiratory depression is a concern in
nonintubated patients. Hypotension may occur in
hemodynamically unstable patients or in hypovolemic patients. A depressed level of consciousness and
hallucinations leading to increased agitation may be
seen in some patients. Gastric retention and ileus
may occur as well.

Renal or hepatic insufficiency may alter opioid
and metabolite elimination. Titration to the desired
response and assessment of prolonged effects are
necessary. Elderly patients may have reduced opioid
requirements. Administration of a reversal agent
such as naloxone is not recommended after prolonged analgesia. It can induce withdrawal and may
cause nausea, cardiac stress, and dysrhythmias.[40]

Fentanyl may also be administered by a transdermal patch in hemodynamically stable patients with
chronic pain. The patch provides consistent drug
delivery, but the extent of absorption varies depending on permeability, temperature, perfusion, and
thickness of the skin. Fentanyl patches are not recommended for acute analgesia because it takes 12 to
24 hours to achieve peak effect and, once the patch
is removed, another 12 to 24 hours until the medication is no longer present in the body.

Preventing pain is more effective than treating
established pain. When patients are administered
opioids on an "as needed" basis, they may receive
less than the prescribed dose, and there may be
delays in treatment. Analgesics should be administered on a continuous or scheduled intermittent
basis, with supplemental bolus doses as required.[40]
Intravenous administration usually requires lower
and more frequent doses than intramuscular administration to achieve patient comfort. Intramuscular
administration is not recommended in hemodynamically unstable patients because of altered perfusion
and variable absorption.[40] A pain management plan
should be established for each patient and reevalu-
ated as the patient's clinical condition changes.

Patient-Controlled Analgesia

Patient-controlled analgesia (PCA) is a medication
delivery system in which the patient is able to control
when medication is given. PCA involves a special
type of infusion pump (Figure 5-7) that has a "locked"
supply of opioid medication. When the patient feels
pain or just before any pain-inducing therapy, the
patient can depress a button on the pump that will
deliver a prescribed bolus amount of medication.
Opioids delivered by PCA pump result in stable drug
concentrations, good quality of analgesia, less sedation, less opioid consumption, and potentially fewer
side effects. PCA has been proven to be a safe and
effective method of pain management.[76]

PCA management is rarely appropriate for critically ill patients because most patients are unable to
depress the button, or they are too ill to manage their

BOX 5-4   Typical Patient Criteria for Patient-Controlled Analgesia Therapy

- An elective surgical procedure
- Large surgical wounds likely to result in pain (e.g., thoracotomy incisions)
- Large traumatic wounds
- Normal cognitive function
- Normal motor skills (able to depress the medication delivery button)

BOX 5-5   Potential Benefits of Epidural Analgesia

System	Response
Pulmonary	↑ Vital capacity
	↑ Functional residual capacity
	Improved airway resistance
Cardiac	Coronary artery vasodilation
	↓ Blood pressure, heart rate
Gastrointestinal	Less nausea and vomiting
	Faster return of gastrointestinal function
Neurological	↓ Total opioid requirement
	↓ Sedation
Activity	Earlier extubation
	Earlier mobilization
	Decreased length of stay

↑, Increased; ↓, decreased
Modified from Alpen, M. A., & Morse, C. (2001). Managing the pain of traumatic injury. *Critical Care Nursing Clinics of North America, 13*(2), 243-257.

pain effectively.[76] However, some patients in the surgical critical care unit after an elective operation may benefit from PCA therapy to manage postoperative incisional pain. Typical patient criteria for PCA therapy are listed in Box 5-4.

Epidural Analgesia

Opioids or local anesthetics can also be delivered through an epidural or intrathecal (subarachnoid space) catheter. The discovery of opioid receptors in the spinal cord is considered a major breakthrough in the management of pain associated with traumatic injury of the chest and abdomen. Patients with such injuries do not want to cough, breathe deeply, ambulate, or participate in pulmonary exercises because these activities are too painful. Eventually, atelectasis, hypoxemia, respiratory failure, and pneumonia result.

The administration of epidural agents has been demonstrated to decrease postoperative analgesic requirements, decrease pain, enable patients to get more rest, allow patients to move within 24 hours after surgery, improve pulmonary function, decrease the number of days patients require mechanical ventilation, and decrease critical care and hospital stays.[1,5,46] Box 5-5 describes further potential benefits of epidural analgesia. A recent advancement in epidural analgesia is the combination of magnesium sulfate ($MgSO_4$) with epidural or intrathecal analgesia.[5] $MgSO_4$ blocks the *N*-methyl-D-aspartate (NMDA) receptor in the spinal cord, which decreases the induction and maintenance of central sensitization, thereby decreasing pain.

Patients receiving epidural analgesia are carefully assessed to determine the appropriateness of spinal analgesia. Contraindications include coagulopathies, cardiovascular instability, sepsis, spine injury, infection or injury to the skin at the proposed insertion site, patient refusal, inability to lie still during catheter insertion, and alcohol or drug intoxication.[1] In addition, it is difficult to place an epidural catheter in obese patients or patients with compression fractures

of the lumbar spine. Because of issues associated with spinal analgesia, research is being conducted to assess outcomes of caudal epidural analgesia as an alternative to spinal epidural analgesia.[46]

Potential side effects of spinal analgesia with opioids include respiratory depression, sedation, nausea and vomiting, and urinary retention. Potential side effects of spinal analgesia with local anesthetics include sympathetic blockade (hypotension, venous pooling), motor weakness, sensory block, and urinary retention.

Nonsteroidal Antiinflammatory Drugs

NSAIDs provide analgesia by inhibiting cyclooxygenase, a critical enzyme in the inflammatory cascade. NSAIDs have the potential to cause significant adverse effects including gastrointestinal bleeding, bleeding secondary to platelet inhibition, and renal insufficiency. The risk of developing NSAID-induced renal insufficiency is higher in patients with hypovolemia or renal hypoperfusion, in the elderly, and in patients with preexisting renal impairment. NSAIDs should not be administered to patients with asthma and aspirin sensitivity.

Administration of NSAIDs may reduce opioid requirements, although the analgesic benefits of NSAIDs have not been studied in critically ill patients. Oral agents are available, and ibuprofen and naproxen are available in liquid form. Ketorolac is the only NSAID available in intravenous form.

Acetaminophen is used to treat mild to moderate pain, such as pain associated with prolonged bed rest, or as an antipyretic. In combination with an opioid, acetaminophen has a greater analgesic effect than higher doses of an opioid alone. Acetaminophen is administered cautiously in patients with renal or hepatic dysfunction.

Sedative Agents

Anxiety in the critical care setting is typically treated with benzodiazepines, propofol, or dexmedetomidine. Both pain and anxiety may exist with evidence of psychotic features (as manifested in delirium). In this situation, neuroleptic agents, antidepressants, and anesthetic agents are administered.

Benzodiazepines are sedatives and hypnotics that block new information and potentially unpleasant experiences at that moment. Although they are not considered an analgesic, they do moderate the anticipatory pain response. Benzodiazepines vary in their potency, onset and duration of action, distribution, and metabolism. The patient's age, prior alcohol abuse, concurrent drug therapy, and current medical condition affect the intensity and duration of drug activity. Elderly patients and patients with renal or hepatic insufficiency exhibit slower clearance of benzodiazepines, a feature contributing to a significant delay in elimination.

Benzodiazepines should be titrated to a predefined end point, for example, a specific level of sedation using a standard sedation scale. Hemodynamically unstable patients may become hypotensive with the initiation of sedation. Sedation may be maintained with intermittent doses of lorazepam, diazepam, or midazolam; however, patients requiring frequent doses to maintain the desired effect may benefit from a continuous infusion by using the lowest effective dose. Patients receiving continuous infusions must be monitored for the effects of oversedation.

Propofol is an intravenous general anesthetic; however, sedative and hypnotic effects are achieved at lower doses. Propofol has no analgesic properties. It has a rapid onset and short duration of sedation once it is discontinued. Adverse effects include hypotension, bradycardia, and pain when the drug is infused through a peripheral intravenous site. Propofol is available as an emulsion in a phospholipid substance, which provides 1.1 kcal/mL from fat, and it should be counted as a caloric source.[40] Long-term or high-dose infusions may result in high triglyceride levels, metabolic acidosis, or dysrhythmias. Propofol requires a dedicated intravenous catheter for continuous infusion because of the risk of incompatibility and infection. The infusion should not hang for more than 12 hours.

Dexmedetomidine is an anesthetic agent with selective alpha-2 agonist properties that is approved for short-term use as a sedative (less than 24 hours) in patients receiving mechanical ventilation. It reduces concurrent analgesic and sedative requirements and produces anxiolytic effects comparable to those of the benzodiazepines. Transient elevations in blood pressure may be seen with rapid administration. Bradycardia and hypotension may develop, especially in the presence of hypovolemia, in patients with severe ventricular dysfunction and in the elderly. The role of this medication in the sedation of critically ill patients is being determined.

Multidisciplinary development and implementation of sedation guidelines have been shown to reduce the cost of sedation medication, the number of hours patients require mechanical ventilation, and the length of time patients spend in the critical care unit.[40] The use of an algorithm assists in this process (Figure 5-8).

Tolerance and Withdrawal

Patients who require more than 1 week of high-dose opioid or sedative therapy may develop physiological dependence. Stopping these medications abruptly could lead to withdrawal symptoms. Opioid withdrawal symptoms include pupillary dilation, sweating, rhinorrhea, tachycardia, hypertension, tachypnea, vomiting, diarrhea, increased sensitivity to pain, restlessness, and anxiety. Signs of benzodiazepine withdrawal include tremor, headache, nausea, sweating, fatigue, anxiety, agitation, increased sensitivity to light and sound, muscle cramps, sleep disturbances, and seizures. Doses should be tapered slowly and systematically.

MANAGEMENT CHALLENGES

Invasive Procedures

Many invasive procedures, including nasogastric tube insertion, tracheal suctioning, central venous catheter insertion, chest tube insertion, wound care; and removal of tubes, lines, and sheaths, take place in the critical care unit. All these invasive procedures have the likelihood of inducing pain or anxiety.[81] If pain or anxiety occurs during a procedure, the length and difficulty of the procedure may be increased, inaccurate data may be obtained, and physical harm can result.[71] To avoid negative outcomes, the patient's comfort and anxiety must be appropriately assessed and managed. Many times, the patient is kept in a conscious state during the procedure to avoid the risk of complications such as respiratory depression and hypotension. Therefore, sedative or analgesic agents, or both, are given in a way that the patient appears sedate yet is able to verbalize. This type of

THE CLEVELAND CLINIC FOUNDATION CICU SEDATION GUIDELINES

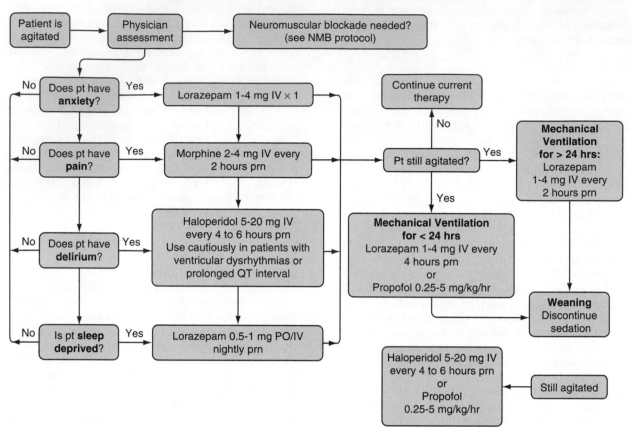

FIGURE 5-8. Sample algorithm of sedation guidelines. *(Courtesy of The Cleveland Clinic Foundation, Cleveland, OH.)*

sedation has been referred to as procedural sedation or conscious sedation.

Typical nursing care during these procedures involves monitoring vital signs including pulse oximetry, ensuring a patent airway, and observing for the adverse effects of medications. Many institutions use specialized flowsheets or forms in which assessment findings are documented during invasive procedures (Figure 5-9). Pain or sedation scales are often included as part of an ongoing assessment so the patient's level of pain or anxiety can be quantified at regular intervals.

Substance Abuse

Critically ill patients who have a history of substance abuse pose special challenges. Several studies have shown that alcoholism increases hospital length of stay because of an increased number of complications. These complications include higher infection rates, sepsis, increased use of restraints, increased

incidence of acute respiratory distress syndrome, and acute delirium.[72,73,75,98]

The pharmacological management of patients in the critical care unit typically involves the administration of sedative and hypnotic medications. Patients with a history of substance abuse may have a higher-than-normal dosage threshold to achieve therapeutic actions with many of these pharmacological agents. If alcoholism or drug abuse is suspected, it may be beneficial to start with higher-than-normal doses of sedative and analgesic medications. Based on the patient's response, it may be necessary to exceed the recommended maximum dosage of a medication.

Alcoholism continues to be an underrecognized problem in many medical centers. Chronic alcoholism that is not recognized, and therefore not treated on hospital admission, predisposes the patient to alcohol withdrawal syndrome. Symptoms of alcohol withdrawal syndrome usually present within 72 to 96 hours after the patient's last alcohol intake. The symptoms may begin as delirium tremens

Nursing Assessment:

NPO since: _____

I.D. Band check (if applicable): _____

Dentures ☐ yes ☐ no ☐ N/A

Glasses ☐ yes ☐ no ☐ N/A

Other: _____

Patient Education re: procedure ☐ yes ☐ no ☐ N/A

Nursing Plan of Care initiated: ☐ yes ☐ no ☐ N/A

Patient Assessment Score	pre	post
Moves 4 extremities voluntarily on command	2	2
Moves 2 extremities voluntarily on command	1	1
Moves 0 extremities voluntarily on command	0	0
Able to breathe deeply & cough freely	2	2
Dyspnea or limited breathing	1	1
Apneic	0	0
Fully awake	2	2
Arousable on calling	1	1
Not responding	0	0
Able to maintain O_2 saturation > 90% on RA	2	2
Needs O_2 to maintain O_2 sat > 90%	1	1
O_2 sat < 90% with O_2	0	0
Able to stand up and walk upright	2	2
Vertigo when erect	1	1
Dizziness when supine	0	0
Non-ambulatory	0	0
TOTAL		

PRE-PROCEDURAL VASCULAR ASSESSMENT ☐ No deferred/ not indicated

PALPABLE: 4+= BOUNDING 3+= normal 2+= decreased 1+= weak 0= absent

Pulses: Pre	F	P	DP	PT	OTHER
RL					
LL					

Prep: _____

Transportation home verified? ☐ yes ☐ no ☐ N/A

IV site: _____

_____Initials _____

INTAKE				
TIME	SOLUTION - ml's/hr		ABSORBED	CREDIT

OUTPUT				
TIME	URINE	EBL		

Procedure Start Time: _____

Procedure Finish Time: _____

Total fluoroscopy time: _____

Dressing: _____

Bovie pad site: _____

Condition of skin upon removal of Bovie: _____

Pre-Procedure Vital Signs: Time: _____ BP: _____ P. _____ R: _____ T. _____ O_2 Sat: _____

TIME	BP	P	R	O_2 SAT	LOC*	MEDS / O_2	NOTES/PAIN ASSESSMENT	INITIALS

*Modified Ramsay Score LOC 1=Anxious 2=Awake, tranquil 3=Drowsy, responds easily to verbal commands 4=Asleep, brisk response to tactile or loud auditory stimulus 5=Asleep, minimal response to tactile or loud auditory stimulus 6=Asleep, no response
Patients should not remain below level 4 for longer than 15 minutes in conscious sedation. Patients with a Ramsay score of 5 or 6 are in deep sedation.

FIGURE 5-9. The Cleveland Clinic Foundation Procedural Sedation Record: Nursing Assessment Page. *(Courtesy of The Cleveland Clinic Foundation, Cleveland, OH.)*

(shaking of the extremities or digits) and can progress to paranoid-like behavior, seizures, convulsions, and even death. Folic acid and thiamine are frequently given to patients with a history of alcoholism to prevent Wernicke's encephalopathy. Research shows that surgical patients who received symptom-oriented bolus titration of intravenous flunitrazepam (agitation), intravenous clonidine (sympathetic hyperactivity), or intravenous haloperidol (productive psychotic symptoms) required fewer days of mechanical ventilation, had a lower incidence of pneumonia, and had shorter ICU stays.[92]

Restraining Devices

Restraining or immobilizing devices are commonly used in the critical care setting to ensure that the patient is unable to disrupt invasive lines or pull at lifesaving devices. The purpose of restraints is to promote patient safety; however, restraints can be dangerous if the patient is not oriented.[23] Use of physical restraint without sedation has been associated with PTSD after critical care unit discharge.[42] The goal of applying restraints is to use the least restrictive device so the patient still has some movement. Commonly used restraining devices are listed in Table 5-12.

A common adverse event associated with restraints involves complications associated with immobility. Patients with restraining devices must be repositioned, and the areas where the restraints are applied are assessed for perfusion and sensation at least every hour. This assessment is documented on the critical care flowsheet.

Effects of Aging

As the population ages, the number of elderly patients admitted to a critical care unit continues to increase. Elderly patients have a high prevalence of pain, and

GERIATRIC CONSIDERATIONS

Strategies for Managing Pain and Anxiety
- Speak slowly and clearly.
- Verify any underlying cognitive deficits (e.g., dementia, Alzheimer disease, cerebrovascular accident).
- Ensure that scales or other assessment tools have a large font/text.
- Stoic behavior may be the patient's normal baseline; therefore, assess for nonverbal cues to pain (facial grimace or withdrawal).
- Observe for changes in behavior, such as confusion or agitation. Elderly patients are at risk of developing delirium.
- Elderly patients may be resistant to taking additional medications; therefore, offer nonpharmacological strategies to manage anxiety or pain.
- Elderly patients may not ask for as-needed medications in a timely fashion. Pain medications should be routinely scheduled.
- Medication dosages may be reduced because of decreased renal and liver clearance.
- Certain medications may have paradoxical effects in the elderly (e.g., benzodiazepines causing agitation).

TABLE 5-12 Common Restraining Devices

Restraint Type	Description
Soft wrist restraints	Constructed from padded foam with Velcro or tie straps. Typically applied around the wrist and tied to the bed frame. Prevents the patient from pulling at items on the upper torso or near the face.
Soft mitts	Constructed from a padded foam material with mesh. Slipped over the hand so the palm rests on a pillow foam. Allows the patient full range of motion with the upper extremities but does not allow a grasping motion with the fingers. Ideal for patients who are "picking" at items such as dressings, intravenous infusion sites, or feeding tubes.
Elbow immobilizer	Large plastic sheath that is soft but does not have any flexion. Slipped over the forearm and placed over the elbow joint. Allows full range of motion at the shoulder and wrist but does not allow the elbow to bend. The patient cannot bring the forearm towards the head. Works well for patients who are attempting to remove an endotracheal tube.
Posey vest	Made from a Teflon-mesh material with straps that can be tied. Typically worn around the upper torso and can be tied to a bed frame or a chair. Keeps the patient bound to the bed or chair. Full range of motion in the lower extremities is possible. Ideal for patients who are sitting in chairs. Prevents the patient from standing unassisted.

they might experience a multitude of painful conditions (neoplasms, injuries and other external causes, and diseases of the musculoskeletal and connective tissues systems). Patients who are older than 65 years pose special concerns because of their physiology, many comorbidities, the multiple medications, physical frailty, and cognitive/sensory deficits. Elderly patients are also more vulnerable to alcohol abuse, substance abuse, and may be more vulnerable to toxicity from analgesics. Elderly patients often have decreased renal function with a reduced creatinine clearance rate, resulting in a longer elimination half-life of analgesic drugs.

Older patients generally receive less analgesia or sedation compared with younger adults, perhaps because of elderly patients' beliefs about their pain and anxiety. Some elderly patients believe that pain is a normal process of aging and is something that they must learn to accept as normal. Elderly patients often believe that complaining of pain to nursing staff will label them as "problem" patients. Finally, elderly patients may comment to their family and friends that the nurse is too busy to listen to their complaints, and they do not want to be a "bother." Refer to Geriatric Considerations for strategies for managing pain and anxiety in the elderly patient.

CASE STUDY

evolve

MB is a 52-year-old man in the surgical intensive care unit after liver transplantation the previous day. He has a 15-year history of hepatic cirrhosis secondary to alcohol abuse. He is intubated and is receiving multiple vasopressor medications for hypotension. At 6:30 AM, he follows simple commands and denies pain or anxiety with simple head nods. At 7:00 AM, MB is kicking his legs and places his arms outside the side rails. Attempts by the nurse to reorient him result in his pulling at his endotracheal tube. His wrists are restrained with soft restraints. At this time, he does not follow any simple commands. He continually shakes his head back and forth. Facial grimacing is noted, and he is biting down on the endotracheal tube, which is causing the ventilator to sound the high-pressure alarm. His blood pressure is now 185/110 mm Hg, with a mean arterial pressure of 135 mm Hg. The monitor displays sinus tachycardia at a rate of 140 beats per minute. Medication infusions include epinephrine (3 mcg/min), norepinephrine (15 mcg/min), dopamine (2 mcg/kg/min), and fentanyl (100 mcg/hr). His only other medications are his immunosuppressive drug regimen.

QUESTIONS

1. Score MB's pain and/or anxiety using the objective tools listed below:

Tool	Score
Behavioral Pain Scale (BPS):	_____
Critical-Care Pain Observation Tool (CPOT):	_____
Richmond Agitation Sedation Scale (RASS):	_____
Ramsay Sedation Scale (RSS):	_____
Sedation-Agitation Scale (SAS):	_____
The Confusion Assessment Method for the Intensive Care Unit (CAM-ICU)	_____

2. Would complementary or alternative medicine therapies be appropriate at this time? If not, what therapies would be appropriate?
3. What type of medication is MB receiving for pain?
4. Is this an appropriate dose of pain medication for MB?
5. What other medications could be given to manage his agitative state?

SUMMARY

Patients admitted to the critical care unit are at an increased risk of developing pain and anxiety. The critical care environment and medical interventions may be the greatest contributing factors in the development of pain and anxiety. The assessment of both is a challenge for the critical care nurse because patients may not be able to communicate. The use of assessment tools designed to recognize pain and anxiety is helpful. Nonpharmacological and pharmacological strategies to relieve pain and anxiety should be used so critical care patients have the best possible outcomes.

CRITICAL THINKING QUESTIONS

evolve

1. Describe factors that increase the risk for pain and anxiety in critically ill patients.
2. Differentiate between subjective and objective tools when assessing pain, and provide examples of each.
3. What is delirium? What are some of the behaviors seen in the hyperacute subtype?

evolve Be sure to check out the bonus material, including free self-assessment exercises, on the Evolve Web site at http://evolve.elsevier.com/Sole.

REFERENCES

1. Alpen, M. A., & Morse, C. (2001). Managing the pain of traumatic injury. *Critical Care Nursing Clinics of North America, 13*, 243-257.
2. Ambuel, B., Hamlett, K. W., Marx, C. M., & Blumer, J. L. (1992). Assessing distress in pediatric intensive care environments: The COMFORT scale. *Journal of Pediatric Psychology, 17*, 95-109.
3. Apkarian, A. V., Bushnell, M. C., Treede, R. D., & Zubieta, J. K. (2005). Human brain mechanisms of pain perception and regulation in health and disease. *European Journal of Pain, 9*, 63-84.
4. Arbour, R. (2000). Sedation and pain management in critically ill adults. *Critical Care Nurse, 20*, 39-56.
5. Arcioni, R., Palmisani, S., Tigano, S., Santorsola, C., Sauli, V., Romano, S., et al. (2007). Combined intrathecal and epidural magnesium sulfate supplementation of spinal anesthesia to reduce post-operative analgesic requirements: A prospective, randomized, double-blind, controlled trial in patients undergoing major orthopedic surgery. *Acta Anaesthesiologica Scandinavica, 51*(5), 482-489.
6. Aspect Medical Systems. (1999). *Overview: The effects of electromyography (EMG) and other high-frequency signals on the bispectral index (BIS)* [pamphlet]. Newton, MA: Aspect Medical Systems, Inc.
7. Balas, M. C., Deutschman, C. S., Sullivan-Marx, E. M., Strumpf, N. E., Alston, R. P., & Richmond, T. S. (2007). Delirium in older patients in surgical intensive care units. *Journal of Nursing Scholarship, 39*, 147-154.
8. Beyea, S. (2002). Guided imagery; intervention for smoking; pagers and bacteria; scissors; abdominal wound separation [compendium]. *AORN Journal, 76*, 520-522.
9. Birka, A. (1999). New perspectives on the use of propofol [commentary]. *Critical Care Nurse, 19*(4), 18-19.
10. Bonnet, F., & Marret, E. (2007). Postoperative pain management and outcome after surgery. *Best Practice & Research. Clinical Anaesthesiology, 21*, 99-107.
11. Breau, L. M., Camfield, C. S., McGrath, P. J., & Finley, G. A. (2004). Risk factors for pain in children with severe cognitive impairments. *Developmental Medicine and Child Neurology, 46*, 364-371.
12. Carroll, K. C., Atkins, P. J., Herold, G. R., Mlcek, C. A., Shively, M., Clopton, P., et al. (1999). Pain assessment and management in critically ill postoperative and trauma patients: A multisite study. *American Journal of Critical Care, 8*, 105-117.
13. Chlan, L. L. (2000). Music therapy as a nursing intervention for patients supported by mechanical ventilation. *AACN Clinical Issues, 11*, 128-138.
14. Chlan, L. L. (2004). Relationship between two anxiety instruments in patients receiving mechanical ventilatory support. *Journal of Advanced Nursing, 48*, 493-499.
15. Closs, S. J., Barr, B., & Briggs, M. (2004). Cognitive status and analgesic provision in nursing home residents. *British Journal of General Practice, 54*, 919-921.
16. Costa, M. G., Chiarandini, P., & Della, R. G. (2006). Sedation in the critically ill patient. *Transplantation Proceedings, 38*, 803-804.
17. Cullen, L., Greiner, J., & Titler, M. G. (2001). Pain management in the culture of critical care. *Critical Care Nursing Clinics of North America, 13*(2), 151-166.
18. De Jong, M. M., Burns, S. M., Campbell, M. L., Chulay, M., Grap, M. J., Pierce, L. N., et al. (2005). Development of the American Association of Critical-Care Nurses' sedation assessment scale for critically ill patients. *American Journal of Critical Care, 14*, 531-544.
19. DeLeo, J. A. (2006). Basic science of pain. *Journal of Bone and Joint Surgery American, 88*(Suppl. 2), 58-62.
20. Ely, E. W., Margolin, R., Francis, J., May, L., Truman, B., Dittus, R., et al. (2001). Evaluation of delirium in critically ill patients: Validation of the Confusion Assessment Method for the Intensive Care Unit (CAM-ICU). *Critical Care Medicine, 29*, 1370-1379.
21. Ely, E. W., Shintani, A., Truman, B., Speroff, T., Gordon, S. M., Harrell, F. E., Jr., et al. (2004). Delirium as a predictor of mortality in mechanically ventilated patients in the intensive care unit. *Journal of the American Medical Association, 291*, 1753-1762.
22. Ely, E. W., Truman, B., Shintani, A., Thomason, J. W., Wheeler, A. P., Gordon, S., et al. (2003). Monitoring sedation status over time in ICU patients: Reliability and validity of the Richmond Agitation-Sedation Scale (RASS). *Journal of the American Medical Association, 289*, 2983-2991.
23. Evans, D., Wood, J., & Lange, P. (2003). Patient injury and physical restraint devices: A systematic review. *Journal of Advanced Nursing, 413*, 282.
24. *Facts and Comparison. Drug Facts and Comparison* (61st ed.). (2007). Philadelphia: Lippincott Williams & Wilkins.
25. Feldt, K. S. (2000). The Checklist of Nonverbal Pain Indicators (CNPI). *Pain Management Nursing, 1*, 13-21.
26. Fraser, G. L., Prato, B. S., Riker, R. R., Berthiaume, D., & Wilkins, M. L. (2000). Frequency, severity, and treatment of agitation in young versus elderly patients in the ICU. *Pharmacotherapy, 20*, 75-82.
27. Fraser, G. L., & Riker, R. R. (2005). Bispectral index monitoring in the intensive care unit provides more signal than noise. *Pharmacotherapy, 25*, 19S-27S.
28. Galli, S. J., Nakae, S., & Tsai, M. (2005). Mast cells in the development of adaptive immune responses. *Nature Immunology, 6*, 135-142.
29. Gelinas, C., Fillion, L., Puntillo, K. A., Viens, C., & Fortier, M. (2006). Validation of the critical-care pain observation tool in adult patients. *American Journal of Critical Care, 15*, 420-427.
30. Gelinas, C., Fortier, M., Viens, C., Fillion, L., & Puntillo, K. (2004). Pain assessment and management in critically ill intubated patients: A retrospective study. *American Journal of Critical Care, 13*, 126-135.

31. Gelinas, C., & Johnston, C. (2007). Pain assessment in the critically ill ventilated adult: Validation of the critical-care pain observation tool and physiologic indicators. *Clinical Journal of Pain, 23,* 497-505.

32. Gordon, D. B., Dahl, J. L., Miaskowski, C., McCarberg, B., Todd, K. H., Paice, J. A., et al. (2005). American Pain Society recommendations for improving the quality of acute and cancer pain management: American Pain Society Quality of Care Task Force. *Archives of Internal Medicine, 165,* 1574-1580.

33. Granja, C., Lopes, A., Moreira, S., Dias, C., Costa-Pereira, A., & Carneiro, A. (2005). Patients' recollections of experiences in the intensive care unit may affect their quality of life. *Critical Care, 9,* R96-R109.

34. Granot, M., Khoury, R., Berger, G., Krivoy, N., Braun, E., Aronson, D., et al. (2007). Clinical and experimental pain perception is attenuated in patients with painless myocardial infarction. *Pain, 133*(1-3), 120-127.

35. Guyton, A. C., & Hall, J. (2006). *Textbook of medical physiology* (11th ed.). Philadelphia: Saunders.

36. Hamill-Ruth, R. J., & Marohn, M. L. (1999). Evaluation of pain in the critically ill patient. *Critical Care Clinics, 15,* 35-54.

37. Herr, K., Bjoro, K., & Decker, S. (2006). Tools for assessment of pain in nonverbal older adults with dementia: A state-of-the-science review. *Journal of Pain and Symptom Management, 31,* 170-192.

38. Herr, K., Coyne, P. J., Key, T., Manworren, R., McCaffery, M., Merkel, S., et al. (2006). Pain assessment in the nonverbal patient: Position statement with clinical practice recommendations. *Pain Management Nursing, 7,* 44-52.

39. Huether, S., & DeFriez, C. B. (2006). Pain, temperature regulation, sleep, and sensory function. In McCance, K.L., & Huether, S.E. (Eds.), *Pathophysiology: The biologic basis for disease in adults and children,* 5th edition (pp. 447-489). St. Louis: Mosby.

40. Jacobi, J., Fraser, G. L., Coursin, D. B., Riker, R. R., Fontaine, D., Wittbrodt, E. T., et al. (2002). Clinical practice guidlines for the sustained use of sedatives and analgesics in the critically ill adult. *Critical Care Medicine, 30,* 119-141.

41. Joint Commission. (2007). *2006 Top standards compliance issues.* Retrieved May 24, 2007, from www.jointcommissionreport.org/performanceresults/top-standards-compliance.aspx.

42. Jones, C., Backman, C., Capuzzo, M., Flaatten, H., Rylander, C., & Griffiths, R. D. (2007). Precipitants of post-traumatic stress disorder following intensive care: A hypothesis generating study of diversity in care. *Intensive Care Medicine, 33,* 978-985.

43. Jones, C., Griffiths, R. D., Humphris, G., & Skirrow, P. M. (2001). Memory, delusions, and the development of acute posttraumatic stress disorder-related symptoms after intensive care. *Critical Care Medicine, 29,* 573-580.

44. Justic, M. (2000). Does "ICU psychosis" really exist? *Critical Care Nurse, 20*(3), 28-39.

45. Katz, W. A., & Rothenberg, R. (2005). Section 3: The nature of pain: Pathophysiology. *Journal of Clinical Rheumatology, 11,* S11-S15.

46. Kita, T., Maki, N., Song, Y. S., Arai, F., & Nakai, T. (2007). Caudal epidural anesthesia administered intraoperatively provides for effective postoperative analgesia after total hip arthroplasty. *Journal of Clinical Anesthesia, 19,* 204-208.

47. Koh, J. L., Fanurik, D., Harrison, R. D., Schmitz, M. L., & Norvell, D. (2004). Analgesia following surgery in children with and without cognitive impairment. *Pain, 111,* 239-244.

48. Kruskamp, T. (2003). The changing face of sedation: Goal-directed care. *AACN News, 20*(11), 12-16.

49. Kshettry, V. R., Carole, L. F., Henly, S. J., Sendelbach, S., & Kummer, B. (2006). Complementary alternative medical therapies for heart surgery patients: Feasibility, safety, and impact. *Annals of Thoracic Surgery, 81,* 201-205.

50. Kupers, R., & Kehlet, H. (2006). Brain imaging of clinical pain states: A critical review and strategies for future studies. *Lancet Neurology, 5,* 1033-1044.

51. Kwekkeboom, K. L., & Herr, K. (2001). Assessment of pain in the critically ill. *Critical Care Nursing Clinics of North America, 13,* 181-194.

52. Langford, RM. Pain management today: What have we learned? *Clinical Rheumatology, 25*(Suppl. 1), S2-S8.

53. Lee, O. K., Chung, Y. F., Chan, M. F., & Chan, W. M. (2005). Music and its effect on the physiological responses and anxiety levels of patients receiving mechanical ventilation: A pilot study. *Journal of Clinical Nursing, 14,* 609-620.

54. Lehne, R. (2007). *Pharmacology for nursing* (6th ed.). Philadelphia: Saunders.

55. Leon-Pizarro, C., Gich, I., Barthe, E., Rovirosa, A., Farrus, B., Casas, F., et al. (2007). A randomized trial of the effect of training in relaxation and guided imagery techniques in improving psychological and quality-of-life indices for gynecologic and breast brachytherapy patients. *Psychooncology, 16*(11), 971-979.

56. Lighthall, G. K., & Pearl, R. G. (2003). Volume resuscitation in the critically ill: Choosing the best solution—How do crystalloid solutions compare with colloids? *Journal of Critical Illness, 18*(6), 252-260.

57. Luer, J. M. (2002). Sedation and neuromuscular blockade in patients with acute respiratory failure: Protocols for practice. *Critical Care Nurse, 22*(5), 70-75.

58. Malarkey, L. M., & McMorrow, M. E. (2000). *Nurse's manual of laboratory tests and diagnostic procedures* (2nd ed.). Philadelphia: Saunders.

59. McCaffery, M. (1979). *Nursing management of the patient with pain* (2nd ed.). Philadelphia: Lippincott.

60. McCartney, J., & Boland, R. (1994). Anxiety and delirium in the intensive care unit. *Critical Care Clinics, 10,* 673-680.

61. McGaffigan, P. (2002). Advancing sedation assessment to promote patient comfort. *Critical Care Nurse, 22,* (Suppl.): 29-36.

62. McHugh, J. M., & McHugh, W. B. (2000). Pain: Neuroanatomy, chemical mediators, and clinical implications. *AACN Clinical Issues, 11,* 168-178.

63. McKenry, L., Tessier, E., & Hogan, M. (2006). *Mosby's pharmacology in nursing*. St. Louis: Mosby.

64. Mechlin, M. B., Maixner, W., Light, K. C., Fisher, J. M., & Girdler, S. S. (2005). African Americans show alterations in endogenous pain regulatory mechanisms and reduced pain tolerance to experimental pain procedures. *Psychosomatic Medicine, 67*, 948-956.

65. Melloni, C., Devivo, P., Launo, C., Mastronardi, P., Novelli, G. P., Romano, E., et al. (2006). Cisatracurium versus vecuronium: A comparative, double blind, randomized, multicenter study in adult patients under propofol/fentanyl/N$_2$O anesthesia. *Minerva Anestesiologica, 72*, 299-308.

66. Merkel, S. I., Voepel-Lewis, T., Shayevitz, J. R., & Malviya, S. (1997). The FLACC: A behavioral scale for scoring postoperative pain in young children. *Pediatric Nursing, 23*(3), 293-297.

67. Merker, B. (2007). Consciousness without a cerebral cortex: A challenge for neuroscience and medicine. *Behavioral and Brain Sciences, 30*, 63-81.

68. Merskey, H., & Bogduk, N. (1994). *Classification of Chronic Pain: Descriptions of Chronic Pain Syndromes and Definitions of Pain Terms* (2nd ed., pp. 209-214). Seattle: IASP Press.

69. Miller, C., & Newton, S. E. (2006). Pain perception and expression: The influence of gender, personal self-efficacy, and lifespan socialization. *Pain Management Nursing, 7*, 148-152.

70. Moalem, G., & Tracey, D. J. (2006). Immune and inflammatory mechanisms in neuropathic pain. *Brain Research. Brain Research Reviews, 51*, 240-264.

71. Moline, L. R. (2006). Patient psychologic preparation for invasive procedures: An integrative review. *Journal of Vascular Nursing, 18*, 117-122.

72. Moss, M., & Burnham, E. L. (2006). Alcohol abuse in the critically ill patient. *Lancet, 368*, 2231-2242.

73. Moss, M., Parsons, P. E., Steinberg, K. P., Hudson L. D., Guidot D. M., Burnham E. L., Eaton S., & Cotsonis G. A. (2003). Chronic alcohol abuse is associated with an increased incidence of acute respiratory distress syndrome and severity of multiple organ dysfunction in patients with septic shock. *Critical Care Medicine, 31*, S207-S212.

74. Nygaard, H. A., & Jarland, M. (2006). The Checklist of Nonverbal Pain Indicators (CNPI): Testing of reliability and validity in Norwegian nursing homes. *Age and Ageing, 35*, 79-81.

75. O'Brien, J. M., Jr., Lu, B., Ali, N. A., Martin, G. S., Aberegg, S. K., Marsh, C. B., et al. (2007). Alcohol dependence is independently associated with sepsis, septic shock, and hospital mortality among adult intensive care unit patients. *Critical Care Medicine, 35*, 345-350.

76. Pasero, C., & McCaffery, M. (2001). Multimodal balanced analgesia in the critically ill. *Critical Care Nursing Clinics of North America, 13*, 195-206.

77. Payen, J. F., Bru, O., Bosson, J. L., Lagrasta, A., Novel, E., Deschaux, I., et al. (2001). Assessing pain in critically ill sedated patients by using a behavioral pain scale. *Critical Care Medicine, 29*(12), 2258-2263.

78. Payen, J. F., Chanques, G., Mantz, J., Hercule, C., Auriant, I., Leguillou, J. L., et al. (2007). Current practices in sedation and analgesia for mechanically ventilated critically ill patients: A prospective multicenter patient-based study. *Anesthesiology, 106*, 687-695.

79. Puntillo, K. (1997). Stitch, stitch . . . creating an effective pain management program for critically ill patients. *American Journal of Critical Care, 6*, 259-260.

80. Puntillo, K. A. (1990). Pain experiences of intensive care unit patients. *Heart and Lung, 19*, 526-533.

81. Puntillo, K. A., Morris, A. B., Thompson, C. L., Stanik-Hutt, J., White, C. A., & Wild, L. R. (2004). Pain behaviors observed during six common procedures: Results from Thunder Project II. *Critical Care Medicine, 32*, 421-427.

82. Puntillo, K. A., Wild, L. R., Morris, A. B., Stanik-Hutt, J., Thompson, C. L., & White, C. (2002). Practices and predictors of analgesic interventions for adults undergoing painful procedures. *American Journal of Critical Care, 11*, 415-429.

83. Rahim-Williams, F. B., Riley, J. L., III, Herrera, D., Campbell, C. M., Hastie, B. A., & Fillingim, R. B. (2007). Ethnic identity predicts experimental pain sensitivity in African Americans and Hispanics. *Pain, 129*, 177-184.

84. Ramsay, M. A., Savege, T. M., Simpson, B. R., & Goodwin, R. (1974). Controlled sedation with alphaxalone-alphadolone. *British Medical Journal, 2*(90), 656-659.

85. Riker, R. R., Fraser, G. L., Simmons, L. E., & Wilkins, M. L. (2001). Validating the Sedation-Agitation Scale with the bispectral index and Visual Analog Scale in adult ICU patients after cardiac surgery. *Intensive Care Medicine, 27*(5), 853-858.

86. Ringdal, M., Johansson, L., Lundberg, D., & Bergbom, I. (2006). Delusional memories from the intensive care unit: Experienced by patients with physical trauma. *Intensive and Critical Care Nursing, 22*, 346-354.

87. Robillard, D., Shim, S., Irwin, R., Katonah, J., Wren, R., Greig, J., et al. (2005). Support services perspective: The Critical Care Family Assistance Program. *Chest, 128*, 124S-127S.

88. Sessler, C. N., Gosnell, M. S., Grap, M. J., Brophy, G. M., O'Neal, P. V., Keane, K. A., et al. (2002). The Richmond Agitation-Sedation Scale: Validity and reliability in adult intensive care unit patients. *American Journal of Respiratory and Critical Care Medicine, 166*, 1338-1344.

89. Setty, A. R., & Sigal, L. H. (2005). Herbal medications commonly used in the practice of rheumatology: Mechanisms of action, efficacy, and side effects. *Seminars in Arthritis and Rheumatism, 34*, 773-784.

90. Shannon, K., & Bucknall, T. (2003). Pain assessment in critical care: What have we learnt from research. *Intensive and Critical Care Nursing, 19*, 154-162.

91. Siegel, M. D. (2003). Management of agitation in the intensive care unit. *Clinics in Chest Medicine, 24*, 713-725.

92. Spies, C. D., Otter, H. E., Huske, B., Sinha, P., Neumann, T., Rettig, J., et al. (2003). Alcohol withdrawal severity is decreased by symptom-orientated adjusted bolus therapy in the ICU. *Intensive Care Medicine, 29*, 2230-2238.

93. Szokol, J. W., & Vender, J. S. (2001). Anxiety, delirium, and pain in the intensive care unit. *Critical Care Clinics, 17*, 821-842.

94. Thomason, J. W., Shintani, A., Peterson, J. F., Pun, B. T., Jackson, J. C., & Ely, E. W. (2005). Intensive care unit delirium is an independent predictor of longer hospital stay: A prospective analysis of 261 non-ventilated patients. *Critical Care, 9*, R375-R381.

95. Truman, B., & Ely, E. W. (2003). Monitoring delirium in critically ill patients: Using the Confusion Assessment Method for the intensive care unit. *Critical Care Nurse, 23*(2), 25-36.

96. Tusek, D. L., & Cwynar, R. E. (2000). Strategies for implementing a guided imagery program to enhance patient experience. *AACN Clinical Issues, 11*(1), 68-76.

97. Twiss, E., Seaver, J., & McCaffrey, R. (2006). The effect of music listening on older adults undergoing cardiovascular surgery. *Nursing in Critical Care, 11*, 224-231.

98. Uusaro, A., Parviainen, I., Tenhunen, J. J., & Ruokonen, E. (2005). The proportion of intensive care unit admissions related to alcohol use: A prospective cohort study. *Acta Anaesthesioogical Scandinavica, 49*, 1236-1240.

CHAPTER 6

Nutritional Support

Melissa L. Hutchinson, MN, RN, CCRN, CWCN

INTRODUCTION

"Let food be thy medicine, and medicine be thy food." The father of medical science, Hippocrates, made this statement around the fifth century BC. Adequate nutrition remains an important part of comprehensive patient care management. More than 50% of hospitalized patients are undernourished on admission, and they often receive suboptimal nutrition throughout their hospitalization.[18] The components of nutrition—proteins, carbohydrates, and fats—are the body's building blocks for maintaining both mental and physical health. Without appropriate nutrition, individuals are at a higher risk for disease and are more prone to complications such as skin breakdown, drug intolerance, and infections while hospitalized.[16]

This chapter reviews the gastrointestinal (GI) system and the basic assessment of a patient's nutritional status. Nutrient additives and formulas, goals of therapy, practice guidelines for enteral and parenteral nutrition, drug-nutrient interactions, and complications related to nutritional therapy are also discussed.

GASTROINTESTINAL TRACT

A functioning GI tract, or gut, is essential to the health and well-being of a critically ill patient. The gut has protective mechanisms that include intestinal permeability and intestinal mucosal defense. Intestinal permeability is controlled by the gut's tight junctions, which prevent passage of molecules into or out of the GI tract. Failure of the junctions related to inflammation or lack of nutrition allows volatile bacteria to escape, which can result in systemic infection. The mucosal defense, regulated by the gut-associated lymphoid tissue, is designed to protect the GI tract from toxic invaders and inflammatory mediators, and prevents passage of these harmful particles into the systemic circulation. When the gut's defense mechanisms are suboptimal, the functional structures (the villi, which absorb and process nutrients) can atrophy. The villi are replenished every 3 to 4 days, and without adequate nutritional stimulation, the cells are not available for nutrition absorption. Dysfunction of the GI tract, or an extended period of hypoperfusion in critical illness, can impair a critically ill patient's recovery by disrupting the gut-associated lymphoid tissue and the tight junctions. Providing and maintaining adequate nutrition is advocated to protect the continuity and function of the GI tract.

UTILIZATION OF NUTRIENTS

The body uses nutrients in a variety of ways. Each cell requires carbohydrates, proteins, fats, water, electrolytes, vitamins, and trace elements to provide fuel for the energy necessary to maintain bodily functions. The proper combination of nutrients necessary to produce the energy requirements is called *metabolism*. When nutrients are ingested, they are broken down to form a food bolus through the mixture of enzymes (salivary amylase, which digests starch) secreted by the salivary glands to create saliva. Saliva is rich in mucus and helps to coat the food bolus. The bolus stimulates peristalsis, the contraction and relaxation of esophageal muscles, which continues until the bolus reaches the esophageal sphincter. Peristalsis causes the esophageal sphincter to relax so the bolus can pass into the stomach. The function of the stomach is to break down larger molecules into smaller ones and to store food before delivery. The stomach produces both acidic and basic secretions. Acidic secretions, produced at a rate of 2 to 3 liters per day, assist in the breakdown of proteins to facilitate digestion. Chyme, which is the mixture of the gastric secretions and the food bolus formed by the stomach for delivery into the small intestine, is very acidic with a pH of around 2. The gastric mucosal cells provide a protective coating to lubricate the stomach lining and shield it from erosion by the harsh acidic secretions. The stomach also secretes intrinsic factor, which is necessary for the absorption of vitamin B_{12} in the ileum. Vitamin B_{12} is critical for the formation of red blood cells. The stomach secretes fluid that is high in sodium, potassium, and other electrolytes. If excessive fluid is lost from the stomach, either from vomiting or from gastric suction, the patient is at risk for fluid and electrolyte imbalances.

The first part of the small intestine is the duodenum, the area where the pancreatic juices and the bile from the liver empty, and minerals such as chloride, sulfate, iron, calcium, and magnesium are absorbed. The duodenum contains mucus-secreting glands called Brunner's glands that produce an alkaline compound. The glands' secretions protect the duodenal wall from the acidic chyme and raise the pH of the chyme to around 7 before it reaches the ileum. The next segment is the jejunum; monosaccharides (sugars), glucose, galactose, and fructose are absorbed in the first part of the jejunum along with the water-soluble vitamins: thiamine, riboflavin, pyridoxine, folic acid, and vitamin C. At the end of the jejunum is the ileum. Protein is broken down into amino acids and absorbed in the first part of the ileum. The fat-soluble vitamins (A, D, E, and K), fat, cholesterol, bile salts, and vitamin B_{12} are absorbed at the end of the ileum. The ileocecal valve located at the end of the ileum helps to prevent reflux of colonic contents from the large intestine into the ileum.

The colon is next and is divided into the ascending, transverse, and descending colon and the rectum. Sodium and potassium are absorbed in the first part of the colon. Vitamin K is formed by bacterial action and is absorbed toward the distal portion of the colon. Water is reabsorbed at the end of the colon. The colon is also a major site for generation and absorption of short-chain fatty acids. These fatty acids are the products of bacterial metabolism of undigested complex carbohydrates such as fruits and vegetables.

The pancreas aids in digestion, has both exocrine and endocrine functions, and secretes bicarbonate and enzymes into the first part of the duodenum. Exocrine digestive enzymes (trypsinogen and chymotrypsinogen) are secreted in an inactive form to prevent autodigestion of the pancreas. Bicarbonate is also secreted by the pancreas and aids in neutralizing the pH of gastric chyme. The endocrine function produces insulin and glucagon.

The contraction of the gallbladder and the relaxation of the sphincter of Oddi control the bile flow that is secreted into the duodenum. The body produces anywhere from 400 to 800 mL of bile per day. Bile helps to emulsify and absorb fats, and provides the primary route for the breakdown and elimination of cholesterol.

The largest solid organ in the body is the liver. It aids in digestion by filtering out bacteria and foreign material, and also secretes bile. The liver is important in lipid and vitamin A metabolism, synthesis of clotting factors, and synthesis of most circulating proteins and albumin. It detoxifies ammonia (a byproduct of the breakdown of amino acids) by combining it with carbon dioxide, producing urea and releasing it into the bloodstream. The liver is also responsible for more than half of the body's lymph production. It is important to note this lymph production by the liver because during liver dysfunction, lymph may be forced into the abdominal cavity because of decreased liver blood flow and increased hepatic pressure.

Metabolism is a key function of the liver. Protein metabolism occurs through amino acid synthesis, which converts to glucose and lipids. Fatty acids are synthesized from carbohydrate precursors and are generally stored in the form of triglycerides to be metabolized later by other tissues. Carbohydrate metabolism helps maintain normal blood glucose concentrations. When glucose levels fall, glucose, stored in the form of glycogen, is readily transported back to the cells as needed for energy. Another pathway that generates glucose is gluconeogenesis, carried out only in the liver and the renal cortex. Gluconeogenesis creates glucose from other substrates (amino acids) when glycogen reserves are depleted.

ASSESSMENT OF NUTRITIONAL STATUS

The nurse is the first line of defense when assessing a patient for nutritional deficits. Evaluating nutritional status is essential to determine whether a hypermetabolic and catabolic state related to critical illness, minimal nutritional intake, or both, are present. Nutritional status is the balance between a patient's current nutritional supply and demand. A comprehensive approach to determining nutritional status evaluates several criteria: medical history and examination, medication history, physical assessment, anthropometric measurements, and laboratory data.[1] The data are organized and evaluated to form a professional opinion regarding the patient's nutritional status and needs during hospitalization. The purpose of a nutritional assessment in the critically ill patient is to document baseline subjective and objective nutritional parameters, determine nutritional risk factors, identify nutritional deficits, establish nutritional needs for patients, and identify medical, psychosocial, and socioeconomic factors that may influence the administration of specialized nutritional support (SNS).[17] (See Geriatric Considerations.)

Assessment of the critically ill patient begins with the subjective assessment of data. The nurse determines whether the patient is alert and oriented, has an adequate gag reflex, and is able to swallow without difficulty. Overly sedated or intubated patients are not candidates for oral feedings until their mental or respiratory status improves. If an oral diet is appropriate, the ability to tolerate a variety of textures is determined in part by adequate dentition and also by the adequacy of saliva production, which is demonstrated by a pink, moist oral mucosa. Extra fluids may be required to facilitate easier swallowing if dryness is apparent. Additional assessments that assist in determining nutritional deficits include muscle or adipose tissue loss, the appearance of wasting associated with chronic disease (e.g., cancer, multiple sclerosis), and whether the patient is retaining fluid, which could be related to a protein deficit. The patient's medical history provides objective data demonstrating the presence of malabsorptive syndromes that can impair the patient's ability to utilize nutrients. These conditions include short bowel syndrome, a history of radiation to the bowel, the presence of an ileus, intestinal pseudo-obstruction, persistent vomiting, Crohn's disease, diverticulosis, or gastroparesis.

OVERVIEW OF NUTRITIONAL SUPPORT

Enteral Nutrition

Patients who are not able to meet their needs orally for more than 3 days require enteral nutrition.[12,16] Enteral nutrition refers to the delivery of nutrients into the GI tract, which is the preferred route of nutrient administration unless contraindicated. Large-bore nasogastric tubes can be used for medication administration, decompression of the gut, gastric suction, or drainage. A flexible small-bore tube (usually 5 to 12 French) is often inserted in place of large-bore tubes to initiate feedings. The small-bore tube is better tolerated because of its size and flexibility; it also reduces the risk of nasal tissue necrosis. Nasally inserted small-bore tubes (nasogastric, nasojejunal) can be used in short-term situations, usually no more than 6 weeks, but may not be beneficial in patients at high risk for aspiration. Feeding tubes directly inserted into the stomach or jejunum (e.g., gastrojejunostomy or jejunostomy) are chosen for long-term access, especially for patients at high risk of aspiration pneumonia. A percutaneous endoscopic gastrostomy (PEG) tube is often inserted because placement does not require general anesthesia, and allows for feedings to begin soon after placement. A jejunostomy tube must be placed during a laparotomy.

Parenteral Nutrition

Parenteral nutrition refers to the infusion of nutrient solutions into the bloodstream by some form of central intravenous access catheter. A central catheter (or central line) is defined as a line placed in the superior vena cava, right atrium, or inferior vena cava. The central catheter options include a peripherally inserted central catheter (PICC); an external, tunneled catheter; or a subcutaneous port. Placement of these lines is verified by chest x-ray immediately after insertion. There are two options for parenteral nutrition administration: peripheral parenteral nutrition (PPN) or total parenteral nutrition (TPN) solutions. Solution concentration is the main determinant of administration site, specifically the carbohydrate concentration. Isotonic parenteral solutions

---

GERIATRIC CONSIDERATIONS

- Elderly patients (older than 65 years) are at a higher risk for altered nutrition due to:
  - Chronic diseases that affect the appetite or the ability to obtain and prepare appropriate and adequate caloric intake—dementia, chronic obstructive pulmonary disease, osteoarthritis, heart failure, and impaired mobility.
  - Decreased intake due to poor fitting dentures or missing teeth.
  - Decreased income levels, which may lead to food choices based on cost rather than nutritional value.
  - Social isolation. Older adults living alone are more likely to experience hunger.
  - Inability to obtain food because of lack of transportation or minimal access to Meals-on-Wheels type of program.
- Potential drug-nutrient interactions are assessed in all elderly patients. A person who takes multiple daily medications is at a higher risk for nutritional alterations due to medication side effects, which may alter appetite.

Data from A.S.P.E.N. Board of Directors and the Clinical Guidelines Task Force. (2002). Guidelines for the use of parenteral and enteral nutrition in adult and pediatric patients. *Journal of Parenteral and Enteral Nutrition, 26S*, 61SA-96SA.

EVIDENCE-BASED PRACTICE

PROBLEM

Early initiation of enteral nutrition is recommended for critically ill patients. Research findings regarding outcomes associated with enteral nutrition often vary.

QUESTION

Does administration of enteral nutrition influence clinical outcomes?

REFERENCE

Koretz, R. L., Avenell, A., Lipman, T. O., Braunschweig, C. L., & Milne, A. C. (2007). Does enteral nutrition affect clinical outcomes? A systematic review of randomized trials. *American Journal of Gastroenterology, 102*, 412-429.

EVIDENCE

The authors evaluated 82 randomized clinical trials that evaluated outcomes of enteral nutrition in a variety of patient populations, including patients with pancreatitis, perioperative, and critical illness. They reviewed trials that compared administration of enteral nutrition or nutritional supplements versus no artificial nutrition or parenteral nutrition. Conduct of studies was varied, making comparison across populations difficult. They found that administration of enteral nutrition versus no support decreased the length of stay and the time patients required mechanical ventilation. Infection rates were found to be reduced in those who received enteral nutrition, and those with burns had fewer episodes of sepsis. Early administration of enteral feedings (within 1-2 days of admission) resulted in better survival in some studies. Enteral nutrition was associated with fewer metabolic complications (e.g., hyperglycemia) when compared with parenteral nutrition; no statistically significant differences were noted between the two in mortality or length of stay. In patients with pancreatitis, mixed findings were noted when comparing enteral versus parenteral nutrition. The authors concluded that there is reasonable evidence for giving enteral nutrition in perioperative and critically ill patients, but the quality of most studies was weak.

IMPLICATIONS FOR NURSING

Despite many randomized clinical trials, the evidence for administration of enteral nutrition in critically ill patients is often mixed. Based on results of this systematic review, it is important to initiate early enteral feeding to patients. If glycemic control is an issue, enteral nutrition is preferred over parenteral nutrition. Nurses can assist in monitoring outcomes of nutritional support within their facility. In particular, outcomes related to the incidence of infections and sepsis should be monitored. Since results in patients with pancreatitis are mixed, nurses can expect to be administering either enteral or parenteral nutrition to this patient population until more evidence is produced.

are appropriate for peripheral administration (PPN). Hypertonic parenteral solutions (TPN) can only be administered centrally because of the risk of phlebitis and the potential for vascular damage.

Parenteral nutrition is a successful way to provide nutrients to patients who are unable to tolerate enteral therapy because of a GI obstruction, intractable vomiting or diarrhea, or because they must have *nothing by mouth* for an extended period of time, usually for greater than one week. Factors for deciding which therapy to use are based on the length of time the patient will receive parenteral nutrition, as well as the patient's vascular access history, venous anatomy, and coagulation status related to central line site selection.

Nutritional Additives

During the last 10 years, specialized nutritional formulas, specifically immune-enhancing formulas, have generated interest and debate regarding their treatment benefit for critically ill patients. Immune-enhancing formulas have been demonstrated to decrease length of stay, hospital costs, and infection risk, and improve wound healing in certain patient populations. Several immune-enhancing formulas are available and are listed in Table 6-1.

NUTRITIONAL THERAPY GOAL

The goal of nutritional therapy is to provide nutritional support consistent with specific metabolic needs and disease processes, to avoid complications of feedings, and ultimately to improve patient outcomes. This is accomplished by creating a *nutrition care plan*. A multidisciplinary approach, which includes a registered dietitian, is used to analyze the patient information, including nutrient requirements and intake targets, the route of SNS administration, and measurable short- and long-term goals of care. The first step in formulating the nutrition care plan is to estimate the patient's calorie and protein requirements (Table 6-2).

Parenteral nutrition support is usually individualized, and a pharmacist often assists in determining the prescription that best meets the patient's nutritional needs. The usual recommendations for fatty acids are that 1% to 2% of daily energy requirements

TABLE 6-1 Components of Immune-Enhancing Formulas

Component	Action	Population Benefited	Example
Arginine	Decreases T suppressor cells Increases T-helper cells Improves wound healing Substrate used for nitric oxide production	Postoperative patients, especially abdominal surgeries Mild sepsis Trauma ARDS	Juven Immun-Aid Impact Extra Vivonex Plus
Glutamine	Essential acid at times of stress and hypercatabolism May diminish atrophy of GI tract mucosa and bacterial translocation Stimulates protein synthesis and inhibits protein breakdown Acts as fuel for antiinflammatory cells such as colonocytes, enterocytes, and macrophages	Burn patients Trauma patients Wound healing	AlitraQ Juven Vivonex Plus
Omega-3 fatty acids	Important for cell membrane stabilization Improves immune function Antiinflammatory properties especially to the lungs Reduces the hypermetabolic response	Postoperative patients, especially abdominal surgeries Mild sepsis Trauma ARDS	Oxcepa Impact Extra
Branched-chain amino acids	Supplies fuel to skeletal muscle during times of stress Important defense mechanism for infection, especially for patients with hepatic dysfunction Improves protein synthesis Improves nitrogen balance	Stressed patients with hepatic dysfunction ARDS	Oxcepa Impact Immun-Aid
Nucleotides	Increases protein synthesis Aids in the immune function and helps fight infection. Aids in preventing immunosuppression Essential for protein, carbohydrate, and fat synthesis	Mild sepsis Trauma ARDS Lactose-free Kosher Malabsorption	Impact Vivonex Plus
Vitamin A	Improves immune response, particularly in conjunction with arginine	Wound healing Critical illness	Replete Vivonex Plus NutriHeal
Vitamin C	Traps free radicals Increases antibody production and lymphocyte response Promotes collagen formation and improves wound healing	Wound healing Critical illness	Vivonex Plus NutriHeal
Vitamin E	Antioxidant properties Cytoprotective, protects red cells from destruction	Wound healing Critical illness	Vivonex Plus

ARDS, Acute respiratory distress syndrome.
From Kudsk, K. A. (2006). Immunonutrition in surgery and critical care. *Annual Review of Nutrition, 26,* 463-479.

should be provided in the form of lipids to prevent essential fatty acid deficiency.[3] Sources of amino acids for parenteral nutrition are synthetic crystalline and essential and nonessential amino acids. The standard dosing ranges for parenteral electrolytes assume normal organ function without abnormal losses and follow the recommended dietary allowances and dietary reference intakes (RDA/DRI).

Enteral nutrition is preferred to parenteral nutrition in most cases in order to preserve gut mucosa.[2]

TABLE 6-2   Estimation of Nutrient Needs

Caloric Requirements	Protein Requirements	Patient Appearance
Normal nonstressed 25 kcal/kg/day	0.8 g/kg/day	Normal
Mildly stressed 25-30 kcal/kg/day	0.8-1.0 g/kg/day	May appear malnourished Postoperative or acutely ill
Moderately stressed 30-35 kcal/kg/day	1.0-1.5 g/kg/day	May appear malnourished May have trouble with absorption Signs of sepsis Recent major surgery
Severely stressed 35 kcal/kg/day	1.0-2.0 g/kg/day	Likely to be underweight Major procedure with a septic event Catabolic state Unable to meet nutritional needs by oral intake alone

It is commonly selected for patients with neuromuscular impairment, patients who cannot meet their nutritional needs by oral intake alone, patients who are hypercatabolic, or patients who are unable to eat as a result of their underlying illness, such as those receiving mechanical ventilation or those with hypoperfusion states. Enteral feeding is associated with a significantly lower risk for infection; it is relatively inexpensive; and placement of a feeding tube in the correct site is relatively easy.[4] An enteral formula is selected that most closely meets the patient's current requirements for type and location of enteral tube. Consideration of how the gut is functioning is weighed along with other underlying medical problems, such as gastroparesis. Administration of enteral feedings, even if the gut cannot handle a full enteral feeding schedule, is advantageous because it prevents bacterial overgrowth and potential bacterial migration across the intestinal wall and into the bloodstream.[7] These benefits are crucial in critically ill patients. Enteral feedings have been used successfully in almost all situations, including the presence of ileus and pancreatitis.[14] TPN can be used in combination with enteral nutrition to meet the nutritional needs of the patient whose GI tract cannot accommodate the full caloric load of enteral feeding.

Various enteral formulas are marketed (Table 6-3). Standard formulas are typically 1 kcal/mL and are not designed for any specific disease state (e.g., Osmolite). Complete protein sources include soy protein isolate, calcium caseinate, sodium caseinate, and milk protein concentrate. The protein may be prepared as a form of hydrolyzed protein, which is broken down into smaller components to aid in digestion. In addition, the protein can be in the form of an elemental protein (e.g., Criticare HN), which is completely broken down and ready for absorption. Patients with short bowel syndromes or malabsorption may benefit from elemental protein formulas. Fat sources include canola oil, a medium-chain triglyceride oil, sunflower oil, safflower oil, soy, and lecithin. Lipids provide 30% to 50% of the total kilocalories. There are two primary lipid forms: the long-chain triglycerides (a major source of essential fatty acids and fat-soluble vitamins) and the medium-chain triglycerides. The medium-chain triglycerides foster the absorption of fat better than the long-chain triglycerides, but have side effects of nausea, vomiting, abdominal distention, and diarrhea.[16] Carbohydrates are the most easily digested and absorbed component of enteral formulas.[16] Sources include corn syrup, hydrolyzed cornstarch, and maltodextrin. The carbohydrates are not usually from lactose to minimize complications related to lactose intolerance. Fiber can also be added to improve blood glucose control, reduce hyperlipidemia, and improve diarrhea symptoms (e.g., Jevity).

Vitamins and trace elements are essential nutrients that act as coenzymes and cofactors involved in metabolism. For enteral nutrition, recommendations are based on the RDA/DRI levels. Dosing beyond the RDA/DRI values is not generally supported by experimental data for most patients requiring SNS. The dosing guidelines for parenteral vitamins and trace elements are considered as approximations of need during critical illness.

TABLE 6-3   Enteral Formulas

Generic Description	Sample Product	Indications
Elemental/predigested 1 kcal/mL 45 g Pro/L Free Amino Acids	Perative Criticare HN	GI dysfunction: short bowel syndrome, impaired digestion
Standard isotonic 1 kcal/mL 37 g Pro/L	Osmolite Nutren 1.0 Isosource	Normal GI function
High protein 1 kcal/mL 62.5 g Pro/L	Promote	Normal GI function with need for increased protein because of catabolism—burns, critical illness
Fiber enriched 1 kcal/mL 44 g Pro/L	Jevity	Normal GI function Need for increased fiber for diarrhea or constipation
Calorie dense 2 kcal/mL 70 g Pro/L	Two Cal HN	Heart failure Liver disease
Wound healing Includes high protein, vitamins, some with arginine, glutamine, and/or omega-3 fatty acids	Replete with Fiber Juven Immun-Aid	Used with wounds, trauma, burns
Oral supplements 1.06 kcal/mL 54.9 g Pro/L	Ensure Boost	Inability to consume enough orally

GI, Gastrointestinal; *Pro*, protein.

PRACTICE GUIDELINES

Enteral Nutrition

Decisions regarding access for enteral nutrition should take into account the effectiveness of gastric emptying, GI anatomy, and aspiration risk. In addition, enteral nutrition depends on an intact bowel that is able to absorb nutrients. Feedings into the small bowel (postpyloric) are often initiated within 24 hours of the onset of injury or illness. Nutrients are usually well absorbed in the small bowel. Feedings delivered into the small intestine are delivered by continuous infusion via an enteral feeding pump because the intestinal mucosa normally receives nutrients from the stomach in peristaltic waves and does not tolerate large-volume intermittent feedings. Nasoenteric tube placement is attempted at the bedside; if this is unsuccessful, fluoroscopic or endo-scopic guidance is used. Radiographic confirmation of the feeding tube tip position is obtained after placement of a nasogastric or nasojejunal tube before initiating feedings.

Although many critically ill patients receive feedings into the small intestine, outcomes of patients who receive gastric feedings versus postpyloric feedings are similar.[15] An analysis of nine studies conducted in medical, neurosurgical, and trauma patients found no difference in the incidence of pneumonia, the length of stay, or the mortality. Feedings were started earlier in those receiving gastric feedings, because delays are often associated with proper placement of feeding tubes into the small intestine.[15]

Feeding tubes are routinely flushed with 20 to 30 mL of warm water every 4 hours during the continuous feedings, and before and after intermittent feedings and medication administration.[4] When patients receive enteral feedings, the gastric residuals are checked every 4 hours. Clinical judgment is used when assessing residuals. Recent research demonstrates that elevated residuals, when examined alone, are a poor indicator of tube feeding tolerance and the potential risk of aspiration. Monitoring for gradually increasing residual volumes and assessing for other signs of intolerance are recommended before holding tube feedings.[13,16] Current recommendations are to stop tube feedings if residuals are greater than 250 mL. Residuals should be rechecked every 2 hours, and feedings can resume when residuals are less than 250 mL (or other ordered amount). Tolerance of feedings includes the auscultated presence of bowel sounds in four quadrants, the presence of bowel motility or bowel movements, palpation of a soft abdomen, and percussion of the abdomen revealing tympanic findings. Signs of intolerance include the presence of nausea, vomiting, absent bowel sounds, abdominal distention, or cramping. Complications of enteral feedings are summarized in Table 6-4. See also the Clinical Alert.

Parenteral Nutrition

Each parenteral nutrition formulation that is compounded is inspected for signs of gross particulate contamination, discoloration, particulate formation, and phase separation at the time of compounding.[5] Maintaining the sterility of the setup is essential. All tubing is changed every 24 hours. The TPN/PPN line is a dedicated line for only parenteral nutrition; no intravenous push or infusion medications are given in this line except lipid infusions. Intravenous site care must be meticulous because of the infection risk related to the administration of a hyperosmolar solution. Monitoring for fluid and electrolyte imbalance, including chemistry panels and glucose, and monitoring for early signs of infection are important aspects of nursing care because of the potential for adverse outcomes. Patients receiving parenteral nutrition should have blood glucose monitoring at least every 6 hours. Insulin therapy is usually administered subcutaneously according to a sliding scale. Insulin is also added to the TPN solution; the amount of insulin is adjusted daily based on the patient's laboratory values over the previous 24 hours.

Drug-Nutrient Interactions

Medication profiles of patients receiving SNS are reviewed for potential effects on nutritional and metabolic status.[5] Medications that are coadministered with enteral nutrition are reviewed periodically for potential incompatibilities. Whenever medications are administered via an enteral feeding tube, the tube should be flushed with 30 mL of warm water before and after each medication is administered.

Bioavailability of some medications (e.g., phenytoin) is reduced when administered with enteral feedings. Current recommendations for administration of phenytoin are to stop enteral feedings 1 to 2 hours before dosing and resume 1 to 2 hours after dosing.[9] This method may not always be optimal, especially for malnourished patients. Another option is to monitor and adjust phenytoin dosages based on serum drug levels while the patient is receiving enteral nutrition. Once enteral nutrition is discontinued, the drug dosage is readjusted.

Liquid medication formulations are preferred for administration via the enteral feeding tube. Pharmacists can often order and/or prepare many medications in liquid form upon request. Sustained-release medications must not be crushed and given via a feeding tube because of the potential for overdose. Patients receiving enteral nutrition who develop diarrhea are evaluated for antibiotic-associated causes, particularly *Clostridium difficile*.

The coadministration of an admixture of medications known to be incompatible with parenteral nutrition must also be prevented. In the absence of reliable information concerning compatibility of a specific drug with an SNS formula, the medication is administered separately from the SNS.

Monitoring Nutritional Status and Monitoring for Complications

Malnourished patients are at risk for refeeding syndrome, which leads to sudden electrolyte abnormalities and fluid shifts. Glucose and electrolytes (sodium, chloride, potassium, magnesium, and phosphorus) should be monitored regularly until stable. This is

CLINICAL ALERT
Assessment of Feeding Tube Placement

Misplacement of feeding tubes increases the risk of complications including nutrition delays, aspiration pneumonia, and pneumothorax. X-ray confirmation of correct tube placement is expected before initiation of tube feedings or administration of medications. Tube placement must also be verified if the tube becomes dislodged and requires reinsertion. Auscultatory methods for assessing tube placement are unreliable. Patients with the highest risk of placement complications are intubated patients, those with an altered level of consciousness and an impaired gag reflex.[10]

TABLE 6-4   Tube Feeding Complications and Nursing Interventions

Complication	Nursing Interventions
Mechanical	
Tube obstruction	• Flush feeding tube with at least 30 mL of warm water every 4 hours during continuous feeding, after medications, after intermittent feedings, and before and after gastric residuals are checked. • Administer medications in elixir form whenever possible. • Irrigate tube with warm water or pancreatic enzymes to relieve obstruction.
Pulmonary	
Improper tube placement	• Verify the position of all feeding tubes by x-ray prior to initiating feedings; auscultatory methods of assessment are often inaccurate. • Identify patients at risk for malposition of the tube, such as those with impaired gag/cough reflex, those who are obtunded or heavily sedated, and those receiving neuromuscular blocking agents.
Aspiration	• Attempting to aspirate gastric contents may be difficult as small-bore tubes collapse easily. • Monitor residuals every 4 hours and temporarily discontinue feedings if volume is >250 mL; recheck every 2 hours until residuals are <250 mL, and then restart feedings. • Do not use blue dye in enteral formulas to assess for aspiration; it is an unreliable indicator. • To prevent reflux, keep head of bed elevated at least 30 degrees during feedings; stop feedings for 10-15 minutes before patient is turned or bed is flattened for therapies. • Position flat for therapies. • Monitor for abdominal girth measurements for abdominal distention. • Assess bowel sounds. • Mark feeding tube at exit site to monitor for proper tube placement.
Gastrointestinal	

Diarrhea	• Review medications that may increase the likelihood of diarrhea: sorbitol, laxatives, digitalis, antibiotics.
	• Assess for *Clostridium difficile*; obtain order for stool sample culture.
	• If infection is not the cause of the diarrhea, administer fiber-enriched formulas or bulking agents to normalize stool consistency (e.g., Metamucil).
	• Prevent bacterial contamination:
	  • When possible, use full-strength, ready-to-use formula.
	  • Use meticulous hand-washing techniques prior to handling formulas and supplies.
	  • Avoid touching the inside of delivery sets.
	  • Rinse delivery sets with warm (preferably soapy) water after feedings.
	  • Change administration sets every 24 hours.
	  • Limit hanging time of formulas at room temperature to 8 hours. Exception: prefilled sets; read manufacturer recommendations and follow institutional policy.

Dumping syndrome	• Limit bolus feedings to <300 mL. • Slow the rate and frequency of feeding bolus if abdominal distention or cramping occurs.
Metabolic	
Hyperglycemia	• Monitor blood glucose level at least every 6 hours, or per institution policy. • Administer insulin as ordered, usually per sliding scale.
Electrolyte imbalance	• Monitor fluid status closely. • Monitor electrolytes for changes.

especially important in patients with diabetes or in those who have risk factors for glucose intolerance. Patients receiving intravenous fat emulsion require serum triglyceride levels to be evaluated and monitored until stable. Additional monitoring is needed when changes are made to the lipid content, such as administration of propofol, a lipid-based sedative-anesthetic agent. Liver function tests are performed and trended to assess for changes in patients receiving PPN or TPN.

LABORATORY ALERT

Lab Test	General Critical Values*	Significance
Prealbumin	<16 mg/dL	• 1.9-day half life makes it a sensitive indicator of protein synthesis and catabolism • Decreased in protein deficiency • Decreased in response to increased catabolism
Albumin	<3.5 g/dL	• Decreased in liver disease • Decreased in protein deficiency
Triglycerides	>400 mg/dL	• If elevated, evaluate feeding route and formula • Dosages of propofol and/or lipids may need to be adjusted
Sodium	<120 mEq/L >150 mEq/L	• Low levels can affect neurological status • Elevated indicates free water excess, which can exacerbate heart failure
Potassium	<3.0 mEq/L >6.0 mEq/L	• Hypokalemia; can cause dysrhythmias • Hyperkalemia; can cause dysrhythmias, may be due to dehydration or renal impairment
Magnesium	<1.9 mEq/L	• May indicate malnutrition and/or malabsorption
Phosphate	<1 mg/dL	• Can be due to malnutrition, sepsis, increased calcium delivery (calcium and phosphate are inversely related)
Glucose	>200 mg/dL	• Indicates inability to tolerate glucose in parenteral nutrition and/or carbohydrate load in enteral nutrition formulas • Additional administration of insulin required to achieve glycemic control
BUN	>100 mg/dL	• Indicates inability of kidneys to tolerate TPN or enteral nutrition • May be elevated in dehydration
Creatinine	>2.0 mg/dL	• May need to reassess formula selection, additives, and electrolyte combinations • Indicates overall renal function

BUN, Blood urea nitrogen.
*Depends on facility laboratory ranges.

MONITORING AND EVALUATING THE NUTRITION CARE PLAN

Documentation of daily weights, tolerance to eating, and evaluation of enteral or parenteral intake is important.[11] Tests commonly ordered to assess nutritional status include complete blood count, chemistry panels, and liver function tests (triglycerides, albumin, and prealbumin levels). Any changes in medications are reviewed, and decisions are made regarding whether the patient is meeting intermediate outcomes toward the goals of nutritional support. (See Laboratory Alert.) If goals are not being met, reassessment of the plan is necessary to help the patient to achieve optimal nutritional goals. Assessment of weight loss, elevated glucose levels, or the appearance of dehydration or fluid overload are indicators that the nutritional care plan may need to be adjusted.

CASE STUDY

Mr. Howard is at postoperative day 7 after coronary artery bypass graft surgery. He has not eaten any significant calories since the operation. He does not like hospital food and has trouble chewing because of poor dentition. He appears depressed and has lost 15 pounds since admission. Objective data include the following: height, 6 feet; weight, 135 pounds; and a history of a 20-pound weight loss in the last month. Laboratory data include a prealbumin level of less than 7.4 g/dL (normal values, 16.4-38 g/dL) and an albumin level of 1.6 g/dL (normal values, 3.5-5 g/dL); urine output has been adequate, and he has hypoactive bowel sounds.

Estimation of the patient's calorie and protein needs are noted using data in Table 6-2. Based on the subjective and objective data presented, Mr. Howard is a combination of moderately stressed to severely stressed. His kilocalorie intake requirements are 35 kcal/kg/day, and his protein requirements are approximately 1.5 to 2.0 g/kg/day.

Another patient, Mr. Johnson, is a 67-year-old man admitted for pneumonia who has a history of chronic obstructive pulmonary disease. He is alert and oriented. He has not eaten for the past 10 days and says that when he tries to swallow, food gets caught in his throat. His physical appearance is of a man who appears older than his stated age. He has extensive muscle wasting and poor skin turgor, his oral mucosa appears dry, and he is missing teeth. He has faint bowel sounds. His current diet order is

nothing by mouth, and he is being assessed for the potential for aspiration. He is 6 feet tall and weighs 120 pounds. Current medications include furosemide (Lasix), potassium chloride, and phenytoin (Dilantin). He is admitted to the critical care unit. Within the first 24 hours, he is unable to maintain adequate oxygenation on supplemental oxygen, and he requires intubation.

His initial serum chemistry laboratory values are normal. Of note, his albumin level is 4.0 g/dL, and his sodium concentration is 148 mg/dL. He is receiving an infusion of 5% dextrose and half-normal saline with 20 mEq of potassium chloride at 75 mL/hour. His intake is greater than his output, and he has lower extremity edema. The health care team decides to start nutritional support. A small-bore feeding tube is inserted, and placement is verified with a KUB x-ray. Mr. Johnson is evaluated to be moderately to severely stressed, and he requires kilocalorie and protein requirements similar to those for Mr. Howard.

QUESTIONS

1. What combination of assessment findings determines the patient's nutritional status in these case studies?
2. How do you justify the preferred route of intake in the critically ill patient?
3. What laboratory data best determine the patient's state within a nutritional context?
4. What is the overall goal of nutritional therapy?

SUMMARY

Patients with critical illness are at high risk for nutritional deficits. SNS is initiated early for critically ill patients who may be unable to meet nutrient needs orally for more than 7 days. Enteral nutrition is the preferred route for SNS, and parenteral nutrition is reserved for patients in whom enteral nutrition is not

possible.[6] Nutritional support is critical for optimal outcomes and successful management of critically ill patients. Adequate nutrition provides for the basic metabolic needs of the critically ill patient and aids in wound healing, tissue repair, and immune function, while minimizing muscle wasting. Assessment of patients' nutritional status by the critical care nurse and timely intervention by the interdisciplinary health care team can optimize and improve patients' outcomes.

CRITICAL THINKING QUESTIONS

1. What factors are considered when selecting a type of enteral tube for feedings?
2. What assessment findings are indicative of a patient's intolerance to feedings, both enteral and parenteral?
3. What factors would you consider in selecting an enteral formula?
4. Do any drug interactions form potential complications with either enteral or parenteral formulas?

> **evolve** Be sure to check out the bonus material, including free self-assessment exercises, on the Evolve Web site at http://evolve.elsevier.com/Sole.

REFERENCES

1. A.S.P.E.N. Board of Directors and the Clinical Guidelines Task Force. (2002). Section III: Nutrition assessment: Adults. Guidelines for the use of parenteral and enteral nutrition in adult and pediatric patients. *Journal of Parenteral and Enteral Nutrition, 26S,* 9SA-12SA.
2. A.S.P.E.N. Board of Directors and the Clinical Guidelines Task Force. (2002). Section V: Administration of specialized nutrition support. Guidelines for the use of parenteral and enteral nutrition in adult and pediatric patients. *Journal of Parenteral and Enteral Nutrition, 26S,* 18SA-21SA.
3. A.S.P.E.N. Board of Directors and the Clinical Guidelines Task Force. (2002). Section VI: Normal requirements: Adults. Guidelines for the use of parenteral and enteral nutrition in adult and pediatric patients. *Journal of Parenteral and Enteral Nutrition, 26S,* 22SA-24SA.
4. A.S.P.E.N. Board of Directors and the Clinical Guidelines Task Force. (2002). Section VIII: Access for administration of nutrition support. Guidelines for the use of parenteral and enteral nutrition in adult and pediatric patients. *Journal of Parenteral and Enteral Nutrition, 26S,* 33SA-41SA.
5. A.S.P.E.N. Board of Directors and the Clinical Guidelines Task Force. (2002). Section IX: Drug-nutrient interactions. Guidelines for the use of parenteral and enteral nutrition in adult and pediatric patients. *Journal of Parenteral and Enteral Nutrition, 26S,* 42SA-44SA.
6. A.S.P.E.N. Board of Directors and the Clinical Guidelines Task Force. (2002). Section X: Life cycle and metabolic conditions. Guidelines for the use of parenteral and enteral nutrition in adult and pediatric patients. *Journal of Parenteral and Enteral Nutrition, 26S,* 45SA-60SA.
7. A.S.P.E.N. Board of Directors and the Clinical Guidelines Task Force. (2002). Section XI: Specific guidelines for disease: Adults. Guidelines for the use of parenteral and enteral nutrition in adult and pediatric patients. *Journal of Parenteral and Enteral Nutrition, 26S,* 61SA-96SA.
8. Ackley, B. J., & Ladwig, G. B. (2008). *Nursing diagnosis handbook* (8th ed.). St. Louis: Mosby.
9. Au Yeung, S. C., & Ensom, M. H. (2000). Phenytoin and enteral feedings: Does evidence support an interaction? *Annals of Pharmacotherapy, 34*(7), 896-905.
10. de Aguilar-Nascimento, J. E., & Kudsk, K. A. (2007). Use of small-bore feeding tubes: Successes and failures. *Current Opinion in Clinical Nutrition and Metabolic Care, 10*(3), 291-296.
11. Heitz, U. E., & Horne, M. M. (2005). *Pocket guide to fluid, electrolyte, and acid-base balance* (5th ed.). St. Louis: Mosby.
12. Kattelmann, K. K., Hise, M., Russell, M., et al. (2006). Preliminary evidence for a medical nutrition therapy protocol: Enteral feedings for critically ill patients. *Journal of the American Dietetic Association, 106*(8), 1226-1241.
13. Koretz, R. L., Avenell, A., Lipman, T. O., Braunschweig, C. L., & Milne, A. C. (2007). Does enteral nutrition affect clinical outcome? A systematic review of the randomized trials. *American Journal of Gastroenterology, 102,* 412-429.
14. Kreymann, K. G., Bergen, N. E. P., Deutz, M., et al. (2006). ESPEN guidelines on enteral nutrition: Intensive care. *Clinical Nutrition, 25,* 210-223.
15. Marik, P. E., & Zaloga, G. P. (2003). Gastric versus post-pyloric feeding: A systematic review. *Critical Care, 7*(3), R46-R51.
16. McClave, S. A., Lukan, J. K., Stefater, J. A., et al. (2005). Poor validity of residual volumes as a marker for risk of aspiration in critically ill patients. *Critical Care Medicine, 33*(2), 324-330.
17. Russell, M. K., Andrews, M. R., Brewer, C. K., Rogers, J. Z., & Seidner, D. L. (2002). Standard for specialized nutrition support: Adult hospitalized patients. *Nutrition in Clinical Practice, 16,* 385-386.
18. Sullivan, D. H., Sun, S., & Walls, R. C. (1999). Protein-energy undernutrition among elderly hospitalized patients: A prospective study. *JAMA, 281,* 2013-2019.

CHAPTER 7

Dysrhythmia Interpretation and Management

Susan Loyola, MSN, RN

INTRODUCTION

The ability to analyze and interpret dysrhythmias is a fundamental skill that is required of the critical care nurse. The goal of this chapter is to provide a basic understanding of electrocardiography for the purpose of analyzing and interpreting cardiac dysrhythmias. Electrocardiography is the process of creating a visual tracing of the electrical activity of the cells in the heart. This tracing is called the *electrocardiogram* (ECG). The critical care nurse must have a clear understanding of cardiac monitoring, lead selection, and rhythm interpretation. Critical care nurses are expected to perform at high levels of expertise, accurately interpreting dysrhythmias to assess, intervene early, and improve patient outcomes. Part of the difficulty in learning rhythm interpretation is that many of the terms used are synonymous. Throughout this chapter those terms will be clarified. This chapter discusses general concepts of dysrhythmia interpretation.

Practice standards for ECG monitoring in hospital settings have been developed by experts in the field of electrocardiology and cardiac monitoring. A rating system was devised and consists of the following categories:[3,4,8,10]

Class I: cardiac monitoring is indicated in most, if not all patients in this group. Critically ill patients are considered Class I.

Class II: cardiac monitoring may be of benefit in some patients but is not considered essential for all patients.

Class III: cardiac monitoring is not indicated because a patient's risk of a serious event is so low.

BASIC ELECTROPHYSIOLOGY

Automaticity

The ECG tracing provides evidence that the cardiac muscle is generating electrical activity. The basis for this electrical activity is *automaticity*. Automaticity means that the cardiac muscle can generate its own electrical activity, even during brief times when blood supply or nervous stimulation is absent. Special groups of cells generate automatic impulses for the purpose of exciting the remainder of the heart's muscle cells. Although this process is facilitated by blood flow from the coronary arteries and stimulation from the sympathetic and parasympathetic nervous systems, the heart can continue to generate electrical activity for a brief time after blood and nervous supply have ceased.

The Cardiac Cycle

The cardiac cycle is composed of both the electrical activity caused by automaticity and the mechanical, or muscular, response known as *contraction*. The electrical activity is divided into two phases: depolarization and repolarization. *Depolarization* is the active phase of electrical activity and is associated with systole. *Repolarization* is the resting phase and is associated with diastole. Electrical activity precedes mechanical activity. The mechanical response is divided into systole and diastole.

Cardiac Action Potential

Cardiac muscle cells are capable of generating an electrical current. This mechanism is known as the *cardiac action potential.* This is especially noted in a small group of special cardiac cells located in the posterior wall of the right atrium—the sinoatrial node (SA node).

Depolarization and repolarization occur as a result of an exchange of electrolytes across the cell membrane. Before depolarization, sodium is mostly outside the cell, and potassium is found predominantly inside the cell. This initial state causes the myocardial cell membrane to be negatively charged, thus setting up the cardiac action potential. The initial phase is known as the cardiac cell resting membrane potential. It begins at −90 mV for the cardiac conduction system. However, the resting membrane potential for the SA and atrioventricular (AV) nodes is −65 mV, which allows these special cells to initiate the electrical impulse earlier than the other cells. These specialized cells are referred to as pacemaker cells.

When a cell is stimulated, the permeability of the myocardial cell membrane changes. Large amounts of sodium enter the cell and cause it to have a more positive value, thus initiating the electrical process known as depolarization. Following this, calcium ions slowly enter the cell through special calcium channels. This prolongs depolarization and allows for cardiac muscle contraction. Toward the end of depolarization, sodium ceases its movement into the cardiac cell. Potassium continues to leak to the outside of the cardiac cell. To return to the resting membrane potential, sodium moves back out of the cell and potassium back into the cell by means of a pump. The pump requires energy in the form of adenosine triphosphate, or ATP. The energy generated by this pump aids in removing calcium from the cell. The net result is restoration of the normal resting membrane potential of −90 mV for nonpacemaker cells and −65 mV for pacemaker cells, and the resting phase, or repolarization, begins. This state of repolarization stimulates the next depolarization (Figure 7-1).

The goal of the conduction system is to transfer the electrical stimulation that begins in the SA node down to the Purkinje fibers. Normally, a cardiac action potential originates in the SA node, spreads through the heart, and initiates the electrical activity of the heart. However, if the SA node fails to generate an electrical impulse, another area of the cardiac muscle will generate an impulse and take control of the heartbeat, as discussed later in this chapter. Many antidysrhythmic drugs affect the cardiac action potential by altering the sodium, potassium, and calcium gradients across the cardiac cell membrane (Table 7-1 and Clinical Alert: Antidysrhythmic Drugs).

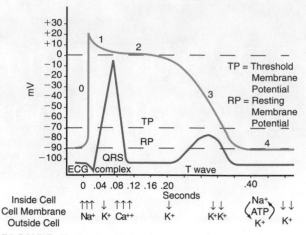

FIGURE 7-1. Cardiac action potential with the electrocardiogram and movement of electrolytes. *ATP,* Adenosine triphosphate; *Ca,* calcium; *K,* potassium; *Na,* sodium. *(From American Heart Association. [1997]. Advance cardiac life support textbook. Dallas: Author.)*

Relationship Between Electrical Activity and Muscular Contraction

Under normal circumstances, depolarization is followed by contraction of a cardiac muscle fiber. The term *systole* refers to this contraction. Repolarization of the cardiac cell leads to a resting state for the muscle, or *diastole.* During repolarization the ventricles fill with blood from the atria. A sufficient time of rest is necessary for the ventricles to be adequately filled before the next depolarization and subsequent systole occur.

The ECG tracing is evidence of electrical activity only. The presence of an ECG pattern does not necessarily ensure that the patient's heart is also contracting. For confirmation that cardiac contractions are occurring, a clinically detectable pulse and an adequate blood pressure must be present. If no pulse is detected, cardiopulmonary resuscitation is begun unless there is a "do not resuscitate" order for the patient. The condition of electrical activity without mechanical activity (contractility) is known as pulseless electrical activity. For the best chance of survival, the cause of pulseless electrical activity must be quickly identified and treated. The most common conditions impairing contractile function include hypovolemia, hypoxemia, electrolyte imbalances, hypothermia, tension pneumothorax, cardiac tamponade, massive myocardial infarction, drug overdose, acidosis, trauma, hypoglycemia, and pulmonary emboli.[1] Pulseless electrical activity is discussed in greater depth in Chapter 10, "Code Management."

PHARMACOLOGY

TABLE 7-1 Antidysrhythmic Drug Classifications

Class*	Description	Examples
IA	Inhibits the fast sodium channel Prolongs repolarization time Used to treat atrial and ventricular dysrhythmias	Quinidine, disopyramide, procainamide
IB	Inhibits the fast sodium channel Shortens the action potential duration Used to treat ventricular dysrhythmias only	Lidocaine, phenytoin, mexiletine, tocainide
IC	Inhibits the fast sodium channel Shortens the action potential duration of only Purkinje fibers Controls ventricular tachydysrhythmias resistant to other drug therapies Has proarrhythmic effects	Flecainide, propafenone
II	Causes beta-adrenergic blockade	Esmolol, propranolol, sotalol
III	Lengthens the action potential Acts on the repolarization phase	Amiodarone, sotalol, dofetilide; ibutilide
IV	Blocks the slow inward movement of calcium to slow impulse conduction, especially in the atrioventricular node Used for treatment of supraventricular tachycardias	Diltiazem, verapamil
IVb-like	Opens the potassium channel	Adenosine, ATP

*Class I, sodium channel blockers; Class II, beta-adrenergic blockers; Class III, potassium channel blockers; Class IV, calcium channel blockers.
Modified from Opie, L. H., & Gersh, B. J. (2001). *Drugs for the heart* (5th ed.). Philadelphia: Saunders.

CLINICAL ALERT
Antidysrhythmic Drugs

Some antidysrhythmic drugs are proarrhythmic. These drugs tend to have serious side effects and become less effective over time. The rhythm control drugs are Class I and Class III (see Table 7-1). Class I procainamide can cause lupus. Quinidine increases the risk of death with long-term use. Disopyramide, flecainide, and propafenone should be avoided for patients with structural heart disease or patients who have had a myocardial infarction. These drugs may worsen heart failure. Class III amiodarone can cause serious injury to the liver, lungs, thyroid, and eyes. Dofetilide and ibutilide can cause torsades de pointes, so it is important to check potassium levels. Sotalol can cause life-threatening ventricular dysrhythmias and thrombocytopenia. These antidysrhythmic drugs can aggravate existing dysrhythmias or cause new ones. Monitor cardiac rate and rhythm continuously when therapy starts or anytime the dosage is adjusted.

Because of the heart's ability to initiate electrical activity, an ECG tracing may be noted after a person is pronounced to be clinically dead. Once death is declared, the cardiac monitor can be turned off. The length of time that the heart can continue to create an electrical activity varies, but it usually ceases within minutes.

Normal Cardiac Conduction Pathway

Theoretically, any cardiac cell can generate an electrical impulse. However, under normal conditions, special groups of cardiac cells are responsible for impulse generation and conduction. These special cells make up the cardiac conduction pathway (Figure 7-2). The cardiac cells are networked so depolarization can spread easily from cell to cell. Depolarization normally begins in the SA node, a special group of cardiac cells located high in the right atrium. The SA node is often referred to as the "master," or "dominant," pacemaker of the heart. This dominance results from the SA node's anatomical position and its

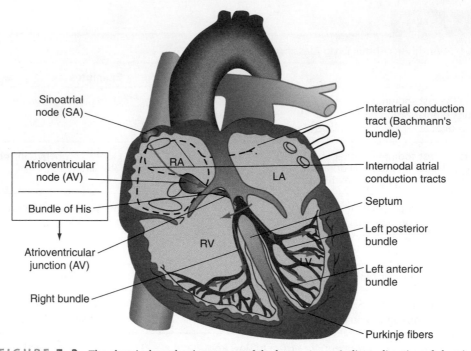

FIGURE 7-2. The electrical conduction system of the heart. *Arrows* indicate direction of electrical currents. The ECG represents the net sum of these currents. *RA,* Right atrium; *RV,* right ventricle; *LA,* left atrium; *LV,* left ventricle. *(Modified from Paul, S., & Hebra, J. [1998]. The nurse's guide to cardiac rhythm interpretation: Implications for patient care. Philadelphia: Saunders.)*

intrinsic ability to generate 60 to 100 beats per minute under normal circumstances. Once the impulse is formulated in the SA node, it is conducted through the atria by the internodal pathways. These pathways connect the SA and AV nodes and are responsible for conducting the impulse throughout the right and left atria. The atria serve as reservoirs that collect blood returning from the head, body, and lungs. The right atrium receives deoxygenated blood from the head through the superior vena cava and from the body through the inferior vena cava. The left atrium receives oxygenated blood that is returning from the lungs through the pulmonary veins.

Atrial depolarization precedes atrial contraction. The time during which atrial depolarization occurs correlates with the time when the atria drain their blood into the ventricles. Most of this process occurs as a result of gravity flow. However, as depolarization ends, the atria contract, emptying any remaining blood into the ventricles. Contraction of the atria results in roughly a 30% increase in the volume of blood sent to the ventricles, thereby dramatically affecting stroke volume and cardiac output for the next ventricular systole. The final phase of atrial systole is known as the *atrial kick.*

From the atria, depolarization proceeds to the AV node, which is located between the atria and the ventricles. The AV node has two important func-

tions. First, the AV node delays entry of the electrical impulse into the ventricles. If the impulse immediately proceeded into the ventricle, contraction would occur before the ventricles have adequate time to fill with blood from the atria. The result would be a decreased stroke volume for the next systole and a decrease in cardiac output. This delay in impulse conduction is very short, only 0.02 seconds.

A second important function of the AV node is to act as a backup pacemaker for the heart should the SA node fail. When acting as the backup pacemaker, the AV node generates 40 to 60 beats per minute under normal conditions. The AV node can emerge as the dominant pacemaker when the SA node's rate falls to less than 40 beats per minute or when automaticity is increased in the AV node. Stress, caffeine, and nicotine may increase automaticity.

Once ventricular filling has been accomplished, the impulse leaves the AV node and moves down into the ventricles through the common bundle of His. The bundle of His is a thick cord of nerve fibers that runs down the first third of the ventricular septum. The common bundle then divides into the right and left bundle branches. The right bundle branch runs down the right side of the ventricular septum, and the left bundle branch runs down the left side. The bundle branches have divisions known as *fascicles.* The right bundle branch has one fascicle. The left bundle branch divides into two fascicles, the anterior-superior and the posterior-inferior fascicles. The large muscle mass of the left ventricle requires two fascicles for adequate depolarization, whereas the smaller right ventricle requires only one (see Figure 7-2). The impulse first enters the left ventricle through the left bundle branch and then moves across the septum for conduction down the right bundle branch. The impulse enters the left ventricle first, to allow more time for its depolarization. However, despite this slight lead time, the overall effect is virtually simultaneous depolarization of both ventricles. From the bundle branches, the electrical impulse is carried deep within the ventricular muscle by fine conductive fibers known as *Purkinje fibers*. The Purkinje fibers also act as a final backup pacemaker for the heart. Should both the SA and the AV nodes fail, the Purkinje fibers can generate an intrinsic rhythm of 15 to 40 beats per minute.

Any change in the normal generation or conduction of impulses leads to the development of dysrhythmias. Therefore, a thorough understanding of the normal conduction pathway and of its intrinsic capabilities is prerequisite knowledge.

THE 12-LEAD ELECTROCARDIOGRAPHY SYSTEM

The 12-lead ECG system includes 3 standard limb leads, 3 augmented limb leads, and 6 precordial leads. It is useful to think of the 12-lead ECG as depicting the cardiac rhythm from 12 different views. Waveforms, particularly the QRS complex, thus vary according to the lead monitored. In some leads, the QRS complex is normally upright above the isoelectric line, whereas in other leads it is negative, deflected below the isoelectric line. The summation of the electrical current of the heart depolarizes right to left, with the exception of the septum, which depolarizes left to right (see Figure 7-2). Therefore, the QRS complex is upright in leads at which depolarization is in the direction of the positive electrode, such as leads II and V_5, and is negative in leads at which depolarization is going away from the positive electrode, such as aV_R and V_1.

Standard Limb Leads

The first leads used in the early 1900s were devised by Einthoven. These are the standard three limb leads I, II, and III. Limb leads are placed on the arms and legs, with leg leads placed below the level of the umbilicus. These leads are bipolar, meaning that a positive lead is placed on one limb and a negative lead on another.

Electricity flows from negative to positive. Lead I records the flow of electricity from the negative lead on the right arm to the positive lead on the left arm. Lead II records activity between the negative lead on the right arm and the positive lead on the left leg. Lead III records activity from the negative lead on the left arm to the positive lead on the left leg (Figure 7-3 and 7-4). The normal ECG waveforms are upright in the limb leads, with lead II producing the most upright waveforms.

Augmented Limb Leads

To provide more views of cardiac electrical activity, augmented voltage limb leads aV_R, aV_L, and aV_F were added. These leads are unipolar, meaning that they record electrical flow in only one direction. A reference point is established in the center of the heart, and electrical flow is recorded from that reference point toward the right arm (aV_R), the left arm (aV_L), and the left foot (aV_F) (Figure 7-5). The *a* in the names of these leads means augmented, and because these leads produce small ECG complexes, they must be augmented or enlarged for analysis. The ECG machine increases the size of these complexes 1.5-fold. The augmented leads are monitored by using the electrodes already in place for the limb leads.

The triaxial diagrams (Figures 7-4 and 7-5) shows that leads I and AV_L are close in proximity, as are leads II, III, and AV_F. Therefore, the QRS patterns of leads within close proximity of each other appear similar. Leads II and aV_R point in opposite directions, thereby creating a negative deflection for aV_R and a positive deflection in lead II.

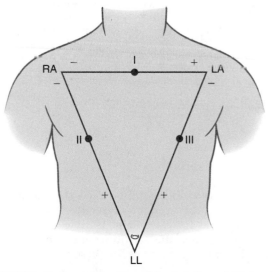

FIGURE 7-3. Orientation of leads I, II, and III. Lead I records the difference in electrical potentials between the left arm and right arm. Lead II records it between the left leg and right arm. Lead III records it between the left leg and left arm. *(Adapted from Goldberger, A. L. [2006]. Clinical electrocardiography: A simplified approach [7th ed., p. 23]. St. Louis: Mosby.)*

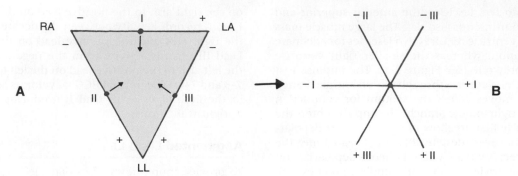

FIGURE 7-4. A, Einthoven's triangle. **B,** The triangle is converted to a triaxial diagram by shifting leads I, II, III that they intersect at a common point. *(From Goldberger, A. L. [2006]. Clinical electrocardiography: A simplified approach [7th ed., p. 25]. St. Louis: Mosby.)*

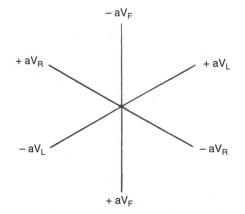

FIGURE 7-5. Triaxial lead diagram showing the relationship of the three augmented (unipolar) leads aV_R, aV_L, and aV_F. Notice that each lead is represented by an axis with a positive and negative pole. The term unipolar was used to mean that the leads record the voltage in one location relative to about zero potential instead of relative to the voltage in one other extremity. *(From Goldberger, A. L. [2006]. Clinical electrocardiography: A simplified approach [7th ed., p. 26]. St. Louis: Mosby.)*

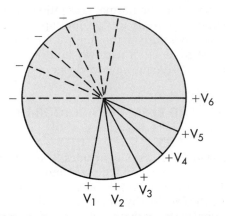

FIGURE 7-6. The precordial leads. The positive poles of the chest leads point anteriorly and the negative poles *(dashed lines)* point posteriorly. *(From Goldberger, A. L. [2006]. Clinical electrocardiography: A simplified approach [7th ed., p. 28]. St. Louis: Mosby.)*

Precordial Leads

The six precordial leads (also called chest leads) are positioned on the chest wall directly over the heart. The landmarks for placement of these leads are the intercostal spaces, the sternum, and the clavicular and axillary lines. Positions for these six leads are as follows:

V_1: Fourth intercostal space, right sternal border
V_2: Fourth intercostal space, left sternal border
V_3: Halfway between V_2 and V_4
V_4: Fifth intercostal space, left midclavicular line

V_5: Fifth intercostal space, left anterior axillary line
V_6: Fifth intercostal space, left midaxillary line

The precordial leads are unipolar, with a positive electrode and the heart as a center reference (Figure 7-6). The precordial leads are useful in the localization of septal, anterior, and lateral myocardial ischemia, injury, and infarction of the left ventricle. Because these leads lie directly over the surface of the heart, changes in the normal ECG can indicate which areas of the heart have sustained insult. V_1 lies over the anterior or frontal surface of the right ventricle and septum. V_2 lies over the septum and the anterior part of the left ventricle. V_3 and V_4 lie over the anterior, or frontal, surface of the left ventricle, and V_5 and V_6 lie over the lateral, or side, surface of

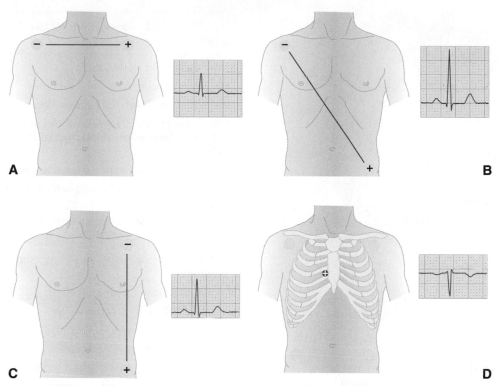

FIGURE 7-7. Limb leads and V₁ electrode placement and their respective waveforms: **A,** Lead I; **B,** lead II; **C,** lead III; and **D,** lead V₁. *(From Paul, S., & Hebra, J. [1998]. The nurse's guide to cardiac rhythm interpretation: Implications for patient care. Philadelphia: Saunders.)*

the left ventricle. None of the 12 leads records activity directly over the posterior, or back side, of the heart. In some situations, right chest leads are placed to obtain additional views of the right side of the heart. These leads are V₁R through V₆R and are useful in identifying right ventricular infarction. Table 7-2 describes recommendations for monitoring different clinical conditions. Figure 7-7 shows electrode placement and waveforms for leads I, II, III, and V₁.

Continuous Cardiac Monitoring

In most settings a 6-second strip of the patient's rhythm is obtained and documented in the patient's chart every 4 hours. In addition to scheduled times, a rhythm strip should be obtained when a different nurse assumes care of a patient and when a patient experiences any change in cardiac rhythm or has chest pain.

Most critical care units use five-lead systems capable of monitoring multiple leads. Other units, such as telemetry units or emergency departments, may use a three-lead system for cardiac monitoring. Whatever type of monitoring system is used, proper lead placement is necessary for the production of high-quality ECG tracings.

TABLE 7-2 Recommended Electrocardiographic Monitoring Leads for Specific Clinical Incidents

Clinical Incident	ECG Monitoring Leads
Atrial flutter	II, III, aV$_F$
New-onset bundle branch block	V₁, V₆
Acute coronary syndrome	III, V₃ (ideally, continuous 12-lead ST-segment monitoring is recommended)
Dysrhythmias	V₁
Broad QRS tachycardia, cardiac dysrhythmias	V₁, V₂, V₆
Anterior MI—Left anterior descending artery	V, V₂, V₃
Inferior MI—Right coronary artery	II, III, aV$_F$
Lateral MI—Circumflex or right coronary artery	No definitive lead; consider V₅, V₆
Posterior MI—Right coronary artery	Reciprocal leads: V₁, V₂, V₃

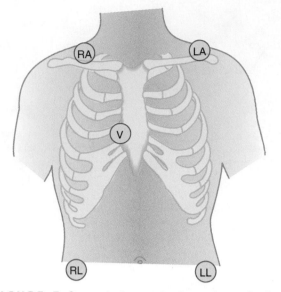

FIGURE 7-8. Lead placement when using a five-lead cable. The chest lead is shown in the V₁ position.

Figure 7-8 shows correct lead placement for a five-lead system. Limb leads are placed on the body close to where the limbs join the torso. The right and left arm leads are placed at the shoulder, above the clavicle or scapula, where the arms join the body. The right and left leg leads are placed on the lower abdomen, below the umbilicus, close to where the legs join the torso. The left leg lead is the most often misplaced lead and must be placed lower than the umbilicus, or the anatomical view for the three leads dependent on this lead will not be depicted as expected. The chest lead (V lead) can be placed to monitor any of the V leads.

In the clinical setting, most monitors are capable of viewing two leads simultaneously. Many monitors have ST-segment monitoring capabilities to identify ischemia, assess effectiveness of therapy such as thrombolytics or percutaneous coronary intervention, and facilitate rapid intervention should acute changes occur. It is recommended that nurses use both leads III and V₃ to detect acute ischemic changes.[4]

Some newer monitors have the capability of performing 12-lead ECGs. Research recommends continuous ST-segment monitoring of all 12 leads to detect ischemia accurately.[5,6,9]

A complete 12-lead ECG is usually obtained daily in patients with cardiac disease and when the patient experiences a change in cardiac status, particularly chest pain. Notably, there are *best practice standards* for electrocardiographic monitoring in hospital settings. Table 7-3 lists priority patient populations for dysrhythmia monitoring.[3,4,8,10]

TABLE 7-3   Indications for Cardiac Dysrhythmia Monitoring[3]
Resuscitated from cardiac arrest
Early phase of acute coronary syndromes
Newly diagnosed high-risk coronary lesions
After cardiac surgery (record atrial electrogram from epicardial pacer wires with tachycardias of unknown origin)
After nonurgent percutaneous coronary intervention
After implantation of automatic defibrillator or pacemaker leads
Temporary or transcutaneous pacemaker
AV block
Dysrhythmias complicating Wolff-Parkinson-White syndrome
Drug-induced long QT syndrome
Intraaortic balloon counterpulsation
Acute heart failure, pulmonary edema
Conditions requiring intensive care admission
Procedures that require conscious sedation or anesthesia

ANALYZING THE BASIC ELECTROCARDIOGRAPHIC TRACING

Measurements

ECG paper has standard measures, whether a single-lead or a 12-lead rhythm strip is obtained (Figure 7-9). The horizontal boxes measure time, and the vertical boxes measure voltage or amplitude.

When ECG paper is used to measure time, the least unit of measure is the small box, which is equal to 0.04 seconds, or 40 milliseconds. The next greater unit of measure is the large box, which contains five small boxes. One large box represents 0.20 seconds, or 200 milliseconds. Five large boxes represent 1 second, or 1000 milliseconds.

The largest unit of measure is in seconds and is marked off at the top of the ECG paper by vertical hatch marks (see Figure 7-9). There may be 1, 2, or 3 seconds between two hatch marks. Five large boxes between hatch marks equal 1 second. Ten large boxes between hatch marks equal 2 seconds. Fifteen large boxes between hatch marks equal 3 seconds. In the clinical setting, it is standard for 6-second rhythm strips to be obtained for analysis and

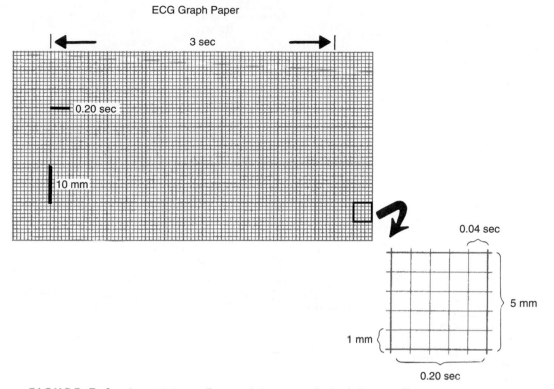

FIGURE 7-9. The ECG is usually recorded on a graph divided into millimeter squares, with darker lines marking 5-mm squares. Time is measured on the horizontal axis. With a paper speed of 25 mm/sec, each small (1-mm) box side equals 0.04 second and each larger (5-mm) box side equals 0.2 second. The amplitude of any wave is measured in millimeters on vertical axis. *(From Goldberger, A. L. [2006].* Clinical electrocardiography: A simplified approach *[7th ed., p. 10]. St. Louis: Mosby.)*

mounting in the patient's chart. To obtain a 6-second strip, the clinician counts off the appropriate number of hatch marks. The value of measuring time on the ECG tracing is that speed of depolarization and repolarization in the atria and ventricles can be determined when printed at 25 mm/sec.

Amplitude is measured on the vertical axis of the ECG paper (see Figure 7-9). Each small box is equal to 0.1 mV in amplitude. Waveform amplitude indicates the amount of electrical voltage being generated in the various areas of the heart. Waveforms from small muscles manifest as low-voltage waveforms. Waveforms representing large muscle mass are manifested as large-voltage waveforms. Low-voltage and small waveforms are expected from the small muscle mass of the atria. Large-voltage and large waveforms are expected from the larger muscle mass of the ventricles. However, if a patient has had a myocardial infarction (necrotic muscle tissue), voltage might be low because electrical voltage is not generated in necrotic myocytes.

Waveforms and Intervals

The normal ECG tracing is composed of P, Q, R, S, and T waves (Figure 7-10). These waveforms emerge from a flat baseline called the *isoelectric line. Isoelectric* means neither positive nor negative, that is, a flat line in the horizontal direction. Any waveform that projects above the isoelectric line is considered positive (upward), meaning the wave of depolarization spreads toward the positive pole of that lead. If the waveform projects below the line it is considered negative (downward), meaning the wave of depolarization spreads away from the positive pole. If the wave of depolarization goes perpendicular to any lead, a biphasic deflection occurs (Figure 7-11).

P Wave
The P wave is an indication of atrial depolarization. It is usually upright in leads I and II and has a rounded configuration. The amplitude of the P wave is measured at the center of the waveform and

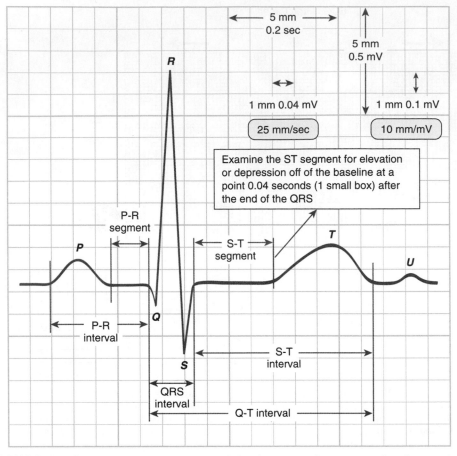

FIGURE 7-10. The P wave represents atrial depolarization. The PR interval is the time from initial stimulation of the atria to initial stimulation of the ventricles. The QRS represents ventricular depolarization. The ST segment, T wave, and U wave are produced by ventricular depolarization.

normally does not exceed three boxes, or 3 mm, in height. The P wave is normally symmetrical.

Normally, a P wave indicates that the SA node initiated the impulse that depolarized the atrium. However, a change in the form of the P wave can indicate that the impulse did not come from the SA node but from an alternate pacemaking site, such as the atria or AV node.

PR Interval

The P wave is connected to the next set of waveforms, the QRS complex, by the PR interval. The interval is measured from the beginning of the P wave, in which the positive deflection of the P wave leaves the isoelectric line, to where the QRS complex begins. The PR interval measures the time it takes for the impulse to depolarize the atria, travel to the AV node, and then dwell there briefly before entering the bundle of His. The normal PR interval is 0.12 to 0.20 second, which is three to five small boxes wide (see Figure 7-10). When the PR interval is

longer than normal, the speed of conduction is abnormally slow. When the PR interval is shorter than normal, the speed of conduction is abnormally fast.

QRS Complex

The QRS complex is a set of three distinct waveforms that are indicative of ventricular depolarization (see Figure 7-10). The classic QRS complex begins with a negative, or downward, deflection immediately after the PR interval. The first negative deflection after the P wave is named the Q wave. Sometimes a Q wave is not present.

The first positive, or upright, waveform that follows the PR interval is the R wave. A Q wave may or may not be present before the R wave. The amplitude of the R wave varies across leads. The R wave is normally tall and positive in lead II. Leads V_4 to V_6 usually have the tallest R waves because they measure electricity in the large muscle mass of the left ventricle.

Three Basic Laws of Electrocardiography

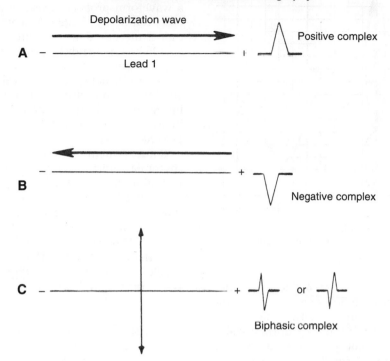

FIGURE 7-11. **A,** A positive complex is seen in any lead if the wave of depolarization spreads toward the positive pole of the lead. **B,** A negative complex is seen if the depolarization wave spreads toward the negative pole (away from the positive pole) of the lead. **C,** A biphasic (partly positive, partly negative) complex is seen if the mean direction of the wave is at right angles. These apply to the P wave, QRS, and T wave. *(From Goldberger, A. L. [2006]. Clinical electrocardiography: A simplified approach [7th ed., p. 34]. St. Louis: Mosby.)*

The S wave is a negative waveform that follows the positive waveform or R wave. In an S wave, the waveform must go below the isoelectric line. The amplitude of the S wave is measured from the point at which it leaves the isoelectric line to its deepest point.

Some patients may have a second positive waveform in their QRS complex. If so, then that second positive waveform is called *R prime (R′)*.

The term *QRS complex* is imprecise. The QRS complex is a generic term for the waveforms that indicate ventricular depolarization. However, many people do not have all three distinct waveforms, Q, R, and S. Figure 7-12 depicts variations of the QRS complex.

If present, the Q wave is assessed for abnormalities. When a Q wave is 0.04 seconds in width and measures more than one fourth of the R wave amplitude, it is abnormal. This is referred to as a *pathological Q wave* or a *significant Q wave*. Pathological Q waves are found on ECGs of patients who have had myocardial infarctions. The deep Q wave in these patients indicates that an area of myocardial tissue has died (Figure 7-13).

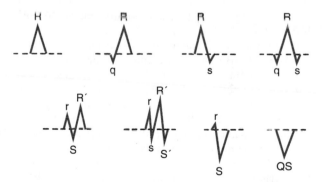

FIGURE 7-12. Different types of QRS complexes. An R wave is a positive waveform. A negative deflection before the R wave is a Q wave. The S wave is a negative deflection after the R wave. If the waveform is tall or deep, the letter naming the waveform is a capital letter. If the waveform is small in either direction, the waveform is labeled with a lower case letter.

QRS Interval

The QRS interval is measured from the beginning to the end of the QRS complex (see Figure 7-10). Whichever waveform begins the QRS complex (whether it is a Q or an R) marks the beginning of

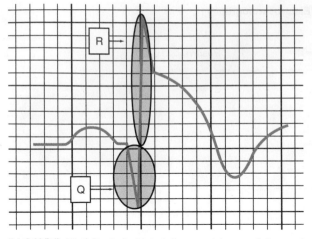

FIGURE 7-13. Pathological Q wave (abnormal Q wave) 0.04 seconds wide and at least one fourth the height of the R wave.

the interval. Therefore, the first deflection, either negative or positive, that follows the P wave indicates the beginning of the interval. The final deflection may be an R or an S wave. The normal width of the QRS complex is 0.06 to 0.10 seconds. This width equates to 1.5 to 2.5 small boxes in length.

When the QRS width is greater than 0.10 second, the patient is suspected of having a bundle branch block (BBB), or an intraventricular conduction delay. The delay in conduction is most commonly caused by coronary artery disease. Either one or both of the bundle branches can be blocked. A complete BBB will have a QRS width of 0.12 seconds or greater. An incomplete BBB has a width from 0.10 to 0.11 seconds and the characteristics of either right BBB or left BBB. A BBB causes a change in the normal conduction of impulses through the ventricles, hence the prolonged interval. BBBs also result in a change in the QRS complex morphology (Figure 7-14).

A right BBB usually produces a QRS that has two distinct R waves (rSR′) in V₁. The second R wave results from delayed conduction through the right ventricle. Normally, the QRS complex is evidence of biventricular depolarization. However, in right BBB, the first R wave is evidence of septal and then left ventricular depolarization, and the second R (R′) wave is evidence of the delayed right ventricular depolarization.

A left BBB usually produces a wide, negative QRS complex in V₁. The widening of the QRS complex occurs because of a delay of the impulse's entry into the left ventricle.

T Wave

The T wave represents ventricular repolarization (see Figure 7-10). Note that a waveform indicating atrial repolarization is not described in this chapter. Such a waveform probably exists, but it is thought to be obscured by the large QRS complex. T-wave amplitude is measured at the center of the waveform and should be no greater than five small boxes, or 5 mm, high. P waves are usually symmetrical, whereas T waves are usually asymmetrical. Changes in T-wave amplitude can indicate electrical disturbances resulting from an electrolyte imbalance or a myocardial infarction. For example, hyperkalemia can cause tall, peaked T waves.

Some students who are beginning to learn dysrhythmia interpretation state that they have problems differentiating the P wave from the T wave. This differentiation should not be a problem because the P wave normally precedes the QRS complex, and the T wave normally follows the QRS complex. In addition, the T wave is usually of greater size and amplitude than the P wave. This is because the atria are smaller muscle masses and therefore produce smaller waveforms than do the larger ventricles.

ST Segment

The ST segment connects the QRS complex to the T wave. The ST segment is usually isoelectric, or flat. However, in some conditions the segment may be depressed (falling below baseline) or elevated (rising above baseline). The point at which the QRS complex ends and the ST segment begins is called the J (junction) point. ST-segment change is measured 0.04 seconds after the J point. It is imperative that ST displacement above or below the isoelectric line be reported and documented. To identify ST-segment elevation, use the PR segment as a reference for baseline. Next, check to see whether the ST segment is level with the PR segment (see Figure 7-10). If the ST segment is above or below the baseline, count the number of small boxes above or below at 0.04 seconds after the J point. A displacement in the ST segment can indicate myocardial ischemia or injury.[1]

ECG monitors should be set to alarm to detect ST-segment changes. Current bedside monitors have the software capability to monitor continuously for ST-segment changes. The leads identified to best monitor for ST-segment changes are both III and V₃ when the ideal continuous 12-lead technology is not available (see Table 7-2 and Clinical Alert: ST Segment Ischemia Monitoring Practice Standards).

QT Interval

The QT interval (QTI) is measured from the beginning of the QRS complex to the end of the T wave (Figure 7-15). This interval measures the time taken for ventricular depolarization and repolarization. The QTI occurs during the relative refractory period where the heart is most vulnerable to any ectopic

Right Bundle Branch Block

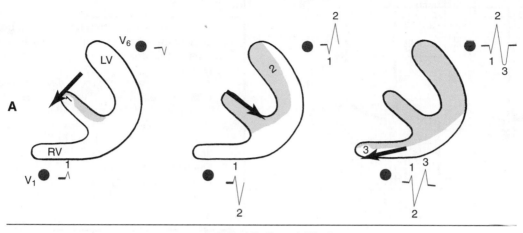

Left Bundle Branch Block

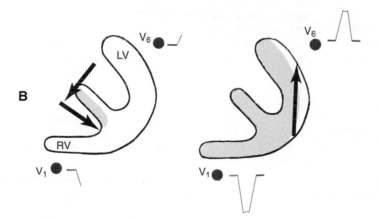

FIGURE 7-14. **A,** Step-by-step sequence of ventricular depolarization in right bundle branch block. **B,** The sequence of ventricular depolarization in left bundle branch block produces a wide QS complex in lead V_1 and a wide R wave in lead V_6. *LV,* Left ventricle; *RV,* right ventricle. *(From Goldberger, A. L. [2006]. Clinical electrocardiography: A simplified approach [7th ed., pp. 74, 77] St. Louis; Mosby.)*

CLINICAL ALERT

ST Segment Monitoring Practice for Ischemia[2]

Class I	Patients in the early phase of acute coronary syndromes (ST-elevation or non–ST-elevation myocardial infarction), unstable angina, rule out myocardial infarction
Class II	Patients at high risk for ischemia or infarction
Class III	ST monitoring unnecessary in patients with left bundle branch block, ventricular-paced rhythms, and patients who are agitated and who have other dysrhythmias that obscure the ST segment

foci. An accurate measure is important, as a prolonged QTI may cause monomorphic ventricular tachycardia, polymorphic ventricular tachycardia (torsades de pointes), and sudden cardiac death.[13] No standard QTI exists. Normal QTIs are based on heart rate. The slower the heart rate is, the longer the normal QTI, and the faster the rate is, the shorter the normal QTI. The QTI is normally longer in females. A QT chart is used to determine the outer limits for normal intervals. Generally, the QTI is less than half the R-R interval (see Figure 7-15). Another method to determine the QTI is the QTc. QTc = QTI divided by the square root of the R to R interval:

$$QTc = \frac{QT}{\sqrt{RR}}$$

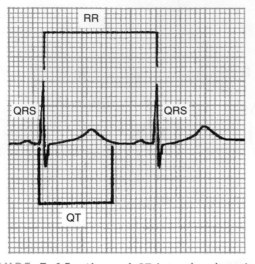

FIGURE 7-15. Abnormal QT interval prolongation in patient taking quinidine. The QT interval (0.6 seconds) is markedly prolonged for the heart rate (65/min) and the QT interval is greater than one half the R-R interval. *(From Goldberger, A. L. [2006]. Clinical electrocardiography: A simplified approach [7th ed., p. 15]. St. Louis: Mosby.)*

CLINICAL ALERT
QT Interval and ECG Monitoring for Detection of Proarrhythmias[2]

Class I	Patients administered an antidysrhythmic drug known to cause *torsades de pointes*
Class II	Patients who require treatment with antipsychotics with possible risk of *torsades de pointes*. Patients who have new-onset bradydysrhythmias (e.g., complete heart block, long sinus pauses). Patients who have severe hypokalemia or hypomagnesemia.
Class III	ECG monitoring unnecessary in patients without baseline QT prolongation

The QTc should be ≤0.44 seconds in men and ≤0.45 seconds in females. (See Clinical Alert: QT Interval and ECG Monitoring for Detection of Proarrhythmias.)

A final waveform that may be noted on the ECG is the U wave. The U wave is a small waveform of unknown origin. If present, it immediately follows the T wave and is of the same deflection (see Figure 7-10). In other words, if the T wave is positive, the U wave is also positive. U waves may be seen in patients with electrolyte imbalances, particularly hypokalemia, and in those who have had a myocar-

1. Is the underlying rhythm regular or irregular? Look at the atrial and ventricular rhythms.
2. What is the atrial rate? What is the ventricular rate?
3. Are there P waves? Do the P waves precede the QRS complex? Are the P waves consistent in appearance? What is the PR interval?
4. What is the QRS complex duration and configuration? Is the QRS complex consistent in appearance?
5. Examine the ST segment and T waves for signs of myocardial injury or ischemia.
6. Using rules for interpretation, what is the rhythm?

dial infarction. However, the U wave is sometimes a normal finding, indicative of late repolarization of the Purkinje fibers; therefore, diagnosis of disease should be dependent on more specific indicators.

SYSTEMATIC INTERPRETATION OF DYSRHYTHMIAS

This section proposes a systematic approach for the analysis and interpretation of dysrhythmias (Box 7-1). Systematic analysis focuses attention on the following areas:
- Assessment of rhythmicity, both atrial and ventricular
- Assessment of rate, both atrial and ventricular
- Assessment of waveform configuration and location
- Assessment of intervals

Rhythmicity

Rhythmicity refers to the regularity or pattern of the heartbeats. P waves are used to establish atrial rhythmicity, and R waves establish ventricular rhythmicity. When an atrial rhythm is perfectly regular, each P wave is an equal distance from the next P wave. When a ventricular rhythm is perfectly regular, each R wave is an equal distance from the next R wave. Systematic interpretation of rhythm strips requires looking at both atrial and ventricular rhythmicities.

Rhythmicity can be established through the use of calipers or paper and pencil, and must be analyzed in both the atria and the ventricles. Establishing atrial rhythmicity requires placing one caliper point

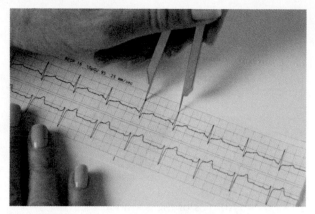

FIGURE 7-16. Establishing ventricular rhythmicity with calipers.

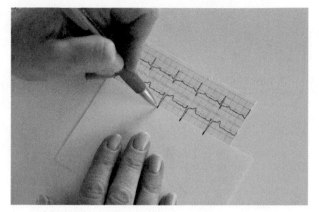

FIGURE 7-17. Establishing ventricular rhythmicity with paper and pencil.

on one P wave and the other caliper point on the next consecutive P wave. The second point is left stationary, and the calipers are flipped over. If the first caliper point lands exactly on the next P wave, the atrial rhythm is perfectly regular. If the point lands one small box or less away from the next P or R wave, the rhythm is essentially regular. If the point lands more than one small box away, the rhythm is considered irregular.

The same process is followed for assessing ventricular rhythmicity, except that the caliper points are placed on R waves. For establishment of ventricular rhythmicity, one caliper point is placed on one R wave and the other caliper point on the next consecutive R wave. The second point is left stationary, and the calipers are flipped over. If the first caliper point lands exactly on the next R wave, the ventricular rhythm is perfectly regular (Figure 7-16).

Rhythmicity can also be established by using paper and pencil. A piece of blank paper is slid over the rhythm strip, and the straight edge is placed along the peak of the P wave to assess atrial rhythmicity or along the peak of the R wave to assess ventricular rhythmicity. With the pencil, the peak of either the P or the R wave is marked on the paper. Without moving the paper, another mark is made on the next P or R wave. The paper is then slid over to the next P or R waveform. If the pencil mark lands exactly on the next P or R wave, the rhythm is perfectly regular. If the pencil mark is one small box or less away from the next P or R wave, the rhythm is essentially regular. If the pencil mark lands more than one small box away from the next P or R wave, the rhythm is irregular (Figure 7-17). Irregular rhythms can be regularly irregular or irregularly irregular. Regularly irregular rhythms have a pattern. Irregularly irregular rhythms have no pattern and no predictability. Atrial fibrillation is an example of an irregularly irregular rhythm.

Rate

The rate equals how fast the heart is depolarizing. Under normal conditions, the atria and the ventricles depolarize at the same rate. However, each can depolarize at a different rate. An important part of systematic analysis is calculation of both the atrial and the ventricular rates. P waves are used to calculate the atrial rate, and R waves are used to calculate the ventricular rate. Rate can be assessed in various ways. Although many methods for assessing heart rate exist, this text addresses the following two popular methods:

1. The rule of 1500 is used to calculate the *exact* rate of a *regular* rhythm. In this method, 2 consecutive P and R waves are located. The number of small boxes between the highest points of 2 consecutive P waves is counted, and that number of small boxes is divided into 1500 to determine the atrial rate in beats per minute. The number of small boxes between the highest points of 2 consecutive R waves is counted, and that number of small boxes is divided into 1500 to determine the ventricular rate (Figure 7-18). This method is accurate only if the rhythm is regular. Charts are available to calculate heart rate based on the rule of 1500.

2. The rule of 10 is a popular method for calculating the *approximate* rate. This method can be used for either regular or irregular rhythms. The rule of 10 is accomplished by counting the number of P or R waves in a 6-second strip and then multiplying that number by 10. This equation yields an approximate heart rate for 60 seconds, or 1 minute. For example, if 6 R waves are found on a 6-second strip, those 6 complexes are multiplied by 10 for an approximate rate of 60 ventricular beats per minute. This method is used when a quick assessment of rate is needed or when a patient is having an irregular rhythm.

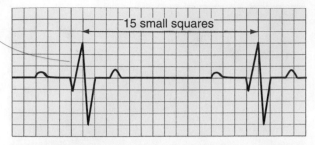

15 small squares

FIGURE 7-18. Calculating ventricular rate with the rule of 1500. Count the number of small boxes between QRS complexes. In this strip there are 15 small squares between QRS complexes; 1500 divided by 15 equals a heart rate of 100. *(From Paul, S., & Hebra, J. D. [1998]. The nurse's guide to cardiac rhythm interpretation: Implications for patient care. Philadelphia: Saunders.)*

Cardiac monitors continuously display heart rates. However, these monitor-calculated rates may be inaccurate and should always be verified by one of the aforementioned rate-calculation methods.

Waveform Configuration and Location

In the systematic analysis of ECG rhythms, configuration and location of the normal P, Q, R, S, and T waveforms are very important.

Configuration

Each cardiac cell, once depolarized, creates a distinct waveform on the ECG rhythm strip. Changes in the shape and appearance of a waveform are often the first clue in the assessment of dysrhythmias. Once a clinician is knowledgeable regarding normal waveform configuration, abnormal waveforms can easily be discerned. No systematic analysis and interpretation are complete without careful study and comparison of each waveform on the 6-second strip, in which both normal and abnormal configurations are assessed.

Location

Location of waveforms is very important for a systematic analysis of dysrhythmias. The normal waveforms P, Q, R, S, and T should occur in their natural order. A P wave should precede each QRS; QRS complexes should be followed by T waves; and T waves should be followed by the P wave of the next complex. In the later discussion of the basic dysrhythmias, several rhythms are characterized by abnormal location or sequencing of waveforms, such as the P waves in complete heart block.

Intervals

A final important aspect of the systematic analysis of rhythm strips is the assessment of the intervals dis-

cussed previously. No rhythm strip analysis is complete and no interpretation is possible without the assessment of the PR, QRS, and QT intervals.

Basic Dysrhythmias

The word *dysrhythmia* refers to an abnormal cardiac rhythm. People also speak of cardiac arrhythmias. The word *arrhythmia* means no rhythm. Therefore, dysrhythmia is a more useful and descriptive term and is used throughout this text.

The basic dysrhythmias are classified by the following anatomical areas:

• Dysrhythmias of the SA node
• Dysrhythmias of the atria
• Dysrhythmias of the AV node
• Dysrhythmias of the ventricles
• AV blocks

A section has been developed for each anatomical area and includes rhythm strip examples of common dysrhythmias. It is important to know the characteristics that make each dysrhythmia unique and recognizable. These characteristics are listed as the criteria for the diagnosis of that particular dysrhythmia. The most critical criteria for diagnosis are listed first.

These critical criteria eliminate the confusion surrounding dysrhythmia analysis and interpretation. The practitioner must learn the criteria for each rhythm and then make a diagnosis based on the criteria.

Those beginning the study of basic electrocardiography should memorize these critical criteria or keep them in a notebook for easy reference. Initially, the task seems overwhelming, and much information must be learned. Focusing on the critical criteria helps one to organize the information for easier analysis and interpretation.

The criteria become easier to remember as the clinician encounters patients with the dysrhythmia. Dysrhythmia analysis and interpretation are skills that develop through practice.

Each dysrhythmia has an impact on the body's ability to maintain a normal hemodynamic status and adequate cardiac output. The hemodynamic effects of each dysrhythmia are discussed. The treatments for the dysrhythmias are discussed at the end of the chapter.

Normal Sinus Rhythm

The most important rhythm of this chapter, normal sinus rhythm, is the rhythm against which all others are compared (Figure 7-19). Without a thorough understanding of the characteristics of a normal rhythm, abnormal rhythms cannot be understood.

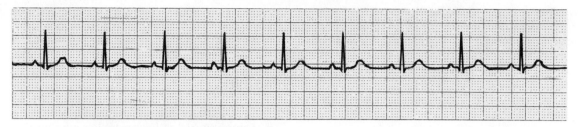

FIGURE 7-19. Normal sinus rhythm. Rhythm strip generated by the AA-700 Rhythm Simulator. *(Courtesy of Armstrong Medical Industries, Lincolnshire, IL.)*

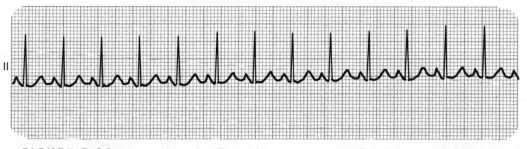

FIGURE 7-20. Sinus tachycardia. *(From Goldberger, A. L. [2006]. Clinical electrocardiography: A simplified approach [7th ed., p. 158]. St. Louis: Mosby.)*

Initial analysis of a rhythm strip should determine whether the rhythm is normal sinus rhythm or a dysrhythmia that requires further analysis.

The SA node is the master pacemaker of the heart. This special group of cardiac cells generates an electrical impulse that is conducted down the normal conduction pathway, thereby depolarizing all cardiac cells.

Critical Criteria for Diagnosis of Normal Sinus Rhythm
- Rhythm is regular or essentially regular.
- Both the atrial rate and the ventricular rate are the same, and that rate is between 60 and 100 beats per minute.
- Upright, small, rounded P waves are present in lead II.
- P waves precede each QRS complex.
- The PR interval is 0.12 to 0.20 seconds in duration.
- The QRS interval is 0.06 to 0.10 seconds in duration.

Hemodynamic Effects. Normal sinus rhythm is the optimal cardiac rhythm for the maintenance of adequate cardiac output.

Dysrhythmias of the Sinoatrial Node

Sinus Tachycardia
Tachycardia is defined as a rapid heart rate. Sinus tachycardia results when the SA node generates more than 100 beats per minute (Figure 7-20). Sinus tachycardia is a normal response to stimulation of the sympathetic nervous system. Sinus tachycardia is also a normal finding in children younger than 6 years. Several other processes can lead to sinus tachycardia including exercise, use of stimulants, increased body temperature, and alterations in fluid status. Therefore, the goal in sinus tachycardia is to identify the cause and correct the underlying problem.

Exercise. Exercise is a natural stimulant to the heart. The heart rate increases as the body's oxygen demand and consumption increase.

Stimulants. Many types of stimulants increase the heart rate. Commonly used and abused drugs such as caffeine and nicotine stimulate the heart rate. Drugs such as decongestants and appetite suppressants can markedly increase the heart rate. Stress and pain also stimulate the sympathetic nervous system, resulting in a faster heart rate.

Increased Body Temperature. Elevation in body temperature causes an increase in heart rate.

Alterations in Fluid Status. Both hypovolemia and hypervolemia can result in an increased heart rate. When the circulating blood volume is low, such as in dehydration or after hemorrhage, the heart rate increases to maintain adequate cardiac output. When the circulating blood volume is increased, the heart rate increases to compensate for the increased blood volume returning to the heart.

Critical Criteria for Diagnosis of Sinus Tachycardia
- Same criteria as for normal sinus rhythm except the heart rate is greater than 100 beats per minute.

Hemodynamic Effects. Sinus tachycardia leads to a decrease in ventricular filling time, less blood volume in the ventricle for the next systole, and consequently lower cardiac output. Another consequence of sinus tachycardia is increased myocardial oxygen consumption. This condition is especially detrimental in the patient with inadequate coronary artery perfusion.

Sinus Bradycardia

Bradycardia is defined as a slowed heart rate. Sinus bradycardia results when the SA node generates fewer than 60 beats per minute (Figure 7-21). Several processes can lead to sinus bradycardia.

Bradycardia as a Normal Finding. Athletes and others who are physically fit may have a slower-than-normal heart rate. Physical conditioning leads to increased strength of the cardiac muscle and therefore increased effectiveness of the heart as a pump. An effective pump can deliver adequate amounts of blood to the body at a slower heart rate.

Increased Vagal Stimulation. The parasympathetic nervous system influences the heart rate through the vagus nerve. When the vagus nerve is stimulated, an impulse is sent to the heart, and the heart rate is decreased. The Valsalva maneuver, as well as coughing, gagging, suctioning, and vomiting, can stimulate the vagus nerve and cause sinus bradycardia.

Drug Effects. Many of the drugs administered to patients with cardiac disease decrease the heart rate. This slowing in heart rate is often a desired result of treatment. When a patient's heart beats at a slower rate, oxygen demands are lessened. When bradycardia occurs as a side effect of a drug, the drug is said to have a negative chronotropic effect (Box 7-2).

SA Node Ischemia. When the patient has myocardial ischemia, injury, or infarction in the area surrounding the SA node, the node may become less able to generate impulses. Bradycardia can result.

Effects of Hypoxemia. Sinus bradycardia can occur during episodes of hypoxemia. Hypoxemia may result from both acute and chronic conditions, or procedures such as endotracheal suctioning.

Increased Intracranial Pressure. Cushing's reflex is a hemodynamic response to increased intracranial pressure. The heart rate decreases and often becomes irregular.

Critical Criteria for Diagnosis of Sinus Bradycardia

* Same criteria as for normal sinus rhythm except that the heart rate is less than 60 beats per minute.

Hemodynamic Effects. Patients demonstrate various hemodynamic responses to sinus bradycardia. Many patients continue to maintain adequate cardiac output, despite a lowered heart rate. This ability to compensate is better in patients with a healthy heart. Other patients experience a decrease in cardiac output and related symptoms and require treatment (Box 7-3).

BOX 7-2   Categories of Drugs

* **Dromotropic:** Drugs that affect speed or velocity of conduction
* **Chronotropic:** Drugs that affect the heart rate
* **Inotropic:** Drugs that affect contractility

BOX 7-3   Symptoms of Decreased Cardiac Output

* Decreased level of consciousness
* Hypotension
* Chest pain
* Shortness of breath
* Pulmonary congestion; crackles
* Syncope

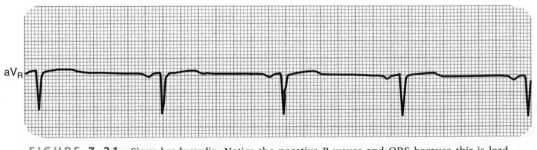

FIGURE 7-21. Sinus bradycardia. Notice the negative P waves and QRS because this is lead aV_R. *(From Goldberger, A. L. [2006]. Clinical electrocardiography: A simplified approach [7th ed., p. 158]. St. Louis: Mosby.)*

Sinus Dysrhythmia

Sinus dysrhythmia is a cardiac rhythm disturbance that is associated with respiration. During inspiration, air is brought into the lungs by a negative intrathoracic pressure. Because the heart lies within the thoracic cavity, this negative intrathoracic pressure causes more blood to return to the right atrium from the superior and inferior vena cava. The heart rate increases to compensate for this increased volume. During expiration, the intrathoracic pressure changes to positive, and air is forced from the lungs. The flow of blood into the heart returns to normal, as does the heart rate.

The ECG tracing demonstrates an alternating pattern of faster heart rate, which is associated with inspiration, then slower heart rate, which is associated with exhalation (Figure 7-22). This rhythm is considered a normal phenomenon; however, certain conditions such as increased intracranial pressure, increased vagal tone, and myocardial ischemia can also cause the rhythm changes.

Critical Criteria for Diagnosis of Sinus Dysrhythmia

- Same criteria as for normal sinus rhythm except for a cyclical increasing and decreasing of the heart rate.
- Changes in heart rate are associated with respiration.
- The rhythm is usually regularly irregular.

Hemodynamic Effects. Significant changes in cardiac output rarely occur with sinus dysrhythmia. It is normally tolerated well unless it is associated with bradycardia or tachycardia.

Sinus Pauses and Sinus Arrest

Occasionally, the SA node temporarily fails as the dominant pacemaker. This failure may be caused by an inability of the sinus node to generate an electrical impulse (sinus arrest), or the impulse may be generated but blocked from exiting the SA node (sinus exit block). The end result is that no atrial or ventricular depolarization occurs for one heartbeat or more. In determining the difference between sinus arrest and sinus block, note that the P-P interval of the underlying rhythm remains undisturbed in sinus block, whereas in sinus arrest the P-P interval is reset by the arrest and changes (Figure 7-23).

This loss of the normal waveform (depolarization) creates a pause of varying length on the ECG tracing. A pause is a long flat line between two beats that exceeds the normal amount of space found between other beats. If this pause is long enough and results in a decrease in the heart rate to less than 60 beats per minute, the AV node or the Purkinje fibers may serve as a backup pacemaker to generate an escape beat. The escape beat is so named because it allows the patient to escape the slowed heart rate, thus preventing further compromise. Sinus arrest or sinus exit block may be caused by enhanced vagal tone, coronary artery disease, or use of certain drugs.

Enhanced Vagal Tone. The Valsalva maneuver, coughing, gagging, or vomiting may temporarily suppress

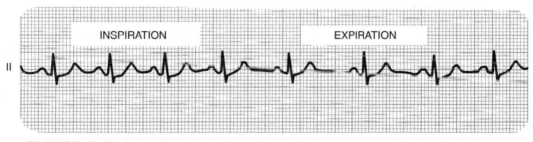

FIGURE 7-22. Sinus dysrhythmia. Normally, the heart rate increases slightly with inspiration and decreases slightly with expiration. *(From Goldberger, A. L. [2006]. Clinical electrocardiography: A simplified approach [7th ed., p. 159]. St. Louis: Mosby.)*

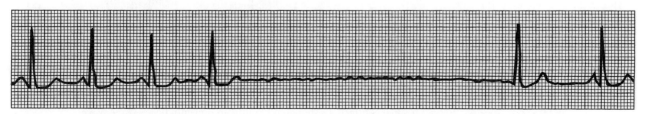

FIGURE 7-23. Sinus arrest/sinus exit block. Note the junctional escape beat at the end of the pause. *(From Huszar, R. J. [2002]. Basic dysrhythmias interpretation & management [3rd ed., p. 104]. St. Louis: Mosby.)*

impulse generation in, or conduction from, the SA node.

Coronary Artery Disease. Coronary artery disease can lead to decreased perfusion of the SA node, resulting in impaired performance.

Effects of Drugs. Administration of various cardiac drugs that slow the heart rate can lead to episodes of sinus arrest and exit block.

Critical Criteria for Diagnosis of Sinus Arrest and Sinus Exit Block

- The heart rate can be normal (60 to 100 beats per minute) or slower than normal.
- Pauses caused by missed beats are noted on the ECG.
- The rhythm is irregular as the result of missed beats.
- Pauses may be interrupted by an escape beat from the AV node or the Purkinje fibers.

Hemodynamic Effects. The hemodynamic effects of sinus arrest or sinus exit block depend on the number of sinus beats that are arrested or blocked, and the length of the resulting pause. Changes in cardiac output depend on how low the heart rate falls. When multiple beats are arrested or blocked, asystole results. The patient ceases to have any cardiac output.

Dysrhythmias of the Atria

Normally, the SA node is the intrinsic pacemaker initiating the heart rate; however, stimuli within the atria can also initiate the heart rate. The term *supraventricular* refers to those nonsinus impulses arising above the ventricle. Increased automaticity in the right atrium, the left atrium, or both atria can result in abnormal cardiac rhythms. Severe conditions can affect automaticity.

Stress. The stress response causes the liberation of epinephrine and norepinephrine, increasing automaticity in the atria. Drugs that stimulate the sympathetic nervous system, such as amphetamines, cocaine, and decongestants, can also cause atrial dysrhythmias.

Electrolyte Imbalances. Electrolyte imbalances, particularly hypokalemia, can result in increased automaticity in the atria.

Hypoxemia. The atria become irritable when they are deprived of oxygen. Patients with chronic obstructive pulmonary disease are at high risk for atrial dysrhythmias.

Injury to the Atria. When the atria are injured, such as with trauma related to cardiac surgery, they are more prone to generate ectopic beats.

Digitalis Toxicity. Administration of digitalis in toxic doses stimulates the myocardium, particularly the atria. Digitalis may convert atrial dysrhythmias to sinus rhythm, or it may only slow the ventricular response to atrial tachycardias. Toxicity should be suspected in patients receiving digoxin who develop atrial tachycardia. Subsequent doses should be withheld until digoxin toxicity is ruled out.

Hypothermia. Lowered body temperature predisposes a patient to atrial dysrhythmias.

Hyperthyroidism. Hyperthyroidism places a patient in a metabolic state that is very similar to the stress response. The hormones produced by the thyroid gland have a stimulating effect on the heart.

Alcohol Intoxication. Alcohol is a cardiac stimulant that has an irritating effect on the heart.

Pericarditis. When the pericardial lining surrounding the heart is inflamed or infected, the atria become more irritable. Atrial dysrhythmias may be one of the first signs of pericarditis.

Premature Atrial Contractions

Premature atrial contractions (PACs) are common dysrhythmias and are usually seen in the setting of normal sinus rhythm (Figure 7-24). PACs are generated very near the SA node. The terms premature atria contractions, atrial premature beats, and atrial extrasystoles are used interchangeably. The generation of PACs near the SA node frequently leads to depolarization of the tissue surrounding the SA node

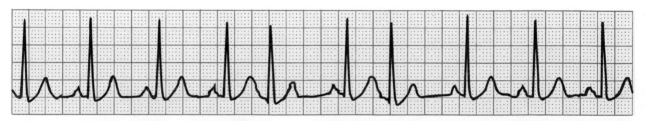

FIGURE 7-24. Premature atrial contractions shown in the fifth and seventh beats. The P wave occurs on the T wave for these premature atrial contractions. *(From Paul, S., & Hebra, J. D. [1998]. The nurse's guide to cardiac rhythm interpretation: Implications for patient care. Philadelphia: Saunders.)*

and causes a pause on the ECG. This pause is usually noncompensatory. Box 7-4 discusses determining compensatory versus noncompensatory pauses (Figure 7-25).

Critical Criteria for Diagnosis of Premature Atrial Contractions

- The ectopic beats are premature.
- The PR interval is usually normal but often differs from the PR interval seen during normal sinus rhythm.
- PACs are usually followed by a noncompensatory pause.
- The P wave of the premature beat may be found in the T wave just before the premature beat. When this occurs, the T wave of the preceding beat is distorted. The T wave of the beat preceding the premature beat can be compared with other normal T waves on the ECG strip.

Occasionally, a PAC is generated and conducted down to the AV node just after a normal impulse has been conducted. The PAC arrives at the AV node when the bundle of His and its branches are refractory to, or unable to conduct, the premature impulse. The impulse is blocked and is not allowed to enter the ventricle. This blocked PAC can be detected as a pause on the ECG. Before the pause, a different-looking T wave can usually be noted. The unusual T wave is caused by the premature P wave of the PAC imposed on the normal T wave (Figure 7-26).

Critical Criteria for Diagnosis of Blocked Premature Atrial Contractions

- A pause is noted on the ECG tracing.
- A premature P wave, which differs from the normal P wave, is found in the T wave or just after the T wave of the last normal beat before the pause.

Hemodynamic Effects. PACs do not usually alter cardiac output. However, many patients report having pal-pitations. Increasing numbers of PACs may herald the development of atrial fibrillation or flutter.

Atrial Tachycardia

Atrial tachycardia is a rapid rhythm that arises from the atria muscle. Because of the fast rate, atrial tachycardia can be a life-threatening dysrhythmia. It is usually seen in patients with cardiac disease; however, it may also occur in healthy patients. In some instances, increased numbers of PACs precede the onset of atrial tachycardia. Sometimes the atria generate impulses more rapidly than the AV node can conduct while still in the refractory phase from

---

BOX 7-4 Compensatory versus Noncompensatory Pause

- A rhythm strip with a premature beat is analyzed using calipers or paper and pencil.
- Two consecutive normal beats are located just before the premature beat, and the caliper points or pencil marks are placed on the R wave of each normal beat.
- The calipers are flipped over, or the paper is slid over, to where the next normal beat should have occurred. The premature beat occurs early.
- Now, with care taken not to lose placement, the calipers are flipped, or the paper is slid over, one more time. If the point of the calipers or the mark on the paper lands exactly on the next normal beat's R wave, the sinus node compensated for the one premature beat and kept its normal rhythm (Figure 7-25).
- If the caliper point or pencil mark does not land on the next normal beat's R wave, then the sinus node did not compensate and had to establish a new rhythm, resulting in a noncompensatory pause.

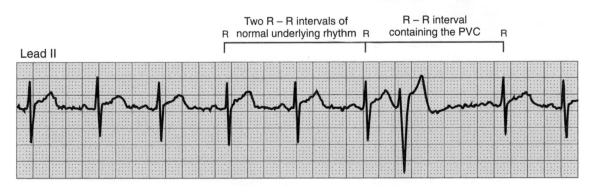

FIGURE 7-25. Compensatory pause. *PVC,* Premature ventricular contraction. *(From Paul, S., & Hebra, J. D. [1998]. The nurse's guide to cardiac rhythm interpretation: Implications for patient care. Philadelphia: Saunders.)*

the previous impulse, and these impulses are not transmitted to the ventricles. This refractoriness serves as a safety mechanism to prevent the ventricles from depolarizing and contracting too rapidly. The AV node may block impulses in a set pattern, such as every second, third, or fourth beat. However, if the ventricles respond to every ectopic atrial impulse, it is called 1:1 conduction, one P wave for each QRS complex.

Some clinicians refer to an atrial tachydysrhythmia as a *supraventricular tachycardia* (Box 7-5). When the patient experiences tachycardia, the nurse must assess the patient for symptoms of low cardic output (Figure 7-27).

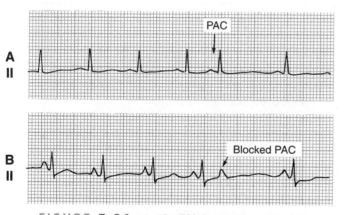

A II

B II

FIGURE 7-26. A, The fifth beat is an atrial premature contraction. **B,** Blocked premature atrial contraction (PAC). *(From Goldberger, A. L. [2006]. Clinical electrocardiography: A simplified approach [7th ed., p. 164]. St. Louis: Mosby.)*

BOX 7-5 Supraventricular Tachycardia

- **Definition:** Supraventricular tachycardia describes any tachycardia that originates from a site above the ventricles, usually the atria, at a rate of greater than 150 beats per minute.
- **Paroxysmal:** Refers to supraventricular tachycardia that starts suddenly.

Two other types of atrial tachycardia are *AV nodal reentrant tachycardia* and *atrial ventricular reentrant tachycardia*. An example of AV nodal reentrant tachycardia is atrial flutter/atrial fibrillation. An example of atrial ventricular reentrant tachycardia is Wolff-Parkinson-White (WPW) syndrome (Figure 7-28). WPW syndrome is related to the presence of a bypass tract that connects the atria and ventricles, "bypassing" the AV node. WPW syndrome is discussed in more advanced ECG courses.

Critical Criteria for Diagnosis of Atrial Tachycardia
- The rhythm is absolutely regular.
- The heart rate is usually 150 to 250 beats per minute.
- It occurs suddenly, usually without warning.
- P waves, if present, usually merge with the preceding T waves, thereby altering the appearance of the T wave.
- AV block that may be of a fixed or varying degree is present.
- The width of the QRS complex is usually normal.
  Hemodynamic Effects. The hemodynamic effects of atrial tachycardia can vary from none to shock. The faster the heart rate, the less time there is for ventricular filling. At faster rates, cardiac output can be severely compromised.

Wolff-Parkinson with Preexcitation Patterns (Figure 7-29)
- The QRS complex may be widened, giving the appearance of a bundle branch block.
- The PR is shortened (but not always <0.12 seconds) because of ventricular preexcitation.
- The QRS upstroke may be slurred or notched, which is called a delta wave and may be more visible in some leads than others.
- If a patient has atrial fibrillation with WPW, the rhythm will be irregular.

Wandering Atrial Pacemaker
Wandering atrial pacemaker is a dysrhythmia characterized by varied pacemaking activity throughout the atria. For the criteria of this rhythm to be met,

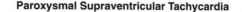

Paroxysmal Supraventricular Tachycardia

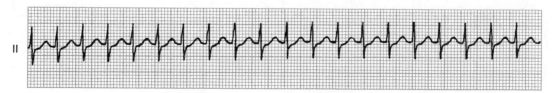

II

FIGURE 7-27. Notice the marked regularity of rhythm in this paroxysmal supraventricular tachycardia (PSVT). The rate is 170 beats per minute. *(From Goldberger, A. L. [2006]. Clinical electrocardiography: A simplified approach [7th ed., p. 168]. St. Louis: Mosby.)*

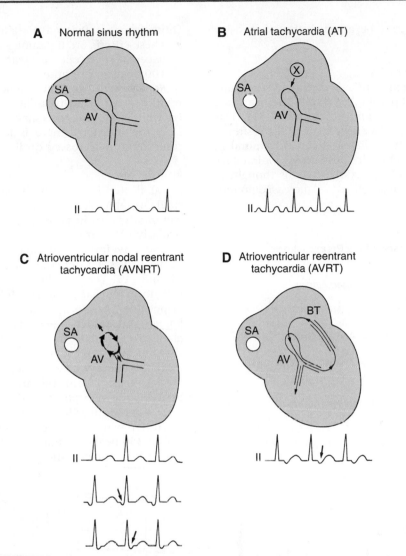

A Normal sinus rhythm

B Atrial tachycardia (AT)

C Atrioventricular nodal reentrant tachycardia (AVNRT)

D Atrioventricular reentrant tachycardia (AVRT)

FIGURE 7-28. A, Normal sinus rhythm. **B,** With atrial tachycardia (AT), a focus (X) outside the sinoatrial (SA) node fires off automatically at a rapid rate. **C,** With atrioventricular (AV) nodal reentrant tachycardia (AVNRT), the cardiac stimulus originates as a wave of excitation that spins around the AV nodal (junctional) area. As a result, retrograde P waves may be buried in the QRS or appear immediately before or just after the QRS complex *(arrows)* because of nearly simultaneous activation of the atria and ventricles. **D,** A similar type of reentrant (circus movement) mechanism in Wolff-Parkinson-White syndrome. This mechanism is referred to as atrioventricular reentrant tachycardia (AVRT). Note the P wave in lead II somewhat after the QRS complex. *(From Goldberger, A. L. [2006]. Clinical electrocardiography: A simplified approach [7th ed., p. 166]. St. Louis: Mosby.)*

at least three sites of atrial pacemaking must be documented.

When impulses are generated from different pacemaking sites, different P-wave morphologies are present on the ECG. The P waves look different in shape, slope, or orientation. P waves in wandering atrial pacemaker can be upright, inverted, flat, pointed, notched, and/or slanted in different directions. The PR interval varies because the impulses originate from different locations within the atria,

taking various times to reach the AV node (Figure 7-30).

Critical Criteria for Diagnosis of Wandering Atrial Pacemaker
- The rhythm is usually irregular.
- The heart rate is less than 100 beats per minute.
- At least three different-looking P waves are seen.
- The PR intervals vary.

Hemodynamic Effects. Wandering atrial pacemaker may result in less effective atrial depolarization.

Ventricular filling may be affected, thus decreasing cardiac output.

Multifocal Atrial Tachycardia

Multifocal atrial tachycardia is essentially the same as wandering atrial pacemaker, except the heart rate exceeds 100 beats per minute (Figure 7-31). This type of atrial tachycardia arises from multiple sites of atrial stimulation. It is almost exclusively found in the patient with chronic obstructive pulmonary disease. The cause of the dysrhythmia is thought to be right atrial dilation secondary to increased pulmonary pressures.[7]

Critical Criteria for Diagnosis of Multifocal Atrial Tachycardia

- These criteria are the same as for wandering atrial pacemaker except the heart rate is greater than 100 beats per minute.

Hemodynamic Effects. The hemodynamic effects of multifocal atrial tachycardia are the same as those for wandering atrial pacemaker. The faster the heart rate, the less time there is for ventricular filling, resulting in a decreased cardiac output.

Atrial Flutter

Atrial flutter is a dysrhythmia that arises from a single irritable focus in the atria. Atrial flutter is most commonly seen in patients with heart disease, particularly valvular disease.[1]

The waveforms associated with atrial flutter are flutter waves. Flutter waves are best seen in leads II, III, and aVF. They are biphasic: the first part of the waveform is negative, and it is followed by an upright, or positive, waveform (Figure 7-32). This waveform has an appearance much like the teeth of a saw's blade. To calculate the atrial flutter rate, find the sharpest point of two consecutive flutter waves. Mark the points with a pencil mark or with the point of a caliper. Count the number of small boxes between the two points and divide the number of small boxes into 1500.

Flutter waves are usually generated at a rate of 250 to 350 beats per minute with perfect regularity. The irritable focus in the atria never stops firing. This

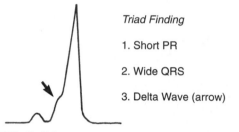

Wolff-Parkinson-White Preexcitation

Triad Finding

1. Short PR

2. Wide QRS

3. Delta Wave (arrow)

FIGURE 7-29. Preexcitation via the bypass tract in the Wolff-Parkinson White (WPW) pattern is associated with a triad finding. *(From Goldberger, A. L. [2006]. Clinical electrocardiography: A simplified approach [7th ed., p. 148]. St. Louis: Mosby.)*

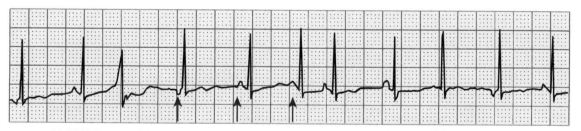

FIGURE 7-30. Wandering atrial pacemaker. Note the varying P-wave morphologies. *(From Paul, S., & Hebra, J. D. [1998]. The nurse's guide to cardiac rhythm interpretation: Implications for patient care. Philadelphia: Saunders.)*

Multifocal Atrial Tachycardia

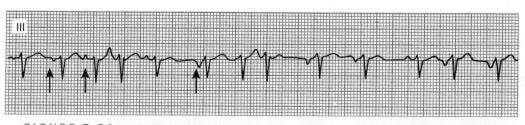

FIGURE 7-31. Multifocal atrial tachycardia. *(From Goldberger, A. L. [2006]. Clinical electrocardiography: A simplified approach [7th ed., p. 241]. St. Louis: Mosby.)*

means that the flutter waves continue throughout the ECG strip and often alter the appearance of the QRS complex and the T wave (Figure 7-33). The AV node is physiologically unable to conduct all these impulses. Therefore, as in paroxysmal atrial tachycardia, the AV node selectively conducts a given number of flutter waves down to the ventricle. For example, if the atrial focus generates 300 beats per minute, the AV node may be able to conduct every third beat. This would be a 3:1 ratio of conduction, and the resultant ventricular rate would be 100 beats per minute (300 ÷ 3 = 100).

Critical Criteria for Diagnosis of Atrial Flutter

- The atrial rate is usually 250 to 350 beats per minute. The ventricular rate varies with the degree of AV block.
- The onset is usually rapid.

Hemodynamic Effects. The hemodynamic effects of atrial flutter are dependent on the ventricular rate, sometimes called the *ventricular response*. Patients who sustain atrial flutter with a fast ventricular response often have symptoms of low cardiac output. Patients whose AV nodes are blocking greater numbers of the atrial impulses, and who maintain a heart rate between 60 and 100 beats per minute, tend to maintain a more normal cardiac output.

Atrial Fibrillation

Atrial fibrillation is the most common clinically important rhythm disturbance encountered with respect to treatment, morbidity, mortality, and eco-

nomic effects on society. This dysrhythmia is characterized by erratic impulse formation throughout the atria, classically described as "irregularly irregular." Widespread irritability and increased automaticity lead to a chaotic state of impulse formation (Figure 7-34). Atrial fibrillation produces a wavy baseline with no discernible P wave. As the AV node is bombarded with rapidly fired atrial impulses, it conducts impulses to the ventricles in an unpredictable fashion, and the result is an irregularly irregular ventricular rhythm. (See Evidence-Based Practice feature.)

As the AV node attempts to regulate the movement of impulses into the ventricle, it may conduct an atrial impulse before the bundle of His and the branches are able to conduct. The right bundle branch requires a longer time to repolarize than the left bundle. If the right bundle branch is still repolarizing, the impulse must cross the ventricular septum and move down the left bundle branch first and then crosses back over the septum and depolarizes the right ventricle. Depolarization of the ventricles takes longer, resulting in a widened QRS complex. When this event occurs, the impulse is said to be aberrantly conducted (Figure 7-35).

In atrial fibrillation, aberrantly conducted beats are referred to as *Ashman's beats*. Ashman's beats are more likely to occur when an atrial impulse arrives at the AV node just after a previously conducted impulse (Figure 7-36). Ashman's beats are often seen when the rate changes from slower to faster, which is referred to as a long-short cycle. Ashman's beats are not clinically significant.

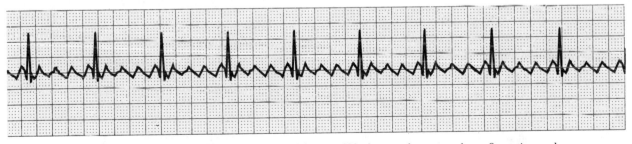

FIGURE 7-32. Atrial flutter with a fixed degree of block. Note the sawtooth configuration and the negative orientation of the flutter waves. Rhythm generated by the AA-700 Rhythm Simulator. *(Courtesy of Armstrong Medical Industries, Lincolnshire, IL.)*

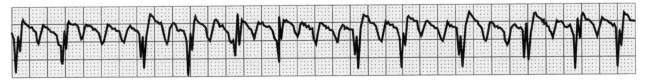

FIGURE 7-33. Atrial flutter with varying degrees of block. *(From Paul, S., & Hebra, J. D. [1998]. The nurse's guide to cardiac rhythm interpretation: Implications for patient care. Philadelphia: Saunders.)*

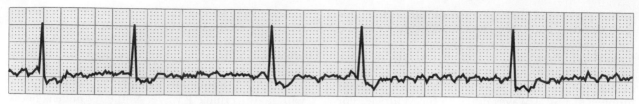

FIGURE 7-34. Atrial fibrillation. *(From Paul, S., & Hebra, J. D. [1998].* The nurse's guide to cardiac rhythm interpretation: Implications for patient care. *Philadelphia: Saunders.)*

EVIDENCE-BASED PRACTICE

PROBLEM

After cardiac surgery, there is a significant risk of dysrhythmias, especially atrial fibrillation. Interventions are rendered to reduce this risk.

REFERENCE

Shiga, T., Wajima, Z., & Inoue, T., et al. (2004). Magnesium prophylaxis for arrhythmias after cardiac surgery: A meta-analysis of randomized controlled trials. *American Journal of Medicine, 117,* 325-333.

QUESTION

What is the effect of prophylactic treatment with magnesium on reducing dysrhythmias after cardiac surgery?

EVIDENCE

Atrial dysrhythmias occur in 11% to 40% of patients after coronary artery bypass graft surgery and 50% of patients after valvular surgery. Ventricular dysrhythmias are rare, but if they occur, the prognosis is poor. The authors searched the literature from 1966-2003 for all randomized controlled trials in any language that tested the effects of prophylactic magnesium compared with those of treatments without magnesium, on dysrhythmias after cardiac surgery.

Meta-analysis confirmed that prophylactic magnesium reduced the risk of supraventricular dysrhythmias after cardiac surgery by 23%, atrial fibrillation by 29%, and ventricular dysrhythmias by 48%. Hypomagnesemia occurs after cardiac surgery because of the use of the cardiopulmonary bypass machine and diuretics that deplete the body of magnesium.

IMPLICATIONS FOR NURSING

This meta-analysis is important to nurses caring for cardiac patients. The findings show outcomes and risk considerations. Other medications used to treat these dysrhythmias are associated with more side effects; therefore prophylactic magnesium is a reasonable approach. Magnesium alteration has no effect on length of stay, myocardial infarction, or mortality.

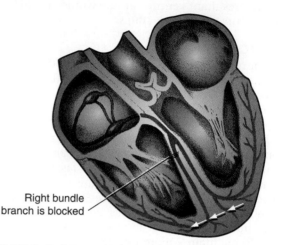

Right bundle branch is blocked

FIGURE 7-35. Aberrancy is most likely to result when the right bundle branch blocks. The impulse must depolarize the left side of the heart first. The impulse then crosses the septum and abnormally depolarizes the right side of the heart. This results in a widened QRS complex.

One complication of atrial fibrillation is thromboembolism. The blood that collects in the atria is agitated by fibrillation, and normal clotting is accelerated. Small thrombi, called *mural* thrombi, begin to form along the walls of the atria. These clots may dislodge, resulting in pulmonary embolism or stroke.

For this reason, if a patient has been in atrial fibrillation for less than 48 hours and if the blood pressure is stable, the patient should receive anticoagulation therapy before any attempt is made to convert atrial fibrillation to normal sinus rhythm (see Clinical Alert). Intravenous heparin or subcutaneous low molecular weight heparin is administered for anticoagulation. If atrial fibrillation persists or is recurrent, long-term warfarin (Coumadin) therapy is usually prescribed to diminish the risk of thromboembolism.[11,14,15]

Critical Criteria for Diagnosis of Atrial Fibrillation

- An irregularly irregular ventricular rhythm exists.
- A wavy baseline exists with no discernible P waves.

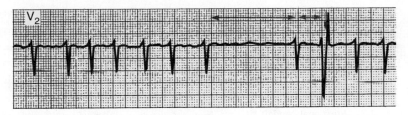

FIGURE 7-36. Atrial fibrillation. Note Ashman's beat, following a long-short cycle. *(From Laver, J. [1992]. Electrical activity of the heart and dysrhythmias. In C. Guzzetta & B. Dossey [Eds.], Cardiovascular nursing: Body mind tapestry. St. Louis: Mosby.)*

CLINICAL ALERT

In patients older than 65 years, administration of rate control drugs has resulted in better outcomes than those achieved with cardioversion.[11,14,15]

- The width of the QRS complex may vary between normal and slightly widened.
- Ashman's beats may be present.

Hemodynamic Effects. In atrial fibrillation, the atria are never fully depolarized and therefore do not contract. Therefore, patients lose atrial kick. The hemodynamic effects of atrial fibrillation also relate to the ventricular response time. Patients with markedly slower or faster rates are more likely to experience a decrease in cardiac output.

Dysrhythmias of the Atrioventricular Node

Junctional Rhythm

Dysrhythmias of the AV node are called *junctional rhythms*. The term nodal rhythms is also used. The AV node is located in the middle of the heart between the atria and the ventricles. The tissue immediately surrounding the AV node is referred to as junctional tissue. Both the AV node itself and the junctional tissue are capable of generating cardiac rhythms.

The following are the two primary causes of junctional rhythms:

1. Dysrhythmias can originate in the AV node or the junctional tissue surrounding it. When a singular beat or ongoing rhythm originates in an area other than the sinus node, that beat or rhythm is considered *ectopic*. Ectopic means out of the normal place. Ectopic rhythms are usually caused by increased automaticity. Increased automaticity is commonly caused by stress or the use of nicotine or caffeine. It can also result from myocardial ischemia, injury, or infarction. Digitalis toxicity can produce all forms of junctional rhythms. At toxic levels, digitalis can suppress the heart rate or can act as a myocardial stimulant.

2. Escape rhythms can be generated from the AV node should the sinus node fail. The AV node is capable of generating 40 to 60 beats per minute as a backup pacemaker.

Several ECG changes are common to all the junctional dysrhythmias. These changes include P-wave abnormalities and PR-interval changes.

P-Wave Changes. Because of the location of the AV node—in the center of the heart—impulses generated may be conducted forward, backward, or both. Like ripples from a rock thrown into a pool of water, the impulse can radiate both forward and backward. With the potential of forward, backward, or bidirectional impulse conduction, three different P waveforms may be associated with junctional rhythms:

1. When the AV node impulse moves forward, *P waves may be absent* because the impulse enters the ventricle first. The atria receives the wave of depolarization at the same time as the ventricles; thus due to the larger muscle mass of the ventricles, no P wave exists (Figure 7-37).

2. When the AV node impulse is conducted backward, the impulse enters the atria first. Conduction back toward the atria allows for at least partial depolarization of the atria. When depolarization occurs in a backward fashion, an inverted P wave is created. Once the atria have been depolarized, the impulse then moves down the bundle of His and depolarizes both ventricles normally (Figure 7-38). A short PR interval (<0.12 second) is noted.

3. When the impulse is conducted in both a forward and a backward fashion, *P waves may be present after the QRS*. In this type of conduction, the impulse first moves into the ventricles, depolarizing them and creating a QRS complex. Because the impulse is also conducted backward, some atrial depolarization occurs, and a late P wave is noted after the QRS complex (Figure 7-39).

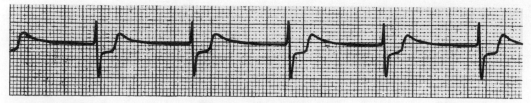

FIGURE 7-37. Junctional (nodal) rhythm. Note absence of P waves. *(From Lewis, S., Collier, I. C., & Heitkemper, M. M. [1996]. Medical-surgical nursing: Assessment and management of clinical problems [4th ed.]. St. Louis: Mosby.)*

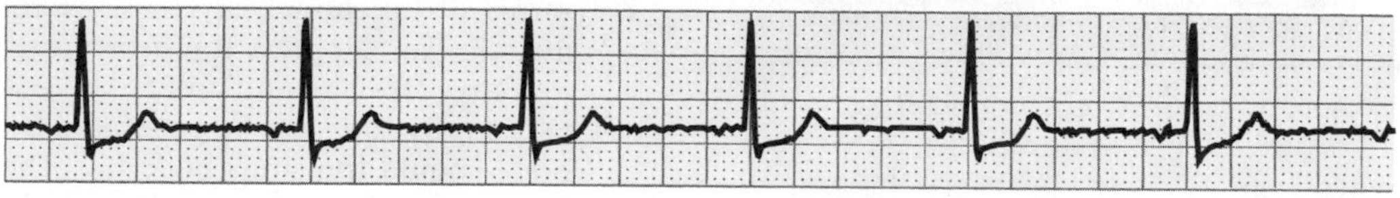

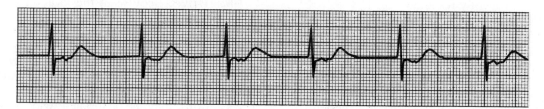

FIGURE 7-38. Junctional (nodal) rhythm. Note the inverted P wave and the shortened PR interval. *(From Paul, S., & Hebra, J. D. [1998]. The nurse's guide to cardiac rhythm interpretation: Implications for patient care. Philadelphia: Saunders.)*

FIGURE 7-39. Junctional (nodal) rhythm. Note the P waves after the QRS complex. *(From Patel, J., McGowan, S., & Moody, L. [1989]. Arrhythmias: Detection, treatment, and cardiac drugs. Philadelphia: Saunders.)*

Critical Criteria for Diagnosis of Junctional Rhythm

- The rhythm is usually regular.
- The heart rate is 40 to 60 beats per minute.
- P waves may be absent, inverted, or follow the QRS complex.
- The PR interval is at the low end of normal or shorter than normal.
- The QRS complex is of normal width.

Hemodynamic Effects. In junctional rhythms, atrial depolarization (atrial kick) is usually less effective or absent, resulting in decreased ventricular filling. Diminished cardiac output may occur.

Accelerated Junctional Rhythm and Junctional Tachycardia

The normal intrinsic rate for the AV node and junctional tissue is 40 to 60 beats per minute, but rates can accelerate. Accelerated junctional rhythms have a rate between 60 and 100 beats per minute, whereas junctional tachycardia (rates faster than 100 beats per minute) can reach the upper rate capability for the AV node of 150 (Figure 7-40).

Critical Criteria for Diagnosis of Accelerated Junctional and Junctional Tachycardia

These criteria are the same as for junctional rhythm except for the following:

- The heart rate is between 60 and 100 beats per minute for an accelerated junctional rhythm.
- The heart rate is between 100 and 150 beats per minute for a junctional tachycardia.

Hemodynamic Effects. The hemodynamic effects of junctional tachycardia are the same as for a junctional rhythm. However, ventricular filling may be further compromised by the faster heart rate. Conversely, the acceleration in heart rate may actually improve cardiac output if stroke volume is decreased.

Premature Junctional Contractions

Irritable areas in the AV node and junctional tissue can generate beats that are earlier than the next expected beat (Figure 7-41). These premature beats

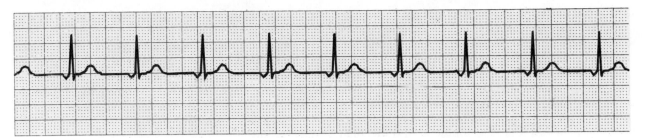

FIGURE 7-40. Junctional tachycardia. Note the short PR interval and heart rate of 70 beats per minute. Rhythm generated by the AA-700 Rhythm Simulator. *(Courtesy of Armstrong Medical Industries, Lincolnshire, IL.)*

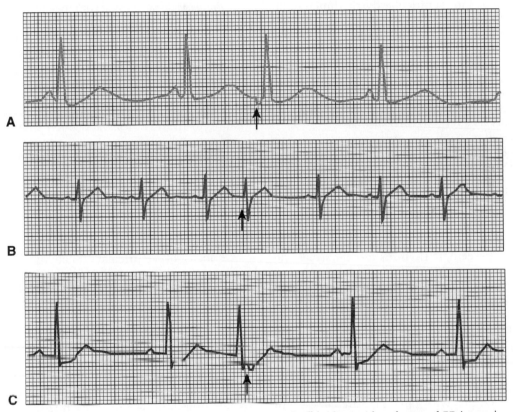

FIGURE 7-41. Premature junctional contractions. **A,** Third beat with a shortened PR interval and an inverted P wave. **B,** Fourth beat, no P waves visible. **C,** Third beat with a retrograde P wave. *(From Conover, M. B. [1996]. Understanding electrocardiography [7th ed.]. St. Louis: Mosby.)*

most often occur in normal sinus rhythm and temporarily upset rhythmicity.

Either a compensatory or noncompensatory pause may occur after a premature junctional contraction. The closer the site of premature impulse generation is to the sinus node, the less likely it is that the SA node will compensate. When a premature impulse fires close to the SA node, a wave of depolarization moves backward toward the sinus node and excites the tissue of the SA node. After

depolarization has occurred, the sinus node requires time for repolarization before generating the next beat. This delay usually creates a noncompensatory pause on the ECG.

Critical Criteria for Diagnosis of Premature Junctional Contractions

- The ectopic beats are premature.
- P waves may be absent or inverted or may occur after the QRS complex

- If a P wave is present before the QRS complex, the PR interval is usually shorter than normal.
- Premature junctional contractions are usually followed by a noncompensatory pause.

Hemodynamic Effects. Premature junctional contractions do not usually alter the cardiac output. However, many patients report having palpitations. Increasing numbers of premature junctional contractions may herald the development of junctional tachycardia.

Dysrhythmias of the Ventricle

Because impulses for ventricular dysrhythmias originate in the lower portion of the heart, depolarization occurs in an abnormal way. The impulse must travel in a backward or sideways fashion to depolarize the ventricles. This abnormal flow of electricity lengthens the time interval in which depolarization of the ventricles occurs. The result is a widened QRS complex. The QRS interval extends beyond the normal interval of 0.06 to 0.10 seconds.

Depolarization from abnormal ventricular beats rarely moves as far backward as the atria. Therefore, most ventricular dysrhythmias have no evident P waves. However, if a P wave is present, it is usually seen in the T wave of the following beat. Two types of ventricular dysrhythmias, ectopic and escape, exist:

1. Ectopic means occurring outside of the normal place. The ectopic rhythms are abnormal and disturb or override the normal sinus rhythm. These ectopic rhythms are capable of firing at fast rates and may be life-threatening.
2. The escape rhythm is seen when the Purkinje backup pacemaker fires if should the SA and AV nodes fail. The Purkinje fibers can generate an escape rhythm of 15 to 40 beats per minute. Although this is a very slow intrinsic rate, many patients are able to maintain an adequate cardiac output with rates that are close to 40 beats per minute.

Severe conditions are associated with ventricular dysrhythmias.[1]

Myocardial Ischemia, Injury, and Infarction. When blood supply is decreased to an area of the ventricle, the blood-deprived area becomes irritable and is more likely to have increased automaticity. Prolonged ischemia can lead to permanent injury to the area, creating an even greater potential for ectopic impulse formation.

Hypokalemia. Low serum potassium levels facilitate the development of ventricular dysrhythmias. As discussed earlier, potassium plays an important role in the normal depolarization/repolarization process.

Hypomagnesemia. Low serum magnesium levels have been correlated with the development of ventricular dysrhythmias, in particular torsades de pointes.[1] Torsades de pointes is a type of ventricular tachycardia in which the QRS complex changes polarity from negative to positive, manifesting as twisting of the points.

Hypoxemia. Inadequate amounts of oxygen are irritating to the ventricles and often stimulate ectopic and escape beats.

Acid-Base Imbalances. Both alkalosis and acidosis can stimulate ventricular ectopy.

Premature Ventricular Contractions

Premature ventricular contractions (PVCs) are a common ventricular dysrhythmia. The beats can be generated anywhere in the ventricles. When only one focus of ventricular irritability exists, all the ectopic beats appear the same. Ventricular beats coming from one area are called *unifocal PVCs* (Figure 7-42). Because PVCs are generated in the ventricles, a considerable distance from the SA node, the SA node is usually able to compensate for the premature beat. This compensation is noted on the ECG tracing as a compensatory pause that follows the PVC.

There can also be multiple areas, or foci, of ventricular irritability. When ventricular ectopic beats come from multiple areas, each QRS looks different (Figure 7-43). These PVCs are called *multifocal.*

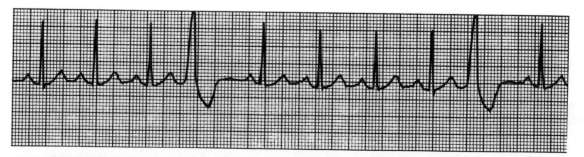

FIGURE 7-42. Unifocal premature ventricular contractions. *(From Patel, J., McGowan, S., & Moody, L. [1989].* Arrhythmias: Detection, treatment, and cardiac drugs. *Philadelphia: Saunders.)*

PVCs may also occur in a predictable pattern. For example, PVCs may occur every other beat, every third beat, or every fourth beat. When PVCs occur every other beat, the pattern is referred to as *bigeminy* (Figure 7-44). When the PVCs occur every third beat, the pattern is called *trigeminy*, and every fourth beat, *quadrigeminy*. PVCs can also occur sequentially. Two PVCs in a row are termed a *couplet* when the morphology of each beat is different, whereas they are termed a *pair* when the morphology is similar (Figure 7-45). Three PVCs in a row are termed a *triplet* or *salvo* (Figure 7-46).

From the peak of the T wave through the downslope of the T wave is considered the *vulnerable period*. If a PVC is generated during this time, ventricular tachycardia may occur. This is referred to as the *R-on-T phenomenon*; the R wave of a PVC falls on the T wave of a normal beat (Figure 7-47). The R-on-T phenomenon occurs frequently in the clinical setting.

Isolated (<6 PVCs per minute) PVCs are rarely treated. Rather, PVCs are considered signs of underlying disease that requires attention—for example, hypoxemia, ischemia, or electrolyte imbalance. PVCs

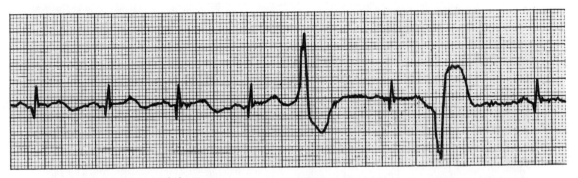

FIGURE 7-43. Multifocal premature ventricular contractions. Note the compensatory pause. *(From Patel, J., McGowan, S., & Moody, L. [1989]. Arrhythmias: Detection, treatment, and cardiac drugs. Philadelphia: Saunders.)*

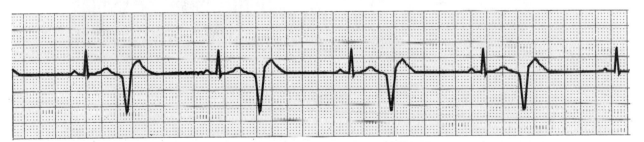

FIGURE 7-44. Premature ventricular contractions in a bigeminal pattern. Rhythm strip generated by the AA-700 Rhythm Simulator. *(Courtesy of Armstrong Medical Industries, Lincolnshire, IL.)*

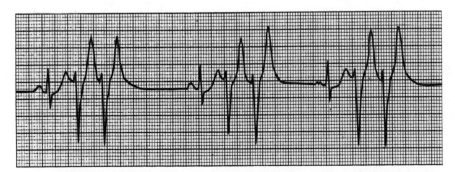

FIGURE 7-45. Two premature ventricular contractions in a row (pair). *(From Patel, J., McGowan, S., & Moody, L. [1989]. Arrhythmias: Detection, treatment, and cardiac drugs. Philadelphia: Saunders.)*

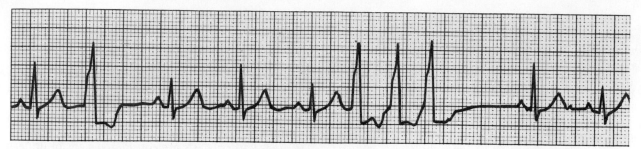

FIGURE 7-46. Three premature ventricular contractions in a row (triplet). *(From Patel, J., McGowan, S., & Moody, L. [1989]. Arrhythmias: Detection, treatment, and cardiac drugs. Philadelphia: Saunders.)*

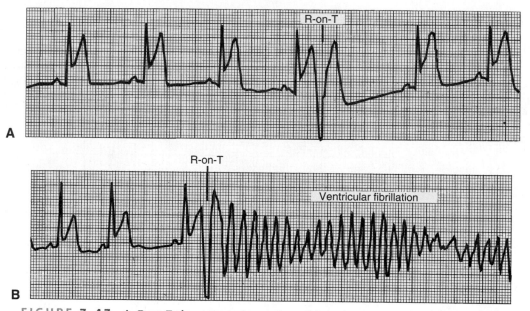

FIGURE 7-47. A, R-on-T phenomenon in a patient with an acute myocardial infarction. **B,** In the same patient, the R-on-T phenomenon causes ventricular fibrillation. *(From Conover, M. B. [1996]. Understanding electrocardiography [7th ed.]. St. Louis: Mosby.)*

in the patient with myocardial infarction are treated when associated with such symptoms as angina or hypotension.[1]

PVCs, couplets, the R-on-T phenomenon, and multifocal ventricular ectopy should be considered warning dysrhythmias. The nurse should assist in identifying causative factors and be alert for the development of worsening dysrhythmias.

Critical Criteria for Diagnosis of Premature Ventricular Contractions

- The rhythm is irregular as a result of the premature beats. However, the premature beats may occur in a regular pattern.
- The ectopic beat occurs prematurely, before the next anticipated sinus beat.
- P waves are usually absent before the ectopic beat.
- The premature beat is usually followed by a compensatory pause.

- The QRS complex of the premature beat is wider than 0.12 seconds.
- The T wave of the PVC is in the opposite direction of the QRS of the PVC. In other words, if the QRS complex of the PVC is upright, or positive, then the T wave is downward, or negative (see Figure 7-42).
- PVCs may be unifocal or multifocal and may occur in tandem as couplets or triplets.

Hemodynamic Effects. The hemodynamic effects associated with PVCs are varied. Some patients may be asymptomatic, whereas others may report having palpitations and lightheadedness. Symptoms usually worsen with an increase in the number of PVCs.

Ventricular Tachycardia

Ventricular tachycardia is a rapid, life-threatening dysrhythmia that originates in the ventricles. It is characterized by at least three premature ventricular

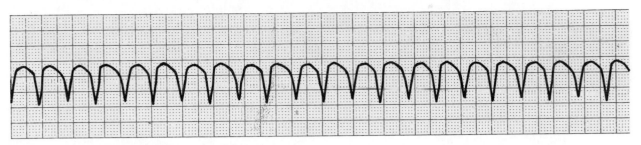

FIGURE 7-48. Ventricular tachycardia. Rhythm strip generated by the AA-700 Rhythm Simulator. *(Courtesy of Armstrong Medical Industries, Lincolnshire, IL.)*

complexes in a row. Ventricular tachycardia occurs at a rate greater than 100 beats per minute. The site of irritability in the ventricle is usually unifocal; therefore, all waveforms usually appear the same. Depolarization of the ventricles occurs in an abnormal way, producing a widened QRS complex (Figure 7-48).

The wave of depolarization associated with ventricular tachycardia rarely reaches the atria. Therefore, P waves are usually absent. If P waves are present, they have no association with the QRS complex. The sinus node may continue to depolarize at its normal rate, unaware that the ventricle is being depolarized abnormally by an ectopic pacer. P waves may appear to be randomly scattered throughout the rhythm, but the P waves are actually being fired at a consistent rate from the sinus node.

Critical Criteria for Diagnosis of Ventricular Tachycardia
- The heart rate is faster than 100 beats per minute.
- The QRS complex width is greater than 0.12 seconds.
- The occurrence of more than three PVCs in a row is considered ventricular tachycardia.
- P waves may or may not be visible. If visible, P waves appear to be scattered throughout the rhythm and have no relationship with the QRS complex.

Hemodynamic Effects. Hemodynamic effects associated with ventricular tachycardia may vary. Most patients have a significant loss of cardiac output, with a resultant low blood pressure. Many patients become pulseless, with no obtainable blood pressure. However, in rare instances, some patients maintain a pulse and a blood pressure while experiencing ventricular tachycardia. Treatment of the dysrhythmia is dependent on the presence or absence of a pulse and blood pressure.[1]

Ventricular Fibrillation
Ventricular fibrillation is a chaotic rhythm characterized by a quivering of the ventricles that results in total loss of cardiac output. Patients experiencing ventricular fibrillation are in a state of clinical death. Clinical death means that the patient's heart has

stopped contracting; therefore, there is no blood flow to the vital organs.

Ventricular fibrillation can occur without a known cause. Ventricular fibrillation that occurs without the presence of cardiac disease or other explainable cause is referred to as *primary ventricular fibrillation*. More commonly, however, fibrillation occurs secondary to the processes listed under the discussion of PVCs.

The electrical energy created by ventricular fibrillation varies in amplitude. When voltage is low in the fibrillating ventricle, the result is a small-amplitude waveform. This form of ventricular fibrillation is referred to as *fine* (Figure 7-49).

When voltage is greater in the fibrillating ventricle, the result is a larger-amplitude waveform. This form of ventricular fibrillation is referred to as *coarse* (Figure 7-50). Coarse ventricular fibrillation responds better to defibrillation than does fine ventricular fibrillation.[1]

Because a loose lead or electrical interference can produce a waveform similar to ventricular fibrillation, it is always important to confirm ventricular fibrillation in at least two leads and to assess the patient's condition.

Critical Criteria for Diagnosis of Ventricular Fibrillation
- A fluctuating, jagged baseline exists. No discernible P, Q, R, S, and T waves are present.
- Ventricular fibrillation may be coarse or fine.

Hemodynamic Effects. All atrial and ventricular contractions cease, leading to total loss of cardiac output. No palpable pulse is present, and no blood pressure can be obtained. Brain death occurs within 4 to 6 minutes if life support is not instituted.

Idioventricular Rhythm
Idioventricular rhythm is an escape rhythm that is generated by the Purkinje fibers. This rhythm emerges only when the SA and AV nodes have failed. The Purkinje fibers are capable of an intrinsic rate of 15 to 40 beats per minute. Because this rhythm originates in the deepest portion of the ventricles, normal depolarization is impossible, and aberrant conduction results. Therefore, the QRS of the

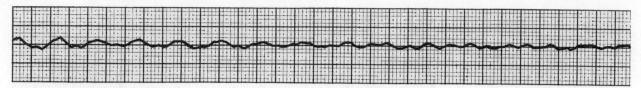

FIGURE 7-49. Fine ventricular fibrillation. *(From Patel, J., McGowan, S., & Moody, L. [1989].* Arrhythmias: Detection, treatment, and cardiac drugs. *Philadelphia: Saunders.)*

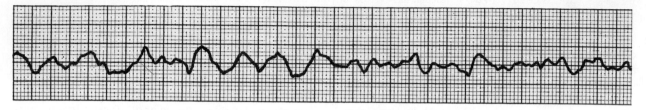

FIGURE 7-50. Coarse ventricular fibrillation. *(From Patel, J., McGowan, S., & Moody, L. [1989].* Arrhythmias: Detection, treatment, and cardiac drugs. *Philadelphia: Saunders.)*

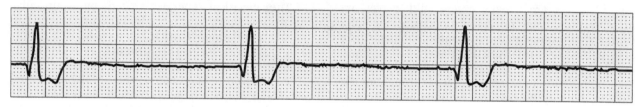

FIGURE 7-51. Idioventricular rhythm. *(From Paul, S., & Hebra, J. D. [1998].* The nurse's guide to cardiac rhythm interpretation: Implications for patient care. *Philadelphia: Saunders.)*

idioventricular rhythm is wider than normal. Because of the distance of the impulse formation from the atria, atrial depolarization is not likely to occur. Usually, no evidence of P waves is present on the ECG strip (Figure 7-51).

Some patients with cardiac disease may experience idioventricular rhythm while they are sleeping. During deep sleep the metabolic demands of the body are diminished, and the heart rate decreases. If the patient is in sinus bradycardia, this further slowing can encourage competition between the SA node and the Purkinje fibers, resulting in an idioventricular rhythm. The rhythm disappears on awakening as the release of epinephrine and nor-epinephrine causes an increase in heart rate.

Critical Criteria for Diagnosis of Idioventricular Rhythm
- The heart rate is 15 to 40 beats per minute and regular.
- A widened QRS interval is present, usually 0.12 seconds or greater.
- P waves are not usually visible.

Hemodynamic Effects. Hemodynamic effects vary with the idioventricular rhythm. Some patients are able

to maintain adequate cardiac output, whereas others become hypotensive.

Accelerated Idioventricular Rhythm
Accelerated idioventricular rhythm is the same as that discussed for idioventricular rhythm, except the rate exceeds 40 beats per minute. The faster rate is the result of increased automaticity in the Purkinje fibers. This effect is most often caused by myocardial ischemia, injury, or infarction, but it can also be caused by hypokalemia, digitalis toxicity, or various forms of heart disease (Figure 7-52).

Critical Criteria for Diagnosis of Accelerated Idioventricular Rhythm
- These criteria are the same as for idioventricular rhythm, except the heart rate is greater than 40 beats per minute but less than 100 beats per minute.

Hemodynamic Effects. The hemodynamic effects of accelerated idioventricular rhythm correspond to the heart rate. If the rate decreases or increases significantly, the patient can experience a compromise in hemodynamic status.

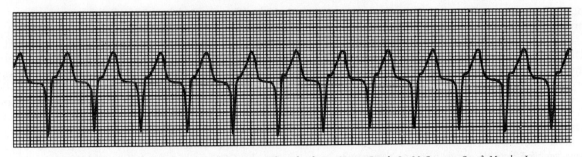

FIGURE 7-52. Accelerated idioventricular rhythm. *(From Patel, J., McGowan, S., & Moody, L. [1989]. Arrhythmias: Detection, treatment, and cardiac drugs. Philadelphia: Saunders.)*

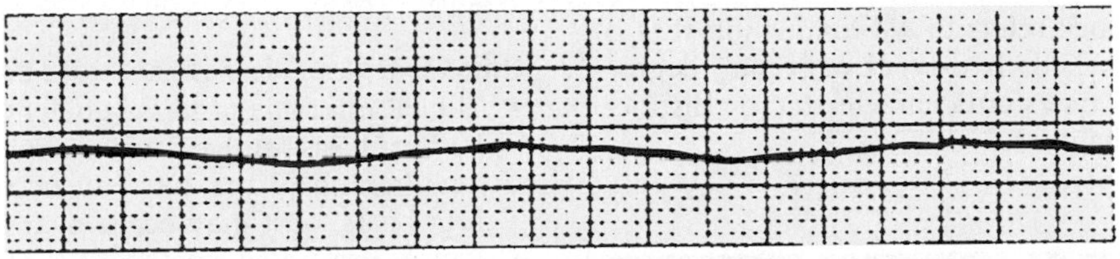

FIGURE 7-53. Ventricular standstill or asystole. *(From Fenstermacher, K. [1989]. Dysrhythmia recognition and management. Philadelphia: Saunders.)*

Ventricular Standstill (Asystole)

Ventricular standstill is characterized by complete cessation of all electrical activity. A flat baseline is seen, without any evidence of P, Q, R, S, or T waveforms. Ventricular standstill is also called *asystole* because all contraction of the heart muscle stops (Figure 7-53).

Asystole may occur as the end result of a severe bradycardia or sinus arrest. In the evaluation of asystole, the nurse should *always* check to see that the patient's electrodes and ECG connections are intact. For patient safety, asystole should be confirmed in two leads.

Critical Criteria for Diagnosis of Ventricular Standstill (Asystole)

- A flat baseline is observed, with no evidence of P, Q, R, S, or T waveforms in two leads.

Hemodynamic Effects. The hemodynamic effects are the same as for ventricular fibrillation. The patient loses all cardiac output, and death occurs without intervention.

Atrioventricular Blocks

AV block refers to impairment in the conduction of impulses from the atria to the ventricles. This impairment may cause slowed conduction of impulses, intermittent blockage of impulses, or complete blockage of impulse conduction from the atria to the ventricles. The following discussion describes the most common causes of impaired impulse conduction.

Coronary Artery Disease. Coronary artery disease robs the AV node conduction pathway of its normal blood supply, thereby impairing impulse generation and conduction.

Infectious and Inflammatory Processes. Infectious and inflammatory processes can damage the AV node conduction pathway and can lead to impairment or blockage of impulses. These processes include systemic lupus erythematosus and myocarditis.

Enhanced Vagal Tone. When the vagus nerve is stimulated, the heart rate decreases, and a transient impairment in AV node impulse conduction may occur.

Effects of Drugs. Many cardiac drugs have a negative dromotropic effect; that is, they slow down conduction of impulses from the atria to the ventricles. This is often a desired effect, in that a slower heart rate decreases the myocardial oxygen demand.

Four types of AV block exist, each categorized in terms of degree. The four types of block are first-degree, second-degree type I, second-degree type II, and third-degree. The greater the degree of block is, the more severe are the consequences. First-degree block has minimal consequences, whereas third-degree block may be life-threatening.

First-Degree Block

First-degree AV block is delayed conduction through the AV junction. It is shown on the ECG as a prolonged PR interval.

First-degree block is a common dysrhythmia in the elderly and in patients with cardiac disease. As the normal conduction pathway ages or becomes diseased, impulse conduction becomes slower than normal (Figure 7-54). (See Geriatric Considerations.)

Critical Criteria for the Diagnosis of First-Degree Block

- The underlying rhythm is usually normal sinus rhythm.
- The PR interval is longer than 0.20 seconds.
- The PR interval of each beat is the same.
- First-degree block is often accompanied by sinus bradycardia.

Hemodynamic Effects. Hemodynamic changes do not usually occur with first-degree block.

Second-Degree Block

Second-degree block refers to AV conduction that is intermittently blocked. Two types of second-degree block exist. Both types are characterized by distinctive criteria for diagnosis.

GERIATRIC CONSIDERATIONS

- The sinoatrial node becomes fibrotic with aging.
- The number of pacemakers located in the sinoatrial node decreases with age.
- By the age of 75 years, only 10% of the normal number of pacemaker cells may remain.
- The PR interval, QRS complex, and QT interval are increased.
- The amplitude of the QRS complex is increased because of left ventricular wall thickening.
- Atrial fibrillation occurs frequently in the elderly as a result of fibrosis and cellular alteration.
- Elderly persons are susceptible to dysrhythmias.
- Peak heart rate declines with age, and elderly persons must rely on increased stroke volume to increase cardiac output.
- Elderly persons are less dependent on rapid filling of the heart, but they are more dependent on active filling (atrial kick) to maintain stroke volume and cardiac output.

Second-Degree Block Type I: Mobitz I or Wenckebach's Phenomenon

Second-degree AV block type I usually occurs at the level of the AV node and is characterized by a steadily lengthening PR interval. The AV node becomes progressively more fatigued as it conducts each beat. Therefore, each beat takes longer to conduct through the AV node, resulting in a longer PR interval. Ultimately, the AV node is unable to conduct one or more beats. When conduction fails, a P wave is seen on the ECG that is not followed by a QRS complex. By not conducting this one beat, the AV node is able to recover and then conduct the next atrial impulse (Figure 7-55).

Critical Criteria for Diagnosis of Second-Degree Block Type I

- The PR interval progressively lengthens on a beat-by-beat basis until a P wave is not conducted. The lengthening of the PR may occur over three to four beats, or it may occur over fewer beats.
- Pauses are noted on the ECG after the nonconducted P waves.
- A pattern or group of beats appears before each missed beat.
- P to P intervals are usually regular.
- R to R intervals are usually irregular.
- QRS width is usually normal.

Hemodynamic Effects. Second-degree block type I is considered a self-limiting rhythm and rarely progresses to a higher or more severe degree of block.[1] Hemodynamic effects rarely occur unless the underlying rhythm is slow. Bradycardia with this block may result in decreased cardiac output.

Second-Degree Block Type II: Mobitz II

Second-degree block type II is a more severe form of AV block. The conduction delay occurs below the AV node, often at the level of the bundle branches. The SA node generates impulses, so P waves occur at regular intervals. In Mobitz II block, impulses are occasionally blocked, resulting in a P wave with no QRS after it (Figure 7-56). Mobitz II block is often

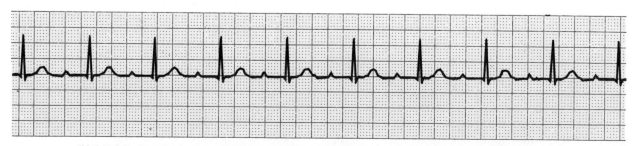

FIGURE 7-54. First-degree block. Rhythm strip generated by the AA-700 Rhythm Simulator. *(Courtesy of Armstrong Medical Industries, Lincolnshire, IL.)*

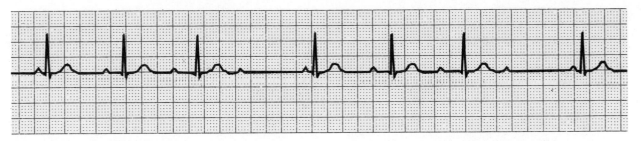

FIGURE 7-55. Second-degree block, Mobitz type I, or Wenckebach's phenomenon. Note the steadily lengthening PR interval. Rhythm strip generated by the AA-700 Rhythm Simulator. *(Courtesy of Armstrong Medical Industries, Lincolnshire, IL.)*

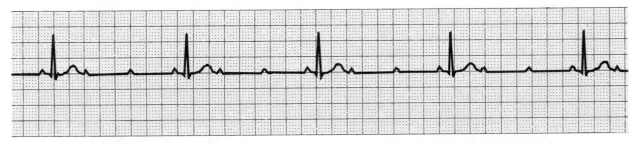

FIGURE 7-56. Second-degree block, Mobitz type II. Note the fixed PR interval. Rhythm strip generated by the AA-700 Rhythm Simulator. *(Courtesy of Armstrong Medical Industries, Lincolnshire, IL.)*

associated with a BBB of abnormal conduction through the ventricles. Second-degree block type II may progress to the more clinically significant third-degree block.

Critical Criteria for Diagnosis of Second-Degree Block Type II

- Occasional P waves are not followed by a QRS complex. These unconducted P waves may occur in a regular pattern, such as every other beat, or they may occur randomly, without a pattern.
- The PR interval of conducted beats is consistently the same, or fixed.
- The P to P interval is regular.
- The condition may be associated with a BBB.

Hemodynamic Effects. The hemodynamic effects of second-degree block type II correspond to the decrease in rate caused by the nonconducted beats. The greater the number is of nonconducted beats, the greater the impact is on the cardiac output. Patients with second-degree block type II may require a temporary or permanent pacemaker, or both, if the cardiac output is compromised. Patients must be observed for progression to third-degree block.

Third-Degree Block (Complete Heart Block)

Third-degree block is often called complete heart block because *no* atrial impulses are conducted down to the ventricles. The block in conduction can occur at the level of the AV node, the bundle of His, or the bundle branches.

With complete heart block, the atria and ventricles beat independently of each other. The atria beat at one rate, and the ventricles beat at a different rate. No communication exists between the two. For this reason, third-degree block is sometimes called AV dissociation.

In third-degree block, the atria are paced by the SA node, usually at a rate of 60 to 100 beats per minute. However, the atrial impulses are blocked from entering the ventricles. When the ventricles do not receive an impulse from the atria, either the AV node or the Purkinje fibers can generate an escape rhythm. If the AV node becomes the secondary pacemaker, a junctional escape rhythm will be noted. A third-degree block may also be associated with a ventricular escape rhythm (Figure 7-57).

One hallmark of third-degree heart block is an abnormal sequencing of the P wave, QRS complex, and T wave. P waves are not related to the QRS complex because of the blocked conduction. Whenever a strip appears to have no consistent, predictable relationship between P waves and QRS complexes, third-degree block should be considered.

Critical Criteria for Diagnosis of Third-Degree Block (Complete Heart Block)

- A difference exists between the atrial and ventricular heart rates. The atrial rate is usually greater than the ventricular rate.
- The P to P intervals are regular.

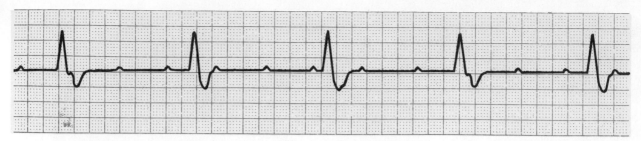

FIGURE 7-57. Third-degree block with ventricular escape. Rhythm strip generated by the AA-700 Rhythm Simulator. *(Courtesy Armstrong Medical Industries, Lincolnshire, IL.)*

- The R to R intervals are regular.
- No true PR interval exists.
- P waves are not related to the QRS complex.
- Either a junctional or a ventricular escape rhythm is present.

Hemodynamic Effects. The hemodynamic effects of third-degree block depend on the ventricular rate. Cardiac output decreases if the heart rate is low. Transcutaneous pacing is often warranted for symptomatic third-degree block.

INTERVENTIONS FOR DYSRHYTHMIAS

Dysrhythmias must be treated if the patient has symptoms of decreased cardiac output. Treatments for dysrhythmias are addressed in depth in Chapter 12.

Tachydysrhythmias

Treatment of symptomatic tachycardia may include the following:
1. The effects of the sympathetic nervous system are mediated through stress reduction techniques, avoiding caffeine and nicotine, and relief of pain.
2. Vagal maneuvers are used to stimulate the parasympathetic nervous system (and slow the heart rate). Carotid massage and the Valsalva maneuver are two strategies for stimulating the vagus nerve that may be ordered by the physician. To perform carotid massage, the physician exerts gentle, downward pressure on one carotid artery. The procedure can lead to cerebral insufficiency in patients with carotid occlusive disease, so the patient's neurological status must be closely monitored. The Valsalva maneuver is performed by asking the patient to "bear down." As vagal maneuvers are performed, the cardiac rhythm is closely monitored for the rhythm to return to a more normal rate. If the rhythm does not respond to vagal stimulation, medications and/or electrical cardio-

version may be needed. Drugs should not be used to manage patients with unstable tachycardias; instead immediate cardioversion is necessary.
3. Intervention with appropriate cardiac drugs (see Table 7-1 and Chapter 10).
   a. Adenosine can be given for narrow complex (QRS complex is 0.06-0.10 seconds) supraventricular tachycardias.
   b. Calcium channel blockers or beta blockers can be effective in slowing down the heart rate.
   c. Amiodarone can be used if there is uncertainty about whether the rhythm is originating from the ventricle or the atrium.
4. Electrical energy (cardioversion or defibrillation) is used to convert the rhythm to a slower, more normal rhythm (see Chapter 16). Recurrent life-threatening tachycardias may need to be treated with an implantable cardioverter-defibrillator, a permanent device.
5. Overdrive cardiac pacing is used to interrupt a rapid rhythm.
6. Radiofrequency ablation is used to destroy abnormal pathways in the conduction system.

Bradydysrhythmias

Treatment of symptomatic bradycardia may include the following:
1. The parasympathetic nervous system is suppressed (and the heart rate is increased). Strategies include avoiding activities that increase vagal tone, such as vomiting, gagging, Valsalva maneuver, or endotracheal suctioning.
2. Intervening with an appropriate cardiac drug, such as atropine.
3. Cardiac pacing is used.

ELECTRICAL PACEMAKERS

An electrical pacemaker delivers electrical current to stimulate depolarization. A pacemaker may be required to treat symptomatic bradycardia, second-degree block type II, and third-degree block. Pacemakers can also be set at a fast rate to overdrive or interrupt a symptomatic tachycardia. The need for the pacemaker may be temporary (e.g., after an acute myocardial infarction or cardiac surgery) or permanent. Battery-operated, external pulse generators are used to provide electrical energy for temporary pacemakers. Internal pulse generators with long-life batteries provide electrical stimulation for permanent pacing.

Methods for temporary pacing include the following:

- Transcutaneous: Electrical stimulation is delivered through external electrode pads connected to an external pacemaker or pacemaker-defibrillator (see Chapter 10).
- Transvenous: A pacemaker catheter is inserted into the right ventricle, where it contacts the endocardium near the ventricular septum; it is connected to a small external pulse generator.
- Epicardial: Pacing wires are inserted into the epicardial wall of the heart during cardiac surgery; wires are brought through the chest wall and can be connected to a pulse generator if needed.

Methods for permanent pacing include transvenous and epicardial. Transvenous pacing is more commonly used. Many implantable cardioverter-defibrillators also have pacemaker capabilities and are known as pacemaker cardioverter-defibrillators.

Pacemakers may be used to stimulate the atrium, ventricle, or both chambers (dual-chamber pacemakers). Atrial pacing is used to mimic normal conduction and to produce the atrial kick. Ventricular pacing stimulates ventricular contraction; it is commonly used in emergency situations. Dual-chamber pacing allows for stimulation of both atria and ventricles as needed to produce a near-normal cardiac contraction.

Permanent pacemakers have the ability to be programmed in a variety of ways. The International Commission on Heart Disease Code is a method for programming pacemakers; it is described in Chapter 12. It is important to know the programming information for the pacemaker to assess proper functioning on the rhythm strip. Other terms used in describing pacemaker function are *rate*, *mode*, *electrical output*, *sensitivity*, *sense-pace indicator*, and *AV interval*.

Rate. The rate control determines the number of impulses delivered per minute to the atrium, the ventricle, or both. The rate is set to produce effective cardiac output and to reduce symptoms.

Mode. Pacemakers can be operated in a *demand* mode or *asynchronous* mode. The demand mode paces the heart based on need. For example, the rate control is set at 60 beats per minute. The pacemaker will generate a beat only if the patient's rate drops to less than 60. The asynchronous mode paces the heart at a set rate, independent of any activity the patient's heart generates. The asynchronous mode may compete with the patient's own rhythm and deliver an impulse on the T wave (R on T), with the potential for producing ventricular tachycardia or fibrillation. The demand mode is safer and is the mode of choice.

Electrical Output. The electrical output is the amount of electrical energy needed to stimulate depolarization. The output is measured in *milliamperes*, which varies depending on the type of pacing. Transcutaneous pacing requires higher amounts of milliamperes than transvenous or epicardial pacing, because the electrical energy must be delivered through the chest wall.

Sensitivity. The sensitivity is the ability of the pacemaker to recognize the body's intrinsic electrical activity (heartbeat). It is measured in *millivolts*. Some temporary pacemakers have a *sense-pace indicator*. When the generator delivers a paced beat, the "pace" light comes on. If the generator detects the patient's own beat, the "sense" indicator should light. Temporary pacemakers have settings for adjusting sensitivity.

AV Internal. The AV indicator is used to determine the interval between atrial and ventricular stimulation. It is used only in dual-chamber pacemakers.

Pacemaker Rhythms. Pacemaker rhythms are usually easy to note on the cardiac monitor or rhythm strip. The electrical stimulation is noted by an electrical artifact called the pacer spike. If the atrium is paced, the spike appears before the P wave (Figure 7-58). If the ventricle is paced, the spike appears before the QRS complex (Figure 7-59). If both the atrium and ventricle are paced, spikes will be noted before both the P wave and the QRS complex (Figure 7-60). The heart rate is carefully assessed on the rhythm strip. The rate should not be lower than the rate set on the pacemaker.

The pacemaker spike is usually followed by a larger-than-normal P wave in atrial pacing or a widened QRS complex in ventricular pacing. Sometimes the P wave is not seen even though an atrial pacer spike is present. Because the heart is paced in an artificial or abnormal fashion, the path of depolarization is altered, resulting in waveforms and intervals that are also altered.

Pacemaker Malfunction. Three primary problems can occur with a temporary pacemaker. These problems include *failure to pace*, *failure to capture*, and *failure to sense*.

Failure to Pace. Failure to pace occurs when the pacemaker fails to initiate an electrical stimulus

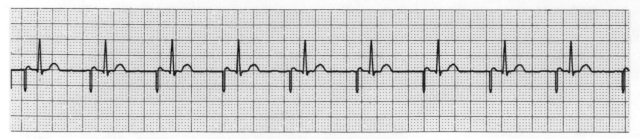

FIGURE 7-58. Paced rhythm: atrial. Note the spike in front of the P wave. Rhythm strip generated by the AA-700 Rhythm Simulator. *(Courtesy of Armstrong Medical Industries, Lincolnshire, IL.)*

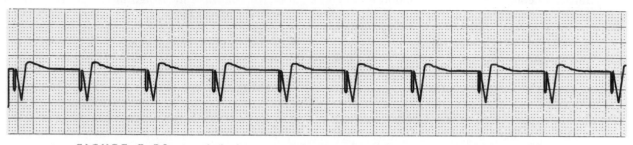

FIGURE 7-59. Paced rhythm: ventricular. Note the spike in front of the QRS complex. Rhythm strip generated by the AA-700 Rhythm Simulator. *(Courtesy of Armstrong Medical Industries, Lincolnshire, IL.)*

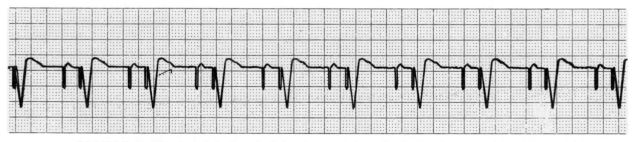

FIGURE 7-60. Paced rhythm: dual chamber. Note the spikes before the P wave and the QRS complex. Rhythm strip generated by the AA-700 Rhythm Simulator. *(Courtesy of Armstrong Medical Industries, Lincolnshire, IL.)*

when the pacemaker is due to fire. It is noted by absence of pacer spikes on the rhythm strip. Causes of failure to pace include battery or pulse generator failure, fracture or displacement of a pacemaker wire, loose connections, or electromagnetic interference.

Failure to Capture. When the pacemaker generates an electrical impulse (pacer spike) and no depolarization is noted, it is known as failure to capture. On the ECG, a pacer spike is noted, but it is not followed by a P wave (atrial pacemaker) or a QRS complex (ventricular pacemaker) (Figure 7-61). Common causes of failure to capture include output (milliamperes) set too low or displacement of pacing lead wire from the myocardium (transvenous or epicardial leads). Other causes of failure to capture include

battery failure, fracture of the pacemaker wire, or increased pacing threshold as a result of medication or electrolyte imbalance. Adjusting the milliamperes and placing the patient on his or her left side are nursing interventions to treat failure to capture. Turning the patient onto the left side facilitates contact of a transvenous pacing wire with the endocardium and septum.

Failure to Sense. When the pacemaker does not sense the patient's own cardiac rhythm and initiates an electrical impulse, it is called failure to sense. Failure to sense manifests as pacer spikes that fall too closely to the patient's own rhythm, earlier than the programmed rate (Figure 7-62). The most common cause is displacement of the electrode. Repositioning the patient (left side) and adjusting the sensitivity are

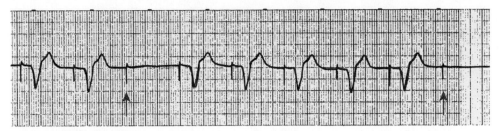

FIGURE 7-61. Paced rhythm with failure to capture. *(From Smith, L. F., & Fish, F. H. [1995]. Pure practice for ECGs. Philadelphia: Saunders.)*

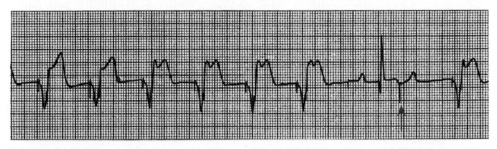

FIGURE 7-62. Paced rhythm with failure to capture (seventh spike) and failure to sense, note *arrow* (eighth spike). *(From Smith, L. F., & Fish, F. H. [1995]. Pure practice for ECGs. Philadelphia: Saunders.)*

nursing interventions to use when failure to sense occurs.

Biventricular Pacemaker

Biventricular pacemaker implantation, also known as *cardiac resynchronization therapy*, can produce dramatic results in patients with advanced congestive heart failure. Those with advanced heart failure can exhibit interventricular conduction delay, also known as *ventricular dyssynchrony*. This results in an abnormal contraction of the heart along with abnormal septal wall motion, reduced cardiac contractility, decreased diastolic filling time, and mitral regurgitation. Increased morbidity and mortality have been reported with these abnormalities. In addition, these patients have a high propensity for conduction disturbances that can result in sudden cardiac death from ventricular tachycardia or ventricular fibrillation.

Right and left pacemaker wires are placed in the heart. One pacing wire is placed in the right ventricle. The other is skillfully placed in the outside of the left posterior ventricular wall by way of the tortuous coronary sinus (Figure 7-63). Results are often immediate, with patients experiencing improvement within a day of the procedure (Figure 7-64). This device not only helps the heart to pump more effectively, but it also treats life-threatening dysrhythmias.[12]

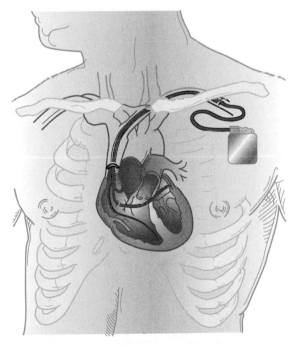

FIGURE 7-63. Biventricular pacing with wires of the right atrium/ventricle and left ventricle. *(Courtesy of Guidant Corporation, St. Paul, MN.)*

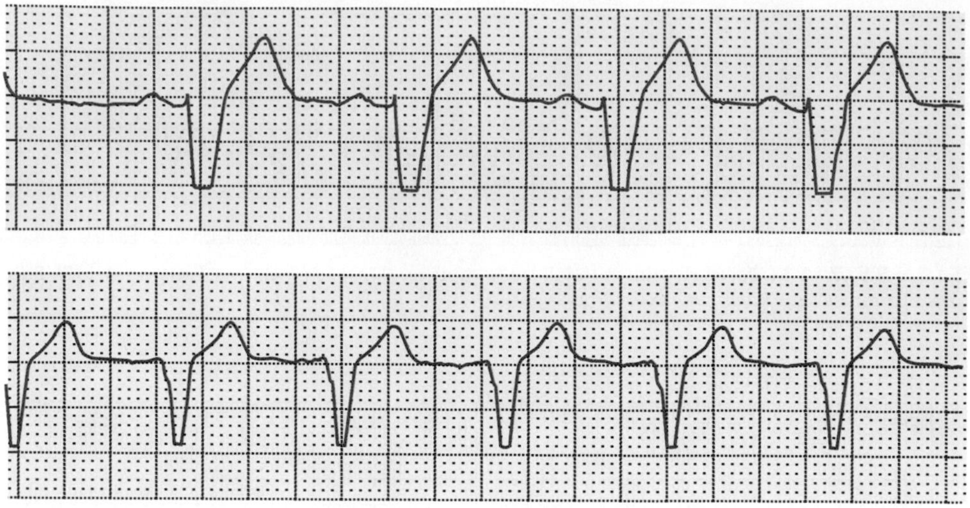

FIGURE 7-64. Patient's actual rhythm (**top strip,** note the wide QRS). Biventricular pacing of right and left ventricle (**bottom strip,** note the QRS is not as wide as the top strip). *(Courtesy of Guidant Corporation, St. Paul, MN.)*

NURSING CARE PLAN

NURSING DIAGNOSIS

Alteration in tissue perfusion related to dysrhythmias

PATIENT OUTCOMES
Maintains optimal cardiac output

- Strong peripheral pulses
- Blood pressure within normal limits for patient
- Skin warm and dry
- Lungs clear bilaterally
- Urine output greater than 30 mL/hr
- Regular cardiac rhythm

NURSING INTERVENTIONS	RATIONALES
• Monitor for tachycardia or bradycardia and irregularity and check vital signs for alteration in perfusion	• Assess for rate, regularity, and perfusion
• Assess for signs of reduced cardiac output: rapid, slow, or weak pulse; hypotension; dizziness; syncope; shortness of breath; chest pain; fatigue; and restlessness	• Detect symptoms of decreased cardiac output Many dysrhythmias affect cardiac output
• Determine acuteness or chronicity of dysrhythmia	• Assess and guide treatment
• Review history and assess for causative factors	• Identify factors causing dysrhythmias that can be eliminated or corrected
• Determine specific type of dysrhythmia	• Guide assessment and treatment
• Evaluate rhythm from monitor leads that show the most prominent findings	• Differentiate atrial from ventricular and lethal from nonlethal dysrhythmias; detect changes in ST segment that may indicate ischemia, injury, or infarct

NURSING CARE PLAN—cont'd

NURSING INTERVENTIONS	RATIONALES
• Monitor for side effects of medication therapy	• Medications prescribed to "treat" dysrhythmias can themselves be proarrhythmogenic
• If the patient is asymptomatic, provide reassurance if the dysrhythmia is not life-threatening. Ensure that monitoring will be ongoing	• Provide psychosocial support to the patient
• Provide oxygen therapy	• Relieve dysrhythmias associated with hypoxemia
• If the patient has a new-onset acute dysrhythmia, obtain an ECG immediately to document it before the rhythm reverts to baseline	• Guide diagnosis and treatment
• Assess urine output	• Assess adequacy of perfusion to kidneys

CASE STUDY

evolve

A 56-year-old patient was *fast tracked* to the ventilator weaning protocol and was successfully extubated 4 hours after coronary artery bypass graft surgery. However, 2 hours later, the patient complains of his heart racing, and it is determined that he has palpitations. The heart rate on the bedside monitor is 168 beats/min, blood pressure is 100/60, and respiratory rate is 26. The ECG now shows an irregularly irregular rhythm, which is a change from the sinus rhythm noted at the last assessment.

QUESTIONS
1. What complications could occur?
2. What clinical data would lead you to believe this complication could occur?
3. What data are you going to give the physician?
4. What orders do you expect to get?
5. What nursing actions do you need to take and why?
6. What are some of the etiologies of this rhythm interpretation?

SUMMARY

Interpretation of cardiac rhythms is a basic skill that develops only through practice. For the beginning student, the critical criteria for diagnosis provide the structure by which rhythms are analyzed. The initial effort should be the memorization of these criteria. It is hoped that this chapter will be a valuable reference in the delivery of high-quality care to patients with cardiac dysrhythmias and to their families. Care for a patient with dysrhythmias is summarized in the nursing care plan.

CRITICAL THINKING QUESTIONS

evolve

1. You are working in the critical care unit and your patient's heart rate suddenly decreases from 88 to 50 beats per minute. What may be some of the reasons for the decreased heart rate? What assessments will you make?
2. Discuss why patients with pulmonary disease are prone to atrial dysrhythmias.
3. A 65-year-old woman with type 2 diabetes presents to the emergency department; she is short of breath and complaining of neck and shoulder pain. Her blood pressure is 185/95 mm Hg, and her heart rate is 155 beats/min. How will you initially manage this patient? What medical intervention would you anticipate? List serious signs and symptoms of hemodynamic instability in a patient with a tachydysrhythmia.
4. Why does tachycardia sometimes lead to heart failure?

evolve Be sure to check out the bonus material, including free self-assessment exercises, on the Evolve Web site at http://evolve.elsevier.com/Sole.

REFERENCES

1. American Heart Association (AHA). (2005). *Textbook of advanced cardiac life support*. Dallas, TX: Author.
2. Drew, B. J. (2002). Celebrating the 100th birthday of the electrocardiogram: Lessons learned from research in cardiac monitoring. *American Journal of Critical Care, 11*, 378-386.
3. Drew, B. J., Califf, R. M., Funk, M., Kaufman, E. S., Krucoff, M. W., Laks, M. M., et al. (2004). Practice standards for electrocardiographic monitoring in hospital settings. Circulation, *110*, 2721-2746.
4. Drew, B. J., & Funk, M. (2006). Practice standards for ECG monitoring in hospital settings: Executive summary and guide for implementation. *Critical Care Nursing Clinics of North America, 18*(2), 157-168.
5. Drew, B. J., & Krucoff, M. W. (1999). Multilead ST-segment monitoring in patients with acute coronary syndromes: A consensus statement for healthcare professionals. ST-Segment Monitoring Practice Guideline International Working Group. *American Journal of Critical Care, 8*, 372-386.
6. Flanders, S. A. (2006). Continuous ST-segment monitoring: Raising the bar. *Critical Care Nursing Clinics of North America, 18*(2), 169-177.
7. Goldberger, A. L. (2006). *Clinical electrocardiography: A simplified approach* (7th ed.). St. Louis: Mosby.
8. Kligfield, P., Gettes, L. S., Bailey, J. J., Childers, R., Deal, B. J., Hancock, E. W., et al. (2007). Recommendations for the standardization and interpretation of the electrocardiogram. Part I: The electrocardiogram and its technology. *Journal of the American College of Cardiology, 49*(10), 1109-1127.
9. Leeper, B. (2003). Continuous ST-segment monitoring. *AACN Clinical Issues, 14*(2), 145-154.
10. Mason, J. W., Hancock, E. W., Gettes, L. S., Bailey, J. J., Childers, R., Deal, B. J., et al. (2007). Recommendations for the standardization and interpretation of the electrocardiogram. Part II: The electrocardiography diagnostic statement list. *Journal of the American College of Cardiology, 49*(10), 1128-1135.
11. Rowan, S. B., Bailey, D. N., Bublitz, C. E., & Anderson, R. J. (2007). Trends in anticoagulation for atrial fibrillation in the U.S. *Journal of American College of Cardiology, 49*, 1561-1565.
12. Saul, S. (2007). Cardiac resynchronization therapy. *Critical Care Nursing Quarterly, 30*(1), 58-66.
13. Sha, R. (2005). Drugs, QTc interval prolongation and final ICH E14 guideline: An important milestone with challenges ahead. *Drug Safety, 28*(11), 1009-1028.
14. Vidallet, H., & Greenlee, R. (2005). Rate control versus rhythm control. *Current Opinion in Cardiology, 20*, 15-20.
15. Wyse, D. G., & the AFFIRM Investigators. (2002). A comparison of rate control and rhythm control on patients with atrial fibrillation. *New England Journal of Medicine, 347*(23), 1825-1832.

CHAPTER 8

Hemodynamic Monitoring

Jana L. Nohrenberg, MSN, APRN-BC, CCNS
Marthe J. Moseley, PhD, RN, CCRN, CCNS, CNL
Mary Lou Sole, PhD, RN, CCNS, CNL, FAAN

INTRODUCTION

Critical care units contain an array of monitors and equipment. Among the most complex are those designed to provide information regarding the hemodynamic status of the patient. Hemodynamic monitoring studies the dynamic physiological relationship between several variables including heart rate, blood flow, oxygen delivery, and tissue perfusion. While gathering the physiological data is relatively easy with the advances in technology, ensuring that the data are accurate, and analyzing and interpreting the data, are more complex skills. The interpretation requires the clinician to have a broad theoretical knowledge base and the ability to apply that knowledge to the clinical situation. Competency in noninvasive and invasive hemodynamic monitoring techniques is essential for critical care nurses. This chapter reviews the basics of cardiovascular anatomy and physiology, the fundamentals of hemodynamic monitoring, and various modalities available to the clinician to assess hemodynamic status.

REVIEW OF ANATOMY AND PHYSIOLOGY

Cardiovascular System Structure

The cardiovascular system is a closed network of arteries, capillaries, and veins through which blood, oxygen, hormones, and nutrients are delivered to the tissues by the pumping action of the heart (Figure 8-1). Metabolic wastes are removed from the circulating blood via the venous conduits to the liver and kidneys. The major components of the cardiovascular system are described.

Heart

The heart is a four-chambered organ that weighs approximately 1 lb, is the size of a human fist, and lies obliquely in the thoracic cavity. The heart is responsible for pumping oxygenated blood forward through the arterial vasculature and receiving deoxygenated blood via the venous vasculature. Blood flow through the heart itself is regulated by four one-way valves. Two atrioventricular (AV) valves (tricuspid and mitral) open during ventricular diastole allowing blood to flow from the atria into the ventricles. As the ventricles begin to contract in systole, the atrioventricular valves close and the semilunar valves (pulmonic and aortic) open, allowing blood to flow into the pulmonary and systemic vasculature. At the end of ventricular systole, the semilunar valves close and the cycle begins again (Figure 8-2).

Arteries

Arteries are the tough, elastic vessels that carry blood away from the heart. The elasticity of the vessels allows them to expand to accommodate volumetric changes that result with the contraction and relaxation of the heart. When the artery diameter is less than 0.5 mm, it is termed an arteriole. The arterial system is a high-pressure, low-volume, high-resistance circuit responsible for delivering nutrient rich blood to the capillary system.

Capillaries

The capillaries are composed of a network of low-pressure, thin-walled vessels allowing for easy passage of hormones, nutrients, and oxygen to the target tissues. They also receive metabolic wastes from the tissues and begin the process of returning deoxygenated blood to the venous portion of the cardiovascular system.

141

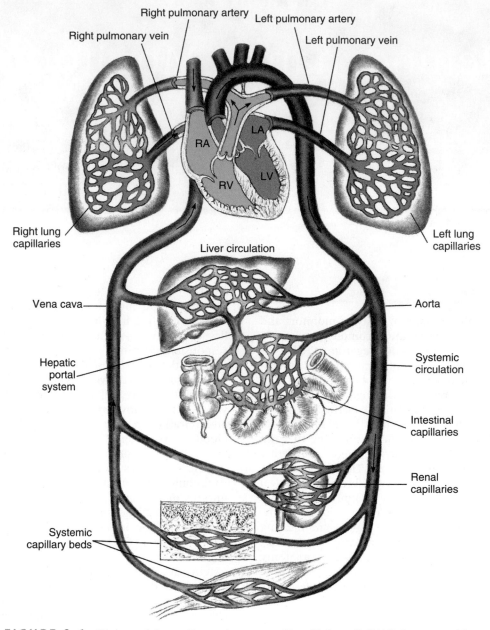

FIGURE 8-1. Diagram of the cardiovascular system. *(From McCance, K. [2006]. Structure and function of the cardiovascular and lymphatic systems. In K. McCance, & S. Huether [Eds.], Pathophysiology: The biologic basis for disease in adults and children [5th ed., p. 1030]. St. Louis: Mosby.)*

Veins

Compared with the arterial system, veins are thin-walled, less elastic, fibrous, and larger in diameter. Veins of the extremities contain valves to assist with maintaining a one-way flow of deoxygenated blood returning to the heart. The venous system has the ability to respond to metabolic needs by vasodilatation or vasoconstriction, thereby increasing or decreasing flow from the target organs. Approximately 70% of the circulating blood volume is located in the venous system at any given time.

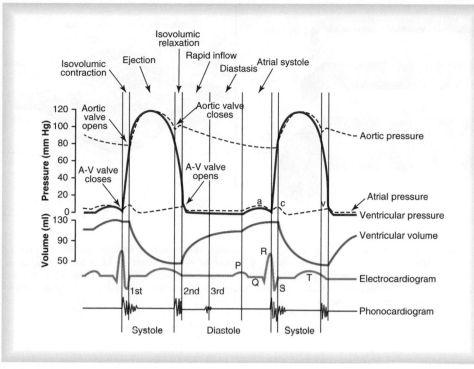

FIGURE 8-2. Cardiac cycle. *(From Guyton, A. C., & Hall, J. E. [2006]. Heart muscle: The heart as a pump and function of the heart valves. In A. C. Guyton, & J. E. Hall [Eds.],* Textbook of medical physiology *[11th ed., p. 107]. Philadelphia: Elsevier.)*

Blood

Under normal circumstances, the human body contains a fixed volume of blood. The fluid component, or plasma, makes up approximately 60% of the blood volume. The remaining 40% consists of the cellular component—erythrocytes (red blood cells), leukocytes (white blood cells), and platelets. The more viscous the blood, the greater the turbulence in blood flow, resulting in a reduction in flow in the microcirculation. The cellular component of the blood is crucial for oxygen delivery to the tissues. A reduction in oxygen delivery or an increase in oxygen consumption directly impacts the hemodynamic responses of the body.

Principles of Physics

According to Poiseuille's law, the rate of flow of a fluid through a vessel is determined by the pressure difference between the two ends of the vessel and the resistance within the lumen.[13] Mathematically, this is represented as:

$$Flow(Q) = \frac{Pressure\ difference\ (\Delta P)}{Resistance\ (R)}$$

For any fluid to flow within a circuit, a difference in pressures within the circuit must exist. In the cardiovascular system, the driving pressure is generated by the contractile force of the heart. There is a continuous drop in pressure from the left ventricle to the tissues, and further reduction in pressure from the tissue bed to the right atrium. Without these pressure gradients, no flow occurs.

Resistance is a measure of the ease with which the fluid flows through the lumen of a vessel. It is essentially a measure of friction, which is dependent upon *viscosity* of the fluid, and radius and length of the vessel. A vessel with a small diameter has a greater resistance than one with a larger diameter (Figure 8-3). Longer vessels have greater resistance to the flow of fluid within the vessel. Increased viscosity of a fluid results in increased friction within the fluid; rate of flow is inversely proportional to the fluid viscosity.

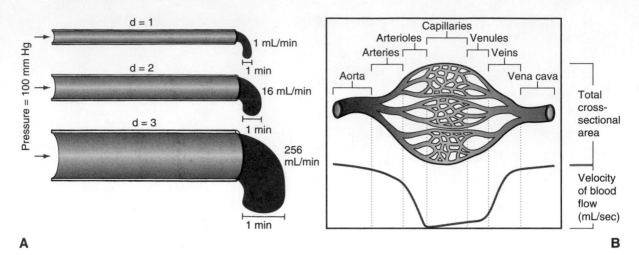

FIGURE 8-3. Relationship between vessel diameter, flow, and resistance. **A,** Effect of lumen diameter on flow through vessel. *d,* Diameter. **B,** Blood flows with great speed in the large arteries. However, branching of arterial vessels increases the total cross-sectional areas of the arterioles and capillaries, thus reducing the flow rate. *(**A** from McCance, K., & Huether, S. [Eds.]. [2006]. Pathophysiology: The biologic basis for disease in adults and children [5th ed., p. 1058]. St. Louis: Mosby; **B** from Thibodeau, G., & Patton, K. [2004]. Anatomy and physiology [5th ed.]. St. Louis: Mosby.)*

Highly compliant systems have low resistance; therefore, if resistance increases, compliance decreases. For example, an atherosclerotic vessel has a reduced capacitance and compliance, leading to increased resistance and hypertension.

The body's response to metabolic demands alters the flow of blood to and from the target tissues. In response to increased metabolic demands, the circulatory system increases the volume of blood flow to the target tissues by increasing the diameter of the vessel, thereby reducing the resistance within the vessel.

Another determinant of flow rate is the degree of turbulence within a vessel. The rate of fluid movement in laminar flow is greater fluid movement than in turbulent flow. A vessel lining that has excess plaque accumulation or calcification results in more turbulence, reduced flow, and reduced tissue perfusion.

Components of Cardiac Output

Cardiac output (CO) is determined by heart rate and stroke volume. Stroke volume is affected by preload, afterload, and contractility (Figure 8-4). Comprehending hemodynamics requires having a working knowledge of normal intracardiac pressures, as each chamber of the heart has a unique pressure (Figure 8-5). In addition, a familiarity with the cardiac cycle (see Figure 8-2) assists in understanding hemodynamic concepts. Relevant concepts are defined below.

Systole is the excitation or pumping portion of the cardiac cycle. Left ventricular systole usually occurs slightly before right ventricular systole.

Diastole is the relaxation or filling part of the cardiac cycle. The majority of ventricular diastole is a passive event that occurs as the AV valves open. However, as the atria contract, they force the remaining atrial blood into the ventricles—this is commonly referred to as the "atrial kick" and contributes up to 30% of the CO.

Preload is the degree of ventricular stretch before the next contraction. The degree of stretch is directly impacted by the amount of blood volume present in the ventricles at end-diastole. In hemodynamic monitoring, preload is quantified by measuring ventricular end-diastolic pressures. Based on the Frank-Starling law, when ventricular fibers are at maximal stretch, maximal CO results. Too much end-diastolic volume in the right ventricle results in congestion of the systemic vasculature, and too much end-diastolic volume in the left ventricle results in a backing up of fluid into the pulmonary vasculature. Too little blood at end-diastolic

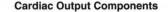

Cardiac Output Components

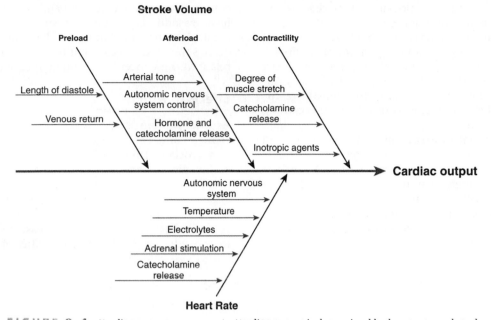

FIGURE 8-4. Cardiac output components. Cardiac output is determined by heart rate and stroke volume.

FIGURE 8-5. Normal blood flow through the heart and intrachamber pressures; *arrows* indicate the normal direction of blood flow. This schematic representation of the heart shows all four chambers and valves visible in the anterior view to facilitate conceptualization of blood flow. *(Modified from Darovic, G. [2002]. Hemodynamic monitoring: Invasive and noninvasive clinical application [3rd ed., p. 64]. Philadelphia: Saunders.)*

volume results in a reduction in CO. Optimizing preload or ventricular filling is the goal of many therapeutic interventions in critical care.

Afterload is the amount of resistance the ventricles must overcome to deliver the stroke volume into the receiving vasculature (pulmonary for the right ventricle and systemic via the aorta for the left ventricle). Arterial systemic tone, blood viscosity, flow patterns (laminar versus turbulent), and valve competency all affect the degree of afterload the ventricle must overcome.

Contractility is the strength of myocardial muscle fiber shortening during the systolic phase of the cardiac cycle. It is the force with which the heart propels the stroke volume forward into the vasculature. The preload influences contractility, as optimizing the preload ensures maximal stretch of the myocardial fibers according to the Frank-Starling law. Contractility is not directly measured; however, it can be expressed by the calculated values of right or left ventricular stroke work index.

Regulation of Cardiovascular Function

Cardiovascular anatomy and physiology were described in Chapter 7. Sympathetic nervous system activity enhances myocardial performance by shortening the conduction time through the AV node and enhancing rhythmicity of the AV pacemaker cells. Parasympathetic nervous system activity via the vagus nerve results in blocking of cardiac action potentials initiated by the atria.

The cardiac system has biochemical and hormonal influences that also assist in regulation of cardiovascular function. Norepinephrine increases the heart rate and myocardial contractility, and causes vasoconstriction. Epinephrine dilates the hepatic vasculature and skeletal muscle tissues while also causing vasoconstriction.

The hormonal influence on blood pressure and CO regulation is complex and not completely understood. Adrenocortical hormones potentiate the effects of catecholamines. Thyroid hormones influence sympathetic activity by an as yet undefined mechanism, which promotes an increase in CO. Intravascular fluid balance is affected by antidiuretic hormone and aldosterone balance. Several hormones (i.e.,

endothelin-1, serotonin, and thromboxane A_2) are released at the local tissue level and result in vasoconstriction of the vascular bed.[13] Other hormones have vasodilatory properties such as nitric oxide, prostaglandins, bradykinin, and kallidin.[13] Figure 8-6 depicts the many factors that regulate blood flow and relate to the concepts of hemodynamic monitoring.

Effects of Aging

As the human body ages, normal physiological changes and changes associated with disease processes occur. Differentiating between normal and pathological changes is difficult and poses a challenge in the management of the elderly patient. As elasticity and compliance decrease, the pressure within the arterial system increases, resulting in systemic hypertension. The increase in impedance to the left ventricular ejection often leads to left

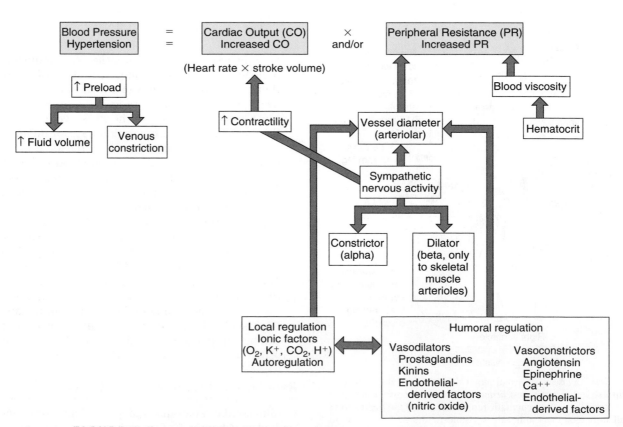

FIGURE 8-6. Factors regulating blood flow. *(From McCance, K. [2006]. Structure and function of the cardiovascular and lymphatic systems. In K. McCance, & S. Huether [Eds.],* Pathophysiology: The biologic basis for disease in adults and children *[5th ed., p. 1062]. St. Louis: Mosby.)*

ventricular hypertrophy. As the left ventricle stiffens, diastolic filling is impaired, leading to diastolic heart failure. The number and sensitivity of β-adrenoreceptors in the sinoatrial node decrease, resulting in a decreased intrinsic and maximal heart rate. Fibrosis of the cardiac structures and conduction system can lead to heart block and valvular dysfunction. All of these changes significantly impact hemodynamic functioning. Figure 8-7 highlights the age-related changes on the cardiac system.

HEMODYNAMIC MONITORING MODALITIES

Hemodynamic monitoring is part of a comprehensive assessment of the critically ill patient. Hemodynamic assessment aids in detecting an impending cardiovascular crisis before any end organ damage occurs. The information gathered is used to titrate therapies to a specific end point (e.g., mean arterial pressure, CO), detect inadequate tissue perfusion, quantify severity of disease, guide therapy, and assist in differential diagnosis. Normal hemodynamic values are described in Table 8-1; however, these values only provide a guideline to assist in the interpretation of assessment findings. The primary goal of hemodynamic monitoring is to assess and trend adequacy of tissue perfusion, rather than to compare a patient's values to so-called normal parameters.

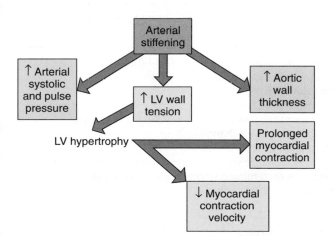

FIGURE 8-7. Impact of age-related changes on cardiac function. *(Adapted from McCance, K. [2006]. Structure and function of the cardiovascular and lymphatic systems. In K. McCance, & S. Huether [Eds.], Pathophysiology: The biologic basis for disease in adults and children [5th ed., p. 1075]. St. Louis: Mosby.)*

Noninvasive Monitoring

Many critically ill patients can be adequately assessed and managed with noninvasive hemodynamic monitoring. Two frequently applied noninvasive modalities are noninvasive blood pressure (NIBP) measurement and assessment of jugular venous pressure as an estimation of central venous pressure (CVP). In addition, measurement of serum lactate levels provides data about tissue perfusion.

Noninvasive Blood Pressure

Since 1962, clinicians have used NIBP monitoring to assess patients.[9] The NIBP is readily available and easy to use. However, obtaining accurate and reliable readings requires an understanding of the science of pressure measurement and attention to detail. It is critical that the proper size cuff be selected. If the cuff size is too small for the patient, the pressures recorded will be falsely elevated; if the cuff size is too large, the resulting pressures will be falsely low. In addition, the patient's arm should be positioned at the level of the heart. Patients who are hemodynamically unstable—either profoundly hypotensive or hypertensive—cannot be adequately assessed using the NIBP. In the profoundly obese patient with conically shaped upper arms, it is technically difficult to measure an NIBP because the cuff will not fit appropriately or stay positioned properly. Blood pressure readings are also affected by cardiac dysrhythmias, respiratory variation, shivering, seizures, external cuff compression, and patient talking or movement during the measurement. Routine calibration of the NIBP equipment is required to ensure accurate measurement. The nurse must also understand that isolated blood pressure readings are not used to guide patient management; trending of values over a period of time and assessing the response to interventions are critical interventions.

Jugular Venous Pressure

Assessment of the jugular veins provides a method for the clinician to estimate intravascular volume and pressure. Because the internal jugular vein is in direct communication with the right atrium, it can serve as a manometer and provide an estimate of the CVP. Jugular venous distention occurs when the CVP is elevated, which can occur in fluid overload or right ventricular dysfunction. The technique for assessing jugular venous pressure is outlined in Figure 8-8.

Lactate

Anything that deprives the tissues of oxygen disrupts the Kreb's cycle, resulting in anaerobic metabolism and lactic acidosis. High serum lactate levels are

TABLE 8-1   Normal Hemodynamic Values

Hemodynamic Parameter	Significance	Normal Range
Cardiac output (CO)	Amount of blood pumped out by a ventricle every minute	4-8 L/min
Cardiac index (CI)	CO individualized to patient body surface area (size)	2.5-4.2 L/min/m^2
Central venous pressure (CVP)	Pressure created by volume of blood in right heart; used to guide assessment of fluid balance and responsiveness	2-6 mm Hg
Right atrial pressure (RAP)	Used interchangeably with CVP	2-6 mm Hg
Left atrial pressure (LAP)	Pressure created by volume of blood in left heart; used after open heart surgery to evaluate ability of left ventricle to eject blood volume ($\uparrow$LAP = $\downarrow$Ejection fraction)	8-12 mm Hg
Pulmonary artery occlusive pressure (PAOP)	Pressure created by volume of blood in left heart	8-12 mm Hg
Stroke volume (SV)	Amount of blood ejected from the ventricle with each contraction	60-130 mL/beat
Stroke volume index (SI)	SV individualized to patient size	30-65 mL/beat/m^2
Systemic vascular resistance (SVR)	Resistance that the left ventricle must overcome to eject a volume of blood; generally as SVR increases, CO falls	770-1500 dynes/sec/cm^{-5}
Systemic vascular resistance index (SVRI)	SVR individualized to patient size	1680-2580 dynes/sec/cm^{-5}/m^2
Pulmonary vascular resistance (PVR)	Resistance that the right ventricle must overcome to eject a volume of blood, normally one sixth of SVR	20-120 dynes/sec/cm^{-5}
Pulmonary vascular resistance index (PVRI)	PVR individualized to patient size	69-177 dynes/sec/cm^{-5}/m^2
Right cardiac work index (RCWI)	Amount of work the right ventricle performs each minute when ejecting blood; increases or decreases depending upon changes in volume (CO) or pressure (PA mean)	0.54-0.66 kg-m/m^2
Right ventricular stroke work index (RVSWI)	Amount of work the right ventricle performs with each heartbeat; increases or decreases depending upon changes in volume (SV) or pressure (PA mean); quantifies contractility	7.9-9.7 g-m/beat/m^2
Left cardiac work index (LCWI)	Amount of work the left ventricle performs each minute when ejecting blood; increases or decreases depending upon changes in volume (CO) or pressure (MAP)	3.4-4.2 kg-m/m^2
Left ventricular stroke work index (LVSWI)	Amount of work the left ventricle performs with each heartbeat; increases or decreases depending upon changes in volume (SV) or pressure (MAP); quantifies contractility	50-62 g-m/beat/m^2

TABLE 8-1   Normal Hemodynamic Values—cont'd

Hemodynamic Parameter	Significance	Normal Range
Right ventricular end-diastolic volume (RVEDV) and pressure (RVEDP)	Measures right ventricular preload	100-160 mL 0-8 mm Hg
Left ventricular end diastolic volume (LVEDV) and pressure (LVEDP)	Measures left ventricular preload	4-12 mm Hg
Mixed venous oxygen saturation (SvO$_2$)	Provides an assessment of balance between oxygen supply and demand. Measured in the pulmonary artery; increased values indicate ↑ supply and ↓ demand, or ↓ ability to extract oxygen from blood. Decreased values indicate ↓ oxygen supply from low hemoglobin, low CO, low SaO$_2$ and/or ↑ consumption	60%-75%
Central venous oxygen saturation (ScvO$_2$)	Similar to SvO$_2$ but measured in the distal portion of the subclavian vein before right atrium and before the point where the cardiac sinus returns deoxygenated blood from the myocardium, thus the reason for the discrepancy between SvO$_2$ and ScvO$_2$ normal ranges	65%-80%

CO, Cardiac output; SV, stroke volume.

noted in patients with hypoperfusion, such as in shock states. Normal arterial lactate levels are less than 1 mEq/L. In lactic acidosis the lactate level is at least 4 to 5 mEq/L and commonly 10 to 30 mEq/L. While not a specific marker for assessing hemodynamic status, lactate level may be useful in guiding fluid resuscitation in the hypoperfused patient.

Invasive Hemodynamic Monitoring

Indications
Invasive methods of hemodynamic monitoring are used to obtain more detailed physiological information. Common indications for invasive monitoring are outlined in Box 8-1. The majority of these medical diagnoses can be summarized by three nursing diagnoses:
- Ineffective tissue perfusion
- Decreased CO
- Fluid volume excess or deficit

BOX 8-1   Indications for Invasive Hemodynamic Monitoring

Arterial Lines
- Hemodynamic instability
- Assess efficacy of vasoactive medications
- Frequent arterial blood gas analysis

Central Venous Catheter
- Measure right heart filling pressures
  - Estimate fluid status
  - Guide volume resuscitation
- Assess central venous oxygen saturation—ScvO$_2$
- Administer large-volume fluid resuscitation or irritant medications
- Access to place transvenous pacemaker

Pulmonary Artery Catheter
- Hemodynamic instability
- Assess pulmonary artery pressures
- Assess mixed venous oxygen saturation—SvO$_2$
- Directly measure cardiac output

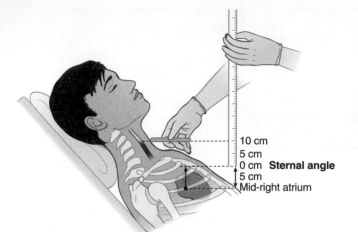

10 cm
5 cm
0 cm **Sternal angle**
5 cm
Mid-right atrium

FIGURE 8-8. Assessment of jugular venous pressure:
1. Place the patient in a supine position with the head of bed elevated 30 to 45 degrees.
2. Position yourself at the patient's right side.
3. Have the patient turn head slightly to the left.
4. If you cannot readily identify the jugular vein, place light pressure with your fingertips across the sternocleidomastoid muscle just superior and parallel to the clavicle. This pressure obstructs the external jugular vein and allows it to fill. Shine a pen light tangentially across the neck to accentuate the pulsations.
5. Assess for jugular venous distention at end exhalation.
6. Any fullness in the vein extending >3 cm above the sternal angle or angle of Louis is considered elevated jugular venous pressure. The higher the degree of elevation, the higher the central venous pressure.
7. Observe the highest point of pulsation in the internal jugular vein at end exhalation.
8. Measure the vertical distance between this pulsation and the angle of Louis in centimeters.
9. Add 5 cm to this number for an estimation of central venous pressure.
10. Normal is 7 to 9 cm.

Understanding these three major indications assists the critical care nurse in identifying the rationale for interventions and anticipating potential complications (Box 8-2).

Equipment Common to All Intravascular Monitoring

The basic hemodynamic monitoring system has five major components: (1) the invasive catheter, (2) noncompliant pressure tubing, (3) the transducer (and stopcocks), (4) a pressurized flush system, and (5) the bedside monitoring system (Figure 8-9).

The *invasive catheter* varies depending upon the type of catheter, purpose, and location of insertion. The catheter can be placed into an artery, a vein, or the heart. An arterial catheter consists of a relatively small-gauge, short, pliable catheter that is placed over a guidewire or in a catheter-over-needle system.

BOX 8-2   Complications of Invasive Hemodynamic Monitoring Devices

- Vascular complications
  - Thrombosis
  - Hematoma
- Infection
- Bleeding
- Pneumothorax and/or hemothorax
- Cardiac dysrhythmias
- Pericardial tamponade

CVP or oxygen saturation monitoring is done via a central catheter placed into the superior vena cava; therefore, it requires a longer catheter that may have multiple ports (Figure 8-10). Pulmonary artery (PA) pressure and mixed venous oxygen saturation (SvO_2) monitoring requires a longer catheter that is placed into the PA (Figure 8-11).

Noncompliant pressure tubing designed specifically for hemodynamic monitoring is used to minimize artifact and increase the accuracy of the data. Noncompliant tubing allows for the efficient and accurate transfer of intravascular pressure changes to the transducer and the monitoring system. The tubing should be no longer than 36 to 48 inches, with a minimum number of additional stopcocks.

The *transducer* (Figure 8-12) translates intravascular pressure changes into waveforms and numeric data. Most institutions use disposable transducer systems available from commercial vendors. A stopcock attached to the transducer is generally used as the reference point for zeroing and leveling the system. This is referred to as the *air-fluid interface* or the *zeroing stopcock*. Discussion of these concepts follows.

The *flush system* maintains patency of the pressure tubing and catheter. A solution of 0.9% normal saline is recommended for the flush system. Heparin may be added to the solution (1 unit/mL) to minimize thrombi and maintain patency of the system. The flush solution is placed in a pressure bag that is inflated to 300 mm Hg to ensure a constant flow of fluid through the pressure tubing. The rate of fluid administration varies from 2 to 5 mL/hr per lumen. Several years ago, the American Association of Critical-Care Nurses conducted a large multicenter study of the patency of intravascular monitoring devices with and without heparinization. The study found that catheters had a greater chance of remaining patent if the flush system was heparinized, but that catheters could be maintained without heparin.[3] The ultimate recommendation was that the

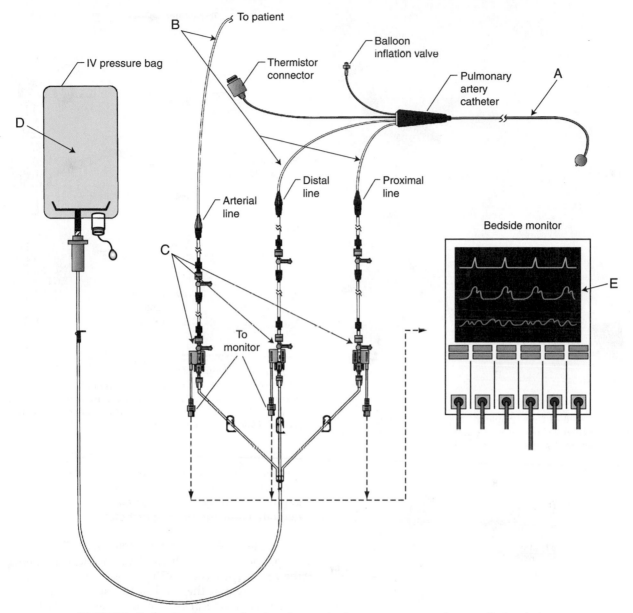

FIGURE 8-9. Components of an invasive monitoring system connected to one flush solution. **A**, Invasive catheter. **B**, Noncompliant pressure tubing. **C**, Transducer and zeroing stopcock. **D**, Pressurized flush system. **E**, Bedside monitoring system. (Not to scale)

risk-benefit ratio needs to be considered for the use of heparin in flush systems.

Bedside *monitoring systems* vary in accessories and capabilities, but all have the same general function and purpose. They provide the visual display of the signal information provided by the transducer, and the ability to store and record the data. Interpretation of the data is the responsibility of the clinician.

Nursing Implications

Accuracy in hemodynamic monitoring is essential for ensuring clinically relevant decision making and proper patient management (see Clinical Alert for Hemodynamic Monitoring). Four major components for validating the accuracy of hemodynamic monitoring systems are (1) leveling the air-fluid interface (zeroing stopcock) to the phlebostatic axis, (2) patient

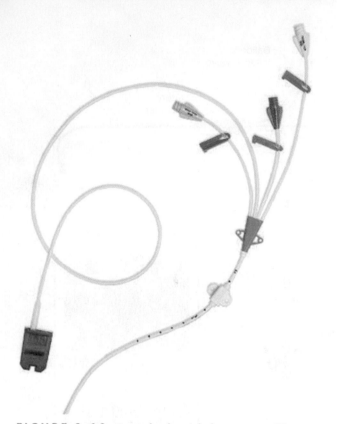

FIGURE 8-10. Example of a triple-lumen central line to measure central venous pressure and oxygen saturation. *(Courtesy of Edwards Lifesciences, Irvine, CA.)*

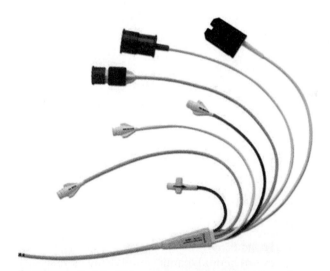

FIGURE 8-11. Example of a pulmonary artery catheter with capability of monitoring mixed venous oxygenation. *(Courtesy of Edwards Lifesciences, Irvine, CA.)*

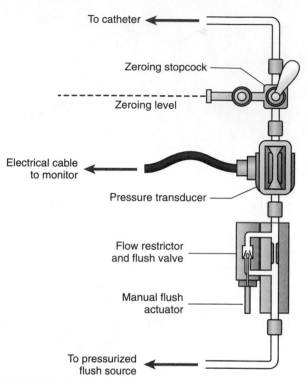

FIGURE 8-12. A schematic of a typical pressure transducer. *(From Kruse, J. A. [2003]. Fast flush test. In J. A. Kruse, M. P. Fink, & R. W. Carlson [Eds.],* Saunders manual of critical care *[p. 779]. Philadelphia: Saunders.)*

positioning, (3) zeroing the transducer, and (4) assessing dynamic responsiveness (performing the *square wave test*). Prevention of infection is another key nursing intervention for patients with invasive hemodynamic monitoring catheters.

Leveling the Air-Fluid Interface (Zeroing Stopcock)

To provide accurate hemodynamic measurements, the zeroing stopcock of the transducer system must be positioned at the level of the atria and PA. This external anatomical location is termed the *phlebostatic axis,* and is located by identifying the fourth intercostal space at the midway point of the anterior-posterior diameter of the chest wall (Figure 8-13). Once the level of the phlebostatic axis is identified, the transducer and zeroing stopcock can be secured to the chest wall or to a standard intravenous pole positioned near the patient. If the transducer is affixed to the chest wall, it is important to monitor skin integrity because skin breakdown can occur. An indelible marker can be used to mark the location of the phlebostatic axis on the patient to ensure future measurements are done using the same reference point.

Due to the effects of hydrostatic pressure on the fluid-filled monitoring system, variations in the height of the transducer system by as little as 1 cm

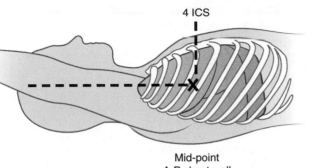

FIGURE 8-13. Locating the phlebostatic axis in the supine position.

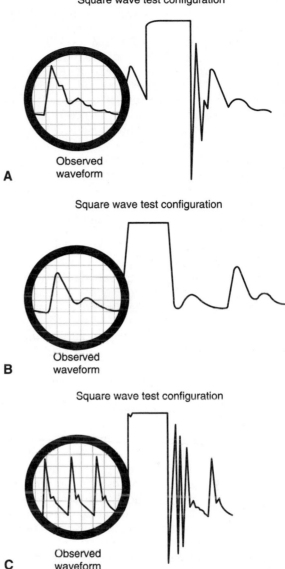

FIGURE 8-14. A, Optimal Dynamic Response Test. **B,** Overdamped Dynamic Response Test. **C,** Underdamped Dynamic Response Test.

below the phlebostatic axis can result in a false elevation by as much as 0.73 mm Hg. Conversely, if the transducer is above the phlebostatic axis, a falsely low reading results. Therefore, the location of the zeroing stopcock must be monitored on a regular basis and releveled with each change in the patient's position (Figure 8-14).

Patient Position

Assessment of hemodynamic status would be easier if patients remained in the supine, flat position all the time. However, most patients are more comfortable with the head of the bed (HOB) elevated, and elevation of the HOB is a key factor in the prevention of complications, such as ventilator-associated pneumonia. Hemodynamic parameters can be accurately measured and trended with the HOB elevated up to 45 degrees as long as the zeroing stopcock is properly leveled to the phlebostatic axis.

CLINICAL ALERT

Hemodynamic Monitoring

Keys to success in hemodynamic monitoring are ensuring the data are accurate, conducting waveform analysis, and integrating the data with other assessment variables. Clinical decision making should never be based solely on one variable.

No hemodynamic parameter should be interpreted in isolation. Integration of clinical data, patient presentation, and subjective assessment are crucial to making relevant clinical decisions that will improve patient outcomes.

Accurate hemodynamic data can also be obtained in lateral positions from 30 to 90 degrees, although it is technically more difficult to level the transducer to the atria. In the 30-degree lateral position, the transducer is placed half the distance from the surface of the bed to the left sternal border. The patient must be positioned *exactly* at a 30-degree lateral position for this method to be accurate. If the patient is in a 90-degree right lateral position, the transducer is leveled to the fourth intercostal space, midsternum. If the patient is in a 90-degree left lateral position, the transducer is leveled to the fourth intercostal space, left parasternal border.[15] The clinician should document patient position (e.g., HOB angle, lateral rotation) with each hemodynamic measurement.

Zero Referencing

The effects of atmospheric pressure on the fluid-filled hemodynamic monitoring system must be negated for accurate measurements. At sea level the atmospheric pressure exerts a force of 760 mm Hg on any object on the earth's surface. To eliminate the impact of the atmospheric pressure on the physiological variables, the transducer system is "zeroed" at the level of the phlebostatic axis. To accomplish this task, the zeroing stopcock of the transducer is opened to air (closed to the patient), and the monitoring system is programmed to read a pressure of 0 mm Hg. Each computer system has a zeroing function that is easy to perform. Zero referencing is done at the time of catheter insertion, at the beginning of each shift, and with significant changes in hemodynamic status.

Dynamic Response Testing

Fluid-filled monitoring systems rely on the ability of the transducer to translate the vascular pressure into waveforms and numeric data. To verify the accurate functioning of the transducer system, the responsiveness of the system is tested by performing the dynamic response or *square wave* test. This test is done by recording the pressure waveform while activating the fast flush valve/actuator on the pressure tubing system for at least 1 second. The resulting graph should depict a rapid upstroke from the baseline with a plateau before returning to the baseline (i.e., *square wave*). Upon the return of the pressure tracing to the baseline, a small undershoot should occur below the baseline, along with one or two oscillations, within 0.12 seconds prior to resuming the pressure waveform. If the dynamic response test meets these criteria, the system is optimally damped (Figure 8-14, *A*), and the resulting waveforms and numeric data can be interpreted as accurate. The dynamic response test should be performed after catheter insertion and at least once every 8 hours. It is a simple, but crucial test that must be incorporated into routine hemodynamic assessment.

The system is overdamped if the dynamic response test results in no oscillations, the upstroke is slurred, or a small undershoot is not produced (Figure 8-14, *B*). An overdamped system can result in a systolic pressure that is falsely low and a diastolic pressure that is falsely elevated.

Conversely, the system is underdamped if the dynamic response test results in excessive oscillations (Figure 8-14, *C*). The displayed pressure waveform and numeric data will show erroneously high systolic pressures and low diastolic pressures. Box 8-3 describes causes of abnormal dynamic response test results and interventions for troubleshooting systems that are overdamped or underdamped.

BOX 8-3   Abnormal Dynamic Response Test: Causes and Interventions

Overdamped system
- Blood clots, blood left in the catheter after obtaining a blood sample, air bubbles at any point between the catheter tip and transducer
  - Flush the system or aspirate, disconnecting from the patient if needed to adequately flush the system to remove clots or air bubbles
- Compliant tubing
  - Change to noncompliant tubing or commercially available tubing system
- Loose connections
  - Ensure all connections are secure
- Kinks in the tubing system
  - Straighten tubing

Underdamped system
- Excessive tubing length (>36-48 inches)
  - Remove extraneous tubing, stopcocks, or extensions
- Small bore tubing
  - Replace small bore tubing with a larger bore set
- Cause unknown
  - Add a damping device into the system to reduce artifact

Infection Control

Since invasive catheters are direct portals into the circulating blood volume, strict infection control measures must be implemented to reduce catheter-related bloodstream infections. Infection prevention measures include strict hand washing whenever handling, accessing, or manipulating the system; proper site maintenance, cleaning, and dressing; strict sterile technique during placement including maximal barrier precautions; and minimizing the number of times the system is opened by changing the tubing system and flush bag no more frequently than every 72 to 96 hours.[6] Institutional policies dictate the frequency of tubing change. Another consideration is the location of central venous catheter placement. Whenever possible, the subclavian vein is preferred for cannulation. This site affords the clinician a greater ability to maintain an intact dressing and provides the distance necessary to avoid contamination.[6] Box 8-4 describes general strategies for managing hemodynamic monitoring systems.

BOX 8-4   General Nursing Strategies for Managing Hemodynamic Monitoring Systems

- Document insertion date
- Change dressings according to institutional policy
  - Assess for signs of infection
  - Date dressing changes
- Maintain patency of the flush system
  - Flush the system after each use of a port
  - Clear any blood from the tubing, ports, and/or stopcocks
  - Maintain a pressure of 300 mm Hg on the flush solution using a pressure bag
  - Ensure adequate amount of flush solution in the intravenous bag
- Ensure tightened connections in the tubing and flush system
- Keep tubing free of kinks
- Minimize excess tubing and the number of stopcocks
- Place sterile caps on stopcock openings
- Ensure that alarm limits are set on the monitor and alarms are turned on
- Limit disconnecting or opening the system

BOX 8-5   Allen's and Modified Allen's Test Procedure

Allen's Test
- The patient forms a tight fist with the wrist in a neutral position
- The clinician occludes the radial artery by applying pressure with the thumb for approximately 1 minute
- Patient opens fist while the clinician maintains thumb pressure on radial artery
- Ulnar circulation is adequate if blanching resolves within 5 seconds, inadequate if hand remains pale for >10 seconds

Modified Allen's Test
- The patient forms a tight fist with the wrist in a neutral position
- Clinician occludes radial and ulnar arteries for approximately 1 minute
- Patient opens fist, revealing a blanched hand
- Clinician releases pressure on ulnar artery, maintaining pressure on radial artery
- Ulnar circulation is adequate if blanching resolves within 5 seconds, inadequate if hand remains pale for >10 seconds

Arterial Pressure Monitoring

Direct measurement of arterial blood pressure is a common procedure in critical care. Arterial pressure monitoring involves cannulation of an artery and recording pressures with the fluid-filled monitoring system. Radial artery placement is the site of choice because of its ready accessibility, collateral perfusion to the hand via the ulnar artery, and compressibility of the location. Alternative sites include the femoral and brachial arteries. Prior to cannulation of the radial artery, it is common to perform an Allen's test or a modified Allen's test to detect the presence or absence of collateral arterial flow to the distal extremity (Box 8-5). However, recent studies indicate that the Allen's test has poor interrater reliability and questionable definitions of an abnormal test, and may be a poor predictor of ischemia after removal of the catheter.[4]

Arterial pressure monitoring provides the most accurate reflection of the systemic blood pressure. This method of measuring blood pressure allows for continuous, beat-to-beat analysis of the arterial pressure. It is the method of choice in assessing blood pressure in the hemodynamically unstable patient. An additional benefit in having an indwelling arterial catheter is the ability to perform frequent, painless blood sampling for analysis of blood counts, chemistries, gases, and drug levels.

The normal arterial waveform (Figure 8-15) consists of a sharp upstroke, the peak of which represents the systolic pressure. After this systolic peak, the force is decreased as the pressure drops. This downstroke contains a dicrotic notch reflecting aortic valve closure and the beginning of diastole. The remainder of the downstroke is arterial distribution of blood flow through the arterial system. The lowest point on the waveform represents the diastolic pressure value.

Complications

The major complications of arterial pressure monitoring include thrombosis, embolism, blood loss, and infection. Embolism may occur as a result of small clot formation around the tip of the catheter or from air entering the system. Thrombosis (clot) may occur if a continuous flush solution is not used properly. Blood loss results from sudden dislodgment of the catheter from the artery or from a disconnection in the tubing. Rapid blood loss may occur (because this is in an artery, not a vein) if either of these occurrences is not promptly recognized. Infection may occur if the catheter is left in place for a prolonged

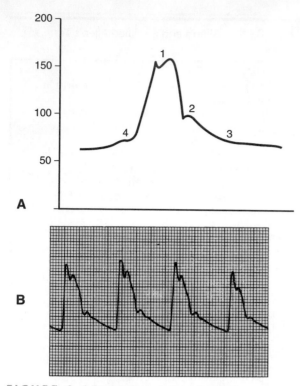

FIGURE 8-15. **A,** Normal arterial pressure tracing; *1,* peak systolic pressure; *2,* dicrotic notch; *3,* diastolic pressure; *4,* anacrotic notch. **B,** Arterial pressure waveform obtained from arterial line.

period; however, routine replacement of the catheter is not recommended.

Clinical Considerations

The invasive method of obtaining blood pressure is considered to be more accurate than noninvasive methods because it gives beat-by-beat information instead of measuring vibrations (Korotkoff's sounds) of the arterial wall over several beats. In patients who are hypotensive, a serious discrepancy may exist between the blood pressures obtained by invasive and noninvasive means. The cuff pressure may be significantly lower, leading to dangerous mistakes in the treatment of such a patient. Under normal circumstances, a difference of 5 to 20 mm Hg or more between invasive and noninvasive blood pressure is expected, with the invasive blood pressure generally higher than the noninvasive value. This difference may vary substantially from the invasive blood pressure determination, and, for this reason, treatment should never be based on the measurement of a single determination of NIBP. When the noninvasive value is higher than the invasive number, one must suspect equipment malfunction or technical error. Box 8-6 lists the possible causes.

BOX 8-6   Causes of Higher Noninvasive versus Invasive Blood Pressure

- Air bubbles
- Failure to *zero* the transducer air-fluid interface
- Blood in the catheter system
- Blood clot at the catheter tip
- Kinking of the tubing system
- Catheter tip lodging against the arterial wall
- Soft, compliant tubing
- Long tubing (>48 inches)
- Too many stopcocks (>3)
- Improper cuff size
- Improper cuff placement

Nursing Implications

Standard management of all invasive hemodynamic systems was described in Box 8-4. Additional interventions specific to management of the intraarterial catheter include:

- Document assessment of the extremity every 2 hours for perfusion: color, temperature, sensation, pulse, and capillary refill.
- Keep the patient's wrist in a neutral position and/or place it on an armboard (radial artery catheters).
- When the catheter is removed, ensure that adequate pressure is applied to the site of insertion until hemostasis is obtained (for a minimum of 5 minutes for radial artery catheters). The time required varies, depending on the type, size, and location of the catheter and the patient's coagulation status.

Right Atrial Pressure/Central Venous Pressure Monitoring

CVP has been used as a method to assess central venous blood volume for many years. The CVP is obtained from a central line inserted into the superior or inferior vena cava. When the pressure is obtained from the right atrial port of a PA catheter (PAC), it is called right atrial pressure (RAP). Because no valves are present between the vena cavae and right atrium, both the CVP and RAP are essentially equal pressures. Both terms refer to pressures from the right side of the heart and are often used interchangeably. The term RAP is used most of the time in this textbook. Normal CVP/RAP ranges from 2 to 6 mm Hg.

Several sites may be used for RAP line insertion; the subclavian and internal jugular veins are commonly used sites. Catheters used for RAP measurement are generally stiff and radiopaque. They vary in length and diameter depending on the vein that is used. Shorter catheters are inserted into the subclavian and internal jugular veins, and longer catheters are used for insertion into the upper extremities or femoral vein. Central venous catheters often have multiple lumens that facilitate pressure monitoring, administration of several types of fluids, and blood sampling. Insertion is similar to that for PACs, which is described later in the chapter.

Figure 8-16 shows a position of a central venous catheter in the right atrium along with the corresponding waveform. During right ventricular diastole, the tricuspid valve is open, thereby allowing a clear passage for blood to flow from the right atrium to the right ventricle. Because of this fact, the RAP provides a reliable measurement of right ventricular preload.

Although RAP is often used to determine right ventricular preload, the response to the administration of fluids, or both, the measurement may not always be accurate, especially in critically ill patients.[17] A primary reason for the inaccuracy is the inconsistent methods of obtaining the numeric value. There is far more to assessing RAP than recording the digital value on the bedside monitor. The zeroing stopcock must be properly leveled and zero referenced, since the normal value of RAP is low and within a narrow range. Every centimeter that the zeroing stopcock is off from the phlebostatic axis dramatically affects the reading.

The bedside monitor displays a mean value as opposed to a true reading of RAP.[2] For accuracy, the RAP must be measured at end expiration and at the end of ventricular diastole. Simultaneous graphing of the cardiac rhythm (ECG), RAP, and respiratory tracing (if available) is done to obtain an accurate measurement of RAP. The RAP tracing is composed of 3 major waveforms: a, c, and v waves (Figure 8-16). The a wave is produced by atrial contraction and follows the P wave on the ECG tracing. The c wave is produced by closure of the tricuspid valve and follows the R wave. Finally, the v wave correlates with right atrial filling; it follows the T wave on the ECG.[2]

To measure the RAP, the a, c, and v waves of the RAP tracing at end expiration are identified (Figure 8-17). The RAP is measured at end expiration to ensure that pleural pressure changes do not skew the numeric value. True RAP is best measured by locating the c wave and identifying the value immediately preceding the c wave (termed the pre-c measurement). Alternatively, the average of the a waves may be computed, or the z-point method may be implemented. The z-point method consists of identifying the RAP by locating the end of the QRS complex and using that as the reference point on the tracing. Box 8-7 outlines circumstances for using the different methods for determining RAP.[11]

Complications

Nurses assist in insertion of central lines. Infection prevention is essential because catheter-related bloodstream infections are common with central lines, which increases the risk of sepsis. Other complications may occur during insertion. These include

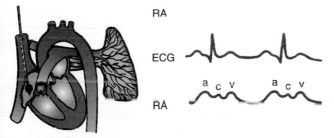

FIGURE 8-16. Position of central venous catheter in right atrium along with associated waveforms.

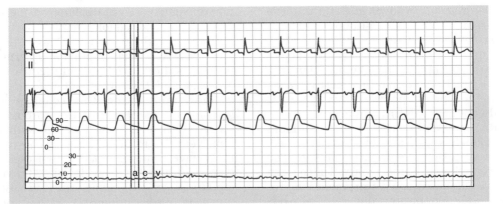

FIGURE 8-17. Identifying the a, c, and v waveforms to determine right atrial pressure.

BOX 8-7   Methods for Determining Accurate Right Atrial Pressure

Pre-c method
- Most accurate measure of right-sided preload; method of choice for numeric assessment
- Represents the last atrial pressure before ventricular contraction
- Difficult to use because often the *c* wave is unidentifiable

Mean of the *a* waves
- Clinically significant as the *a* wave results from atrial contraction
- Used if the *c* wave cannot be identified
- Obtain the numeric for the top and bottom of the *a* wave. Calculate the sum and divide by 2.

Z-point method
- Used when *a–v* synchrony is not present; atrial fibrillation 3rd degree heart block.
- Standardized approach results in the most reproducible results between clinicians
- Does not account for hemodynamic effects on kidneys or liver that result from the prominent *a* or *v* waves
- Locate the end of the QRS complex, use the numeric at the exact point of intersection of the *RA* wave.

carotid puncture, pneumothorax, hemothorax, perforation of the right atrium or ventricle, and cardiac dysrhythmias. A chest x-ray is obtained after insertion to confirm placement and detect complications.

Clinical Considerations

Abnormalities in RAP are generally caused by any condition that alters venous tone, blood volume, or right ventricular contractility. For example, a patient with a low RAP may be hypovolemic because of dehydration or traumatic blood loss. Low pressures are also seen in relative hypovolemia as a result of vasodilation from rewarming, medications, or sepsis. In all of these conditions, RAP reflects blood return to the heart that is insufficient to meet the body's requirements. Confounding the interpretation of a low RAP is that the value may be negative in an individual in the upright position even if cardiac function and volume status are normal.[11]

A high RAP measurement indicates conditions that reduce the right ventricle's ability to eject blood, thereby increasing right ventricular pressure and RAP. Such conditions include hypervolemia (seen with aggressive administration of intravenous fluids), severe vasoconstriction, or any condition that overloads the ventricle so it is unable to eject properly.

Other examples include pulmonary hypertension and right-sided heart failure (often seen in cardiac ischemia of the right heart, which reduces the contractile ability of the right ventricle during systole, causing a backup of blood into the right side of the heart).

Nursing Implications

The critical care nurse is responsible for collecting and recording patient data, ensuring the accuracy of the data, and reporting abnormal findings and trends to the physician. Analyzing the various hemodynamic parameters is a collaborative responsibility between the medical and nursing staff so that prompt and appropriate treatments occur. Measurements of RAP are most valuable when they are compared with other physiological parameters and physical assessment.

Pulmonary Artery Pressure Monitoring

The ability to measure pressures in the PA and the left side of the heart became reality after the development of the flow-directed PAC by Drs. Jeremy Swan and William Ganz in 1970.[1] Prior to this development, the only direct cardiac pressure measurement available was the RAP, which provides no indication of function of the left side of the heart. The PAC became the *gold standard* in hemodynamic management.

Determining PA pressures (PAPs) is done via a specialized catheter placed directly into the PA (Figure 8-18). The PAC is a long, flexible, multilumen catheter that measures a variety of hemodynamic parameters. The proximal lumen is situated in the right atrium and measures RAP; the distal lumen measures PAPs; and the thermistor is used to determine thermodilution CO. Many catheters have an additional proximal infusion port for fluid and medication administration. The balloon inflation lumen provides the ability to inflate the small-volume (approximately 1.5 mL) balloon at the distal tip of the catheter. The balloon is inflated to facilitate insertion of the catheter and to measure PA occlusion pressure (PAOP), which provides information about the function of the left side of the heart.

Specialized PACs are also designed for the purpose of transvenous pacing. This technique involves the insertion of pacemaker wires through additional lumina in the PAC, which exit the catheter into the right ventricle to provide ventricular pacing. Other PACs have continuous CO (CCO) capabilities. This type of catheter was developed to provide ongoing monitoring of CO. Some catheters also have the capability of measuring SvO$_2$. Continuous monitoring of SvO$_2$ is through a fiberoptic network housed

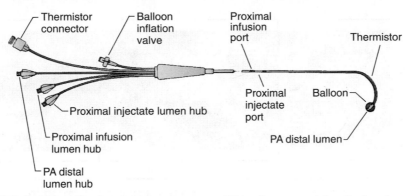

FIGURE 8-18. A five-lumen pulmonary artery (PA) catheter containing the four-lumen components in addition to a second proximal lumen for infusion of fluid or medications. *(Courtesy of Edwards Lifesciences, Irvine, CA.)*

inside a conventional PAC. The concepts of CCO and SvO_2 are discussed later in this chapter.

Nurses assist during PAC insertion, and nursing interventions include patient education and advocacy. While it is the physician's responsibility to obtain the informed consent for insertion of the PAC, the critical care nurse provides much of the education regarding patient positioning and what the patient may feel or experience during the procedure, as well as allaying the patient's anxiety before and during the procedure.

The PAC is usually inserted into the subclavian, internal jugular, or external jugular vein. The patient's bed is placed in Trendelenburg position to promote venous filling in the upper body for easier insertion of the catheter. This position can also prevent air embolism during insertion. If Trendelenburg position is contraindicated, a blanket roll can be placed between the patient's shoulder blades to facilitate insertion. The skin is cleaned and draped and is then injected with a local anesthetic. A needled syringe is used to puncture the vessel and to confirm placement by backward flow of blood into the syringe. The syringe is removed, and a guidewire is threaded through the needle into the vessel. The needle is then removed so a hollow tube, called an introducer, may be passed over the guidewire. The wire is then removed, and the PAC is passed freely into the vessel through the introducer. The physician inserting the catheter will instruct the nurse (or other professional helping during insertion) to inflate and deflate the balloon during the procedure to facilitate flow from the right atrium to the PA. The insertion technique may vary according to physician preference, brand of equipment used, and the patient's anatomy.

During the PAC insertion, the critical care nurse is responsible for monitoring and recording heart rate and rhythm, recognizing dysrhythmias, and monitoring blood pressure. Ventricular dysrhythmias often occur as the PAC passes through the right ventricle into the PA. The nurse may assist with balloon inflation during the procedure. As the catheter passes through each chamber, the nurse observes the waveform characteristics and records pressure values: RAP, right ventricular pressure, PAP, and PAOP (Figure 8-19, *A* and *B*). The PAOP waveform signals the end of insertion, at which time the balloon is deflated. Once the balloon is deflated, the tip of the catheter falls back into position in the PA (Figure 8-19, *C*). After the catheter is inserted and placement is verified, the balloon is only inflated to obtain periodic PAOP measurements (Figure 8-19, *D*); otherwise it remains deflated to prevent complications (e.g., pulmonary infarction, PA rupture). It is important for the nurse to identify and recognize typical waveforms. Graphing the pressure waveforms and ECG tracing is also recommended.

As patient advocate, the critical care nurse is responsible for promoting patient safety throughout the procedure. This includes ensuring that sterility is maintained, patient monitoring, and assisting with balloon inflation and deflation. Because PAC insertion involves certain risks, emergency medications and equipment must be readily available. Complications of insertion include hemothorax, pneumothorax, perforation of the vein or cardiac chamber, and cardiac dysrhythmias—especially as the PAC passes through the right ventricle. After the procedure, a chest x-ray is obtained to verify placement and to assess for complications (i.e., pneumothorax, hemothorax). Once position is radiographically verified, the nurse should document the depth of catheter insertion; depth markings are noted on the PAC.

Hemodynamic Parameters Monitored via the PAC
Several pressures are measured by the PAC: systolic, diastolic, and mean. The PA systolic pressure is the peak pressure as the right ventricle ejects its stroke

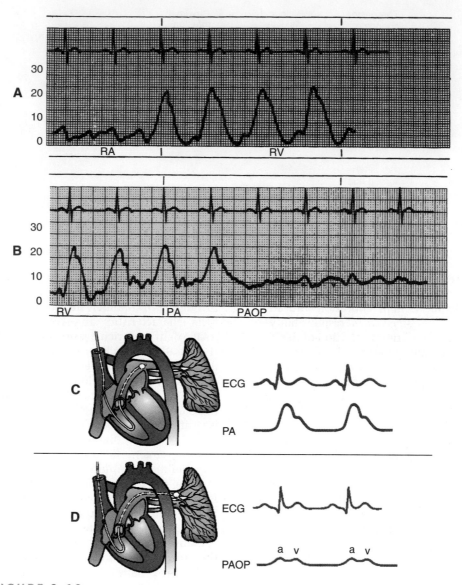

FIGURE 8-19. Position of pulmonary artery (PA) catheter and associated waveforms. **(A)** Dual-channel tracing of cardiac rhythm with pressure waveforms obtained as the PA catheter is inserted into the right atrium (RA) and right ventricle (RV); **(B)** dual-channel tracing of cardiac rhythm with RV, PA, and pulmonary artery occlusion pressure (PAOP) waveforms as the catheter is floated into proper position; **(C)**, PA catheter in pulmonary artery; **(D)** PA catheter floating into pulmonary capillary with balloon inflated for PAOP measurements.

volume, and reflects the amount of pressure needed to open the pulmonic valve and eject blood into the pulmonary vasculature. The PA diastolic pressure (PADP) represents the resistance of the pulmonary vascular bed as measured when the pulmonic valve is closed and tricuspid valve is opened. The PA mean pressure is the average pressure exerted on the pulmonary vasculature. The normal PAP is approximately 25/10 mm Hg, and the mean pressure is 15 mm Hg.

Another parameter that is obtained by the PAC is the PAOP. When the balloon is inflated and the PA is occluded, the resulting pressure reflects the left atrial pressure and left ventricular end-diastolic pressure when the mitral valve is open. When properly assessed, the PAOP is a reliable indicator of left ventricular function. Normal PAOP is 8 to 12 mm Hg. The PAOP is measured at regular intervals as ordered by the physician, or in accordance with unit protocols. The measurement is obtained by inflating the balloon with no more than 1.5 mL of air, for no longer than 8 to 10 seconds, while noting the waveform change from the PAP to the PAOP (Figure 8-19, *D*). To obtain accurate measurement of the

PAOP, the critical care nurse must print the PAOP waveform as well as the ECG and respiratory patterns. Similar to RAP, PAP and PAOP measurements must be obtained at end expiration. In the patient who is spontaneously breathing, pressures are highest at end expiration and decline with inhalation (Figure 8-20, A). Measurements are obtained from the waveform just before pressures decline. In the mechanically ventilated patient, pressures increase with inhalation, and decrease with exhalation (Figure 8-20, B). Measurements are obtained just before the increase in pressures during inhalation (www.pacep.org).

Clinical Considerations

Trending of PAPs provides an indirect measure of left ventricular function. The PAOP provides more specific information to guide treatment and monitor the patient's response. The PAOP reflects the pressure ahead of the catheter—both the left atrial pressure and the left ventricular end-diastolic pressure when the mitral valve is open. Thus, the PAOP is a reliable indirect measurement of left ventricular function. In the absence of valvular disease and pulmonary vascular congestion, the PADP also closely approximates left ventricle function because the mitral valve is open during end diastole. The PADP is often used as an indirect measurement of PAOP.

An increase in left ventricular end-diastolic pressure (and therefore PAOP) indicates an increase in left ventricular blood volume to be ejected with the next systole. Increased PAOP may occur in patients who have fluid volume excess resulting from overzealous administration of intravenous fluid, as well as in those with renal dysfunction. An increase in PAOP also provides the clinician with early information about impending left ventricular failure, as may be seen with myocardial infarction.

A decrease in left ventricular end-diastolic pressure (and a subsequently low PAOP) signals a reduction in left ventricular blood volume available for the next contraction. Conditions causing a low PAOP include those that cause fluid volume deficit, such as dehydration, excessive diuretic therapy, and hemorrhage. Through monitoring of changes and trends, the PAOP can be invaluable in determining appropriate therapy, as well as the effectiveness of that therapy.

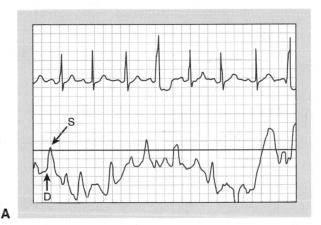

A

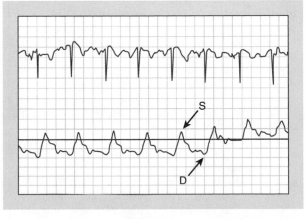

B

FIGURE 8-20. Effect of respiration on pulmonary artery waveforms in patients with spontaneous breathing (A) and mechanical ventilation (B).

Nursing Implications

Patients with prolonged PA catheterization must be carefully examined for signs or symptoms of infection. Nurses regularly monitor RAP, PAP, and PAOP to identify trends and the clinical significance of the values. The catheter position must be maintained in the PA; the nurse assesses placement by reviewing results of chest x-rays, observing for normal waveforms, and ensuring that the balloon is deflated except during PAOP measurements.

It is helpful to know how much air is needed to obtain the PAOP (≤1.5 mL). If the PAOP is obtained with a much smaller amount of air, the catheter may have migrated into the PA. The nurse never forces the balloon to inflation if resistance is met. If the PAOP is not noted with inflation of 1.5 mL, the catheter may have been pulled out of position, or the balloon may have ruptured. In both of these situations, verification of proper positioning by a chest x-ray and observation of the PAP waveform are important interventions. The nurse should also make periodic comparisons of the PADP and PAOP to assess the accuracy of the PAOP measurement, especially in patients having acute hemodynamic changes. When it is determined that the PAC is no longer needed, nurses who are specially trained in withdrawing the PAC often perform the procedure.

Controversy Surrounding the PAC

Despite the widespread use of the PAC, in the mid-1990s randomized controlled trials demonstrated that patients with PACs did not necessarily have better outcomes than those managed without them. Patients with PACs tended to have more complications than those managed more conservatively. Some clinicians suggested that outcomes were not improved in patients with a PAC because of a lack of standardized education, a lack of understanding of how to obtain accurate data, and an inability to interpret the findings. These findings became the impetus to develop a multidisciplinary, standardized, Web-based education program, The Pulmonary Artery Catheter Education Project (www.pacep.org), and newer, less invasive means of evaluating cardiac function. (See Evidence-Based Practice.)

Cardiac Output Monitoring

The CO is the amount of blood ejected by the heart each minute and is calculated from the heart rate and stroke volume. Cardiac index (CI) is the CO adjusted for an individual's size or body surface area. Monitoring of CO/CI is done to assess the heart's ability to pump oxygenated blood to the tissues. Causes of low and high COs are outlined in Box 8-8. Two methods are commonly used to evaluate CO via the PAC: thermodilution (TdCO) and CCO.

Thermodilution Cardiac Output

To measure the CO via the TdCO method, the thermistor connector on the PAC is attached to a CO module on the cardiac monitor. A set volume (5 to 10 mL) of room temperature or iced solution (injectate) of 0.9% normal saline or 5% dextrose in water, is injected quickly and smoothly via the proximal port of the PAC. Many institutions use a closed injectate delivery system to facilitate the procedure (Figure 8-21). As the fluid bolus passes into the right ventricle and subsequently the PA, the difference in temperature is sensed by the thermistor located at the distal portion of the catheter (Figure 8-22). The TdCO is calculated as the difference in temperatures on a time versus temperature curve. Normal CO is represented by a smooth curve with a rapid upstroke and slow return to the baseline. The CO module calculates the area under the curve. The CO is inversely proportional to the area under the curve—patients with a high CO have a low calculated area under the curve. Therefore, the TdCO measurement is least accurate in patients with a low CO state and most accurate in high CO states. Several steps must

EVIDENCE-BASED PRACTICE

PROBLEM

Pulmonary artery catheters (PACs) have been used in the management of critically ill patients for more than 30 years. Insertion of these catheters is associated with risks, such as infection. Benefits of the PAC may not outweigh the risks.

QUESTION

What is the effect of pulmonary artery catheterization on patient outcomes?

REFERENCES

Hadian, M., & Pinsky, M. R. (2006). Evidence-based review on the use of the pulmonary artery catheter: Impact data and complications. *Critical Care*, *10*(Suppl. 3), S8, 1-11.

Harvey, S., Young, D., Brampton, W., Cooper, A. B., Doig, G., Sibbald, W., et al. (2007). Pulmonary artery catheters for adult patients in intensive care. *Cochrane Database of Systematic Reviews*, *4*. Retrieved December 3, 2007, from www.cochrane.org.

EVIDENCE

The authors searched the literature published since the PAC was introduced in 1971. Hadian and Pinsky (2006) evaluated the impact of the PAC on clinical outcomes, cost-effectiveness, and complications. Harvey and colleagues (2007) evaluated trials comparing outcomes of patients with and without a PAC. No differences in clinical outcomes were found to result from the insertion of a PAC, including length of stay, faster recovery, or survival. Average costs for patients with a PAC were higher than for those without a PAC. The PAC was associated with more complications, such as dysrhythmias during insertion, infections, thrombotic complications, and rupture of the pulmonary artery (although rare).

IMPLICATIONS FOR NURSING

Many researchers who have evaluated the evidence related to PACs do not recommend routine insertion of PACs. Less invasive methods of hemodynamic monitoring—such as RAP and central venous oxygen saturation ($ScvO_2$) monitoring from a central line—provide data to guide treatment with fewer complications in many patients. Noninvasive methods of hemodynamic monitoring may also be considered as newer modalities are developed and tested in the critically ill patient. Additional research is needed to determine which patients benefit most from PAC insertion, such as those with sepsis. Nurses must be aware of the current evidence related to hemodynamic monitoring and become knowledgeable and skilled in newer modalities of assessment and monitoring.

BOX 8-8 Interpretation of Abnormal Cardiac Output/Index Values

Low Cardiac Output/Index
- Heart rate that is too fast or too slow leading to inadequate ventricular filling
- Stroke volume reduction as a result of:
  - Decreased preload
    Hemorrhage
    Hypovolemia from diuresis, dehydration, etc.
    Vasodilatation
    Fluid shifts (i.e., third spacing) outside the intravascular space
  - Increased afterload
    Vasoconstriction
    Increased blood viscosity
  - Decreased contractility
    Myocardial infarction or ischemia
    Heart failure
    Cardiomyopathy
    Cardiogenic shock
    Cardiac tamponade

High Cardiac Output/Index
- Heart rate elevation secondary to:
  - Increased activity
  - Anemia
  - Metabolic demands
  - Adrenal disorders
  - Fever
  - Anxiety
- Stroke volume increase as a result of:
  - Increased preload
    Fluid resuscitation
    Alteration in ventricular compliance
  - Decreased afterload
    Vasodilatation in sepsis
    Decreased blood viscosity (anemia)
    Increased contractility
    Hypermetabolic states
    Medication therapy

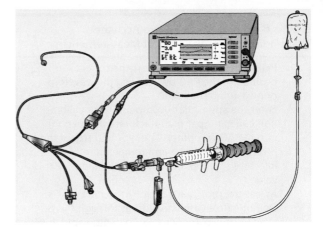

FIGURE 8-21. Illustration of the closed injectate delivery system (room temperature fluids) for thermodilution cardiac output measurement.

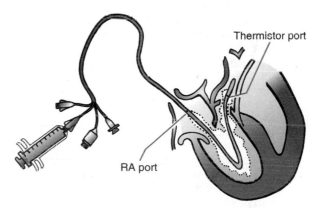

FIGURE 8-22. Illustration of injection of fluid into the right atrium (RA) for cardiac output measurement.

be taken to obtain accurate TdCO measurements. Box 8-9 describes these important points.

Continuous Cardiac Output

The CCO method is based on the same theory as TdCO. The CCO system uses a modified PAC and a CO computer specific to the device. The PAC has a copper filament near the distal end that delivers pulses of energy at prescribed time intervals and warms the blood in the right ventricle. This temperature change is detected by the thermistor at the tip of the PAC about every 30 to 60 seconds. The computer interprets the temperature change and aver-

ages the CO measurements over the previous 3 to 6 minutes. Figure 8-23 shows an example of a computer interface for CCO and other hemodynamic parameters. Patients with a CCO device can be positioned supine with the HOB elevated up to 45 degrees. Removing the operator error potential makes the CCO method attractive to the bedside clinician. Other advantages of CCO are that no extra fluid is administered to the patient, data are available for trending throughout the shift, and there is no need to change the computation constant. Drawbacks to CCO include that the device may not sense the CCO in the patient whose body temperature is greater than 40° C to 43° C, as the thermal filament heats to a maximum of 44° C. CCO does not reflect acute changes in CO. Since the measurements provide an average of CO over several minutes, a delay of 10 minutes or more is common to detect a change in CO of 1 L/min.

BOX 8-9 Steps to Ensure Accurate Thermodilution Cardiac Output Measurements

- Before the procedure, assess the correct position of the PAC by verifying the waveform or measuring the PAOP.
- Enter the appropriate computation or calibration constant (per manufacturer's instruction) into the CO computer. The type and size of the PAC, and the volume and temperature of the injectate solution are factors that determine this value.
- Assess the proximal port for the patency.
- Do not infuse vasoactive drugs through the port used to obtain TdCO measurements. Rapid infusion of the injectate solution for the TdCO will result in delivery of these medications beyond the recommended dosage and cause potentially harmful side effects.
- Position the patient in the supine position with the backrest elevation 0 to 30 degrees.
- Room temperature injectate is acceptable as long as there is at least a 10-degree difference between the temperature of the injectate and the patient's temperature.
- Inject the solution smoothly and rapidly (within 4 seconds) at the end of expiration to reduce the impact of chest wall motion and intrathoracic pressure changes.
- Obtain three CO measurements, and calculate the average CO (a feature on the CO computer averages the measurements). Values should be within 10% of each other. Measurements outside of 10% agreement should be discarded and repeated before averaging the results.
- The first CO is usually the most variable.

PAC, Pulmonary artery catheter; *PAOP,* pulmonary artery occlusion pressure; *CO,* cardiac output; *TdCO,* thermodilution cardiac output.

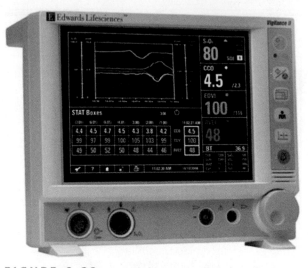

FIGURE 8-23. A sample monitor interface displaying hemodynamic parameters and trends, including continuous cardiac output (CCO) and mixed venous oxygen saturation (SvO$_2$). *(Courtesy of Edwards Lifesciences, Irvine, CA.)*

Oxygen Delivery and Consumption

One of the key indices of adequate CO is the ability of the cardiovascular system to meet the metabolic needs of the tissues. Venous oxygen saturation is the percent of hemoglobin saturation in the central venous circulation and provides an assessment of the amount of oxygen extracted by the tissues. Oxygenated arterial blood passes through the capillary network to deliver oxygen and nutrients to the tissues; however, not all the oxygen is used, and residual oxygen bound to the hemoglobin is returned to the central circulation to be reoxygenated. The oxygen saturation of this *mixed venous* blood from various organs and tissues that have different metabolic needs provides a global picture of oxygen delivery and oxygen consumption. Factors that affect venous oxygen saturation include CO, hemoglobin, arterial oxygen saturation, and tissue metabolism.

Oxygen delivery and consumption can be calculated by a variety of formulas (Table 8-2). Two invasive techniques are also available for clinical determination of venous oxygen saturation: SvO$_2$ and central venous oxygen saturation (ScvO$_2$). SvO$_2$ is measured in the PA, and ScvO$_2$ is measured in the central venous system, usually the superior vena cava. Both SvO$_2$ and ScvO$_2$ methods use fiberoptic catheters that are connected to monitors/computers with an optical module (see Figure 8-11). Calibration of the system is usually done upon insertion, and if the system becomes disconnected from the optical module. A blood sample is obtained from either the PAC (SvO$_2$) or central venous catheter (ScvO$_2$), and a blood gas analysis is done. Oxygen saturation results from this analysis are used to calibrate the equipment. Figure 8-23 shows an example of the clinical information provided by one monitoring device.

Monitoring of SvO$_2$ and ScvO$_2$ is indicated for any critically ill or injured patient who has the potential to develop an imbalance between oxygen delivery and demand by the tissues. Patients with trauma, acute respiratory distress syndrome, and septic shock, and those undergoing complex cardiac surgery may benefit from venous oxygen saturation monitoring.

TABLE 8-2   Hemodynamic Calculations

Mean arterial pressure	$[\text{Systolic BP} + (2 \times \text{DBP})] \div 3$	70-105 mm Hg
Arterial oxygen content (CaO_2)	$[1.34 \times \text{Hgb (g/dL)} \times SaO_2] + [0.003 \times PaO_2]$	19-20 mL/dL
Venous oxygen content (CvO_2)	$[1.34 \times \text{Hgb (g/dL)} \times SvO_2] + [0.003 \times PvO_2]$	12-15 mL/dL
Oxygen delivery (DO_2)	$\text{CO} \times CaO_2 \times 10$	900-1100 mL/min
Oxygen consumption (VO_2)	$C(a\text{-}v)O_2 \times \text{CO} \times 10$	200-250 mL/min
Oxygen extraction ratio (O_2ER)	$[(CaO_2 - CvO_2)/CaO_2] \times 100$	22%-30%

BP, Blood pressure; *CO*, cardiac output; *Hgb*, hemoglobin; *SaO₂*, arterial oxygen saturation, *SvO₂*, mixed venous oxygen saturation; *PaO₂*, partial pressure of arterial oxygen; *PvO₂*, partial pressure of venous oxygen.

TABLE 8-3   Alterations in Mixed Venous Oxygen Saturation

Alteration	Cause	Possible Etiology
Low SvO₂ (<60%)	↓ O₂ delivery	Hypoxia or hemorrhage, anemic states, hypovolemia, cardiogenic shock, dysrhythmias, myocardial infarction, congestive heart failure, cardiac tamponade, massive transfusions of stored blood, restrictive lung disease, ventilation/perfusion abnormalities
	↑ O₂ consumption	Strenuous activity, fever, pain, anxiety or stress, hormonal imbalances, increased work of breathing, bathing, septic shock (late), seizures, shivering
High SvO₂ (>75%)	↑ O₂ delivery	Increase in FiO₂, hyperoxygenation
	↓ O₂ consumption	Hypothermia, anesthesia, hypothyroidism, neuromuscular blockade, early stages of sepsis
High SvO₂ (>80%)	Technical error	PA catheter in wedged position, fibrin clot at end of catheter, computer needs to be recalibrated

FiO₂, Fractional concentration of oxygen in inspired gas; *O₂*, oxygen; *PA*, pulmonary artery; *SvO₂*, mixed venous oxygen saturation.

An SvO₂ between 60% and 75% indicates an adequate balance between supply and demand. The normal range for ScvO₂ (65% to 85%) is slightly higher because the measurement is from the blood in the central venous circulation versus the PA.

Many nursing interventions and clinical conditions affect the SvO₂/ScvO₂. Table 8-3 highlights causes for alterations in SvO₂ values. Any changes in arterial oxygen saturation, tissue metabolism, hemoglobin, or CO affect the values. For example, endotracheal suctioning may cause a transient decrease in the SvO₂/ScvO₂ values if arterial oxygen saturation decreases during the procedure. Factors that increase the metabolic rate, such as shivering, can also lead to a dramatic decrease in SvO₂/ScvO₂.

SvO₂/ScvO₂ values in the normal range can be misleading to clinicians and like all other hemodynamic parameters should not be assessed in isolation.

Integration of clinical data is crucial to ensure good clinical decision making. Decreased SvO₂/ScvO₂ values result from a failure to deliver adequate oxygen to the tissues or increased oxygen consumption. Elevated SvO₂/ScvO₂ values indicate that the tissues are not utilizing the oxygen delivered, which is related to four physiological reasons:

1. Shunting, either intravascular or intracardiac, does not allow the tissues to be exposed to the oxygen being delivered to the tissue bed.
2. A shift of the oxyhemoglobin dissociation curve to the left results in an increased affinity of hemoglobin for oxygen.
3. An increased diffusion distance between the capillaries and cells is present due to interstitial edema.
4. Cells are unable to take up or use the oxygen being delivered, or both, a frequent phenomenon in sepsis.

BOX 8-10   Esophageal Doppler Monitoring
Indications and Contraindications

Indications
- States of hypoperfusion (hypovolemia, hemor-rhagic shock, septic shock)
- Hemodynamic monitoring and evaluation of major end organ dysfunction
- Differential diagnosis of hypotensive states
- As an adjunct for diagnosis and management of heart failure, cardiogenic shock, valvular dysfunction, ventricular septal rupture, cardiac rupture with tamponade
- Preoperative, intraoperative, and postoperative management of high-risk cardiac patients undergoing surgical procedures

Contraindications
- Local disease
  - Esophageal stent
  - Carcinoma of the esophagus or pharynx
  - Previous esophageal surgery
  - Esophageal stricture
  - Esophageal varices
  - Pharyngeal pouch
- Aortic abnormalities
  - Intraaortic balloon pump
  - Coarctation of the aorta
- Systemic
  - Severe coagulopathy

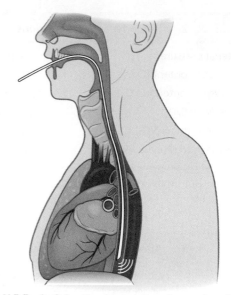

FIGURE 8-24. Esophageal Doppler probe placement. *(Courtesy of Deltex Medical, Inc., Branford, CT.)*

EMERGING TECHNIQUES AND TECHNOLOGIES

In recent years, resources, time, and energy have been devoted to developing less invasive ways of assessing hemodynamic status and adequacy of tissue perfusion. As new technologies emerge, it is important to understand the science behind the method as well as the ability of the new technology to assist in guiding therapies to improve patient outcomes. This continues to be an active area of research and development in critical care.

Esophageal Doppler Monitoring

Optimization of intravenous fluid replacement (colloid or crystalloid solutions) is essential to achieve and maintain adequate organ perfusion. Ideally, this requires measurement of blood pressure and flow. Blood pressure must be sufficient to maintain a patent vessel lumen, and blood flow must be sufficient to deliver adequate oxygen and metabo-

BOX 8-11   Nurse-Driven Protocol Using
Esophageal Doppler Monitoring to Guide Therapy[14]

- Once the probe is properly placed and focused, record the baseline cardiac output, FTc, and stroke volume.
- Administer a fluid challenge of either 250 to 500 mL of crystalloid solution, or 250 mL of 5% albumin.
- Refocus the probe and record the same measurements as done at baseline.
  - If the stroke volume increases by 10%, repeat the fluid challenge up to 4 times or until the stroke volume does not increase by 10%.
  - If the stroke volume increases, but not quite by 10%, and the FTc improves but is still less than 360 milliseconds, consider a repeat bolus.
  - If the stroke volume and FTc do not increase by 10%, the left ventricle is well filled for the present afterload and contractility.

FTc, Corrected flow time.

lites to every cell (as well as remove metabolic byproducts such as carbon dioxide and lactate). If fluid volume is inadequate, hypovolemia, hypotension, and inadequate perfusion of end organs such as kidneys, mesentery, and skin may occur. Conversely, excess administration of fluids may precipitate heart failure, especially in patients with underlying cardiac disease. Clinicians have struggled to find a method to evaluate and assess a patient's clinical volume status.

Doppler techniques for assessing CO and function have been used extensively by cardiologists for

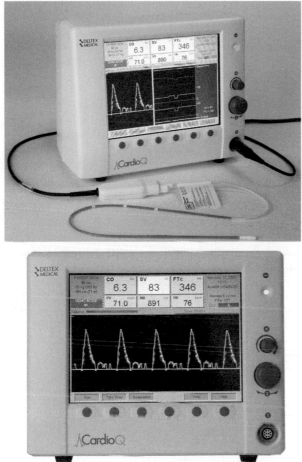

FIGURE 8-25. **A,** CardioQ monitoring system for assessing cardiac output and function via the esophageal Doppler probe. **B,** Numeric and graphic data provided by the CardioQ device. *(Courtesy of Deltex Medical, Inc., Branford, CT.)*

years. The technology for bedside assessment of CO and fluid responsiveness in critically ill patients is rapidly evolving. Esophageal Doppler monitoring (EDM) uses a thin silicone probe placed in the distal esophagus, allowing the clinician to evaluate descending aortic blood flow, to provide an immediate assessment of left ventricular performance (Figure 8-24). EDM provides real-time hemodynamic assessment. The probe is easily placed in a manner similar to an orogastric or nasogastric tube. Some patients may require a small amount of sedation to tolerate the procedure. The probe is lubricated and inserted either orally or nasally with the bevel facing upwards until the depth of the catheter is approximately 35 to 40 cm. Focusing the probe entails rotating, advancing, and/or withdrawing the probe until the loudest sound is heard from the monitor. Box 8-10 outlines indications and contraindications for the EDM.

The monitor interface (Figure 8-25) provides a variety of clinical parameters including CO and stroke volume derived from a proprietary algorithm. The corrected flow time (FTc), peak velocity (PV), and minute distance are obtained from the Doppler velocity measurements.[16] The base of the waveform depicts the FTc and is indicative of left ventricular preload. The height of the waveform represents peak velocity and reflects contractility. Normal FTc is 330 to 360 milliseconds. Normal peak velocity varies by age: 90 to 120 cm/sec for a 20-year-old person, 70 to 100 cm/sec for a 50-year-old person, and 50 to 80 cm/sec for a 70-year-old person.[16] An FTc of less than 330 milliseconds almost always represents an underfilled left ventricle. Critically ill patients often have maximum ventricular filling with an FTc near 400 milliseconds. Normal values are relative and do not replace physiological targets for optimization of fluid administration. Table 8-4 provides interpretation guidelines for waveform and numeric variations. Box 8-11 provides an example of a nurse-driven

Waveform Alteration	Numeric Correlation	Interpretation
↓ Base width	↓ FTc	Hypovolemia
↑ Base width	↑ FTc	Euvolemia
↓ Waveform height	↓ PV/SV	Left ventricular failure
↑ Waveform height	↑ PV/SV	Hyperdynamic state (i.e., sepsis)
↓Waveform height + ↓ base width	↓ FTc ↓ PV/SV	Elevated systemic vascular resistance

TABLE 8-4 Interpretation Guidelines for Esophageal Doppler Monitoring

FTc, Corrected flow time; *PV,* peak velocity; *SV,* stroke volume.

protocol to guide therapy and optimize ventricular filling.[14]

The EDM technology has been demonstrated to reduce intensive care unit length of stay, hospital length of stay, and infectious complications when compared with those patients managed by invasive technologies.[8,14] Because EDM is minimally invasive, the risks to the patient are significantly lower than those with invasive monitoring. In addition, EDM is simple to use and provides a vast amount of clinical information to guide therapy in the critical care environment.

Pulse Contour Cardiac Output Monitoring

Another minimally invasive method of assessing CO, stroke volume, and other hemodynamic parameters is pulse contour analysis. The theory of pulse contour analysis is based on the assumption that the contour of the arterial pressure waveform is proportional to the stroke volume. The CO derived from arterial pulse contour analysis is comparable to that obtained via PAC methods. Presently three devices that use the pulse contour analysis for determining CO are available. The PiCCO (Pulsion Medical Systems, Munich, Germany) uses thermodilution for calibration and requires femoral or axillary arterial cannulation. The FloTrac (Edwards Lifesciences, Irvine,

CA) does not require a calibration process to ensure accuracy; rather it uses a formula to continually update a constant that is used in a proprietary algorithm to determine CO. The PulseCO (LiDCO Ltd., London, UK) uses lithium dilution for calibration, and arterial pulse wave analysis from any arterial measurement site. These devices are promising breakthroughs in hemodynamic assessment and management. However, more clinical research is needed to validate the ability of these devices to reliably and accurately predict preload or fluid volume responsiveness.

For illustration purposes, the LiDCO technology will be used. The LiDCO System CO method provides a bolus indicator dilution method of measuring CO. A small dose of lithium chloride is injected via a central or peripheral venous line; the resulting arterial lithium concentration–time curve is recorded by withdrawing blood past a lithium sensor attached to the patient's existing arterial line (Figure 8-26). The dose of lithium needed (0.15 to 0.3 mmol for an average adult) is very small and has no known pharmacological effects. The PulseCO System software calculates continuous beat-to-beat CO by analysis of the arterial blood pressure trace after calibration with an absolute LiDCO CO value (Figure 8-27). Limited studies demonstrate good correlation between CO readings derived by LiDCO and those measured by traditional TdCO.[10]

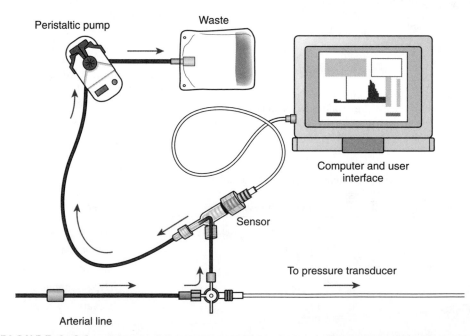

FIGURE 8-26. Schematic of the LiDCO system for assessing cardiac output via the pulse contour analysis method. *(Courtesy of LiDCO, London, UK.)*

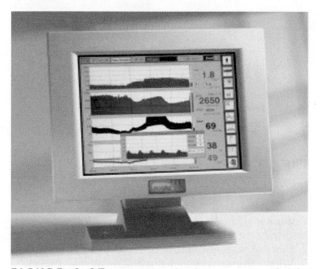

FIGURE 8-27. Example of information provided by LiDCO device. *(Courtesy of LiDCO, London, UK.)*

Keys to successful and accurate readings with the LiDCO device include having a fully functional arterial line with an optimally damped waveform, and calibrating the system with the lithium dilution every 12 to 24 hours, or with significant hemodynamic changes. This device provides the clinician with a beat-to-beat analysis of CO. In addition, it provides a numeric assessment of systolic pressure variability as well as percentage values representing stroke volume and pulse pressure variability.

Assessing Effect of Respiratory Variation on Hemodynamic Parameters

Right Atrial Pressure Variation

While the RAP is less predictive of responsiveness to fluid resuscitation, assessing the degree of change with respiration has the potential to be a useful indicator of responsiveness. A change (Δ) of RAP greater than 1 mm Hg with inspiration is indicative of a positive responder, while a Δ RAP of less than 1 mm Hg is likely to be a nonresponder.[5] Assessment of variation does not require specialized equipment to evaluate (other than a central line connected to a pressure transducer) and can be used on the spontaneously breathing patient. Additional research is needed to validate the usefulness of this assessment.

Systolic Pressure Variation

Patients receiving positive pressure ventilation have a decrease in stroke volume with inspiration that ultimately leads to a decrease in systolic blood pressure. The normal systolic pressure variation (ΔP) is 8 to 10 mm Hg. A ΔP of greater than 10 mm Hg is indicative of a patient who would respond to fluid resuscitation and improve tissue perfusion.[5] The limitation to this strategy is that it requires the patient to be mechanically ventilated in a strict volume control mode. In addition, the predictive capability may be affected if a patient has an alteration of the compliance in the lung or chest wall.

Arterial Pulse Pressure Variation

Arterial pulse pressure is defined as the difference between arterial systolic and diastolic pressure measurements. The arterial pulse pressure is affected by 3 variables: stroke volume, resistance, and compliance.[5] Since arterial resistance and compliance do not change significantly with each breath, the variation in pulse pressure is likely due to variations in stroke volume. A pulse pressure variation of 13% or greater is believed to be predictive of a patient's ability to respond to fluid resuscitation. To be predictive, the patient must be mechanically ventilated in a controlled mode, possibly requiring deep sedation, chemical paralysis, or both. The limited studies that have been conducted used tidal volumes of 10 mL/kg, which may not be feasible or recommended for optimal mechanical ventilation. Efficacy of this strategy with lower tidal volumes (currently used in clinical practice) has not yet been demonstrated.

Stroke Volume Variation

Another potential modality for assessing volume status is analysis of the degree of variation in stroke volume. The dividing line between responders and nonresponders with regards to fluid resuscitation is a stroke volume variability of 9.5%.[5] Assessment of stroke volume variability requires the use of proprietary pulse contour analysis via an arterial line with a specialized transducer. Again, this is only predictive in the patient who is mechanically ventilated in a controlled mode. Also, dysrhythmias affect the ability to consistently quantify the degree of variability, as the dysrhythmia itself can lead to a decreased stroke volume independent of respiratory variability.

While these functional indices show promise for giving the clinician another less invasive mechanism for assessing volume status in the critically ill patient, limitations may hinder their applicability. More research is needed to confirm the predictability and usefulness of these modalities.

CASE STUDY

evolve

J.P., a 44-year-old male with no previous medical history, presents to the emergency department with a chief complaint of severe abdominal pain, fever, and chills. He is subsequently admitted to the critical care unit after an open exploratory laparotomy where it was found that he had a perforated appendix and diffuse peritonitis. Intraoperatively he had an estimated blood loss of 200 mL, and he received 2.5 L of crystalloid solution. He arrives to the critical care unit intubated and sedated with an arterial line, subclavian triple-lumen catheter, indwelling urinary catheter, and esophageal Doppler monitor in place. He is placed on mechanical ventilation with the following settings: assist/control mode at 12 breaths/min; tidal volume, 700 mL; fraction of inspired oxygen, 1.0 (100%); and positive end-expiratory pressure, 5 cm H_2O. His initial vital signs are:

Heart rate	133 beats/min
Blood pressure	88/49 mm Hg
Mean arterial pressure	62 mm Hg
Respiratory rate	12 breaths/min
Right atrial pressure	3 mm Hg
Temperature	39.2° C (102.6° F)
Flow time corrected (FTc)	250 milliseconds
Peak velocity (PV)	130 cm/sec

The physician orders administration of a 250-mL infusion of 5% albumin and to prepare to replace the triple-lumen catheter with an $ScvO_2$ catheter. You administer the albumin and assist with the placement of the $ScvO_2$ catheter. After these interventions, his vital signs are now:

Heart rate	120 beats/min
Blood pressure	94/50 mm Hg
Mean arterial pressure	65 mm Hg
Right atrial pressure	5 mm Hg
Flow time corrected (FTc)	277 milliseconds
Peak velocity (PV)	120 cm/sec
$ScvO_2$	65%

QUESTIONS

1. The 2.5 L of crystalloid solution the patient received during surgery should have provided adequate volume resuscitation. What was the rationale for the albumin bolus?
2. Discuss which hemodynamic parameters would you monitor to assess efficacy of the bolus and why.
3. What advantage would the $ScvO_2$ catheter provide over the traditional triple-lumen catheter?
4. What technical factors would you need to consider ensuring accuracy in the hemodynamic parameters that you are monitoring?
5. Discuss the significance of the $ScvO_2$ value.
6. Recently, you attended an inservice on the Esophageal Doppler monitoring device that your unit uses. The representative stated that the best way to evaluate preload optimization was to assess FTc before and after each intervention. He provided a journal article outlining a study that suggested that you should continue to bolus the patient until you no longer see an increase in the FTc by 10% after each intervention. Given that information, what would you suggest to the physician?

SUMMARY

Hemodynamic monitoring of the critically ill patient is exciting yet challenging. It is important that the clinician remember that no single hemodynamic parameter can be used to determine volume status, contractility, or tissue perfusion. A holistic approach to patient evaluation, assessment, and treatment is vital to ensuring patient outcomes. Understanding the fundamentals of hemodynamic assessment, cardiac anatomy and physiology, and equipment function are critical in accurately evaluating and managing the critically ill or injured patient. The critical care nurse also needs to understand that while there are established normal values for the various hemodynamic parameters, it is more important to optimize a patient's tissue perfusion and clinical stability than to try to attain a normal numeric value for a particular parameter.

The development of new devices to assist in determining hemodynamic function is just the beginning of a revolution in methods for managing critically ill patients. Each new product needs to be critically reviewed and evaluated for efficacy and the ability to impact length of stay and patient outcomes before being applied to the general population. No single instrument will ever replace the vigilant clinician with strong assessment skills and the ability to critically think and put the clinical puzzle pieces together at the bedside.

CRITICAL THINKING QUESTIONS

evolve

1. How does stroke volume affect CO?
2. Describe how CO affects the delivery of oxygen to tissues. What parameters would be the best to monitor in a patient to assess this influence?
3. If a patient's mean arterial pressure continues to rise significantly, indicating an increase in resistance and an altered ability of the heart to eject blood, what parameters would also be affected as a result?
4. A patient who has undergone surgery has received a bed bath with back care and then undergoes suctioning and is turned. During these care activities, the patient experiences pain. What consequences does this pain have on the patient's SvO_2 status?
5. A patient is bleeding significantly and receives a transfusion of packed red blood cells. You note that the PAOP remains low, and the CI drops again. What is the significance of these alterations? What additional interventions would you expect?

evolve Be sure to check out the bonus material, including free self-assessment exercises, on the Evolve Web site at http://evolve.elsevier.com/Sole.

REFERENCES

1. Adams, K. L. (2004). Hemodynamic assessment: The physiologic basis for turning data into clinical information. *AACN Clinical Issues, 15*(4), 534-546.
2. Ahrens, T. S., & Schallom, L. (2001). Comparison of pulmonary artery and central venous pressure waveform measurements via digital and graphic measurement methods. *Heart and Lung, 30*(1), 26-38.
3. American Association of Critical-Care Nurses. (1993). Evaluation of the effects of heparinized and nonheparinized solutions on the patency of arterial pressure monitoring lines: The AACN Thunder Project. *American Journal of Critical Care, 2*(1), 3-15.
4. Barone, J. E., & Madlinger, R. V. (2006). Should an Allen test be performed before radial artery cannulation? *Journal of Trauma Injury, Infection, and Critical Care, 61*(2), 468-470.
5. Bridges, E. J. (2006). Pulmonary artery pressure monitoring: When, how, and what else to use. *AACN Advanced Critical Care, 17*(3), 286-305.
6. Centers for Disease Control and Prevention (CDC). (2002). Guidelines for the prevention of intravascular catheter-related infections. *MMWR. Recommendations and Reports: Morbidity and Mortality Weekly Report, 51*(RR10), 1-29.
7. Chaney, J. C., & Derdak, S. (2002). Minimally invasive hemodynamic monitoring for the intensivist: Current and emerging technology. *Critical Care Medicine, 30*(10), 2338-2345.
8. Chytra, I., Pradl, R., Bosman, R., Pelnar, P., Kasal, E., & Zidkova, A. (2007). Esophageal Doppler-guided fluid management decreases blood lactate levels in multiple-trauma patients: A randomized controlled trial. *Critical Care, 11*(1), R24.
9. Darovic, G. O. (2002). *Hemodynamic monitoring: Invasive and noninvasive clinical application* (3rd ed.). Philadelphia: Saunders.
10. Jonas, M. M., & Tanser, S. J. (2002). Lithium dilution measurement of cardiac output and arterial pulse waveform analysis: An indicator dilution calibrated beat-by-beat system for continuous estimation of cardiac output. *Current Opinion in Critical Care, 8*(3), 257-261.
11. Magder, S. (2006). Central venous pressure: A useful but not so simple measurement. *Critical Care Medicine, 34*(8), 2224-2227.
12. Magder, S. (2006). Central venous pressure monitoring. *Current Opinion in Critical Care, 12*(3), 219-227.
13. McCance, K. L., & Huether, S. E. (2004). *Pathophysiology. The biologic basis for disease in adults and children* (4th ed.). St. Louis: Mosby.
14. McKendry, M., McGloin, H., Saberi, D., Caudwell, L., Brady, A. R., & Singer, M. (2004). Randomized controlled trial assessing the impact of a nurse delivered, flow monitored protocol for optimization of circulatory status after cardiac surgery. *BMJ, 329*(7463), 258-262.
15. Preuss, T., & Wiegand, D. J. (2005). Single- and multiple-pressure transducer systems. In D. J. Wiegand, & K. K. Carlson (Eds.), *AACN procedure manual for critical care* (5th ed., pp. 591-601). St. Louis: Mosby.
16. Turner, M. A. (2003). Doppler-based hemodynamic monitoring: A minimally invasive alternative. *AACN Clinical Issues, 14*(2), 220-231.

CHAPTER 9

Ventilatory Assistance

Lynelle N. B. Pierce, MSN, RN, CCRN

Mary Lou Sole, PhD, RN, CCNS, CNL, FAAN

INTRODUCTION

Essential nursing interventions for all patients include maintaining an adequate airway, and ensuring adequate breathing (ventilation) and oxygenation. These nursing interventions provide the framework for this chapter. Respiratory anatomy and physiology are reviewed to provide a basis for discussing ventilatory assistance. Assessment of the respiratory system includes physical examination, arterial blood gas (ABG) interpretation, and noninvasive methods for assessing gas exchange. Airway management, oxygen therapy, and mechanical ventilation, important therapies in the critical care unit (CCU), are also discussed.

REVIEW OF RESPIRATORY ANATOMY AND PHYSIOLOGY

The primary function of the respiratory system is gas exchange. Oxygen and carbon dioxide are exchanged via the respiratory system to provide adequate oxygen to the cells and to remove excess carbon dioxide, the byproduct of metabolism, from the cells. The respiratory system is divided into (1) the upper airway, (2) the lower airway, and (3) the lungs. The upper airway conducts gas to and from the lower airway, and the lower airway provides gas exchange at the alveolar-capillary membrane. The anatomical structure of the respiratory system is shown in Figure 9-1.

Upper Airway

The upper airway consists of the nasal cavity and the pharynx. The nasal cavity conducts air, filters large foreign particles, and warms and humidifies air. When an artificial airway is placed, these natural functions of the airway are bypassed. The nasal cavity also is responsible for voice resonance, smell, and sneeze reflexes. The throat, or pharynx, transports both air and food. Air enters the superior part of the pharynx (the nasopharynx) and passes behind the mouth through the oropharynx.

Lower Airway

The lower airway consists of the larynx, trachea, right and left mainstem bronchi, bronchioles, and alveoli. The larynx is the narrowest part of the conducting airways in adults and contains the vocal cords. The larynx is partly covered by the epiglottis, which prevents aspiration of food, liquid, or saliva into the lungs during swallowing. The passage through the vocal cords is the glottis (Figure 9-2).

The trachea warms, humidifies, and filters air. Cilia in the trachea propel mucus and foreign material upward through the airway. At about the level of the fifth thoracic vertebra (sternal angle, or angle of Louis), the trachea branches into the right and left mainstem bronchi, which conduct air to the respective lungs. This bifurcation is referred to as the *carina*. The right mainstem bronchus is shorter, wider, and straighter than the left. The bronchi further branch into the bronchioles and finally the terminal bronchioles, which supply air to the alveoli. Mucosal cells in the bronchi secrete mucus that lubricates the airway and traps foreign materials, which are moved by the cilia upward to be expectorated or swallowed.

The alveoli are the distal airway structures and are responsible for gas exchange at the capillary level. More than 300 million of these tiny air sacs are

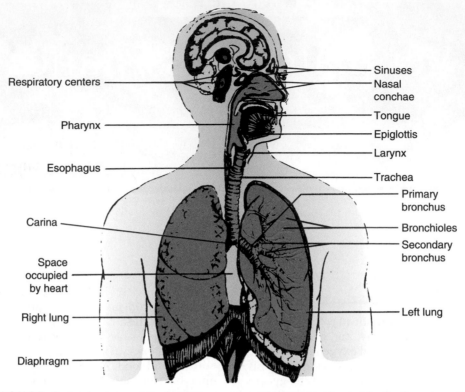

FIGURE 9-1. Anatomy of the respiratory system. The lungs are located in the thoracic cavity. The diaphragm forms the floor of the thoracic cavity and separates it from the abdominal cavity. The internal view of one lung shows air passages. *(From Solomon, E. P. [2003]. Introduction to human anatomy and physiology [2nd ed., p. 220]. Philadelphia: Saunders.)*

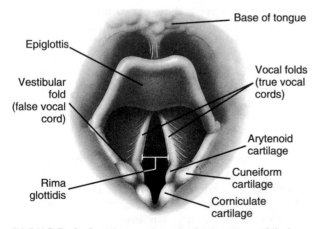

FIGURE 9-2. The vocal cords/glottis. *(From Thibodeau, G. S., & Patton, K. T. [2003]. Anatomy and physiology [5th ed., p. 691]. St. Louis: Mosby.)*

present in the lungs. The alveoli consist of a single layer of epithelial cells and fibers that permit expansion and contraction. The type II cells inside the alveolus secrete surfactant, which coats the inner surface of the alveoli and prevents it from collapsing.

A network of pulmonary capillaries covers the alveoli. Gas exchange occurs between the alveoli and these capillaries.[64] As seen in Figure 9-3, the large combined surface area and single cell layer of the alveoli promote very efficient diffusion of gases.

Lungs

The lungs consist of lobes; the left lung has two lobes, and the right lung has three lobes. Each lobe consists of lobules, or segments, that are supplied by one bronchiole. The top of each lung is the apex, and the lower part of the lung is the base.

The lungs are covered by pleura. The visceral pleura covers the lung surfaces, whereas the parietal pleura covers the internal surface of the thoracic cage. Between these two layers the pleural space is formed, which contains pleural fluid. This thin fluid lubricates the pleural layers as they slide across each other during breathing. It also holds the two pleurae together because it creates surface tension, an attractive force between liquid molecules. It is this surface tension between the two pleurae, opposing the tendency of the elastic lung to want to collapse, that leads to a negative pressure of 5 cm H_2O within the

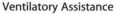

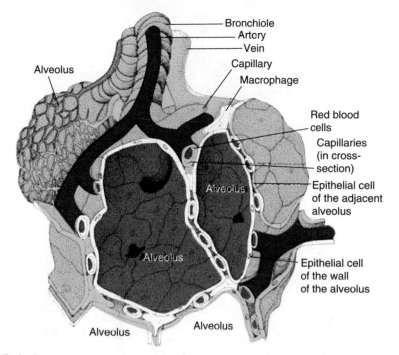

Bronchiole
Artery
Vein
Capillary
Macrophage

Alveolus

Red blood cells

Capillaries (in cross-section)

Epithelial cell of the adjacent alveolus

Alveolus

Epithelial cell of the wall of the alveolus

Alveolus

Alveolus

Alveolus

FIGURE 9-3. Structure and function of the alveolus. *(From Solomon, E. P. [2003].* Introduction to human anatomy and physiology *[2nd ed., p. 222]. Philadelphia: Saunders.)*

pleural space.[22] In disease of the pleural space, such as pneumothorax, this negative pressure is disrupted, leading to collapse of the lung and the need for a chest tube.

PHYSIOLOGY OF BREATHING

The basic principle behind the movement of gas in and out of the lung is that gas travels from an area of higher to lower pressure. During inspiration, the diaphragm lowers and flattens and the intercostal muscles contract, lifting the chest up and outward to increase the size of the chest cavity. Subsequently, intrapleural pressure becomes even more negative than stated above, and intraalveolar pressure (the pressure in the lungs) becomes negative, causing air to flow into the lungs (inspiration). Expiration is a passive process in which the diaphragm and intercostal muscles relax and the lungs recoil. This recoil generates positive intraalveolar pressure relative to atmospheric pressure, and air flows out of the lungs (expiration).

Gas Exchange

The process of gas exchange (Figure 9-4) consists of four steps: (1) ventilation, (2) diffusion at pulmonary capillaries, (3) perfusion (transportation), and (4) diffusion to the cells.[22]

1. Ventilation is the movement of gases (oxygen and carbon dioxide) in and out of the alveoli.
2. Diffusion of oxygen and carbon dioxide occurs at the alveolar-capillary membrane (Figure 9-5). The driving force to move the gas from the alveoli to the capillary and vice versa is the pressure of the gases across the alveolar-capillary membrane. Diffusion is the movement of gas molecules from an area of higher to lower pressure. Oxygen pressure is higher in the alveoli than in the capillaries, thus promoting oxygen diffusion from the alveoli into the blood. Carbon dioxide pressure is higher in the capillaries, thus promoting the diffusion of carbon dioxide into the alveoli for elimination during exhalation.
3. The oxygenated blood in the pulmonary capillary is transported via the pulmonary vein to the left side of the heart. The oxygenated blood is perfused or transported to the tissues.
4. Diffusion of oxygen and carbon dioxide occurs at the cellular level based on pressure gradients. Oxygen diffuses from blood into the cells, and carbon dioxide leaves the cells and diffuses into the blood. This process is called internal respiration. Carbon dioxide is transported via the vena cava to the right side of the heart and into the pulmonary capillaries where it diffuses into the alveoli and is eliminated through exhalation.

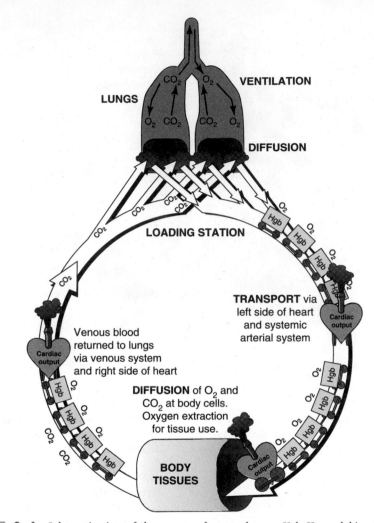

FIGURE 9-4. Schematic view of the process of gas exchange. *Hgb*, Hemoglobin. *(Modified from Alspach, J. [1992]. AACN instructor's resource manual for AACN core curriculum for critical care nursing [4th ed., transparency 29]. Philadelphia: Saunders.)*

Numerous physiological features must be present for optimal gas exchange to occur. These include an intact nervous system, compliant lungs, a sufficient number of functioning alveoli, unencumbered alveolar-capillary membranes, an adequate level of normal hemoglobin, an adequate cardiac output to transport the gases, and patent vasculature.[56]

Regulation of Breathing

The rate, depth, and rhythm of ventilation are controlled by respiratory centers in the medulla and pons. When the carbon dioxide level is high or the oxygen level is low, chemoreceptors in the respiratory center, carotid arteries, and aorta send messages to the medulla to regulate respiration. In persons with normal lung function, high levels of carbon dioxide stimulate respiration. However, patients with chronic obstructive pulmonary disease (COPD) maintain higher levels of carbon dioxide as a baseline, and their ventilatory drive in response to increased carbon dioxide levels is blunted. In these patients, the stimulus to breathe is hypoxemia, a low level of oxygen in the blood.

Respiratory Mechanics

Work of Breathing

The work of breathing (WOB) is the amount of effort required for the maintenance of a given level of

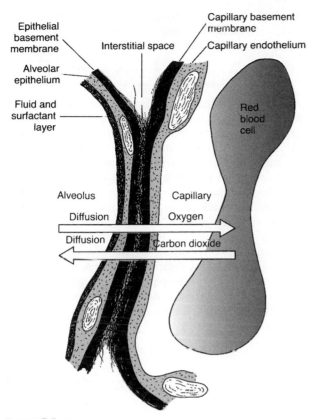

FIGURE 9-5. Diffusion of oxygen and carbon dioxide at the alveolar-capillary membrane. *(From Guyton, A. C., & Hall, J. E. [2006]. Textbook of medical physiology [11th ed., p. 497]. Philadelphia: Saunders.)*

ventilation. When the lungs are not diseased, the respiratory muscles manage the WOB using unlabored respirations. The respiratory pattern changes automatically to manage an increased WOB when lung disease is present, and the patient may use accessory muscles of ventilation. As the WOB increases, more energy is expended for adequate ventilation to be obtained; this increased energy expenditure requires proportionately more oxygen and glucose. If the WOB becomes too high, respiratory failure may ensue and mechanical ventilatory support may be needed.

Compliance

Compliance is a measure of the distensibility, or stretchability, of the lung and chest wall. The lungs are primarily made up of elastin and collagen fibers. In some disease states, these fibers become less elastic, leading to so-called stiff lungs. *Elastic recoil* refers to the ability of the lung tissue to return to its resting position after stretching during inspiration. The lungs have strong elastic recoil and want to continually return to their resting state. *Distensibility* refers to the stretchability of the lung or how easily it can be stretched when the respiratory muscles work and expand the thoracic cavity. Compliance is a measurement of the lung's distensibility. It is defined as the change in lung volume per unit of pressure change.[50,65]

Various pathologic conditions such as pulmonary fibrosis, acute respiratory distress syndrome (ARDS), and pulmonary edema lead to low compliance. In these situations the lungs are stiff and difficult to distend. The patient must generate more work to breathe to create the higher pressures required to inflate the lungs. Severe obesity also decreases compliance because inflating the lungs in the presence of increased chest wall mass is more difficult.

In emphysema, destruction of lung tissue and enlarged air spaces cause the lungs to lose their elasticity. The decrease in elastic recoil causes compliance to be increased, or high. The lungs are more distensible in this situation and require lower pressures for ventilation.

Monitoring changes in compliance provides an objective clinical indicator of changes in the patient's lung condition and ability to ventilate, especially if the patient is requiring mechanical ventilatory support. Compliance of the lung tissue is best measured under conditions of no airflow, and is achieved by instituting a 2-second inspiratory hold maneuver with the mechanical ventilator. The subsequent measurement, called static compliance, is an indicator of the elasticity of the lung. Static compliance in patients with normal lung function usually ranges from 50 to 170 mL/cm H_2O.[52] This means that for every 1-cm H_2O change of pressure in the lungs, the volume of gas increases by 50 to 170 mL. Lung function is altered in most patients requiring mechanical ventilation, resulting in decreased compliance. No single value of compliance is as useful as a trend of the variable with time. Measures are used to quantify the extent of the compliance problem and monitor patient progress after therapy is instituted.

Dynamic compliance is measured while gases are flowing during breathing; therefore it measures not only compliance but also resistance to gas flow. The normal value for dynamic compliance is 50 to 80 mL/cm H_2O. Dynamic compliance is easier to measure because it does not require breath holding or an inspiratory hold; however, it is not a pure measurement of lung compliance. A decrease in dynamic compliance may mean a decrease in compliance or an increase in resistance to gas flow.

The respiratory therapist (RT) or nurse measures compliance in the mechanically ventilated patient to identify trends developing in the patient's condition. Poor compliance requires higher ventilatory pressures for adequate ventilation. Higher ventilatory pressures place the patient at increased risk of complications such as volutrauma. Improved compliance reflects improved pulmonary status.

Resistance

Resistance refers to the opposition to the flow of gases in the airways. Factors that affect airway resistance and thus the flow of gases are airway length, airway radius, and the flow rate of gases. Airway resistance is increased when the airway is lengthened or narrowed, as with an artificial airway, or when the natural airway is narrowed by spasms (bronchoconstriction), the presence of mucus, or edema. Finally, resistance increases when gas flow is increased, as with increased breathing effort or when a patient requires mechanical ventilation. When resistance increases, more effort is required by the patient to maintain gas flow. If the patient is unable to generate the increased WOB, the amount of gas flow the patient produces decreases. Thus

increasing airway resistance may result in reduced lung volume and inadequate ventilation.

LUNG VOLUMES AND CAPACITIES

Air volume within the lung is measured with an instrument called a spirometer. Lung volumes and capacities (two or more lung volumes added together) are important for determining adequate pulmonary function, and are shown graphically in Figure 9-6. Descriptions of the lung volumes and capacities are provided in Table 9-1. Measurements of lung volumes and capacities allow the practitioner to assess baseline pulmonary function and to monitor the improvement or progression of pulmonary diseases and how the patient is responding to therapy. For example, when the patient performs incentive spirometry, the nurse and RT assess the patient's inspiratory capacity and trend its improvement or decline over time and with interventions. Lung capacities decline gradually with aging.

TABLE 9-1   Lung Volumes and Capacities

Name	Definition	Average	Formula
Volumes*			
Tidal volume (V_T)	Volume of a normal breath	500 mL or 5-7 mL/kg	
Inspiratory reserve volume (IRV)	Maximum amount of gas that can be inspired at the end of a normal breath (over and above the V_T)	3000 mL	
Expiratory reserve volume (ERV)	Maximum amount of gas that can be forcefully expired at the end of a normal breath	1200 mL	
Residual volume (RV)	Amount of air remaining in the lungs after maximum expiration	1300 mL	
Capacities			
Inspiratory capacity (IC)	Maximum volume of gas that can be inspired at normal resting expiration; the IC distends the lungs to their maximum amount	3500 mL	$IC = V_T + IRV$
Functional residual capacity (FRC)	Volume of gas remaining in the lungs at normal resting expiration	2500 mL	$FRC = ERV + RV$
Vital capacity (VC)	Maximum volume of gas that can be forcefully expired after maximum inspiration	4700 mL	$VC = V_T + IRV + ERV$
Total lung capacity (TLC)	Volume of gas in the lungs at end of maximum inspiration	6000 mL	$TLC = V_T + ERV + RV$

*Volumes are average in a 70-kg young adult. There is a range of normal values that varies by age, height, body size, and gender. Volumes are less in women than men when height and age are equal.

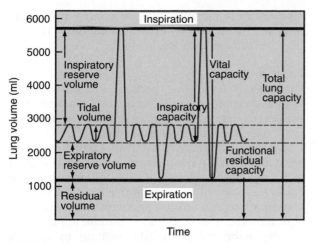

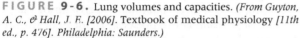

FIGURE 9-6. Lung volumes and capacities. *(From Guyton, A. C., & Hall, J. F. [2006]. Textbook of medical physiology [11th ed., p. 476]. Philadelphia: Saunders.)*

GERIATRIC CONSIDERATIONS

PHYSIOLOGICAL CHANGES WITH AGING

- ↓ Alveolar surface area
- ↓ Alveolar elasticity
- ↓ Chest wall distensibility
- ↓ Physiological compensatory mechanisms (respiratory, renal, cardiac, immune)

ASSESSMENT CHANGES

NORMAL FINDINGS BECAUSE OF AGING PROCESS

- Kyphosis
- Barrel chest
- ↓ Chest expansion
- Lower PaO$_2$ levels on ABG

INCREASED RISK FOR

- Poor gas exchange
- Respiratory distress
- Respiratory failure

ABG, Arterial blood gas; *PaO$_2$*, partial pressure of oxygen in arterial blood.

RESPIRATORY ASSESSMENT

The ability to perform a physical assessment of the respiratory system is an essential skill for the critical care nurse. Assessment findings assist in identifying potential patient problems and in evaluating patient response to interventions. See the Geriatric Considerations box for information related to assessment of elderly patients.

Health History

Critically ill patients are frequently unable to provide health history information because of their physical condition, cognitive condition, or both. Information is often obtained from significant others who know the patient's history. Several questions pertinent to the respiratory system should be asked when the health history is obtained, including the following:

1. Tobacco use: type, amount, and number of pack-years (number of packs of cigarettes per day × number of years smoking)
2. Occupational history such as coal mining, asbestos work, farming
3. History of symptoms such as shortness of breath, dyspnea, cough, anorexia, weight loss, chest pain, or sputum production. Further assessment of sputum including amount, color, consistency, time of day, and whether its appearance is chronic or acute
4. Use of oral and inhalant respiratory medications, such as bronchodilators and steroids
5. Use of over-the-counter or street inhalant drugs
6. Allergies: medication, food, or environmental
7. Dates of last chest radiograph and tuberculosis screening

Physical Examination

Inspection

Inspection provides an initial clue for potential acute and chronic respiratory problems. The head, neck, fingers, and chest are inspected for abnormalities.

The chest is observed for shape, abnormal breathing patterns, use of chest and abdominal accessory muscles, asymmetrical chest wall movement, and abnormal chest excursion. Signs of acute respiratory distress include labored respirations with the use of accessory muscles, asymmetrical chest movements, chest-abdominal asynchrony, open-mouthed breathing, or gasping breaths. Additional signs of acute respiratory distress in pediatric patients include sternal retractions and nasal flaring. Cyanosis is a late sign of hypoxemia and should not be relied on as an early warning of distress. Other indications of respiratory abnormalities include pallor or rubor, pursed-lip breathing, jugular venous distention, prolonged expiratory phase of breaths, poor capillary refill, clubbing of fingers, and a barrel-shaped chest.

The respiratory rate (RR) should be counted for a full minute in critically ill patients. The normal RR is 12 to 20 breaths per minute, and expiration is usually twice as long as inspiration (inspiration-to-expiration ratio, 1:2). The normal breathing pattern

Cheyne-Stokes Respirations gradually increase in depth, then become more shallow; followed by a period of apnea

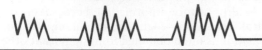

Biot's Highly irregular breathing pattern with abrupt pauses between efforts

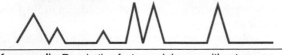

Kussmaul's Respiration faster and deeper without pauses

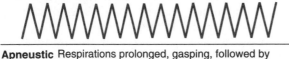

Apneustic Respirations prolonged, gasping, followed by extremely short, inefficient expiration

FIGURE 9-7. Breathing patterns.

is regular and even with an occasional sigh, and is called *eupnea*. *Tachypnea* is defined as an RR of greater than 20 breaths per minute. Tachypnea may occur with anxiety, fever, pain, anemia, low PaO_2, and elevated $PaCO_2$. *Bradypnea* is an RR of less than 10 breaths per minute. Bradypnea may occur in central nervous system disorders; it may also result from administration or ingestion of certain central nervous system depressant medications or alcohol, severe metabolic alkalosis, and fatigue. The depth of respirations is as important as the rate and provides information about the adequacy of ventilation. Alterations from normal rate and depth should be documented and reported.

Several abnormal breathing patterns (Figure 9-7) are possible and should be reported. *Cheyne-Stokes respirations* have a cyclical respiratory pattern. The patient has deep respirations that become increasingly shallow, followed by a period of apnea that lasts approximately 20 seconds. The cycle repeats after each apneic period. The apneic period may vary and progressively lengthen; therefore, the duration of the apneic period is timed for trending. Cheyne-Stokes respirations may occur in central nervous system disorders and congestive heart failure. *Biot's respirations*, or cluster breathing, are cycles of breaths that vary in depth and have varying periods of apnea. Biot's respirations are seen with brain stem injury. *Kussmaul's respirations* are deep, regular, and rapid (usually more than 20 breaths per minute). Kussmaul's respirations commonly occur in diabetic keto-acidosis and other disorders that cause metabolic acidosis. *Apneustic respirations* are gasping inspirations followed by short, ineffective expirations. They are often associated with lesions to the pons.

Palpation

Palpation is frequently performed simultaneously with inspection. Palpation is used to evaluate chest wall excursion, tracheal deviation, chest wall tenderness, subcutaneous crepitus, and tactile fremitus.

During inspiration, chest wall excursion should be symmetrical. Asymmetrical excursion is usually associated with unilateral ventilation problems. The trachea is normally in a midline position; a tracheal shift may occur in tension pneumothorax. The chest wall should not be tender to palpation; tenderness is usually associated with inflammation or trauma, including rib fractures. *Subcutaneous crepitus* or *subcutaneous emphysema* is the presence of air beneath the skin surface that has escaped from the airways or lungs. It is palpated with the fingertips and may feel like crunching Rice Krispies under the skin. The temptation to further palpate should be resisted, as palpation promotes air dissection in the skin layers. Subcutaneous air may result from chest trauma, such as rib fractures, and from barotrauma. It indicates that the lung or airways are not intact.

Tactile fremitus is assessed by palpating the patient's chest wall with the palmar or ulnar surface of the hand. The patient is asked to recite sounds that vibrate, such as "ninety-nine," and the examiner notes vibrations transmitted through the chest wall. The intensity of vibrations is compared bilaterally. Tactile fremitus may be increased over consolidated areas of the lungs; vibrations may be decreased in pleural effusion and pneumothorax.

Percussion

The chest may be percussed to identify respiratory disorders such as hemothorax, pneumothorax, and consolidation. In percussion, the middle finger of one hand is tapped twice by the middle finger of the opposite hand placed against the patient's chest. The vibrations produced by tapping create different sounds, depending on the density of the underlying tissue being percussed. Five sounds may be audible on percussion: resonance, dullness, flatness, hyper-resonance, and tympany. Table 9-2 provides a description of the sounds, their causes, and clinical conditions associated with the sounds.

Auscultation

Lung sounds are routinely assessed every 1 to 4 hours in critically ill patients using the diaphragm of the stethoscope pressed firmly against the chest wall. Attempts should be made to make the environment as quiet as possible by turning off the television or

TABLE 9-2   Percussion of the Chest Wall

Percussion Note	Sounds Like	Causes	Clinical Condition
Resonance	Muffled drum	Produced by normal lung tissue	
Dullness	Dull thud	Tissue is denser than normal	Pleural effusion, hemothorax, consolidation, atelectasis, tumors, and pulmonary fibrosis
Flatness	Extreme dullness	Absence of air in lung tissues	Massive pleural effusion, lung collapse
Hyperresonance	Musical sound like a hollow drum	Increased amount of air	Emphysema, pneumothorax, acute asthma
Tympany	Musical drum-like sound	Large air-filled area	Tension pneumothorax, air filled cavity secondary to infection or abscess, gastric distention

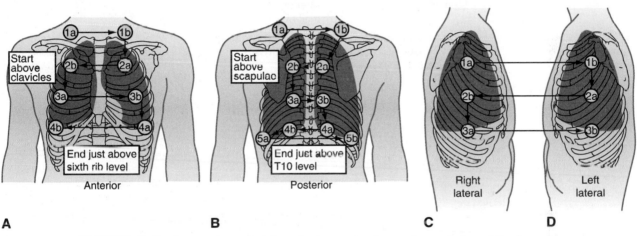

FIGURE 9-8. Systematic method for palpation, percussion, and auscultation of the lungs in anterior (**A**), posterior (**B**), and lateral regions (**C** and **D**). The techniques should be performed systematically to compare right and left lung fields.

radio, and reducing conversation in the room. The stethoscope should be placed directly on the patient's chest; sounds are difficult to distinguish if they are auscultated through the patient's gown or clothing. The friction of chest hair on the stethoscope may mimic the sound of crackles; wetting the chest hair may reduce this sound. In addition, the stethoscope tubing should not rest against skin or objects such as sheets, bed rails, or ventilator circuitry during auscultation.

A systematic sequence should be used during auscultation, with sounds from one side of the chest wall compared with those from the other (Figure 9-8). Auscultation is best performed with the patient sitting in an upright position breathing deeply in and out through the mouth. It may not be feasible for a critically ill patient to assume a sitting position for auscultation. In this circumstance, auscultation of the anterior and lateral chest is often performed. However, every opportunity should be taken to turn the patient and auscultate the chest posteriorly. When the patient has an artificial airway, the trachea should be auscultated for the presence of an air leak.

Breath Sounds

The nurse listens carefully for both normal and abnormal, or adventitious, breath sounds. Types of normal breath sounds include bronchial, bronchovesicular, and vesicular (Table 9-3). Adventitious sounds include crackles, rhonchi, wheezes, pleural friction rub, and stridor (Table 9-4). At times, breath sounds may be decreased. The presence of fluid, air, or increased tissue density can cause decreased breath

TABLE 9-3   Normal Breath Sounds

Sound/Description	Location	Cause	Clinical Significance
Bronchial—tubular, hollow, loud intensity, high pitched	Over large airways, i.e., larynx, trachea	Turbulent flow of air through large airways	None unless heard over peripheral lung fields, which indicates consolidation as in pneumonia.
			Normally, air-filled alveoli filter bronchial sounds from reaching periphery.
			Consolidation creates denser lung tissue, which transmits bronchial sounds to periphery.
Bronchovesicular—hollow, breezy quality	Large central airways, i.e., main-stem bronchi; anteriorly at 1-2 ICS; posteriorly between scapulas	Turbulent flow in central airways; less intense and lower pitched than bronchial because of filtering of sound by chest wall tissue	None unless heard peripherally, which indicates consolidation.
Vesicular—soft, breezy, moderate intensity, low pitched	Peripheral lung fields throughout chest except over central airways	Air movement through smaller airways	When diminished or absent indicates decreased sound *production* (shallow breathing) or decreased sound *transmission* (less dense lung tissue, as in hyperinflation, or partial physical obstruction, such as with mucus).
			Absent vesicular sounds indicate that transmission is blocked, as in pleural effusion, pneumothorax.

ICS, Intercostal space.

sounds. Shallow respirations can also mimic decreased breath sounds; therefore, the patient must take deep breaths during auscultation. The breath sounds should be carefully documented and abnormalities reported.

Arterial Blood Gas Interpretation

The ability to interpret ABG results rapidly is an essential critical care skill. ABG results reflect oxygenation, adequacy of gas exchange in the lungs, and acid-base status. Blood for ABG analysis is obtained from either a direct arterial puncture (radial, brachial, or femoral artery) or an arterial line. ABGs are assessed periodically to aid in patient assessment. However, noninvasive measures of gas exchange have reduced the frequency of ABG measurements. All blood gas findings must be interpreted in conjunction with the patient's physical assessment findings, clinical history, and previous ABG values (Table 9-5).

Oxygenation
The ABG values that reflect oxygenation include the partial pressure of oxygen dissolved in arterial blood (PaO_2) and the arterial oxygen saturation of hemoglobin (SaO_2). Approximately 3% of the available oxygen is dissolved in plasma. The remaining 97% of the oxygen attaches to hemoglobin in red blood cells, forming oxyhemoglobin.

Partial Pressure of Arterial Oxygen. The normal PaO_2 is 80 to 100 mm Hg at sea level. The PaO_2 decreases in the elderly; the value for persons 60 to 80 years of age usually ranges from 60 to 80 mm Hg.

Arterial Oxygen Saturation of Hemoglobin. The SaO_2 refers to the amount of oxygen bound to hemoglobin. The normal saturation of hemoglobin ranges from 92% to 99%. The SaO_2 is very important because most

TABLE 9-4   Adventitious Breath Sounds

Sound/Description	Cause	Clinical Significance	Additional Descriptors/Comments
Crackles—discontinuous, explosive, bubbling sounds of short duration	Air bubbling through fluid or mucus, or alveoli popping open on inspiration	Atelectasis, fluid retention in small airways (pulmonary edema), retention of mucus (bronchitis, pneumonia), interstitial fibrosis	Fine: soft, short duration Coarse: loud, longer duration Wet or dry May disappear after coughing, suctioning, or deep inspiration if alveoli remain inflated
Rhonchi—coarse, continuous, low-pitched, sonorous, or rattling sound	Air movement through excess mucus, fluid, or inflamed airways	Diseases resulting in airway inflammation and excess mucus (e.g., pneumonia, bronchitis, or excess fluid, as in pulmonary edema)	Inspiratory and/or expiratory; may clear or diminish with coughing if caused by airway secretions
Wheezes—high- or low-pitched whistling, musical sound heard during inspiration and/or expiration	Air movement through narrowed airway, which causes airway wall to oscillate or flutter	Bronchospasm, as in asthma, partial airway obstruction by tumor, foreign body or secretions, inflammation, or stenosis	High or low pitched; inspiratory and/or expiratory
Pleural friction rub—coarse, grating, squeaking, or scratching sound, as when two pieces of leather rub together	Inflamed pleura rubbing against each other	Pleural inflammation, as in pleuritis, pneumonia, tuberculosis, chest tube insertion, pulmonary infarction	Occurs during breathing cycle and is eliminated by breath holding Need to discern from pericardial friction rub, which continues despite breath holding
Stridor—high-pitched, continuous sound heard over upper airway; a crowing sound	Air flowing through constricted larynx or trachea	Partial obstruction of upper airway, as in laryngeal edema, obstruction by foreign body, epiglottitis	Potentially life-threatening

oxygen supplied to the tissues is transported via hemoglobin. The SaO_2 is measured in the lab from an arterial blood sample or continuously monitored with the use of a pulse oximeter. The oxygen saturation measured by a pulse oximeter is the SpO_2.

Both the PaO_2 and the SaO_2 are used to assess oxygenation. Decreased oxygenation of arterial blood (PaO_2 <60 mm Hg) is referred to as *hypoxemia*. Hypoxemia is different from *hypoxia*, which is a decrease in oxygen at the tissue level. Symptoms of hypoxemia are described in Box 9-1. A patient with a PaO_2 of less than 60 mm Hg requires immediate intervention with supplemental oxygen to treat the hypoxemia while further assessment is done to identify the cause. A PaO_2 of less than 40 mm Hg is life-threatening because oxygen is not available for metabolism. Without treatment, cellular death will occur.[22,56]

The relationship between the PaO_2 and the SaO_2 is shown in the S-shaped oxyhemoglobin dissociation curve (Figure 9-9). The upper portion of the curve (PaO_2 >60 mm Hg) is flat. In this area of the curve, large changes in the PaO_2 result in only small changes in SaO_2. For example, the normal PaO_2 of 80 to 100 mm Hg is associated with an SaO_2 of 92% to 100%. If the PaO_2 decreases from 80 to 60 mm Hg, the SaO_2 decreases from 92% to 90%. Although this example reflects a drop in PaO_2, the patient is not immediately compromised, because the hemoglobin responsible for carrying oxygen to all the tissues is still well saturated with oxygen.

The critical zone of the oxyhemoglobin dissociation curve occurs when the PaO_2 decreases to less than 60 mm Hg. At this point, the curve slopes sharply, and small changes in PaO_2 are reflected in large changes in the oxygen saturation. These changes in SaO_2 may cause a significant decrease in oxygen delivered to the tissues.[65]

As shown in Figure 9-9, the oxyhemoglobin dissociation curve may shift under certain conditions. When the curve shifts to the right, a decreased hemoglobin affinity for oxygen exists. This means that oxygen is more readily released to the tissues.

TABLE 9-5   Blood Gas Interpretation

Status	pH	PCO_2	HCO_3^-	Base Excess
Respiratory Acidosis				
Uncompensated	↓ 7.35	↑ 45	Normal	Normal
Partially compensated	↓ 7.35	↑ 45	↑ 26	↑ +2
Compensated	7.35-7.45	↑ 45	↑ 26	↑ +2
Respiratory Alkalosis				
Uncompensated	↑ 7.45	↓ 35	Normal	Normal
Partially compensated	↑ 7.45	↓ 35	↓ 22	↓ −2
Compensated	7.40-7.45	↓ 35	↓ 22	↓ −2
Metabolic Acidosis				
Uncompensated	↓ 7.35	Normal	↓ 22	↓ −2
Partially compensated	↓ 7.35	↓ 35	↓ 22	↓ −2
Compensated	7.35-7.45	↓ 35	↓ 22	↓ −2
Metabolic Alkalosis				
Uncompensated	↑ 7.45	Normal	↑ 26	↑ +2
Partially compensated*	↑ 7.45	↑ 45	↑ 26	↑ +2
Compensated*	7.40-7.45	↑ 45	↑ 26	↑ +2
Combined Respiratory and Metabolic Acidosis	↓ 7.35	↑ 45	↓ 22	↓ −2
Combined Respiratory and Metabolic Alkalosis	↑ 7.45	↓ 35	↑ 26	↓ −2

*Partially compensated or compensated metabolic alkalosis generally is rarely seen clinically because of the body's mechanism to prevent hypoventilation.
Modified from Kacmarek, R. M., Dimas, S., & Mack, C. W. (2005). Acid-base balance and blood gas interpretation. In R. M. Kacmarek, S. Dimas, & C. W. Mack (Eds.), *The essentials of respiratory care* (p. 260). St. Louis: Mosby.

Conditions that cause a right shift include acidemia, increased temperature, and increased levels of 2,3-diphosphoglycerate (2,3-DPG), which is a glucose metabolite. Levels of 2,3-DPG are increased in anemia, chronic hypoxemia, and low cardiac output states. When conditions exist where the curve has shifted to the right, for any given SaO_2/SpO_2 value the PaO_2 will be higher than what would be expected at the normal curve.

When the curve shifts to the left, hemoglobin affinity for oxygen increases and hemoglobin clings to oxygen. Conditions that cause a left shift include alkalemia, decreased temperature, high altitude, carbon monoxide poisoning, and a decreased 2,3-DPG level. Common causes of decreased 2,3-DPG include administration of stored bank blood, septic shock, and hypophosphatemia.[22,65] With a left shift,

with any given SaO_2/SpO_2 value, the PaO_2 will be lower than with the normal curve. Therefore, if the patient's SpO_2 is 92%, an ABG should be drawn to assess whether hypoxemia is present.

Ventilation and Acid-Base Status

Blood gas values that reflect ventilation and acid-base or metabolic status include the partial pressure of carbon dioxide ($PaCO_2$), pH, and bicarbonate (HCO_3^-).[22,56,65]

pH. The concentration of hydrogen ions (H^+) in the blood is referred to as the *pH*. The pH is the negative logarithm of the H^+ concentration; therefore, as the H^+ ion concentration increases, the pH decreases and vice versa. The normal range for pH is 7.35 to 7.45 (exact value, 7.40). If the H^+ ions increase, the pH decreases (becomes <7.35) and the patient is

BOX 9-1 Signs and Symptoms of Hypoxemia

Integumentary System
- Pallor
- Cool, dry
- Cyanosis (late)
- Diaphoresis (late)

Respiratory System
- Dyspnea
- Tachypnea
- Use of accessory muscles

Cardiovascular System
- Tachycardia
- Dysrhythmias
- Chest pain
- Hypertension early, followed by hypotension
- Increased heart rate early, followed by decreased heart rate

Central Nervous System
- Anxiety
- Restlessness
- Confusion
- Fatigue
- Combativeness/agitation
- Coma

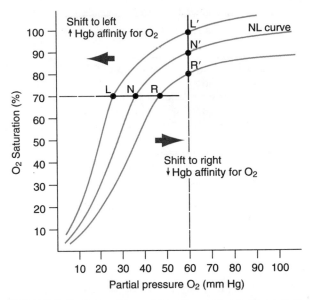

FIGURE 9-9. Oxyhemoglobin dissociation curve. A PaO_2 of 60 mm Hg correlates with an oxygen saturation of 90%. When the PaO_2 falls below 60 mm Hg, small changes in PaO_2 are reflected in large changes in oxygen saturation. Shifts in the oxyhemoglobin curve. *L*, Left shift; *N*, normal; *R*, right shift. *(From Alspach, J. [2001]. AACN instructor's resource manual for AACN core curriculum for critical care nursing [5th ed.]. Philadelphia: Saunders.)*

said to have *acidemia*. Conversely, a decrease in H^+ level results in an increase in the pH (>7.45), and the patient is said to have *alkalemia*. The suffix "emia" is used to refer to the alteration in pH. The suffix "osis" is used to refer to the condition or process that causes the alteration in pH, such as diabetic ketoacidosis.

Partial Pressure of Arterial Carbon Dioxide. $PaCO_2$ is the partial pressure of carbon dioxide (CO_2) dissolved in arterial plasma. CO_2 is considered a volatile acid because it can combine with H_2O to form carbonic acid (H_2CO_3). The $PaCO_2$ is regulated by the lungs and has a normal range of 35 to 45 mm Hg. The respiratory system controls the $PaCO_2$ by regulating ventilation (the patient's rate and depth of breathing). A $PaCO_2$ of less than 35 mm Hg indicates the presence of respiratory alkalosis; a $PaCO_2$ greater than 45 mm Hg indicates the presence of respiratory acidosis. If the patient hypoventilates, carbon dioxide is retained, leading to respiratory acidosis ($PaCO_2$ >45 mm Hg). Conversely, if a patient hyperventilates, excess carbon dioxide is excreted by the lungs, resulting in respiratory alkalosis ($PaCO_2$ <35 mm Hg).

Conditions that cause respiratory acidosis and alkalosis are noted in Box 9-2.

Sodium Bicarbonate. Whereas H^+ ions are an acid in the body, HCO_3^- is a base, a substance that neutralizes or buffers acids. HCO_3^- is regulated by the kidneys. Its normal range is 22 to 26 mEq/L. An HCO_3^- level greater than 26 mEq/L indicates metabolic alkalosis, whereas an HCO_3^- level less than 22 mEq/L indicates metabolic acidosis. Conditions that cause metabolic acidosis and alkalosis are noted in Box 9-2.

Buffer Systems. The body regulates acid-base balance through buffer systems, which are substances that minimize the changes in pH when either acids or bases are added. For example, acids are neutralized through combination with a base, and vice versa. There are various buffer systems in the body. For example, proteins and phosphates are buffers in the cell, and hemoglobin is a buffer in the red blood cell. By far the most important buffering system is the bicarbonate buffer system because it accounts for more than half of the total buffering. The bicarbonate buffer system is activated as the H^+ concentration increases. HCO_3^- combines with H^+ to form carbonic acid (H_2CO_3), which breaks down into carbon dioxide (which is excreted through the lungs) and water

BOX 9-2   Causes of Common Acid-Base Abnormalities

Respiratory Acidosis: Retention of CO_2
- Hypoventilation
- CNS depression (anesthesia, narcotics, sedatives, drug overdose)
- Respiratory neuromuscular disorders
- Trauma: spine, brain, chest wall
- Restrictive lung diseases
- Chronic obstructive pulmonary disease
- Acute airway obstruction (late phases)

Respiratory Alkalosis: Hyperventilation
- Hypoxemia
- Anxiety, fear
- Pain
- Fever
- Stimulants
- CNS irritation (e.g., central hyperventilation)
- Excessive ventilatory support (bag-valve-mask, mechanical ventilation)

Metabolic Acidosis
Increased Acids
- Diabetic ketoacidosis
- Renal failure
- Lactic acidosis
- Drug overdose (salicylates, methanol, ethylene glycol)

Loss of Base
- Diarrhea
- Pancreatic or small bowel fluid loss

Metabolic Alkalosis
Gain of Base
- Excess ingestion of antacids
- Excess administration of sodium bicarbonate
- Citrate in blood transfusions

Loss of Metabolic Acids
- Vomiting
- Nasogastric suctioning
- Low potassium and/or chloride
- Diuretics (loss of chloride and/or potassium)

CNS, Central nervous system; CO_2, carbon dioxide.

(H_2O). The equation for this mechanism is as follows:

$$H^+ + HCO_3^- \rightarrow H_2CO_3 \rightarrow H_2O + CO_2$$

The bicarbonate buffering system operates by using the lungs to regulate CO_2 and the kidneys to regulate HCO_3^-.[34]

Base Excess or Base Deficit. The base excess or base deficit is reported on most ABG results. This lab value reflects the sum of all of the buffer bases in the body, the total buffer base. The normal range for base excess/base deficit is −2 to +2 mEq/L. In pure respiratory acid-base imbalances, the total buffer base remains unchanged. However, in metabolic acidosis, the body's buffers are used up in an attempt to neutralize the acids, and a base deficit occurs. When a condition causing metabolic alkalosis occurs, the total buffer base increases and the patient will have a base excess. All metabolic acid-base disturbances are accompanied by a change in the base excess/base deficit, making it a very reliable indicator of metabolic acid-base disorders.[34] In pure respiratory acid-base disturbances, the base excess/base deficit is normal; however, once compensation occurs, the base excess/base deficit changes (see Compensation).

Compensation. Compensation involves various mechanisms used by the body to normalize the pH when a primary acid-base abnormality occurs. Compensation for primary metabolic acid-base abnormalities is via the respiratory system, which responds quickly to alterations. In metabolic acidosis, the depth and rate of ventilation is increased in an effort to blow off more CO_2 (acid), thereby working to normalize the pH. Conversely in metabolic alkalosis, the rate and depth of ventilation may be decreased in an effort to retain acid; however, respiratory compensation is limited because of the body's mechanism to limit hypoventilation.

Compensation for primary respiratory acid-base abnormalities is via the renal system. The renal system works to balance the pH by excreting excess H^+ and retaining bicarbonate. The renal system activates more slowly and may take up to 2 days to regulate acid-base balance. The kidneys excrete HCO_3^- when respiratory alkalosis is present, and retain HCO_3^- when respiratory acidosis is present.[22,34] The renal and respiratory systems exist in harmony to maintain acid-base balance (Figure 9-10).

Steps in Arterial Blood Gas Interpretation

Systematic analysis of ABG values involves five steps.[50] The oxygenation status is evaluated first. Second, the acid-base status is determined. Third, the primary cause of the acid-base imbalance is determined. Last, an assessment is made for a compensatory response, if any, that originates from the lungs or kidneys attempting to bring the pH back into balance. Table 9-5 lists ranges for interpretation of blood gases. Critical ABG values are noted in the Laboratory Alert feature.

Step 1: Look at Each Number Individually and Label It. Decide whether the value is high, low, or normal and label

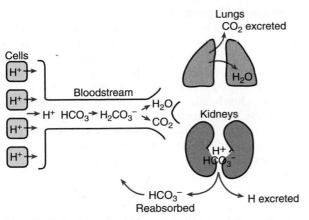

FIGURE 9-10. The kidneys and lungs work together to compensate for acid-base imbalances in the respiratory or metabolic systems. HCO_3^-, Bicarbonate; H_2CO_3, carbonic acid. *(Modified from Harvey, M. A. [2000]. Study guide to the core curriculum for critical care nursing [3rd ed., p. 11]. Philadelphia: Saunders.)*

LABORATORY ALERT
Arterial Blood Gas Critical Values*

PaO_2 <60 mm Hg

$PaCO_2$ >50 mm Hg

pH <7.25 or >7.60

---

*These are critical values only if they differ from baseline values (i.e., an acute change). Some patients with pulmonary disease tolerate highly "abnormal" arterial blood gas values.
$PaCO_2$, Partial pressure of carbon dioxide in arterial blood; *PaO_2*, partial pressure of oxygen in arterial blood.

the finding. For example, a pH of 7.50 is high and labeled as alkalemia.

Step 2: Evaluate Oxygenation. Oxygenation is analyzed by evaluating the PaO_2 and the SaO_2. Hypoxemia is present and considered a significant problem when the PaO_2 falls to less than 60 mm Hg or the SaO_2 falls to less than 90%. A complete assessment must take into account the level of supplemental oxygen a patient is receiving when the ABG is drawn. If the PaO_2 is less than expected for a patient receiving no supplemental oxygen, hypoxemia is classified as follows:[34]

Mild hypoxemia	PaO_2 70 to 79 mm Hg
Moderate hypoxemia	PaO_2 50 to 69 mm Hg
Severe hypoxemia	PaO_2 less than 50 mm Hg

When supplemental oxygen is used the assessment of oxygenation is modified:[34]

Uncorrected	PaO_2 less than 60 mm Hg
Corrected	PaO_2 60 to 100 mm Hg
Overcorrected	PaO_2 greater than 100 mm Hg

Age and disease conditions are considered when evaluating oxygenation. Elderly patients normally have a lower PaO_2 because of the progressive changes in pulmonary physiology associated with the natural process of aging. A "normal" baseline can be estimated for individuals older than 60 years by subtracting 1 mm Hg from the lower limits of mild and moderate hypoxemia for each year greater than 60. However, even for the elderly, a PaO_2 less than 60 mm Hg is always considered hypoxemic.[34] Patients with COPD have chronic hypoxemia.

Step 3: Determine Acid-Base Status. Assess the pH to determine the acid-base status. A pH of less than 7.35 indicates the presence of acidemia; a pH greater than 7.45 indicates the presence of alkalemia. A pH of 7.40 is the absolute normal. If the pH is less than 7.4, the primary disorder is acidosis. If the pH is greater than 7.4, the primary disorder is alkalosis. Therefore, even if the pH is within the normal range, noting whether it is on the acid or alkaline side of 7.40 is important.

Step 4: Determine Whether Primary Acid-Base Disorder Is Respiratory or Metabolic. Assess the $PaCO_2$, which reflects the respiratory system, and the HCO_3^-, which reflects the metabolic system, to determine which one is altered in the same manner as the pH. The ABG results may reflect only one disorder (respiratory or metabolic). However, two primary acid-base disorders may occur simultaneously (mixed acid-base imbalance). For example, during cardiac arrest, both respiratory acidosis and metabolic acidosis commonly occur because of hypoventilation and lactic acidosis. Use the base excess to confirm your interpretation of the primary acid-base disturbance, especially if the disorder is mixed.

Step 5: Determine Whether Any Form of Compensatory Response Has Taken Place. Compensation refers to a return to a normal blood pH by means of respiratory or renal mechanisms. The system opposite the primary disorder attempts the compensation. The kidneys attempt to compensate for respiratory abnormalities, whereas the lungs attempt to compensate for metabolic problems. For example, if a patient has respiratory acidosis, such as occurs in COPD (low pH, high $PaCO_2$), the kidneys respond by retaining more HCO_3^- and excreting H^+. Conversely, if a patient has metabolic acidosis, such as occurs in diabetic ketoacidosis (low pH, low HCO_3^-), the lungs respond by hyperventilation and excretion of carbon dioxide (respiratory alkalosis).

Compensation may be absent, partial, or complete. Compensation is absent if the usual compensatory

BOX 9-3   Examples of Arterial Blood Gases and Compensation

Example 1

PaO_2	80 mm Hg (normal)
pH	7.30 (low; acidosis)
$PaCO_2$	50 mm Hg (high; respiratory acidosis)
HCO_3^-	22 mEq/L (normal)
SaO_2	95% (normal)

Interpretation: Normal oxygenation, respiratory acidosis; no compensation.

Example 2

PaO_2	80 mm Hg (normal)
pH	7.32 (low; acidosis)
$PaCO_2$	50 mm Hg (high; respiratory acidosis)
HCO_3^-	28 mEq/L (high; metabolic alkalosis)
SaO_2	95% (normal)

Interpretation: Normal oxygenation, partly compensated respiratory acidosis. The arterial blood gases are only partly compensated because the pH is not yet within normal limits.

Example 3

PaO_2	80 mm Hg (normal)
pH	7.36 (acid side of normal)
$PaCO_2$	50 mm Hg (high; respiratory acidosis)
HCO_3^-	29 mEq/L (high; metabolic alkalosis)
SaO_2	95% (normal)

Interpretation: Normal oxygenation, completely (fully) compensated respiratory acidosis. The pH is now within normal limits; therefore complete compensation has occurred.

HCO_3^-, Bicarbonate; $PaCO_2$, partial pressure of carbon dioxide in arterial blood; PaO_2, partial pressure of oxygen in arterial blood; SaO_2, saturation of hemoglobin with oxygen in arterial blood.

mechanisms do not occur as expected to correct an acid-base disturbance. If a compensatory mechanism has occurred but the pH is still abnormal, compensation is referred to as partial. Compensation is complete if compensatory mechanisms are present and the pH is within normal range. The body does not overcompensate. Examples of ABG compensation are shown in Box 9-3.

Noninvasive Assessment of Gas Exchange

Intermittent ABG results have been the "gold standard" for the monitoring of gas exchange and acid-base status. Improvements in technology for noninvasive assessment of gas exchange by pulse oximetry and capnography have reduced the numbers of ABG samples obtained in critically ill patients.

Assessment of Oxygenation

Pulse Oximetry. Pulse oximetry measures a value called SpO_2 and reflects the SaO_2. Pulse oximetry uses a light-emitting diode to measure pulsatile flow and light absorption of the hemoglobin. A sensor that measures SpO_2 is placed on the patient's finger, toe, ear, or forehead. To ensure accurate readings, the nurse must ensure that the sensor is placed correctly and an adequate pulsatile signal is detected. Accurate readings are obtained from warm, well-perfused areas. In the critical care unit, most patients have continuous pulse oximetry. SpO_2 values are sometimes "spot checked" in patients who are less acutely ill.

The oxyhemoglobin dissociation curve (see Figure 9-9) shows the relationship between SaO_2 and PaO_2 and provides the basis for pulse oximetry. An SaO_2 of 92% is equivalent to a PaO_2 of 80 mm Hg, whereas an SaO_2 of 90% is equivalent to a PaO_2 of 60 mm Hg unless physiological conditions result in a shift of the oxyhemoglobin dissociation curve. In general, SpO_2 values of less than 90% require further assessment and clinical intervention if the patient is exhibiting symptoms of hypoxemia.[50]

Pulse oximetry values are used to monitor a patient's response to treatment (e.g., ventilator changes, suctioning, inhalation therapy, body position changes) by following trends in oxygen saturation. However, SpO_2 only measures fluctuation in oxygenation and cannot be used to assess carbon dioxide levels.

Several factors affect the accuracy of SpO_2 values. Artifact from patient motion, or edema at the sensor site, may prevent an accurate measurement. The SpO_2 measurements may be lower than the actual SaO_2 if the perfusion to the sensor site is reduced, or in the presence of sunlight, fluorescent light, nail polish or artificial nails, and intravenous dyes. The SpO_2 measurements may be higher than the actual SaO_2 reported by ABG analysis if the patient has an abnormal hemoglobin, such as methemoglobin or carboxyhemoglobin.[20,34]

Assessment of Ventilation

End-Tidal Carbon Dioxide Monitoring. End-tidal carbon dioxide monitoring ($ETCO_2$) is the noninvasive measurement of alveolar CO_2 at the end of exhalation when CO_2 concentration is at its peak. It is used to monitor and assess trends in the patient's ventilatory status. Expired gases are sampled from the patient's airway and are analyzed by a CO_2 sensor that uses infrared light to measure exhaled CO_2 at the end of inspiration. The sensor may be attached to an adaptor on the endotracheal tube (ETT) or the tracheostomy tube.[50,60,61] A nasal cannula with a sidestream capnometer can be used in patients without an artificial airway. The sampling port should be placed as close as possible to the patient's airway. The device must be calibrated periodically for accurate results.

Carbon dioxide, which is a byproduct of metabolism, diffuses from the cells into the blood and is carried to the lungs for elimination. In the lung, CO_2 readily diffuses from the pulmonary capillary into the alveoli; therefore the amount of CO_2 in these two compartments reaches near equilibrium. During exhalation, CO_2 is eliminated from the alveolus, reaching its peak at the end of exhalation. Therefore the measurement of CO_2 at the end of the breath ($ETCO_2$) provides a reflection of the alveolar CO_2, which in turn reflects the arterial CO_2 ($PaCO_2$).

Normally, $PaCO_2$ is 35 to 45 mm Hg, and $ETCO_2$ values average 2 to 5 mm Hg less than the $PaCO_2$ in individuals with normal lung and cardiac function.[34] To determine the baseline correlation between $ETCO_2$ and $PaCO_2$, the $ETCO_2$ is measured at the same time an ABG is obtained. $ETCO_2$ is subtracted from the $PaCO_2$, providing an index known as the $PaCO_2$-$ETCO_2$ gradient. For example, if a blood gas shows that the $PaCO_2$ is 40 mm Hg and simultaneously the $ETCO_2$ is noted to be 36 mm Hg, the $PaCO_2$-$ETCO_2$ gradient is +4. Knowing the gradient allows for non-invasive assessment of the patient's ventilation by trend monitoring the $ETCO_2$ and inferring the $PaCO_2$ by use of the gradient.[68]

$ETCO_2$ monitoring is used to evaluate ventilation when precision is not essential and for trending data. Clinical applications of $ETCO_2$ monitoring include assessment of the patient's response to ventilator changes and respiratory treatments, determining the proper position of the ETT, trending CO_2 in the traumatic brain injury patient, detecting disconnection from the ventilator, and detecting disconnection from anesthesia equipment intraoperatively.[61,68] The most common pitfall of $ETCO_2$ monitoring is believing that the value reflects only the patient's ventilatory status. Changes in exhaled CO_2 may occur because of changes not only in ventilation, but also in CO_2 production (metabolism), transport of CO_2 to the lung, and accuracy of the equipment. For example, a decreased $ETCO_2$ value could indicate decreased alveolar ventilation, a reduction in lung perfusion as in hypotension or pulmonary embolus, a reduction in metabolic production of CO_2 as in hypothermia or return to normothermia after fever, or obstruction of the CO_2 sampling tube.[34,61,68]

Colorimetric Carbon Dioxide Detector. Disposable colorimetric $ETCO_2$ detectors are routinely used after intubation to differentiate tracheal from esophageal intubation (Figure 9-11). The device is placed on the end of the ETT and the patient is given 6 full breaths. At end expiration on the sixth breath the color is

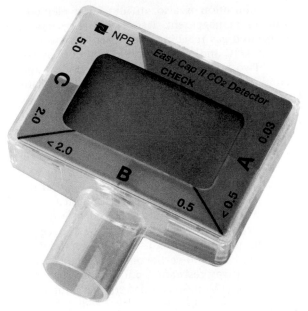

FIGURE 9-11. Disposable colorimetric carbon dioxide (CO_2) detector for confirming endotracheal tube placement. Detection of CO_2 confirms tube placement in the lungs because the only source of CO_2 is the alveoli. *(Courtesy of Nellcor Puritan Bennett, Inc., Pleasanton, CA.)*

read. When CO_2 is detected, the color of the indicator changes from purple to yellow. Detection of CO_2 confirms tube placement in the lungs because the only source of CO_2 is the alveoli.

OXYGEN ADMINISTRATION

Oxygen is administered to treat or prevent hypoxemia. Oxygen may be supplied by various sources such as piped into wall devices, oxygen tanks, or oxygen concentrators. Oxygen delivery devices are categorized by design. Three basic designs exist: low-flow devices (nasal cannula), reservoir systems (simple face mask, partial-rebreather mask, and nonrebreather mask), and high-flow systems (air-entrainment or Venturi mask).[50]

Humidification

Humidification of the oxygen is recommended when O_2 flow is greater than 4 L/min to prevent the mucous membranes from drying. Oxygen delivery at a flow of 4 L/min or less is often provided without humidification. At lower flow rates, the patient's natural humidification system provides adequate humidity.[67]

Humidification is also an important element of ventilator management. It is essential to maintain the inspired gas reaching the patient's airway at as close to 37° C and 100% relative humidity as possible.[7,12] Two approaches are used to supply supplemental humidification with mechanical ventilation. One method functions by actively passing the dry inspired gas through a water-based humidification system before it reaches the patient's airway. This method is often ordered for patients requiring long-term mechanical ventilation. The second method is to attach a heat-moisture exchanger (HME) to the ventilator circuit. The HME functions as an artificial "nose" to warm and humidify the patient's inspired breath with his or her own expired moisture and body heat. The HME must also be inspected regularly for accumulation of patient secretions in the device, which could result in partial or complete obstruction, increased airway resistance, and increased WOB.[67]

During mechanical ventilation, frequent inspection of the humidification unit is needed. The temperature of heated humidification devices is routinely evaluated, and the RT is notified if the heater alarm goes off. Routine checks include maintaining the humidifier water reservoir level and removing condensate from loops in the ventilator circuit. During manipulation of the circuit tubing, it is important to prevent emptying the condensate into the patient's airway. This can lead to contamination of the patient's airway as well as breathing difficulty. The nurse monitors the quantity and quality (consistency) of the patient's secretions to determine the adequacy of humidification. If the secretions are thick despite adequate humidification of the delivered gases, the patient needs systemic hydration.

Picking the Best Device

The successful administration of oxygen therapy is important in treating hypoxemia. When administering oxygen, it is important to consider two components of oxygen therapy: fit and function of a device, and the total flow delivered by a device to the patient.

Fit and Function

Assessing proper fit and functioning of an oxygen device may be forgotten during a clinical crisis. To ensure proper fit and function, the nurse or respiratory care practitioner inspects the patient's face and assesses the location of the oxygen delivery device and how well it is positioned on the patient's face. While doing this, the caregiver determines whether the patient is breathing through an unobstructed airway. The oxygen-connecting tubing is traced back to the gas source origin to ensure that it is connected. Finally, it is important to ensure that the gas source is oxygen and that it is turned on.

Total Flow

Flow is determined by two factors: how much oxygen the device can deliver and whether the delivered oxygen remains fixed or varied under changing patient demands.[28,50,66] The amount of oxygen being administered to the patient, or the oxygen delivery is described as the fraction of inspired oxygen (FiO_2). Devices can deliver low (<35%), moderate (35% to 60%), or high (>60%) oxygen concentrations.[28,66]

The delivery of fixed or variable amounts of oxygen depends on how much of the patient's inspired gas the device supplies. If a device provides all the patient's inspired gas (air-entrainment, or Venturi mask), the FiO_2 remains *fixed* or stable, even if the patient's ventilatory demands change. *Variable-flow* devices (nasal cannula, simple face mask, partial and nonrebreather masks) provide only some of the inspired gases; the patient draws, or entrains, the remainder of inspired gases from the ambient air. With these systems, the FiO_2 delivered to the patient can only be estimated because the actual FiO_2 cannot be precisely controlled. The FiO_2 is determined not only by the amount of oxygen delivered to the patient but also by the ventilatory pattern and the amount of air the patient entrains. For example, if the patient's ventilation increases, the delivered FiO_2 decreases because the patient entrains a larger percentage of room air. Conversely, if a patient draws in less air, the oxygen delivered is less diluted and the FiO_2 rises.[50,67]

Oxygen Delivery Devices

Nasal Cannula (Variable Performance)

A nasal cannula is commonly used to deliver oxygen. The device is relatively comfortable to wear and is easy to secure on the patient. In adult patients, nasal cannulas provide oxygen concentrations between 24% and 44% oxygen at flow rates up to 6 L/min.[28,34] An increase in oxygen flow rate by 1 L/min generally increases oxygen delivery by 4% (e.g., 2 L/min nasal cannula delivers 28% of oxygen, whereas 3 L/min provides 32%). Administering oxygen through a nasal cannula at flow rates higher than 6 L/min is not effective in increasing oxygenation because the capacity of the patient's anatomical reservoir in the nasopharynx is surpassed. Gas flowing into the nasopharynx beyond 6 L/min is diverted away from the patient's anatomical reservoir and is lost to the surrounding environment. An important nursing intervention for patients receiving oxygen via nasal cannula is to assess the skin above the ears for skin breakdown. It may be necessary to pad the tubing over the ear with gauze.

Simple Face Mask (Variable Performance)

The placing of a mask over the patient's face creates an additional oxygen reservoir beyond the patient's natural anatomical reservoir. Because this mask is tight fitting (ideally) and rests on the face, it is important that the flow rate for this device be set to at least 5 L/min to avoid rebreathing carbon dioxide. Oxygen is delivered directly from an oxygen flow meter to the mask at flow rates of 5 to 12 L/min, which provides an FiO_2 of 0.30 to 0.60.[34] The patient should be instructed about the importance of wearing the mask as applied. The inside of the mask should be cleaned as needed, and the skin should be assessed for areas of pressure.[28]

Face Masks with Reservoirs (Variable Performance)

Both the partial rebreathing and nonrebreathing masks are similar to the design of a simple face mask, but with the addition of an oxygen reservoir bag. The addition of the reservoir increases the amount of oxygen available to the patient during inspiration and allows for the delivery of concentrations of 35% to 60% (partial rebreather) or 60% to 80% (nonrebreather) dependent on the flowmeter setting, the fit of the mask, and the patient's respiratory pattern. The main difference between these two devices is that the nonrebreather mask has a one way valve between the mask and reservoir bag and over one of the exhalation ports. These valves ensure the patient breathes a high concentration of oxygen-enriched gas from the reservoir with each breath (Figure 9-12). The flow rate on the meter should be set to prevent the reservoir bag from deflating no more than one half during inspiration for the partial rebreather and to prevent the bag from deflating for the nonrebreather.[28,34] Either mask may be used in the critically ill patient with severe hypoxemia in an effort to prevent the need for endotracheal intubation and mechanical ventilation.

Venturi or Air-Entrainment Mask (Fixed Performance)

The Venturi or air-entrainment mask appears much like a simple face mask; however, it has a jet adapter placed between the mask and the tubing to the oxygen source. The jet adapters come in various sizes and are often color-coded to the FiO_2 they deliver. The appropriate flow rate is often inscribed on the adapter. Air-entrainment devices direct high-pressure oxygen through the jet or small nozzle, which is surrounded by air-entrainment ports. As the oxygen is directed under high pressure through the jet, room air is pulled into the air-entrainment ports on the sides of the adapter (Figure 9-13). The Venturi mask delivers a fixed FiO_2 and therefore provides an accurate delivery of prescribed oxygen to the patient. Because the level of oxygen can be closely regulated, the Venturi mask is commonly used in the hypoxemic patient with chronic pulmonary disease for whom the delivery of excessive oxygen could depress the respiratory drive.[28,34]

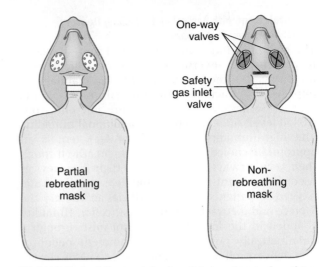

FIGURE 9-12. Partial rebreathing and nonrebreathing oxygen masks. *(From Kacmarek, R. M., Dimas, S., & Mack, C. W. [2005]. Oxygen, helium and nitric oxide therapy [p. 616]. St. Louis: Mosby.)*

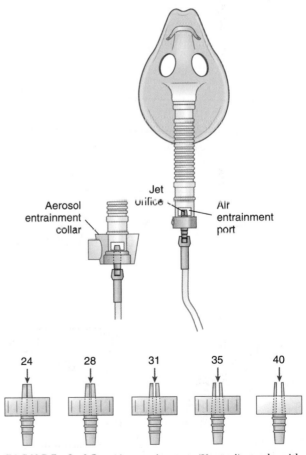

FIGURE 9-13. Air-entrainment (Venturi) mask with various jet orifices. Each orifice provides a specific delivered FiO_2. *(From Kacmarek, R. M., Dimas, S., & Mack, C. W. [2005]. Oxygen, helium and nitric oxide therapy [p. 612]. St. Louis: Mosby.)*

Air Entrainment with Aerosol and Humidity Delivery (Variable or Fixed Performance)

The goal of adding humidity to the inspired gases is to prevent the adverse effects to the patient from breathing dry medical gases and to maintain or improve the function of the normal mucosa of the airway. Sometimes patients require not only controlled levels of oxygen but also additional humidity. The high-humidity face mask or face tent is an appropriate choice for patients who breathe through their own airways (Figure 9-14). High-flow devices used for administering humidified, supplemental oxygen to patients with an artificial airway are the T-piece and the tracheostomy mask/collar. Humidity is added in the form of an aerosol mist through a pneumatically powered, air-entrainment nebulizer that delivers a fixed FiO₂. The desired FiO₂ is chosen by adjusting the air-entrainment port on the top of the nebulizer. The initial flow rate is set at 10 L/min. To ensure the patient's entire ventilatory needs are met, the flow rate is adjusted so that a constant mist can be seen coming from the exhalation port of the chosen device. If the patient has high ventilatory needs and the mist is not evident throughout the respiratory cycle, an additional flowmeter and nebulizer are added with the use of a Y-adapter.[28,34]

Manual Resuscitation Bag (Variable Performance)

A manual resuscitation bag, or bag-valve device, is used to ventilate a patient manually while also providing supplemental oxygen (see Chapter 10). The device is attached to a face mask or connected directly to an ETT or tracheostomy tube to ventilate the patient. When used on an emergency basis, the bag-valve device should have a reservoir attached to increase the FiO₂. The oxygen flowmeter attached to the bag is set at 15 L/min to provide adequate flow of oxygen to meet the inspiratory demands of assisted manual ventilation.

AIRWAY MANAGEMENT

Positioning

A primary nursing intervention with any patient is to maintain an open airway. The first method for maintaining a patent airway is proper head position with the head-tilt/chin-lift or jaw thrust. An airway adjunct such as the oral or nasopharyngeal airway may be needed to help maintain the airway.

Oral Airways

The oropharyngeal airway prevents the tongue from falling back and obstructing the pharynx (Figure 9-15). It is indicated when the patient has a depressed level of consciousness, resulting in loss of muscle tone and airway obstruction. It may also be used to make ventilation with a manual resuscitation bag more effective, or to prevent a patient from biting and occluding an ETT. It is contraindicated in a patient who is awake because it stimulates the gag reflex, resulting in discomfort, agitation, and possibly emesis. Some oral airways are made of rigid plastic, whereas others are made of softer plastic. It is important to choose the proper size airway. An oral airway that is too short forces the patient's tongue back into the pharynx. An airway that is too long stimulates the gag reflex. Additional issues related to oral airway use are trauma to the lips and tongue, and accumulation of secretions in the oropharynx if oral suctioning is not done. The technique for inserting an oral airway is described in Box 9-4.

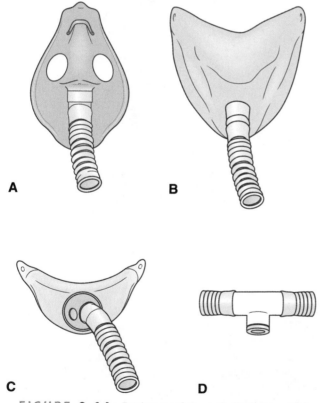

A,   **B,**

C,   **D,**

FIGURE 9-14. Devices used to apply high-flow, high-humidity oxygen therapy. **A,** Aerosol mask. **B,** Face tent. **C,** Tracheostomy collar. **D,** Briggs T-piece. *(From Kacmarek, R. M., Dimas, S., & Mack, C. W. [2005]. Oxygen, helium and nitric oxide therapy [p. 614]. St. Louis: Mosby.)*

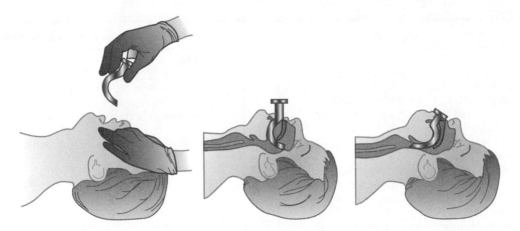

FIGURE 9-15. Maintaining a patent airway with an oral airway. *(From Durbin, C. G. [2004]. Airway management. In J. M. Cairo & S. P. Pilbeam (Eds.), Mosby's respiratory care equipment [7th ed., p. 157]. St. Louis: Mosby.)*

BOX 9-4   Insertion of Oral Airway

1. Choose the proper size by measuring the airway on the patient. Airway should extend from the edge of the patient's mouth to the ear lobe.
2. Suction mucus from the mouth using a tonsil (Yankauer) tip catheter.
3. Turn the airway upside down with its tip against the hard palate and slide airway into mouth until the soft palate is reached; then rotate the airway to match the curvature of the tongue into the proper position.
4. An alternative method to step 3 is to use a tongue blade to depress the patient's tongue while inserting the airway, matching its curvature to that of the tongue.
5. Advance tip to back of mouth. Ensure end of airway rests between the teeth but does not compress the lips against the teeth, which would cause injury.
6. Assess airway patency, breath sounds, and chest movement. Noises indicating upper airway obstruction should be absent.
7. Maintain the patient's proper head alignment after airway insertion.

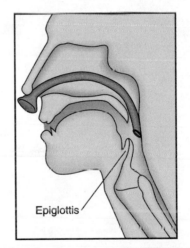

Epiglottis

FIGURE 9-16. The nasopharyngeal airway is used to relieve upper airway obstruction and to facilitate passage of a suction catheter.

Nasopharyngeal Airways

The nasopharyngeal airway, also known as nasal airway or nasal trumpet, is a soft rubber or latex tube placed in the nose and extending to the posterior portion of the pharynx (Figure 9-16). It is indicated when an oropharyngeal airway is contraindicated or too difficult to place, such as when the patient's jaw is tight during a seizure, or if oral trauma is present. Nasopharyngeal airways are better tolerated than oral airways in the conscious patient, are more comfortable, and facilitate the passage of a suction catheter during nasotracheal suctioning.

The procedure for inserting a nasotracheal airway is described in Box 9-5. Complications of nasopharyngeal airways include insertion into the esophagus if the airway is too long, nosebleeds, and ulceration of the nares. Extended use of nasopharyngeal airways is not recommended because of an increased risk for sinusitis or otitis.

BOX 9-5   Insertion of Nasal Airway

1. Choose the proper size by positioning the airway along the side of the head. The proper length airway extends from the nostril to the earlobe, or just past the angle of the jaw.
2. Generously lubricate the tip and sides of the nasal airway with a water-soluble lubricant.
3. If time allows, lubricate the nasal passage with a topical anesthetic.
4. Insert the airway medially and downward, not upward because the nasopharynx lies directly behind the nares. It may be necessary to rotate the airway slightly.
5. After insertion, assess airway patency, breath sounds, and chest movement.

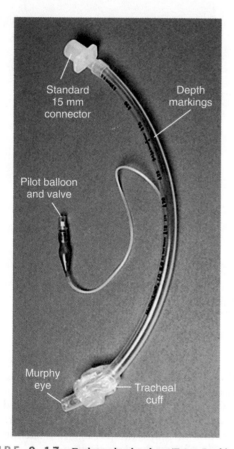

Standard 15 mm connector

Depth markings

Pilot balloon and valve

Murphy eye

Tracheal cuff

FIGURE 9-17. Endotracheal tube. (*From Durbin, C. G.* [2004]. *Airway management. In J. M. Cairo & S. P. Pilbeam (Eds.). Mosby's respiratory care equipment [7th ed., p. 164]. St. Louis: Mosby.*)

BOX 9-6   Oral versus Nasotracheal Intubation

Oral Intubation
Advantages
- Quickly performed, emergency airway
- Larger tube facilitates secretion removal and bronchoscopy; creates less airway resistance
- Less kinking of tube
- Preferred method; less sinusitis and otitis media

Disadvantages
- Discomfort
- Mouth care more difficult to perform
- Impairs ability to swallow
- May increase oral secretion production
- May cause irritation and ulceration of the mouth
- Greater risk of self-extubation
- More difficult to communicate by mouthing words
- Patient may bite on airway, reducing gas flow

Nasotracheal Intubation
Advantages
- Greater patient comfort and tolerance
- Better mouth care possible
- Fewer oral complications
- Less risk of accidental extubation
- Facilitates swallowing of oral secretions
- Communication by mouthing words enhanced

Disadvantages
- More difficult to place
- Possible epistaxis during insertion
- Increases risk for sinusitis and otitis media
- May be more difficult to perform
- Secretion removal more difficult because of smaller tube diameter
- Increases work of breathing associated with smaller diameter tube

Endotracheal Intubation

Intubation refers to the insertion of an ETT into the trachea through either the mouth or the nose. Advantages of oral versus nasal endotracheal intubation are listed in Box 9-6. The ETT (Figure 9-17) is typically made of a polyvinyl chloride or silicone material with a distal cuff that is inflated via a one-way valve pilot balloon. The purpose of the cuff is to facilitate ventilation of the patient by sealing the trachea and allowing air to pass through, not around the ETT. Standard ETT cuffs are the high-volume, low-pressure type, and most cuffs are inflated with air (some tubes have a foam-filled cuff). The pilot balloon is used to monitor cuff pressure and adjust cuff pressure as indicated.

ETTs capable of continuous suctioning of subglottic secretions are used in some facilities. These tubes (e.g., Hi-Lo Evac tube) have an extra suction port just above the cuff for removal of secretions that accumulate above the cuff. Evidence shows a decrease in ventilator-associated pneumonia by nearly 50% when these tubes are used.[12] Additional interventions are required when these tubes are in place. Continuous low-pressure suction not exceeding −20 mm Hg is applied to the suction lumen. The suction lumen must remain patent. Administration of a bolus of air through the suction port is often needed to relieve obstruction and promote continuous suction.

Intubation is performed to establish an airway, assist in secretion removal, protect the airway from aspiration in patients with a depressed cough and gag, and provide mechanical ventilation. Personnel who are trained and skilled in intubation perform the procedure: anesthesiologists, nurse anesthetists, acute care nurse practitioners, emergency department physicians, intensivists, RTs, and some paramedics.[50] Intubation may be performed emergently on a patient in cardiac or respiratory arrest, or electively in a patient with impending respiratory failure.

The nurse must be familiar with and be able to gather quickly the equipment used for intubation. The nurse also needs to know how to connect the laryngoscope blade to the handle, check to see that it illuminates properly, and change the bulb as needed. Intubation equipment is frequently kept together in an emergency cart or special procedures box to facilitate emergency intubation (Figure 9-18). The nurse notifies the RT to obtain a ventilator, explains the procedure to the patient, removes dentures if present, gathers all equipment, and ensures that suction equipment is in working order. The nurse assists in positioning the patient, verifies that the patient has a patent intravenous line for the administration of fluids and medications, and provides the necessary equipment while anticipating the needs of the individual performing the intubation.

Procedure for Oral Endotracheal Intubation

The proper size ETT is chosen; it is important that the ETT not be too small, because a smaller-diameter ETT substantially increases airway resistance and the patient's WOB. Increased WOB negatively affects the patient's efforts to breathe spontaneously and may make weaning from mechanical ventilation difficult. The average-sized ETT ranges from 7.5 to 8.0 mm for

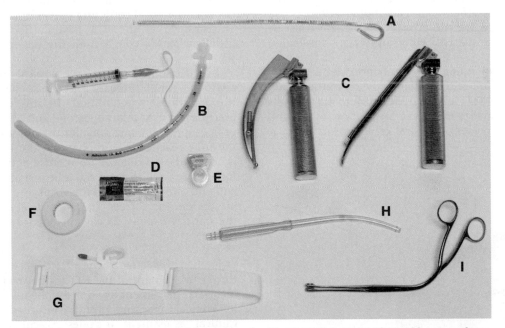

FIGURE 9-18. Equipment used for endotracheal intubation: **A,** stylet (disposable); **B,** endotracheal tube with 10-mL syringe for cuff inflation; **C,** laryngoscope handle with attached curved blade *(left)* and straight blade *(right)*; **D,** water-soluble lubricant; **E,** colorimetric CO_2 detector to check tube placement; **F,** tape or **G,** commercial device to secure tube; **H,** Yankauer disposable pharyngeal suction device; **I,** Magill forceps (optional). Additional equipment, not shown, includes suction source and stethoscope.

women and from 8.0 to 9.0 mm for men.[63] After the proper size ETT is selected, the cuff is inflated to check for symmetry and any leaks. A plastic-coated malleable stylet may be used to stiffen the ETT to facilitate insertion, but it should be carefully placed inside the ETT to avoid its protrusion beyond the end of the ETT. The ETT is lubricated with a water-soluble lubricant to facilitate passage through the structures of the oropharynx.

The laryngoscope is attached to the appropriate size and type of blade (straight or curved). The choice of blades varies based on the patient's anatomy and the preference of the clinician performing the intubation. Blade sizes range from 0 to 4. The average-sized adult is intubated with a size-3 blade.[14] Optional equipment includes a fiberoptic laryngoscope or equipment for video-assisted intubation.

To facilitate intubation, the patient is placed in a "sniffing" position to facilitate visualization of the glottis, or vocal cords. Placing a folded towel or bath blanket under the head may help to achieve this position (Figure 9-19). Time permitting, the patient is premedicated. A sedative and a paralytic agent may be administered to allow for easier manipulation of the mandible and visualization of the glottis. Before intubation is performed, the patient is hyperoxygenated with 100% oxygen by using a bag-valve device connected to a face mask. The intubation procedure should be performed within 30 seconds. If the intubation is difficult and additional attempts are required to secure the airway, the patient must be manually ventilated between each intubation attempt.

The person doing the intubation, while taking care not to damage the patient's teeth or other structures, inserts the laryngoscope blade into the patient's mouth to visualize the vocal cords. If secretions and vomitus are present, the oral cavity is suctioned. A rigid tonsil tip suction (e.g., Yankauer) is very efficient in removing thick secretions and is often used. When the tube is properly inserted about 5 to 6 cm beyond the vocal cords into the trachea, the laryngoscope and stylet are removed and the ETT cuff is inflated.

Procedure for Nasotracheal Intubation

Two approaches to nasal intubation are possible: blind and direct visualization.[57] The equipment for nasotracheal intubation is the same as for oral intubation with the addition of Magill forceps. The nasal intubation procedure differs from oral intubation in that the naris selected for the ETT passage is prepared with a topical vasoconstricting agent to reduce bleeding, and an anesthetic agent. One option is to lubricate the ETT with a water-soluble gel containing 2% lidocaine. The patient is positioned as indicated by the preference of the person performing the intubation: semi-Fowlers, high Fowler's, or supine.

After the patient's naris and the ETT have been prepared, the ETT is inserted "blindly"; that is, no laryngoscope is used to visualize the cords. The ETT is advanced toward the glottis as the intubator listens to the intensity of the patient's breathing. Blind intubation can be performed only in the patient who is capable of spontaneous respirations. The closer the intubator comes to the glottis, the more intense the sound of air movement becomes until the ETT passes through the vocal cords and moves into the trachea. The passage of the ETT beyond the vocal cords usually elicits a cough from the patient and vocal silence.

Because some patients have atypical upper airway anatomy, nasal intubation can also be performed through direct visualization. In this method, the practitioner uses a laryngoscope and Magill forceps, or fiberoptic bronchoscopy, for the procedure. When the tube reaches the oropharynx, the laryngoscope is inserted to visualize the cords, and the Magill forceps are used to grasp the tube just above the ETT cuff and direct it between the vocal cords. With nasal intubation, the correct placement level of the ETT at the naris is usually 28 cm for males and 26 cm for females.

Verification of Endotracheal Tube Placement

Correct placement of the ETT in the trachea (versus incorrect placement in the esophagus) is verified by clinical assessment and confirmation devices. Clinical assessment includes auscultation of the epigastrium and lung fields, and observing for bilateral chest expansion.[63] Failure to hear breath sounds while hearing air over the epigastrium represents esophageal rather than tracheal intubation. Breath sounds are equal bilaterally when the tube is placed

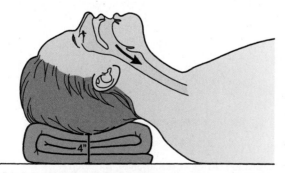

FIGURE 9-19. Elevating the head with a blanket or folded towels places the patient in the "sniffing position" to facilitate endotracheal intubation. *(From Mims, B. C., Toto, K. H., Luecke, L. E., Roberts, M. K., Wilmouth, J. B., & Tyner, T. E. [2003]. Critical care skills [2nd ed., p. 23]. Philadelphia: Saunders.)*

correctly. Intubation of the right mainstem bronchus is common because the right mainstem is straighter than the left, and the ETT is occasionally placed deeper in the trachea during intubation than necessary. Right mainstem bronchus intubation is suspected when unilateral expansion of the right chest is observed during ventilation and the breath sounds are louder on the right than left.

Another method of assessment is done with a confirmation device. Monitoring devices to confirm ETT placement include either a disposable $ETCO_2$ detector or a bulb aspiration device (esophageal detector device). The disposable $ETCO_2$ detector is attached to the end of the ETT. This device changes color when carbon dioxide is detected and is a highly reliable method of confirming tracheal (versus esophageal) intubation.[14,63] Another option is to attach an aspiration device that is similar to a bulb syringe. The device is compressed and deflated and is attached to the ETT. If the tube is in the trachea, the bulb inflates rapidly. If the tube is in the esophagus, filling is delayed. Pulse oximetry also assists in assessment of tube placement. SpO_2 will fall if the esophagus has been inadvertently intubated, and may be decreased in right mainstem intubation. Finally, a portable chest radiograph is ordered to confirm tube placement.

The tip of the ETT should be approximately 3 to 4 cm above the carina.[63] Once the placement is confirmed, the centimeter depth marking at the teeth or naris should be noted in the medical record. An indelible marker can be used to mark the ETT at the lip or naris. These nursing measures assist with ongoing monitoring of proper tube position. The nurse and RT collaborate to ensure the ETT is properly secured with tape or a commercial device to prevent dislodging. Figure 9-20 shows two methods for securing the ETT.

Tracheostomy

A tracheostomy tube provides an airway directly into the anterior portion of the neck. Tracheostomy tubes are indicated for long-term mechanical ventilation, long-term secretion management, protecting the airway from aspiration when the cough and gag reflexes are impaired, bypassing an upper airway obstruction that prevents placement of an ETT, and reducing the WOB associated with an ETT. The tracheostomy tube reduces the WOB because it is shorter than an ETT and airflow resistance is less.[15,50,63]

Several advantages are associated with tracheostomy tubes. Tracheostomy tubes are better tolerated than ETTs; therefore, patients may require less

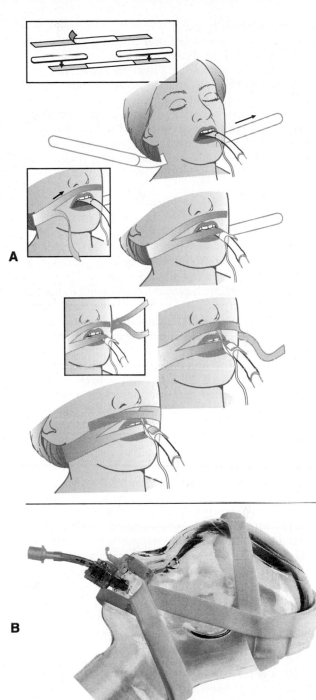

FIGURE 9-20. Two methods for securing the endotracheal tube: tape **(A)** and harness device **(B)**. Harness device shown is the SecureEasy Endotracheal Tube Holder. Nonelastic headgear reduces the risk of self-extubation. A soft bite block prevents tube occlusion. (**A** from Mims, B. C., Toto, K. H., Luecke, L. E., Roberts, M. K., Wilmouth, J. B., & Tyner, T. E. [2003]. Critical care skills [2nd ed., p. 30]. Philadelphia: Saunders; **B** courtesy of Medex, Carlsbad, CA.)

sedation or restraint use. Patients with tracheostomy tubes are often permitted oral intake if swallowing studies demonstrate absence of aspiration. It is easier for the nurse to provide oral hygiene in patients with tracheostomy tubes. Some tracheostomy tube designs allow for talking, facilitating patient communication. A tracheostomy tube can be more securely fixed than an ETT, thus decreasing the incidence of accidental extubation. Once a tracheostomy is performed, many patients are able to transfer to a progressive care unit because the WOB is decreased and mobility is improved.

There is no clearly defined time for when a tracheostomy should be performed in patients with an ETT who require mechanical ventilation. If mechanical ventilation and an artificial airway are projected to be needed for a prolonged period, the decision to perform a tracheostomy should be made.[26]

The tracheostomy has traditionally been a surgical technique performed in the operating room. However, a percutaneous dilatational tracheostomy (PDT) procedure may be performed safely at the bedside by a trained physician.[16] The PDT is performed by making a small incision into the anterior neck down to the trachea. Once this location has been reached, the physician inserts a needle and sheath into the trachea. The needle is removed, and a guidewire is passed through the sheath. Progressively larger dilators are introduced over the guidewire until the patient's stoma is large enough to accommodate a tracheostomy tube.[16]

Collaboratively, the nurse and RT assist in the PDT procedure. Before the procedure, the nurse ensures that intravenous access lines are accessible for administration of sedatives and analgesic medications. The patient is properly positioned, and the height of the bed is adjusted relative to the individual performing the procedure. Sterile supplies are gathered, and sterility is maintained throughout the procedure. Physiological parameters are monitored continuously and documented at least every 15 minutes throughout the PDT, and for a least an hour after the procedure.[50]

The most significant postprocedure complication of PDT is accidental decannulation. When a patient undergoes a surgical tracheostomy, the trachea is surgically attached to the skin. This promotes prompt identification of the tract and reinsertion of the tracheal tube should it become dislodged. With a PDT, the trachea is not secured in this way, and a mature tract takes approximately 2 weeks to form. Accidental decannulation and attempted reinsertion of the airway during this time may result in difficulty securing the airway, bleeding, tracheal injury, and death. Oral intubation may be required if the airway becomes dislodged or needs to be replaced.[50]

Tracheostomy Tube Designs

Tracheostomy tubes come in a variety of sizes and styles, and are primarily made of plastic. Design features are shown in Figure 9-21. The flange lies against the patient's neck and has an opening on both ends for the placement of tracheostomy ties for securing the airway. Similar to the ETT, some tracheostomy tubes have a distal cuff and pilot balloon. An important part of the tracheostomy system is the obturator, which is inserted into the trachea tube during insertion. The rounded end of the obturator extends just beyond the end of the tracheostomy tube and creates a smooth tip, allowing for easy entry into the stoma. The obturator is removed after tube insertion to allow for air passage through the trachea. It must be kept in a visible location in the patient's room should emergency reinsertion of a misplaced tube be necessary.[50]

Cuffed versus Uncuffed Tracheostomy Tubes. Critically ill patients who need mechanical ventilation require cuffed tubes to ensure delivery of ventilation and prevent aspiration. The cuff may be a conventional low-pressure, high-volume type, or it may be constructed of foam. The foam-cuff tube may prevent trauma to the airway because of the low pressure exerted to the airway, and it is sometimes used for patients who have difficulty maintaining a good seal

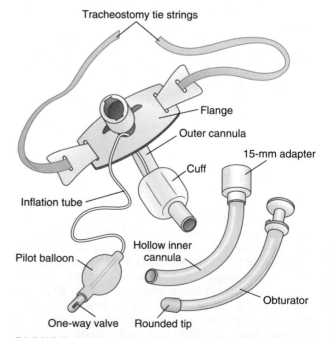

FIGURE 9-21. General design features of the tracheostomy tube. *(From Simmons, K. F., & Scanlan, C. L. [2003]. Airway management. In R. L. Wilkins, J. K. Stoller, & C. L. Scanlan [Eds.], Egans' fundamentals of respiratory care [8th ed., p. 667]. St. Louis: Mosby.)*

with conventional cuffed tracheostomy tubes. Many other types of tracheostomy tubes are available.[62,63] An uncuffed tracheostomy tube is used for long-term airway management in a patient who does not require mechanical ventilation and is at low risk of aspiration. For example, a patient with a neurological injury may require a tracheostomy for airway management and secretion removal. Metal tracheostomy tubes are uncuffed.[63]

Single- versus Double-Cannula Tracheostomy Tubes. Tracheostomy tubes may have one or two cannulas. A single-cannula tube does not have an inner cannula, whereas a double-cannula tube has both an inner and outer cannula. The inner cannula is removable to facilitate cleaning of the inner lumen and to prevent tube occlusion from accumulated secretions. Inner cannulas can be reusable or disposable. Cuffed tracheostomy tubes with disposable inner cannulas are commonplace in the critical care unit.

Fenestrated Tracheostomy Tube. The fenestrated tracheostomy tube has a hole in the outer cannula that allows air to flow above the larynx. The tube functions as a standard tracheostomy tube when the inner cannula is in place. When the inner cannula is removed, the fenestrated tracheostomy tube assists in weaning a patient from the tracheostomy by gradually allowing the patient to breathe through the natural upper airway. The fenestrated tube also allows the patient to emit vocal sounds, thereby facilitating communication.[63] To use a cuffed fenestrated tracheostomy tube for speaking or to promote breathing through the natural airway, the inner cannula is carefully removed and the cuff is deflated. The inner cannula must be reinserted and the cuff reinflated for eating, suctioning, mechanical ventilation, or use of a bag-valve device.[50]

Speaking Tracheostomy Valves. One-way speaking valves are available to allow patients with a tracheostomy an opportunity to speak. These valves can be used in both ventilated and nonventilated patients. However, they can be used only in patients capable of initiating and maintaining spontaneous ventilation.[14,63] Examples of these adjunctive devices include the Passy-Muir valve and the Olympic Trach-Talk.

For the speaking valve to work correctly, the valve is connected to the tracheostomy tube, the cuff on the tracheostomy tube is deflated, and the patient is allowed to breathe and exhale through the natural airway. The valve itself is a one-way device allowing gas to enter through it into the tracheostomy tube, and to the patient. Because this is a one-way valve, exhaled gas exits the trachea via the natural airway, past the deflated cuff of the tracheostomy tube and through the vocal cords.[14]

If a speaking valve is used in conjunction with mechanical ventilation, it must be used with a tracheostomy tube, not an ETT. The delivered tidal volume (V_T) must be increased to ensure an adequate volume to ventilate the patient. This increase in V_T is necessary because a portion of the delivered V_T is lost via the deflated tracheostomy cuff.[27,34] While the valve is in place, the patient should be carefully assessed for respiratory stability and tolerance. Monitoring should include measurements of the patient's SpO_2, heart rate, RR, and blood pressure; observations about the patient's anxiety level and perception of the experience; and assessment of the patient's WOB. Management of secretions is another important nursing intervention.[50]

Endotracheal Suctioning

Patients with an artificial airway need to be suctioned to ensure airway patency because the normal protective ability to cough up secretions is impaired. Suctioning is performed according to a standard procedure to prevent complications such as hypoxemia, airway trauma, infection, and increased intracranial pressure in patients with head injury. Suctioning also stimulates the cough reflex and promotes the mobilization and removal of secretions.

Because suctioning is associated with complications, it is performed only as indicated by physical assessment and not according to a predetermined schedule. Indications for endotracheal suctioning include visible secretions in the tube, frequent coughing, presence of rhonchi, oxygen desaturation, a change in vital signs (e.g., increased or decreased heart rate or RR), dyspnea, restlessness, increased peak inspiratory pressure (PIP), or high-pressure ventilator alarms.[50,63] The number of suction passes is usually 1 to 3; however the patient is suctioned until secretions are removed. Suction duration is limited to 10 to 15 seconds and rest periods are provided between suction passes.

Key points related to endotracheal suctioning are discussed in Box 9-7. Several techniques are implemented to reduce complications associated with suctioning. Hyperoxygenation with 100% oxygen should be performed for 30 seconds before suctioning, during the procedure, and immediately after suctioning.[63] Most ventilators have a built-in suction mode that delivers 100% oxygen for a short period (e.g., 2 minutes). Hyperoxygenation can also be administered with a bag-valve device. If the patient does not tolerate suctioning with hyperoxygenation alone, hyperinflation may be used. Hyperinflation involves the delivery of breaths 1.0 to 1.5 times the V_T and is performed by giving the patient three to five breaths before and between suctioning attempts using either the ventilator or bag-valve device.

BOX 9-7   Key Points for Endotracheal Suctioning

- Suction only as indicated by patient assessment.
- Choose the proper-size device. The diameter of the suction catheter should be no more than half the diameter of the artificial airway.
- Assemble equipment: suction kit with two gloves or closed suction system (CSS), sterile water or saline for rinsing the catheter. The CSS is attached to the ventilator circuit, usually by a respiratory therapist.
- Set the suction regulator at 80 to 120 mm Hg.
- Use sterile technique for suctioning.
- Hyperoxygenate the patient via the ventilator circuit before, between, and after suctioning.
- Gently insert suction catheter until resistance is met, then pull back 1 cm.
- Suction the patient no longer than 10 to 15 seconds while applying intermittent or constant suction.
- Repeat endotracheal suctioning until the airway is clear.
- Rinse the catheter with sterile saline after endotracheal suctioning is performed.
- Suction the mouth and oropharynx with the single-use suction catheter, suction swabs, or a tonsil suction device.
- Auscultate the lungs to assess effectiveness of suctioning, and document findings.
- Document the amount, color, and consistency of secretions.
- *Steps specific to closed suctioning* (in addition to those noted above):
  - Using the dominant hand, insert the suction catheter into the airway until resistance is met. Simultaneously, use the nondominant hand to stabilize the artificial airway.
  - Withdraw the suction catheter while depressing the suction valve; be careful to not angle the wrist of the hand while withdrawing the catheter, as kinking of the catheter and loss of suction may occur.
  - Ensure that CSS catheter is completely withdrawn from the airway. A marking is visible on the suction catheter when it is properly withdrawn.
  - Rinse the catheter after the procedure. Connect a small vial or syringe of normal saline for tracheal instillation (without preservatives) to the irrigation port, and simultaneously instill the saline into the port while depressing the suction control.
  - Keep the CSS suction catheter out of the patient's reach to avoid accidental self-extubation.

The closed tracheal, or in-line, suction catheter is an alternative to the single use suction catheter. The closed tracheal suction system consists of a suction catheter enclosed in a plastic sheath that is attached to the patient's ventilator circuit and airway (Figure 9-22). The device assists in maintaining oxygenation during suctioning, reduces symptoms associated with hypoxemia, maintains positive end-expiratory pressure (PEEP), and protects staff from the patient's secretions; the data are inconsistent regarding its cost-effectiveness.[17,33] Most institutions use closed suctioning for mechanically ventilated patients. At many institutions, all ventilated patients are treated with closed suction devices. Other institutions use these devices for specific patient indications, such as for clinically unstable patients receiving high levels of PEEP, and for those requiring frequent suctioning.[59] (See Evidence-Based Practice feature.)

Saline instillation into the trachea during suctioning should not be routinely performed. Although use of saline has been a common practice for many years, recent studies have found saline instillation to be associated with problems such as oxygen desaturation and patient discomfort.[1,27,46,54] Adequate patient hydration and airway humidification, rather than saline instillation, facilitate secretion removal.

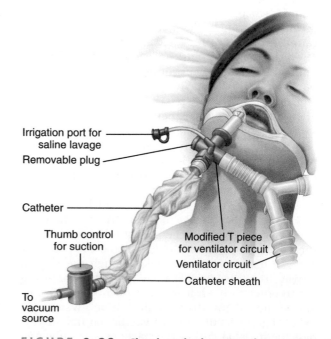

Irrigation port for saline lavage
Removable plug
Catheter
Thumb control for suction
To vacuum source
Modified T piece for ventilator circuit
Ventilator circuit
Catheter sheath

FIGURE 9-22. Closed tracheal suction device. *(From Simmons, K. F., & Scanlan, C. L. [2003]. Airway management. In R. L. Wilkins, J. K. Stoller, & C. L. Scanlan [Eds.], Egans' fundamentals of respiratory care [8th ed., p. 667]. St. Louis: Mosby.)*

EVIDENCE-BASED PRACTICE

PROBLEM

Patients with endotracheal tubes and tracheostomies require endotracheal suctioning to maintain airway patency. Closed tracheal suction devices are commonly used for endotracheal suctioning for their convenience, ability to maintain oxygenation during suctioning, and protecting the health care workers from the patients' secretions. The closed suction devices are used for extended periods and therefore may be associated with higher rates of ventilator-associated pneumonia.

QUESTION

What is the effect of closed tracheal suctioning on the risk for ventilator-associated pneumonia?

REFERENCE

Niel-Weise, B. S., Snoeren, R. L., & van den Broek, P. J. (2007). Policies for endotracheal suctioning of patients receiving mechanical ventilation: A systematic review of randomized controlled trials. *Infection Control and Hospital Epidemiology, 28*, 531.

EVIDENCE

The authors conducted an extensive search of clinical trials that compared outcomes of open versus closed endotracheal suctioning. Ten trials were reviewed; however, the authors noted that the quality of most of the studies was low. The review concluded that the choice of suctioning methods does not affect the incidence for ventilator-associated pneumonia. The authors recommended changing the closed suction devices every 48 hours.

IMPLICATIONS FOR NURSING

The choice of suctioning method should be determined by the needs of the patient and unit protocols. Although closed suction devices are used for extended periods, they are not associated with a higher risk for infection. Additional research is needed regarding the length of time that these devices can be used. Many institutions extend the time beyond 48 hours.

MECHANICAL VENTILATION

Mechanical ventilation is a sophisticated therapy that requires the nurse's constant surveillance and critical assessment. The purpose of mechanical ventilation is to support the respiratory system until the underlying cause of respiratory failure can be corrected. Most ventilatory support requires an artificial airway; however, it may be applied without an artificial airway and is called noninvasive ventilation.

Indications

Mechanical ventilation is warranted for patients who have acute respiratory failure and are unable to maintain normal gas exchange. This inadequacy is reflected in the patient's ABGs. An objective clinical definition of respiratory failure is as follows:

- PaO_2 ≤60 mm Hg on a FiO_2 greater than 0.5 (oxygenation)
- $PaCO_2$ ≥50 mm Hg, with a pH of 7.25 or less (ventilation)[34]

The patient may also demonstrate progressive physiological deterioration such as an increasing RR, a decreasing V_T, and an increase in the WOB as evidenced by increased use of the accessory muscles of ventilation, abnormal breathing patterns, and complaints of dyspnea. As lifesaving therapy, mechanical ventilation is more of a temporary intervention than a means of reversing the acute medical problem.[34,50,52] Ongoing assessment is essential in determining the need for mechanical ventilation so that a treatment plan can be instituted to correct the underlying abnormality.

Positive-Pressure Ventilation

In the acute care setting, most patients are mechanically ventilated with positive-pressure ventilation. This method uses positive pressure to force air into the lungs via an artificial airway. Figure 9-23 illustrates the concept of positive-pressure ventilation. Some degree of positive-pressure ventilation or forward flow of inspired gas is necessary to deliver V_T during the act of ventilation.[34,50] The movement of gases into the lungs through the use of *positive pressure* is opposite of normal spontaneous breathing. The physiology of spontaneous ventilation requires that energy be expended to contract the muscles of respiration. The contraction of the respiratory muscles enlarges the thoracic cavity, increases *negative pressure* within the chest, and results in the flow of air, at atmospheric pressure, into the lungs. If mechanical ventilators could mimic the intrathoracic pressures present during spontaneous ventilation, it would be ideal. Negative-pressure ventilators, which originated with the iron lung, perform in this manner; however, these ventilators are for management of chronic conditions. Many of the complications of mechanical ventilation are related to air being forced into the lungs under positive pressure.

Ventilator Settings

In most institutions in the United States and Canada, ventilators are set up and managed by respiratory therapy personnel. However, the nurse must be familiar with selected values on the control panel or graphic interface unit to assess ventilator settings, patient response to ventilation, and alarms. Representative control panels and screens of ventilators are shown in Figure 9-24. Although the control panel of a microprocessor-type ventilator can appear overwhelming, it is important for the nurse to learn to identify the common screen views that provide the settings and patient data that are integral to patient assessment. The nurse must know the basic ventilator settings of mode of ventilation, FiO_2, V_T, set RR rate, and PEEP. Additional settings of inspiratory-to-expiratory (I:E) ratio, sensitivity, and sigh are also discussed to provide a basis for the nurse to knowledgeably communicate with the RT and physician.

Fraction of Inspired Oxygen

The FiO_2 is the fraction (or percentage) of inspired oxygen delivered to the patient by the ventilator. FiO_2 is set from 0.21 (21% or room air) to 1.00 (100% oxygen). The initial FiO_2 setting is based on the patient's immediate physiological needs. The following equation is used to establish a starting FiO_2 value if an ABG is done to guide treatment:

$$\text{Desired } FiO_2 = \frac{PaO_2 \text{ (desired)} \times FiO_2 \text{ (known)}}{PaO_2 \text{ (known)}}$$

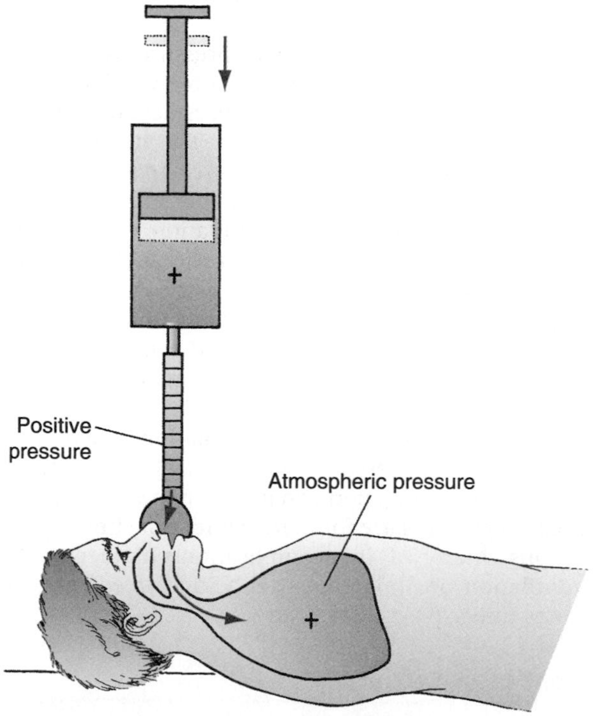

When mechanical ventilation is initiated after emergency intubation, the initial FiO_2 is set between 0.5 and 1.0 to ensure a SpO_2 of 92% or greater to meet the patient's physiological needs. After the patient is stabilized, the setting is adjusted based on ABG or pulse oximetry values.

Tidal Volume

The amount of air delivered with each preset breath is the V_T. The V_T is dictated by body weight and by the patient's lung characteristics (compliance and resistance), and is set to ensure that excessive stretch and pressure on the lung tissue is avoided. The parameters monitored to avoid excessive pressure are the PIP and plateau airway pressure (Pplat). These pressures should remain below 40 cm H_2O and

FIGURE 9-23. Concept of positive-pressure ventilation. *(From Cairo, J. M., & Pilbeam, S. P. [2004]. Mosby's respiratory care equipment [7th ed., p. 322]. St. Louis: Mosby.)*

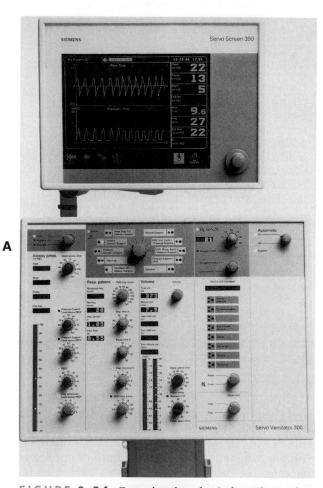

FIGURE 9-24. Examples of mechanical ventilators, their control panels and graphic interface unit (GIU). **A,** Servo ventilator 300A control panel.

30 cm H₂O, respectively. A starting point for the V_T setting is 8 to 10 mL/kg of ideal body weight.[34] Thus a patient who weighs 70 kg would have the V_T set between 560 and 700 mL. The setting can be adjusted if the resulting airway pressures are too high. Conversely, if the airway pressures are acceptable and a larger V_T is needed to remove CO_2, it can be increased. When choosing and adjusting the V_T setting, the goal is to achieve the lowest Pplat while maintaining gas exchange and patient comfort.

Lower V_T settings may be indicated. Recent research has found that lower V_T levels (4 to 8 mL/kg) can provide adequate ventilation while reducing complications associated with mechanical ventilation.[7,29] Large V_T ventilation associated with a Pplat

of greater than 30 cm H₂O increases ventilator days and reduce survival. These studies demonstrate that high priority should be given to ventilator strategies that prevent excessive lung stretch.

Exhaled Tidal Volume. The exhaled V_T (EV_T) is the amount of gas that comes out of the patients lungs on exhalation. This is the most accurate measure of the volume received by the patient. Although the prescribed V_T is set on the ventilator control panel, it is not guaranteed to be delivered to the patient. Volume may be lost because of leaks in the ventilator circuit, around the cuff of the airway, or via a chest tube if there is a pleural air leak.[49] The volume actually received by the patient, regardless of mode of ventilation, must be confirmed by monitoring the EV_T on the display panel of the ventilator. If the EV_T deviates from the set V_T by 50 mL or more, the nurse and RT must troubleshoot the system to identify the source of gas loss.[50]

Respiratory Rate

The RR is the frequency of breaths (f) set to be delivered by the ventilator to the patient. The RR is set as near to physiological rates (14 to 20 breaths/min) as possible. Frequent changes in the RR are often required based on observation of the patient's WOB and comfort, and assessment of the $PaCO_2$ and pH. During initiation of mechanical ventilation, many patients require full ventilatory support. The RR at this time is selected on the basis of the V_T, to achieve a minute ventilation (VE) that maintains an acceptable acid-base status (VE = RR × V_T). As the patient becomes capable of participating in the ventilatory work, the ventilator RR is decreased, or the mode of ventilation is changed, to encourage more spontaneous breathing.

Inspiratory-to-Expiratory Ratio

The I:E ratio is the duration of inspiration in comparison with expiration. In spontaneous ventilation, inspiration is shorter than expiration. When a patient undergoes mechanical ventilation, the I:E ratio is usually set to mimic this pattern of spontaneous ventilation. Generally the I:E ratio is set at 1:2; that is, 33% of the respiratory cycle is spent in inspiration and 66% in the expiratory phase. Longer expiratory times, I:E ratio of 1:3 or 1:4, may be needed in patients with COPD. A longer expiratory time promotes more complete exhalation and reduces air trapping.

Inverse Inspiratory-to-Expiratory Ratio

I:E ratios such as 1:1, 2:1, and 3:1 are called inverse I:E ratios. An inverse I:E ratio is used to improve oxygenation in patients with noncompliant lungs, such as in ARDS. During the traditional I:E ratio of

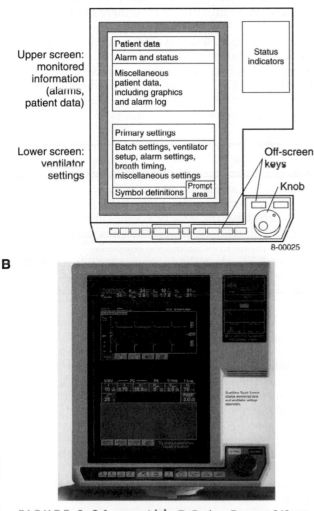

B

FIGURE 9-24, cont'd. B, Puritan Bennett 840 ventilator GIU. *(A courtesy of Siemens-Elma AB, Solna, Sweden; B courtesy of Puritan Bennett, Inc., Pleasanton, CA.)*

1:2, unstable alveoli in noncompliant lungs may not have sufficient time to reopen during the shorter inspiratory phase, and may collapse during the relatively longer expiratory phase. The inspiratory effect of an inverse I:E ratio allows unstable alveoli time to fill. The shortened expiratory phase prevents unstable alveoli from collapsing because the next inspiration begins before the alveoli reach a volume where they can collapse.[34,50]

Positive End-Expiratory Pressure

PEEP is the addition of positive pressure into the airways during expiration. PEEP is measured in cm H_2O. Typical settings for PEEP are 5 to 20 cm H_2O, although higher levels may be used to treat refractory hypoxemia. Because positive pressure is applied at end expiration, the airways and alveoli are held open, and oxygenation improves. PEEP increases oxygenation by preventing collapse of small airways and maximizing the number of alveoli available for gas exchange (Figure 9-25). By recruiting more alveoli for gas exchange and by holding them open during expiration, the functional residual capacity improves, resulting in better oxygenation.

Many mechanically ventilated patients routinely receive 3 to 5 cm H_2O of PEEP, a value often referred to as physiological PEEP. This small amount of PEEP is thought to mimic the normal "back pressure" created in the lungs by the epiglottis in the spontaneously breathing patient that is removed by the displacement of the epiglottis by the artificial airway. A small amount of PEEP may also promote a more normal functional residual capacity.

PEEP is often added to decrease a high FiO_2 that may be required to achieve adequate oxygenation. For example, a patient may require a FiO_2 of 0.80 to maintain a PaO_2 of 85 mm Hg. By adding PEEP, it may be possible to decrease the FiO_2 to a level where oxygen toxicity in the lung is not a concern (<0.5) while maintaining an adequate PaO_2.[52] The nurse monitors the PEEP level by observing the pressure level displayed on the ventilator's analog and graphic displays. When no PEEP is set, the pressure reading on the graphic display should be zero at end expiration. When PEEP is applied, the pressure reading does not return to zero at the end of the breath and the display shows the amount of PEEP.

It is important for the nurse to be aware of the adverse effects of PEEP and how they are prevented or managed. Problems related to PEEP occur as a result of the increase in intrathoracic pressure. These problems include a decrease in cardiac output secondary to decreased venous return, volutrauma or barotrauma, increased intracranial pressure resulting from impedance of venous return from the head, and alterations in renal function caused by reduced renal blood flow. Each time PEEP is increased, the nurse should evaluate the patient's hemodynamic response by physical assessment and by evaluation of the hemodynamic profile in a patient with a pulmonary artery catheter. Management of the adverse effects of PEEP begins by ensuring the patient has adequate intravascular volume (preload). If the cardiac output remains inadequate, an inotropic agent such as dobutamine should be considered. Optimal PEEP is defined as the amount of PEEP that affords the best oxygenation without resulting in adverse hemodynamic effects or pulmonary injury.[50]

Auto-PEEP. Auto-PEEP is the spontaneous development of PEEP caused by gas trapping in the lung resulting from insufficient expiratory time and incomplete exhalation. These trapped gases create positive pressure in the lung. Both set PEEP and auto-PEEP have the same physiological effects; therefore it is important to know when auto-PEEP is present so it can be managed properly.[34,50,52]

Causes of auto-PEEP formation include rapid RR, high VE demand, airflow obstruction, and inverse I:E ratio ventilation. Auto-PEEP cannot be detected by the ventilator pressure manometer until a special maneuver is performed. This maneuver involves instituting a 2-second end-expiratory pause, which allows the ventilator to read the pressure deep in the lung. The airway pressure manometer reading therefore reflects total PEEP, which is the set PEEP and auto-PEEP added together. For determination of auto-PEEP, the following calculation is performed

$$\text{Auto-PEEP} = \text{Total PEEP} - \text{Set PEEP}.$$

Sensitivity

Sensitivity determines the amount of patient effort needed to initiate gas flow through the circuitry on a patient-initiated breath. The sensitivity is set so that the ventilator is "sensitive" to the patient's effort to inspire. If the sensitivity is set too low, the patient

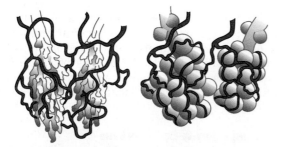

FIGURE 9-25. Effect of application of positive end-expiratory pressure (PEEP) on the alveoli. *(Modified from Pierce, L. N. B. [2007]. Management of the mechanically ventilated patient [p. 205]. St. Louis: Saunders.)*

must generate more work to trigger gas flow. If it is set too high, auto-cycling of the ventilator may occur, resulting in patient-ventilator dyssynchrony, because the ventilator cycles into the inspiratory phase when the patient is not ready for a breath.[50,52]

Sigh

A sigh is a mechanically set breath with greater volume than the preset V_T, usually 1.5 to 2.0 times the V_T. The rationale for using a sigh is to prevent atelectasis, because a ventilated patient is not able to take a natural sigh—a deep spontaneous breath. The sigh mechanism is infrequently used because PEEP achieves the same purpose.

Patient Data

The nurse and RT ensure that the ventilator settings are consistent with the physician's orders. The ventilator control panel or graphic interface unit also provides valuable information regarding the patient's response to mechanical ventilation. These patient data include EV_T, PIP, and total RR.

Peak Inspiratory Pressure

The PIP is the maximum pressure that occurs during inspiration. The amount of pressure necessary to ventilate the patient increases with increased airway resistance (e.g., secretions in the airway, bronchospasm, biting the ETT) and decreased lung compliance (e.g., pulmonary edema, worsening infiltrate or ARDS, pleural space disease). The PIP should never be allowed to rise above 40 cm H_2O, because higher pressures can result in ventilator-induced lung injury.[7,8,34]

The nurse should monitor and record the PIP at least every 4 hours and with any change in patient condition that could increase airway resistance or decrease compliance.[49] Increasing PIP or values greater than 40 cm H_2O should be immediately reported so that interventions can be ordered to improve lung function, ventilator settings can be adjusted to reduce the inspiratory pressure, or both.

Total Respiratory Rate

The total RR equals the number of breaths delivered by the ventilator (set rate) plus the number of breaths initiated by the patient. Assessing the total RR provides data regarding the patient's contribution to the WOB, or whether the ventilator is performing all of the work. It also provides an assessment of the ability of the set RR rate and V_T to meet VE demands. The total RR is a very sensitive indicator of overall respiratory stability.[49] For example, if the patient is on assist/control ventilation at a set RR of 10 breaths/

min, and the total RR for 1 minute is 16, the patient is initiating 6 breaths above the set rate of 10. If the patient is on synchronized intermittent mandatory ventilation at a set RR of 8 breaths/min, and the total RR is 12 breaths/min with good spontaneous V_T for body weight, the patient is tolerating the mode of ventilation. If the patient's total RR increases to 26 breaths/min, this finding indicates that something has changed and the patient needs to be reassessed. For example, the patient may be fatigued and have a lower spontaneous V_T. The increased RR is an attempt to sustain an adequate VE.

Modes of Mechanical Ventilation

Modes of mechanical ventilation are the techniques that the ventilator and patient work together to perform the respiratory cycle. Modes of positive-pressure ventilation are classified as volume-controlled, pressure-controlled, or dual-controlled ventilation. This classification is based on the variable that the ventilator maintains at a preset value during inspiration.[50] In a volume-controlled mode of ventilation, the set V_T is maintained during inspiration. In a pressure-controlled mode of ventilation, pressure is set and does not vary throughout inspiration. An understanding of the volume-controlled and pressure-controlled modes of ventilation provides a solid foundation for the nurse to learn the dual-controlled modes in advanced courses.

Volume-Controlled Ventilation

In volume-controlled ventilation, V_T is constant for every breath delivered by the ventilator. The ventilator is set to allow airflow into the lungs until a preset volume has been reached. A major advantage of this mode is that the V_T is delivered, regardless of changes in lung compliance or resistance. However, the PIP varies in this mode, depending on compliance and resistance. Volume-controlled modes of ventilation include assist/control (A/C) and synchronized intermittent mandatory ventilation (SIMV; Figure 9-26).

Assist/Control Ventilation. The A/C mode of ventilation delivers a preset number of breaths of a preset V_T. The patient may trigger additional spontaneous breaths between the ventilator-initiated breaths. When the patient initiates a breath by exerting a negative inspiratory effort, the ventilator delivers an assisted breath of the preset V_T. The V_T of the assisted breaths does not vary, as the preset V_T is delivered every time the patient initiates a breath. The preset RR ensures that the patient receives adequate ventilation, regardless of spontaneous efforts. The A/C mode is indicated when it is desirable for the

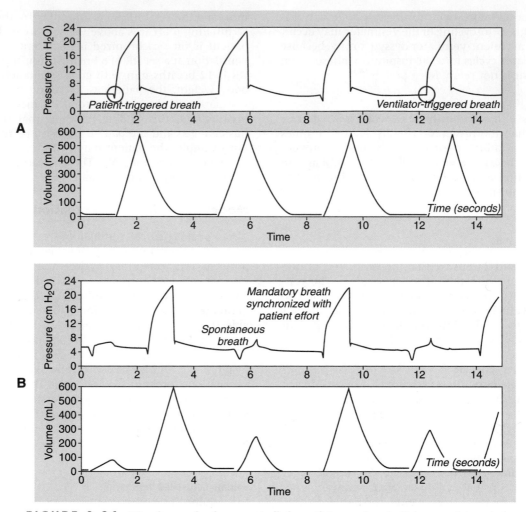

FIGURE 9-26. Waveforms of volume-controlled ventilator modes. **A,** Volume assist control (A/C) ventilation. The patient may trigger additional breaths above the set rate. The ventilator delivers the same volume for ventilator-triggered and patient-triggered (assisted) breaths. **B,** Synchronized intermittent mandatory ventilation (SIMV). Both spontaneous and mandatory breaths are graphed. Mandatory breaths receive the set tidal volume (V_T). V_T of spontaneous breaths depends on work patient is capable of generating, lung compliance, and airway resistance.

ventilator to perform the bulk of the WOB. The only work the patient must perform is the negative inspiratory effort required to trigger the ventilator on the patient-initiated breaths. The A/C mode is useful in a patient with a normal respiratory drive but whose respiratory muscles are too weak or unable to perform the WOB (e.g., patient emerging from general anesthesia or patient with pulmonary disease such as pneumonia).[52] A disadvantage of A/C ventilation is that respiratory alkalosis may develop if the patient has a tendency to hyperventilate because of anxiety, pain, or neurological factors. Respiratory alkalosis is treated or prevented by providing sedation or anal-

gesia as needed, or changing to SIMV.[34] Another disadvantage is that the patient may rely on the ventilator and not attempt to initiate spontaneous breathing if ventilatory demands are met.

During A/C ventilation, the nurse monitors several parameters. These include the total RR, to determine whether the patient is initiating spontaneous breaths; the EV_T, to ensure that the set V_T is delivered; the PIP, to determine whether it is increasing (indicating a change in compliance or resistance, which needs to be further evaluated); the patient's sense of comfort and synchronization with the ventilator; and the acid-base status.[49]

Synchronized Intermittent Mandatory Ventilation. The SIMV mode of ventilation delivers a set number of breaths of a set V_T, and between these mandatory breaths the patient may initiate spontaneous breaths. The depth or volume of the spontaneous breaths depends on the muscular respiratory effort that the patient is able to generate. If the patient initiates a breath near the time a mandatory breath is due, the delivery of the mandatory breath is synchronized with the patient's spontaneous effort to prevent patient-ventilator dyssynchrony. The main difference between the SIMV and A/C modes is the volume of the patient-initiated breaths. Patient-initiated breaths in A/C ventilation result in the patient receiving a set V_T. In SIMV, the V_T of spontaneous breaths is variable because it depends on patient effort and lung characteristics.

The SIMV mode helps to prevent respiratory muscle weakness associated with mechanical ventilation because the patient contributes more to the WOB. SIMV is indicated when it is desirable to allow patients to breathe at their own RR and thus assist in maintaining a normal $PaCO_2$, or when hyperventilation has occurred in the A/C mode. SIMV is also indicated as a mode for weaning patients from mechanical ventilation. As the SIMV rate is lowered, the patient initiates more spontaneous breaths, assuming a greater portion of the ventilatory work. As the patient demonstrates the ability to take on even more WOB, the mandatory breath rate is decreased accordingly. However, compared with other weaning modalities, SIMV is associated with the longest weaning and lowest success rate.[5,19]

During SIMV, the nurse monitors the total RR to determine whether the patient is initiating spontaneous breaths, and the patient's ability to manage the WOB. If the total RR increases, the V_T of the spontaneous breaths is assessed for adequacy. An adequate spontaneous V_T is 5 to 7 mL/kg of ideal body weight. A rising total RR may indicate that the patient is beginning to fatigue, resulting in a more shallow and rapid respiratory pattern. This pattern may lead to atelectasis, a further increase in the WOB, and the need for greater ventilatory support.[49,50] The nurse monitors the EV_T of both the mandatory and spontaneous breaths to ensure that the set V_T is being delivered with the mandatory breaths, and that the spontaneous V_T is adequate. As in A/C ventilation, the nurse assesses the PIP, the patient's sense of comfort and synchronization with the ventilator, and the acid-base status.

Pressure-Controlled Ventilation

In pressure-controlled ventilation, inspiratory pressure levels are constant for every breath. The ventilator is set to allow air to flow into the lungs until a preset pressure has been reached. The V_T the patient receives is variable and depends on the patient's lung compliance, and airway and circuit resistance. Patients with normal lung compliance and low resistance will have better delivery of V_T for the amount of inspiratory pressure set.[34,49,52] An advantage of pressure-controlled modes is that the PIP can be reliably controlled for each breath the ventilator delivers. A disadvantage is that hypoventilation and respiratory acidosis may occur since delivered V_T varies; therefore the nurse must closely monitor EV_T. Pressure modes include continuous positive airway pressure, pressure support, pressure control, pressure-controlled inverse-ratio ventilation, and airway pressure–release ventilation.

Continuous Positive Airway Pressure. Continuous positive airway pressure (CPAP) is positive pressure applied throughout the respiratory cycle to the spontaneously breathing patient (Figure 9-27). The patient must have a reliable respiratory drive and adequate V_T because no mandatory breaths or other ventilatory assistance is given. The patient performs all the WOB. CPAP provides pressure at end expiration, which prevents alveolar collapse and improves the functional residual capacity and oxygenation.[34] CPAP is identical to PEEP in its physiological effects. CPAP is the correct term when the end-expiratory pressure is elevated in the spontaneously breathing patient. PEEP is the term used for the same setting when the end-expiratory pressure is elevated, and the patient is receiving some additional form of respiratory support (e.g., A/C, SIMV, pressure support). CPAP is indicated as a mode of weaning, when the patient has adequate ventilation but requires end-expiratory pressure to stabilize the alveoli and maintain oxygenation, and for obstructive sleep apnea. Because the ventilator is used to deliver CPAP during weaning, the nurse can monitor the adequacy of the patient's EV_T, alarms can be set to detect low EV_T and apnea, and mechanical breaths can be delivered in the event of apnea.

CPAP can also be administered via a nasal or face mask. Typically, a nasal CPAP system is used to keep the airway open in patients with obstructive sleep apnea.

Pressure Support. Pressure support (PS) is a mode of ventilation in which the patient's spontaneous respiratory activity is augmented by the delivery of a preset amount of inspiratory positive pressure. There is no rate set on the ventilator; the patient must generate each breath (Figure 9-28). Typical levels of PS ordered for the patient are 6 to 12 cm H_2O. The positive pressure is applied throughout inspiration, thereby promoting the flow of gas into the lungs, augmenting the patient's spontaneous V_T, and

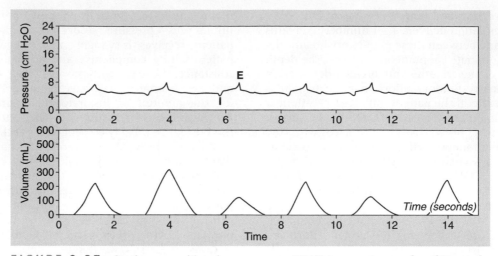

FIGURE 9-27. Continuous positive airway pressure (CPAP) is a spontaneous breathing mode. Positive pressure at end expiration splints alveoli and supports oxygenation. *I,* Inspiration; *E,* Expiration.

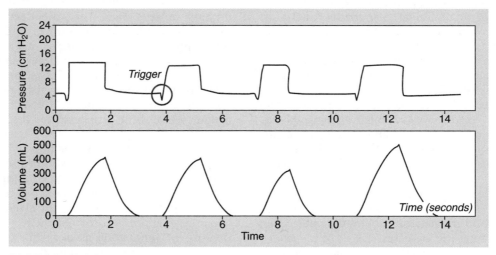

FIGURE 9-28. Pressure support ventilation requires the patient to trigger each breath, which is then supported by pressure on inspiration. Patient may vary amount of time in inspiration, respiratory rate, and tidal volume (V_T).

decreasing the WOB associated with breathing through an artificial airway and the ventilatory circuit.[34,50,52] PS may be used as a stand-alone mode or in combination with other modes, such as SIMV, to augment the V_T of the spontaneous breaths (Figure 9-29). PS may also be used for weaning from mechanical ventilation. The V_T is variable, determined by patient effort, the amount of PS applied, and the compliance and resistance of the patient and ventilator system. EV_T must be closely monitored during PS; if it is inadequate, the level of PS is increased. PS may increase patient comfort because

the patient has greater control over the initiation and duration of each breath. PS promotes conditioning of the respiratory muscles since the patient works throughout the breath; this may facilitate weaning from the ventilator.

Pressure Assist/Control. Pressure assist/control (P-A/C) is a mode of ventilation in which there is a set RR, and every breath is augmented by a set amount of inspiratory pressure. If the patient triggers additional breaths beyond the mandatory breaths, those breaths are augmented by the set amount of inspiratory pressure (Figure 9-30). Just as with PS, there is no set

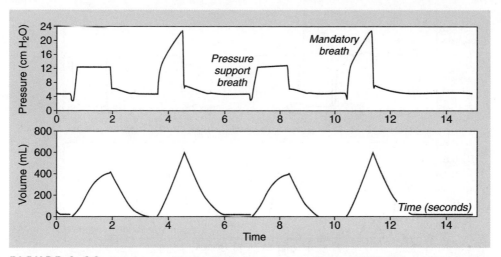

FIGURE 9-29. Synchronized intermittent mandatory ventilation (SIMV) with pressure support (PS). SIMV breaths receive set tidal volume (V_T). Pressure support is applied to the spontaneous, patient-triggered breaths.

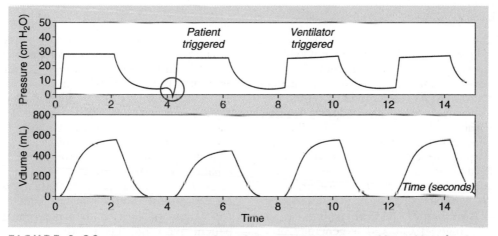

FIGURE 9-30. Pressure assist/control ventilation. Patient can trigger additional breaths above the set rate. Patient- and ventilator-triggered breaths receive the same inspiratory pressure.

V_T. The V_T the patient receives is variable and determined by the set inspiratory pressure, the patient's lung compliance, and circuit and airway resistance. The typical pressure in P-A/C ranges from 15 to 25 cm H_2O, which is higher than a PS level because P-A/C is indicated for patients with ARDS, or those with a high PIP during traditional volume ventilation. Because the lungs are noncompliant in these conditions, higher inspiratory pressure levels are needed to achieve an adequate V_T. P-A/C allows the practitioner to control the PIP and reduce the risk of barotrauma, while maintaining adequate oxygenation and ventilation. During P-A/C, the nurse must be familiar with all the ventilator settings: the level

of pressure, the set RR, the FiO_2, and the level of PEEP. The nurse monitors the total RR to evaluate whether the patient is initiating spontaneous breaths, and EV_T for adequacy of volume.

Pressure-Controlled Inverse-Ratio Ventilation. With pressure-controlled inverse-ratio ventilation (PC-IRV), the patient receives P-A/C ventilation as described, and the ventilator is set to provide longer inspiratory times. The I:E ratio is inversed to increase the mean airway pressure, open and stabilize the alveoli, and improve oxygenation. PC-IRV is indicated for patients with noncompliant lungs such as in ARDS, when adequate oxygenation is not achieved despite high FiO_2, PEEP, or positioning. Because the reverse I:E

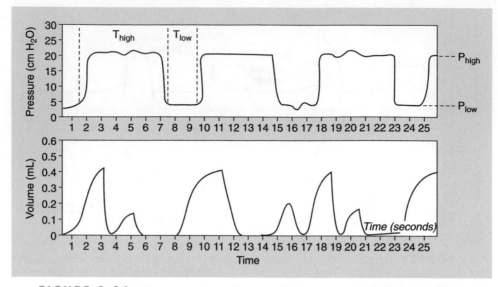

FIGURE 9-31. Airway pressure–release ventilation. See text below for description.

ratio ventilation is uncomfortable, the patient must be sedated and possibly paralyzed to prevent ventilator dyssynchrony and oxygen desaturation.[49,50]

Airway Pressure–Release Ventilation. Airway pressure–release ventilation (APRV) is a mode of ventilation that provides two levels of CPAP, one during inspiration and the other during expiration, while allowing unrestricted spontaneous breathing at any point during the respiratory cycle (Figure 9-31). APRV starts at an elevated pressure, the CPAP level or pressure high (P_{HIGH}), followed by a release pressure, pressure low (P_{LOW}). After the airway pressure release, the P_{HIGH} level is restored.[23] The time spent at P_{HIGH} is known as time high (T_{HIGH}) and is generally prolonged, 4 to 6 seconds. The shorter release period (P_{LOW}) is known as time low (T_{LOW}) and is generally 0.5 to 1.1 seconds. When observing the pressure waveform, APRV is similar to PC-IRV; however, unlike PC-IRV, the patient has unrestricted spontaneous breathing. The patient is more comfortable on APRV, and neither deep sedation nor paralysis is needed. APRV assists in providing adequate oxygenation while lowering PIP. It is indicated as an alternative to A/C or P-A/C for patients with significantly decreased lung compliance, such as those with ARDS.[23,34]

Noninvasive Positive-Pressure Ventilation

Noninvasive positive-pressure ventilation (NPPV) is the delivery of mechanical ventilation without an artificial airway (ETT or tracheostomy tube). NPPV provides ventilation via (1) a face mask that covers the nose, mouth, or both; (2) a nasal mask or pillow; or (3) a full face mask (Figure 9-32). Complications associated with an artificial airway are reduced, such as vocal cord injury and ventilator-associated pneumonia, and sedation needs are less. During NPPV, the patient can eat and speak, and is free from the discomfort of an artificial airway.

NPPV is indicated for the treatment of acute exacerbations of COPD, and may prevent the need for intubation in these patients. Patients with hypoxemic respiratory failure may also benefit from NPPV. NPPV may be applied to avoid reintubation in a patient who has been extubated but is having some respiratory distress. Other indications for NPPV include management of cardiogenic pulmonary edema, obstructive sleep apnea, and early hypoxemic respiratory failure in immunocompromised patients. NPPV may also be used to provide ventilatory support while an acute problem is treated in patients for whom intubation is undesirable, such as those with "do not intubate" orders.[49] Contraindications to NPPV include apnea, cardiovascular instability (hypotension, uncontrolled dysrhythmias, and myocardial ischemia), claustrophobia, somnolence, high aspiration risk, viscous or copious secretions, inability to clear secretions, recent facial or gastroesophageal surgery, craniofacial trauma, and burns.

NPPV can be delivered with critical care ventilators or a ventilator specifically designed to provide NPPV (Figure 9-33). Modes delivered can be pressure or volume; however, pressure modes are better tol-

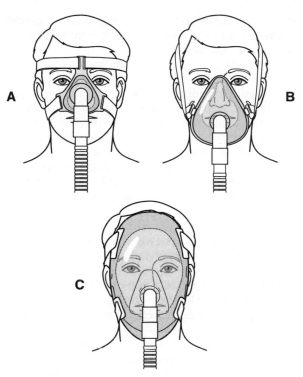

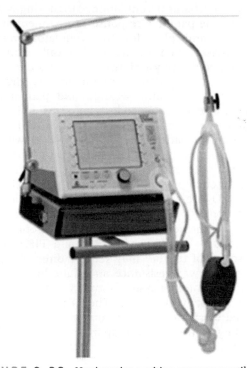

FIGURE 9-32. Masks used for noninvasive positive-pressure ventilation. **A,** Nasal. **B,** Oronasal. **C,** Total face mask. *(From Mims, B. C., Toto, K. H., Luecke, L. E., Roberts, M. K., Wilmouth, J. B., & Tyner, T. E. [2003]. Critical care skills [2nd ed., p. 132]. Philadelphia: Saunders.)*

FIGURE 9-33. Noninvasive positive-pressure ventilation (NIPPV) may be administered through a mask with the BiPAP Vision ventilator. This ventilator is capable of operating in four modes: pressure support (PS); spontaneous/timed (S/T) mode, which is pressure support with back-up pressure control; timed (T), which is pressure control; and continuous positive airway pressure (CPAP). *(Courtesy of Respironics, Murrysville, PA.)*

erated. The most common modes of ventilation delivered via NPPV are pressure support or pressure control with PEEP and CPAP.

During NPPV, it is important for the nurse to work with the RT to ensure the right size and type of mask is chosen, and that it fits snugly enough to prevent air leaks. The nurse monitors the mask and the skin under the mask edges for signs of breakdown. If signs of excess pressure are noted, interventions include repositioning the mask, placing a layer of wound care dressing on the skin as a protective shield, or trying another type of mask. If mouth breathing is a problem with the nasal mask, a chin strap can be applied, or the mask should be changed to an oronasal or full face mask. Leakage of gases around the mask edges may lead to drying of the eyes and the need for eye drops. The mouth and airway passages should be monitored for excessive drying, and a humidification system applied as indicated. The nurse also monitors the total RR, the EV_T to ensure it is adequate, and the PIP.

Advanced Methods and Modes of Mechanical Ventilation

Microprocessor ventilators offer a wide range of options for mechanical ventilation. However, other forms of ventilatory support are available. These advanced techniques are usually ordered to treat patients with respiratory failure that is refractory to conventional treatment. These techniques include, but are not limited to, high-frequency jet or oscillatory ventilation, extracorporeal membrane oxygenation, and inhaled nitric oxide. Specialized equipment and training are essential for these advanced treatments. They are not described in this textbook.

Respiratory Monitoring During Mechanical Ventilation

Nurses and RTs routinely monitor numerous physiological and respiratory parameters while a patient receives mechanical ventilation. Monitoring is done to assess the patient's response to treatment and to anticipate and plan for the ventilator weaning process. Assessment of the mechanically ventilated patient includes physical assessment and the assessment of the ventilator system: airway, circuitry, accuracy of ventilator settings, and patient data. Physical assessment includes vital signs and hemodynamic parameters, patient comfort and WOB, synchrony of patient's respiratory efforts with the ventilator, breath sounds, amount and quality of respiratory secretions, and assessment of the chest drain system if present. ABG results, pulse oximetry, and $ETCO_2$ are evaluated to assess oxygenation and ventilation.[20,50,61] Patient data evaluated from the ventilator include EV_T (mandatory, spontaneous, and assisted breaths), total RR, and PIP. Further assessment of the PIP may require direct measurements of airway resistance and static lung compliance. The ventilator system should be checked by the nurse at least every 4 hours. The RT performs a more detailed assessment of the ventilator's functioning, including alarms and the appropriateness of alarm settings.

Alarm Systems

Alarms are an integral part of mechanical ventilation because this equipment provides vital life support functions. Those who care for patients receiving mechanical ventilation must be knowledgeable about alarms and how to troubleshoot them. Two important rules must be followed to ensure patient safety:
1. Never shut off alarms. It is acceptable to silence alarms for a preset delay while working with a patient, such as during suctioning. However, alarms are never shut off.
2. Manually ventilate the patient with a bag-valve device if unable to troubleshoot alarms quickly or if equipment failure is suspected. A bag-valve device must be readily available at the bedside of every patient who is mechanically ventilated.

All mechanical ventilators provide an array of alarm systems; however, ventilator alarms vary from machine to machine. Therefore the nurse must be familiar with the ventilators used in the facility. Most alarms alert the nurse to changes in volume, pressure, or RR, such as apnea. Examples of alarms include the following:
1. Increased V_T, VE, or RR alarms
2. Decreased V_T, VE, or RR alarms
3. High and low inspiratory pressure alarms
4. High and low PEEP or CPAP alarms
5. Special mode activation alarms (e.g., I:E ratio activation), apnea alarms
6. Loss of power or loss of gas pressure alarms

When an alarm sounds, the nurse must quickly assess whether the patient is being ventilated and is adequately oxygenated. The nurse assesses the patient's airway, RR, oxygen saturation level, heart rate, level of consciousness, color, WOB, chest wall movement, and lung sounds. The ventilator display is observed to identify the status message related to the alarm, and the alarm is silenced while the cause of the alarm is determined. Immediate action is required if the patient is in acute distress with labored respirations, an abnormal breathing pattern, pallor and diaphoresis, deterioration in breath sounds, or decreasing SpO_2.[52] The nurse quickly disconnects the patient from the ventilator and manually ventilates with a bag-valve device while a second caregiver, often the RT, further assesses the problem. Table 9-6 provides an overview of management of common ventilator alarms.

Volume Alarms. Volume alarms are valuable for ensuring adequate alveolar ventilation, particularly in the patient receiving a pressure mode of ventilation where V_T varies. A low–exhaled-volume alarm sounds if the patient is not receiving an adequate V_T. Causes of volume alarms include inadequate spontaneous V_T, or a leak in the circuit and loss of gas from a variety of causes, such as disconnection of the ventilator circuit from the artificial airway, a leak in the ETT or tracheostomy cuff, displacement of the ETT or tracheostomy tube, or disconnection of any part of the ventilator circuit. The nurse quickly conducts a systematic assessment of the patient and ventilator system for these potential causes.

Pressure Alarms. A high-pressure alarm sounds if the amount of pressure needed for ventilating a patient exceeds the preset pressure limit. Several patient factors cause high-pressure alarms to sound: coughing, secretions in the airway, biting on the ETT, gagging, attempting to talk, bronchospasm, or conditions that cause a decrease in pulmonary compliance such as pulmonary edema, pneumothorax, or hemothorax. Kinks in the ventilator circuit can also cause a high-pressure alarm to sound. When a high-pressure alarm sounds, the ventilator terminates the inspiratory phase to avoid causing pressure injury to the patient's lung (barotrauma) by continuing to force gas under high pressure into the lung. The nurse quickly assesses the potential causes and intervenes as relevant, such as suctioning the patient or administering sedative agents.

Apnea Alarm. An apnea alarm sounds if the ventilator does not detect spontaneous respiration within a preset interval. This alarm is very important when the patient is on a spontaneous breathing mode such as PS or CPAP, and no mandatory breaths are set. Causes of the apnea alarm sounding include a diminished level of consciousness, and effects of sedative

TABLE 9-6   Management of Common Ventilator Alarms

Alarm	Intervention
High peak pressure	Assess level of sedation; administer medications if warranted Empty water from water traps if indicated Auscultate lung sounds for need for suctioning Assess for kinks in endotracheal tube or ventilator circuit Assess for worsening pulmonary pathology resulting in reduction in lung compliance Notify RT and/or physician if alarm persists
Low pressure	Assess for leaks in ventilator circuit or disconnection of ventilator circuit from airway; reconnect If malfunction is noted, manually ventilate patient with bag-mask device Notify RT to troubleshoot alarm
Low exhaled volume	Assess for disconnection of ventilator circuit from airway; reconnect Assess for disconnection in any part of the ventilator circuit Assess for leak in cuff of artificial airway by listening for audible sounds around the airway and using device to measure cuff pressure; inflate as needed Assess for changes in lung compliance, increase in airway resistance or patient fatigue in patient on a pressure mode of ventilation
Apnea alarm	Assess patient for spontaneous respiratory effort; encourage patient to take a deep breath Manually ventilate patient while RT and/or physician are notified to modify settings on the ventilator

RT, Respiratory therapist.

or analgesic medications. If the patient fails to initiate a breath for typically 20 seconds, the ventilator alarm alerts the nurse to this potentially dangerous situation. If this alarm sounds, the nurse must immediately assess the patient for apnea. The ventilator settings may need to be adjusted; for example, the ventilator may not be sensitive enough to the patient's respiratory efforts. On many ventilators a back-up mode of ventilation will be activated in the event of an apnea alarm to ensure adequate ventilation.

Complications of Mechanical Ventilation

Numerous complications are associated with intubation and mechanical ventilation. It is imperative that the nurse understand the problems associated with the use of mechanical ventilators. Many complications can be prevented or treated rapidly through vigilant nursing care.[50] It is recommended that the "ventilator bundle" be implemented as a best practice for all mechanically ventilated patients to prevent complications and improve outcomes. (See Clinical Alert.)

Airway Problems
Intubation of Right Mainstem Bronchus. The right mainstem bronchus is straighter than the left. If the ETT is manipulated, such as occurs during changing of the

CLINICAL ALERT
Implementation of the Ventilator Bundle

The "ventilator bundle" of care should be implemented in all patients who receive mechanical ventilation. This bundle is a group of evidence-based recommendations that has been demonstrated to improve outcomes. It is expected that all interventions in the bundle be implemented unless contraindicated:

- Maintain head of bed elevation at 30 to 45 degrees
- Interrupt sedation each day to assess readiness to wean from ventilator
- Provide prophylaxis for deep vein thrombosis
- Administer medications for peptic ulcer disease prophylaxis

tape, it may slip into the right mainstem bronchus. Symptoms include absent or diminished breath sounds in the left lung. Whenever the ETT is manipulated, the nurse must assess for bilateral chest excursion, auscultate the chest for bilateral breath sounds after the procedure, and reassess tube position at the lip.

Endotracheal Tube Out of Position. The ETT can become dislodged if it is not secured properly, during procedures such as changing the tape on the ETT, during transport, or if the patient is anxious or agitated and attempts to pull out the tube. The ETT may be displaced upward, resulting in the cuff being positioned between or above the vocal cords. Conversely, the tube may advance too far into the airway and press on the carina or move into the right mainstem bronchus. A quick check of the centimeter markings can determine whether the tube has advanced or pulled out of proper position. When a serious airway problem cannot be quickly resolved, the nurse attempts to manually ventilate the patient to assess airway patency. If the patient cannot be ventilated and the tube is not obviously displaced or the patient is not biting the airway, the nurse should attempt to pass a suction catheter through the airway to determine whether it is obstructed. If the catheter cannot be passed and the patient has spontaneous respirations, the cuff is deflated to allow air to pass around the tube. If the patient still cannot be adequately ventilated, the airway must be removed and the patient is ventilated with a bag-valve device.[52]

Unplanned Extubation. The patient may intentionally or inadvertently remove the airway. The two most frequent methods by which self-extubation occurs are (1) by using the tongue, and (2) by leaning forward and downward to the restrained hands and manually removing the tube.[4,53] Unplanned extubation can also occur as a result of patient care. For example, the tube can be dislodged if the ventilator circuit or closed suction catheter pulls on the ETT during procedures such as turning. Despite vigilant nursing care, unplanned extubation may result. Strategies for preventing an unplanned extubation are described in Box 9-8.

Laryngeal and Tracheal Injury. Damage to the larynx and trachea can occur because of tube movement and excess pressure exerted by the distal cuff. Preventive measures are implemented to avoid injury to the trachea and vocal cords, and long-term complications. The nurse should prevent the patient from excessive head movement, especially flexion and extension, which result in the tube moving up and down in the airway, causing abrasive injury. An intervention for preventing tracheal damage from the cuff is routine cuff pressure monitoring (Figure 9-34). Pressures should not exceed 25 to 30 cm H_2O (18 to 22 mm Hg).[58,63] Various commercial devices are available to measure cuff pressures quickly and easily. The nurse works with the RT to ensure an appropriate cuff volume and pressure.

Damage to the Oral or Nasal Mucosa. Tape or commercial devices that secure the ETT can cause breakdown of the lip and oral mucosa. Nasal intubation may result in skin breakdown on the nares and also a higher risk of sinusitis. Ongoing assessment and skin care

---

BOX 9-8   Strategies for Unplanned or Self-Extubation

- Provide adequate patient sedation and analgesia.
- Monitor all intubated patients vigilantly; assess for risks for self-extubation.
- Apply protective devices (e.g., soft wrist restraints, arm immobilizers, mitts) according to hospital standards of practice.
- Adequately secure the endotracheal tube around the patient's head, not just to the face.
- Cut the end of the endotracheal tube to 2 inches beyond the fixation point.
- Provide support for the ventilator tubing and closed suction systems; keep these items out of the patient's reach.
- Use two staff members when repositioning an endotracheal tube.
- Educate the family to assist in monitoring the patient.
- Extubate the patient in a timely manner when the patient meets established criteria.

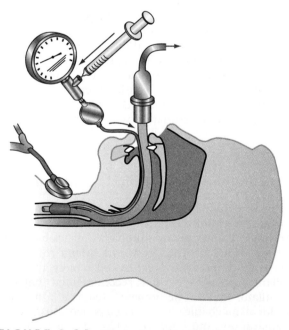

FIGURE 9-34. Monitoring endotracheal tube cuff pressures. *(From Lewis, S. M. [2000]. Lower respiratory problems. In S. M. Lewis, M. M. Heitkemper, & S. R. Dirksen [Eds.], Medical-surgical nursing [5th ed.]. St. Louis: Mosby.)*

assist in preventing damage to the mouth and nose. The ETT should be repositioned daily to prevent pressure necrosis.

Pulmonary System

Trauma. *Barotrauma*, which means pressure trauma, is the injury to the lungs associated with mechanical ventilation. In barotrauma, alveolar injury or rupture occurs as a result of excessive pressure, excessive peak inflating volume (volutrauma), or both.[34] Barotrauma may occur when the alveoli are overdistended, such as with positive-pressure ventilation, PEEP, and high V_T. The alveoli rupture or tear so that air escapes into various parts of the thoracic cavity, causing subcutaneous emphysema (air in the tissue space), pneumothorax or tension pneumothorax, pneumomediastinum, pneumopericardium, or pneumoperitoneum. Signs and symptoms of barotrauma include PIP and mean airway pressures, decreased breath sounds, tracheal shift, subcutaneous crepitus, new air leak or increase in air leak in a chest drainage system, and symptoms associated with hypoxemia.

A life-threatening complication is a tension pneumothorax. When tension pneumothorax occurs, pressurized air enters the pleural space. Air is unable to exit the pleural space and continues to accumulate. Air in the pleural space causes an increase in intrathoracic pressure, increasing amounts of lung collapse, shifting of the heart and great vessels to the opposite thorax (mediastinal shift), and tachycardia and hypotension. Treatment consists of immediate insertion of a chest tube or a needle thoracostomy. Whenever a pneumothorax is suspected in a patient receiving mechanical ventilation, the patient should be removed from the ventilator and ventilated with a bag-valve device until a needle thoracostomy is performed or a chest tube is inserted.

Lung tissue injury induced by local or regional overdistending volume is called *volutrauma*. The damage that occurs to the lung is similar to the pathological findings of early ARDS and is probably the result of local stress and strain on the alveolar-capillary membrane. Volutrauma results in increased permeability of the alveolar-capillary membrane, pulmonary edema, accumulation of white blood cells and protein in the alveolar spaces, and reduced surfactant production. Because it is difficult to determine the exact distribution of volume in a patient's lung, pressure is used as a surrogate for volume. The PIP is kept below 40 cm H_2O and/or the Pplat is kept at less than 30 cm H_2O as lung protective strategies to prevent both volutrauma and barotrauma.[34]

Oxygen Toxicity. The exposure of the pulmonary tissues to high levels of oxygen can lead to pathological changes. The degree of injury is related to the duration of exposure and to the FiO_2, not to the PaO_2. The first sign of oxygen toxicity is caused by irritant effects of oxygen and presents as tracheobronchitis. Prolonged exposure to high FiO_2 may lead to changes in the lung that mimic ARDS. As a general rule, an FiO_2 up to 1.0 may be tolerated for up to 24 hours. However, the goal is to lower the FiO_2 to less than 0.60.[28] Absorption atelectasis is another problem associated with high FiO_2. Nitrogen is needed to prevent collapse of the airway. When the FiO_2 is 1.0, alveolar collapse and atelectasis result from a lack of nitrogen in the distal air spaces.

Respiratory Acidosis or Alkalosis. Acid-base disturbances may occur secondary to V_T and RR settings on the ventilator. For example, if a patient is receiving A/C ventilation set at 10 breaths/min but the patient's RR is 28 breaths/min because of pain or anxiety, respiratory alkalosis may occur. If the ventilator is set at a low RR (e.g., 2 to 6 breaths/min) and the patient does not have an adequate drive to initiate additional breaths, respiratory acidosis may occur. Ideally the V_T and RR are set to achieve a VE that ensures a normal $PaCO_2$ level.

Infection. Patients with artificial airways who are receiving mechanical ventilation are at an increased risk of ventilator-associated pneumonia (VAP) because normal upper airway defense mechanisms are bypassed. About 10% to 20% of ventilated patients develop VAP.[55] The incidence is highest in the first 5 days of mechanical ventilation.[3] The principal mechanism for the development of VAP is aspiration of colonized gastric and oropharyngeal secretions. Factors that contribute to VAP include poor oral hygiene, aspiration, contaminated respiratory therapy equipment, poor hand washing by caregivers, breach of aseptic technique when suctioning, inadequate humidification or systemic hydration, and decreased ability to produce an effective cough because of the artificial airway. Specific strategies to reduce VAP include the following:

- Elevate head of the bed 30 to 45 degrees if not medically contraindicated to prevent reflux and aspiration of gastric contents. Elevation of head of the bed is associated with a 26% risk reduction in pneumonia.[13]
- Prevent drainage of ventilator circuit condensate into the patient's airway. Always discard condensate and never drain it back into the humidifier.
- Practice proper hand hygiene and wear gloves when handling respiratory secretions.
- Use an ETT with a lumen for aspirating subglottic secretions that pool above the airway cuff.[11]
- Ensure secretions are aspirated from above the cuff before cuff deflation or tube removal.

- Provide comprehensive oral hygiene that includes a mechanism for dental plaque removal and reduction of bacterial burden in the oral cavity.[11]
- Use noninvasive mechanical ventilation when possible.

Cardiovascular System

Hypotension and decreased cardiac output may occur with mechanical ventilation and PEEP, secondary to increased intrathoracic pressure, which can result in decreased venous return. The hemodynamic effects of mechanical ventilation are more pronounced in patients with hypovolemia or poor cardiac reserve. Patients with a high PIP and receiving PEEP of greater than 10 cm H_2O may need a pulmonary artery catheter inserted to monitor volume status and cardiac output. Management of hypotension and decreased cardiac output primarily involves the administration of volume to ensure an adequate preload, followed by administration of inotropic agents as necessary.

Gastrointestinal System

Stress ulcers and gastrointestinal bleeding may occur in patients who undergo mechanical ventilation. All patients undergoing mechanical ventilation should receive medications for stress ulcer prophylaxis.[31] Enteral feeding is initiated as soon as possible, and the patient is monitored for gross and occult blood in the gastric aspirate and stools. Other interventions include identification and reduction of stressors, communication and reassurance, and administration of anxiolytic or sedative agents, or both, as necessary based on standardized assessment tools (see Chapter 5).

Nutritional support is required for all patients who require mechanical ventilation. Inadequate nutrition may occur if the patient is not started on early nutritional support or receives inadequate supplemental nutrition.[47] See Chapter 6 for an in-depth discussion of nutritional support. The type of formula may need to be modified for ventilated patients. Excess CO_2 production may occur with high-carbohydrate feedings and place a burden on the respiratory system to excrete the CO_2, increasing the WOB.[47] Formulas developed for the patient with pulmonary disorders may be indicated. Such formulas are higher in fat content.[42]

An essential nursing intervention for the intubated patient who receives enteral nutrition is to reduce the risk of aspiration. The nurse must keep the head of the bed elevated during enteral feeding.

After extubation or tracheostomy, the transition to oral feedings may be indicated. A speech therapy evaluation for swallowing is recommended before oral feedings are initiated because many patients have difficulty with swallowing and are prone to aspiration after prolonged intubation.[2]

Psychosocial Complications

Several psychosocial hazards may occur because of mechanical ventilation. Patients may experience stress and anxiety because they require a machine for breathing. If the ventilator is not set properly or if the patient resists breaths, patient-ventilator dyssynchrony may occur. The noise of the ventilator and the need for frequent procedures, such as suctioning, may alter sleep and wake patterns. In addition, the patient can become psychologically dependent on the ventilator.

NURSING CARE

Nursing care of the patient who requires mechanical ventilation is complex. The nurse must provide care to the patient by using a holistic approach, incorporating competent delivery of a highly sophisticated technology. A detailed plan of care is described in the Nursing Care Plan for the Mechanically Ventilated Patient.

Communication

Communication difficulties are common because of the artificial airway. The lack of vocal expression has been identified by patients as a major stressor that elicits feelings of panic, isolation, anger, helplessness, and sleeplessness.[24] Patients express a need to know, as well as to make themselves understood.[30] They need constant reorientation, reassuring words emphasizing a caregiver's presence, and point-of-care information that painful procedures done to them are indeed necessary and helpful. In addition, touch, eye contact, and positive facial expressions are beneficial in relieving anxiety.[44] Caregivers who attempt to individualize communication with intubated patients by using a variety of methods provide patients a greater sense of control, encourage participation in their own care, and minimize cognitive disturbances.

Gestures are identified as the most frequently used method of nonverbal communication among intubated CCU patients, but they are often inhibited by wrist restraints. Communication with gestures and lip reading can convey some basic needs; however, augmentative communication devices may facilitate even better communication. Although writing is sometimes used, critically ill patients are too weak or poorly positioned to write, or lack the concentration to spell. A picture board with

Text continued on p. 222

NURSING CARE PLAN for the Mechanically Ventilated Patient[21]

NURSING DIAGNOSIS

Impaired spontaneous ventilation related to respiratory muscle fatigue, acute respiratory failure, metabolic factors

PATIENT OUTCOMES

- Spontaneous ventilation with normal ABGs. Free of dyspnea or restlessness
- No complications associated with mechanical ventilation

NURSING INTERVENTIONS	RATIONALES
• Maintain artificial airway; secure ETT or tracheostomy with tape or commercial devices; prevent unplanned extubation (see Box 9-8)	• Maintain an adequate airway to facilitate mechanical ventilation; prevent accidental removal of artificial airway
• Assess position of artificial airway:	• Maintain an adequate airway by ensuring that artificial airway in the proper position
▪ Auscultate for bilateral breath sounds	
▪ Observe for abdominal distention	
▪ Evaluate placement on chest x-ray	
▪ Once proper position is confirmed, mark the position (cm marking) of the ETT with an indelible pen and note position of the tube at the lip line as part of routine assessment	
• Monitor oxygenation and ventilation at all times, and respond to changes:	• Ensure adequate oxygenation and acid-base balance; changes are seen if oxygenation and/or ventilation are impaired
▪ Vital signs	
▪ Total respiratory rate	
▪ Exhaled tidal volume of ventilator-assisted and patient-initiated breaths	
▪ Oxygen saturation	
▪ End-tidal CO_2	
▪ Mental status and level of consciousness	
▪ ABGs	
• Assess respiratory status at least every 4 hours and respond to changes:	• Ensure adequate oxygenation and ventilation; changes are seen if oxygenation and/or ventilation are impaired
▪ Breath sounds anteriorly and posteriorly	
▪ Respiratory pattern	
▪ Chest excursion	
▪ Patient's ability to initiate a spontaneous breath	
▪ Signs and symptoms of hypoxemia	
• Reposition ETT from side to side every 24 hours; assess and document skin condition	• Prevent skin breakdown from tape or devices that secure the airway; reduce aspiration of oral secretions and ventilator-associated pneumonia; and ensure that tube remains in proper position after manipulation
▪ Note placement of tube at lip line	
▪ Use two staff members for procedure	
▪ Suction secretions above the ETT cuff before repositioning tube	
▪ After the procedure, assess position of tube at lip line and auscultate for bilateral breath sounds	
• Have bag-valve device and suctioning equipment readily available	• Maximize effectiveness of mechanical ventilation and promote patient safety

Continued

NURSING INTERVENTIONS

- Maintain integrity of mechanical ventilator circuit; monitor ventilator settings; respond to ventilator alarms; keep tubing free of moisture by draining away from the patient and using devices such as water traps to facilitate drainage of moisture
- Monitor cuff pressure of ETT or tracheostomy and maintain within therapeutic range
- Monitor serial chest x-ray studies

- Implement an interdisciplinary plan of care to maintain patient comfort, mobility, nutrition, and skin integrity; support patient and family involvement in plan of care

RATIONALES

- Maximize ventilation and prevent aspiration of contaminated condensate

- Prevent complications associated with overinflation or underinflation of ETT cuff
- Assess for correct position of ETT and improvement or worsening of pulmonary conditions
- Prevent complications associated with mechanical ventilation and bedrest; foster patient and family well-being

NURSING DIAGNOSIS

Risk for ineffective airway clearance related to ETT, inability to cough, thick secretions, fatigue

PATIENT OUTCOMES

- Airway free of secretions
- Clear lung sounds

NURSING INTERVENTIONS

- Assess need for suctioning (pressure alarm on ventilator, audible secretions, rhonchi on auscultation)
- Suction as needed according to standard of practice (see Box 9-7)
- Assess breath sounds after suctioning

- If tracheal secretions are thick, assess hydration of patient and humidification of ventilator; avoid instillation of normal saline
- Reposition the patient frequently

RATIONALES

- Indicate possibility of airway obstruction with secretions and need for suctioning

- Remove secretions; maintain patent airway; improve gas exchange
- Assess effectiveness of suctioning; breath sounds should improve
- Assist in thinning secretions for easier removal; saline has not shown to be effective and is associated with hypoxemia
- Mobilize secretions

NURSING DIAGNOSIS

Risk for infection related to endotracheal intubation and aspiration of oropharyngeal secretions

PATIENT OUTCOMES

Absence of ventilator-associated pneumonia

NURSING CARE PLAN — for the Mechanically Ventilated Patient—cont'd

NURSING INTERVENTIONS	RATIONALES
• Maintain head of bed at 30 degrees or greater	• Decrease risk for aspiration of oropharyngeal and gastric secretions
• Monitor temperature every 4 hours; assess amount, color, consistency, and odor of secretions; notify physician if secretions change	• Identify signs of infection
• Use good hand-washing techniques; wear gloves for procedures, including closed suctioning; use aseptic technique for suctioning	• Prevent transmission of bacteria to the patient
• Implement a comprehensive oral care protocol that includes oral suction at least every 4 hours and brushing teeth at least every 12 hours	• Remove dental plaque and bacteria from the oropharynx, and prevent aspiration of oral secretions
• Maintain integrity of ETT cuff; keep cuff pressure between 20 and 30 cm H_2O	• Prevent aspiration of oropharyngeal secretions

NURSING DIAGNOSIS

Ineffective protection related to ventilator dependence, PEEP, decreased pulmonary compliance, and issues related to mechanical ventilator (settings, alarms, disconnection)

PATIENT OUTCOME

• Free of ventilator-induced lung injury.

NURSING INTERVENTIONS	RATIONALES
• Assess prescribed ventilator settings every 2 hours (mode, set rate, V_T, FiO_2, PEEP); ensure that alarms are on	• Ensure that patient is receiving therapy as ordered; promote patient safety
• Assess PIP every 2 hours	• Identify elevations in PIP which may indicate worsening lung function, need to adjust pulmonary therapies or ventilator settings
• Assess tolerance to ventilatory assistance and monitor for asynchronous chest movement, subjective report of breathlessness, or high PIP; if symptomatic, remove patient from ventilator and manually ventilate and prepare for chest tube insertion	• Provide cues of condition improving or worsening; may indicate need for suctioning or development of barotrauma complications

• Assess for signs of barotrauma every hour:
  ▪ Subcutaneous crepitus
  ▪ Altered chest excursion
  ▪ Restlessness
  ▪ Increasing PIP
  ▪ Tracheal shift
  ▪ Decreasing SpO_2
	• Assist in detecting barotrauma

• Respond to all ventilator alarms	• Provide immediate intervention in response to specific alarm; promote patient safety

Continued

NURSING CARE PLAN **for the Mechanically Ventilated Patient—cont'd**

NURSING DIAGNOSIS

Anxiety and fear related to need for mechanical ventilation, inability to speak to communicate needs, change in environment, fear of death, unmet needs

PATIENT OUTCOMES

- Calm and cooperative

NURSING INTERVENTIONS

- Assess patient every 4 hours for signs of anxiety; use standardized assessment tools

- Collaborate with physician to develop a sedation plan if anxiety or agitation impairs ventilation
- Assess respiratory pattern for synchrony with ventilator

- Talk to patient frequently; establish method for communication that is appropriate for the patient's native language and abilities; speak slowly and do not shout; expect frustration
  - Yes/no questions
  - Clipboard with paper and pencil
  - Picture communication boards
  - Computerized systems
  - Lip reading
  - Devices that allow the patient to speak
- Implement interventions to reduce anxiety:
  - Simple explanations before and during procedures
  - Call light within reach
  - Family visitation
  - Diversionary activities, such as music or television
- Collaborate with the health care team to develop strategies to reduce anxiety and maximize effectiveness of mechanical ventilation: changes in settings, sedation, analgesia, complementary and alternative therapies

RATIONALES

- Identify presence or absence (or relief) of anxiety; standardized tools facilitate trending of findings
- Promote effectiveness of mechanical ventilation and patient ventilator synchrony
- Respiratory efforts that are asynchronous with the ventilator result in discomfort, anxiety, dyspnea, and abnormal ABGs
- Promote communication with the patient and help to identify needs, assess responses to treatment, and reduce anxiety; strategies must be culturally appropriate to facilitate patient understanding

- Assist in preventing and/or relieving fear and anxiety

- Medications are frequently needed as an adjunct during mechanical ventilation; complementary therapies may also be effective

NURSING DIAGNOSIS

Decreased cardiac output related to effects of positive pressure ventilation, PEEP, volume depletion or overload

PATIENT OUTCOME

- Adequate cardiac output

NURSING CARE PLAN | **for the Mechanically Ventilated Patient—cont'd**

NURSING INTERVENTIONS	RATIONALES
• Assess for hypotension, tachycardia, dysrhythmias, decreased level of consciousness, cool skin, mottling	• Indicate decreased cardiac output
• Measure hemodynamic profile at least every 4 hours if pulmonary artery catheter is in place; reassess after any ventilator setting changes that affect V_T, PEEP, or PIP	• Assess filling pressure and cardiac output, and identify trends
• Alert the physician to changes in cardiac output and hemodynamic profile	• Ventilator settings, especially PEEP, may need to be adjusted
• Maintain optimum fluid balance	• Additional volume may be needed, especially if patient is receiving PEEP; fluid retention may also occur
• Administer other medications as ordered (e.g., inotropic agents or diuretics)	• Medications may be needed to optimize cardiac output and/or relieve fluid retention

NURSING DIAGNOSIS

Dysfunctional ventilatory weaning response related to ineffective airway clearance, sleep-pattern disturbances, inadequate nutrition, pain, and psychological factors

PATIENT OUTCOME
Liberation from

- Mechanical ventilation
- Adequate ABG values
- Respiratory pattern and rate WNL
- Effective secretion clearance

NURSING INTERVENTIONS	RATIONALE
• Assess patient's readiness to wean (see Box 9-10)	• Identify readiness to begin the weaning process using validated parameters
• Provide weaning method based on protocols and research evidence (see Box 9-9)	• Protocol-driven weaning is an effective strategy for systematic weaning that reduces ventilator days, CCU, and hospital length of stay
• Collaborate with the health care team to provide mechanical ventilation and coaching that supports respiratory muscle training	• Promote respiratory conditioning that facilitates weaning
• Promote rest and comfort throughout the weaning process, especially between weaning trials; identify strategies that result in relaxation and comfort; ensure that environment is safe and comfortable	• Facilitate weaning from mechanical ventilation
• Support patients in setting goals for weaning	• Promote rehabilitation and give patients some control in the process
• Collaborate with the health care team to determine the most effective strategies for weaning those with severe dysfunctional breathing patterns	• Various strategies may be needed to wean the patient; ongoing assessment is essential to determine the most effective strategy

Continued

NURSING CARE PLAN for the Mechanically Ventilated Patient—cont'd

NURSING INTERVENTIONS	RATIONALES
• Implement strategies that maximize tolerance of weaning: ▪ Titrate sedation and analgesia to a level at which patient is calm and cooperative with absence of respiratory depression ▪ Schedule when patient is rested ▪ Avoid other procedures during weaning ▪ Promote normal sleep-wake cycle ▪ Limit visitors to supportive persons ▪ Coach through periods of anxiety	• Strategies assist in ensuring that patient is rested, with an adequate level of consciousness and decreased anxiety; weaning efforts will be maximized
• Terminate weaning if patient is unable to tolerate the process (see Box 9-11)	• Maintain adequate ventilation and gas exchange
• Consider referring patients with prolonged ventilator dependence to an alternative setting	• Alternative settings specialize in weaning patients who are "difficult to wean"

ABG, Arterial blood gas; *CCU,* critical care unit; *CO,* cardiac output; CO_2, carbon dioxide; *ETT,* endotracheal tube; FiO_2, fraction of inspired oxygen; *PEEP,* positive end-expiratory pressure; *PIP,* peak inspiratory pressure; *PS,* pressure support; *RR,* respiratory rate; SpO_2, oxygen saturation as measured by pulse oximetry; V_T, tidal volume; *WNL,* within normal limits.

icons representing basic needs and possibly the alphabet that can be easily cleaned between patients should be available in every CCU. A board with pictures improved communication for patients after cardiothoracic surgery and was preferred by a small group of critical care survivors who were interviewed about augmentative communication methods.[48] Family members can serve as a communication link between the patient and the care providers. It is important to reassure the patient that the loss of their voice is temporary and that speech will be possible after the tube is removed.

Medications

Intubation, mechanical ventilation, advanced methods for ventilation (e.g., inverse-ratio ventilation), and suctioning contribute to patient discomfort. Patients often need both pharmacological and nonpharmacological methods to manage discomfort and to treat anxiety. Strategies to promote patient comfort are discussed in-depth in Chapter 5.

Commonly used medications include analgesics, sedatives, and neuromuscular blocking agents; many patients need a combination of these drugs.[38] Medications are chosen based on the hemodynamic stability of the patient, the diagnosis, and the desired patient goals/outcomes. It is very important that the nurse, RT, and physician all use the same objective sedation and analgesia scoring systems to promote unambiguous assessment and communication. In some institutions, nurses use decision trees or

algorithms to guide initiation and titration of medications to a targeted sedation/analgesia goal.[6] Medications are tapered or discontinued when the patient is ready to be weaned from mechanical ventilation.

Analgesics, such as morphine and fentanyl, are administered to provide pain relief. Sedatives, such as benzodiazepines and propofol, are given to sedate the patient, reduce anxiety, and promote comfort. Benzodiazepines also promote amnesia. Patients who have acute lung injury or increased intracranial pressure, or who require nontraditional modes of mechanical ventilation may require deep sedation or therapeutic paralysis with neuromuscular blocking agents. Chemical paralysis must be discontinued before attempting to wean the patient from mechanical ventilation.[32]

Optimal sedation of the mechanically ventilated patient is essential. Insufficient sedation may precipitate ventilator dyssynchrony and physiological alterations in thoracic pressures and gas exchange. Inadequate sedation is also associated with unplanned extubation. Oversedation and prolonged sedation are associated with a longer duration of mechanical ventilation.[35] Prolonged duration of mechanical ventilation predisposes the patient to an increased risk of VAP, lung injury, and other complications. Depth of sedation also contributes to delayed weaning from mechanical ventilation. Since sedation, duration of mechanical ventilation, and ventilator weaning are interrelated, the nurse must ensure that the patient is maintained on the lowest dose and lightest level of sedation as possible. "Daily interruption" or "sedation vacation" to ensure accurate patient assessment, and titration to lowest sedation dose are important nursing interventions.[37] Optimal sedation of the mechanically ventilated patient is present when the patient resides at a state in which patient-ventilator harmony exists and the patient remains capable of taking spontaneous breaths in readiness for weaning, when appropriate.[38,50]

WEANING PATIENTS FROM MECHANICAL VENTILATION

Mechanical ventilation is a therapy designed to support the respiratory system until the underlying disease or indication for mechanical ventilation is resolved. The team caring for a ventilated patient should always be planning for how the patient will be weaned or "liberated" from the ventilator. Another term for liberation is discontinuation of ventilator support. In general, patients who require short-term ventilatory support, defined as 3 days or less of mechanical ventilation, are weaned quickly.[9,40] Conversely, weaning patients who require long-term ventilatory support, is usually a slower process and may be characterized by periods of success as well as setbacks.

Methods for Weaning

Reduction of ventilator support can be done as the patient demonstrates the ability to resume part of or all of the WOB. Four methods of titrating down ventilatory support are used: SIMV, PS, T-piece, or CPAP. Studies do not demonstrate one method to be superior to the others; however, they do show that weaning takes longer with the SIMV method.[5,19,43] Current evidenced-based practice guidelines recommend the use of a spontaneous breathing trial (SBT) for weaning. PS, T-piece and CPAP qualify as spontaneous breathing modes. SIMV, due to the provision of mandatory breaths, does not.

Synchronized Intermittent Mandatory Ventilation

Weaning with SIMV entails a progressive reduction in the number of mandatory breaths, usually in increments of 1 to 2 breaths/min, as the patient is able to take on more of the WOB. For example, the patient may begin on SIMV at a RR of 10 breaths/min. The RR may be reduced in increments of 2 breaths/min.[51] If the patient's spontaneous V_T is less than 5 mL/kg, PS may be added. Significant work is associated with the SIMV weaning method during both the mandatory and spontaneous breaths. The patient's respiratory pattern may be asynchronous with the mandatory breaths because the respiratory centers in the central nervous system are not anticipating a mandatory breath.

Pressure Support

Weaning with PS ventilation involves a gradual reduction in the level of PS while monitoring the patient's ability to maintain an acceptable V_T and RR. PS of 5 cm H_2O is considered the same as spontaneous breathing, as this is just enough inspiratory support to assist the gas flow through the ventilator circuit and artificial airway.[9,51] PS weaning provides endurance conditioning of the respiratory muscles.

T-Piece

A T-piece trial involves disconnecting the patient from the ventilator and connecting supplemental oxygen to the ETT or tracheostomy tube via a T-piece device, as shown in Figure 9-16. During a T-piece trial, the patient breathes without any ventilator support; however, mechanical ventilation can easily be reinitiated should the patient not tolerate the weaning trial. The length of time breathing through the T-piece should increase as the rest periods between the T-piece trials decrease.[9,51] Breathing through the T-piece encourages muscle strengthening.

Continuous Positive Airway Pressure

A CPAP trial is a process similar to a T-piece trial. However, CPAP is useful when the patient still requires PEEP to maintain adequate oxygenation. A CPAP trial is done while the patient is connected to the ventilator system. Therefore the nurse has the advantage of all the alarm systems to provide early warnings of apnea, a high RR, and/or inadequate EV_T. Furthermore, the ventilator can be set to provide a back-up mode of ventilation in the event of apnea. CPAP trials promote respiratory muscle strength.

Approach to Weaning Using Best Evidence

A systematic approach to weaning is indicated for patients. Based on a comprehensive review of the research, evidenced-based guidelines for ventilator weaning were developed.[39-41] Box 9-9 summarizes these guidelines.

Assessment for Readiness to Wean (Wean Screen)

Several physiological parameters are monitored to determine patient readiness to be weaned from the ventilator (Box 9-10). Patients are usually able to wean when the underlying disease process is resolving, they are hemodynamically stable, and they have the capability to initiate an inspiratory effort.[40] Weaning assessment tools are useful in assessing a

BOX 9-9 Evidence-Based Guidelines for Weaning from Mechanical Ventilation[39,40]

1. Identify causes for ventilator dependence if the patient requires ventilation for longer than 24 hours.
2. Conduct a formal assessment to determine a high potential for successful weaning:
   - Evidence of reversal of underlying cause of respiratory failure
   - Adequate oxygenation (PaO_2/FiO_2 >150-200; positive end-expiratory pressure <5-8 cm H_2O; FiO_2 <0.4-0.5) and pH (>7.25)
   - Hemodynamic stability
   - Able to initiate an inspiratory effort
3. Conduct a spontaneous breathing trial (SBT). During the SBT, evaluate respiratory pattern, adequacy of gas exchange, hemodynamic stability, and comfort. Patients who tolerate SBTs for 30 to 120 minutes should be considered for permanent ventilator discontinuation.
4. If a patient fails an SBT, determine the cause for the failed trial. Provide a method of ventilatory support that is nonfatiguing and comfortable. Correct reversible causes, and attempt SBTs every 24 hours if the patient meets weaning criteria.
5. Assess airway patency and the ability of the patient to protect the airway to determine whether to remove the artificial airway from a patient who has been successfully weaned.
6. In postsurgical patients, provide anesthesia/ sedation strategies and ventilator management aimed at early extubation.
7. Develop weaning protocols that the nurse and respiratory therapist can implement.
8. Consider a tracheostomy when it becomes apparent that the patient will require prolonged ventilator assistance (more than 2 weeks). Patients with the following conditions may benefit most from early tracheostomy:
   - High levels of sedation
   - Marginal respiratory mechanics (e.g., tachypnea) associated with work of breathing
   - Psychological benefit from ability to eat and speak
   - Enhanced mobility to promote physical therapy efforts and psychological support
9. Conduct slow-paced weaning in patients requiring prolonged mechanical ventilation. Wean patients to 50% of maximum ventilator support before daily SBTs. Then initiate SBTs with gradual increase in duration of the SBT.
10. Unless evidence of irreversible disease exists (e.g., high cervical spine injury), do not consider a patient to be ventilator dependent until 3 months of weaning attempts have failed.
11. Transfer patients in whom weaning attempts have failed but are medically stable to facilities that specialize in management of ventilator-dependent patients.

PaO_2, Partial pressure of oxygen in arterial blood; FiO_2, fraction of inspired oxygen.

patient's strengths, and factors that may interfere with successful weaning. The decision about what variables to screen depends on whether the patient has been receiving short- or long-term mechanical ventilation. Fewer parameters need to be evaluated if the patient has required ventilatory support for a short duration. Assessment parameters identified in Box 9-10 may provide a sufficient wean screen for this group of patients.

Patients who require long-term mechanical ventilation may have more physiological factors that affect weaning, such as inadequate nutrition and respiratory muscle deconditioning. A tool that provides a more comprehensive or multidimensional assessment of weaning readiness, as well as a baseline score from which to measure patient progress once weaning is begun, is the Burns Wean Assessment Program (BWAP). The BWAP has been scientifically tested in critically ill patients.[10] The BWAP evaluates nonpulmonary factors that impact weaning

success such as hematocrit; fluids, electrolytes, and nutrition; anxiety, pain, and rest; bowel function; and physical conditioning and mobility. Pulmonary factors assessed with the BWAP include RR and pattern; secretions; neuromuscular disease and deformities; airway size and clearance; and ABGs.

The nurse must use data and weaning assessment tools to identify readiness for weaning and factors that may impede successful weaning. When a patient continues to not be ready to wean or is not successful at a weaning trial, these factors should be assessed and optimized to promote patient success in future weaning endeavors.

Weaning Process (Weaning Trial)

Weaning protocols managed by nurses and RTs, as compared with traditional weaning directed by physicians, result in a reduction of ventilator days and shorter stays in the CCU and hospital.[18,36] The

BOX 9-10   Assessment Parameters Indicating Readiness to Wean

Underlying Cause for Mechanical Ventilation Resolved
- Improved chest x-ray findings
- Minimal secretions
- Normal breath sounds

Hemodynamic Stability; Adequate Cardiac Output
- Absence of hypotension
- Minimal vasopressor therapy

Adequate Respiratory Muscle Strength
- Respiratory rate <25-30 breaths/min
- Negative inspiratory pressure or force that exceeds −20 cm H_2O
- Spontaneous tidal volume 5 mL/kg
- Vital capacity 10-15 mL/kg
- Minute ventilation 5-10 L/min
- Rapid shallow breathing index <105

Adequate Oxygenation Without a High FIO_2 and/or a High PEEP
- PaO_2 >60 mm Hg with FiO_2 0.4-0.5
- PaO_2/FiO_2 >150-200
- PEEP <5-8 cm H_2O

Absence of Factors that Impair Weaning
- Infection
- Anemia
- Fever
- Sleep deprivation
- Pain
- Abdominal distention; bowel abnormalities (diarrhea or constipation)

Mental Readiness to Wean: Calm, Minimal Anxiety, Motivated

Minimal Need for Sedatives and Other Medications That May Cause Respiratory Depression

FiO₂, Fraction of inspired oxygen; *PEEP*, positive end-expiratory pressure; *PaO₂*, partial pressure of oxygen in arterial blood.

BOX 9-11   Criteria for Discontinuing Weaning

Respiratory
- Respiratory rate >35 breaths/min or <8 breaths/min
- Spontaneous V_T <5 mL/kg ideal body weight
- Labored respirations
- Use of accessory muscles
- Abnormal breathing pattern: chest/abdominal asynchrony
- Oxygen saturation <90%

Cardiovascular
- Heart rate changes more than 20% from baseline
- Dysrhythmias (e.g., premature ventricular contractions or bradycardia)
- Ischemia: ST-segment elevation
- Blood pressure changes more than 20% from baseline
- Diaphoresis

Neurological
- Agitation, anxiety
- Decreased level of consciousness
- Subjective discomfort

V_T, Tidal volume.

protocol should clearly define the method or screening tool to determine the patient's readiness to wean, the method and duration of the weaning trial, and when to terminate a weaning trial versus proceed with requesting an order for extubation. The weaning plan should include methods to facilitate respiratory muscle work along with adequate rest.[9,40]

The weaning process is challenging for many patients. Patients are assessed and monitored throughout the weaning process. Several steps are followed before and during the weaning trial. The procedure is explained to the patient and family in a manner that reduces anxiety. The patient should be adequately rested and positioned optimally for diaphragm function and lung expansion, such as sitting. Baseline parameters are obtained: vital signs, heart rhythm, ABGs or pulse oximetry/ETCO₂ values, and neurological status. The patient is monitored during the weaning process for tolerance or intolerance to the procedure. Although the patient is required to increase participation in the WOB, caregivers must ensure that the patient does not become fatigued by the weaning effort and become dyspneic or compromised in some other manner.[9,34] Box 9-11 provides a list of physiological changes indicating that the patient is not tolerating the weaning process. If the patient does not tolerate the weaning process, the weaning trial is stopped and mechanical ventilation is resumed at ventilator settings that provide full ventilatory support.

Many respiratory and nonrespiratory factors can impact weaning success. Increased oxygen demands occur with fever, anemia, pain, or asking the patient to perform another activity during the trial, and can impair weaning. Other factors to assess for are decreased lung function, psychological factors, and equipment or technique factors, such as time of day or method for weaning. Decreased lung function may result from malnutrition, overuse of sedatives or hypnotics, and sleep deprivation. Psychological factors to evaluate include apprehension and fear, helplessness, and depression.[25]

Extubation

If the patient demonstrates tolerance to the weaning procedure and can sustain spontaneous breathing for 30 to 120 minutes, the decision may be made to extubate (remove the ETT) the patient. Consideration must be given to the need for the airway for secretion clearance. If the patient has a tracheostomy, the patient may be liberated from the ventilator but the tracheostomy is maintained to facilitated airway clearance. If the decision is made to extubate, the ETT should be suctioned thoroughly before removal. Secretions that may have pooled above the cuff should be aspirated, the balloon of the ETT is deflated, and the ETT is removed during inspiration.[11,50,63] Once extubated, the patient is assessed for stridor, hoarseness, changes in vital signs, or low SpO_2 that may indicate complications.[63] Noninvasive ventilation may be used to avert reintubation in some patients.[39]

CASE STUDY   *evolve*

Mr. P, age 65, was transferred to the CCU from the emergency department after successful resuscitation from a cardiac arrest sustained out of the hospital. Initial diagnosis based on laboratory results and electrocardiography is acute anterior myocardial infarction. It is suspected that Mr. P aspirated gastric contents during the cardiac arrest. He is orally intubated and receiving mechanical ventilation. He is on assist-control ventilation, respirations set at 12 breaths/min, FiO_2 of .40, PEEP 5 cm H_2O. He opens his eyes to painful stimuli. An arterial blood gas is drawn upon arrival to the CCU and shows the following values: pH, 7.33; $PaCO_2$, 40 mm Hg; HCO_3^-, 20 mEq/L; PaO_2, 88 mm Hg; and SaO_2, 99%. A decision is made to maintain the initial ventilator settings. The following day, Mr. P's chest radiograph shows progressive infiltrates. His oxygen saturation is dropping below 90% and he is demonstrating signs of hypoxemia: increased heart rate and premature ventricular contractions. Arterial blood gas analysis at this time shows pH, 7.35; $PaCO_2$, 45 mm Hg; HCO_3^-, 26 mEq/L; PaO_2, 58 mm Hg; and SaO_2, 88%. The physician orders that the respiratory rate on the ventilator be increased to 16 breaths/min, FiO_2 increased to .50, and PEEP increased to 10 cm H_2O.

QUESTIONS
1. What were the results of Mr. P's first arterial blood gas analysis? What factors are contributing to these results?
2. What factor is contributing to Mr. P's worsening condition the day after hospital admission?
3. Interpret the arterial blood gases done the day after the arrest.
4. Why did the physician change the ventilator settings after the second set of arterial blood gases?
5. What must the nurse assess after the addition of the PEEP? Why is this especially important for Mr. P?

SUMMARY

Skills in establishing and maintaining an open airway, initiating mechanical ventilation, and ongoing patient assessment are essential for critical care nurses. Care of the patient requiring mechanical ventilation is common practice in the critical care unit; therefore it is essential that the nurse apply knowledge and skills to effectively care for these vulnerable patients.

CRITICAL THINKING QUESTIONS

1. Based on your knowledge of clinical disorders, identify different clinical conditions that could cause problems with the following steps in gas exchange:
   a. Ventilation
   b. Diffusion
   c. Perfusion (transportation)
2. Your patient has the following arterial blood gas results: pH, 7.28; PaO_2, 52 mm Hg; SaO_2, 84%; $PaCO_2$, 55 mm Hg; HCO_3^-, 24 mEq/L.
   a. What is your interpretation of these arterial blood gases?
   b. What clinical condition or conditions could cause the patient to have these arterial blood gas results?
3. Your patient requires mechanical ventilation for treatment. The pressure alarm keeps going off for a few seconds at a time, even though you have just suctioned the patient. What nursing actions are warranted at this time?
4. You are caring for a patient who has been mechanically ventilated for 2 weeks. Physically, the patient meets all the criteria to begin weaning from mechanical ventilation. What parameters should the nurse monitor to assess tolerance of weaning?
5. Your patient is being ventilated with noninvasive positive-pressure ventilation with a nasal mask. The patient is mouth breathing and the ventilator is alarming low exhaled tidal volume. What interventions should the nurse take to ensure the patient receives adequate ventilation?

---

evolve Be sure to check out the bonus material, including free self-assessment exercises, on the Evolve Web site at http://evolve.elsevier.com/Sole.

REFERENCES

1. Ackerman, M. H., & Mick, D. J. (1998). Instillation of normal saline before suctioning in patients with pulmonary infections: A prospective randomized controlled trial. *American Journal of Critical Care, 7,* 261-266.
2. Ajemian, M. S., Nirmul, G. B., Anderson, M. T., et al. (2001). Routine fiberoptic endoscopic evaluation of swallowing following prolonged intubation: Implications for management. *Archives of Surgery, 136,* 434-437.
3. American Thoracic Society. (2005). Guidelines for the management of adults with hospital-acquired, ventilator-associated, and healthcare-associated pneumonia. *American Journal of Respiratory and Critical Care Medicine, 171,* 388-416.
4. Bouza, C., Garcia, E., Diaz, M., et al. (2007). Unplanned extubation in orally intubated medical patients in the intensive care unit: A prospective cohort study. *Heart and Lung, 36,* 270-276.
5. Brochard, L., Rauss, A., Benito, S., et al. (1994). Comparison of three methods of gradual withdrawal from ventilatory support during weaning from mechanical ventilation. *American Journal of Respiratory and Critical Care Medicine, 150,* 896-903.
6. Brook, A. D., Ahrens, T. S., Schaiff, R., et al. (1999). Effect of a nursing-implemented sedation protocol on the duration of mechanical ventilation. *Critical Care Medicine, 27,* 2609-2615.
7. Brower, R., Matthay, M., Morris, A., et al. (2000). Ventilation with lower tidal volumes as compared with traditional tidal volumes for acute lung injury and the acute respiratory distress syndrome: The acute respiratory distress syndrome network. *New England Journal of Medicine, 342,* 1301-1308.
8. Brower, R. G. (2001). Ventilation in acute lung injury and ARDS 6 ml/kg. End of the story? *Minerva Anestesiologica, 67,* 248-251.
9. Burns, S. M. (2007). AACN protocols for practice: Weaning from mechanical ventilation. In S. M. Burns (Ed.), *AACN protocols for practice: Care of the mechanically ventilated patient* (2nd ed., pp. 97-160). Boston: Jones and Bartlett.
10. Burns, S. M., Earven, D., & Fisher, C. (2003). Implementation of an institutional program to improve clinical and financial outcomes of patients requiring mechanical ventilation: One year outcomes and lessons learned. *Critical Care Medicine, 31,* 2752-2763.
11. Centers for Disease Control. (2004). Guidelines for preventing health-care associated pneumonia. *MMWR. Morbidity and Mortality Weekly Report, 53*(RR-3).
12. Dezfulian, C., Shojania, K., Collard, H. R., et al. (2005). Subglottic secretion drainage for preventing ventilator-associated pneumonia: A meta-analysis. *American Journal of Medicine, 118,* 11-18.
13. Drakulovic, M. B., Torres, A., Bauer, T. T., et al. (1999). Supine body position as a risk factor for nosocomial pneumonia in mechanically ventilated patients: A randomised trial. *Lancet, 354,* 1851-1858.
14. Durbin, C. G. (2004). Airway management. In J. Cairo, S. P. Pilbeam (Eds.), *Mosby's respiratory care equipment.* St. Louis: Mosby.
15. Durbin, C. G., Jr. (2005). Indications for and timing of tracheostomy. *Respiratory Care, 50,* 483-487.
16. Durbin, C. G., Jr. (2005). Techniques for performing tracheostomy. *Respiratory Care, 50,* 488-496.

17. El Masry, A., Williams, P. F., Chipman, D. W., et al. (2005). The impact of closed endotracheal suctioning systems on mechanical ventilator performance. *Respiratory Care, 50,* 345-353.

18. Ely, E. W., Bennett, P. A., Bowton, D. L., et al. (1999). Large scale implementation of a respiratory therapist-driven protocol for ventilator weaning. *American Journal of Respiratory and Critical Care Medicine, 159,* 439-446.

19. Esteban, A., Frutos, F., Tobin, M. J., et al. (1995). A comparison of four methods of weaning patients from mechanical ventilation. Spanish Lung Failure Collaborative Group. *New England Journal of Medicine, 332,* 345-353.

20. Grap, M. J. (2006). Pulse oximetry. In S. M. Burns (Ed.), *AACN protocols for practice: Noninvasive monitoring* (2nd ed.). Boston: Jones and Bartlett.

21. Gulanick, M., & Myers, J. L. (2007). *Nursing care plans: Nursing diagnosis and intervention* (6th ed.). St. Louis: Mosby.

22. Guyton, A. C., & Hall, J. E. (2006). *Textbook of medical physiology* (11th ed.). Philadelphia: Saunders.

23. Habashi, N. M. (2005). Other approaches to open-lung ventilation: airway pressure release ventilation. *Critical Care Medicine, 33,* S228-S240.

24. Happ, M. B. (2001). Communicating with mechanically ventilated patients: State of the science. *AACN Clinical Issues, 12,* 247-258.

25. Happ, M. B., Swigart, V. A., Tate, J. A., et al. (2007). Family presence and surveillance during weaning from prolonged mechanical ventilation. *Heart and Lung, 36,* 47-57.

26. Heffner, J. (1999). Tracheostomy: Indications and timing. *Respiratory Care, 44,* 759-772.

27. Hess, D. R. (2001). The evidence for secretion clearance techniques. *Respiratory Care, 46,* 1276-1293.

28. Heuer, A. J., & Scanlan, C. L. (2003). Medical gas therapy. In R. L. Wilkins, J. K. Stoller, & C. L. Scanlan (Eds.), *Egan's fundamentals of respiratory care* (8th ed., pp. 827-858). St. Louis: Mosby.

29. Hickling, K. G. (2000). Lung-protective ventilation in acute respiratory distress syndrome: Protection by reduced lung stress or by therapeutic hypercapnia? *American Journal of Respiratory and Critical Care Medicine, 162,* 2021-2022.

30. Hupcey, J. E. (2000). The need to know: Experiences of critically ill patients. *American Journal of Critical Care, 9,* 192-198.

31. Institute for Healthcare Improvement. (2007). Getting started kit: Prevent ventilator associated pneumonia. *How to Guide.* Available at www.ihi.org.

32. Jacobi, J., Fraser, G. L., Coursin, D. B., et al. (2002). Clinical practice guidelines for the sustained use of sedatives and analgesics in the critically ill adult. *Critical Care Medicine, 30,* 119-141.

33. Jongerden, I. P., Rovers, M. M., Grypdonck, M. H., et al. (2007). Open and closed endotracheal suction systems in mechanically ventilated intensive care patients: A meta-analysis. *Critical Care Medicine, 35,* 260-270.

34. Kacmarek, R. M., Dimas, S., & Mack, C. W. (2005). *The essentials of respiratory care.* St. Louis: Mosby.

35. Kollef, M. H., Levy, N. T., Ahrens, T. S., et al. (1998). The use of continuous I.V. sedation is associated with prolongation of mechanical ventilation. *Chest, 114,* 541-548.

36. Kollef, M. H., Shapiro, S. D., Silver, P., et al. (1997). A randomized, controlled trial of protocol-directed versus physician-directed weaning from mechanical ventilation. *Critical Care Medicine, 25,* 567-574.

37. Kress, J. P., & Hall, J. B. (2006). Sedation in the mechanically ventilated patient. *Critical Care Medicine, 34,* 2541-2546.

38. Luer, J. (2007). Sedation and neuromuscular blockade in the mechanically ventilated patient. In S. M. Burns (Ed.), *AACN protocols for practice: Care of the mechanically ventilated patient* (2nd ed., pp. 253-284). Boston: Jones and Bartlett.

39. MacIntyre, N. (2007). Discontinuing mechanical ventilatory support. *Chest, 132,* 1049-1056.

40. MacIntyre, N., Cook, D., & Ely, E. (2001). Evidence-based guidelines for weaning and discontinuing mechanical ventilatory support: A collective task force facilitated by the American College of Chest Physicians; the American Association for Respiratory Care; and the American College of Critical Care Medicine. *Chest, 120,* 375S-395S.

41. MacIntyre, N. R. (2004). Evidence-based ventilator weaning and discontinuation. *Respiratory Care, 49,* 830-836.

42. Malone, A. M. (2004). The use of specialized enteral formulas in pulmonary disease. *Nutrition in Clinical Practice, 19,* 557.

43. Meade, M., Guyatt, G., & Cook, D. (2001). Weaning from mechanical ventilation: The evidence from clinical research. *Respiratory Care, 46,* 1408.

44. Menzel, L. (1999). Ventilated patients' self-esteem during intubation and after extubation. *Clinical Nursing Research, 8,* 51-68.

45. Niel-Weise, B. S., Snoeren, R. L., & van den Broek, P. J. (2007). Policies for endotracheal suctioning of patients receiving mechanical ventilation: A systematic review of randomized controlled trials. *Infection Control and Hospital Epidemiology, 28,* 531.

46. O'Neal, P. V., Grap, M. J., Thompson, C., et al. (2001). Level of dyspnoea experienced in mechanically ventilated adults with and without saline instillation prior to endotracheal suctioning. *Intensive and Critical Care Nursing, 17,* 356-363.

47. Parrish, C. R., Krenitsky, J., & Willcutts, K. (2007). Nutritional support for mechanically ventilated patients. In S. M. Burns (Ed.), *AACN protocols for practice: Care of the mechanically ventilated patient* (2nd ed., pp. 191-244). Boston: Jones and Bartlett.

48. Patak, L., Gawlinski, A., Fung, N. I., et al. (2006). Communication boards in critical care: Patients' views. *Applied Nursing Research, 19,* 182-190.

49. Pierce, L. N. B. (2007). Invasive and noninvasive modes and methods of mechanical ventilation. In S. M. Burns (Ed.), AACN *protocols for practice: Care of the mechanically ventilated patient* (2nd ed., pp. 59-89). Boston: Jones & Bartlett.

50. Pierce, L. N. B. (2007). *Management of the mechanically ventilated patient* (2nd ed.). Philadelphia: Saunders.

51. Pilbeam, S. P. (2006). Discontinuation of and weaning from mechanical ventilation. In S. P. Pilbeam, & J. M. Cairo (Eds), *Mechanical ventilation: Physiological and clinical applications* (4th ed., pp. 443-471). St. Louis: Mosby.

52. Pilbeam, S. P., & Cairo, J. M. (2006). *Mechanical ventilation: Physiological and clinical applications* (4th ed.). St. Louis: Mosby.

53. Richmond, A. L., Jarog, D. L., & Hanson, V. M. (2004). Unplanned extubation in adult critical care. Quality improvement and education payoff. *Critical Care Nurse, 24*, 32-37.

54. Ridling, D. A., Martin, L. D., & Bratton, S. L. (2003). Endotracheal suctioning with or without instillation of isotonic sodium chloride solution in critically ill children. *American Journal of Critical Care, 12*, 212-219.

55. Safdar, N., Dezfulian, C., Collard, H. R., et al. (2005). Clinical and economic consequences of ventilator-associated pneumonia: A systematic review. *Critical Care Medicine, 33*, 2184-2193.

56. Scanlan, C. L., & Wilkins, R. L. (2003). Gas exchange and transport. In R. L. Wilkins, J. K. Stoller, & C. L. Scanlan (Eds.), *Egan's fundamentals of respiratory care* (8th ed., pp. 229-254). St. Louis: Mosby.

57. Simmons, K. F., & Scanlan, C. L. (2003). Airway management. In R. L. Wilkins, J. K. Stoller, & C. L. Scanlan (Eds.), *Egan's fundamentals of respiratory care* (8th ed., pp. 653-704). St. Louis: Mosby.

58. Skillings, K., & Curtis, B. (2005). Tracheal tube cuff care. In D. Lynn-McHale Wiegand, K. Carlson (Eds.) *AACN procedure manual for critical care* (pp. 653-704). Philadelphia: Saunders.

59. Sole, M. L., Byers, J. F., Ludy, J. E., et al. (2003). A multisite survey of suctioning techniques and airway management practices. *American Journal of Critical Care, 12*, 220-230.

60. St. John, R. E. (2004). Airway management. *Crit Care Nurse, 24*, 93-96.

61. St. John, R. E. (2006). End-tidal CO_2 monitoring. In S. M. Burns (Ed.), *AACN protocols for practice: Noninvasive monitoring* (2nd ed.). Boston: Jones and Bartlett.

62. St. John, R. E., & Malen, J. F. (2004). Contemporary issues in adult tracheostomy management. *Critical Care Nursing Clinics of North America, 16*, 413-430.

63. St. John, R. E., & Seckel, M. A. (2007). Airway management. In S. M. Burns (Ed.), *AACN protocols for practice: Care of the mechanically ventilated patient* (2nd ed.). Boston: Jones and Bartlett.

64. Thibodeau, G. A., & Patton, K. T. (2003). Anatomy of the respiratory system. In G. A. Thibodeau, & K. T. Patton (Eds.), *Anatomy and physiology* (pp. 684-705). St. Louis: Mosby.

65. West, J. B. (2005). *Respiratory physiology: The essentials* (7th ed.). Baltimore, MD: Lippincott Williams and Wilkins.

66. Wilkins, R. L., Sheldon, R. L., & Krider, S. J. (2005). *Clinical assessment in respiratory care* (5th ed.). St. Louis: Mosby.

67. Wissing, D. R. (2004). Humidity and aerosol therapy. In J. M. Cairo, & S. P. Pilbeam (Eds.), *Mosby's respiratory care equipment* (7th ed.). St. Louis: Mosby.

68. Zwerneman, K. (2006). End-tidal carbon dioxide monitoring: A vital sign worth watching. *Critical Care Nursing Clinics of North America, 18*, 217-225.

CHAPTER 10

Code Management

Deborah G. Klein, MSN, RN, CCRN, CS

INTRODUCTION

Code, code blue, code 99, and *Dr. Heart* are terms frequently used in hospital settings to refer to emergency situations that require lifesaving resuscitation and interventions. Codes are called when patients have a cardiac and/or respiratory arrest or a life-threatening cardiac dysrhythmia that causes a loss of consciousness. (The generic term *arrest* is used in this chapter to refer to these conditions.) Regardless of cause, patient survival and positive outcomes depend on prompt recognition of the situation and immediate institution of basic and advanced life support measures. *Code management* refers to the initiation of a code and the lifesaving interventions performed when a patient arrests.

This chapter discusses the roles of the personnel involved in a code and identifies equipment that must be readily available during a code. Basic and advanced life support measures are presented, including medications commonly used during a code. For the most up-to-date information, the reader should contact the American Heart Association (AHA) for current recommendations for basic and advanced cardiac life support (www.americanheart.org/cpr). Supporting family members during a code is discussed along with patient management after a code, including the use of induced hypothermia. Prevention of cardiopulmonary arrest by activation of rapid response teams is also described.

In the absence of a written order from a physician to withhold resuscitative measures, cardiopulmonary resuscitation (CPR) and a code must be initiated when a patient has a cardiopulmonary arrest. Ideally, the physician, family, and patient (if possible) make the decision whether CPR is to be performed before resuscitative measures are needed. However, it is the physician who makes the decision to terminate resuscitation efforts in progress. Decisions about resuscitation status often create ethical dilemmas for the nurse, patient, and family (see Chapter 3).

All personnel involved in hospital patient care should have basic life support (BLS) training, including how to operate an automated external defibrillator (AED). This training is also recommended for the lay public through the "Heartsaver" course. Advanced cardiac life support (ACLS) provider training is available through the AHA and is strongly recommended for anyone working in critical care.

ROLES OF CAREGIVERS IN CODE MANAGEMENT

Prompt recognition of a patient's arrest and rapid initiation of BLS and ACLS measures are essential for improved patient outcomes. The first person to recognize that a patient has had an arrest should call for help, instruct someone to "call a code," call for a defibrillator, and begin CPR. One-person CPR is continued until additional help arrives.

Code Team

Key personnel are notified to assist with code management. An overhead paging system or individual pagers may be used to contact personnel, depending on hospital policies. Most hospitals have code teams that are designated to respond to codes (Table 10-1). The code team usually consists of a physician, a critical care or emergency department nurse, a nursing supervisor, a nurse anesthetist or anesthesiologist, a respiratory therapist, a pharmacist or pharmacy technician, an electrocardiogram (ECG) technician, and a chaplain. The code team responds to the code and works in conjunction with the patient's nurse and primary physician, if present. If a code team does not exist, any available trained personnel usually respond.

Leader of the Code

The person who directs, or "runs," the code is responsible for making diagnoses and treatment

TABLE 10-1   Roles and Responsibilities of Code Team Members

Team Member	Primary Role
Leader of the code (usually a physician)	Directs code Makes diagnoses and treatment decisions
Primary nurse	Provides information to code leader Measures vital signs Assists with procedures Administers medications
Second nurse	Coordinates use of the crash cart Prepares medications Assembles equipment (intubation, suction)
Nursing supervisor	Controls the crowd Contacts the attending physician Assists with medications and procedures Ensures that a bed is available in critical care unit Assists with transfer of patient to critical care unit
Nurse or assistant	Records events on designated form
Anesthesiologist, nurse anesthetist	Intubates patient Manages airway and oxygenation
Respiratory therapist	Assists with ventilation and intubation Obtains blood sample for ABG analysis Sets up respiratory equipment/mechanical ventilator
Code management pharmacist or technician	Assists with medication preparation Prepares intravenous infusions
ECG technician	Obtains 12-lead ECG
Chaplain	Supports family

ABG, Arterial blood gas; *ECG*, electrocardiogram.

decisions. The leader is usually a physician who is preferably experienced in code management, such as an intensivist or emergency department physician. However, the leader may be the patient's primary physician or another physician who is available and qualified for the task. If several physicians are present, one should assume responsibility for being the code team leader and should be the only person giving orders for interventions, to avoid confusion and conflict. In some small hospitals, codes may be directed by a nurse trained in ACLS. In this situation, standing physician orders are needed to guide and support the nurse's decision making.

The leader of the code needs as much information about the patient as possible to make treatment decisions. Necessary information includes the reason for the patient's hospitalization, the patient's current treatments and medications, the patient's code status, and the events that occurred immediately before the code. If possible, the code leader should not perform CPR or other tasks. The leader should give full attention to assessment, diagnosis, and treatment decisions to direct resuscitative efforts.

Code Nurses

Primary Nurse. The patient's primary nurse should be free to relate information to the person directing the code. The primary nurse may also start intravenous (IV) lines, measure vital signs, administer emergency medications, assist with procedures, or defibrillate the patient as directed by the code leader (if the primary nurse is qualified).

Second Nurse. The major task of the second nurse present is to coordinate the use of the crash cart. This nurse must be thoroughly familiar with the layout of the cart and the location of items. This nurse locates, prepares, and labels medications and IV fluids, and also assembles equipment for intubation, suctioning, and other procedures, such as central line insertion. An additional nurse or assistant records the code events on a designated form.

Nursing Supervisor. The nursing supervisor responds to the code to assist in whatever manner is needed. Frequently, more people respond to a code than are needed. One job of the supervisor is to limit the number of people in the code to only those necessary and those there for learning purposes. This approach decreases crowding and confusion. Other responsibilities may include contacting the patient's primary physician, relaying information to the staff and family, and ensuring that all the necessary equipment is present and functioning. If the patient must be transferred to the critical care unit, the supervisor may also ensure that a critical care bed is available and coordinate the transfer.

Anesthesiologist or Nurse Anesthetist

The anesthesiologist or nurse anesthetist assumes control of the patient's ventilation and oxygenation. This team member intubates the patient to ensure an adequate airway and to facilitate ventilation. The primary or second nurse assists with the setup and checking of intubation equipment.

Respiratory Therapist

The respiratory therapist usually assists with manual ventilation of the patient before and after intubation. The therapist may also obtain a blood sample for arterial blood gas analysis, set up oxygen and ventilation equipment, and suction the patient. In some institutions, the therapist performs intubation.

Pharmacist or Pharmacy Technician

In some hospitals, a pharmacist or pharmacy technician responds to codes. This person may prepare medications and mix IV infusions for administration during the code. The pharmacist may also calculate appropriate medication doses based on the patient's weight. Frequently, pharmacy staff members are also responsible for bringing additional medications. At the termination of the code, pharmacy staff may replenish the crash cart medications and ensure pharmacy charges to the patient's account.

Electrocardiogram Technician

In some hospitals, an ECG technician responds to codes. This person is available to obtain 12-lead ECGs that may be ordered to assist with diagnosis and treatment.

Chaplain

As a code team member, the hospital chaplain can be very helpful in comforting and waiting with the patient's family. The chaplain or other support person usually takes the family to a quiet, private area for waiting and remains with them during the code. This person may also be able to check on the patient periodically to provide the family a progress report.

Other Personnel

Other personnel should be available to run errands, such as taking blood samples to the laboratory or obtaining additional supplies. Meanwhile, other patients need monitoring and care. Only staff members necessary for the code should remain; others should attend to the other patients.

EQUIPMENT USED IN CODES

While the first person to recognize a code calls for help and begins life support measures, another team member immediately brings the crash cart and defibrillator to the patient's bedside (Figure 10-1). Crash carts vary in organization and layout, but they all contain the same basic emergency equipment and medications. Many hospitals have standardized crash carts, so anyone responding to a code is familiar with

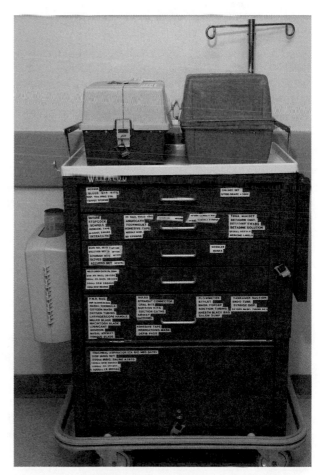

FIGURE **10-1.** A typical crash cart.

the location of the items on the cart. In other hospitals, the makeup and organization of the crash cart are unique to each unit. Whether carts are standardized or unique to an individual unit, nurses responding to codes must be familiar with them.

Most carts have equipment stored on top and in several drawers. Table 10-2 lists equipment on a typical crash cart. Equipment such as back boards and portable suction machines may be attached to the cart. Larger equipment is stored on the top of the cart or in a large drawer; smaller items, such as medications and IV equipment, are in the smaller drawers.

A back or "cardiac" board is usually located on the back or side of the cart. It is placed under the patient as soon as possible to provide a hard, level surface for the performance of chest compressions. Alternatively, some hospital bed headboards are removable for use as a cardiac board. The patient is either lifted up or log-rolled to one side for placement of the board. Care should be taken to protect the patient's cervical spine if injury is suspected.

A monitor-defibrillator is located on top of the cart or on a separate cart. The patient's cardiac rhythm is monitored via the leads and electrodes or through adhesive electrode pads on this machine. A "quick look" at the patient's cardiac rhythm can also be obtained by placing the defibrillation paddles on the chest. In the hospital setting, continuous monitoring via the electrodes is preferable to intermittent use of the defibrillation paddles for a quick look at the rhythm. The monitor must have a strip chart recorder for documenting the patient's ECG rhythm for the cardiac arrest record. A transcutaneous pacemaker is often part of the monitor/defibrillator unit. Some patient care units may use an AED for initial code management.

A bag-valve device (BVD) with an attached face mask and oxygen tubing is usually kept on the crash cart. The tubing is connected either to a wall oxygen inlet or to a portable oxygen tank on the crash cart. Supplemental oxygen is always used with the BVD. Airway management supplies are located in one of the drawers. Some institutions

---

TABLE 10-2   Typical Contents of a Crash Cart

Main Items	Specific Supplies
Back	
Cardiac board	
Side	
Portable suction machine, bag-valve device, and oxygen tubing	Suction canister and tubing, face mask, and oxygen tank Container for disposing of needles, syringes, and other sharp items
Top	
Monitor-defibrillator with recorder, clipboard with code record and drug calculation reference sheets	ECG leads, electrodes, conductive gel or adhesive code electrode pads; possible transcutaneous pacemaker or combination unit
Airway equipment drawer or box	Oral and nasal airways, ETTs, stylet, laryngoscope handle and curved and straight blades, Magill forceps, lubricating jelly, 10 mL syringes, and tape
IV equipment drawer	IV catheters of various sizes, tape, syringes, needles and needleless adaptors, IV fluids (NS, Ringer's lactate solution, and D_5W); and IV tubing
Medication drawer or box	All IV push emergency medications in prefilled syringes if available, sterile water and NS for injection, and IV infusion emergency medications (see Table 10-4)
Miscellaneous supply drawer	Sterile and nonsterile gloves, suction catheters, nasogastric tubes, chest tubes, blood pressure cuff, blood collection tubes, sutures, pacemaker magnet, extra ECG recording paper, gauze pads, face masks
Procedure kits	Arterial blood gas, tracheostomy, intraosseous insertion kit, central line insertion kit, chest tube tray

D_5W, 5% Dextrose in water; *ECG*, electrocardiogram; *ETTs*, endotracheal tubes; *IV*, intravenous; *NS*, normal saline.

have a separate box containing airway management supplies.

Another drawer contains IV supplies and solutions. Normal saline (NS) and Ringer's lactate solution are the IV fluids most often used. A 5% dextrose in water solution (D_5W) in 250- and 500-mL bags is used to prepare vasoactive infusions.

Emergency medications fill another drawer or may be located in a separate box. These include IV push medications and medications that must be added to IV fluids for continuous infusions. Most IV push medications are available in prefilled syringes. Several drugs that are given via a continuous infusion (e.g., lidocaine, dopamine) are also available as premixed bags. Medications are discussed in depth later in the Pharmacological Intervention during a Code section of this chapter.

Other important items on the cart include a suction setup and suction catheters, nasogastric tubes, and a blood pressure cuff. Various kits used for tracheotomy, central line insertion, and intraosseous insertion are also frequently kept on the crash cart.

The crash cart and defibrillator are usually checked by nursing staff at designated time intervals (every shift or every 24 hours) to ensure that all equipment and medications are present and functional. Once the cart is fully stocked, it should be kept locked, to prevent borrowing of supplies and equipment.

The nurse can become familiar with the location of items on the cart by being responsible for checking it. Management of the code is more efficient when the nurse knows where items are located on the crash cart, as well as how to use them. Many institutions require nursing staff to participate in periodic "mock" codes to assist in maintaining skills.

RESUSCITATION EFFORTS

The flow of events during a code is the result of a concentrated team effort. BLS is provided until the code team arrives. Once help has arrived, CPR is continued by use of the two-person technique. Priorities during cardiac arrest are high-quality CPR and early defibrillation. Other tasks such as connecting the patient to an ECG monitor, starting IV lines, attaching an oxygen source to the BVD, and setting up suction are performed by available personnel as soon as possible. The activities that occur during the code are summarized in Table 10-3. Often, several activities are performed simultaneously.

TABLE 10-3	Flow of Events during a Code	
Priorities	**Equipment from Cart**	**Intervention**
Recognition of arrest		Assess code status, call for help, initiate CPR
Arrival of resuscitation team, emergency cart, monitor-defibrillator, AED	Cardiac board Mouth-to-mask or bag-valve-mask unit with oxygen tubing Oral airway Oxygen and regulator if not already at bedside	Place patient on cardiac board Ventilate with 100% oxygen with oral airway and mouth-to-mask or bag-valve-mask device Continue chest compressions
Identification of team leader		Assess patient Direct and supervise team members Solve problems Obtain patient history and determine events leading up to the code
Rhythm diagnosis	Cardiac monitor with quick-look paddles—defibrillator AED 12-Lead ECG machine	Apply quick-look paddles first Attach limb leads, or adhesive electrode pads, but do not interrupt CPR
Prompt defibrillation if indicated	Defibrillator/AED	Use correct algorithm

Continued

TABLE 10-3   Flow of Events during a Code—cont'd

Priorities	Equipment from Cart	Intervention
Intubation (if ventilation inadequate and trained personnel available)	Suction equipment Laryngoscope Endotracheal tube and other intubation equipment Stethoscope Exhaled CO_2 or esophageal detectors	Connect suction equipment Intubate patient (interrupt CPR no more than 30 seconds) Confirm tube position: listen over epigastrium; listen over bilateral lung fields; confirm with secondary measure Secure tube Hyperoxygenate
Venous access	Peripheral or central IV equipment IV tubing, infusion fluid (NS)	Insert peripheral IV into antecubital sites Central line may be inserted by physician
Drug administration	Drugs as ordered (and in anticipation, based on algorithms)	Use correct algorithm

Ongoing assessment of the patient's response to therapy during resuscitation		Assess frequently:
		    Pulse generated with CPR
		    Adequacy of artificial ventilation
		    Arterial blood gases or other laboratory studies
		    Spontaneous pulse after any intervention or rhythm change
		    Spontaneous breathing with return of pulse
		    Blood pressure, if pulse is present
		    Decision to stop, if no response to therapy

Drawing arterial and venous blood specimens	Arterial puncture and venipuncture equipment	Draw specimens Treat as needed, based on results
Documentation	Code record	Accurately record events while resuscitation is in progress Record rhythm strips during the code
Controlling or limiting crowd		Dismiss those not required for bedside tasks
Family notification		Keep family informed of patient's condition Notify outcome with sensitivity
Transfer of patient to critical care unit		Ensure bed assigned for patient Transfer with adequate personnel and emergency equipment
Critique		Evaluate events of code and express feelings

AED, Automated external defibrillator; *CO₂*, carbon dioxide; *CPR*, cardiopulmonary resuscitation; *ECG*, electrocardiogram; *IV*, intravenous; *NS*, normal saline.
Data from American Heart Association. (2005). 2005 American Heart Association guidelines for cardiopulmonary resuscitation and emergency cardiovascular care. *Circulation, 112*(24 Suppl.), IV-1–IV-211; and American Heart Association. (2006). *ACLS provider manual*. Dallas, TX: Author.

The code team should be alerted to the patient's code status. Individuals may have a living will documenting their wishes. This document provides instructions to family members, physicians, and other health care providers. (See Chapter 3.)

Many states have implemented "no CPR" options. The patient, who usually has a terminal illness, signs a document requesting "no CPR" if there is a loss of pulse or if breathing stops. In some states, this document directs the patient to wear a "no CPR" identification bracelet. In the event of a code, the bracelet alerts the responders that CPR efforts are prohibited. The responders should respect the person's wishes.

Basic Life Support

The goal of BLS is to support or restore effective oxygenation, ventilation, and circulation with return of spontaneous circulation. Early CPR and early defibrillation with an AED are stressed.[3] CPR must be initiated immediately in the event of an arrest to improve the patient's chance of survival.

The ABCDs of BLS are airway, breathing, circulation, and determining whether defibrillation is needed. Assessment is a part of each step, and the steps are performed in order (Box 10-1). The following summary is adapted from the AHA standards.[4]

Airway

An open airway is essential. The first intervention is to assess unresponsiveness by tapping or shaking a patient and shouting, "Are you OK?" If the patient is unresponsive, the nurse calls for help by shouting to fellow caregivers or by using the nurse-call system. The patient is positioned on his or her back, and the airway is opened by use of the head-tilt/chin-lift method (Figure 10-2). If the patient must be turned to the supine position, the head and body are turned as a unit to prevent possible injury.

Breathing

The second step of CPR is to assess breathing and to initiate rescue breathing if necessary. Early initiation of rescue breathing may prevent a cardiac arrest in a patient who stops breathing but still has a pulse (e.g., a patient with hypercapnia). To assess breathing, the nurse looks, listens, and feels for breathing while maintaining an open airway. The nurse looks at the chest wall to see whether it is moving up and down, listens for air movement, and feels for exhaled air. Rescue breathing, or ventilation, is initiated if the patient is not breathing.

BOX 10-1 Steps in Basic Cardiac Life Support

Airway
- Determine unresponsiveness.
- Call for help.
- Position patient on back.
- Open airway using head-tilt/chin-lift technique.

Breathing
- Assess breathing (look, listen, feel).
- If breathing present, maintain airway.
- If breathing absent, give two slow breaths.

Circulation
- Determine pulselessness.
- If pulse present, give 1 breath every 5-6 seconds.
- If pulse absent, perform chest compressions at rate of 100 beats/min (30 compressions and 2 breaths).

Defibrillation
- If no pulse, check for shockable rhythm with a defibrillator or AED.
- Provide shocks as indicated.

From American Heart Association. (2006). *BLS for healthcare providers.* Dallas, TX: Author.

If possible, the code team is notified of the arrest at this time. The first person who arrives to help should "call the code." Some units and emergency departments have an emergency call system that can be activated from the patient's room by the pressing of a button. If the nurse is alone and an emergency call system is not available, the nurse presses the nurse-call system and begins CPR. When the call is answered the nurse states, "Call a code!"

In mouth-to-mouth resuscitation, the open airway is maintained, and the nurse seals his or her mouth over the patient's mouth, pinches off the patient's nose, and gives two slow breaths to the patient. If the nurse experiences difficulty in ventilating the patient, the patient's head should be repositioned, because an improperly opened airway is the most common cause of an inability to ventilate.

If the patient has a mouth injury or the nurse has difficulty maintaining a good seal, mouth-to-nose ventilation can be performed. Mouth-to-stoma ventilation is performed when the patient has a tracheal stoma or laryngectomy.

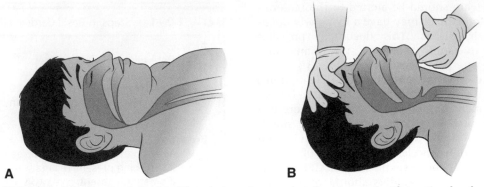

FIGURE 10-2. Head-tilt/chin-lift technique for opening the airway. **A,** Obstruction by the tongue. **B,** Head-tilt/chin-lift maneuver lifts tongue relieving airway obstruction.

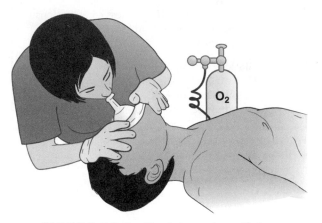

FIGURE 10-3. Mouth-to-mask ventilation.

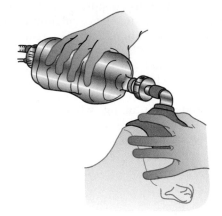

FIGURE 10-4. Rescue breathing with bag-valve device.

Although health care providers should be able to provide mouth-to-mouth breathing, mouth-to-nose breathing, and mouth-to-stoma breathing, barrier devices must be available in the workplace for individuals who are expected to perform CPR. In the hospital setting, these include a BVD and a face mask. Many hospitals have a pocket mask at every patient's bedside. In addition, most critical care units have a BVD at every patient's bedside.

The mouth-to-mask technique involves placing a mask over the patient's mouth and breathing through a mouthpiece connected to the mask (Figure 10-3). Masks have a one-way valve that protects the nurse from the patient's exhalation. Some masks have an oxygen inlet for administration of supplemental oxygen. When oxygen is available, a minimum flow rate of 10 to 12 L/min should be provided.

Ventilation of the patient with a BVD and face mask requires that an open airway be maintained.

Frequently, an oral airway is used to keep the airway patent and to facilitate ventilation. The BVD is connected to an oxygen source set at 15 L/min. The face mask is positioned and sealed over the patient's mouth and nose. The patient is manually ventilated with the BVD (Figure 10-4). Personnel should be properly trained to use the BVD effectively.

Circulation

The third step of CPR is to ensure adequate circulation. After the initial two breaths are given, the nurse assesses the patient to determine the presence or absence of a pulse. (NOTE: The pulse check is no longer recommended for lay rescuers.[4]) The pulse is assessed even if the patient is attached to a cardiac monitor because artifact or a loose lead may mimic a cardiac dysrhythmia. The nurse checks the patient's carotid pulse on the side nearest the nurse. The pulse is assessed for at least 5 seconds but no longer than 10 seconds to detect bradycardia.

If a pulse is present, the nurse continues to perform rescue breathing at a rate of 8 to 10 breaths per minute, or 1 breath every 6 to 8 seconds. The pulse should be assessed every 2 minutes for no longer than 10 seconds.

If the pulse is absent, the nurse begins cardiac compressions. The patient is placed supine on a firm surface (cardiac board). Proper hand position is essential for performing compressions. The location for compressions is the lower half of the sternum in the center of the chest between the nipples. The heel of one hand is placed on the lower half of the sternum. The heel of the second hand is placed on top of the first hand so the hands are overlapped and parallel. Using both hands, the nurse begins compressions by depressing the sternum 1.5 to 2.0 inches for the average adult and then letting the chest return to its normal position. Compressions are performed at a rate of 100 per minute at a ratio of 30 compressions to 2 breaths (30:2). Every effort is made to minimize any interruptions in chest compressions. CPR is continued until an AED arrives, electrode pads are placed, and the AED is ready to analyze the rhythm. With two-person CPR, one person performs compressions while the other person maintains the airway and performs rescue breathing at the same 30:2 ratio at a rate of 100 compressions per minute ("hard and fast").

Advanced Cardiac Life Support

For cardiac or respiratory emergencies, many institutions follow the AHA standards for ACLS. The conceptual tools of management are the BLS primary survey followed by the ACLS secondary survey.[5]

Primary Survey
The BLS primary survey focuses on early CPR and early defibrillation. The ABCs of ACLS are the same as for BLS: airway, breathing, and circulation. "D" refers to early defibrillation that can be accomplished with an AED or a conventional defibrillator. It is a requirement that BLS providers be trained in the use of an AED. The AED is discussed in more detail later in the Electrical Therapy section of this chapter.

Secondary Survey
At the time of defibrillation, the secondary survey is initiated. The ABCD (airway, breathing, circulation, differential diagnosis) in the ACLS secondary survey involves the performance of more in-depth assessments and interventions.

Airway
Airway management involves reassessment of original techniques established in BLS. Endotracheal intubation provides definitive airway management and should be performed if needed by properly trained personnel as soon as possible during any resuscitation effort.[3] Endotracheal intubation is associated with the following advantages:

1. Keeps the airway patent.
2. Enables the administration of a high concentration of oxygen.
3. Ensures delivery of a selected tidal volume to maintain adequate lung inflation.
4. Protects the patient from gastric distention and aspiration of stomach contents.
5. Permits effective suctioning of the trachea.
6. Provides a route for administration of certain medications.

During a cardiopulmonary arrest, CPR should not be disrupted for longer than 10 seconds except as needed for interventions such as intubation. Techniques of endotracheal intubation are discussed in Chapter 9. Once intubated, the patient is manually ventilated with a BVD attached to the endotracheal tube (ETT; Figure 10-5). The BVD should have a reservoir and be connected to an oxygen source to deliver 100% oxygen while providing a tidal volume of 6-7 mL/kg. Chest compressions are not stopped for ventilations. Chest compressions are delivered continuously at a rate of 100 per minute. Ventilations are delivered one breath every 6 to 8 seconds or approximately 8 to 10 breaths per minute.

Breathing
Breathing assessment determines whether the ventilatory efforts are causing the chest to rise. After

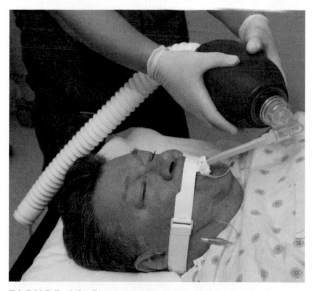

FIGURE 10-5. Ventilation with a bag-valve device connected to endotracheal tube.

intubation, the nurse first auscultates the epigastrium. If stomach gurgling is heard in this area and no chest expansion is present, the ETT has mistakenly been placed in the esophagus and is removed immediately. ETT placement should be confirmed by bilateral breath sounds and observation of chest movement with ventilation. A secondary method of assessing ETT placement must be done with an exhaled carbon dioxide detector or esophageal detector device (Figure 10-6).[3] A chest x-ray study confirms placement after the code.

Circulation

Circulation focuses on IV access, attachment of monitor electrodes and leads, rhythm identification, blood pressure measurement, and medication administration. A patent IV is necessary during an arrest for the administration of fluids, medications, or both. Intraosseous (IO) cannulation may be performed when IV access is not available, and is now recommended by the AHA as the primary alternative to IV access. Commercially available kits can facilitate IO access in adults. Endotracheal administration may be considered; however, tracheal absorption of medications is poor, and optimal dosing is not known. Medications that can be administered through the ETT until IV access is established are epinephrine, lidocaine, vasopressin, and atropine.[3]

Most critically ill patients already have IV access. If the patient does not have IV access, or needs additional IV access, a large-bore IV should be inserted. The antecubital vein should be the first target for IV access. Other areas for IV insertion include the dorsum of the hands and the wrist. If a peripheral IV cannot be started, the physician inserts a central line

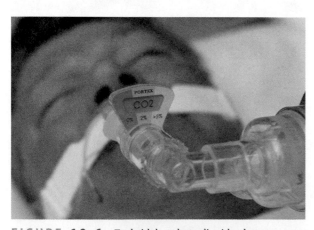

FIGURE 10-6. End-tidal carbon dioxide detector connected to an endotracheal tube. Exhaled carbon dioxide reacts with the device to create a color change indicating correct endotracheal tube placement.

for IV access. The IO route is an option if IV access is difficult.

NS is the preferred IV fluid because it expands intravascular volume better than dextrose. When any medication is administered by the peripheral IV route, it is best followed with a 20-mL bolus of IV fluid and elevation of the extremity for about 10 to 20 seconds to enhance delivery to the central circulation.

Differential Diagnosis

Differential diagnosis involves investigation into the cause of the arrest. If a reversible cause is identified, a specific therapy can be initiated. Cardiac dysrhythmias that result in cardiac arrests have many possible causes. The lethal dysrhythmias include ventricular fibrillation/ventricular tachycardia (VF/VT), asystole, and pulseless electrical activity (PEA). Other dysrhythmias that may lead to a cardiopulmonary arrest include symptomatic bradycardias and symptomatic tachycardias. Algorithms for treating these rhythm disorders have been established by the AHA.[3] Because these algorithms periodically change, critical actions in the management of these dysrhythmias are summarized.

Recognition and Treatment of Dysrhythmias

Ventricular Fibrillation and Pulseless Ventricular Tachycardia

The most common initial rhythms in witnessed sudden cardiac arrest are VF or pulseless VT. When VF is present, the heart quivers and does not pump blood. The treatment for VF and pulseless VT is the same.

Critical Actions

- Initiate the ABCDs of the primary survey. Initiate CPR until a defibrillator is available. Defibrillate as soon as possible because early defibrillation and CPR increase the chance of survival.
- Give one shock and resume CPR beginning with chest compressions. If a biphasic defibrillator is available, use the dose at which that defibrillator has been shown to be effective for terminating VF (typically 120 joules [J] to 200 J). If the dose is not known, use 200 J. If a monophasic defibrillator is available, use an initial shock of 360 J and use 360 J for subsequent shocks. Resume CPR immediately beginning with chest compressions for 5 cycles or about 2 minutes. After 5 cycles of CPR, check rhythm. (Monophasic versus biphasic defibrillation is discussed later in the Electrical Therapy section of this chapter.)
- If VF/VT persists, continue CPR, charge the defibrillator, intubate at once, and obtain IV access. Intubation optimizes airway management and provides a route for some medication administration. Give

one shock (biphasic defibrillator, use same joules as first shock or higher; monophasic defibrillator, use 360 J). Resume CPR immediately for 5 cycles or about 2 minutes.

- Administer epinephrine, 1 mg IV push every 3 to 5 minutes, if VF persists. One dose of vasopressin, 40 units IV push, may be given to replace the first or second dose of epinephrine. Check rhythm and if VF/VT persists, resume CPR immediately for 5 cycles or 2 minutes, and charge the defibrillator.
- Give one shock (biphasic defibrillator, use same joules as first shock or higher; monophasic defibrillator, use 360 J). Resume CPR immediately for 5 cycles or about 2 minutes.
- Administer antidysrhythmic medications during CPR. These medications include amiodarone, lidocaine, and magnesium sulfate. Dosages and administration are discussed later in the Pharmacological Intervention during a Code section of this chapter.
- Reassess the patient frequently. Check for return of pulse, spontaneous respirations, and blood pressure. Resume CPR if appropriate.

Pulseless Electrical Activity and Asystole

The goal in treating any rhythm without a pulse is to determine and treat the probable underlying cause of this condition. PEA is often associated with clinical conditions that can be reversed if they are identified early and treated appropriately.[3] Asystole is the absence of electrical activity on the ECG and has a poor prognosis. The rescuer must focus aggressively on the differential diagnosis of the secondary survey.

Critical Actions

- Initiate the ABCDs of the primary and secondary survey. Initiate CPR for 5 cycles or 2 minutes. The patient is intubated, and IV access is obtained.
- Consider possible causes. Some of the causes of PEA include hypovolemia, hypoxia, cardiac tamponade, tension pneumothorax, drug overdose, pulmonary embolism, acidosis, massive myocardial infarction, hyperkalemia or hypokalemia, hypoglycemia, trauma, and hypothermia.
- Confirm asystole by ensuring lead and cable connections are correct, ensuring that the power is on, and verifying asystole in another lead. An additional lead confirms or rules out the possibility of a fine VF.
- Check rhythm for no longer than 10 seconds. If no rhythm is present (e.g., asystole), resume CPR for 5 cycles or 2 minutes. If organized electrical activity is present, palpate a pulse for at least 5 seconds but no longer than 10 seconds. If no pulse is present (e.g., PEA), resume CPR

starting with chest compressions for 5 cycles or 2 minutes.

- During CPR, administer epinephrine, 1 mg IV push every 3 to 5 minutes, or vasopressin, 40 units IV, to replace the first or second dose of epinephrine. CPR is not stopped for drug administration. Consider atropine, 1 mg IV every 3 to 5 minutes (up to three doses) for asystole or slow PEA rate.
- Resume CPR for 5 cycles or 2 minutes, and then check the rhythm and pulse.
- Continue the ABCDs of the secondary survey while identifying underlying causes and initiating related interventions.
- Consider termination of resuscitative efforts if a reversible cause is not rapidly identified and the patient fails to respond to the BLS primary survey and ACLS secondary survey.

Symptomatic Bradycardia

This category encompasses two types: classic bradycardia (i.e., a heart rate <60 beats/min that causes symptoms) or any heart rhythm that is slow enough to cause hemodynamic compromise (Box 10-2). The cause of the bradycardia must be considered. For example, hypotension associated with bradycardia may be caused by dysfunction of the myocardium or hypovolemia, rather than by a conduction system or autonomic nervous system disturbance.

Critical Actions

- Assess the ABCDs of the BLS primary and ACLS secondary survey. Secure the airway, administer oxygen, obtain IV access, and assess vital signs. The use of a pulse oximeter is encouraged. A 12-lead ECG should be obtained to identify the rhythm.

BOX 10-2 Signs and Symptoms of Low Cardiac Output Associated with Bradycardia

- Chest pain
- Shortness of breath
- Decreased level of consciousness
- Weakness
- Fatigue
- Dizziness
- Hypotension
- Diaphoresis
- Pulmonary congestion
- Pulmonary edema

- Administer atropine, 0.5 mg IV every 3 to 5 minutes to a total dose of 3 mg. Atropine is not indicated in second-degree atrioventricular (AV) block type II or third-degree AV block.
- Identify the causative rhythm. Symptomatic bradycardias include sinus rhythm with a rate of less than 60 beats per minute, second-degree AV block types I or II, and third-degree AV block.
- Prepare for transcutaneous pacing for all symptomatic bradycardias. If used, analgesics or sedatives may need to be given because patients often find the pacing stimulus that is delivered with this therapy uncomfortable.
- Consider epinephrine or dopamine infusion while awaiting pacemaker or if pacing is not effective. Dopamine infusion is acceptable if low blood pressure is associated with the bradycardia. An epinephrine infusion may be administered instead if clinical symptoms are severe.

Unstable Tachycardia

Unstable tachycardia occurs when the heart beats too fast for the patient's clinical condition. The treatment of this group of dysrhythmias involves the rapid assessment of the patient and identification of the dysrhythmia. Synchronized cardioversion and antidysrhythmic therapy may be needed.[3]

Critical Actions
- Initiate the BLS primary and ACLS secondary ABCD survey. Assess the patient and recognize the signs and symptoms of cardiovascular instability including chest pain, hypotension, altered mental status, shortness of breath, and syncope, and signs of shock. Provide supplemental oxygen, establish IV access, and prepare suction and intubation equipment. Assess vital signs including oxygen saturation.
- Identify the unstable tachycardia. This group of dysrhythmias includes narrow-complex tachycardias (atrial fibrillation and flutter) and wide-complex tachycardia (VT).
- Prepare for synchronized cardioversion. Premedicate with sedation or analgesia whenever possible. Cardioversion is an uncomfortable procedure, and a fully conscious patient is sedated before electrical intervention.
- Perform synchronized cardioversion at the appropriate energy level. Supraventricular tachycardia and atrial flutter often respond to energy levels as low as 50 J. Cardioversion for the other tachydysrhythmias should be initiated at 100 J, increasing to 200 J, 300 J, and 360 J monophasic for subsequent attempts. Clinically equivalent biphasic energy doses have not yet been determined; however, 100 to 200 J biphasic may be effective.[2]

- Reassess the patient and rhythm, and consider the need for follow-up monitoring and antidysrhythmic therapy including adenosine, verapamil, diltiazem, and amiodarone.

Electrical Therapy

The therapeutic use of electrical current has expanded over the past several years with the addition and increased use of the AED. This section addresses the use of electricity in code management for the purposes of defibrillation, cardioversion, and transcutaneous (external) pacing. Defibrillation of the patient with an implantable cardioverter-defibrillator (ICD) is also discussed.

Defibrillation

The only effective treatment for VF and pulseless VT is defibrillation. VF deteriorates into asystole if not treated. VF may occur as a result of coronary artery disease, myocardial infarction, electrical shock, drug overdose, near drowning, and acid-base imbalance.

Definition. Defibrillation is the delivery of an electrical current to the heart through the use of a defibrillator (Figure 10-7). The current can be delivered through the chest wall by use of external paddles or adhesive electrode pads ("hands off" defibrillation) connected to cables. Smaller internal paddles may be used to deliver current directly to the heart during cardiac surgery when the chest is open and the heart is visualized. Defibrillation works by completely depolarizing the heart and disrupting the impulses that are causing the dysrhythmia. Because the heart is completely depolarized, the sinoatrial node or

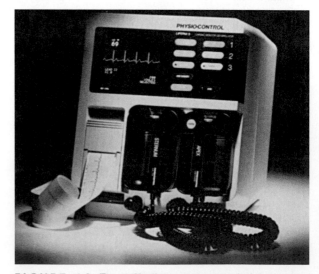

FIGURE 10-7. Defibrillator. *(Courtesy of Philips Medical Systems, Bothell, WA.)*

other pacemaker can resume control of the heart's rhythm.

Defibrillation delivers energy or current in waveforms. *Monophasic* waveforms deliver current in one direction. More recently, defibrillators have been developed that deliver biphasic current. *Biphasic* waveforms deliver current that flows in a positive direction for a specified duration and then reverses and flows in a negative direction. As a result, less joules are needed for defibrillation. Biphasic defibrillation appears to work at least as effectively as monophasic defibrillation, and in some reports is more effective in converting VF with fewer shocks.[3]

Procedure. Two methods exist for paddle placement for external defibrillation. The standard or anterior paddle placement is used most often. In the anterior method, one paddle or adhesive electrode pad is placed at the second intercostal space to the right of the sternum, and the other paddle or adhesive electrode pad is placed at the fifth intercostal space, midaxillary line, to the left of the sternum (Figure 10-8). The alternative method is anteroposterior placement. Adhesive electrode pads are used because of the difficulty in correctly placing the paddles. The anterior adhesive electrode pad is placed at the left anterior precordial area, and the posterior electrode pad is placed at the left posterior-infrascapular area or at the posterior-infrascapular area (Figure 10-9). Refer to the manufacturer's instructions for exact placement of the electrode pads.

The amount of energy delivered is referred to as joules, or watt-seconds (w-s). For monophasic defibrillation, 360 J is used for all shocks. For biphasic defibrillation, refer to the manufacturer's instructions for the amount of joules to be delivered to the patient. If the effective dose range of the defibrillator is not known, deliver 200 J for the first shock and an equal or higher dose for subsequent shocks.[2]

For the shock to be effective, some type of conductive medium is placed between the paddles and the skin. In the past, gel has been used to conduct the electricity. If gel is used, it is important to cover the paddles completely with the gel. Commercially-prepared defibrillator gel pads are available that facilitate defibrillation and also prevent burns on the patient's skin when paddles are used. Adhesive electrode pads used in "hands off" defibrillation also have conductive gel.

The defibrillator is charged to the desired setting. The paddles are placed firmly on the patient's chest.

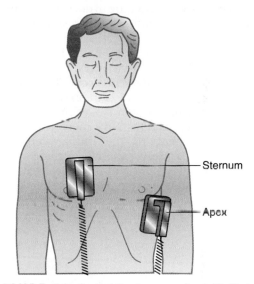

FIGURE 10-8. Paddle placement for defibrillation.

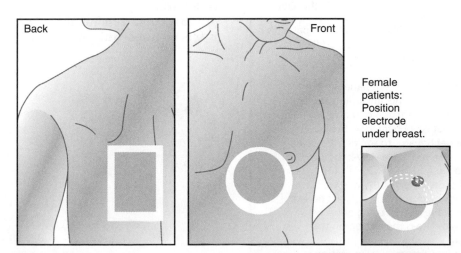

FIGURE 10-9. Anteroposterior placement of adhesive electrode pads for defibrillation or transcutaneous pacing.

Firm pressure is needed to facilitate skin contact and to reduce the impedance to the flow of current. Safety is essential during the procedure to prevent injury to the patient and the personnel assisting with the procedure. The person performing the defibrillation ensures that all personnel are standing clear of the bed and visually checks to see that no one is in contact with the patient or bed. It is important that this step not be omitted when "hands off" defibrillation is used. Using a mnemonic, such as "I'm clear, you're clear, everybody's clear," provides an audible check that no one is touching the patient. The shock is then delivered. CPR is resumed immediately beginning with chest compressions for 5 cycles or 2 minutes. Then the patient's rhythm and pulse are checked. Rhythm strips are recorded during the procedure to document response. The procedure for defibrillation is summarized in Box 10-3.

Complications of defibrillation include burns on the skin and damage to the heart muscle. Arcing of electricity or a spark can occur if the paddles are not firmly placed on the skin, excessive conductive gel is used, or the skin is wet. Arcing has also been noted when patients have medication patches with aluminized backing (i.e., nitroglycerin, nicotine, pain medication); therefore these patches should be removed and the area cleansed before defibrillation. Body jewelry such as nipple rings should also be removed before defibrillation to reduce the risk for arcing of electricity during the procedure.

Automated External Defibrillation

The AED extends the range of personnel trained in the use of a defibrillator and shortens the time between code onset and defibrillation. The AED is considered an integral part of emergency cardiac care.

Definition. The AED is an external defibrillator with rhythm analysis capabilities (Figure 10-10). It is used to achieve early defibrillation. Because of the ease of use, AEDs may be placed on medical-surgical patient units, emergency response vehicles, and in public places.

Indications. The AED should be used only when a patient is in cardiac arrest (unresponsive, no effective breathing, no signs of circulation including no pulse). Confirmation that the patient is in cardiac arrest must be obtained before attaching the AED.[4]

Procedure. The AED is attached to the patient by two adhesive pads and connecting cables. Correct placement of each adhesive pad is displayed on each adhesive pad. These pads serve a dual purpose: recording the rhythm and delivering the shock. The AED eliminates the need for training in rhythm recognition because these microprocessor-based devices analyze the surface ECG signal. The AED "looks" at the patient's rhythm numerous times to confirm the presence of a rhythm for which defibrillation in indicated. The semiautomatic "shock advisory" AED charges the device and "advises" the operator to press a button to defibrillate. The fully automated AED requires only that the operator attach the defibrillation pads and turn on the device (Box 10-4). Both models deliver AHA-recommended energy levels for the treatment of VF/pulseless VT. They are not designed to deliver synchronous shocks and will shock VT if the rate exceeds preset values.

Cardioversion

Definition. Cardioversion is the delivery of a shock that is synchronized with the patient's cardiac rhythm.

BOX 10-3   Procedure for External Defibrillation

- Apply adhesive defibrillator pads to the patient's chest (or apply conductive gel to paddles).
- Turn on the defibrillator.
- Select the energy level.
- Position the paddles on the patient's chest.
- Ensure that all personnel (including yourself) are clear of the patient, the bed, and any equipment that is connected to the patient.
- Charge the defibrillator to the desired setting.
- Shout "I'm clear, you're clear, everybody's clear," and look to verify.
- Apply firm pressure on both paddles.
- Deliver shock by depressing buttons on each paddle simultaneously. If using adhesive electrode pads, press the button on the defibrillator.
- Resume cardiopulmonary resuscitation.

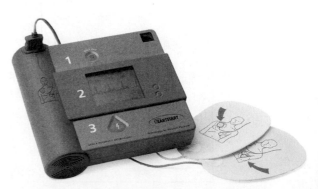

FIGURE 10-10. Automatic external defibrillator. *(Courtesy of Laerdal Medical Corporation, Wappingers Falls, NY.)*

BOX 10-4 Procedure for Automated External Defibrillator Operation

- Turn the power on.
- Attach the AED connecting cables to the AED "box."
- Attach the adhesive electrode pads to the patient:
  Place one electrode pad on the upper right sternal border directly below the clavicle.
  Place the other electrode pad lateral to the left nipple with the top margin of the pad a few inches below the axilla.
  The correct position of the electrode pads is often marked on the electrode pads.
- Attach the AED connecting cables to the adhesive electrode pads.
- "Clear" personnel from the patient (no one should be touching the patient), and press the "analyze" button to start rhythm analysis.
- Listen or read the message "shock indicated" or "no shock indicated."
- "Clear" personnel from the patient, and press the "shock" button if shock is indicated.

AED, Automated external defibrillator.

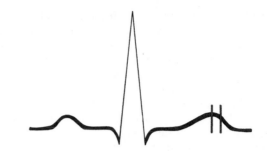

FIGURE 10-11. Approximate location of the vulnerable period. *(From Conover, M. B. [2003]. Understanding electrocardiography [8th ed.]. St. Louis: Mosby.)*

BOX 10-5 Procedure for Synchronous Cardioversion

- Ensure that emergency equipment is readily available.
- Explain the procedure to the patient.
- Sedate the conscious patient unless unstable or rapidly deteriorating.
- Attach monitor leads to the patient. Ensure that the monitor displays the patient's rhythm clearly without artifact.
- Apply the defibrillator pads or adhesive electrode pads to the patient's chest (or apply conductive gel to the paddles).
- Turn on the defibrillator to "synchronous" mode.
- Observe the rhythm on the monitor to determine that the R wave is properly sensed and marked (usually with a spike) (Figure 10-12).
- Select the appropriate energy level.
- Position the paddles on the patient's chest and apply firm pressure.
- Ensure that all personnel (including yourself) are clear of the patient, the bed, and any equipment that is connected to the patient.
- Charge the defibrillator.
- Shout "I'm clear, you're clear, everybody's clear," and look to verify.
- Deliver synchronized shock by depressing the buttons on each paddle simultaneously. Or press the button on the defibrillator if using adhesive electrode pads. Keep the buttons depressed until the shock has been delivered.
- After the cardioversion, observe the patient's heart rhythm to determine effectiveness.

The purpose of cardioversion is to disrupt an ectopic pacemaker that is causing a dysrhythmia and to allow the sinoatrial node to take control of the rhythm. During an emergency situation, cardioversion is used to treat patients with VT or supraventricular tachycardia who have a pulse but are developing symptoms related to a low cardiac output, such as hypotension and a decreased level of consciousness. Elective cardioversion is used to treat atrial flutter and atrial fibrillation.

Cardioversion is similar to defibrillation, except the delivery of energy is synchronized to occur during ventricular depolarization (QRS complex). The rationale for delivering the shock during the QRS complex is to prevent the shock from being delivered during repolarization (T wave), often termed the vulnerable period. If a shock is delivered during this vulnerable period (Figure 10-11), VF may occur. Because the purpose of cardioversion is to disrupt the rhythm rather than completely depolarize the heart, less energy is usually required. Cardioversion can be performed with energy levels as low as 50 J. The amount of energy is gradually increased until the rhythm is converted.

Procedure. The procedure for cardioversion (Box 10-5) is similar to that for defibrillation. However, the defibrillator is set in the "synchronous" mode for the cardioversion. The R waves are sensed by the machine and are noted by "spikes" or other markings on the monitor of the defibrillator (Figure 10-12). It is important to assess that all R waves are properly sensed. When it is time to deliver the shock, the buttons on the paddles must remain depressed until the shock is delivered because energy is discharged only during the QRS complex. When a patient is undergoing cardioversion on a nonemergency basis, sedation is given before the procedure. Rhythm strips are recorded during cardioversion to document response.

Special Situations

Patients at risk for sudden cardiac death may have an implanted ICD/permanent pacemaker that delivers shocks directly to the heart muscle. These devices are easily identified because they create a hard lump beneath the skin of the upper chest or abdomen. When a patient with a permanent pacemaker or ICD requires defibrillation, placing the paddle near the generator is avoided. Although damage to the device rarely occurs, the device can absorb much of the current of defibrillation from the pads or paddles, block the shock delivery, and reduce the chance of success.[2] The paddle or adhesive electrode pad should be placed at least one inch away from the device.

A patient may have an ICD with dual-chamber pacing capabilities. Nurses should become familiar, whenever possible, with the type of therapy the patient's device has been programmed to deliver. By the time VF/VT is recognized on the monitor, the rhythm should also have been recognized by the ICD. If a successful shock by the ICD has not occurred when the rhythm is noted on the monitor, one should proceed with standard code management. If external defibrillation is unsuccessful, the location of the paddles or adhesive electrode pads on the chest should be changed. Anterior-posterior placement may be more effective than anterior-apex placement. External defibrillation of a patient while the ICD is firing does not harm the patient or the ICD. ICDs and permanent pacemakers are insulated from damage caused by conventional external defibrillation. There is no danger to personnel if the ICD discharges while staff members are touching the patient. However, the shock may be felt and has been compared to the sensation of contact with an electrical outlet. The pacing and sensing thresholds of the pacemaker or ICD are assessed after external defibrillation.

Transcutaneous Cardiac Pacing

Definition. Transcutaneous (external noninvasive) cardiac pacing is used during emergency situations to treat symptomatic bradycardia (hypotension, altered mental status, angina, pulmonary edema) that has not responded to atropine. Transcutaneous pacing is not recommended for asystole. In this method of pacing, the heart is stimulated with externally applied, cutaneous adhesive electrodes that deliver the electrical impulse. Impulse conduction occurs across the chest wall to stimulate the cardiac contraction.

The transcutaneous pacemaker may be a freestanding unit with a monitor and a pacemaker. Most models incorporate a monitor, a defibrillator, and an external pacemaker into one system (Figure 10-13). The advantages of transcutaneous pacemakers include easy operation in an emergent situation, minimal training, and none of the risks associated with invasive pacemakers.

Procedure. The procedure (Box 10-6) for transcutaneous pacing involves the placement of adhesive

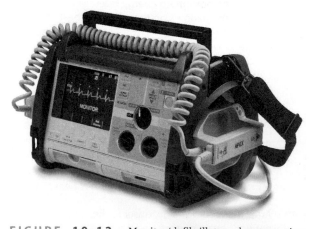

FIGURE 10-12. Monitor/defibrillator demonstrating marked R waves for cardioversion. *(Courtesy of Zoll Medical, Burlington, MA.)*

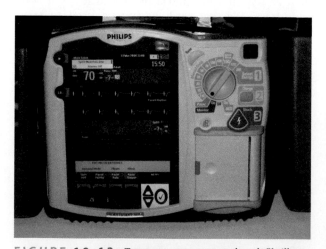

FIGURE 10-13. Transcutaneous pacemaker-defibrillator. *(Courtesy of Philips Medical Systems, Bothell, WA.)*

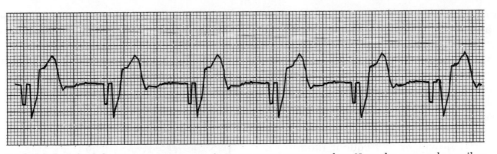

FIGURE 10-14. Electrical capture of transcutaneous pacemaker. Note the pacemaker spikes followed by a wide QRS complex and a tall T wave.

BOX 10-6 Procedure for Transcutaneous Pacemaker

- Obtain the transcutaneous pacemaker, pacemaker electrodes, and emergency equipment.
- If the patient is alert, explain the procedure.
- Clip excess hair from the patient's chest. Do not shave hair.
- Apply the anterior electrode to the chest. The electrode is centered at the fourth intercostal space to the left of the sternum.
- Apply the posterior electrode on the patient's back to the left of the thoracic spine.
- Connect the electrode cable to the pacemaker generator.
- Turn the unit on. Choose pacing mode (if applicable).
- Set the pacemaker parameters for mode, heart rate, and output (mA) according to the manufacturer's instructions.
- Assess the adequacy of pacing:
  Pacemaker spike and QRS complex (capture)
  Heart rate and rhythm
  Blood pressure
  Level of consciousness
- Observe for patient discomfort. The patient may need sedation and/or analgesia.
- Anticipate follow-up treatment (e.g., insertion of a temporary transvenous pacemaker).

---

electrode pads anteriorly and posteriorly on the patient (see Figure 10-9). The electrodes are connected to the external pacemaker allowing for "hands off" pacing. The pacemaker is set in either asynchronous or demand modes. Some devices permit only demand pacing. In the asynchronous mode, the pacemaker generates a rhythm without regard to the patient's own rhythm. In the demand mode, the pacemaker fires only if the patient's heart rate falls below a preset limit determined by the operator (e.g., 60 beats/min). The milliamperes (mA) output is adjusted to stimulate a paced beat, usually 2 mA above the dose at which consistent capture is observed.

The electrical and mechanical effectiveness of pacing is assessed. The electrical activity is noted by a pacemaker "spike" that indicates that the pacemaker is initiating electrical activity. The spike is followed by a broad QRS complex (Figure 10-14). Mechanical activity is noted by palpating a pulse during electrical activity. In addition, the patient has signs of improved cardiac output, including increased blood pressure and improved skin color and skin temperature. If the external pacemaker is effective, the patient may need to have a temporary transvenous pacemaker inserted, depending on the cause of the bradycardia.

The alert patient who requires transcutaneous pacing may experience some discomfort. Because the skeletal muscles are stimulated, as well as the heart muscle, the patient may experience a tingling, twitching, or thumping feeling that ranges from mildly uncomfortable to intolerable. Sedation, analgesia, or both may be indicated.

PHARMACOLOGICAL INTERVENTION DURING A CODE

Medications that are administered during a code depend on several factors: the cause of the arrest, the patient's cardiac rhythm, the physician's preference, and the patient's response. The goals of treatment are to reestablish and maintain optimal cardiac function, to correct hypoxemia and acidosis, and to suppress dangerous cardiac ectopic activity. In addition, medications are used to achieve a balance between myocardial oxygen supply and demand, to maintain adequate blood pressure, and to relieve congestive heart failure. Because of the rapid and profound effects these drugs can have on cardiac activity and hemodynamic function, continuous ECG monitoring is essential, and hemodynamic monitoring should be instituted as soon as possible after the code. If IV push medications are given peripherally, they should be flushed with at least 20 mL of IV fluid to ensure central circulation. In addition, because of the precise dosages and careful administration required with these medications, infusion pumps should be used when continuous infusions are given. IV infusion rates are tapered slowly, with frequent monitoring of clinical effectiveness.

The following drugs are included in ACLS guidelines and represent those drugs most frequently used in code management.[2] Indications, mechanisms of action, and dosages for each drug, as well as side effects and nursing implications, are discussed in this section and are summarized in Table 10-4.

Oxygen

Oxygen is essential to resuscitation and has several pharmacological considerations. Oxygen is used to treat hypoxemia, which exists in any arrest situation as a result of lack of adequate gas exchange, inadequate cardiac output, or both. Artificial ventilation without supplemental oxygen does not correct hypoxemia. In addition, the success of other medications and interventions, such as defibrillation, depends on adequate oxygenation and normal acid-base status.

Oxygen can be delivered via mouth to mask, BVD with mask, BVD to ETT, or other airway adjuncts. During an arrest, 100% oxygen is administered.

Epinephrine (Adrenalin)

Epinephrine is a potent vasoconstrictor. Because of its alpha-adrenergic and beta-adrenergic effects (Box 10-7), epinephrine increases systemic vascular resistance and arterial blood pressure, as well as heart rate, contractility, and automaticity of cardiac pacemaker cells. Because of peripheral vasoconstriction, blood is shunted to the heart and brain. Epinephrine also increases myocardial oxygen requirements.

Epinephrine is indicated for the restoration of cardiac electrical activity in an arrest. In addition, epinephrine increases automaticity and the force of contraction, an effect that makes the heart more susceptible to successful defibrillation. Epinephrine is used to treat VF or pulseless VT that is unresponsive to initial defibrillation, asystole, and PEA.

During a code, epinephrine may be given by the IV or IO route or through an ETT. The IV dosage is 1.0 mg (10 mL of a 1:10,000 solution) and is repeated every 3 to 5 minutes as needed. When given through

---

BOX 10-7   Effects of Adrenergic Receptor Stimulation

Alpha
- Vasoconstriction
- Increased contractility

Beta₁
- Increased heart rate
- Increased contractility

Beta₂
- Vasodilation
- Relaxation of bronchial, uterine, and gastrointestinal smooth muscle

---

the ETT, 2 to 2.5 mg is diluted in 10 mL of NS or sterile water.

Epinephrine may be administered by continuous infusion to increase the heart rate or blood pressure. Dilution is 1 mg in 250 or 500 mL of D₅W or NS. The infusion is started at 1 mcg/min and is titrated according to the patient's response in a range of 2 to 10 mcg/min. In a situation other than cardiac arrest, because epinephrine increases myocardial oxygen requirements, the nurse must monitor the patient closely for signs of myocardial ischemia.

Vasopressin

Vasopressin is recommended as an alternative to epinephrine administration in VF unresponsive to shock.[2] At high doses, vasopressin is a potent vasoconstrictor. A single dose of 40 units IV/IO is recommended. Repeat doses are not necessary because of its 10- to 20-minute half-life. Administration of the drug is not recommended for conscious patients with coronary artery disease because severe angina can result from the vasoconstriction.

Atropine

Atropine is used to increase the heart rate by decreasing the vagal tone. It is indicated for patients with symptomatic bradycardia. In an arrest, atropine may be used for asystole because it may initiate electrical activity or restore conduction through the AV node.

For symptomatic bradycardia, atropine 0.5 mg IV is given and repeated every 3 to 5 minutes as needed (for a total of 3 mg) to maintain a heart rate greater than 60 beats per minute or until adequate tissue perfusion is achieved as indicated by blood pressure and level of consciousness. If atropine is ineffective

Text continued on p. 252

PHARMACOLOGY

TABLE 10-4 Drugs Frequently Used in Code Management

Drug	Indication	Mechanism of Action	Dosage/Route	Side Effects	Nursing Implications
Adenosine (Adenocard)	Initial drug of choice for supraventricular dysrhythmias	Slows conduction in AV node and interrupts AV nodal reentry circuits	6 mg rapid IV bolus over 1-3 seconds, followed by 20-mL rapid flush; if no response in 1-2 minutes, give 12 mg repeat dose and flush; may repeat 12 mg dose if necessary	Headache, facial flushing, dyspnea, and chest pain; may cause asystole up to 15 seconds	Half-life 10 seconds; higher dose needed with theophylline, lower dose with dipyridamole or after cardiac transplantation
Amiodarone (Cordarone)	Treatment and prophylaxis of recurrent VF and hemodynamically unstable VT; rapid atrial dysrhythmias	↓ Membrane excitability, prolongs action potential to terminate VT or VF	*Cardiac arrest:* 300 mg IV/IO push followed by dose of 150 mg in 3 to 5 minutes (maximum dose, 2.2 g/24 hr) NS or D₅W *Recurrent VF/VT:* 150 mg IV over 10 minutes followed by 360 mg (1 mg/min) infusion for 6 hours, then 540 mg for next 18 hours (0.5 mg/min) for a maximum dose of 2.2 g over 24 hours	Bradycardia, hypotension; use with caution on preexisting conduction system abnormalities	Monitor for symptomatic sinus bradycardia, PR prolongation
Atropine	Symptomatic bradycardia, asystole, bradycardic pulseless electrical activity	↑ SA node automaticity and AV node conduction activity	*Bradycardia:* 0.5-1 mg IV every 3-5 minutes to maximum dose of 3 mg *Asystole:* 1 mg IV/IO push every 3-5 minutes to maximum dose of 3 mg or 3 doses 2-3 mg in 10 mL NS may be given via ETT	Tachycardia, increased myocardial oxygen consumption and ischemia	Consider transcutaneous pacing if atropine is ineffective
Calcium chloride	Acute hyperkalemia, hypocalcemia, calcium channel blocker toxicity	↑ Myocardial contractility	8-16 mg/kg of 10% solution slow IV push; 10 mL of 10% solution = 100 mg/mL; repeat as needed		Rapid administration can slow heart rate

Continued

PHARMACOLOGY

TABLE 10-4 Drugs Frequently Used in Code Management—cont'd

Drug	Indication	Mechanism of Action	Dosage/Route	Side Effects	Nursing Implications
Dopamine (Intropin)	Hypotension not related to hypovolemia	*Moderate doses (5-10 mcg/kg/min):* ↑ Contractility and cardiac output *High doses (10-20 mcg/kg/min):* vasoconstriction and ↑ systemic vascular resistance	IV infusion, 2-5 mcg/kg/min initially and titrated as needed	Tachycardia, increased dysrhythmias	Extravasation may cause necrosis and sloughing; dilution, 400-800 mg in 250 mL D_5W = 1600-3200 mcg/mL
Epinephrine (Adrenalin)	VF, pulseless VT, pulseless electrical activity, asystole	↑ Contractility, automaticity, systemic vascular resistance, and arterial blood pressure; improves coronary and cerebral perfusion	1 mg IV/IO, or 2-2.5 mg in 10 mL via ETT; may repeat every 3-5 minutes	Tachycardia, hypertension	In a cardiac arrest may be used as a continuous infusion for hypotension; dilution, 1 mg/250 mL NS; infuse at 1-10 mcg/min and titrate as needed
Lidocaine (Xylocaine)	VF, VT, PVCs	Suppresses ventricular dysrhythmias, raises fibrillation threshold	*VF:* 1-1.5 mg/kg IV/IO, followed by 0.5-0.75 mg/kg every 5-10 minutes to maximum of 3 doses of 3 mg/kg; may be given by ETT at dose of 2-4 mg/kg; follow with continuous IV infusion at 2-4 mg/min	Neurological toxicity if drug level excessive	Lower dose if impaired hepatic blood flow; dilution, 1 g in 250 mL or 2 g/500 mL = 4 mg/mL
Magnesium	Torsades de pointes, hypomagnesemia	Essential for enzyme reactions and sodium-potassium pump, ↓ postinfarction dysrhythmias	*Cardiac arrest:* 1-2 g in 10 mL of D_5W IV/IO over 5-20 min *Nonarrest:* 1-2 g in 50-100 mL of D_5W IV, over 5-60 min followed by infusion of 0.5 to 1 g/hr	Flushing, bradycardia, hypotension	Monitor serum levels

Drug	Indications	Action	Dosage	Side Effects	Nursing Considerations
Norepinephrine (Levophed)	Hypotension uncorrected by other drugs	Alpha-, beta$_1$-agonist, causes arterial and venous vasoconstriction, some ↑ in myocardial contractility	Continuous IV infusion at 0.5-1 mcg/min, titrated upward as needed to maximum of 30 mcg/min Dilution: 4 mg/250 mL D$_5$W	Myocardial ischemia	Administer through central line, if possible; extravasation may cause necrosis and sloughing
Oxygen	Cardiopulmonary arrest, chest pain, hypoxemia	↑ Arterial oxygen content and tissue oxygenation	100% in a code via bag-valve device with mask		Monitor pulse oximetry values
Procainamide (Pronestyl)	PVCs, VT uncontrolled by lidocaine, occasionally supraventricular dysrhythmias	↓ Automaticity of ectopic pacemakers; slows intraventricular conduction	Administer 20 mg/min until dysrhythmia is suppressed, hypotension occurs, or the QRS widens by >50% of original width, or 17 mg/kg has been administered, followed by a continuous infusion of 1-4 mg/min	Hypotension, heart block	Do not exceed recommended infusion rate; dilution; 1 g/250 mL = 4 mg/mL; decrease dose with cardiac or renal dysfunction
Sodium bicarbonate	Preexisting metabolic acidosis, hyperkalemia, or tricyclic antidepressant overdose	Counteracts metabolic acidosis by binding with hydrogen ions to produce water and carbon dioxide	1 mEq/kg IV push initially, subsequent doses based on bicarbonate levels		Ensure adequate CPR, oxygenation, and ventilation
Vasopressin	Alternative vasopressor to epinephrine in VF	Nonadrenergic, peripheral vasoconstriction	40 units IV/IO push (one dose only)	Cardiac ischemia	May also be useful in place of epinephrine in asystole, pulseless electrical activity, VF, or pulseless VT

ABG, Arterial blood gas; *AV*, atrioventricular; *CPR*, cardiopulmonary resuscitation; *D$_5$W*, 5% dextrose in water; *ETT*, endotracheal tube; *IO*, intraosseous; *IV*, intravenous; *NS*, normal saline; *PVC*, premature ventricular contraction; *SA*, sinoatrial; *VF*, ventricular fibrillation; *VT*, ventricular tachycardia.
Data from American Heart Association. (2005). 2005 American Heart Association guidelines for cardiopulmonary resuscitation and emergency cardiovascular care. *Circulation, 112*(24 Suppl.), IV-1–IV-211; Hodgson, B. B., & Kizior, R. J. (2007). *Saunders nursing drug handbook.* St. Louis: Saunders.

in maintaining the heart rate and adequate tissue perfusion, consider transcutaneous pacing.

In asystole, 1.0 mg IV is given and repeated every 3 to 5 minutes, if necessary, up to the maximum total of 3 doses or 3 mg. If necessary, atropine may be given via an ETT. The dose for ETT administration is 2 to 3 mg diluted in 10 mL of NS or sterile water.

Amiodarone (Cordarone)

Amiodarone is a unique antidysrhythmic possessing some characteristics of all groups of antidysrhythmic drugs. It reduces membrane excitability, and by prolonging the action potential and retarding the refractory period it facilitates the termination of VT and VF. It also has alpha-adrenergic and beta-adrenergic blocking properties. Many antidysrhythmic agents, despite their effectiveness in suppression of dysrhythmias, also have a propensity to exacerbate dysrhythmias. This property is known as proarrhythmia or prodysrhythmia. Administration of amiodarone is rarely associated with prodysrhythmias. It is less likely to produce hypotension and myocardial depression than is procainamide. Amiodarone has the added benefit of dilating coronary arteries and increasing coronary blood supply. Amiodarone also decreases systemic vascular resistance, and in patients with impaired left ventricular function it can improve cardiac pump function.

IV amiodarone is indicated for treatment and prophylaxis of recurring VF and unstable VT refractory to other treatment. It is also used in supraventricular tachycardia for rate control or conversion of atrial fibrillation or flutter, especially in patients with heart failure. Bolus and infusion rates are described in Table 10-4. During cardiac arrest it may be administered as a 300-mg IV/IO loading bolus. If VF/pulseless VT persists, a second loading dose of 150 mg IV/IO may be given in 3 to 5 minutes. For recurrent VF/pulseless VT, a bolus dose of 150 mg IV/IO may be administered over 10 minutes, followed by an infusion of 360 mg over the next 6 hours (1 mg/min), and then a maintenance infusion of 540 mg over the next 18 hours (0.5 mg/min). Adverse reactions include hypotension and bradycardia, which can be prevented by slowing the infusion rate or treating the patient with fluids, vasopressors, chronotropic medications, or temporary pacing.

Lidocaine (Xylocaine)

Lidocaine is an antidysrhythmic drug that suppresses ventricular ectopic activity. It depresses the ventricular conduction system and reduces automaticity. Lidocaine is used as an alternative to amiodarone in treating ventricular ectopy (premature ventricular contractions), VT, and VF.

During a code, a bolus dose of 1 to 1.5 mg/kg of lidocaine is administered by IV/IO push. Additional boluses of 0.5 to 0.75 mg/kg may be administered every 5 to 10 minutes, as needed, until a maximum of 3 doses or 3 mg/kg has been given. If IV or IO access is not available, 2 to 4 mg/kg of lidocaine may be given through the ETT.

If lidocaine is successful in treating the cardiac dysrhythmia, a continuous infusion should be started at 2 to 4 mg/min. Dilution is 1 g mixed in 250 mL of D_5W, or 2 g can be mixed in 500 mL. Both solutions deliver 4 mg/mL, the standard dilution.

Dosages of lidocaine should be decreased in patients with impaired hepatic blood flow (as occurs in congestive heart failure, acute myocardial infarction, shock) and in elderly patients. Blood levels are monitored, and the patient is assessed for central nervous system disturbances that may indicate lidocaine toxicity. Common side effects of lidocaine include lethargy, confusion, tinnitus, muscle twitching, seizures, bradycardia, and paresthesias.

Procainamide (Pronestyl)

Procainamide is an antidysrhythmic drug that suppresses both atrial and ventricular dysrhythmias by slowing conduction in myocardial tissue. It is used to treat ventricular ectopy and VT that is uncontrolled by lidocaine. It may also be used to treat supraventricular dysrhythmias. Procainamide is not used initially in VF because of the length of time needed to achieve adequate blood levels; however, it may be used for recurrent VF.

Procainamide is given IV in 100-mg doses (diluted in 10 mL of sterile water for injection) at a rate of 20 mg/min until the dysrhythmia is suppressed, the patient becomes hypotensive, the QRS widens by 50% of its original width, or a total of 17 mg/kg has been given. If procainamide successfully controls the dysrhythmia, a continuous infusion is given at a rate of 1 to 4 mg/min for maintenance. The infusion is prepared by mixing 1 g of procainamide in 250 mL of fluid, yielding 4 mg/mL. As with lidocaine, serum levels should be monitored. It should be administered in reduced dosages to patients with left ventricular dysfunction or renal failure.

Hypotension may occur after rapid injection of procainamide. Procainamide may also cause widening of the QRS interval and prolongation of PR or QT intervals, resulting in AV conduction disturbances, cardiac arrest, or both.

Adenosine (Adenocard)

Adenosine is the initial drug of choice for the diagnosis and treatment of supraventricular dysrhythmias. Adenosine slows conduction through the AV node and interrupts AV node reentrant electrical conduction, which is the cause of most supraventricular dysrhythmias. It is effective in restoring normal sinus rhythm in patients with paroxysmal supraventricular tachycardia, including that caused by Wolff-Parkinson-White syndrome. Adenosine does not convert supraventricular rhythms that do not involve the sinoatrial or AV node, such as atrial fibrillation, atrial flutter, atrial tachycardia, and VT. However, adenosine may produce a brief AV node block, thereby assisting with the diagnosis of these rhythms (Figure 10-15).

Adenosine has an onset of action of 10 to 40 seconds and a duration of 1 to 2 minutes; therefore it is administered rapidly. The initial dose is a 6 mg IV push over 1 to 3 seconds, followed by a 20-mL rapid saline flush. A period of asystole lasting as long as 15 seconds may be seen after adenosine administration that reflects the suppression of AV node conduction. A second and third dose of 12 mg may be given 1 to 2 minutes later if the first dose is ineffective in converting the rhythm. Common side effects include transient facial flushing (from mild dilation of blood vessels in the skin), dyspnea, coughing (from mild bronchoconstriction), and chest pain.

Magnesium

Magnesium is essential for many enzyme reactions and for the function of the sodium-potassium pump. It also acts as a calcium channel blocker and slows neuromuscular transmission. Hypomagnesemia is associated with a high frequency of cardiac dysrhyth-mias, including refractory VF. Magnesium administered IV may terminate or prevent recurrent torsades de pointes in patients who have a prolonged QT interval. Torsades de pointes is a form of VT characterized by QRS complexes that change amplitude and appearance (polymorphic) and appear to twist around the isoelectric line (Figure 10-16). The QRS complexes may deflect downward for a few beats and then upward for a few beats. When VF/pulseless VT cardiac arrest is associated with torsades de pointes, 1 to 2 g of magnesium sulfate diluted in 10 mL of D_5W is given IV/IO over 5 to 20 minutes. In nonarrest situations, a loading dose of 1 to 2 g mixed in 50 to 100 mL of D_5W is given over 5 to 60 minutes. Slower rates are recommended in a stable patient. The side effects of rapid magnesium administration include hypotension, asystole, flushing, and sweating. Serum magnesium levels are monitored to avoid hypermagnesemia.

Sodium Bicarbonate

A patient who has experienced an arrest quickly becomes acidotic. The acidosis results from two sources: (1) no blood flow during the arrest, and (2) no blood flow during CPR. Effective ventilation with supplemental oxygen and rapid restoration of tissue perfusion by CPR and spontaneous circulation are the best mechanisms to correct these causes of acidosis.

Limited data support the administration of sodium bicarbonate during cardiac arrest.[2] Sodium bicarbonate buffers the increased numbers of hydrogen ions

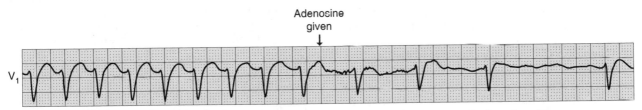

FIGURE 10-15. Atrioventricular block after intravenous administration of adenosine. *(From Paul, S., & Hebra, J. D. (1998). The nurse's guide to cardiac rhythm interpretation: Implications for patient care. Philadelphia: W. B. Saunders.)*

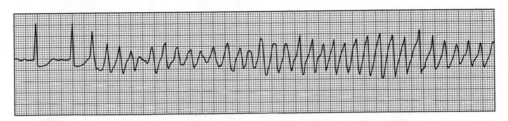

FIGURE 10-16. Torsades de pointes. The QRS complex seems to spiral around the isoelectric line. *(From Urden, L. D., Stacy, K. M., & Lough, M. E. [2006]. Thelan's critical care nursing. St. Louis: Mosby.)*

present in metabolic acidosis. It is beneficial in treating preexisting metabolic acidosis, hyperkalemia, or tricyclic antidepressant overdose.

The initial dosage of sodium bicarbonate is 1 mEq/kg by IV push. When possible, bicarbonate therapy should be guided by the bicarbonate concentration or calculated base deficit from arterial blood gas analysis or laboratory measurement. Sodium bicarbonate should not be mixed or infused with any other medication because it may precipitate or cause deactivation of other medications.

Dopamine (Intropin)

The indication for dopamine is symptomatic hypotension in the absence of hypovolemia. Its effects are dose related. At rates of 5 to 10 mcg/kg/min, myocardial contractility increases from alpha- and beta-adrenergic stimulation, causing enhanced cardiac contractility, increased cardiac output, increased heart rate, and increased blood pressure. At rates greater than 10 mcg/kg/min, systemic vascular resistance markedly increases as a result of generalized vasoconstriction produced from alpha-adrenergic stimulation. At doses greater than 20 mcg/kg/min, marked vasoconstriction and increases in myocardial contractility occur. Myocardial workload is increased without an increase in coronary blood supply, a situation that may cause myocardial ischemia.

Dopamine is administered by continuous IV infusion starting at 5 mcg/kg/min, and the dose is titrated upward. A dilution of 400 to 800 mg of dopamine in 250 to 500 mL of D_5W delivers 1600 to 3200 mcg/mL. The lowest dose necessary for blood pressure control should be used to minimize side effects and to ensure adequate perfusion of vital organs.

In addition to causing myocardial ischemia, dopamine may also cause cardiac dysrhythmias, such as tachycardia and premature ventricular contractions. Necrosis and sloughing of tissue may occur if the drug infiltrates; therefore it should be infused into a central line if possible. Phentolamine, 5 to 10 mg in 10 to 15 mL of NS, can be injected into the infiltrated area to prevent necrosis.

Calcium Chloride

Calcium increases the force of myocardial contraction. The only use of calcium chloride in a code is the treatment of underlying hypocalcemia, hyperkalemia, or calcium channel blocker toxicity that may be a cause of the cardiac arrest. Unless these conditions are present, calcium chloride should not be used in resuscitation efforts.

For hyperkalemia and calcium channel blocker overdose in a code, 8 to 16 mg/kg of a 10% solution is administered via IV push. (A 10-mL prefilled syringe of 10% calcium chloride yields 100 mg/mL.) This dose may be repeated if necessary. Calcium must be administered slowly to prevent bradycardia. Ventricular irritability and coronary or cerebral vasospasm may also occur after administration.

SPECIAL PROBLEMS DURING A CODE

In addition to electrical and pharmacological interventions carried out in a code, immediate treatment of the underlying cause of the arrest may be necessary. Tension pneumothorax and cardiac tamponade are two such problems that require rapid invasive therapeutic techniques.

GERIATRIC CONSIDERATIONS

- Many elderly patients in the hospital would not want their stated resuscitation preferences followed if they were to lose their decision-making capacity. They would prefer that their family and physician make resuscitation decisions for them.[21]
- Elderly patients have an increased incidence of complications from chest compressions, including rib fractures, sternal fractures, pneumothorax, and hemothorax.
- Declines in hepatic and renal functioning occur in the elderly that may result in higher-than-desired serum drug concentrations and adverse drug reactions with standard therapeutic dosing regimens.
- Beta-adrenergic receptors on the myocardium in the elderly are less responsive to changes in heart rate and cardiac contractility. Heart rate responses to beta-blocker (propranolol, metoprolol) and parasympathetic (atropine) medications are less.
- A decline in heart rate and slowing of conduction through the atrioventricular node result in a narrow therapeutic range for cardiovascular medications.
- Cardiopulmonary resuscitation is less likely to be effective in patients older than 70 years with comorbidities, unwitnessed arrest, terminal arrhythmias (asystole, pulseless electrical activity), cardiopulmonary resuscitation duration greater than 15 minutes, metastatic cancer, sepsis, pneumonia, renal failure, trauma, and acute and sustained hypotension.[22]

Tension Pneumothorax

A tension pneumothorax occurs when air enters the pleural space but cannot escape (Figure 10-17). Pressure increases in the pleural space and causes the lung to collapse. Tension pneumothorax is a life-threatening emergency. It may be caused by barotrauma from mechanical ventilation, blunt or penetrating trauma, or invasive procedures (i.e., placement of a central venous catheter) that inadvertently cause air to enter the pleural space. Symptoms of a tension pneumothorax include dyspnea, chest pain, tachypnea, tachycardia, and jugular venous distention. On assessment, breath sounds on the affected side are diminished, and the trachea may shift to the opposite side. If left untreated, the tension pneumothorax may progress and cause cardiovascular collapse and cardiac arrest. It is one of the causes of PEA, and therefore prompt assessment and treatment is essential. Because little time exists for radiographic confirmation, a needle may be inserted into the second or third anterior intercostal space on the affected side if tension pneumothorax is suspected. If air is under pressure in the pleural space, it will escape through the needle and make a hissing noise. As soon as possible after needle placement, a chest tube must be inserted to restore negative pressure in the chest and to reexpand the lung.

Pericardial Tamponade

Pericardial tamponade is the accumulation of fluid in the pericardial sac. The fluid causes a decrease in ventricular filling and results in decreased cardiac output. PEA or cardiac arrest may follow. Cardiac tamponade can be caused by such events as trauma, pericarditis, CPR, or invasive procedures. The patient with cardiac tamponade has increased central venous pressure, hypotension with narrowing of the arterial pulse pressure, and paradoxical pulse. Paradoxical pulse is the exaggerated fluctuation of arterial pressure during the respiratory cycle. It is defined as a peak systolic blood pressure drop of greater than 10 mm Hg during normal inspiration. Further assessment may reveal distant or muffled heart tones. Pericardiocentesis, or needle aspiration of pericardial fluid, is performed to alleviate the pressure around the heart. In addition, rapid administration of IV fluids (to increase preload and stroke volume) and drugs such as epinephrine or isoproterenol may be used temporarily to increase stroke volume and cardiac output.

DOCUMENTATION OF CODE EVENTS

A detailed chronological record of all interventions must be maintained during a code.[16] One of the first actions of the nurse team leader or nursing supervisor is to ensure that someone is assigned to record information throughout the code. Documentation includes the time the code is called, the time CPR is started, any actions that are taken, and the patient's response (e.g., presence or absence of a pulse, heart rate, blood pressure, cardiac rhythm). Intubation and defibrillation (and the energy used) must be

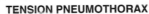

TENSION PNEUMOTHORAX

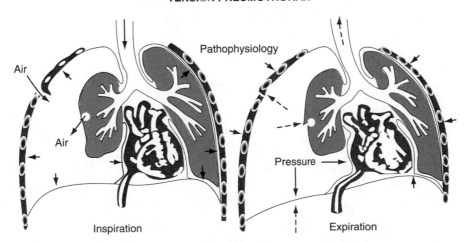

FIGURE 10-17. Tension pneumothorax. On inspiration, air enters the pleural space. On expiration, air is unable to escape the pleural space. Pressure increases, causing the lung on the affected side to collapse and the trachea to shift to the opposite side. *(From Alspach, J. G. [Ed.]. [2001]. AACN instructor's resource manual for the AACN core curriculum for critical care nursing [5th ed.]. Philadelphia: Saunders.)*

documented, along with the patient's response. The time and sites of IV initiations, types and amounts of fluids administered, and medications given to the patient are all accurately recorded. Rhythm strips are recorded to document events and response to treatment. Many hospitals have standardized code records (Figure 10-18) that list actions and medications and include spaces for the time of interventions and any comments. It is best if information can be recorded directly on the code record during the code to ensure that all information is obtained. The code record is signed by the code team and becomes part of the patient's permanent record.

CARE OF THE PATIENT AFTER RESUSCITATION

The survivor of a cardiac or respiratory arrest requires intensive monitoring and care. If not already in a critical care unit, the patient is transferred to one as soon as possible. Postresuscitation goals include optimizing tissue perfusion by airway and blood pressure maintenance, oxygenation, and control of dysrhythmias. Underlying abnormalities that may have caused the arrest, such as hypokalemia and myocardial ischemia, are corrected. See the Laboratory Alerts box, which summarizes critical electrolyte values associated with these conditions. These values are assessed and treated.

Oxygenation and acid-base status must also be assessed. Oxygen is given at a concentration of 100%. It is adjusted according to arterial blood gas and pulse oximetry values. A 12-lead ECG and chest x-ray study are done and compared with previous results. Dopamine or other pharmacological interventions may be required to maintain the systolic blood pressure at 90 mm Hg or greater. Blood pressure and heart rate are recorded at least every 30 minutes during continuous infusions of vasoactive medications. If antidysrhythmic drugs were used successfully during the code, additional doses may be repeated to achieve adequate blood levels, or continuous infusions may be administered for 24 hours. Other drugs may be given to improve cardiac output and myocardial oxygen supply. An arterial line and

---

LABORATORY ALERTS

Laboratory Test	Critical Value	Significance
Sodium (Na)	<136 or >145 mEq/L	Implications for polarization of heart muscle via Na-K pump

Potassium (K)	<3.5 or >5.3 mEq/L	Affects cardiac conduction and contraction
		Maintains cardiac cell homeostasis
		ECG:
		  Hypokalemia: depressed ST segments, flat or inverted T wave, presence of U wave
		  Hyperkalemia: tall, peaked T waves, disappearance of P waves, widening of QRS; can progress to asystole

Calcium (Ca)	<8.8 or >10.2 mg/dL	Affects cardiac cell action potential and contraction
		ECG:
		  Hypocalcemia: prolonged QT interval
		  Hypercalcemia: shortened QT interval

Magnesium (Mg)	<1.3 or >2.5 mEq/L	Affects contraction of cardiac muscle and promotes vasodilation that may reduce preload, alter cardiac output, and reduce systemic blood pressure
		ECG:
		  Hypomagnesemia: flat or inverted T waves, ST segment depression, prolonged QT interval
		  Hypermagnesemia: peaked T waves, bradycardia, signs of depressed contractility

ECG, Electrocardiogram.

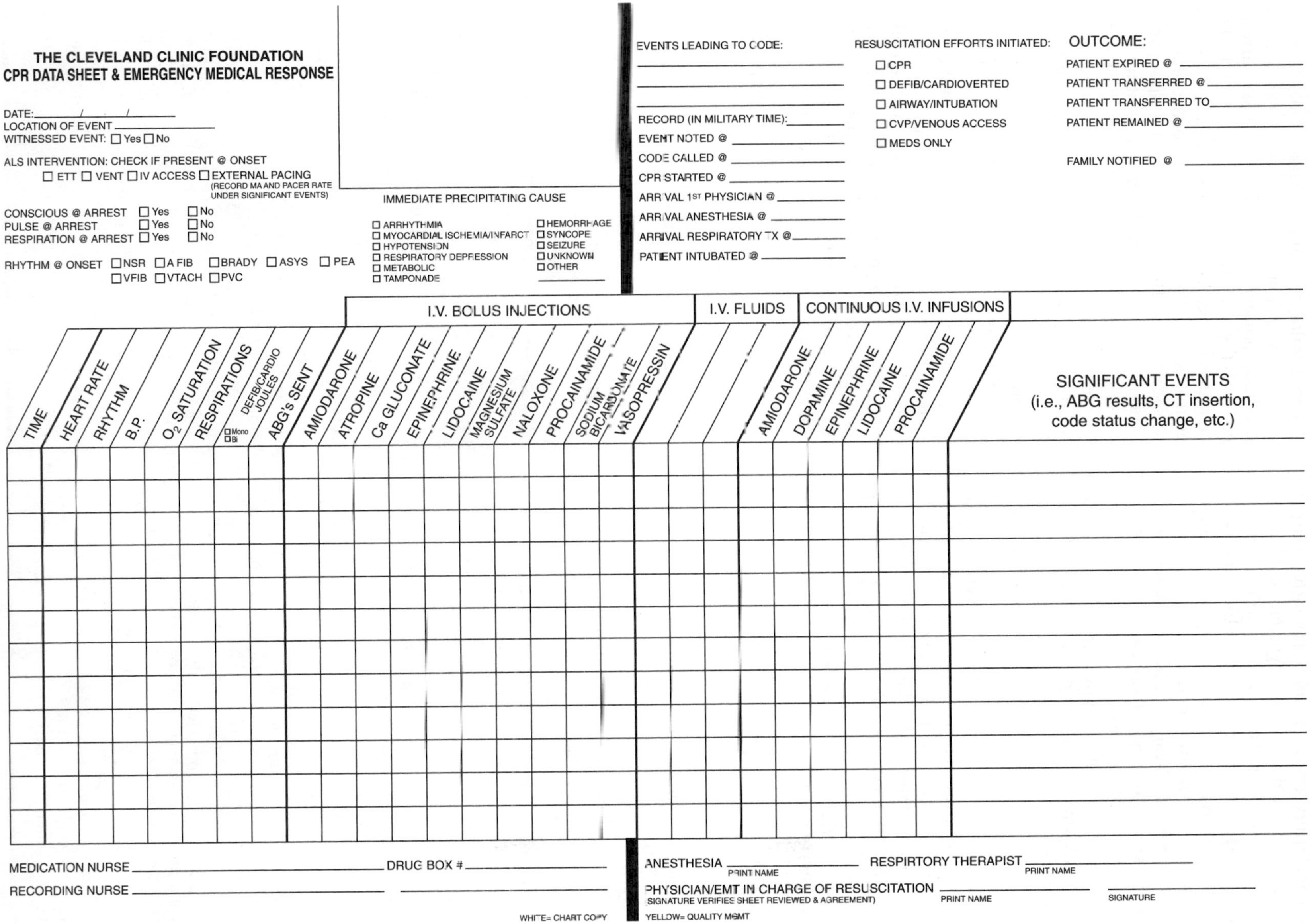

THE CLEVELAND CLINIC FOUNDATION
CPR DATA SHEET & EMERGENCY MEDICAL RESPONSE

DATE: _____
LOCATION OF EVENT: _____
WITNESSED EVENT: ☐ Yes ☐ No

ALS INTERVENTION: CHECK IF PRESENT @ ONSET
☐ ETT ☐ VENT ☐ IV ACCESS ☐ EXTERNAL PACING
(RECORD MA AND PACER RATE UNDER SIGNIFICANT EVENTS)

CONSCIOUS @ ARREST ☐ Yes ☐ No
PULSE @ ARREST ☐ Yes ☐ No
RESPIRATION @ ARREST ☐ Yes ☐ No

RHYTHM @ ONSET ☐ NSR ☐ A FIB ☐ BRADY ☐ ASYS ☐ PEA
☐ VFIB ☐ VTACH ☐ PVC

EVENTS LEADING TO CODE:
_____

RECORD (IN MILITARY TIME):
EVENT NOTED @ _____
CODE CALLED @ _____
CPR STARTED @ _____
ARRIVAL 1ST PHYSICIAN @ _____
ARRIVAL ANESTHESIA @ _____
ARRIVAL RESPIRATORY "X @ _____
PATIENT INTUBATED @ _____

IMMEDIATE PRECIPITATING CAUSE
☐ ARRHYTHMIA ☐ HEMORRHAGE
☐ MYOCARDIAL ISCHEMIA/INFARCT ☐ SYNCOPE
☐ HYPOTENSION ☐ SEIZURE
☐ RESPIRATORY DEPRESSION ☐ UNKNOWN
☐ METABOLIC ☐ OTHER
☐ TAMPONADE

RESUSCITATION EFFORTS INITIATED:
☐ CPR
☐ DEFIB/CARDIOVERTED
☐ AIRWAY/INTUBATION
☐ CVP/VENOUS ACCESS
☐ MEDS ONLY

OUTCOME:
PATIENT EXPIRED @ _____
PATIENT TRANSFERRED @ _____
PATIENT TRANSFERRED TO _____
PATIENT REMAINED @ _____
FAMILY NOTIFIED @ _____

SIGNIFICANT EVENTS
(i.e., ABG results, CT insertion, code status change, etc.)

I.V. BOLUS INJECTIONS
I.V. FLUIDS
CONTINUOUS I.V. INFUSIONS

TIME
HEART RATE
RHYTHM
B.P.
O₂ SATURATION
RESPIRATIONS
DEFIB/CARDIO JOULES
ABG's SENT
AMIODARONE
ATROPINE
CA GLUCONATE
EPINEPHRINE
LIDOCAINE
MAGNESIUM SULFATE
NALOXONE
PROCAINAMIDE
SODIUM BICARBONATE
VASOPRESSIN
AMIODARONE
DOPAMINE
EPINEPHRINE
LIDOCAINE
PROCAINAMIDE

DRUG BOX # _____

MEDICATION NURSE _____
RECORDING NURSE _____

ANESTHESIA _____ RESPIRTORY THERAPIST _____
PRINT NAME   PRINT NAME
PHYSICIAN/EMT IN CHARGE OF RESUSCITATION _____
SIGNATURE VERIFIES SHEET REVIEWED & AGREEMENT)   PRINT NAME   SIGNATURE
YELLOW= QUALITY MGMT

WHITE= CHART COPY

FIGURE 10-18. Sample of a code record used for documenting activities during a code. (Courtesy of Cleveland Clinic, Cleveland, OH.)

pulmonary artery catheters are frequently inserted after a code to facilitate hemodynamic assessment and patient treatment. An indwelling urinary catheter is inserted to monitor urinary output hourly. A nasogastric tube is inserted if bowel sounds are absent and in patients with a decreased level of consciousness who are mechanically ventilated. Management of patient care continues to focus on the differential diagnosis to identify reversible causes of the arrest and the underlying pathophysiology.

Emotional support is an important aspect of care after an arrest. Fear of death or of a recurrence of the arrest is common. Survivors often feel the need to discuss their experience in depth, and nurses should listen objectively and provide psychological support. In addition to the patient, many other people are affected when a code occurs. Family members, roommates and other patients, and staff members are all affected by the emergency.

Therapeutic Hypothermia After Cardiac Arrest

Studies have indicated that fever resulting from brain injury or ischemia exacerbates the degree of permanent neurological damage after cardiac arrest and contributes to an increased length of stay. The higher the body temperature is after a cardiac arrest, the poorer is the neurological recovery. Lower body temperature after cardiac arrest is associated with better neurological recovery.[27] (See Evidence-Based Practice feature on Therapeutic Hypothermia.) Induced hypothermia to a core body temperature of 32°C to 34°C for 12 to 24 hours may be beneficial in reducing neurological impairment after cardiac arrest.[6,23] Hypothermia decreases the metabolic rate by 6% to 7% for every decrease of 1°C in temperature. Because cerebral metabolic rate for oxygen is the main determinant of cerebral blood flow, inducing hypothermia may improve oxygen supply and reduce oxygen consumption in the ischemic brain. The AHA advocates induction of hypothermia after a cardiac arrest if a patient is unresponsive but has adequate blood pressure.[2] Patients may be cooled with ice packs, cooling blankets, specialized cooling pads that adhere to the skin, and cool IV fluids, or through an endovascular device using a femoral catheter and an external heat exchange system. Although hypothermia should be initiated as soon as possible after resuscitation, the optimal duration of hypothermia has not been

EVIDENCE-BASED PRACTICE
Therapeutic Hypothermia

PROBLEM

Patients often suffer neurological damage after surviving cardiac arrest, despite resuscitative efforts. Therapeutic hypothermia has been increasingly used in survivors of cardiac arrest.

QUESTION

Does induced hypothermia improve neurological recovery in patients who survive a cardiac arrest.

REFERENCES

Cheung, K.W., Green, R. S., & Magee, K. D. (2006). Systematic review of randomized controlled trials of therapeutic hypothermia as a neuroprotectant in post cardiac arrest patients. Canadian Journal of Emergency Medicine, 8, 329-337.

Holzer, M., Bernard, S. A., Hachimi-Idrissi, S., et al. (2005). Hypothermia for neuroprotection after cardiac arrest: Systematic review and individual patient data meta-analysis. *Critical Care Medicine, 33,* 414-418.

EVIDENCE

Cheung and colleagues reviewed the results of four studies that evaluated a total of 436 patients; 232 received therapeutic hypothermia. Hypothermia was defined as cooling to a temperature of 32 to 34 degrees Celsius. Results found that hypothermia reduced in-hospital mortality by 25% (RR = .75) and the incidence of poor neurological outcome (RR = .74). Similarly, Holzer and colleagues evaluated three randomized trials on therapeutic hypothermia. In addition to finding that more patients were discharged with better neurological recovery, they reported that one study showed survival to six months with favorable neurological recovery (RR = 1.44).

IMPLICATIONS FOR NURSING

Patients who survive cardiac arrest but remain comatose may benefit from early intervention with therapeutic hypothermia. Nurses must assist in identifying candidates who meet criteria for this intervention. In addition, they must be knowledgeable of the preferred methods for cooling in their institution, cool the patient to the desired level of hypothermia, provide medications to support patient comfort during hypothermia, and rewarm the patient gradually according to established protocols. Skills in neurological assessment before, during, and after the procedure are also essential.

defined. Rewarming should proceed slowly to avoid sudden vasodilation, hypotension, and shock.[13] Refer to Chapter 13 for more discussion on therapeutic hypothermia.

Family Presence during Resuscitation

In the past, family members were not given the opportunity to be present at the bedside during resuscitation. However, research now supports the benefits of family presence during a code. Families who have been present during a code describe the benefits as knowing that everything possible was being done for their loved one, feeling supportive and helpful to the patient and staff, sustaining patient-family relationships, providing a sense of closure on a life shared together, and facilitating the grief process.[2,10,11,19,20] In a prospective study by Meyers and colleagues[20] and Eichhorn and associates,[9] approximately one third of patients' family members did not want to be present during resuscitation in the emergency department. However, 100% of those who were present said that they would choose to do it again. Many health care providers are uncomfortable with having patients' families present during a code, but they often support the practice after they have experienced it. (See Evidence-Based Practice feature on Code Management.)

Several organizations have made formal statements in support of family presence during

---

EVIDENCE-BASED PRACTICE
Code Management

PROBLEM

Family presence during cardiopulmonary resuscitation has been advocated by many professional organizations as well as family members. Nurses and other health care providers are not always in support of this recommendation.

QUESTION

What are the outcomes and issues associated with family presence during cardiopulmonary resuscitation?

REFERENCES

Critchell, C. D., & Marik, P. E. (2007). Should family members be present during cardiopulmonary resuscitation? A review of the literature. *American Journal of Hospice and Palliative Care Medicine, 24,* 311-317.
Fullbrook, P., Latour, J., Albarran, J., de Graaf, W., Lynch, F., Devictor, D., et al. (2007). The presence of family members during cardiopulmonary resuscitation: European Federation of Critical Care Nursing Associations, European Society of Paediatric and Neonatal Intensive Care and European Society of Cardiology Council on Cardiovascular Nursing and Allied Professions joint position statement. *Nursing in Critical Care, 12,* 250-252.
Halm, M. (2005). Family presence during resuscitation: A critical review of the literature. *American Journal of Critical Care, 14,* 494-512.

EVIDENCE

Numerous research studies, both qualitative and quantitative, were evaluated by these research teams. Issues addressed by health care team members include lack of space, violation of patient's confidentiality, not enough staff, stress on staff, family members losing control or the event being too traumatic, difficulty terminating resuscitation efforts, and increased risk for litigation. Most of the concerns have not been substantiated in studies. Many benefits of family presence have been reported for the staff: increased professional behavior of staff members during codes, increased staff member involvement with family members, and increased opportunities to provide family support. Family members have benefited most from their presence, including participating in care at end of life, removing doubt about the circumstances of the code, better grieving and acceptance of death, and a sense of closure.

NURSING IMPLICATIONS

Programs that allow the family to be present during codes will continue to be implemented in hospitals. Family members will likely expect to be present during codes (and invasive procedures) as more research is disseminated. Protocols and procedures must be developed that include a mechanism for supporting the family while allowing essential team members to implement resuscitation efforts. Family members should be offered a choice and not be mandated to be present during a code, and adequate psychosocial support must be available to them throughout the code. The European position statement is applicable to practice in the United States. That statement advocates the following: patients have the right to family presence; family members should be offered the opportunity to be present during a code; one code team member should be available to provide psychosocial support to family members; counseling should be available to family members who have witnessed resuscitation efforts; and debriefing should be available to all health care professionals who participated in the code efforts.

resuscitation.[1,2,8,10,11,14] These organizations advocate a carefully structured protocol that supports family presence during CPR and invasive procedures and supports the patient's wishes, if known, not to have family members present. The protocol should designate a specially trained staff member to prepare families for being at the bedside and supporting them before, during, and after the event, including handling untoward reactions by family members.

Decisions regarding family presence should be made on an individual basis, considering individual preferences and assessment of coping mechanisms.[10,11,25] If family members are not in the patient's room during resuscitation, a staff member, chaplain, volunteer, or friend should remain with them during this time and keep them informed of the patient's progress. Honesty is crucial, and it is important that they know that their family member is receiving the best possible care. If the family is not in the facility during the code, the next of kin should be called as soon as possible and informed of the patient's critical status.

If the patient is successfully resuscitated, the family should be allowed to see the patient as soon as is feasible. Communication regarding the events and status of the patient is extremely important. If the patient does not survive, the family should be encouraged to see the patient if they were not present during the code to facilitate the grief process.

All efforts should be made to remove roommates from the scene. If this is not feasible, the curtains should be drawn. These patients may experience fear and usually want to talk about the experience. As do the survivor and family members, they require emotional support. Patient privacy must also be protected; it suffices to tell curious patients that an emergency is in progress. It is also easy to overlook other patients and their needs during a code. If staff members are not performing a specific role in the code, they should clear the area and tend to other patients.

Staff members are also affected by a code. In addition to the grief that may be felt over the loss of a patient, guilt, anger, and anxiety may also be felt. Debriefings are helpful for the staff involved in a code. In these sessions, feelings and thoughts can be discussed. This is also an opportunity to critique the code and to learn what may be useful next time.

Rapid Response Teams

Rapid response teams (RRTs) or medical emergency teams focus on addressing changes in a patient's clinical condition before a cardiopulmonary arrest occurs. Research has demonstrated that up to 80% of patients having an in-hospital cardiac arrest have signs of physiological instability as evidenced by changes in heart rate, blood pressure, and/or respiratory status in the 24 hours before cardiac arrest.[12,15,18] Implementation of RRTs has been identified to prevent in-hospital arrests, improve patient outcomes, and prevent avoidable deaths.[17]

The goal of the RRT is to ensure that interventions are available quickly when patient conditions become unstable before an actual cardiac arrest. RRT staff should be available in the hospital 24 hours a day, 7 days a week to assess and intervene on patients outside the critical care unit, as well as support and educate the nursing staff in these areas.[24] Composition of the RRT can vary— some are composed of a critical care nurse, a respiratory therapist, and a physician. Other members may include an acute care nurse practitioner, a clinical nurse specialist, or a physician assistant. The RRT may be called upon any time a staff member is concerned about a patient's condition, such as changes in heart rate, systolic blood pressure, respiratory rate, pulse oximetry saturation, mental status, urinary output, or changes in laboratory values. Some institutions encourage family members to activate the RRT if they identify a change in the patient's condition.

The development of criteria to facilitate early identification of physiological deterioration helps nurses to determine whether the RRT should be called for a bedside consultation. ACLS algorithms, standing medical orders, and evidence-based protocols guide interventions used by the RRT. Research on the use of RRTs has demonstrated a reduction in cardiac arrests, a reduction in critical care unit length of stay, and a reduction in the incidence of acute illness, such as respiratory failure, stroke, severe sepsis, and acute renal failure.[5,7,26]

SUMMARY

Positive patient outcomes depend on the health care team members' ability to recognize problems rapidly and to intervene effectively. When a patient has a cardiac or respiratory arrest, or both, in the hospital, BLS and ACLS measures must be initiated immediately. How the code team functions and how interventions are carried out affect the patient's potential for recovery. Thus code management is an important topic for anyone involved in the care of patients, especially those in critical care areas.

CRITICAL THINKING QUESTIONS evolve

1. Discuss nursing strategies to be implemented during and after a code to provide psychosocial support to family members of patients suffering a cardiopulmonary arrest.
2. A surgical patient on a general nursing unit has just been successfully defibrillated with the use of an AED by the nursing staff. He is being manually ventilated with a BVD. Identify the current nursing priorities and their rationales.
3. You are the second nurse to respond to a code. The first nurse is administering CPR. Describe your first actions and their rationales.
4. Your patient has a permanent pacemaker or ICD. How would care and treatment of this patient differ in a code situation?
5. Some hospitals are now considering allowing family members to be present during a code.
   a. How could the presence of family members affect the management of the code?
   b. What factors should you consider before permitting family members to be present?

---

evolve Be sure to check out the bonus material, including free self-assessment exercises, on the Evolve Web site at http://evolve.elsevier.com/Sole.

REFERENCES

1. AACN. (2004). *AACN practice alert: Family presence during CPR and invasive procedures*. Retrieved October 22, 2007, from www.aacn.org/AACN/practiceAlert. nsf/Files/Family%20Presence%20During%20CPR%20and%20Invasive%20Procedures/$file/AACN.PracticeAlert.Family%20Presence.
2. American Heart Association. (2005). 2005 American Heart Association guidelines for cardiopulmonary resuscitation and emergency cardiovascular care. *Circulation, 112*(24 Suppl.), IV-1–IV-211.
3. American Heart Association. (2006). *Advanced cardiac life support provider manual*. Dallas, TX: Author.
4. American Heart Association. (2006). *BLS for healthcare providers*. Dallas, TX: Author.
5. Bellomo, R., Goldsmith, D., Uchino, S., et al. (2004). Prospective controlled trial of effect of an emergency team on postoperative morbidity and mortality rates. *Critical Care Medicine, 32*(4), 916-921.
6. Bernard, S. A., Gray, T. W., Buist, M. D., et al. (2002). Treatment of comatose survivors of out-of-hospital cardiac arrest with induced hypothermia. *New England Journal of Medicine, 346*(8), 557-563.
7. Buist, M. D., Moore, G. E., Bernard, S. A., et al. (2002). Effect of a medical emergency team on reduction of incidence of and mortality from unexpected cardiac arrests in hospital: Preliminary study. *British Medical Journal, 324*(7334), 387-390.
8. Davidson, J. E., Powers, K., Hedayat, K. M., et al. (2007). Clinical practice guidelines for support of the family in the patient-centered intensive care unit: American College of Critical Care Medicine Task Force 2004-2005. *Critical Care Medicine, 35*(2), 605-622.
9. Eichhorn, D. J., Meyers, T. A., Guzzetta, C. E., et al. (2001). Family presence during invasive procedures and resuscitation: Hearing the voice of the patient. *American Journal of Nursing, 101*(5), 48-55.
10. Emergency Nurses Association. (2001a). *Family presence at the bedside during invasive procedures and/or resuscitation* [ENA position statement]. Des Plaines, IL: Author.
11. Emergency Nurses Association. (2001b). *Presenting the option for family presence* (2nd ed.). Des Plaines, IL: Author (www.ena.org).
12. Franklin, C., & Mathew, J. (1994). Developing strategies to prevent in-hospital cardiac arrest: Analyzing responses of physicians and nurses in the hours before the event. *Critical Care Medicine, 22*(2), 244-247.
13. Geocadin, R. G., Koenig, M. A., Stevens, R. D., et al. (2007). Intensive care for brain injury after cardiac arrest: Therapeutic hypothermia and related neuroprotective strategies. *Critical Care Clinics, 22*, 619-636.
14. Halm, M. A. (2005). Family presence during resuscitation: A critical review of the literature. *American Journal of Critical Care, 14*(6), 494-511.
15. Hillman, K. M., Bristow, P. J., Chey, T., et al. (2001). Antecedents to hospital deaths. *Internal Medicine Journal, 31*, 343-348.
16. Howard, P. K. (2005). Documentation of resuscitation events. *Critical Care Nursing Clinics of North America, 17*(1), 39-43.
17. Institute for Healthcare Improvement. *Rapid response teams*. Retrieved October 25, 2007, from www.ihi.org/IHI/Programs/Campaign/Campaign.htm.
18. Krause, J., Smith, G., Prytherch, D., et al. (2004). A comparison of antecedents to cardiac arrests, deaths, and emergency intensive care admissions in Australia, New Zealand, and the United Kingdom. The ACA-DEMIA study. *Resuscitation, 62*(3), 275-282.
19. MacLean, S. L., Guzzetta, C. E., White, C., et al. (2003). Family presence during cardiopulmonary resuscitation and invasive procedures: Practices of critical care and emergency nurses. *American Journal of Critical Care, 12*(3), 246-257.

20. Meyers, T. A., Eichhorn, D. J., Guzzetta, C. E., et al. (2000). Family presence during invasive procedures and resuscitation: The experience of family members, nurses, and physicians. *American Journal of Nursing, 100*(2), 32-42.

21. Puchalski, C. M., Zhong, Z., Jacobs, M. M., et al. (2000). Patients who want their family and physician to make resuscitation decisions for them: Observations from SUPPORT and HELP. *Journal of the American Geriatrics Society, 48*(Suppl. 5), S84-S90.

22. Robinson, E. M. (2002). Ethical analysis of cardiopulmonary resuscitation for elders in acute care. *AACN Clinical Issues, 13*(1), 132-144.

23. The Hypothermia after Cardiac Arrest Study Group. (2002). Mild therapeutic hypothermia to improve the neurologic outcome after cardiac arrest. *New England Journal of Medicine, 346*(8), 549-556.

24. Thomas, K., Force, M. V., Rasmussen, D., et al. (2007). Rapid response teams: Challenges, solutions, and benefits. *Critical Care Nurse, 27*(1), 20-27.

25. Tucker, T. L. (2002). Family presence during resuscitation. *Critical Care Clinics of North America, 14*(2), 177-185.

26. Winters, B. D., Pham, J. C., Hunt, E. A., et al. (2007). Rapid response systems: A systematic review. *Critical Care Medicine, 35*(5), 1238-1243.

27. Zeiner, A., Holzer, M., Sterz, F., et al. (2001). Hyperthermia after cardiac arrest is associated with an unfavorable neurologic outcome. *Archives of Internal Medicine, 161*(16), 2007-2012.

PART III

Nursing Care during Critical Illness

CHAPTER 11

Shock, Sepsis, and Multiple Organ Dysfunction Syndrome

Robin Donohoe Dennison, DNP, RN, CCNS

INTRODUCTION

Shock is a clinical syndrome characterized by inadequate tissue perfusion that results in cellular, metabolic, and hemodynamic derangements. Impaired tissue perfusion occurs when there is an imbalance between cellular oxygen supply and cellular oxygen demand. Shock can result from ineffective cardiac function, inadequate blood volume, or inadequate vascular tone. The effects of shock are not isolated to one organ system; instead, all body systems may be affected. Shock can progress to organ failure and death unless compensatory mechanisms reverse the process, or clinical interventions are successfully implemented. Shock frequently results in systemic inflammatory response syndrome (SIRS) and multiple organ dysfunction syndrome (MODS). There are many different causes of shock and a variety of clinical manifestations. Patient responses to shock and treatment strategies vary, thus presenting a challenge to the health care team in assessment and management.

This chapter discusses the various clinical conditions that create the shock state including hypovolemia, cardiogenic shock, distributive shock (anaphylactic, neurogenic, and septic shock), and obstructive shock. The progression of shock to SIRS and MODS is also described. The pathophysiology, clinical presentation, and definitive and supportive management of each type of shock state are reviewed.

REVIEW OF ANATOMY AND PHYSIOLOGY

The cardiovascular system is a closed, interdependent system composed of the heart, blood, and vascular bed. Arteries, arterioles, capillaries, venules, and veins make up the vascular bed. The micro-circulation, the portion of the vascular bed between the arterioles and the venules, is the most significant portion of the circulatory system for cell survival. Its functions are the delivery of oxygen and nutrients to cells, the removal of waste products of cellular metabolism, and the regulation of blood volume. In addition, the vessels of the microcirculation constrict or dilate selectively to regulate blood flow to cells in need of oxygen and nutrients.

The structure of the microcirculation differs according to the function of the tissues and organs it supplies; however, all of the vascular beds have common structural characteristics (Figure 11-1). As oxygenated blood leaves the left side of the heart and enters the aorta, it flows through progressively smaller arteries until it flows into an arteriole. Arterioles are lined with smooth muscle, which allows these small vessels to change diameter and, as a result, to direct and adjust blood flow to the capillaries. From the arteriole, blood enters a metarteriole, a smaller vessel that branches from the arteriole at right angles. Metarterioles are partially lined with smooth muscle, which also allows them to adjust diameter size and to regulate blood flow into capillaries.

Blood next enters the capillary network by passing through a muscular precapillary sphincter. Capillaries are narrow, thin-walled vascular networks that branch off the metarterioles. This network configuration increases the surface area to allow for greater fluid and nutrient exchange. It also decreases the velocity of the blood flow to prolong transport time through the capillaries. Capillaries have no contractile ability and are not responsive to vasoactive chemicals, electrical or mechanical stimulation, or pressure across their walls. The precapillary sphincter is the only means of regulating blood flow into a capillary. When the precapillary sphincter constricts, blood flow is diverted away from a capillary bed and directed to one that supplies tissues in need of oxygen and nutrients. The capillary bed lies close to the cells of the body, a position that facilitates the delivery of oxygen and nutrients to the cells.

Once nutrients are exchanged for cellular waste products in the capillaries, blood enters a venule. These small muscular vessels are able to dilate and constrict, offering postcapillary resistance for the regulation of blood flow through capillaries. Blood then flows from the venule and enters the larger veins of the venous system. Another component of the microcirculation consists of the arteriovenous anastomoses that connect arterioles directly to venules. These muscular vessels are able to shunt blood away from the capillary circulation and send it directly to tissues in need of oxygen and nutrients.

Blood pressure is determined by cardiac output and systemic vascular resistance (SVR). Blood pressure is decreased whenever cardiac output (hypovolemic, cardiogenic, or obstructive shock) or SVR (neurogenic, anaphylactic, or septic shock) is decreased. Changing pressures within the vessels as blood moves from an area of high pressure within the arteries and passes to the venous system, which has lower pressures, facilitate the flow of blood. The force of resistance opposes blood flow; thus as resistance increases, blood flow decreases. Resistance is determined by three factors: (1) vessel length, (2) blood viscosity, and (3) vessel diameter. Increased resistance occurs with increased vessel length, increased blood viscosity, and decreased blood vessel diameter. Vessel diameter is the most important determinant of resistance.

As the pressure of blood within the vessel decreases, the diameter of the vessel decreases, resulting in decreased blood flow. The critical closing pressure and the resultant cessation of blood flow occur when blood pressure decreases to a point at which it is no longer able to keep the vessel open.

The delivery of oxygen to tissues and cells is required for the production of cellular energy (adenosine triphosphate [ATP]). The delivery of oxygen (DO_2) requires an adequate hemoglobin level to carry oxygen, adequate functioning of the lungs to oxygenate the blood and saturate the hemoglobin (SaO_2), and adequate cardiac functioning (cardiac output) to transport the oxygenated blood to the tissues and cells. Any impairment in the DO_2, or any increase in the consumption of oxygen by the tissues (VO_2), causes a decrease in oxygen reserve (as indicated by the mixed venous oxygen saturation [SvO_2]), which may result in tissue hypoxia, depletion of the supply of ATP, lactic acidosis, organ dysfunction, and potentially death.

Pathophysiology

Diverse events can initiate the shock syndrome. Shock begins when the cardiovascular system fails to function properly because of an alteration in at least one of the four essential circulatory components: blood volume, myocardial contractility, blood flow, or vascular resistance. Under healthy circumstances, these components function together to maintain circulatory homeostasis. When one of these components fails, the others compensate. However, as compensatory mechanisms fail, or if more than one of the circulatory components is affected, a state of shock ensues. Shock states are classified according to which one of these components is adversely affected (Table 11-1).

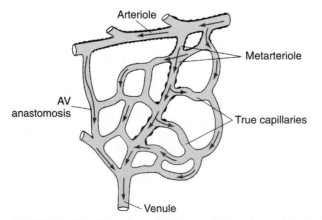

FIGURE 11-1. Microcirculation. *AV*, Arteriovenous. *(From Perry, A. G., & Potter, P. A. [1983]. Shock: Comprehensive nursing management. St. Louis: Mosby.)*

TABLE 11-1	Classification of Shock
Type of Shock	**Physiological Alteration**
Hypovolemic	Inadequate intravascular volume
Cardiogenic	Inadequate myocardial contractility
Obstructive	Obstruction of blood flow

Distributive
  Anaphylactic
  Neurogenic
  Septic
	Inadequate vascular tone

Shock is not a single clinical entity but a life-threatening response to alterations in circulation resulting in impaired tissue perfusion. As the delivery of adequate oxygen and nutrients decreases, impaired cellular metabolism occurs. Cells convert from aerobic to anaerobic metabolism. Less energy in the form of ATP is produced. Lactic acid, a byproduct of anaerobic metabolism, causes tissue acidosis. Cells in all organ systems require energy to function, and this resultant tissue acidosis causes impaired cellular metabolism. Shock is not selective in its effects—all cells, tissues, and organ systems suffer as a result of the physiological response to the stress of shock and decreased tissue perfusion. The end result is organ dysfunction because of decreased blood flow through the capillaries that supply the cells with oxygen and nutrients (Figure 11-2).

Stages of Shock

Although the response to shock is highly individualized, a pattern of stages progresses at unpredictable rates. If each stage of shock is not recognized and treated promptly, progression to the next stage occurs. The pathophysiological events and associated clinical findings for each stage are summarized in Table 11-2.

Stage I: Initiation
The process of shock is initiated by subclinical hypoperfusion that is caused by inadequate DO_2, inadequate extraction of oxygen, or both. No obvious clinical indications of hypoperfusion are noted in this stage although hemodynamic alterations, such as a decrease in cardiac output, are noted if invasive hemodynamic monitoring is used for patient assessment.

Stage II: Compensatory Stage
The sustained reduction in tissue perfusion initiates a set of neural, endocrine, and chemical compensatory mechanisms in an attempt to maintain blood flow to vital organs and to restore homeostasis. During this stage, symptoms become apparent, but shock may still be reversed with minimal morbidity if appropriate interventions are initiated.

Neural Compensation. Baroreceptors (which are sensitive to pressure changes) and chemoreceptors (which are sensitive to chemical changes) located in the carotid sinus and aortic arch detect the reduction in arterial blood pressure. Impulses are relayed to the vasomotor center in the medulla oblongata, stimulating the sympathetic branch of the autonomic nervous system to release epinephrine and norepinephrine from the adrenal medulla. In response to this catecholamine release, the heart rate and contractility increase to improve cardiac output. Dilation of the coronary arteries occurs to increase perfusion to the myocardium to meet the increased demands for oxygen. Systemic vasoconstriction and redistribution of blood occurs. Arterial vasoconstriction improves blood pressure, whereas venous vasoconstriction augments venous return to the heart, increasing preload and cardiac output. Blood is shunted from the kidneys, gastrointestinal tract, and skin to the heart and brain. Bronchial smooth muscles relax, and respiratory rate and depth are increased, improving gas exchange and oxygenation. Additional catecholamine effects include increased blood glucose levels as the liver is stimulated to convert glycogen to glucose for energy production; dilation of pupils; and peripheral vasoconstriction and increased sweat gland activity resulting in cool, moist skin.

Endocrine Compensation. In response to the reduction in blood pressure, messages are also relayed to the hypothalamus, which stimulates the anterior and posterior pituitary gland. The anterior pituitary gland releases adrenocorticotropic hormone (ACTH), which acts on the adrenal cortex to release glucocorticoids and mineralocorticoids (i.e., aldosterone). Glucocorticoids increase the blood glucose level by increasing the conversion of glycogen to glucose (glycogenolysis) and causing the conversion of fat and protein to glucose (gluconeogenesis). Mineralocorticoids act on the renal tubules causing the reabsorption of sodium and water, resulting in increased intravascular volume and blood pressure. The renin-angiotensin-aldosterone system (Figure 11-3) is stimulated by a reduction of pressure in the renal arterioles of the kidneys and/or by a decrease in sodium levels as sensed by the kidney's juxtaglomerular apparatus. In response to decreased renal perfusion, the juxtaglomerular apparatus releases renin. Renin circulates in the blood and reacts with angiotensinogen to produce angiotensin I. Angiotensin I circulates through the lungs, where it forms angiotensin II, a potent arterial and venous vasoconstrictor that increases blood pressure and improves venous return to the heart. Angiotensin II also activates the adrenal cortex to release aldosterone.

Antidiuretic hormone (ADH) is released by the posterior pituitary gland in response to the increased osmolality of the blood that occurs in shock. The overall effects of endocrine compensation result in an attempt to combat shock by providing the body with glucose for energy and by increasing the intravascular blood volume.

Text continued on p. 270

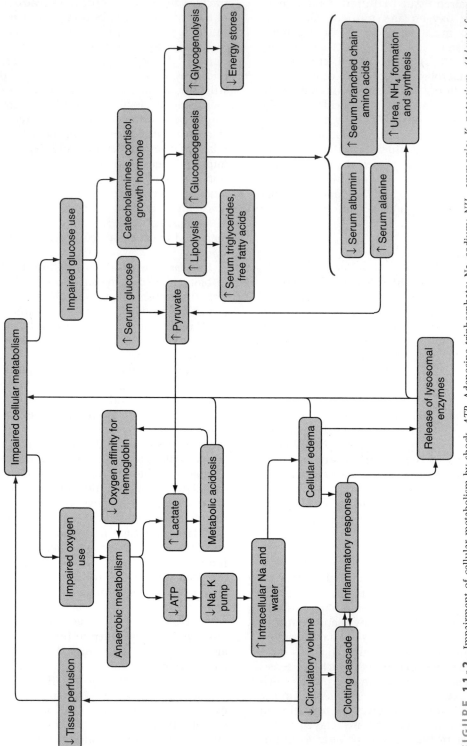

FIGURE 11-2. Impairment of cellular metabolism by shock. *ATP,* Adenosine triphosphate; Na, sodium; *NH₄,* ammonia; *K,* potassium. *(Adapted from McCance, K. L., & Huether, S. E. [2006]. Pathophysiology. The biologic basis for disease in adults and children [5th ed.]. St. Louis: Mosby.)*

TABLE 11-2 Stages of Shock

Stage of Shock	Physiological Events	Clinical Presentation

I: Initiation	↓ Tissue oxygenation caused by:
	  ↓ Intravascular volume (hypovolemic)
	  ↓ Myocardial contractility (cardiogenic)
	  Obstruction to blood flow (obstructive)
	  ↓ Vascular tone (distributive)
	  Septic (mediator release)
	  Anaphylactic (histamine release)
	  Neurogenic (suppression of SNS)
		No observable clinical indications
		↓ CO may be noted with invasive hemodynamic monitoring

II: Compensatory	Neural compensation by SNS
	  ↑ Heart rate and contractility
	  Vasoconstriction
	  Redistribution of blood flow from nonessential to essential organs
	  Bronchodilation
	Endocrine compensation (RAAS, ADH, glucocorticoids release)
	  Renal reabsorption of sodium, chloride, and water
	  Vasoconstriction
	  Glycogenolysis and gluconeogenesis
	Chemical compensation
		↑ Heart rate (except neurogenic)
		Narrowed pulse pressure
		Rapid, deep breathing causing respiratory alkalosis
		Thirst
		Cool, moist skin
		Oliguria
		Diminished bowel sounds
		Restlessness progressing to confusion
		Hyperglycemia
		↑ Urine specific gravity and ↓ creatinine clearance

III: Progressive	Progressive tissue hypoperfusion Anaerobic metabolism with lactic acidosis Failure of sodium-potassium pump Cellular edema	Dysrhythmias ↓ BP with narrowed pulse pressure Tachypnea Cold, clammy skin Anuria Absent bowel sounds Lethargy progressing to coma Hyperglycemia ↑ BUN, creatinine, and potassium Respiratory and metabolic acidosis
IV: Refractory	Severe tissue hypoxia with ischemia and necrosis Worsening acidosis SIRS MODS	Life-threatening dysrhythmias Severe hypotension despite vasopressors Respiratory and metabolic acidosis Acute respiratory failure Acute respiratory distress syndrome Disseminated intravascular coagulation Hepatic dysfunction/failure Renal failure Myocardial ischemia/infarction/failure Cerebral ischemia/infarction

ADH, Antidiuretic hormone; *BP*, blood pressure; *BUN*, blood urea nitrogen; *CO*, cardiac output; *MODS*, multiple organ dysfunction syndrome; *RAAS*, renin-angiotensin-aldosterone system; *SIRS*, systemic inflammatory response syndrome; *SNS*, sympathetic nervous system.

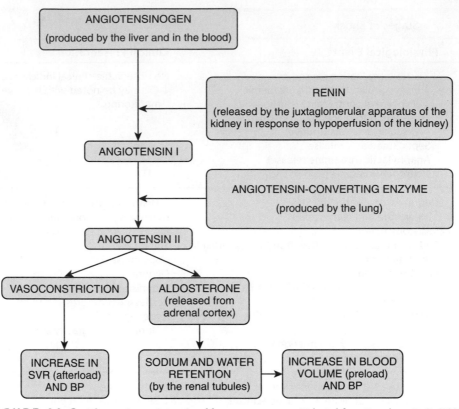

FIGURE 11-3. The renin-angiotensin-aldosterone system. *(Adapted from Dennison, R. D. [2007]. Pass CCRN! [3rd ed.]. St. Louis: Mosby.)*
BP, Blood pressure; *SVR,* systemic vascular resistance.

Chemical Compensation. As pulmonary blood flow is reduced, ventilation-perfusion imbalances occur. Initially alveolar ventilation is adequate, but the perfusion of blood through the alveolar capillary bed is decreased. Chemoreceptors located in the aorta and carotid arteries are stimulated in response to this low oxygen tension in the blood. Consequently, the rate and depth of respirations increase. As the patient hyperventilates, carbon dioxide is excreted and respiratory alkalosis occurs. A reduction in carbon dioxide levels and the alkalotic state cause vasoconstriction of cerebral blood vessels. This vasoconstriction, coupled with the reduced oxygen tension, may lead to cerebral hypoxia and ischemia. The overall effects of chemical compensation result in an attempt to combat shock by increasing oxygen supply; however, cerebral perfusion may decrease.

Stage III: Progressive Stage

If the cause of hypoperfusion is not corrected or if the compensatory mechanisms continue without reversing the shock, profound hypoperfusion results, with further patient deterioration. The systemic circulation continues to vasoconstrict. Although this effect shunts blood to vital organs, the decrease in blood flow leads to ischemia in the extremities, weak or absent pulses, and altered body defenses. Prolonged vasoconstriction results in decreased capillary blood flow and cellular hypoxia. The cells convert to anaerobic metabolism, producing lactic acid, which leads to metabolic acidosis. Anaerobic metabolism produces less ATP than aerobic metabolism, which reduces the energy available for cellular metabolism. The lack of ATP also causes failure of the sodium-potassium pump. Sodium and water accumulate within the cell, resulting in cellular swelling and a further reduction in cellular function.

The microcirculation exerts the opposite effect and dilates to increase the blood supply to meet local tissue needs. Whereas the arterioles remain constricted in an attempt to keep vital organs perfused, the precapillary sphincters relax, allowing blood to flow into the capillary bed. Meanwhile, postcapillary sphincters remain constricted. As a result, blood flows freely into the capillary bed but accumulates in the capillaries as blood flow exiting the capillary bed is impeded. Capillary hydrostatic pressure increases, and fluid is pushed from the capillaries into the interstitial space, causing interstitial edema. This intravascular to interstitial fluid shift is further aggravated by the release of histamine and other inflammatory mediators that increase capillary permeability, along with the loss of proteins through enlarged capillary pores, which decreases capillary oncotic pressure. As intravascular blood volume decreases, the blood becomes more viscous and blood flow is slowed. This situation causes capillary sludging as red blood cells, platelets, and proteins clump together. The loss of intravascular volume and capillary pooling further reduce venous return to the heart and cardiac output.

Coronary artery perfusion pressure is decreased. Myocardial depressant factor (MDF) is released by the ischemic pancreas, causing a decrease in myocardial contractility. Cardiac output, blood pressure, and tissue perfusion continue to decrease, contributing to worsening cellular hypoxia. At this point, the patient shows classic signs and symptoms of shock. This phase of shock responds poorly to fluid replacement alone and requires aggressive interventions if it is to be reversed.

Stage IV: Refractory Stage

Prolonged inadequate tissue perfusion that is unresponsive to therapy ultimately contributes to multiple organ dysfunction and death. A large volume of the blood remains pooled in the capillary bed, and the arterial blood pressure is too low to support perfusion of the vital organs.

Dysrhythmias occur because of the failure of the sodium-potassium pump, resulting from decreased ATP, hypoxemia, ischemia, and acidosis. Cardiac failure may occur because of ischemia, acidosis, and the effects of MDF.

Endothelial damage in the capillary bed and precapillary arterioles, along with damage to the type II pneumocytes, which make surfactant, leads to acute respiratory distress syndrome (ARDS). Hypoxemia causes hypoxemic vasoconstriction of the pulmonary circulation and pulmonary hypertension. Ventilation-perfusion mismatch occurs because of disturbances in both ventilation and perfusion. Pulmonary edema may result from disruption of the alveolar-capillary membrane, ARDS, heart failure, or overaggressive fluid resuscitation.

When cerebral perfusion pressure is significantly impaired, loss of autoregulation occurs, resulting in brain ischemia. Cerebral infarction may occur. Sympathetic nervous system dysfunction results in massive vasodilation, depression of cardiac and respiratory centers results in bradycardia and bradypnea, and impaired thermoregulation results in poikilothermism.

Renal vasoconstriction and hypoperfusion of the kidney decreases the glomerular filtration rate. Prolonged ischemia causes acute tubular necrosis and renal failure. Metabolic acids accumulate in the blood, worsening the metabolic acidosis caused by lactic acid production during anaerobic metabolism.

Hypoperfusion damages the reticuloendothelial cells, which recirculate bacteria and cellular debris, thereby predisposing the patient to bacteremia and sepsis. Damage to hepatocytes causes the liver to be unable to detoxify drugs, toxins, and hormones, conjugate bilirubin, or synthesize clotting factors. Hepatic dysfunction causes a decreased ability to mobilize carbohydrate, protein, and fat stores, which results in hypoglycemia.

Pancreatic enzymes are released by the ischemic and damaged pancreas. Pancreatic ischemia causes the release of MDF, which impairs cardiac contractility. Hyperglycemia may occur because of endogenous corticosteroids, exogenous corticosteroids, or insulin resistance. This hyperglycemia results in dehydration and electrolyte imbalances related to osmotic diuresis; impairment of leukocyte function causing decreased phagocytosis and increased risk of infection; depression of the immune response; impairment in gastric motility; shifts in substrate availability from glucose to free fatty acids or lactate; negative nitrogen balance; and decreased wound healing.

Ischemia and increased gastric acid production caused by glucocorticoids increase the risk of stress ulcer development. Prolonged vasoconstriction and ischemia lead to the inability of the intestinal walls to act as intact barriers to prevent the migration of bacteria out of the gastrointestinal tract. This may result in the translocation of bacteria from the gastrointestinal tract into the lymphatic and vascular beds, increasing the risk for sepsis.

Hypoxia and release of inflammatory cytokines impair blood flow and result in microvascular thrombosis. Sluggish blood flow, massive tissue trauma, and consumption of clotting factors may cause disseminated intravascular coagulation (DIC). The bone marrow mobilizes the release of white blood cells, causing leukocytosis early in shock and then leukopenia as depletion of white blood cells in blood and in bone marrow occurs. Massive tissue injury caused by widespread ischemia stimulates the development of a SIRS with a massive release of mediators of the inflammatory process.

Poor renal function, respiratory failure, and impaired cellular function aggravate the existing state of acidosis, which contributes to further fluid shifts, loss of vasomotor tone, and relative hypovolemia. Alterations in the cardiovascular system and continued acidosis cause a reduction in heart rate, impaired myocardial contractility, and a further decrease in cardiac output and tissue perfusion. Cerebral ischemia occurs because of the reduction in cerebral blood flow. Consequently, the sympathetic nervous system is stimulated, an effect that aggravates the existing vasoconstriction, increasing afterload and decreasing cardiac output. Prolonged cerebral ischemia eventually causes the loss of sympathetic nervous system response, and vasodilation and bradycardia result. The patient's decreasing blood pressure and heart rate cause a lethal decrease in tissue perfusion, multisystem organ failure that is unresponsive to therapy, and ultimately brain death and cardiopulmonary arrest.

Systemic Inflammatory Response Syndrome (SIRS)

SIRS is widespread inflammation that can occur in patients with diverse disorders such as infection, trauma, shock, pancreatitis, or ischemia.[8] It may result from or lead to MODS. SIRS is most frequently associated with sepsis. Sepsis is defined as infection associated with SIRS.[8]

The inflammatory cascade maintains homeostasis through a balance between proinflammatory and antiinflammatory processes. Inflammation is normally a localized process; SIRS is a systemic response associated with the release of mediators. These mediators cause an increase in the permeability of the endothelial wall, shifting fluid from the intravascular space into extravascular spaces, including the interstitial space. Intravascular volume is reduced, resulting in a condition of relative hypovolemia. Other mediators cause microvascular clotting, impaired fibrinolysis, and widespread vasodilation.

Effects of Aging

The effects of aging diminish the body's ability to tolerate shock states. As the body ages, the left ventricular wall thickens, ventricular compliance decreases, and calcification and fibrosis of the heart valves occur. Stroke volume and, resultantly, cardiac output are reduced. There is a decreased sensitivity of the baroreceptors and a diminished heart rate response to sympathetic nervous system stimulation in the early stage of shock. Older adults are more

likely to be prescribed beta-blockers, which also decrease the heart rate response. Arterial walls lose elasticity causing an increase in SVR, which increases the myocardial oxygen demand and decreases the responsiveness of the arterial system to the effects of catecholamines.

Aging causes decreased lung elasticity, decreased alveolar perfusion, decreased alveolar surface area, and thickening of the alveolar-capillary membrane. These changes limit the body's ability to increase blood oxygen levels during shock states. The ability of the kidney to concentrate urine decreases with age, which limits the body's ability to conserve water when required.

The immune system loses effectiveness with age, referred to as immunosenescence. This increases the risk of infection and sepsis, especially with illness, injury, or surgery. Older adults are also at greater risk for anaphylaxis since they have been exposed to more antigens and, therefore, have antibodies to more antigens.

ASSESSMENT

An understanding of the pathophysiology of shock and identification of patients at risk are essential for the prevention of shock. Assessment focuses on three areas: history, clinical presentation, and laboratory studies. The logical approach is to review the history of the patient and then assess the systems most sensitive to a lack of oxygen and nutrients. The patient's history may include an identifiable predisposing factor or cause of the shock state.

Clinical Presentation

Multiple body systems are affected by the shock syndrome. The clinical presentation specific to each classification of shock is discussed later (see also Clinical Alert).

Central Nervous System

The central nervous system is the most sensitive to changes in the supply of oxygen and nutrients. It is the first system affected by changes in cellular perfusion. Initial responses of the central nervous system to shock include restlessness, agitation, and anxiety. As the shock state progresses, the patient becomes confused and lethargic because of the decreased perfusion to the brain. As shock progresses, the patient becomes unresponsive.

Cardiovascular System

A major focus of assessment is blood pressure. It is important for the nurse to know the patient's

CLINICAL ALERT

Assessment	Significance
Change in vital signs, hemodynamic parameters, sensorium	Secondary to decreased tissue perfusion and initiation of compensatory mechanisms
Decreased urine output, rising BUN and creatinine levels	Secondary to initiation of compensatory mechanisms and decreased renal perfusion
Tachypnea, hypoxemia, worsening chest x-ray	Related to development of acute respiratory distress syndrome secondary to hypoperfusion
Petechiae, ecchymosis, bleeding from puncture sites, overt or occult blood in urine, stool, gastric aspirate, tracheal aspirate	Related to development of disseminated intravascular coagulation secondary to shock, SIRS
Hypoglycemia, increase in liver enzymes	Related to hepatic dysfunction secondary to hypoperfusion

BUN, Blood urea nitrogen; *SIRS*, systemic inflammatory response syndrome.

baseline blood pressure. During the compensatory stage, innervation of the sympathetic nervous system results in an increase in myocardial contractility and vasoconstriction, which results in a normal or slightly elevated systolic pressure, an increased diastolic pressure, and a narrowed pulse pressure. As the shock state progresses, the systolic blood pressure decreases, but the diastolic pressure remains normal, resulting in a narrowed pulse pressure. This narrowed pulse pressure may precede changes in heart rate.[10]

Definitions vary, but a decrease in systolic blood pressure to less than 90 mm Hg is considered hypotensive. For hypertensive patients, a decrease in systolic pressure of 40 mm Hg from their usual systolic pressure is considered severely hypotensive. Auscultated blood pressure in shock may be significantly inaccurate because of peripheral vasoconstriction. If blood pressure is not audible, the approximate systolic pressure can be assessed by palpation or ultrasound (Doppler) devices. If the brachial pulse is readily palpable, the approximate systolic pressure is 80 mm Hg. Corresponding blood pressure for the

femoral and carotid pulses is 70 and 60 mm Hg, respectively. Intraarterial pressure monitoring may be indicated to directly measure blood pressure.

The rate, quality, and character of major pulses (i.e., carotid, radial, femoral, dorsalis pedis, and posterior tibial) are evaluated. In shock states, the pulse is often weak and thready. The pulse rate is increased, usually greater than 100 beats per minute, through stimulation of the sympathetic nervous system as a compensatory response to the decreased cardiac output and increased demand of the cells for oxygen. In later stages of shock, the pulse slows, possibly from release of MDF.

Normal compensatory responses to shock may be altered if the patient is taking certain medications. Negative inotropic agents, such as propranolol and metoprolol, are widely used in the treatment of angina, hypertension, and dysrhythmias. These agents work primarily by blocking the effects of the beta branch of the sympathetic nervous system, and cause a decrease in heart rate and cardiac output. A patient who is taking these medications has an altered ability to respond to the stress of shock and may not exhibit the typical signs and symptoms such as tachycardia and anxiety.

Assessment of the jugular veins provides information regarding the volume and pressure in the right side of the heart. It is an indirect method of evaluating the central venous pressure. Neck veins are distended in patients with obstructive or cardiogenic shock and are flat in hypovolemic shock.

Capillary refill assesses the ability of the cardiovascular system to maintain perfusion to the periphery. The normal response to pressure on the nail beds is blanching, the color returns to a normal pink hue 1 to 2 seconds after the pressure is released. A delay in the return of color indicates peripheral vasoconstriction. Capillary refill provides a quick assessment of the patient's overall cardiovascular status, but this assessment is not reliable in a patient who is hypothermic or has peripheral circulatory problems.

A central venous catheter may be inserted to aid in the differential diagnosis of shock, to administer and monitor therapies, and to evaluate the preload of the heart. Normally, the central venous pressure (or right atrial pressure [RAP]) is 2 to 6 mm Hg. When blood volume decreases (hypovolemic shock), or the vascular capacitance increases (distributive shock), the central venous pressure decreases. In cardiogenic shock, the central venous pressure is increased because of poor myocardial contractility and high filling pressure in the ventricles. In obstructive shock secondary to cardiac tamponade or tension pneumothorax, the central venous pressure is high.

A pulmonary artery catheter is one of the most useful tools for diagnosing and treating the patient in shock. The catheter can give information regarding cardiac dynamics, fluid balance, and effects of vasoactive agents. Preload, which is measured by RAP for the right ventricle and by the pulmonary artery occlusive pressure (PAOP) for the left ventricle, is used to assess fluid balance. The pulmonary artery catheter also allows measurement of cardiac output, which is then divided by the patient's body surface area for calculation of the cardiac index. (Refer to Chapter 8.) Table 11-3 describes hemodynamic values and alterations in each classification of shock.

Vascular resistance or afterload is assessed by the SVR, a calculated value that offers information on the workload of the left ventricle, and by the pulmonary vascular resistance (PVR), which measures right ventricular workload. Two other calculated parameters, left ventricular stroke work index and right ventricular stroke work index, reflect myocardial contractility. Cardiac output and cardiac index are affected by heart rate and stroke volume. Stroke volume is determined by preload, afterload, and contractility. These same factors

TABLE 11-3   Hemodynamic Alterations in Shock States

Hemodynamic Parameter, Normal Value	Hypovolemic	Cardiogenic	Obstructive	Distributive		
				Septic	Anaphylactic	Neurogenic
Heart rate 60-100/min	High	High	High	High	High	Normal or low
Blood pressure	Normal → Low	Normal → Low	Normal → Low	Normal → Low	Normal → Low	Normal → Low
Cardiac output 4-8 L/min	Low	Low	Low	High then low	Normal → Low	Normal → Low
Cardiac index 2.5-4.0 L/min/m²	Low	Low	Low	High then low	Normal → Low	Normal → Low
RAP 2-6 mm Hg	Low	High	High	Low to variable	Low	Low
PAOP 8-12 mm Hg or PADP 8-15 mm Hg	Low	High	High if impaired diastolic filling or high LV afterload; low if high RV afterload	Low to variable	Low	Low
SVR 770-1500 dynes/sec/cm⁻⁵	High	High	SVR Low PVR High	Low to variable	Low	Low
SvO2 60-75%	Low	Low	Low	High then low	Low	Low

LV, Left ventricular; *PADP*, pulmonary artery diastolic pressure; *PAOP*, pulmonary artery occlusion pressure; *PVR*, pulmonary vascular resistance; *RAP*, right atrial pressure; *RV*, right ventricular; *SvO₂*, mixed venous oxygen saturation; *SVR*, systemic vascular resistance.

also determine myocardial oxygen consumption. Critical care management involves optimizing cardiac output, and minimizing myocardial oxygen consumption.

Special oximetric pulmonary artery catheters measure the oxygen saturation in the pulmonary artery, referred to as the mixed venous oxygen saturation (SvO_2). The SvO_2 reflects the amount of oxygen bound to hemoglobin in the venous circulation and reflects the balance between the DO_2 and VO_2. If the SvO_2 is less than 60%, either the DO_2, which is affected by the hemoglobin level, SaO_2, and cardiac output, is inadequate; or the VO_2 is excessive. The SvO_2 is reduced in all forms of shock except in early septic shock, where the poor oxygen extraction causes SvO_2 to be high. The SvO_2 is useful in identifying the type of shock and in evaluating the effectiveness of treatment.

Respiratory System

In the early stage of shock, respirations are rapid and deep. The respiratory center responds to shock and metabolic acidosis with an increase in respiratory rate to eliminate carbon dioxide. Direct stimulation of the medulla by chemoreceptors alters the respiratory pattern. As the shock state progresses, metabolic wastes accumulate and cause generalized muscle weakness, resulting in shallow breathing with poor gas exchange.

Pulse oximetry is frequently used to measure arterial oxygen saturation (SpO_2). It must be used with caution in patients in shock because decreased peripheral circulation may result in inaccurate readings. Arterial blood gas analysis provides a more accurate assessment of oxygenation.

Renal System

Renal hypoperfusion and decreased glomerular filtration rate cause oliguria (urine output <0.5 mL/kg/hr). The renin-angiotensin-aldosterone system is activated, which promotes the retention of sodium and the reabsorption of water in the kidneys, further decreasing urinary output. This prerenal failure is manifested by concentrated urine and an increased blood urea nitrogen level, while the serum creatinine level remains normal. If the decreased perfusion is prolonged, acute tubular necrosis, a form of intrarenal failure, occurs and creatinine levels increase.

Gastrointestinal System

Hypoperfusion of the gastrointestinal system results in a slowing of intestinal activity with decreased bowel sounds, distention, nausea, and constipation. Paralytic ileus and ulceration with bleeding may occur with prolonged hypoperfusion. Damage to the microvilli allows translocation of bacteria from the gastrointestinal tract to the lymphatic and systemic circulation, increasing the risk of infection and sepsis in the already compromised critically ill patient.

Hypoperfusion of the liver leads to decreased function and alterations in liver enzyme levels such as lactate dehydrogenase and aspartate aminotransferase. If decreased perfusion persists, the liver is not able to produce coagulation factors, detoxify drugs, or neutralize invading microorganisms. Clotting disorders, drug toxicity concerns, and increased susceptibility for infection occur.

Hematological System

The interaction between inflammation and coagulation enhances clotting and inhibits fibrinolysis, leading to clotting in the microcirculatory system and bleeding. An increased consumption of platelets and clotting factors occurs, causing a consumptive coagulopathy. The inability of the liver to manufacture clotting factors also contributes to the coagulopathy. A decreased platelet count, decreased clotting factors, and prolonged clotting times are seen with coagulopathy. Petechiae and ecchymosis may occur, along with blood in the urine, stool, gastric aspirate, and/or tracheal secretions. The clotting in the microcirculation causes peripheral ischemia manifested by acrocyanosis and necrosis of digits and extremities. Leukocytosis frequently occurs, especially in early septic shock. Leukopenia occurs later because of consumption of white blood cells.

Integumentary System

Skin color, temperature, texture, turgor, and moisture level are evaluated. Cyanosis may be present; however, it is a late and unreliable sign. The patient may exhibit central cyanosis, seen in the mucous membranes of the mouth and nose, or peripheral cyanosis, evident in the nails and earlobes. While turgor is frequently used to determine the presence of interstitial dehydration, elderly adults have decreased skin elasticity, making this evaluation misleading.

Laboratory Studies

Laboratory studies assist in the differential diagnosis of the patient in shock (see Laboratory Alerts). However, by the time many of the laboratory values are altered, the patient is in the later stages of shock. The clinical picture is often more useful for early diagnosis and immediate treatment.

LABORATORY ALERTS
Shock

Diagnostic Study	Critical Value	Significance
		Chemistry Studies
Glucose	<70 or >105 mg/dL	Frequently ↑ early shock, ↓ late shock ↑ Impairs immune response
Blood urea nitrogen	>20 mg/dL	↑ Hypoperfusion (prerenal failure) ↑ Gastrointestinal bleeding and catabolism
Creatinine	>1.2 mg/dL	↑ Acute renal failure
Sodium	<136 or >145 mEq/L	↓ Hemodilution from replacement of excessive hypotonic fluid ↑ Hemoconcentration from fluid loss
Chloride	>107 mEq/L	↑ Excess infusion of normal saline; may cause hyperchloremic acidosis
Potassium	<3.5 or >5.0 mEq/L	↓ Excessive loss of potassium ↑ Impaired elimination from renal failure Observe for cardiac dysrhythmias
Lactate	>2 mEq/L	↑ Hypoxia leading to anaerobic metabolism and production of lactic acid
AST	>20 units/L	↑ Hepatic impairment
LDH	>102 units/L	↑ Hepatic impairment, renal impairment, intestinal ischemia, or myocardial infarction
		Hematology Studies
WBCs	<4000 or >12,000/mm^3	↑ Stress response; significant increase indicates infection ↓ Late shock due to consumption of WBCs
Hemoglobin	<12 g/dL	↓ Blood loss
Hematocrit	<35%	↓ Blood loss ↑ Dehydration and hemoconcentration
		Arterial Blood Gases
pH	<7.35 or >7.45	↑ Early shock—respiratory alkalosis due to hyperventilation ↓ Late shock—metabolic acidosis due to lactic acidosis
PaCO$_2$	<35 or >45 mm Hg	↓ Early shock—respiratory alkalosis due to hyperventilation
PaO$_2$	<60 mm Hg	↓ Hypoxemia; may indicate pulmonary edema or ARDS
HCO$_3^-$	<22 mEq/L	↓ Late shock—metabolic acidosis caused by hypoxia, anaerobic metabolism, and lactic acidosis

↑, Increased; ↓, decreased; *ARDS*, acute respiratory distress syndrome; *AST*, aspartate aminotransferase; *HCO$_3^-$*, bicarbonate; *LDH*, lactate dehydrogenase; *PaCO$_2$*, partial pressure of arterial carbon dioxide; *PaO$_2$*, partial pressure of arterial oxygen; *WBCs*, white blood cells.

A measure of the overall state of shock, regardless of the cause of inadequate perfusion, is the serum lactate level. Lactate level has been used as an indicator of decreased oxygen delivery to the cells and of the adequacy of resuscitation in shock, and as an outcome predictor. Elevated levels of lactate produce an acidic environment and decrease arterial pH. The serum lactate level correlates with the degree of hypoperfusion. Elevations in lactate occur only after maximal oxygen extraction by the cells.

MANAGEMENT

Management of the patient in shock consists of finding and treating the cause of the shock as rapidly as possible. Care is directed toward correcting or reversing the altered circulatory component (e.g., blood volume, myocardial contractility, obstruction, or vascular resistance) and reversing tissue hypoxia. A combination of fluid, pharmacological, and mechanical therapies are implemented to maintain tissue perfusion and improve oxygen delivery. These interventions include increasing the cardiac output and cardiac index, increasing the hemoglobin level, and increasing the arterial oxygen saturation. Efforts are also aimed toward minimizing oxygen consumption. Specific management for each classification of shock is discussed later.

Maintenance of Circulating Blood Volume and Adequate Hemoglobin Level

Regardless of the cause, shock produces profound alterations in fluid balance. Therefore, patients experiencing absolute hypovolemia (hypovolemic shock) or relative hypovolemia (distributive shock) require the administration of intravenous (IV) fluids to restore intravascular volume, maintain oxygen-carrying capacity, and establish the hemodynamic stability necessary for optimal tissue perfusion. The choice of fluid and the volume and rate of infusion depend on the type of fluid lost, the patient's hemodynamic status, and coexisting conditions.

Benefits of IV fluid administration include increased intravascular volume, increased venous return to the right side of the heart, optimal stretching of the ventricle, improved myocardial contractility, and increased cardiac output. However, these effects may be dangerous to the patient in cardiogenic shock because large volumes of fluid overwork an already failing heart. Instead, cardiogenic shock is managed primarily with medications that reduce both preload and afterload.

Fluid administration is adjusted based on changes in blood pressure, urine output, hemodynamic values, diagnostic test results, and the clinical picture of the patient's response to treatment. Generally, volume replacement continues until an adequate mean arterial pressure (65 to 70 mm Hg) is achieved and evidence of end-organ tissue perfusion is reestablished, as evidenced by improvement in the level of consciousness, urinary output, and peripheral perfusion.

Patients in severe shock may require immediate, rapid volume replacement. The IV infusion rate can be increased by using a blood pump to administer fluids under pressure, by using large-bore infusion tubing, or by using a rapid-infusion device. Infusion pumps are used to rapidly and accurately administer large volumes of fluids. Administration of large volumes of room-temperature fluids can rapidly drop core body temperature and cause hypothermia. Fluid-related hypothermia causes alterations in cardiac contractility and coagulation. For this reason, large volumes of fluids should be infused through warming devices.

Intravenous Access

IV access is needed to administer fluids and medications. The patient in shock requires a minimum of two IV catheters, one in a peripheral vein and one in a central vein. Peripheral access via a large-gauge catheter (14- or 16-gauge) in a large vein in the antecubital fossa provides a route for rapid administration of fluids and medications. Establishing IV routes in a patient in shock is challenging because peripheral vasoconstriction and venous collapse make access difficult.

A central venous access is established for large-volume replacement and can be used to monitor central venous pressure or place a pulmonary artery catheter to guide fluid replacement. Central venous catheters are commonly inserted into the subclavian, internal jugular, or femoral veins. Multilumen catheters, which provide multiple access ports, allow the concurrent administration of fluid, medication, and blood products.

Fluid Challenge

Once IV access is established, a fluid challenge may be performed to assess the patient's hemodynamic response to fluid administration. Various methods for administering a fluid challenge exist. Typically, a rapid infusion of 250 mL (up to 2 L) of a crystalloid solution is initiated first. Nursing responsibilities include obtaining the baseline hemodynamic measurements, administering the fluid challenge, and assessing the patient's response. A fluid challenge algorithm is helpful in guiding fluid resuscitation (Figure 11-4).

Types of Fluids

The choice of fluids depends on the cause of the volume deficit, the patient's clinical status, and the physician's preference. Although the nurse is not responsible for selecting the infusion or transfusion, an understanding of the rationale for the prescribed fluid and the expected effects is needed to assess patient outcomes. The nurse carefully monitors the patient's response to fluid therapy. (See Evidence-Based Practice feature.)

Blood, blood products, crystalloids, and colloids are used alone, or in combination, to restore intravascular volume. Crystalloids are infused until diagnostic testing and blood typing and crossmatching are completed. Colloids are avoided in situations where there is an increase in capillary permeability,

as in sepsis and septic shock, anaphylactic shock, and early burns. A systematic review of 30 randomized controlled trials found no benefit in giving colloids over crystalloids, and recommended against the administration of colloids in most patient populations. In critically ill patients with hypovolemia, administration of albumin was associated with a higher risk of death.[9]

Crystalloids are inexpensive and readily available. Crystalloids are classified by tonicity. Isotonic solutions have approximately the same tonicity as plasma (osmolality, 250 to 350 mOsm/L). Lactated Ringer's (LR) solution and 0.9% normal saline are isotonic solutions that are commonly infused. These solutions move freely from the intravascular space into the tissues. Traditionally, 3 mL of crystalloid solution is

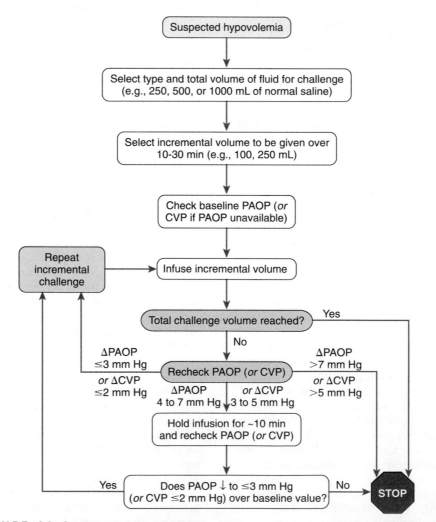

FIGURE 11-4. Fluid challenge algorithm. *CVP*, Central venous pressure; *PAOP*, pulmonary artery occlusion pressure. *(Adapted from Kruse, J. A., Fink, M. P., & Carlson, R. W. [2003]. Saunders manual of critical care. Philadelphia: Saunders.)*

EVIDENCE-BASED PRACTICE

PROBLEM

Massive bleeding is associated with hypovolemic shock. Patients require treatment with transfusions of blood and blood products for hemodynamic stability. Complications are associated with massive transfusions, such as acute respiratory distress syndrome.

QUESTION

Are there options to blood transfusions in the management of hypovolemic shock associated with hemorrhage?

REFERENCES

Franchini, M., Manzato, F., Salvagno, G. L., & Lippi, G. (2007). Potential role of recombinant activated factor VII for the treatment of severe bleeding associated with disseminated intravascular coagulation: A systematic review. *Blood Coagulation and Fibrinolysis, 18*(7), 589-593.

Levy, M., Peters, M., & Buller, H. R. (2005). Efficacy and safety of recombinant factor VIIa for treatment of severe bleeding: A systematic review. *Critical Care Medicine, 33*(4), 883-890.

Warren, O., Mandal, K., Hadjianastassiou, V., Knowlton, L., Panesar, S., John, K., et al. (2007). Recombinant activated factor VII in cardiac surgery: A systematic review. *Annals of Thoracic Surgery, 83*(2), 707-714.

EVIDENCE

Recombinant activated factor VII (rFVIIa) is a hemostatic agent that was developed and approved for treatment of hemophilia. The agent has been used in many "off-label" situations to treat hemorrhage, such as occurring with trauma or surgery. It has also been used off-label to treat disseminated intravascular coagulation. These three teams of researchers conducted systematic reviews of research related to the administration of rFVIIa in a variety of critical care situations. Large randomized clinical trials were lacking for all these conditions. However, the research teams all concluded that administration of rFVIIa shows promise in the treatment of severe bleeding without preexisting coagulation disorders (Levy et al.); in disseminated intravascular coagulation, especially associated with postpartum hemorrhage (Franchini et al.); and in extensive bleeding associated with cardiac surgery (Warren et al.). The main side effect of rFVIIa administration is a low (1% to 2%) incidence of thrombotic complications. All agree that additional controlled trials are necessary to assess the efficacy, safety, dosing regimens, and cost-effectiveness of administering rFVIIa for the treatment of hemorrhage associated with a variety of conditions.

IMPLICATIONS FOR NURSING

At the present time, rFVIIa may be considered for off-label use to treat hemorrhage associated with a variety of critical care conditions. Consent for administration must be obtained by the physician to use the drug in these situations. Nurses must be aware of potential indications and side effects of administration of the drug. Nurses may be assisting research teams in future trials of the medication.

---

administered to replace each 1 mL of blood loss. LR solution closely resembles plasma and may be the only fluid replacement required if blood loss is less than 1500 mL. LR solution contains lactate, which is a salt that the liver converts to bicarbonate, so it counteracts metabolic acidosis if the liver function is normal. LR should not be infused in patients with impaired liver function or severe lactic acidosis. Although 0.9% normal saline is an isotonic solution, its side effects include hypernatremia, hypokalemia, and hyperchloremic metabolic acidosis. Solutions of 5% dextrose in water and 0.45% normal saline are hypotonic and are not used for fluid resuscitation. Hypotonic solutions rapidly leave the intravascular space, causing interstitial and intracellular edema.

When large volumes of crystalloids are infused, the patient is at risk of developing hemodilution of red blood cells and plasma proteins. Hemodilution of red blood cells impairs oxygen delivery if the hematocrit value is decreased and the cardiac output cannot increase enough to compensate. Hemodilution of plasma proteins decreases colloidal osmotic pressure and places the patient at risk of developing pulmonary edema. Elderly patients are at increased risk of developing pulmonary edema and may require invasive hemodynamic monitoring to guide fluid resuscitation.

Colloids contain proteins that increase osmotic pressure. Osmotic pressure holds and attracts fluid into blood vessels, thereby expanding plasma volume. Because colloids remain in the intravascular space longer than crystalloids, smaller volumes of colloids are given in shock states. Albumin and plasma protein fraction (Plasmanate) are naturally occurring colloid solutions that are infused when the volume loss is caused by a loss of plasma rather than blood, such as in burns, peritonitis, and bowel obstruction. Typing and crossmatching of albumin and plasma protein fraction are not required. Pulmonary edema is a potential complication of colloid administration, resulting from increased pulmonary capillary permeability or increased capillary hydrostatic pressure in the pulmonary vasculature created by rapid plasma expansion.

Hetastarch (Hespan) is a synthetic colloid solution that acts as a plasma expander but carries less risk for pulmonary edema. Side effects include altered prothrombin time (PT) and activated partial thromboplastin time (aPTT) and the potential for circulatory overload. No more than 1 L should be administered in a 24-hour period.

Blood products—packed red blood cells, fresh frozen plasma, and platelets—are administered to treat major blood loss. Typing and crossmatching of these products are performed to identify the patient's blood type (A, B, AB, O) and Rh factor, and to ensure compatibility with the donor blood to prevent transfusion reactions. In extreme emergencies, the patient may be transfused with type-specific or O-negative blood, which is considered the universal donor blood type.

Transfusions require an IV access with at least a 20-gauge, preferably an 18-gauge or larger, catheter (a 22- or 23-gauge needle or catheter may be used in children or adults with small veins). Solutions other than 0.9% normal saline are not infused with blood because they cause red blood cells to aggregate, swell, and burst. In addition, IV medications are never infused in the same port with blood. Appropriate patient and blood identification is necessary before starting any transfusion.

Transfusions are administered with a blood filter to trap debris and tiny clots. Frequent patient assessment is necessary during a blood transfusion to monitor for adverse reactions. In the event of a reaction, the transfusion is stopped, the transfusion tubing is disconnected from the IV access site, and the vein is kept open with an IV of 0.9% normal saline solution. The patient is assessed, and the physician and laboratory are notified. All transfusion equipment (bag, tubing, and remaining solutions) and any blood or urine specimens obtained are sent to the laboratory according to hospital policy. The events of the reaction, interventions used, and patient response to treatment are documented.

The transfusion administration time varies with the particular blood product used and the individual patient circumstances. Documentation of the transfusion includes the blood product administered, baseline vital signs, start and completion time of the transfusion, volume of blood and fluid, assessment of the patient during the transfusion, and any nursing actions taken.

Packed red blood cells increase the blood volume and oxygen-carrying capacity with a decreased risk for volume overload. One unit of packed red blood cells increases the hematocrit value by about 3% and the hemoglobin value by 1 g/dL. Typing and crossmatching of packed red blood cells are required. Red blood cells tend to aggregate because of the fibrinogen coating; therefore, washed red blood cells may be given. Acidosis, hyperkalemia, and coagulation problems are associated with transfusions of banked blood older than 24 hours. Massive transfusion (approximately 10 units) is associated with decreased 2,3-diphosphoglycerate (2,3-DPG), causing a shift of the oxyhemoglobin dissociation curve to the left, which impairs the delivery of oxygen to the tissues.

Fresh frozen plasma is administered to replace all clotting factors except platelets. When massive transfusions are infused, fresh frozen plasma is given rapidly to restore coagulation factors. One unit of fresh frozen plasma is given for every 4 to 5 units of packed red blood cells transfused. Typing and crossmatching of fresh frozen plasma are required.

Platelets are given rapidly to help control bleeding caused by low platelet counts (usually <50,000/mm^3). Typing of platelets, but not crossmatching, is required.

Hemoglobin substitutes may be an alternative. Human polymerized hemoglobin (PolyHeme) is a substitute for packed red blood cells that is universally compatible and pathogen-free.[13] Hemoglobin substitutes do not require crossmatching, have a long shelf-life, and eliminate the risk of diseases associated with blood transfusion.[14]

Maintenance of Arterial Oxygen Saturation and Ventilation

Airway maintenance is the top priority. The airway is maintained by proper head position, use of oral or nasopharyngeal airways, or intubation, depending on the patient's condition. Suctioning and chest physical therapy facilitate secretion removal and help to maintain a patent airway.

Oxygen is administered to elevate the arterial oxygen tension, thereby improving tissue oxygenation. Oxygen is administered by methods ranging from nasal cannula to mechanical ventilation, depending on the patient's condition.

Mechanical ventilation is used to maintain adequate ventilation as reflected by a normal partial pressure of arterial carbon dioxide (PaCO$_2$) level. Another benefit of mechanical ventilation in a patient with shock is to reduce the work of breathing and the associated oxygen consumption. Tidal volumes and inspiratory pressures are kept low to prevent ventilator-induced lung injury. Tidal volumes are generally between 4 and 8 mL/kg of ideal body weight, and the inspiratory plateau pressures are maintained at less than 30 cm H_2O.[34] Positive end-expiratory pressure (PEEP) is used to maintain alveolar recruitment and may protect against ventilator-induced lung injury by preventing the repetitive opening and collapsing of the alveoli.[26] Newer ventilator modes, such as the pressure-regulated volume-controlled mode, aid in keeping inspiratory pressures low.

Sedation or neuromuscular blockade is considered to reduce the oxygen consumption. Arterial blood gases, pulse oximetry, and hemodynamic monitoring aid in the evaluation of oxygen consumption and delivery.

Pharmacological Support

Pharmacological management of shock is based on the manipulation of the determinants of cardiac output: heart rate, preload, afterload, and contractility. Figure 11-5 describes therapies used to manipulate these parameters. These drugs are preferably administered through a central venous catheter. Hemodynamic monitoring is often used to assess the effectiveness of medications. Older adults are particular sensitive to the physiologic impact of medications and the deleterious effects of polypharmacy. Table 11-4 describes medications that are commonly administered in shock.

Cardiac Output

Low or high heart rates and dysrhythmias decrease cardiac output. Chronotropic drugs and antidysrhythmic agents are given as indicated. In neurogenic shock, sinus bradycardia secondary to cervical spinal cord injury does not usually require therapy.

Text continued on p. 285

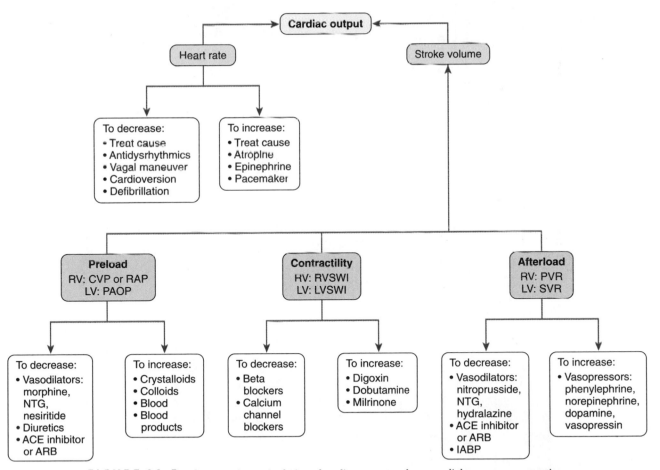

FIGURE 11-5. Therapeutic manipulation of cardiac output and myocardial oxygen consumption. *ACE,* Angiotensin converting enzyme; *ARB,* angiotensin receptor blocker; *CI,* cardiac index; *CO,* cardiac output; *CVP,* central venous pressure; *IABP,* intra-aortic balloon pump; *LR,* lactated Ringer's; *LV,* left ventricle; *LVSWI,* left ventricular stroke work index; *NS,* normal (0.9%) saline; *NTG,* nitroglycerin; *PAOP,* pulmonary artery occlusive pressure; *PDE,* phosphodiesterase; *PVR,* pulmonary vascular resistance; *RAP,* right atrial pressure; *RV,* right ventricle; *RVSWI,* right ventricular stroke work index; *SVR,* systemic vascular resistance. *(Adapted from Dennison, R. D. [2007]. Pass CCRN! [3rd ed.]. St. Louis: Mosby.)*

PHARMACOLOGY

TABLE 11-4   Medications Commonly Used in Shock

Drug	Action	Indication	Dosage/Route	Standard Concentration	Adverse Effects	Nursing Implications
Dobutamine (Dobutrex)	Stimulates primarily beta$_1$ receptors of SNS to ↑ contractility and ↑ heart rate and cause vasodilation	Low CO states	2-20 mcg/kg/min IV infusion Central venous catheter preferred	500 mg in 250 mL NS or D$_5$W Do not administer with alkaline solutions	Tachycardia Dysrhythmias Hypotension Nausea, vomiting Dyspnea Headache Anxiety Paresthesia Palpitations Chest pain	Monitor BP, HR, ECG, PAP, PAOP, SVR, CO, and CI Use cautiously in patients with hypertension or ventricular dysrhythmias Replace volume before initiation of infusion
Dopamine (Intropin)	Dose-dependent effect At ~5 mcg/kg/min stimulates beta$_1$ receptors of SNS to ↑ contractility and ↑ HR At 5-20 mcg/kg/min stimulates alpha receptors to cause vasoconstriction	Low CO states Vasodilatory states (distributive shock) to restore vascular tone	5-20 mcg/kg/min IV infusion (maximum dose 50 mcg/kg/min) Central venous catheter preferred	400 mg/250 mL NS or D$_5$W Do not administer with alkaline solutions	↑ HR Dysrhythmias Nausea, vomiting Dyspnea Headache Palpitations Chest pain in patients with coronary artery disease Tissue necrosis with high dosages or extravasation	Monitor HR, BP, ECG, PAP, PAOP, SVR, CO, CI, and urine output Treat cause of ↓ BP before initiating (e.g., hypovolemia treated with fluid resuscitation) Wean slowly Treat extravasation with phentolamine (Regitine)

Medication	Action	Use	Dosage	Preparation	Adverse Effects	Nursing Considerations
Norepinephrine (Levophed)	Stimulates alpha receptors to cause vasoconstriction. Mild stimulation of beta receptors to ↑ contractility and ↑ heart rate	Vasodilatory states (distributive shock) to restore vascular tone	2-12 mcg/kg/min IV infusion Central venous catheter preferred	4 mg in 250 mL NS or D5W Do not administer with alkaline solutions	↓ HR Ventricular dysrhythmias Hypertension Anxiety Headache Tremor Dizziness Chest pain Metabolic (lactic) acidosis Severe vasoconstriction may cause renal or mesenteric necrosis Tissue necrosis with high dosages or if infusion infiltrates	Monitor BP, HR, ECG, urine output, and neurological status Treat extravasation with phentolamine (Regitine)
Phenylephrine (Neosynephrine)	Stimulates alpha receptors to cause vasoconstriction	Vasodilatory states (distributive shock) to restore vascular tone	2-10 mcg/kg/min IV infusion Central venous catheter preferred	30 mg in 500 mL NS or D5W	Reflex bradycardia Ventricular dysrhythmias Hypertension Nausea, vomiting Paresthesia Palpitations Anxiety Restlessness Headache Tremor Chest pain	Monitor HR, BP, and ECG Treat reflex bradycardia with atropine
Vasopressin	Vasoconstriction via smooth muscle contraction of all parts of capillaries, arterioles, and venules	Vasodilatory states (distributive shock) to restore vascular tone	0.01 to 0.03 unit/min IV infusion Central venous catheter preferred	100 units in 100 mL of NS or D5W	↓ HR ↑ BP Fever Water intoxication (SIADH), hyponatremia Nausea, abdominal cramps Tremor Headache Seizures Coma Chest pain and myocardial ischemia	Monitor HR, BP, daily weight, and serum sodium Use cautiously in patients with coronary artery disease

Continued

PHARMACOLOGY

TABLE 11-4 Medications Commonly Used in Shock—cont'd

Drug	Action	Indication	Dosage/Route	Standard Concentration	Adverse Effects	Nursing Implications
Nitroglycerin	Dose-dependent effect Vasodilation by direct smooth muscle relaxation, predominantly venous Arterial dilation only if infusion >1 mcg/kg/min	Preload and/or afterload reduction (cardiogenic shock)	Initial dose 5-10 mcg/min IV infusion, increase by 5-10 mcg/min every 5 minutes until desired results are achieved (control of chest pain and decreased preload)	50 mg in 250 mL NS or D₅W Administer in glass bottle via non–polyvinyl chloride tubing	↑ or ↓ HR ↑ or ↓ BP Palpitations Weakness Apprehension Flushing Dizziness Syncope Headache	Monitor HR, BP, and urine output Monitor RAP, PAP, PAOP, SVR, CO, and CI if pulmonary artery catheter present Use cautiously in hypotension
Nitroprusside (Nipride)	Vasodilation by direct smooth muscle relaxation, predominantly arterial	Preload and/or afterload reduction (cardiogenic shock)	0.5-10 mcg/kg/min IV infusion	50 mg in 250 mL D₅W Protect from light by wrapping aluminum foil around bag	Nausea, vomiting, abdominal pain Headache Tinnitus Dizziness Diaphoresis Apprehension Hypotension Tachycardia Palpitations Hypoxemia (nitroprusside-induced intrapulmonary thiocyanate toxicity)	Monitor HR, BP, urine output, and neurological status Monitor for patient thiocyanate toxicity (metabolic acidosis, confusion, hyperreflexia, and seizures) Serum thiocyanate levels drawn daily if drug is used longer than 72 hours Treatment includes amyl nitrate, sodium nitrate, and/or sodium thiosulfate

All medications should be administered via volumetric infusion pump.

BP, Blood pressure; *CI,* cardiac index; *CO,* cardiac output; *D₅W,* 5% dextrose in water; *ECG,* electrocardiogram; *HR,* heart rate; *IV,* intravenous; *NS,* normal (0.9%) saline; *PAOP,* pulmonary artery occlusive pressure; *PAP,* pulmonary artery pressure; *RAP,* right atrial pressure; *SIADH,* syndrome of inappropriate secretion of ADH; *SNS,* sympathetic nervous system; *SVR,* systemic vascular resistance.

However, if the bradycardia is significant and results in decreased perfusion, atropine or a temporary pacemaker may be required.

Preload

In hypovolemic and distributive shock, fluid administration is the primary treatment to increase preload. In cardiogenic shock, the myofibrils are overstretched and the preload needs to be reduced. Venous vasodilators or diuretics are administered to reduce preload.

Afterload

Afterload is low in distributive shock. In this situation, agents that cause vasoconstriction are administered to increase vascular tone and tissue perfusion pressure. Examples of vasoconstrictive drugs include phenylephrine, norepinephrine, epinephrine, or vasopressin. These drugs increase blood pressure and SVR. A negative effect of drugs that increase afterload is an increase in the myocardial oxygen demand. Accurate measurement/calculation of SVR and PVR via a pulmonary artery catheter assists in assessment.

Vasopressors should not be administered in hypovolemic shock because these patients require volume replacement. Administration of vasopressors in hypovolemia causes vasoconstriction and further diminishes tissue perfusion.

In cardiogenic shock, the afterload needs to be reduced. The use of arterial vasodilators to reduce afterload may be limited by the patient's blood pressure. In situations where hypotension prevents the use of arterial vasodilators, an intraaortic balloon pump is used to decrease afterload.

Contractility

Drugs that increase contractility, such as dobutamine, may be administered in cardiogenic shock. Although drugs that decrease contractility (e.g., betablockers) may be used to decrease myocardial oxygen consumption in patients with coronary artery disease, they are contraindicated in a patient in shock.

Other Medications

Other drugs used to manage shock include sedatives, analgesics, insulin, corticosteroids, antibiotics, and sodium bicarbonate. Sodium bicarbonate may be given for the treatment of severe metabolic acidosis (pH <7.0) associated with lactic acidosis. Sodium bicarbonate combines with hydrogen ions to form water and carbon dioxide to buffer metabolic acidosis. Sodium bicarbonate is administered cautiously because the carbon dioxide produced crosses rapidly into the cells and may cause a paradoxical worsening of intracellular hypercarbia and acidosis. While respiratory acidosis is treated by improving ventilation, metabolic acidosis caused by lactic acidosis is best treated by improving the aspects of DO_2: SaO_2, hemoglobin level, and cardiac output. These measures should be implemented before the consideration of sodium bicarbonate. Arterial blood gas analysis is used to guide treatment.

Hyperglycemia is common in patients in shock, especially patients with septic shock. Data suggest that intensive insulin therapy to maintain serum glucose levels less than 150 mg/dL reduces morbidity and mortality in critically ill patients.[36]

Low–molecular weight heparin is frequently prescribed for deep vein thrombosis prophylaxis. An H_2-receptor antagonist (ranitidine [Zantac] or proton pump inhibitor (pantoprazole [Protonix]) is frequently prescribed for peptic ulcer prophylaxis.

Maintenance of Body Temperature

Care is directed toward maintaining normal body temperature. Hypothermia depresses cardiac contractility and impairs cardiac output and oxygen delivery. Hypothermia also impairs the coagulation pathway, which can result in a significant coagulopathy. The patient's temperature is monitored frequently. Hypothermia is anticipated when fluids are infused rapidly, and use of a fluid warmer should be considered. Patients should be kept warm and comfortable, but not overly warmed. Excessive warmth increases the oxygen demand on an already stressed cardiovascular system.

Nutritional Support

Nutritional support is essential for patient survival. The goals of nutritional support are to initiate enteral intake as soon as possible and to maintain sufficient caloric intake to assist in the healing process. Early enteral feeding decreases hypermetabolism, minimizes bacterial translocation, decreases diarrhea, and decreases length of stay. Nutritional requirements of the patient in shock are highly variable depending on the degree of hemodynamic stability, the cause of shock, and the patient's age, gender, and preexisting diseases. Enteral feeding is the preferred method, and immune-boosting formulas may be prescribed. Administration of enteral nutrition may be limited by paralytic ileus, gastric dilation, or both, which are common in shock. Total parenteral nutrition is given if patients are unable to tolerate enteral feeding (see Chapter 6).

Maintenance of Skin Integrity

The decreased peripheral perfusion seen in shock can precipitate injury to the skin. Meticulous skin care is required to promote skin integrity. The patient is turned at frequent intervals, and lotion is applied. Pressure-relieving devices, such as therapeutic beds or mattresses, may be indicated.

Psychological Support

Nursing interventions also focus on identifying the impact of the illness on the patient and the family. Nursing interventions include providing information, which is essential for the psychological well-being of the patient and the family, and may help to give them a sense of understanding and control of the situation. Since shock has a high mor-

tality, a discussion should be initiated regarding life-sustaining therapies.

NURSING DIAGNOSIS

The primary nursing diagnosis for all patients in shock is altered tissue perfusion. This diagnosis may be related to decreased tissue perfusion, myocardial contractility, vascular resistance, obstruction, or a combination of these. The nurse provides care to support tissue perfusion of the patient in shock until definitive care is underway. Supportive care is aimed at maintenance of organ function (see Nursing Care Plan).

NURSING CARE PLAN   for the Patient in Shock

NURSING DIAGNOSIS

Altered tissue perfusion related to decreased blood volume (hypovolemic shock); decreased myocardial contractility (cardiogenic shock); impaired circulatory blood flow (obstructive shock); and widespread vasodilatation (septic, anaphylactic, or neurogenic shock)

PATIENT OUTCOMES
Adequate tissue perfusion

- Alert and responsive
- Skin warm and dry with good turgor
- Moist mucous membranes
- Capillary refill less than 2 seconds
- Jugular neck veins 1-2 cm above the angle of Louis
- Vital signs and hemodynamic parameters within normal limits (see Table 11-3)
- Pulses 2+ and regular
- Balanced intake and output
- Stable body weight
- Urine output at least 0.5 mL/kg/hr
- Normal serum and urine laboratory values and ABG results
- Adequate pain management
- Absence of complications (ARDS, DIC, renal failure, hepatic failure, MODS)

NURSING INTERVENTIONS	RATIONALES
• Monitor for early symptoms of shock (see Table 11-2)	• Initiate early support to improve outcomes and reduce risk of complications, organ failure, and death
• Establish or maintain patent airway	• Provide adequate gas exchange
• Monitor oxygenation: pulse oximetry, ABGs, SvO$_2$; administer oxygen to maintain SpO$_2$ at least 90%	• Assess for need for supplemental oxygen; ensure adequate oxygen delivery to the tissues
• Prepare for intubation and mechanical ventilation as needed	• Mechanical ventilation is frequently required to ensure adequate ventilation and reduce the work of breathing
• Establish intravenous access; use large-bore catheters (14 or 16 gauge); obtain central venous access, if possible	• Provide rapid fluid administration; central IV access allows for fluid and drug administration without the concerns of peripheral infiltration and irritation

NURSING CARE PLAN for the Patient in Shock—cont'd

NURSING INTERVENTIONS	RATIONALES
• Control bleeding through the application of pressure or surgical intervention	• Prevent blood loss
• Administer fluids as ordered (crystalloids, colloids, blood products)	• Maintain tissue perfusion
• Consider warming fluids before infusing	• Reduce hypothermia and its complications
• Replace blood components as indicated; obtain laboratory specimen for type and crossmatch	• Replace volume loss associated with blood loss; prevent transfusion reaction
• Evaluate patient's response to fluid challenges and blood product administration: improved vital signs, level of consciousness, urinary output, hemodynamic values, and serum and urine laboratory values	• Monitor response to treatment
• Monitor for clinical indications of fluid overload (↑ HR, ↑ RR, dyspnea, crackles) when fluids are administered rapidly	• Assess for signs of volume overload in response to treatment
• Monitor cardiopulmonary status: HR, RR, BP, MAP, skin color, temperature, and moisture, capillary refill, hemodynamic values, cardiac rhythm, neck veins, lung sounds	• Monitor response to treatment
• Monitor level of consciousness	• Assess perfusion of the central nervous system
• Monitor gastrointestinal status: abdominal distention, bowel sounds, gastric pH, vomiting, large enteral feeding residual	• Assess perfusion of the gastrointestinal system and prevent potential complications
• Monitor fluid balance: I&O, daily weights, amount and type of drainage (chest tube, nasogastric, wounds)	• Evaluate need for continued fluid volume support
• Monitor serial serum values: Hct, Hgb, PT, aPTT, fibrin degradation products, fibrinogen, platelets, ABGs, chemistry profile, lactate, cultures	• Evaluate response to treatment
• Assess and treat pain and discomfort: monitor pain level; administer analgesics; implement comfort and relaxation measures (turning, repositioning, skin care, music); maintain appropriate room temperature; evaluate patient's response	• Promote patient comfort and evaluate response to pain management
• Administer medications as prescribed and specific for the classification of shock (see Table 11-4)	• Improve outcomes and reduce complications
• Provide wound care as indicated and evaluate healing	• Promote wound healing and prevent infection
• Provide adequate nutritional support; collaborate with dietitian about patient's nutritional needs; promote early enteral feed (if tolerated)	• Promote optimum cell function and healing; reduce complications
• Provide psychological support for patient, family, and others	• Reduce the stress response and physiological demand; promote family functioning
• Evaluate patient response to interventions and adjust treatments accordingly; monitor for complications	• Monitor patient response to determine need for modification of treatment and/or nursing care

ABG, Arterial blood gas; *aPTT*, activated partial thromboplastin time; *ARDS*, acute respiratory distress syndrome; *BP*, blood pressure; *DIC*, disseminated intravascular coagulation; *Hct*, hematocrit; *Hgb*, hemoglobin; *HR*, heart rate; *I&O*, intake and output; *MAP*, mean arterial pressure; *MODS*, multiple organ dysfunction syndrome; *SvO₂*, mixed venous oxygen saturation; *PT*, prothrombin time; *RR*, respiratory rate; *SpO₂*, oxygen saturation by pulse oximetry.

SPECIFIC CLASSIFICATIONS OF SHOCK

Table 11-5 provides a summary of the classifications of shock.

Hypovolemic Shock

Hypovolemic shock occurs when the circulating blood volume is inadequate to fill the vascular network. Intravascular volume deficits may be caused by external or internal losses of either blood or fluid. In these situations, the intravascular blood volume is depleted and unavailable to transport oxygen and nutrients to tissues. The severity of hypovolemic shock is dependent upon the volume deficit, the acuity of volume loss, the type of fluid lost, and the age and preinjury health status of the patient.[14]

External volume deficits include loss of blood, plasma, or body fluids. The most common cause of hypovolemic shock is hemorrhage. External loss of

TABLE 11-5   Summary of Classifications of Shock

Classification	Possible Causes	Clinical Presentation	Management

Hypovolemic shock	External loss of blood:
	  GI hemorrhage
	  Surgery
	  Trauma
	External loss of fluid:
	  Diarrhea
	  Diuresis
	  Burns
	Internal sequestration of blood fluid:
	  Hemoperitoneum
	  Retroperitoneal hemorrhage
	  Hemothorax
	  Hemomediastinum
	  Dissecting aortic aneurysm
	  Femur or pelvic fracture
	  Ascites
	  Pleural effusion
		↑ HR
		↓ BP
		Tachypnea
		Oliguria
		Cool, pale skin
		↓ Mentation
		Flat neck veins
		↓ CO, CI, RAP, PAP, PAOP
		↑ SVR
		↓ SvO$_2$
		↑ Hematocrit: if from dehydration
		↓ Hematocrit: if from blood loss
			Eliminate and treat the cause
			Replace lost volume with appropriate fluid

Cardiogenic shock	Myocardial infarction Myocardial contusion Cardiomyopathy Myocarditis Severe heart failure Dysrhythmias Valvular dysfunction Ventricular septal rupture	↑ HR; dysrhythmias ↓ BP Chest pain Tachypnea Oliguria Cool, pale skin ↓ Mentation Left ventricular failure Right ventricular failure ↓ CO, CI ↑ RAP, PAP, PAOP, SVR ↓ SvO$_2$	Improve contractility with inotropic agents Mechanical support as appropriate and available or emergency revascularization Reduce preload Reduce afterload Prevent/treat dysrhythmias

TABLE 11-5 Summary of Classifications of Shock—cont'd

Classification	Possible Causes	Clinical Presentation	Management

Obstructive shock	Impaired diastolic filling:
	  Cardiac tamponade
	  Tension pneumothorax
	  Constrictive pericarditis
	  Compression of great veins
	Increased right ventricular afterload:
	  Pulmonary embolism
	  Severe pulmonary hypertension
	  High intrathoracic pressure
	Increased left ventricular afterload:
	  Aortic dissection
	  Systemic embolization
	  Aortic stenosis
	  Abdominal hypertension
		↑ HR; dysrhythmias
		↓ BP
		Chest pain
		Dyspnea
		Oliguria
		Cool, pale skin
		↓ Mentation
		Jugular venous distention
		Cardiac tamponade: muffled heart sounds, pulsus paradoxus
		Tension pneumothorax: diminished breath sounds on affected side, tracheal shift away from affected side
		Pulmonary embolism: right ventricular failure
		Aortic dissection: ripping chest pain, pulse differences between left and right side, widened mediastinum
		↓ CO, CI
		↑ or normal RAP, PAP, PAOP
		↑ PVR, ↓ SVR
		↓ SvO$_2$
			Eliminate source of obstruction or compression
			Pericardiocentesis for cardiac tamponade
			Fibrinolytics, anticoagulants for PE
			Surgery to remove intracardiac tumor
			Surgical repair of interventricular septum for ventricular septal rupture
			Emergency decompression for tension pneumothorax

Anaphylactic shock	*Foods:* fish, shellfish, eggs, milk, wheat, strawberries, peanuts, tree nuts (pecans, walnuts), food additives *Drugs:* antibiotics, ACE inhibitors, aspirin, local anesthetics, narcotics, barbiturates, contrast media, blood and blood products, allergic extracts *Bites or stings:* venomous snakes, wasps, hornets, spiders, jellyfish, stingrays, deer flies, fire ants *Chemicals:* latex, lotions, soap, perfumes, iodine-containing solutions	↑ HR; dysrhythmias ↓ BP Chest pain Tachypnea Flushed, warm to hot skin Oliguria Restlessness, change in LOC, seizures Nausea, vomiting, abdominal cramping, diarrhea Dyspnea, cough, stridor, wheezing, dysphagia Urticaria, angioedema, hives ↓ CO, CI ↓ RAP, PAP, PAOP, SVR ↓ SvO$_2$ ↑ IgE	Remove offending agent or slow absorption: remove stinger; apply ice to sting or bite; discontinue drug, dye, blood; lavage stomach if antigen ingested; flush skin with water Maintain airway, oxygenation, and ventilation; intubation may be necessary Modify or block the effects of mediators: epinephrine, antihistamines, steroids Maintain MAP
Neurogenic shock	General or spinal anesthesia Epidural block Cervical spinal cord injury *Drugs:* barbiturates, phenothiazines, sympathetic blocking agents	↓HR ↓BP Hypothermia Warm, dry, flushed skin Oliguria Neurological deficit ↓ CO, CI ↓ RAP, PAP, PAOP, SVR ↓ SvO$_2$	Eliminate and treat the cause Maintain MAP Maintain adequate heart rate DVT prophylaxis

Continued

TABLE 11-5   Summary of Classifications of Shock—cont'd

Classification	Possible Causes	Clinical Presentation	Management

Septic shock	Immunosuppression:
	  Extremes of age
	  Malnutrition
	  Alcoholism or drug abuse
	  Malignancy
	  History of splenectomy
	  Chronic health problems
	  Bone marrow depression
	  Immunosuppressive therapies
	Significant bacteremia:
	  Invasive procedures and devices
	  Traumatic wounds or burns
	  GI infection or untreated disease
	  Peritonitis
	  Food poisoning
	  Prolonged hospitalization
	  Translocation of GI bacteria
	    (associated with NPO status)
		Early, hyperdynamic, warm:
		  ↑ HR
		  Normal or ↓ BP
		  ↑ Pulse pressure
		  Skin warm, flushed
		  Confusion
		  Oliguria
		  Hyperthermia
		  ↑ CO, CI
		  ↓ RAP, PAP, PAOP, SVR
		  ↑ SvO$_2$
		Late, hypodynamic, cold:
		  ↑ HR
		  ↓ BP
		  ↓ Pulse pressure
		  Skin cool, pale
		  ↓ LOC
		  Anuria
		  Hypothermia
		  ↓ CO, CI
		  Variable RAP, PAP, PAOP, SVR
		  ↓ SvO$_2$
		  Positive culture
			Good hand-washing techniques
			Avoid invasive procedures
			Identify source of infection
			Meticulous oral and airway care
			Meticulous catheter and wound care
			Avoid NPO status: initiate and maintain enteral nutrition
			Antibiotics as indicated by culture results
			Activated protein C (Xigris)
			Control hyperthermia
			Maintain MAP

ACE, Angiotensin-converting enzyme; *bi-VAD,* biventricular assist device; *BP,* blood pressure; *CI,* cardiac index; *CO,* cardiac output; *CRRT,* continuous renal replacement therapy; *CT,* computed tomography; *DVT,* deep venous thrombosis; *GI,* gastro-intestinal; *HR,* heart rate; *IABP,* intraaortic balloon pump; *LOC,* level of consciousness; *LVAD,* left ventricular assist device; *MAP,* mean arterial pressure; *NPO,* nothing by mouth; *PAOP,* pulmonary artery occlusive pressure; *PAP,* pulmonary artery pressure; *PE,* pulmonary embolism; *RAP,* right atrial pressure; *SvO$_2$,* mixed venous oxygen saturation; *SVR,* systemic vascular resistance.

blood may occur after traumatic injury, surgery, or obstetrical delivery or with coagulation alterations (hemophilia, thrombocytopenia, DIC, and anticoagulant medications). External plasma losses may be seen in patients with burn injuries who have significant fluid shifts from the intravascular space to the interstitial space (see Chapter 20). Excessive external loss of fluid may occur through the gastrointestinal tract via suctioning, upper gastrointestinal bleeding, vomiting, diarrhea, reduction in oral fluid intake, or fistulas; through the genitourinary tract as a result of excessive diuresis, diabetes mellitus with polyuria, diabetes insipidus, or Addison's disease; or through the skin secondary to diaphoresis without fluid and electrolyte replacement.

Blood or body fluids may be sequestered within the body outside the vascular bed. Internal sequestration of blood may be seen in patients with a rup-

tured spleen or liver, hemothorax, hemorrhagic pancreatitis, fractures of the femur or pelvis, and dissecting aneurysm. Internal sequestration of body fluids includes ascites, peritonitis, and peripheral edema. Fluid sequestration is also seen in patients with intestinal obstruction, which causes fluid to leak from the intestinal capillaries into the lumen of the intestine.

Fluid losses may be obvious or subtle. Assessment includes weighing dressings; measuring drainage from chest or nasogastric tubes; monitoring potential sites for bleeding, such as surgical wounds, or IV or intraarterial catheter sites after removal; and considering insensible losses, such as perspiration. Abdominal girth is measured periodically in patients in whom occult bleeding may be suspected or in those with ascites. Daily weights are obtained by using the same scale with the patient wearing the same clothing at approximately the same time each day. Evaluation of the hematocrit is useful in determining whether blood or fluid was lost. In a patient with blood loss, the hematocrit will be decreased, whereas in a patient with fluid loss, the hematocrit will be increased.

Hypovolemic shock results in a reduction of intravascular volume and a decrease in venous return to the right side of the heart. Ventricular filling pressures (preload) are reduced, resulting in a decrease in stroke volume and cardiac output. As the cardiac output decreases, blood pressure decreases and tissue perfusion decreases. Figure 11-6 summarizes the pathophysiology of hypovolemic shock.

Patients with hypovolemic shock present with signs and symptoms as a result of poor organ perfusion, including altered mentation ranging from lethargy to unresponsiveness; rapid, deep respirations; cool, clammy skin with weak, thready pulses; tachy-cardia; and oliguria. Hypovolemic shock resulting from hemorrhage is classified according to the volume of blood lost and the resultant effects on the level of consciousness, vital signs, and urine output (Table 11-6).

A diagnostic peritoneal lavage may be performed to assess for abdominal bleeding. Ultrasonography is also used to diagnose hypovolemic shock secondary to abdominal bleeding. In some facilities, ultrasonography has eliminated the need for diagnostic peritoneal lavage because it is less invasive and can be performed rapidly and repeatedly at the bedside. Abdominal girth is also measured. An increase in the girth may be an indicator of abdominal bleeding or fluid loss into the abdomen. Computed tomography also assists with the differential diagnosis of shock since it can pinpoint sources of bleeding (hypovolemic shock) or abscess formation, which can cause sepsis.

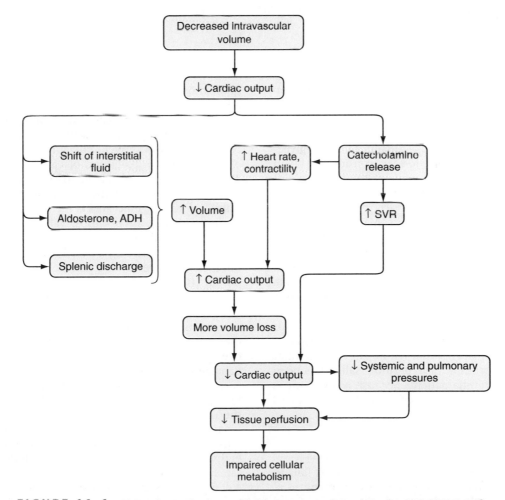

FIGURE 11-6. Hypovolemic shock. *(Modified from McCance, K. L., & Huether, S. E. [2006]. Pathophysiology. The biologic basis for disease in adults and children [5th ed.]. St. Louis: Mosby.)*

TABLE 11-6 Severity of Hemorrhagic Shock

Indicators	Class I	II	III	IV
Blood loss (% blood volume)	<15%	15%-30%	30%-40%	>40%
Blood loss (mL)	<750	750-1500	1500-2000	>2000
Heart rate per minute	<100	>100	>120	>140
Blood pressure	Normal	Normal	Decreased	Decreased
Pulse pressure	Normal or increased	Decreased	Decreased	Decreased
Capillary refill	Normal	Delayed	Delayed	Delayed or absent
Skin appearance	Cool, pink	Cool, pale	Cold, moist, pale	Cold, clammy, cyanotic
Respiratory rate per minute	14-20	20-30	30-40	>35
Urine output (mL/hr)	>30	20-30	<20	Negligible
CNS/mental status	Slightly anxious	Mildly anxious	Anxious, confused	Confused, lethargy

CNS, Central nervous system.
Adapted from American College of Surgeons' Committee on Trauma. (2004). *Advanced trauma life support (ATLS) program for doctors student manual* (7th ed.). Chicago: American College of Surgeons.

Management of hypovolemic shock focuses on identifying, treating, and eliminating the cause of the hypovolemia and replacing lost fluid. Examples of treating the cause include surgery, antidiarrheal medication for diarrhea, and insulin for hyperglycemia. The type of fluid lost is considered when determining fluid replacement. Isotonic crystalloids such as normal saline are generally used first, although blood and blood products may be administered if the patient is bleeding. A guideline that is frequently used is referred to as the 3-for-1 rule. This rule recommends the replacement of 300 mL of isotonic solution for every 100 mL of blood lost. Hemodynamic monitoring provides objective data to guide fluid replacement. Patients receiving blood replacement are likely to require less than 3 times the lost volume.[2] Hypertonic saline (3%) expands the intravascular volume by creating an osmotic effect that displaces water from the intracellular space. Administration of hypertonic saline has been advocated in trauma patients because less volume is required and it is associated with less neutrophil activation.[24,29]

Cardiogenic Shock

Cardiogenic shock can occur when the heart fails to act as an effective pump. A decrease in myocardial contractility results in decreased cardiac output and impaired tissue perfusion. Cardiogenic shock is one of the most difficult types of shock to treat and carries a hospital mortality of 50%.[5]

The most common cause of cardiogenic shock is an extensive left ventricular myocardial infarction. A correlation exists between the amount of myocardial damage and the likelihood of cardiogenic shock. If 40% or more of the left ventricle is damaged, the likelihood of cardiogenic shock increases. Other causes of cardiogenic shock include dysrhythmias, cardiomyopathy, myocarditis, valvular dysfunction, severe heart failure, and structural disorders.

The pathophysiology of cardiogenic shock can be understood by reviewing cardiac dynamics. Cardiac output is determined by heart rate and stroke volume. Stroke volume is determined by preload, afterload, and contractility. Ventricular filling pressure or preload is the pressure in the ventricles as they fill. Afterload is the pressure the heart must overcome to empty the ventricles effectively. When damage to the myocardium occurs, contractile force is reduced and stroke volume decreases. Ventricular filling pressures increase because blood remains in the cardiac chambers. Cardiac output and ejection fraction decrease causing hypotension. This hypotension brings about a reflex compensatory peripheral vasoconstriction and increased afterload. At the same time, backup of blood into the pulmonary circulation causes decreased oxygen perfusion across alveolar membranes, thus reducing the oxygen tension in the blood and decreasing cellular metabo-

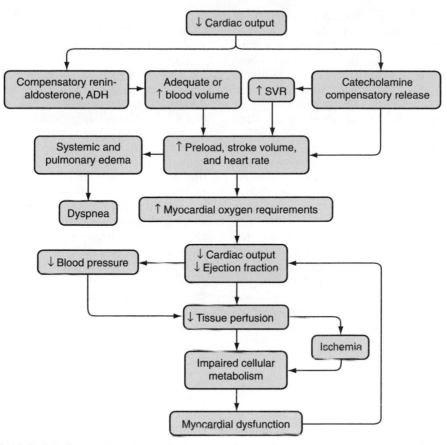

FIGURE 11-7. Cardiogenic shock. *ADH*, Antidiuretic hormone; *SVR*, systemic vascular resistance. *(Modified from McCance, K. L., & Huether, S. E. [2006]. Pathophysiology. The biologic basis for disease in adults and children [5th ed.]. St. Louis: Mosby.)*

lism. Figure 11-7 summarizes the pathophysiology of cardiogenic shock.

An increased demand is placed on the myocardium as it attempts to increase perfusion to the cells. The heart rate increases as a compensatory mechanism, resulting in an increased oxygen demand on an overworked myocardium. In patients with cardiogenic shock secondary to acute myocardial infarction, the increased demand may increase infarction size (Figure 11-8).

The clinical presentation of cardiogenic shock includes manifestations of left ventricular failure (S_3 heart sound, crackles, dyspnea, hypoxemia) and right ventricular failure (jugular venous distention, peripheral edema, hepatomegaly). A pulmonary artery catheter is useful in trending hemodynamic parameters. In cardiogenic shock, cardiac output and cardiac index decrease; however, RAP, pulmonary artery pressure (PAP), and PAOP increase as pressure and volume back up into the pulmonary circulation and the right side of the heart.

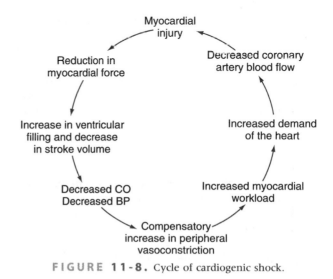

FIGURE 11-8. Cycle of cardiogenic shock.

Prevention of cardiogenic shock is aimed at promoting myocardial contractility, decreasing the myocardial oxygen demand, and increasing the oxygen supply to the damaged tissue. Aggressive management after a myocardial infarction includes percutaneous coronary interventions with transluminal coronary angioplasty, intracoronary stent placement, or both, fibrinolytic agents when primary percutaneous coronary intervention is not available, glycoprotein IIb/IIIa inhibitors, and beta-blockers to limit the size of the infarction. Pain relief and rest reduce the workload of the heart and the infarct size. Oxygen administration increases oxygen delivery to the ischemic muscle and may help save myocardial tissue.

Pharmacological agents are administered to decrease preload (RAP, PAOP), decrease afterload (SVR), increase stroke volume, increase cardiac index, and increase contractility (see Table 11-4). Diuretics (e.g., furosemide) and venous vasodilators (e.g., morphine, nitroglycerin, nitroprusside) reduce preload and venous return to the heart. Nitroglycerin at low doses (<1 mcg/kg/min) causes venous vasodilation to decrease preload. At higher doses (>1 mcg/kg/min) arterial vasodilation decreases afterload. These drugs must be used cautiously because they may cause hypotension, thereby contributing to further cellular hypoperfusion.

Positive inotropic agents (e.g., dobutamine) are given to increase the contractile force of the heart. As contractility increases, ventricular emptying improves, filling pressures decrease (RAP, PAOP), and stroke volume improves. The improved stroke volume increases cardiac output and improves tissue perfusion. However, positive inotropic agents also increase myocardial oxygen demand and must be used cautiously in patients with myocardial ischemia.

Afterload reduction may be achieved by the cautious administration of arterial vasodilators (e.g., nitroprusside) to decrease SVR, increase stroke volume, and increase cardiac index. Blood pressure must be carefully monitored to keep the mean arterial pressure above 65 mm Hg to ensure organ perfusion. Significant hypotension may limit the use of arterial vasodilators, as coronary artery perfusion pressure may be reduced and worsen myocardial ischemia. In this situation, afterload reduction is achieved through the insertion of an intraaortic balloon pump (IABP).

The IABP is a cardiac assist device that provides counterpulsation therapy concurrently with pharmacological support. IABP therapy is initiated by inserting a dual-chambered balloon into the descending thoracic aorta via the femoral artery. The balloon is inserted percutaneously at the patient's bedside or under fluoroscopy. The tip of the balloon is positioned just distal to the left subclavian artery (Figure 11-9). Correct placement is verified by chest x-ray.

The IABP improves coronary artery perfusion, reduces afterload, and improves perfusion to vital organs. The balloon is inflated mechanically with helium. Inflation and deflation are automatically timed with the cardiac cycle. The IABP inflates during diastole when the aortic valve is closed. The inflation cycle displaces blood backward and forward simultaneously. The backward flow increases perfusion to the coronary arteries, and the forward flow increases perfusion to vital organs. Balloon deflation occurs just before systole and left ventricular ejection. This sudden deflation, along with the displacement of blood that occurred during diastole, reduces the pressure in the aorta and decreases afterload and myocardial oxygen demand. Desired outcomes for a patient in cardiogenic shock with an IABP include decreased SVR, diminished symptoms of myocardial ischemia (chest pain, ST-segment elevation), and increased stroke volume and cardiac output.

Counterpulsation therapy with an IABP requires a high degree of nursing skill because of the complexity of the equipment and the need for frequent monitoring. Many institutions require nurses to be credentialed in managing the patient with an IABP. Limb ischemia and embolic phenomena are potential complications that must be assessed. Other complications include dissection of the aorta, infection, ineffective pumping, and technical problems. Use of the IABP is contraindicated in patients with aortic valve insufficiency or aortic aneurysm.

Ventricular assist devices (VADs) may be used temporarily to support a failing ventricle that has not responded to IABP therapy and pharmacological

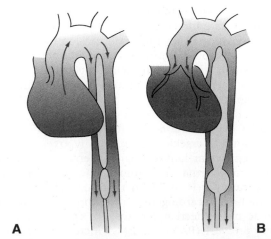

A   **B**

FIGURE 11-9. Intraaortic balloon pump. The balloon is deflated during systole (**A**) and inflated during diastole (**B**).

therapy. VADs are used to treat cardiogenic shock by allowing the ventricle to recover or to support the patient awaiting cardiac transplant as a bridge to transplant. They can be used to support the left ventricle, the right ventricle, or both ventricles. VADs vary in design and technology. In general, they consist of an external pump, which diverts blood from the failing ventricle or ventricles and pumps it back into the aorta (left VAD [LVAD]), the pulmonary artery (right VAD [RVAD]), or both great vessels (Bi-VAD). The use of VADs requires extensive training and advanced nursing care. These devices are not typically available in community hospitals.

Obstructive Shock

Obstructive shock (also known as extracardiac obstructive shock) occurs when there is a physical impairment to adequate circulatory blood flow. Causes of obstructive shock include impaired diastolic filling (cardiac tamponade, tension pneumothorax, constrictive pericarditis, compression of the great veins), increased right ventricular afterload (pulmonary embolism, severe pulmonary hypertension, increased intrathoracic pressures), and increased left ventricular afterload (aortic dissection, systemic embolization, aortic stenosis). Obstruction of the heart or great vessels either impedes venous return to the right side of the heart or prevents effective pumping action of the heart. This results in decreased cardiac output, hypotension, decreased tissue perfusion, and impaired cellular metabolism (Figure 11-10).

Common clinical findings in obstructive shock include chest pain, dyspnea, jugular venous distention, and hypoxia. Other findings are dependent on the cause. Cardiac tamponade is manifested by muffled heart sounds, hypotension, and pulsus paradoxus. Pulsus paradoxus is a decrease in systolic blood pressure of more than 10 mm Hg during inspiration. Tension pneumothorax is manifested by diminished breath sounds on the affected side and tracheal shift away from the affected side. Massive pulmonary embolism is manifested by clinical indications of right ventricular failure (jugular venous distention, peripheral edema, hepatomegaly). Aortic dissection is manifested by complaints of ripping chest pain that radiates to the back, pulse differences between the left and right side, and a widened mediastinum on chest x-ray, echocardiogram, or computed tomography scan.

Obstructive shock may be prevented or treated, or both, by aggressive interventions to relieve the source of the compression or obstruction. Cardiac tamponade may be relieved by a pericardiocentesis, or the removal of fluid from the pericardial sac. A tension

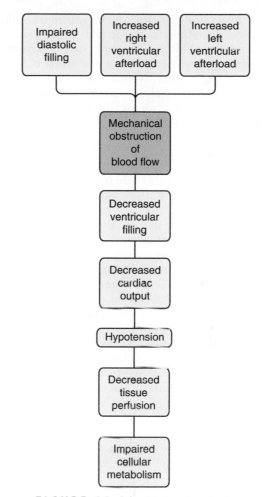

FIGURE 11-10. Obstructive shock.

pneumothorax from blunt or penetrating chest injuries may be relieved by a needle thoracentesis to remove the accumulated intrathoracic pressure. The risk of pulmonary embolism may be reduced by early surgical reduction of long bone fractures, devices to enhance circulation in immobile patients (antiembolism hose or sequential compression device, range-of-motion exercises), and prophylactic anticoagulant therapy.

Distributive Shock

Neurogenic, anaphylactic, and septic shock are forms of distributive shock. Distributive shock, also known as vasogenic shock, describes several different types of shock that present with widespread vasodilation and decreased SVR. Vasodilation increases the vascular capacity; however, the blood volume is unchanged, resulting in a relative hypovolemia. This causes a decrease in venous return to the right side of the heart and a reduction in ventricular filling pressures. Anaphylactic shock and septic shock are also complicated by an increase in capillary permeability, which decreases intravascular volume, further compromising venous return. Eventually, in all forms of distributive shock, stroke volume, cardiac output, and blood pressure decrease, resulting in decreased tissue perfusion and impaired cellular metabolism.

Neurogenic Shock

Neurogenic shock occurs when a disturbance in the nervous system affects the vasomotor center in the medulla. In healthy persons, the vasomotor center initiates sympathetic stimulation of nerve fibers that travel down the spinal cord and out to the periphery. There, they innervate the smooth muscles of the blood vessels to cause vasoconstriction. In neurogenic shock, there is an interruption of impulse transmission or a blockage of sympathetic outflow resulting in vasodilation, inhibition of baroreceptor response, and impaired thermoregulation. Consequently, these reactions create vasodilation with decreased SVR, venous return, preload, and cardiac output and a relative hypovolemia. Figure 11-11 summarizes the pathophysiology of neurogenic shock.

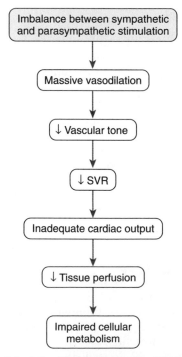

FIGURE 11-11. Neurogenic shock. *SVR,* Systemic vascular resistance. *(Modified from McCance, K. L., & Huether, S. E. [2006]. Pathophysiology. The biologic basis for disease in adults and children [5th ed.]. St. Louis: Mosby.)*

Causes of neurogenic shock include injury or disease of the upper spinal cord, spinal anesthesia, nervous system damage, administration of ganglionic and adrenergic blocking agents, and vasomotor depression. Patients who have a cervical spinal cord injury may experience a permanent or temporary interruption in sympathetic nerve stimulation. Spinal anesthesia may extend up the spinal cord and may block sympathetic nerve impulses from the vasomotor center. Vasomotor depression may be seen with deep general anesthesia, injury to the medulla, administration of drugs, severe pain, and hypoglycemia.

The most profound features of neurogenic shock are bradycardia with hypotension from the decreased sympathetic activity. The skin is frequently warm, dry, and flushed. Hypothermia develops from uncontrolled heat loss. Venous pooling in the lower extremities promotes the formation of deep vein thrombosis, which can result in pulmonary embolism. A neurological deficit may be evident.

Management focuses on treating the cause, including reversal of offending drugs or glucose administration for hypoglycemia. Immobilization of spinal injuries with traction devices (halo brace to maintain alignment) or surgical intervention to stabilize the injury assists in preventing severe neurogenic shock. Patients receiving spinal anesthesia positioned with the head of the bed elevated may prevent the progression of the spinal blockade up the cord. IV fluids are infused to treat hypotension; however, they must be given cautiously to prevent fluid overload and cerebral or spinal cord edema.[6] Vasopressors are frequently required to maintain perfusion. Alpha- and beta-adrenergic agents, such as dopamine or norepinephrine, are preferred since pure alpha-adrenergic agents, such as phenylephrine, are associated with persistent bradycardia.[18] Hypothermia is common so the patient is rewarmed slowly, as rapid rewarming may cause vasodilation and worsen the patient's hemodynamic status. Atropine is used for symptomatic bradycardia; however, a temporary or permanent pacemaker may be required.

Anaphylactic Shock

A severe allergic reaction can precipitate a second form of distributive shock known as anaphylactic shock. Antigens, which are foreign substances to which someone is sensitive, initiate an antigen-antibody response. Table 11-5 lists some common antigens causing anaphylaxis.

Once an antigen enters the body, antibodies (immunoglobulin E [IgE]) are produced that attach to mast cells and basophils. The greatest concentrations of mast cells are found in the lungs, around blood vessels, in connective tissue, and in the uterus.

Mast cells are also found to a lesser extent in the kidneys, heart, skin, liver, and spleen and in the omentum of the gastrointestinal tract. Basophils circulate in the blood. Both mast cells and basophils contain histamine and histamine-like substances, which are potent vasodilators.

The initial exposure (primary immune response) to the antigen does not usually cause any harmful effects; however, subsequent exposures to the antigen may cause an anaphylactic reaction (secondary immune response). The antigen-antibody reaction causes cellular breakdown and the release of powerful vasoactive mediators from the mast cells and basophils. These mediators cause bronchoconstriction, excessive mucus secretion, vasodilation, increased capillary permeability, inflammation, gastrointestinal cramps, and cutaneous reactions that stimulate nerve endings, causing itching and pain. Figure 11-12 summarizes the pathophysiology of anaphylactic shock. The combined effects result in decreased blood pressure, relative hypovolemia caused by the vasodilation and fluid shifts, and symp-toms of anaphylaxis that primarily affect the skin, respiratory, and gastrointestinal systems.

Obtaining a thorough history of allergies and drug reactions, especially reactions to drugs with similar structures, is an important strategy to prevent anaphylactic shock. For example, if patients are allergic to penicillin, they are likely to have a reaction to ampicillin (Principen), carbenicillin (Geopen), or nafcillin sodium. The response to IV administration of medications, particularly antibiotics, is monitored. Injecting small amounts of a drug before the entire dose is given is recommended to assist in detecting a possible reaction. Care is taken during the transfusion of blood or blood products, which can result in allergic reactions. The patient receiving any of these products is observed closely for any signs of an allergic reaction.

The clinical presentation of anaphylactic shock includes flushing, pruritus, urticaria, and angioedema (swelling of eyes, lips, tongue, hands, feet, genitalia). Cough, runny nose, nasal congestion, hoarseness, dysphonia, and dyspnea are common

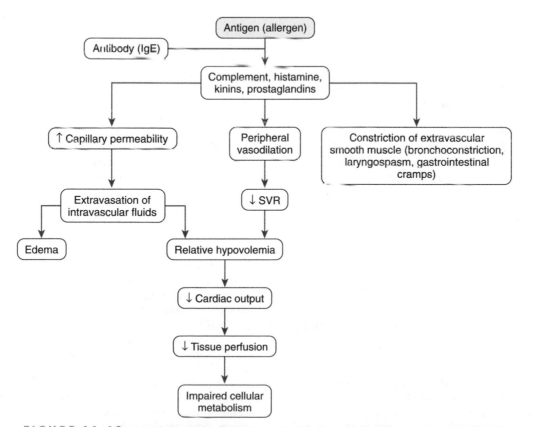

FIGURE 11-12. Anaphylactic shock. *IgE,* Immunoglobulin E; *SVR,* systemic vascular resistance. *(Modified from McCance, K. L., & Huether, S. E. [2006]. Pathophysiology. The biologic basis for disease in adults and children [5th ed.]. St. Louis: Mosby.)*

because of upper airway obstruction from edema of the larynx, epiglottis, or vocal cords. Stridor may occur as a result of laryngeal edema. Lower airway obstruction may result from diffuse bronchoconstriction and cause wheezing and chest tightness. Tachycardia and hypotension occur, and the patient may show signs of pulmonary edema. Gastrointestinal symptoms of nausea, vomiting, cramping, abdominal pain, and diarrhea may also occur. Neurological symptoms include lethargy and decreased consciousness. Elevated levels of IgE are seen on laboratory analysis.

Goals of therapy are to remove the antigen, reverse the effects of the mediators, and promote adequate tissue perfusion. If the anaphylactic reaction results from medications, contrast dye, or blood or blood products, the infusion is immediately stopped. Airway, ventilation, and circulation are supported. Laryngeal edema may be severe enough to require intubation or cricothyrotomy if swelling is so severe that an endotracheal tube cannot be placed. Oxygen is administered to keep the SpO_2 greater than 90%. Removal of the offending agent is achieved by removal of the stinger, administration of antivenom, stopping the drug, gastric lavage, or flushing the skin.

Epinephrine is the drug of choice for treating anaphylactic shock. Epinephrine is an adrenergic agent that promotes bronchodilation and vasoconstriction. For mild reactions, epinephrine 0.3 to 0.5 mg (0.3 to 0.5 mL of a 1:1000 solution) is administered intramuscularly or subcutaneously. The dose may be repeated at 5- to 15-minute intervals until anaphylaxis is resolved. For anaphylaxis with hypotension, 0.3 to 0.5 mg (3 to 5 mL of 1:10,000 solution) is administered IV. The dose may be repeated every 15 minutes if needed. If the patient has been receiving beta-blockers, there may be a limited response to epinephrine, and glucagon 5 to 15 mcg/min IV may be administered instead. To block histamine release, diphenhydramine (Benadryl), an H_1-receptor blocker, is administered IV in a dosage of 1 to 2 mg/kg (maximum, 50 mg) every 4 to 8 hours, and ranitidine (Zantac), an H_2-receptor blocker, is administered IV in a dosage of 50 mg every 6 to 8 hours. Corticosteroids such as methylprednisolone (Solu-Medrol) are used to reduce inflammation. Fluid replacement, positive inotropic agents, and vasopressors may be required.

Septic Shock

Septic shock is one component of a continuum of progressive clinical insults including SIRS, sepsis, and MODS. In the past, there has been confusion about what these various syndromes represented. Because of this confusion and the complexity of these syndromes, consensus definitions were identified in 1992[8] and were reviewed in 2001.[21] The 2001 consensus group took the definitions a step further by identifying diagnostic criteria for sepsis. The intent of the criteria is to provide a tool to recognize and diagnose sepsis quickly and therefore to prompt the search for an infectious source to initiate the appropriate therapy. None of the diagnostic criteria are specific for sepsis because these parameters can be altered by other conditions. The definitions and diagnostic criteria are presented in Table 11-7. Invasion of the host by a microorganism or an infection begins the process that may progress to sepsis, followed by severe sepsis and septic shock, which progresses to MODS.

Once a microorganism has invaded a host, an inflammatory response is initiated to restore homeostasis. SIRS occurs, leading to release of inflammatory mediators or cytokines, which are produced by the white blood cells. SIRS can also occur as a result of trauma, shock, pancreatitis, or ischemia.[8] For reasons not completely understood, SIRS may progress to septic shock and MODS (Figure 11-13). Cytokines are proinflammatory or antiinflammatory. Proinflammatory cytokines including tumor necrosis factor, interleukin-1α, and interleukin-β produce pyrogenic responses and initiate the hepatic response to infection. Antiinflammatory cytokines including nitric oxide, lipopolysaccharide, and interleukin-1–receptor antagonist are compensatory, ensuring that the effect of the proinflammatory mediators does not become destructive. In sepsis, continued activation of proinflammatory cytokines overwhelms the antiinflammatory cytokines and excessive systemic inflammation results.

A state of enhanced coagulation occurs through stimulation of the coagulation cascade, with a reduction in the levels of activated protein C and antithrombin III. This results in the generation of thrombin and the formation of microemboli that impair blood flow and organ perfusion. Fibrinolysis is activated in response to the activation of the coagulation cascade to promote clot breakdown. However, activation is followed by inhibition, further promoting coagulopathy. This imbalance among inflammation, coagulation, and fibrinolysis results in systemic inflammation, widespread coagulopathy, and microvascular thrombi that impair tissue perfusion, leading to MODS.

These inflammatory mediators also damage the endothelial cells that line blood vessels, producing profound vasodilation and increased capillary permeability. Initially, this results in tachycardia, hypotension, and low SVR. Although norepinephrine and the renin-angiotensin-aldosterone system are activated in response to this clinical state, they are unable to enter the cells, and hypotension and vasodilation persist. In contrast, the plasma levels of the

TABLE 11-7 Clinical Condition, Diagnostic Criteria, and Management in the Continuum of Sepsis

Clinical Condition and Definition	Diagnostic Criteria	Management
Infection: Inflammatory response to microorganisms	Fever	Administer antibiotics Surgical excision or drainage of source of infection
SIRS: Systemic inflammatory response to a clinical insult including infection, pancreatitis, ischemia, trauma, or hemorrhagic shock	Tachycardia (HR >90 beats/min) Respiratory rate >20 breaths/min or PaCO₂ <32 mm Hg Temperature >38°C (hyperthermia) or <36°C (hypothermia)	Administer antibiotics Remove source of infection Maintain adequate ventilation and oxygenation Replace fluid
Sepsis: Systemic response to infection manifested by two or more of the symptoms noted with SIRS	Leukocytosis (WBC count >12,000 cells/mm³) or leukopenia (WBC count <4000 cells/mm³) or >10% immature bands	Antipyretics
Severe sepsis: Sepsis associated with organ dysfunction, hypoperfusion, or hypotension	As above with evidence of impaired systemic perfusion and organ function, possibly including lactic acidosis, oliguria, or acute change in mental status	Administer antibiotics Remove source of infection Maintain adequate ventilation and oxygenation Maximize oxygen delivery, minimize oxygen demand Replace fluid Administer vasoactive medications Correct acid-base abnormalities Monitor and support organ function
Septic shock: Sepsis with hypotension despite adequate fluid resuscitation, along with perfusion abnormalities	Hypotension Lactic acidosis, oliguria, acute change in mental status Patients receiving inotropic agents or vasopressors may not exhibit hypotension	Administer antibiotics Maintain adequate ventilation and oxygenation Maximize oxygen delivery, minimize oxygen demand Replace fluid Administer vasoactive medications Correct acid-base abnormalities Monitor and support organ function
MODS: Altered organ function in acutely ill patients	See Table 11-9	Maintain adequate ventilation and oxygenation Maximize oxygen delivery, minimize oxygen demand Perform dialysis Monitor and support organ function Monitor clotting studies and bleeding

HR, Heart rate; *PaCO₂*, partial pressure of arterial carbon dioxide; *MODS*, multiple organ dysfunction syndrome; *SIRS*, systemic inflammatory response syndrome; *WBC*, white blood cell.
Definitions modified from Levy, M. M., Fink, M. P., Marshall, J. C., Abraham, E., Angus, D., Cook, D., et al. (2003). 2001 SCCM/ESICM/ACCP/ATS/SIS International Sepsis Definitions Conference. *Critical Care Medicine, 31*(4), 1250-1256.

antidiuretic hormone (ADH or vasopressin) are low despite the presence of hypotension. The exact mechanism that creates this low concentration is not known; however, administering a continuous infusion significantly increases blood pressure in septic shock.

Once sepsis is present, it can progress to septic shock. Septic shock is sepsis with hypotension that is unresponsive to fluid resuscitation along with signs of inadequate organ perfusion such as metabolic acidosis, acute encephalopathy, oliguria, hypoxemia, or coagulation disorders. The clinical course of septic shock is frequently differentiated between the early (warm, hyperdynamic) phase and the late (cold, hypodynamic) phase (Table 11-8).

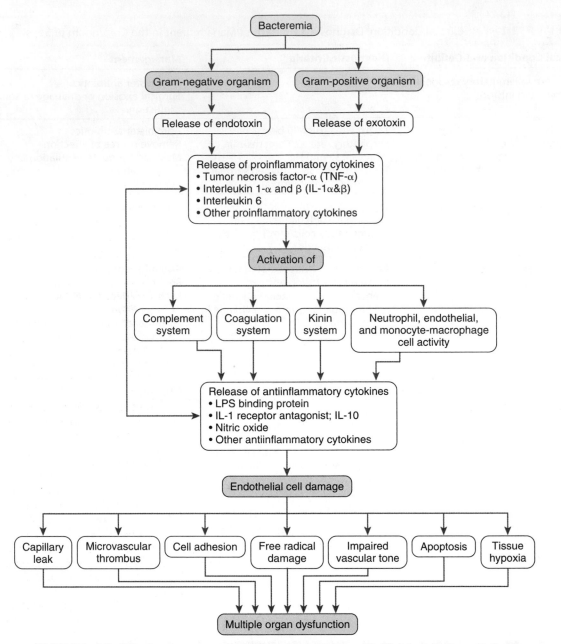

FIGURE 11-13. Sepsis and septic shock pathophysiology. *(Modified from McCance, K. L., & Huether, S. E. [2006]. Pathophysiology. The biologic basis for disease in adults and children [5th ed.]. St. Louis: Mosby.)*

Factors that increase the risk of developing sepsis are categorized as either situations that cause immunosuppression or situations that cause significant bacteremia (see Table 11-5). Sepsis is infection with SIRS and is the systemic response to infection. SIRS is present if two or more of the clinical manifestations of SIRS are identified (see Table 11-7). Sepsis can advance to severe sepsis with hypotension, chills, decreased urine output, decreased skin perfusion, poor capillary refill, skin mottling, decreased platelets, petechiae, hyperglycemia, and unexplained changes in mental status.[15]

Prevention of sepsis is promoted by preventing infections, including proper hand washing, use of aseptic technique, and awareness of the patient at risk. The critically ill patient is debilitated and has

TABLE 11-8 Stages of Septic Shock

Early (Hyperdynamic; Looks Like Infection)	Late (Hypodynamic; Looks Like Shock)
Clinical Presentation	
Tachycardia	Tachycardia
Pulses bounding	Pulses weak and thready
Blood pressure: normal or low	Hypotension
Wide pulse pressure	Narrow pulse pressure
Skin warm, flushed	Skin cool, pale
Hyperpnea	Bradypnea or tachypnea
Change in mental status (irritability and confusion)	↓ Level of consciousness (lethargy or coma)
Oliguria	Anuria
Hyperthermia	Hypothermia
Hemodynamic Parameters	
↑ CO/CI	↓ CO/CI
↓ RAP/PAP/PAOP	RAP/PAP/PAOP variable
↓ SVR	SVR variable
↑ SvO$_2$	↓ SvO$_2$
Diagnostic Findings	
ABGs: respiratory alkalosis with hypoxemia	ABGs: metabolic acidosis with hypoxemia
↑ PT and aPTT	↑ PT and aPTT
↓ Platelets	↓ Platelets
↑ WBC count	↓ WBC count
↑ Glucose	↓ Glucose
	↑ BUN, creatinine
	↑ Serum arterial lactate
	↑ Amylase, lipase
	↑ AST, ALT, LDH

ABGs, Arterial blood gases; *ALT*, alanine aminotransferase; *aPTT*, activated partial thromboplastin time; *AST*, aspartate aminotransferase; *BUN*, blood urea nitrogen; *CI*, cardiac index; *CO*, cardiac output; *LDH*, lactic dehydrogenase; *PAOP*, pulmonary artery occlusive pressure; *PAP*, pulmonary artery pressure; *PT*, prothrombin time; *RAP*, right atrial pressure; *SvO$_2$*, oxygen saturation of venous blood; *SVR*, systemic vascular resistance; *WBC*, white blood cell.

many potential portals of entry for bacterial invasion. Meticulous technique is required during procedures such as suctioning, dressing changes, and wound care and when handling catheters or tubes. Frequent assessment of temperature, wounds, and laboratory results including white blood cell count, differential counts, and cultures is important for the identification of infection.

Gram-negative bacteria such as *Escherichia coli*, *Klebsiella* species, or *Pseudomonas* species are a common cause of infections in adults. Common sites of infection include the pulmonary system, urinary tract, gastrointestinal system, and wounds.

Gram-positive bacteria such as *Staphylococcus aureus* can also lead to sepsis and septic shock. These bacteria release a potent toxin that exerts its effects within hours. Gram-positive infection has been associated with the use of tampons in menstruating women (known as toxic shock syndrome); however, it is also seen after vaginal and cesarean delivery and in patients with surgical wounds, abscesses, infected burns, abrasions, insect bites, herpes zoster, cellulitis, septic abortion, and osteomyelitis, as well as in some newborns in whom the bacteria are transmitted from the mother. Management includes antimicrobial therapy, removal of the source of infection if one is found, fluid resuscitation, and vasoactive medication to improve cardiac performance.

Pneumonia is a common trigger for sepsis. Ventilator-associated pneumonia is a significant risk factor for the development of sepsis. Several strategies have been identified that reduce the risk of ventilator-associated pneumonia and are easily implemented. These include maintaining the head of the bed at 30-degree elevation or greater, providing frequent oral care, and reducing the number of ventilator circuit changes.[1] Another strategy is the use of an endotracheal tube with a dorsal lumen to allow continuous suction of secretions from the subglottic area.[16]

Timely identification of the causative organism and the initiation of appropriate antibiotics improve survival of patients with sepsis or septic shock.[17] Any catheter suspected to be a source of infection should be removed. Surgery may be required to locate the source of infection, drain an abscess, and/or debride any necrosis.

Before antibiotic therapy is initiated, culture and sensitivity tests of blood, urine, sputum, wound, tip of a catheter, and any suspicious site are obtained. This helps to identify the source of the infection, the type of organisms, and which antibiotics should be used.[25] However, the need for early administration of antibiotics, preferably within 1 hour, requires the initial antibiotic selection be directed toward the most likely organism, and frequently empirical and broad-spectrum antibiotics are initiated.[12] Antibiotics may be changed after Gram stain results (approximately 4 hours) or culture and sensitivity results (approximately 72 hours) are available. Antibiotics are discontinued if the cause of the sepsis is not bacterial. Unfortunately, antibiotics do not act on the immune response to infection and do not directly improve tissue perfusion.

Early goal-directed therapy has been shown to decrease mortality in patients with severe sepsis and septic shock, and is advocated for the first 6 hours of sepsis resuscitation.[27,35] Early goal-directed therapy includes administration of IV fluids to keep the central venous pressure at 8 mm Hg or greater (but not >15 mm Hg) and the heart rate at less than 110 beats/min, administration of vasopressors to keep the mean arterial pressure at 65 mm Hg or greater, and administration of dobutamine, packed red blood cells, or both to keep the central venous oxygen saturation ($ScvO_2$) at 70% or greater.[12,35,39] $ScvO_2$ correlates to SvO_2 but is measured with a fiberoptic central venous catheter rather than a pulmonary artery catheter; therefore, assessment of this parameter is easier to obtain in emergent situations.[28]

Isotonic crystalloid solutions are infused for fluid resuscitation. Colloids are likely to leak out of the vascular bed into the interstitium because of increased capillary permeability. Vasopressors, frequently norepinephrine or dopamine, are used to increase SVR and mean arterial pressure. Vasopressin may be added to norepinephrine, especially when high doses of norepinephrine are required.[23] Advantages of vasopressin include decreasing exogenous catecholamines and increasing the release of cortisol and ACTH.[12,20] In addition, vasopressin causes vasoconstriction without the adverse effects of tachycardia and ventricular ectopy seen with catecholamines such as dopamine or norepinephrine. Dobutamine may be used to increase the myocardial contractility and improve the cardiac index and DO_2 in patients with a decreased $ScvO_2$. If the patient's hematocrit is less than 30%, the administration of packed red blood cells is advocated to increase DO_2.[30]

Elevated cardiac troponin levels and elevated brain natriuretic peptide (BNP) indicate left ventricular dysfunction and a poor prognosis in patients with sepsis and septic shock.[22,37] ACTH-stimulated cortisol levels may be measured since poor ACTH-cortisol responses are associated with a high mortality.[11] Corticosteroids have been shown to reduce mortality for those patients with sepsis or septic shock who have an inadequate response to the ACTH stimulation test.[4] Routine use of corticosteroids, however, is not recommended because of the effects on glucose homeostasis, the risk for infection, and the potential for myopathy.[33]

In severe sepsis, the patient has excessive coagulation, inflammation, and impaired fibrinolysis. Recombinant human activated protein C (drotrecogin alfa [Xigris]) is an antiinflammatory, antithrombotic, and profibrinolytic agent that reduces the inflammatory, clotting, and bleeding responses to sepsis. It has been shown to reduce mortality in patients with severe sepsis with dysfunction of two organ systems.[7] The medication is administered as an IV infusion over 96 hours at a dosage of 24 mcg/kg/hr. Patients are monitored for bleeding during the infusion, as it is a profibrinolytic and antithrombotic agent.[38]

Hyperglycemia and insulin resistance are common in the patient with sepsis. Frequent glucose testing and intensive IV insulin protocols to maintain blood glucose levels at less than 150 mg/dL reduces morbidity and mortality in all critically ill patients. The effect is even more significant in patients with MODS caused by sepsis.[31,36]

While pyrogens (polypeptides that produce fever) aid in activation of the immune response, temperature reduction is considered for core body temperatures of 41°C or higher because of the significant increase in oxygen consumption. Treatment of fever includes physiological cooling (ice packs, tepid baths, cooling blanket, or misting) along with administration of antipyretics (acetaminophen, ibuprofen, or aspirin). Care must be taken to avoid overcooling since hypothermia adversely affects oxygen delivery and may result in shivering, which increases oxygen consumption.

Many experimental therapies have been advocated for sepsis and septic shock. Plasmapheresis may remove endotoxin and other harmful substances produced by either the infective organism or the inflammatory process.[19] Immunoglobulins may also be prescribed, especially in patients who are immunocompromised.[19]

MULTIPLE ORGAN DYSFUNCTION SYNDROME

MODS is the progressive dysfunction of two or more organ systems as a result of an uncontrolled inflammatory response to severe illness or injury. Organ dysfunction can progress to organ failure and death. The most common causes of MODS are sepsis and septic shock; however, MODS can occur after any severe injury or disease process that activates a massive systemic inflammatory response including any classification of shock. The immune system and the body's response to stress can cause maldistribution of circulating volume, global tissue hypoxia, and metabolic alterations that result in damage to organs. Failure of two or more organs is associated with an estimated 45% to 55% mortality, 80% mortality when three or more organ systems fail, and 100% mortality if three or more organ systems fail for longer than 4 days.[3]

Damage to organs may be primary or secondary. In primary MODS there is direct injury to an organ from shock, trauma, burn injury, or infection with impaired perfusion that results in dysfunction. Decreased perfusion may be localized or systemic. As a result of this insult, the stress response and inflammatory response are activated with the release of catecholamines and activation of mediators that affect cellular activity (Figure 11-14).

Secondary MODS is a consequence of widespread systemic inflammation that results in dysfunction of organs not involved with the initial insult. It occurs in response to altered regulation of the acute immune and inflammatory responses. Failure to control the inflammatory response leads to excessive production of inflammatory cells and biochemical mediators that cause widespread damage to vascular endothelium and organ damage. The interaction of injured organs then leads to self-perpetuating inflammation with maldistribution of blood flow and hypermetabolism.

Maldistribution of blood flow refers to the uneven distribution of flow to various organs and between the large vessels and capillary beds. It is caused by vasodilation, increased capillary permeability, selective vasoconstriction, and impaired microvascular circulation. This impaired blood flow leads to impaired tissue perfusion and a decreased oxygen supply to the cells. The organs most severely affected are the lungs, splanchnic bed, liver, and kidneys.

Hypermetabolism with altered carbohydrate, fat, and lipid metabolism is initially compensatory to meet the body's increased demands for energy. Eventually, hypermetabolism becomes detrimental, placing tremendous demands on the heart as cardiac output increases up to twice the normal value. Hyperglycemia occurs as gluconeogenesis by the liver increases and glucose use by the cells decreases.

The decreased oxygen delivery to the cells (from maldistribution of blood flow) and increased oxygen needs of the cells (from hypermetabolism) create an imbalance in oxygen supply and demand. In MODS, the amount of oxygen consumed becomes dependent on the amount of oxygen that can be delivered to the cells. Hypoxemia, cellular acidosis, and impaired cellular function result with the development of multiple organ failure.

The clinical presentation of MODS is caused by inflammatory mediator damage, tissue hypoxia, and hypermetabolism. Damage to the organs is usually sequential rather than simultaneous. The first system frequently affected is the pulmonary system, with acute ARDS developing within 12 to 24 hours after the initial insult. Coagulopathy frequently develops, followed by renal, hepatic, and intestinal impairment.[32] Failure of the cardiovascular system, neurologic system, or both, are frequently fatal events. MODS progresses from minor dysfunction of one or multiple organs to multiple organs requiring support.

Criteria used in the diagnoses of organ dysfunction are described in Table 11-9. Pulmonary dysfunction is manifested by tachypnea, hypoxemia despite high levels of supplemental oxygen, and chest x-ray changes. Hematologic dysfunction is manifested by petechiae, bleeding, thrombocytopenia, prolonged PT and aPTT, increased fibrin split products, and a positive D-dimer. The earliest sign of hepatic dysfunction is hypoglycemia, which is followed by jaundice, increased liver enzymes and bilirubin, prolonged PT, and decreased albumin. The first indication of intestinal dysfunction is frequently intolerance of enteral feedings with abdominal distention and increased retention volumes. Renal dysfunction is evidenced by oliguria to anuria, increased blood urea nitrogen and creatinine, and fluid and electrolyte imbalance. Tachycardia (frequently with dysrhythmias), hypotension, and hemodynamic alterations indicate cardiovascular dysfunction. Finally, cerebral dysfunction is manifested by a change in level of consciousness, confusion, and focal neurologic signs such as hemiparesis. The final response to MODS is hypotension that is unresponsive to fluids and vasopressors, and cardiac arrest.

Management of MODS focuses on prevention and support. The initial source of inflammation must be eliminated or controlled. A secondary insult must be avoided. Potential sites of infection are removed, including debriding necrotic tissue, draining abscesses, reducing the number of invasive procedures performed, and removing hematomas. Goals are to control infection, provide adequate tissue oxygenation, restore intravascular volume, and support organ function. Antibiotics are administered. SpO_2 is maintained between 88% and 92%, hemoglobin levels should be above 7 to 9 g/dL, and an SvO_2 greater than 70% is desired. Aggressive fluid therapy with isotonic crystalloid solutions is

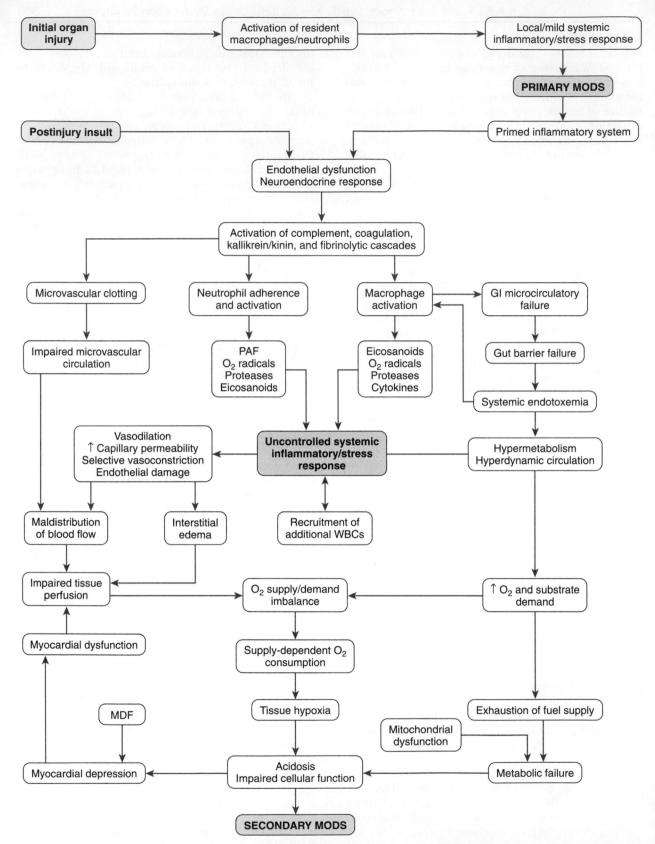

FIGURE 11-14. Pathogenesis of multiple organ dysfunction syndrome. *MODS*, Multiple organ dysfunction syndrome; *GI*, gastrointestinal; *PAF*, platelet activating factor; *WBCs*, white blood cells; *MDF*, myocardial depressant factor. *(Modified from McCance, K. L., & Huether, S. E. [2006]. Pathophysiology. The biologic basis for disease in adults and children [5th ed.]. St. Louis: Mosby.)*

initiated early during systemic vasodilation to promote oxygen delivery to the tissues.

Support for each organ must be provided. Respiratory failure is managed with mechanical ventilation with low tidal volumes, high oxygen concentrations, and positive end-expiratory pressures (see Chapter 14). Adequate nutrition and metabolic support is provided with enteral feedings (see Chapter 6). Renal failure is managed with continuous renal replacement therapies or hemodialysis (see Chapter 15). Inotropic drugs (low-dose dopamine or dobutamine) or vasopressors (norepinephrine or vasopressin) may be needed to maximize cardiac contractility and maintain cardiac output.

PATIENT OUTCOMES

The expected outcome for the patient in shock is that the patient will have improved tissue perfusion. Specific patient outcomes include alertness and orientation; normotension; warm, dry skin; adequate urine output; hemodynamic and laboratory values within normal limits; absence of infection; and intact skin. The patient should be resting quietly.

TABLE 11-9   Multiple Organ Dysfunction Syndrome

System	Dysfunction	Clinical Presentation
Pulmonary	ARDS	Predisposing factor such as shock or sepsis Unexplained hypoxemia ($\downarrow$ PaO_2, $\downarrow$ SaO_2) Dyspnea Tachypnea PaO_2/FiO_2 ratio <300 for acute lung injury and <200 for ARDS Bilateral pulmonary infiltrates on chest x-ray PAOP <18 mm Hg
Cardiovascular	Hyperdynamic or hypodynamic	See Table 11-8
Hematologic	DIC	Fibrin split products >1:40 or D-dimer >2 mg/L Thrombocytopenia Prolonged PT and aPTT INR >1.2 Bleeding Petechiae
Renal	Acute tubular necrosis	Oliguria $\uparrow$ Serum creatinine, $\uparrow$ BUN Urinary sodium >20 mEq/L
Liver	Hepatic dysfunction/failure	$\uparrow$ Serum bilirubin $\uparrow$ AST, ALT, LDH Jaundice Hepatomegaly $\uparrow$ Serum ammonia $\downarrow$ Serum albumin
Central nervous system	Cerebral ischemia/infarction	Lethargy Altered level of consciousness Fever
Metabolic	Lactic acidosis	$\uparrow$ Serum lactate level

aPTT, Activated partial thromboplastin time; *ALT*, alanine transaminase; *ARDS*, acute respiratory distress syndrome; *AST*, aspartate transaminase; *BUN*, blood urea nitrogen; *DIC*, disseminated intravascular coagulation; *FiO₂*, fraction of inspired oxygen; *INR*, international normalized ratio; *LDH*, lactic dehydrogenase; *PaO₂*, partial pressure of arterial oxygen; *PAOP*, pulmonary artery occlusive pressure; *PT*, prothrombin time; *SaO₂*, arterial oxygen saturation.

CASE STUDY

W. R., a 33-year-old man, was involved in a motor vehicle crash in which he sustained chest injuries. W. R., the driver, was not wearing his seat belt, and the steering wheel was bent. At the scene, W. R. was unresponsive. After placing a cervical collar to stabilize his neck, the paramedics performed endotracheal intubation and provided ventilation with 100% oxygen via a bag-valve device. Vital signs included a palpable systolic blood pressure (BP) of 60 mm Hg and a heart rate of 136 beats/min. W. R.'s skin was pale, cold, and clammy with a delay in capillary refill. Peripheral pulses were weak and thready. Two 14-gauge peripheral intravenous catheters were inserted, and lactated Ringer's solution was infused at a wide open rate. He was transported to the emergency department on a backboard. The initial assessment in the emergency department noted that his palpable BP had increased to 90 mm Hg and heart rate was 125 beats/min. He was restless in response to pain, with no other purposeful responses. Pupils were equal and reactive to light. Chest expansion was unequal, and breath sounds were markedly diminished on the right side. A chest x-ray documented a 70% hemopneumothorax on the right side, and a 36-French chest tube was inserted at the eighth intercostal space at the right midaxillary line. Immediately, 2000 mL of blood was drained from the chest, and an additional 500 mL of drainage was recorded in the next 30 minutes. Initial laboratory results were:

Hemoglobin: 9 g/dL
Prothrombin time: 15 seconds
Hematocrit: 31%
Partial thromboplastin time: 47 seconds
Platelets: 274,000/microliter
Red blood cells: 2.9 million/microliter
White blood cells: 5300/microliter

An indwelling urinary catheter was inserted, and 80 mL of clear, yellow urine immediately drained. Fluid resuscitation was continued to maintain a systolic BP at 90 to 100 mm Hg. W. R. was taken immediately to the operating room, where a right thoracotomy was performed, with repair of the right axillary artery. In the operating room, his vital signs remained stable with continued fluid resuscitation of crystalloids, blood, and fresh frozen plasma.

After surgery, he was admitted to the critical care unit, where his BP was 116/70 mm Hg, heart rate was 90 beats/min, and respiration rate was 24 breaths/min on the ventilator (assist/control mode with a rate of 20 breaths/min). He was responsive to commands and denied pain. He was medicated with morphine, 4 mg intravenous push every hour for pain. Laboratory results were:

Hemoglobin: 11 g/dL
Prothrombin time: 18.7 seconds
Hematocrit: 34%
Partial thromboplastin time: 71.7 seconds
Platelets: 180,000/microliter
Fibrinogen: 76 mg/dL
Red blood cells: 4.8 million/microliter
White blood cells: 5300/microliter
Arterial blood gases (on assisted ventilation with a FiO_2 .60):
pH: 7.30
$PaCO_2$: 40 mm Hg
PaO_2: 90 mm Hg
SaO_2: 92%
HCO_3^-: 17 mEq/L

QUESTIONS

1. What type of shock did W. R. demonstrate at the scene, and what components of his assessment supported this diagnosis?
2. W. R.'s initial assessment indicates that he is in which stage of shock?
3. In the emergency department, W. R. received lactated Ringer's solution for fluid resuscitation. Is this the appropriate solution at this time?
4. Explain W. R.'s arterial blood gas results. What treatment is indicated?
5. Describe the nursing care W. R. will receive in the first 24 hours after his surgery.
6. Describe the risk factors W. R. has for developing sepsis.

SUMMARY

The risk of shock is a common threat for all patients. Its causes are many, and treatment for shock is varied and complex. Complications of shock are related to the metabolic and tissue changes that result. If the normal compensatory mechanisms are not supported by effective therapeutic interventions, the pathological consequences perpetuate a vicious cycle of shock. The cycle is initiated by ischemia to the cells. Ischemia results in anaerobic metabolism, which leads to an accumulation of lactic acid and metabolic acidosis. This acidosis potentially leads to irreversible changes in the cells, organ failure, multiorgan failure, and death.

Prevention is the primary goal; it is accomplished through the identification of high-risk patient conditions and early interventions. Successful management relies on accurate nursing assessments, data analysis, implementation of definitive interventions, and evaluation of patient response to treatment. Shock is a crisis for the patient, family, nurse, and health care team. A multidisciplinary approach of clinical expertise combined with caring assists the patient in reaching a positive outcome.

CRITICAL THINKING QUESTIONS

1. Several people are admitted to the critical care unit, including (1) a 79-year-old man with a small anterior myocardial infarction and no prior cardiac history, (2) a 47-year-old man being given contrast media during a diagnostic procedure, (3) a 17-year-old adolescent with a cervical spine injury after a diving accident, and (4) a 72-year-old woman who was admitted with a bowel perforation caused by intestinal malignancy. Discuss what additional assessment information is needed to determine which of these patients has the potential to develop shock and the rationale for your decision.

2. A patient was admitted from the emergency department after a motorcycle crash in which he sustained blunt abdominal trauma. IV access was established in the internal jugular and left antecubital veins, and lactated Ringer's solution was infused. The results of initial computed tomography scan of the abdomen were negative. On admission to the critical care unit, you review the following results of the hematological profile:
   a. Hemoglobin: 9.1 g/dL
   b. Hematocrit: 31.1%
   c. Platelets: 274,000/microliter
   d. Red blood cells: 2.9 million/microliter
   e. White blood cells: 9800/microliter
   f. Prothrombin time: 15 seconds
   g. Activated partial thromboplastin time: 38 seconds
   Explain the rationale for the alterations in these values.

3. Describe factors in the critically ill patient that increase susceptibility to the development of severe sepsis and septic shock. Describe how these can be prevented.

4. Differentiate between the early, hyperdynamic phase and the late, hypodynamic phase of septic shock.

5. Which type of shock is associated with the following hemodynamic changes?
   a. Bradycardia, decreased SVR, decreased SvO_2
   b. Increased RAP, PAP, PAOP, increased SVR, increased SvO_2
   c. Tachycardia, decreased SVR, increased SvO_2
   d. Decreased RAP, PAP, PAOP, increased SVR, decreased SvO_2
   e. Tachycardia, decreased SVR, decreased SvO_2

evolve Be sure to check out the bonus material, including free self-assessment exercises, on the Evolve Web site at http://evolve.elsevier.com/Sole.

REFERENCES

1. Ahrens, T., & Vollman, K. (2003). Severe sepsis management: Are we doing enough? *Critical Care Nurse*, 23(Suppl. 5), 2-15.

2. American College of Surgeons' Committee on Trauma. (2004). *Advanced trauma life support (ATLS) for doctors student manual* (7th ed.). Chicago: American College of Surgeons.

3. Angus, D. C., Linde-Zwirble, W. T., Lidicker, J., Clermont, G., Carcillo, J., & Pinsky, M. R. (2001). Epidemiology of severe sepsis in the United States: Analysis of incidence, outcome, and associated costs of care. *Critical Care Medicine*, 29(7), 1303-1310.

4. Annane, D., Sebille, V., Charpentier, C., Bollaert, P. E., Francois, B., Korach, J. M., et al. (2002). Effect of treatment with low doses of hydrocortisone and fludrocortisone on mortality in patients with septic shock. *Journal of the American Medical Association*, 288(7), 862-871.

5. Babaev, A., Frederick, P. D., Pasta, D. J., Every, N., Sichrovsky, T., & Hochman, J. S. (2005). Trends in management and outcomes of patients with acute myocardial infarction complicated by cardiogenic shock. *JAMA*, 294(4), 448-454.

6. Barker, E. (2007). *Neuroscience nursing. A spectrum of care* (3rd ed.). St. Louis: Mosby.

7. Bernard, G. R., Vincent, J.-L., Laterre, P.-F., LaRosa, S. P., Dhainaut, J.-F., Lopez-Rodriguez, A., et al. (2001). Efficacy and safety of recombinant human activated protein C for severe sepsis. *New England Journal of Medicine*, 344(10), 699-709.

8. Bone, R., Sprung, C., & Sibbald, W. (1992). Definitions for sepsis and organ failure. *Critical Care Medicine*, 20(6), 724.

9. Cochrane Injuries Group Albumin Reviewers. (1998). Human albumin administration in critically ill patients: Systematic review of randomized controlled trials. *British Medical Journal*, 317, 235-240.

10. Cottingham, C. (2006). Resuscitation of traumatic shock. *AACN Advanced Critical Care*, 17(3), 317-326.

11. deJong, M. F. C., Beishuizen, A., Spijkstra, J.-J., & Groeneveld, A. B. J. (2007). Relative adrenal insufficiency as a predictor of disease severity, mortality, and beneficial effects of corticosteroid therapy in septic shock. *Critical Care Medicine*, 35(8), 1-8.

12. Dellinger, R. P., Levy, M. M., Carlet, J. M., Bion, J., Parker, M., Jaeschke, R., et al. (2008). Surviving Sepsis Campaign: International guidelines for management of severe sepsis and septic shock: 2008. *Critical Care Medicine*, 36(1), 298-327.

13. Gould, S. A., Moore, E. E., Hoyt, D. B., Ness, P. M., Norris, E. J., Carson, J. L., et al. (2002). The life-sustaining capacity of human polymerized hemoglobin when red cells might be unavailable. *Journal of the American College of Surgeons*, 195(4), 445-452.

14. Kelley, D. M. (2005). Hypovolemic shock. An overview. *Critical Care Nursing Quarterly*, 28(1), 2-19.

15. Kleinpell, R. M. (2003). The role of the critical care nurse in the assessment and management of the patient with severe sepsis. *Critical Care Nursing Clinics of North America, 15*(1), 27-34.

16. Kollef, M. H. (2004). Prevention of hospital-associated pneumonia and ventilator-associated pneumonia. *Critical Care Medicine, 32*(6), 1396-1405.

17. Kortgen, A., Niederprum, P., & Bauer, M. (2006). Implementation of an evidence-based "standard operating procedure" and outcome in septic shock. *Critical Care Medicine, 34*(3), 943-949.

18. Kruse, J. A., Fink, M. P., & Carlson, R. W. (2003). *Saunders manual of critical care.* Philadelphia: Saunders.

19. Kyles, D. M., & Baltimore, J. (2005). Adjunctive use of plasmapheresis and intravenous immunoglobulin therapy in sepsis: A case report. *American Journal of Critical Care, 14*(2), 109-112.

20. Lee, C. S. (2006). Role of exogenous arginine vasopressin in the management of catecholamine-refractory septic shock. *Critical Care Nurse, 26*(6), 17-23.

21. Levy, M. M., Fink, M. P., Marshall, J. C., Abraham, E., Angus, D., Cook, D., et al. (2003). 2001 SCCM/ESICM/ACCP/ATS/SIS International Sepsis Definitions Conference. *Critical Care Medicine, 31*(4), 1250-1256.

22. Maeder, M., Fehr, T., Rickli, H., & Ammann, P. (2006). Sepsis-associated myocardial dysfunction: Diagnostic and prognostic impact of cardiac troponins and natriuretic peptides. *Chest, 129*(5), 1349-1366.

23. Martin, G. S. (2004). *An evidence-based approach to the therapy of sepsis.* CME activity adapted from a presentation at the CHEST 2004: 70th Annual Meeting of the American College of Chest Physicians. Retrieved July 29, 2007, from www.medscape.com/viewprogram/3628_pnt.

24. Moore, F. A., McKinley, B. A., & Moore, E. E. (2004). The next generation in shock resuscitation. *Lancet, 363,* 1988-1996.

25. Picard, K. M., O'Donoghue, S. C., Young-Kershaw, D. A., & Russell, K. J. (2006). Development and implementation of a multidisciplinary sepsis protocol. *Critical Care Nurse, 26*(3), 43-54.

26. Plotz, F. B., Slutsky, A. S., van Vught, A. J., & Heijnen, C. J. (2004). Ventilator-induced lung injury and multiple system organ failure: A critical review of facts and hypotheses. *Intensive Care Medicine, 30*(10), 1865-1872.

27. Rivers, E., Nguyen, B., Havstad, S., Ressler, J., Muzzin, A., Knoblich, B., et al. (2001). Early goal-directed therapy in the treatment of severe sepsis and septic shock. *New England Journal of Medicine, 345*(19), 1368-1377.

28. Rivers, E. P., Ander, D. S., & Powell, D. (2001). Central venous oxygen saturation monitoring in the critically ill patient. *Current Opinion in Critical Care, 7*(3), 204-211.

29. Rizoli, S. B., Rhind, S. G., Shek, P. N., Inaba, K., Filips, D., Tien, H., et al. (2006). The immunomodulatory effects of hypertonic saline resuscitation in patients sustaining traumatic hemorrhagic shock: A randomized, controlled, double-blinded trial. *Annals of Surgery, 243*(1), 47-57.

30. Shapiro, N. I., Howell, M., & Talmor, D. (2005). A blueprint for a sepsis protocol. *Academy of Emergency Medicine, 12*(4), 352-359.

31. Shapiro, N. I., Howell, M. D., Talmor, D., Lahey, D., Ngo, L., Buras, J., et al. (2006). Implementation and outcomes of the Multiple Urgent Sepsis Therapies (MUST) protocol. *Critical Care Medicine, 34*(4), 1025-1032.

32. Sharma, S., & Kumar, A. (2003). Septic shock, multiple organ failure, and acute respiratory distress syndrome. *Current Opinion in Pulmonary Medicine, 9*(3), 199-209.

33. Shorr, A. (2007). *Clinical challenges in critical care medicine. Managing severe sepsis.* CME activity adapted from American Thoracic Society (ATS) 103rd International Conference May 18-23, 2007, San Francisco, CA. Retrieved November 25, 2007, from www.medscape.com/viewprogram/7302_pnt.

34. The Acute Respiratory Distress Syndrome Network. (2000). Ventilation with lower tidal volumes as compared with traditional tidal volumes for acute lung injury and the acute respiratory distress syndrome. *New England Journal of Medicine, 342,* 1301-1308.

35. Trzeciak, S., Dellinger, R. P., Abate, N. L., Cowan, R. M., Stauss, M., Kilgannon, J. H., et al. (2006). Translating research to clinical practice: A 1-year experience with implementing early goal-directed therapy for septic shock in the emergency department. *Chest, 129*(2), 225-232.

36. van den Berghe, G., Wouters, P., Weekers, F., Verwaest, C., Bruyninckx, F., Schetz, M., et al. (2001). Intensive insulin therapy in critically ill patients. *New England Journal of Medicine, 345*(19), 1359-1367.

37. Varpula, M., Pulkki, K., Karlsson, S., Ruokonen, E., & Pettila, V. (2007). Predictive value of N-terminal pro-brain natriuretic peptide in severe sepsis and septic shock. *Critical Care Medicine, 35*(5), 1277-1283.

38. Vincent, J. L., Bernard, G. R., Beale, R., Doig, C., Putensen, C., Dhainaut, J. F., et al. (2005). Drotrecogin alfa (activated) treatment in severe sepsis from the global open-label trial ENHANCE: Further evidence for survival and safety and implications for early treatment. *Critical Care Medicine, 33*(10), 2266-2277.

39. Vincent, J. L., & Gerlach, H. (2004). Fluid resuscitation in severe sepsis and septic shock: An evidence-based review. *Critical Care Medicine, 32*(Suppl.), S451-S454.

CHAPTER 12

Cardiovascular Alterations

Marthe J. Moseley, PhD, RN, CCRN, CCNS, CNL

INTRODUCTION

Care of the seriously ill patient with alterations in cardiac status includes those cardiac patients at risk for an uncertain prognosis. The critical care nurse needs theoretical knowledge and practice-related understanding of the common cardiac diseases to have the sound clinical judgment necessary for making rapid and accurate decisions. The purpose of this chapter is to identify and explore common cardiac alterations that are likely to be encountered by the critical care nurse caring for adult patients with compromised cardiac status, and to describe the nursing care to optimize the patient's outcome.

NORMAL STRUCTURE AND FUNCTION OF THE HEART

The heart muscle is approximately the size of a person's closed fist and lies within the mediastinal space of the thoracic cavity between the lungs, directly under the lower half of the sternum, and above the diaphragm (Figure 12-1). It is covered by the pericardium, which has an inner visceral layer and an outer parietal layer. Certain diseases can cause this covering to become inflamed and can subsequently diminish the effectiveness of the heart as a pump. Several cubic milliliters of lubricating fluid are present between these layers. Some pathological conditions can increase the amount and the consistency of this fluid, affecting the pumping ability of the heart. The heart muscle itself is composed of three layers. The outer layer, or epicardium, covers the surface of the heart and extends to the great vessels; the middle, muscular layer, or myocardium, is responsible for the heart's pumping action; and the inner endothelial layer, or endocardium, covers the heart valves and the small muscles associated with the opening and closing of those valves. These layers are damaged or destroyed when a patient has a myocardial infarction (MI).

Functionally, the heart is divided into right-sided and left-sided pumps that are separated by a septum. The right side is generally considered to be a low-pressure system, whereas the left side is a high-pressure system. Each side has an atrium that receives the blood and a ventricle that pumps it out. The right atrium receives deoxygenated blood from the body through the superior and inferior venae cavae. Blood travels from the atrium to the ventricles by means of a pressure gradient between the chambers. The right ventricle pumps the deoxygenated blood to the lungs through the pulmonary artery for oxygen and carbon dioxide exchange. The left atrium receives the newly oxygenated blood by way of the pulmonary veins from the lungs, and the left ventricle pumps the oxygenated blood through the aorta to the systemic circulation (Figure 12-2).

The four cardiac valves maintain the unidirectional blood flow through the chambers of the heart. The four valves also assist in producing the pressure gradient needed between the chambers for the blood to flow through the heart. There are two types of valves: the atrioventricular (AV) valves, which separate the atria from the ventricles, and the semilunar valves, which separate the pulmonary artery from the right ventricle and the aorta from the left ventricle (Figure 12-3). The AV valves are the tricuspid valve, which lies between the right atrium and the right ventricle, and the mitral valve, located between the left atrium and the left ventricle. Each AV valve is anchored by chordae tendineae to the papillary muscles on its ventricular floor. The semilunar valves are the pulmonic valve, which lies between the right ventricle and the pulmonary artery, and the aortic valve, located between the left ventricle and the aorta. These semilunar valves are not anchored by chordae tendineae. Instead, their closing is passive and is caused by differences in pressure between the chamber and the respective great vessel.

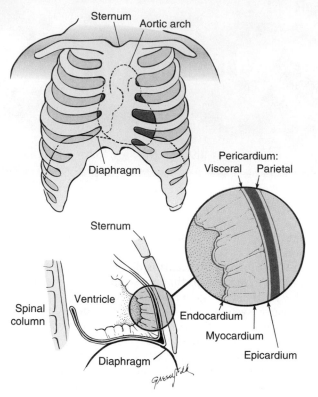

FIGURE 12-1. The heart lies in the mediastinum, between the lungs. Its apex rests on the diaphragm. The heart is covered by the pericardium. The *inset* shows the layers of the heart muscle and the pericardium. *(From Price, S. A., & Wilson, L. M. [2003].* Pathophysiology: Clinical concepts of disease processes *[6th ed.]. St. Louis: Mosby.)*

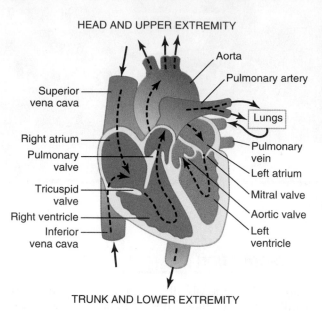

FIGURE 12-2. Structure of the heart and course of blood flow through the heart chambers. *(From Guyton, A. C., & Hall, J. E. [2001].* Textbook of medical physiology *[10th ed.]. Philadelphia: Saunders.)*

Autonomic Control

The autonomic nervous system (sympathetic and parasympathetic) exerts control over the cardiovascular system. The sympathetic nervous system releases norepinephrine, which has two effects. Alpha-adrenergic effects cause arterial vasoconstriction. Beta-adrenergic effects increase sinus node discharge (positive chronotropic), increase the force of contraction (positive inotropic), and accelerate the AV conduction time (positive dromotropic).

The parasympathetic nervous system releases acetylcholine through stimulation of the vagus nerve. It causes a decrease in the sinus node discharge and slows conduction through the AV node.

In addition to this innervation, receptors help to control cardiovascular function. The first receptors are the chemoreceptors, which are sensitive to changes in the partial pressure of arterial oxygen (PaO_2), the partial pressure of arterial carbon dioxide ($PaCO_2$), and pH blood levels. Chemoreceptors stimulate the vasomotor center in the medulla; this center controls vasoconstriction and vasodilation.

Second are baroreceptors, which are sensitive to stretch and pressure. If blood pressure increases, the baroreceptors cause the heart rate to decrease. If the blood pressure decreases, the baroreceptors stimulate an increase in heart rate (Figure 12-4).

Coronary Circulation

Many cardiac problems result from a complete or a partial occlusion of a coronary artery. The blood supply to the myocardium is derived from the coronary arteries that branch off the aorta immediately above the aortic valve (Figure 12-5). Two major branches exist: the right coronary artery and the left coronary artery, which splits into two branches, the left anterior descending and the left circumflex. Knowledge of the portion of the heart that receives its blood supply from a particular coronary artery allows the nurse to anticipate problems related to occlusion of that vessel (Box 12-1). Variations in the branching and the exact placement of the coronary arteries are common.

Blood flow to the coronary arteries occurs during diastole, when the aortic valve is closed and the sinuses of Valsalva are filled with blood. Myocardial fibers are relaxed at this time, thus promoting blood flow through the coronary vessels. The coronary veins return blood from the coronary circulation back into the heart through the coronary sinuses to the right and left atria.

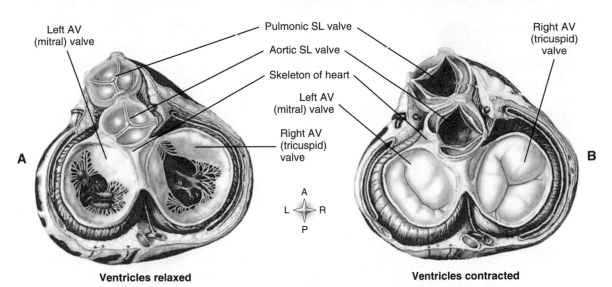

Left AV (mitral) valve

Pulmonic SL valve

Aortic SL valve

Skeleton of heart

Left AV (mitral) valve

Right AV (tricuspid) valve

Right AV (tricuspid) valve

A

B

A
L ✦ R
P

Ventricles relaxed

Ventricles contracted

FIGURE 12-3. A, The atrioventricular (AV) valves in the open position and the semilunar (SL) valves in the closed position. **B,** The AV valves in the closed position and the SL valves in the open position. *(From Thibodeau, G. A. & Patton, K. T. [2003]. Anatomy and physiology [5th ed.]. St. Louis: Mosby.)*

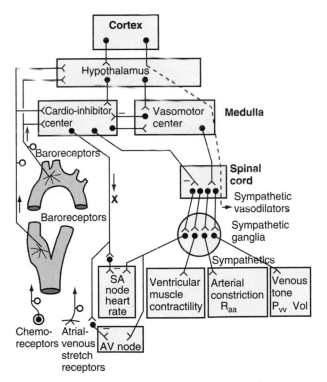

FIGURE 12-4. Autonomic control of circulation. *AV,* Atrioventricular; P_{vv}, pulmonary venules; R_{aa}, renal arterioles; *SA*, sinoatrial.

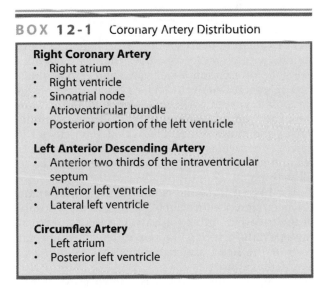

BOX 12-1 Coronary Artery Distribution

Right Coronary Artery
- Right atrium
- Right ventricle
- Sinoatrial node
- Atrioventricular bundle
- Posterior portion of the left ventricle

Left Anterior Descending Artery
- Anterior two thirds of the intraventricular septum
- Anterior left ventricle
- Lateral left ventricle

Circumflex Artery
- Left atrium
- Posterior left ventricle

Other Cardiac Functions

Knowledge of properties of cardiac muscle and the normal conduction system of the heart is essential since many patients have cardiac dysrhythmias (see Chapter 7). Hemodynamics of the cardiovascular system are also important in understanding pathologic disorders such as heart failure (HF). (Refer to Chapter 8 for hemodynamic content.)

Heart Sounds

The vibrations produced by vascular walls, flowing blood, heart muscle, and heart valves create sound

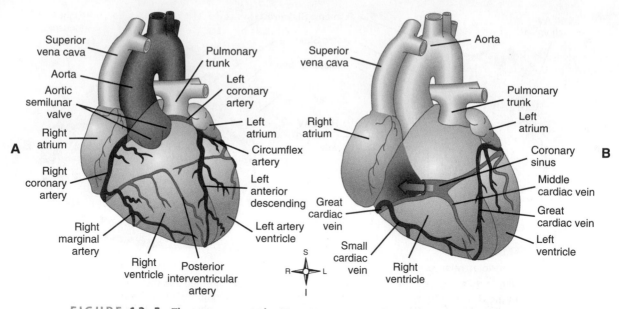

FIGURE 12-5. The coronary vessels. *(From McCance, K. L., & Huether, S. E. [Eds.]. [2002]. Pathophysiology: The biologic basis for disease in adults and children [4th ed.]. St. Louis: Mosby.)*

waves known as heart sounds. Auscultation of these sounds with a stethoscope over the heart provides valuable information about valve and cardiac function (Figure 12-6). Ventricular systole occurs when the pulmonic and aortic valves open to allow blood to be pumped to the lungs (right ventricle-pulmonic valve) and systemic circulation (left ventricle-aortic valve). Ventricular diastole occurs when the tricuspid and mitral valves open to allow the ventricles to fill with blood.

The first heart sound is known as S_1. This sound has been described as "lubb." It is caused by closure of the tricuspid and mitral valves. It is best heard at the apex (fifth intercostal space, left midclavicular line) of the heart and represents the beginning of ventricular systole.

The second heart sound is known as S_2. It has been described as "dubb" and is caused by closure of the pulmonic and aortic valves. It is best heard at the second intercostal space at the left or right sternal border and represents the beginning of ventricular diastole. The first and second heart sounds are best heard with the diaphragm of the stethoscope.

A third heart sound, S_3, usually represents a pathological process in the adult. The sound may be produced at the time when the heart is already overfilled or poorly compliant. The S_3 sound is low pitched and can best be heard with the bell of the stethoscope at the fifth intercostal space, at the left midclavicular line. It occurs immediately after S_2. Together with S_1 and S_2, S_3 produces a "lubb-dubba" or "ken-**tuk**'e"

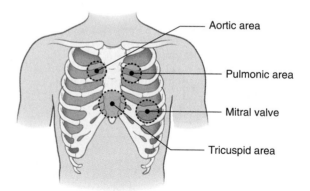

FIGURE 12-6. Chest areas from which each valve sound is best heard. *(Modified from Guyton, A. C., & Hall, J. E. [2001]. Textbook of medical physiology [10th ed.]. Philadelphia: Saunders.)*

sound. S_3 is often heard in patients with HF or fluid overload.

A fourth heart sound, S_4, is produced from atrial contraction that is more forceful than normal. Together with S_1 and S_2, S_4 produces a "te-lubb-dubb" or "**ten**'-ne-see" sound. S_4 can be normal in elderly patients, but it is often heard after an MI, when the atria contract more forcefully against ventricles distended with blood. In the severely failing heart, all four sounds (S_4, S_1, S_2, and S_3) may be heard, producing a "gallop" rhythm, so named because it sounds like the hoof beats of a galloping horse. It can best be

TABLE 12-1   Grading of Heart Murmurs

Intensity of Murmur Graded from I to VI Based on Increasing Loudness

Grade I	Lowest intensity, usually not audible by inexperienced providers
Grade II	Low intensity, usually audible by inexperienced providers
Grade III	Medium intensity without a thrill
Grade IV	Medium intensity with a thrill
Grade V	Loudest murmur audible when stethoscope is placed on the chest; associated with a thrill
Grade VI	Loudest intensity, audible when stethoscope is removed from chest; associated with a thrill

heard with the bell of the stethoscope at the fifth intercostal space, at the left midclavicular line. In addition, it is often documented S_4, S_1, S_2, S_3 because of the order in which the nurse hears the sound.

Heart Murmur

A heart murmur is a sound caused by turbulence of blood flow through the valves of the heart. Murmurs are audible when a septal defect is present; when a valve (usually aortic or mitral) is narrow, inflamed, stenosed, or incompetent; or when the valve leaflets fail to approximate (valve insufficiency). The presence of a new murmur warrants special attention, particularly in a patient with an acute MI (AMI). A papillary muscle may have ruptured, causing the valve to not close correctly, which can be indicative of severe damage and impending complications (HF and pulmonary edema). A murmur is usually a rumbling, blowing, harsh, or musical sound. It is important to distinguish the sound, anatomical location, loudness, and intensity of a murmur and determine whether extra heart sounds are heard. Table 12-1 gives a grading of heart murmurs. Auscultation of heart sounds is a skill developed from practice in listening to many different patients' hearts and in correlating the sounds heard with the patients' pathological conditions.

CORONARY ARTERY DISEASE

Coronary artery disease (CAD) is a broad term used to refer to the narrowing or occlusion of the coronary arteries. Blood supply to the coronary arteries is reduced as a result of CAD. Other terms used to describe CAD include coronary heart disease and atherosclerotic heart disease.

Pathophysiology

CAD is the progressive narrowing of one or more coronary arteries by atherosclerosis. CAD results in ischemia when the internal diameter of the coronary vessel is reduced by 45% to 60% (Figure 12-7).[18]

Atherosclerosis is an inflammatory disease progressing from endothelial injury.[6] The dysfunctional formation of a fatty streak leads to the presence of fibrotic plaque, leading to complicated lesion formation. The injury results from platelet aggregation that attaches to endothelium. Foamy macrophages ingest lipids. Smooth muscle migration occurs into the intima and results in lipid accumulation, thereby releasing fibroblasts. Lipoproteins entering the intima result in fatty streak formation. The monocytes in the fatty streak are transformed into macrophages that develop receptors for engulfing lipids, especially low-density lipoproteins (LDLs). Lipid-rich "foam cells" develop. Foam cells progress to form a fibrous plaque or atheroma. Damage to the intima liberates platelet-derived growth factor, which stimulates migration of smooth muscle cells from the media to the intima of the coronary artery and forms the atheroma. Over time, a fibrous cap is formed from connective tissue (fibroblasts and macrophages) and LDLs.

Many plaques often rupture, producing a thrombus. The thrombus can occlude a coronary artery, with resulting injury and infarction. Rupture of the plaque also initiates the coagulation cascade with the initiation of thrombin production, the conversion of fibrinogen to fibrin, and platelet aggregation at the site.

Possible causes of endothelial injury include the presence of risk factors (Box 12-2). After injury to the endothelium, platelets are exposed to proteins that bind to receptors, causing adhesion of platelets at the site of injury. Next, the platelets are activated and change shape. They release thromboxane A_2 and serotonin. Each platelet has thousands of glycoprotein IIb/IIIa (Gp IIb/IIIa) receptors that are activated and bind with von Willebrand's factor and fibrinogen, which is converted to fibrin strands. At the same time, the platelets aggregate with one another. This process of adhesion, activation, and aggregation causes a rapidly growing thrombus that compromises coronary blood flow.[6]

Assessment

Patient Assessment

A thorough history and cardiovascular assessment provide data to develop a comprehensive plan of care

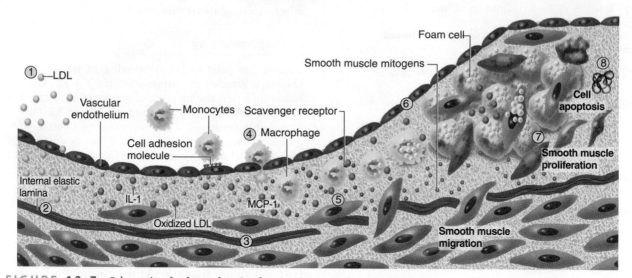

FIGURE 12-7. Schematic of atherosclerotic plaque. *1.* Accumulation of lipoprotein particles in the intima. *2.* Oxidative stress. *3.* Induction of the cytokines and movement into the intima. *4.* Blood monocytes encounter stimuli that augment their expression of scavenger receptors. *5.* Scavenger receptors mediate the uptake of modified lipoprotein particles and promote the development of foam cells. Cytokines and superoxide anion (O_2^-). *6.* Smooth muscle cells divide and migrate into the intima from the media. *7.* Smooth muscle cells promote extracellular atherosclerotic plaque growth. Fatty streaks evolve into fatty lesions. *8.* Calcification can occur and fibrosis continues. *(From Libby, P. [2005]. The vascular biology of atherosclerosis. In D. P. Zipes, P. Libby, R. O. Bonow, & E. Braunwald [Eds.],* Braunwald's heart disease: A textbook of cardiovascular medicine *[7th ed., p. 925]. Philadelphia: Saunders.)*

for the patient with cardiovascular disease. The history includes subjective data regarding medical history, prior hospitalizations, allergies, and family medical history. A previous medical history of both pediatric and adult illnesses is of particular interest and includes a positive history for rheumatic fever, diabetes mellitus, hypertension, asthma, renal disease, or stroke. Knowledge of prior hospitalizations is also important so records can be obtained for review. Information regarding the patient's current medications, both prescription and over-the-counter, should include information about the patient's understanding and use of these medications. A history of the patient's use of sildenafil citrate (Viagra) or similar medications taken for erectile dysfunction is necessary to know when considering nitroglycerin (NTG) administration. These medications potentiate the hypotensive effects of nitrates; thus concurrent use is contraindicated. It is also important to determine whether the patient has any food or drug allergies.

A psychosocial or personal history is also important for the planning of the patient's care. This history includes major stress events and everyday stressors.

Additional information regarding activities for stress reduction is obtained (Box 12-3).

Before beginning the physical examination, the nurse determines recent and recurrent symptoms that may be related to the patient's current problems. Such information gathering includes the presence or absence of fatigue, fluid retention, dyspnea, irregular heartbeat (palpitations), and chest pain (see Clinical Alert: Assessment of the Patient with Chest Pain [PQRST]). The physical examination itself encompasses all the body systems and is not limited to the cardiovascular system, because all the body systems are interrelated and interdependent. Although it is imperative that a total evaluation is completed regarding the physical status of the patient, patients whose primary problems are cardiovascular most commonly exhibit alterations in circulation and oxygenation. Thus, all systems should be examined from this perspective.

The examination is performed in an orderly, organized manner and involves the techniques of inspection, palpation, percussion, and auscultation. A baseline assessment is provided in Table 12-2.

BOX 12-2 Risk Factors for Coronary Artery Disease

Several risk factors predispose persons to coronary artery disease (CAD). Some risk factors cannot be changed (e.g., gender, heredity, and age). Other risk factors are modifiable: smoking, high blood cholesterol, high blood pressure, physical inactivity, overweight or obesity, and diabetes.[2]

Gender
Men have a greater risk of heart attacks than women and have heart attacks earlier in life.

Heredity
Family history of early heart disease is an unmodifiable risk for CAD. A positive history is defined as having a blood-related parent, sister, brother, or child with CAD, with CAD having been diagnosed before age 55 years in a father or brother and before age 65 years in a mother or sister.

Age
Men in their mid 40s and women once they reach menopause are considered at higher risk for CAD.

Smoking
Smokers have a higher risk of CAD. Smoking increases low-density lipoprotein (LDL) levels and damages the endothelium of coronary vessels. These are predisposing factors for the development of atherosclerosis. Smoking also causes vasoconstriction of coronary vessels, thus decreasing blood supply.

Blood Cholesterol
Serum cholesterol or lipid levels play a key role in the development of atherosclerosis. Elevated total cholesterol (>200 mg/dL) is considered a risk factor for CAD. Cholesterol is insoluble in plasma and must be transported by lipoproteins that are soluble. High-density lipoproteins (HDLs) are considered the good cholesterol. HDLs assist in transporting cholesterol to the liver for removal. A high HDL level (>40 mg/dL for men and >50 mg/dL for women) may reduce the incidence of CAD, whereas a low HDL level (<40 mg/dL) is considered a risk factor for developing CAD.

LDLs are considered the bad cholesterol. LDLs transport and deposit cholesterol to the arterial vessels, thus facilitating the process of atherosclerosis. An LDL level of less than 100 mg/dL is optimal. Other non-HDL lipoproteins also contribute to the development of CAD. Very low density lipoproteins are largely composed of triglycerides and contribute to an increased risk of CAD.

High Blood Pressure
A blood pressure greater than 120/80 mm Hg is considered prehypertension and greater than 140/89 or taking antihypertensive medication is a risk factor for CAD. Hypertension causes direct injury to the vasculature, leading to the development of CAD. Oxygen demands are also increased in patients with hypertension. The heart muscle enlarges and weakens over time, thereby increasing the workload of the heart.

Physical Inactivity
Lack of physical activity is a risk factor for CAD. Regular aerobic exercise reduces the incidence of CAD. Exercise also helps to control other risk factors such as high blood pressure, diabetes, and obesity.

Overweight and Obesity
Obesity increases the atherogenic process and predisposes persons to CAD. In addition, obesity is related to hypertension and diabetes, two other major risk factors. Persons with a greater proportion of fat through the abdomen ("apple-shaped") have been shown to have a higher incidence of CAD than those with greater fat distribution over the hips ("pear-shaped"). The waist-to-hip ratio is used to help identify this risk. Body mass index is another way to determine the degree of overweight.

Diabetes
Diabetes is associated with increased levels of LDL and triglycerides. Glycation associated with diabetes decreases the uptake of LDL by the liver and increases the hepatic synthesis of LDL.

BOX 12-3 Questioning of Activities for Stress Reduction

- What, if any, is the patient's exercise routine, including the type, amount, and regularity of the activity?
- What is the patient's daily food pattern and intake?
- What is the patient's sleep pattern?
- What are the patient's habitual social patterns in using tobacco, alcohol, drugs, coffee, tea, and caffeinated sodas?

CLINICAL ALERT
Assessment of the Patient with Chest Pain (PQRST)

P	Provocation
Q	Quality
R	Region/Radiation
S	Severity
T	Timing (when began) and Treatment

TABLE 12-2   Major Systems Assessment

System	Assessment
Neurological	Level of consciousness, orientation to person, place, time, events; presence of hallucinations, depression, withdrawal, trembling; pupils (size, equality, response); paresthesias; eye movements; restlessness, apprehensiveness, irritability, cooperativeness; hand grips (strength and equality); leg movement; response to tactile stimuli; type, location of pain; how pain is relieved; patient's complaints
Skin	Color, temperature, dryness, turgor, presence of rashes, broken areas, pressure areas, urticaria, incision site, wounds
Cardiovascular	BP (bilaterally); apical and radial pulses; pulse deficit; monitor leads on patient in correct placement; rhythm, presence of ectopy; PR interval, QRS, and QT intervals; heart sounds; presence of abnormalities (e.g., rubs, gallops); neck vein distention with head of bed at what angle; edema (sacral and dependent); calf pain; varicosities; presence of pulses: bilateral carotid, radial, femoral, posterior tibial, dorsalis pedis; capillary refill in extremities; hemodynamic measurements; temporary pacemaker settings; medications to maintain BP or rhythm
Respiratory	Rate, depth, and quality of respirations; oxygen; accessory muscle use; cough, sputum: type, color, suctioning frequency; symmetry of chest expansion and breath sounds, describe breath sounds; current ABGs; chest tube with description of drainage, fluctuation in water seal, bubbling, suction applied; tracheostomy or endotracheal tube; ventilator used; ventilator settings; ventilator rate versus patient's own breaths; patient's spontaneous tidal volume
Gastrointestinal	Abdominal size and softness, bowel sounds, nausea and vomiting, bowel movement, dressing and/or drainage, NG tube with description of drainage, feeding tube: type and frequency of feedings, drains
Genitourinary	Foley or voiding, urine color, quality; vaginal or urethral drainage
Intravenous	Volume of fluid, type of solution, rate; intravenous site condition
Wounds	Dry or drainage, type, color, amount, odor; hematoma, inflamed, drains, hemovac, dressing changes, cultures

ABG, Arterial blood gas; *BP*, blood pressure; *NG*, nasogastric.

Diagnostic Studies

Certain diagnostic studies are fundamental for the care and treatment of patients with CAD. The following sections contain brief descriptions of common diagnostic studies the cardiac patient may encounter.[8]

12-Lead Electrocardiography.

This noninvasive test is usually preliminary to most other tests performed. It is used as a baseline for many other tests and often as a comparison of pretest and posttest changes. This test is useful in identification of rhythm disturbances, and myocardial ischemia, injury, or infarct.

Holter Monitor.

This noninvasive test is used to detect suspected dysrhythmias. The patient is connected to a small portable recorder (about the size of a pocket radio) by three to five electrodes; the recorder is worn for 24 to 48 hours. The patient engages in normal daily activities, and keeps a log of all activities and symptoms during the monitoring period. The recording is then analyzed for abnormalities and correlated with the documented activities and symptoms.

Exercise Tolerance Test (ETT) or Stress Test.

This is a noninvasive test in which the patient is connected to an electrocardiogram (ECG) machine while exercising for 3-minute intervals (putting stress on the heart and vascular system). Physical stress causes an increase in myocardial oxygen consumption. If oxygen demand exceeds supply, ischemia may result. The stress test is used to document exercise-induced ischemia, and it can identify those individuals prone to cardiac ischemia during activity when resting ECGs are normal. The exercise usually involves pedaling a stationary bike or walking on a treadmill. The patient is constantly monitored, the pulse and blood pressure are checked at intervals, and the ECG printout is analyzed at the end of the testing period. Patients return to their room or go home after the heart rate returns to baseline.

If a patient is unable physically to perform the exercise, a pharmacological stress test can be done. For example, adenosine can be administered to mimic increased cardiac workload. Adenosine is usually preferred over dobutamine because adenosine has a short duration of action and does not require reversal agents.

Chest X-ray. This noninvasive procedure is usually performed in the anteroposterior view. The chest x-ray study is used for detecting cardiomegaly, cardiac positioning, degree of fluid infiltrating the pulmonary space, and other structural changes that may affect the physical ability of the heart to function in a normal manner.

Echocardiography. This is a noninvasive, acoustic imaging procedure and involves the use of ultrasound to visualize the cardiac structures and the motion and function of cardiac valves and chambers. A transducer placed on the chest wall sends ultrasound waves at short intervals. The reflected sound waves, termed echoes, are displayed on a graph for interpretation. Echocardiography is used to assess valvular function, evaluate congenital defects, measure size of cardiac chambers, evaluate cardiac disease progression, evaluate ventricular function, diagnose myocardial tumors and effusions, and, to a lesser degree, measure cardiac output. Ventricular function is evaluated by obtaining an ejection fraction. The ejection fraction is the percentage of blood ejected from the left ventricle during systole, normally 60% to 70%.

Transesophageal Echocardiography. This test provides ultrasonic imaging of the heart from a view behind the heart. In transesophageal echocardiography (TEE), an ultrasound probe is fitted on the end of a flexible gastroscope, which is inserted into the posterior pharynx and advanced into the esophagus. TEE shows a clear picture because the esophagus is against the back of the heart and parallel to the aorta. TEE is indicated to visualize prosthetic heart valves, mitral valve function, aortic dissection, vegetative endocarditis, congenital heart defects in adults, cardiac masses and tumors, and embolic phenomena. It is also used intraoperatively to assess left ventricular function. Patients should fast (except for medications) for 6 to 8 hours before the examination. During the procedure, vital signs, cardiac rhythm, and oxygen saturation are monitored. After the procedure, the patient is unable to eat until the gag reflex returns. A rare complication of TEE is esophageal perforation, with signs of sore throat, dysphagia, stiff neck, and epigastric or substernal pain that worsens with breathing and movement or pain in the back, abdomen, or shoulder.

Diagnostic Heart Scans. Noninvasive scanning is often used to assess the heart. Injection of a radiopharmaceutical contrast agent assists in visualization of heart structures.

Technetium-99m Stannous Pyrophosphate. Technetium-99m stannous pyrophosphate scanning is used to assess AMI. The technetium combines with calcium in damaged myocardial cells to form spots on the scan. The spots begin within 12 hours of AMI and are prominent within 48 to 72 hours. They disappear within a week after the AMI unless myocardial damage continues.

Thallium-201. The thallium-201 scan is used to assess AMI, CAD, or the effectiveness of coronary interventions such as angioplasty. The isotope is absorbed into healthy myocardium while avoiding damaged tissue, forming spots on the scan. Areas of myocardial damage are then visualized. The test may be performed as part of an exercise tolerance test. It may also be used in conjunction with dipyridamole administration because the drug causes greater uptake of thallium. The combination test is useful in individuals who cannot tolerate exercise testing with the scan.

Multigated Blood Pool Study. The multigated blood pool study (MUGA) scan is used to assess left ventricular function. An isotope is injected and images of the heart are taken during systole and diastole to assess the ejection fraction of the heart. An ejection fraction of 60% to 70% and symmetrical contraction of the left ventricle are considered normal test results. This test may be done under stress.

Nitroglycerin MUGA. The NTG scan is an additional feature of the MUGA scan. Another series of images is taken to evaluate the effectiveness of sublingual NTG administration. This test may be performed under stress.

Sestamibi Exercise Testing and Scan. This is used to evaluate cardiac perfusion before and after a treadmill exercise test. The injected radiopharmaceutical technetium-99m pertechnetate (sestamibi) is taken up by ischemic or infarcted cardiac cells that did not improve in perfusion with exercise and is seen as a "hot spot" in nuclear imaging.

The sestamibi-dipyridamole stress test and scan is for patients who cannot walk on a treadmill or pedal a bicycle because of physical limitations. Dipyridamole is an antiplatelet drug used in nuclear medicine for its coronary artery vasodilatory action causing an effect on the perfusion of the heart muscle similar to that of an exercise test. Tests are compared before and after the tracer and dipyridamole injections. The areas that vasodilate can draw blood flow from less perfused areas; thus the test can cause ischemia and infarction.

Single Photon Emission Computed Tomography. The single photon emission computed tomography (SPECT) scan uses another form of technetium that is injected. A camera is then used to reproduce visual images taken along several planes of the heart. This nuclear medicine procedure can produce clearer, more accurate images.

Cardiac Catheterization and Arteriography. This is an invasive procedure that can be divided into two stages (right-sided and left-sided catheterization). Cardiac catheterization is used to confirm and evaluate the severity of lesions within the coronary arteries, to assess left ventricular function, and to measure pressures in the chambers of the heart, cardiac output, and blood gas content.

Right-sided catheterization is performed by placement of a pulmonary artery catheter in the femoral or brachial vein that is carefully advanced into the right atrium, right ventricle, and pulmonary artery. The practitioner measures pressures in the right atrium, right ventricle, and pulmonary artery, and the pulmonary artery occlusion pressure. Oxygen saturations can be measured if indicated (i.e., valve disease or septal defect).

Left-sided catheterization is performed to visualize coronary arteries, to note the area and extent of lesions within the vessel walls, to evaluate CAD and angina-related spasms, to locate areas of infarct through the use of radioisotopes, and to perform interventions such as percutaneous angioplasty or stent placement.

Left-sided catheterization is performed by cannulation of a femoral or brachial artery. The procedure entails positioning a catheter into the aorta at the proximal end of the coronary arteries. Dye is then injected into the arteries, and a radiographic picture (arteriography) is recorded as the dye progresses or fails to progress through the coronary circulation. In addition, dye is injected into the left ventricle, and the amount of dye ejected with the next systole is measured to determine the ejection fraction.

After the procedure the catheters are removed. To prevent bleeding from the arterial site, a vascular sealing device made of collagen (e.g., AngioSeal) or a stitch device (e.g., Perclose) may be used to close the puncture site in the artery. If the sealing or stitch device is not used, firm pressure is applied for 15 to 30 minutes. Commercial devices (e.g., FemoStop) (Figure 12-8) are available to assist in applying pressure to the site. Depending on the diagnostic study results, patients are usually discharged within 6 to 8 hours of completion of the test.

Nursing care for a patient undergoing cardiac catheterization and arteriography involves the preprocedure instruction (the procedure will be performed using local anesthesia, and the patient may feel a warm or hot *flush* sensation or flutter of the catheter as it moves about) and the postprocedure instruction. The postprocedure routine is noted in Box 12-4.

Magnetic Resonance Imaging. Magnetic resonance imaging (MRI) is a noninvasive test used to detect tissues, structures, and blood flow. For example, MRI is used to detect aortic aneurysms and pericardial tumors. MRI is a technique that uses magnetic resonance to create images of hydrogen. These images

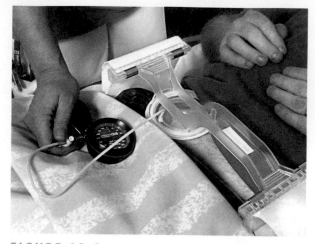

FIGURE 12-8. FemoStop in correct position. *(Courtesy of RADI Medical Systems, Inc. Sweden.)*

BOX 12-4   Nursing Care after Cardiac Catheterization and Arteriography

- Maintain the patient on bed rest (time varies depending on method for preventing arterial bleeding).
- Keep the extremity used for catheter insertion immobile.
- Observe the insertion site for bleeding or hematoma, especially if the patient is receiving postprocedure anticoagulant therapy.
- Mark the hematoma with a marker around outer perimeter, to aid in assessing for an increase in bleeding.
- Maintain head-of-bed elevation no higher than 30 degrees.
- Monitor peripheral pulses, color, and sensation of the extremity distal to insertion site (every 15 minutes × 4, every 30 minutes × 4, every 1 hour × 4, then every 2 hours). In addition, monitor the opposite extremity pulse to assess for presence of equal pulses and color and sensation bilaterally.
- Observe cardiac rhythm.
- Encourage fluid intake.
- Monitor intake and output.
- Observe for an adverse reaction to dye (arteriography).

---

are created as the ions are emitted, picked up, and fed into a computer that reconstructs the image that then can differentiate between healthy and ischemic tissue. Newer enhancements of MRI include the use of diffusion-weighted imaging, functional MRI, and fast MRI. In diffusion-weighted MRI, the intracellular and extracellular spaces are compared for the degree of diffusion of water molecules contained within them. Brighter areas indicate restricted diffusion. In functional MRI, successive images are taken in rapid succession while the patient follows commands. The images are compared. Fast MRI allows shortened breath-holding time frames, better resolution, and procedure completion in 30 minutes or less. The newest equipment is called dual mode imaging, which combines MRI with functional imaging such as positron emission tomography (PET) or SPECT for improved imaging results.

Electrophysiology Study. An electrophysiology study is an invasive procedure that involves the introduction of an electrode catheter percutaneously from a peripheral vein or artery into the cardiac chamber or sinuses and the performance of programmed electrical stimulation of the heart. Electrophysiology studies aid in recording intracardiac ECGs, diagnosing cardiac conduction defects, evaluating the effectiveness of antidysrhythmic medications, determining the proper choice of pacemaker programming, and mapping the cardiac conduction system before ablation.

Laboratory Diagnostics

Other diagnostic measures include the evaluation of serum electrolyte studies and cardiac enzymes. Because many manuals are available regarding the reading and interpretation of laboratory values, this section presents a brief overview of the more important blood studies.[8]

Serum Electrolytes. Electrolytes are important in maintaining the function of the cardiac conduction system. Imbalances in sodium, potassium, calcium, and magnesium can result in cardiac dysrhythmias. There-fore, analysis of serum electrolytes is a routine part of the assessment and treatment of the cardiac patient. Table 12-3 reviews ECG changes that may alert the nurse to possible electrolyte abnormalities.

Serum Enzymes. Enzymes are proteins that are produced by all living cells and released into the bloodstream. When cells are injured or diseased, more enzymes are released. Assessments of enzyme levels released from cardiac muscle are useful in the diagnosis of AMI.[8]

- *Creatine kinase (CK)* enzymes increase within 2 to 6 hours after the onset of myocardial muscle damage. Peak levels occur within 18 to 36 hours, and levels return to baseline in 3 to 6 days. Total CK can be elevated from a variety of diseases and conditions and is nonspecific.
- *CK_2-MB (heart)* is a fraction of the total CK that is specific for cardiac muscle. Normal values of CK_2-MB are 0% to 6% of the total CK or 0.3 to 4.9 ng/mL. Values are elevated after AMI, cardiac surgery, and blunt cardiac trauma. The initial rise in CK_2-MB levels after an AMI occurs within 4 to 8 hours after the onset of damage. Peak levels occur in 18 to 24 hours, and levels return to baseline within 3 days. Total CK and CK_2-MB are usually ordered at the initial assessment and at 8, 16, and 24 hours after the onset of chest pain to assist in the diagnosis of AMI.
- *Troponin I and troponin T.* Serum troponin levels are useful in the early diagnosis of AMI. Levels are normally undetectable in healthy people and elevate as early as 1 hour after myocardial cell injury. Troponin I has a greater specificity than CK_2-MB in the diagnosis of AMI at 7 to 14 hours after the onset of chest pain. Testing for troponin can be done quickly in the field or the emergency department and aids in the

TABLE 12-3   ECG Changes Associated with Electrolyte Imbalances

Electrolyte Imbalance	Panic Value	Manifestations
Hypokalemia	<2.5 mEq/L	U wave, increased ventricular ectopy
Hyperkalemia	>6.6 mEq/L	Tall, peaked T waves, conduction blocks, ventricular fibrillation
Hypocalcemia	<7 mg/dL	Prolonged ST segment and QT interval
Hypercalcemia	>12 mg/dL	Shortened ST segment and QT interval
Hypomagnesemia	<0.5 mEq/L	Prolonged PR and QT intervals, broad, flat T waves, PVCs, ventricular tachycardia or fibrillation
Hypermagnesemia	>3.0 mEq/L	Prolonged PR and QT intervals, widened QRS

PVCs, Premature ventricular contractions.
Modified from Chernecky, C. C., & Berger, B. J. (2008). *Laboratory tests and diagnostic procedures* (5th ed.). Philadelphia: Saunders.

early diagnosis of AMI. The normal value of troponin I is less than 0.5 mcg/L, and that of troponin T is less than 0.1 mcg/L.

- *Myoglobin*. Serum myoglobin is released within 30 to 60 minutes after AMI. Normal values are less than 72 ng/mL in men and less than 58 ng/mL in women. Myoglobin levels rise before CK and CK_2-MB and are useful in the early diagnosis of AMI. Myoglobin alone is not specific for AMI, but when used in combination with other tests, it can aid in the diagnosis. Some institutions order myoglobin levels every 2 hours. A doubling of levels from one sample to the next sample is indicative of AMI.

Nursing Diagnoses

CAD is a broad diagnostic area, and thus several nursing diagnostic categories apply. With the complications of CAD, such as angina, MI, and HF, the diagnostic categories are more specific. Nursing diagnoses of patients with CAD include the following:

- Pain related to decreased coronary artery tissue perfusion
- Anxiety/fear related to treatments and invasive procedures used for diagnostic testing
- Knowledge deficit related to understanding of anatomy and pathophysiology of the heart and its functions; complexity of treatment; new condition; emotional state
- Health-seeking behaviors related to desire for information regarding altered health status, or a disease process or condition

Interventions

Nursing Interventions

Nursing interventions are patient centered and encompass health assessment and patient education. The psychosocial and family support assessment, as well as the patient's history and physical examina-tion findings, are used. The nurse instructs the patient about risk factor modification and signs and symptoms of progression of CAD that warrant medical treatment.

Medical Management

The goals of medical management are to achieve target levels of LDL. The National Cholesterol Education Project of the National Heart, Lung, and Blood Institute recommends that an optimal LDL level is less than 100 mg/dL, but the target level should be adjusted in relation to the patient's number of major risk factors for CAD.[23] These include family history, age, smoking, hypertension, and diabetes. The key to lessening the burden of coronary heart disease in the United States is primary prevention, and one way this can be accomplished is through thorough management of cholesterol levels (see Laboratory Alerts for LDLs, high-density lipoproteins [HDLs], and triglycerides).

Strategies for risk factor modification include a low-fat, low-cholesterol diet, exercise, weight loss, smoking cessation, and control of other risks such as diabetes and hypertension. If LDL levels are not at target values after 6 months of risk factor modification, patients are started on lipid-lowering drugs.

Medications to Reduce Serum Lipid Levels. Lipid-lowering drugs include statins, bile acid resins, and nicotinic acid (Table 12-4). The statins are officially classified as 3-hydroxy-3-methylglutaryl-coenzyme A (HMG-CoA) reductase inhibitors. The statins have been found to lower LDL more than other types of lipid-lowering drugs. They work by slowing the production of cholesterol and increasing the liver's ability to remove LDL from the body. Some commonly used drugs are lovastatin, atorvastatin, pravastatin, and simvastatin. The drugs are well tolerated by most patients. It is recommended that statins be given as a single dose in the evening because the body makes more cholesterol at night. LDL levels are reassessed in 4 to 6 weeks, and dosages are adjusted as needed.[14]

LABORATORY ALERT

Risks	Target Low-Density Lipoprotein Level	Target High-Density Lipoprotein Level	Target Triglyceride Level
No CAD; 0-1 risk factors	<160 mg/dL	>60 mg/dL	<190 mg/dL
No CAD; 2 or more risk factors	<130 mg/dL	>60 mg/dL	<160 mg/dL
CAD or CAD risk equivalent (other atherosclerotic disease, diabetes, multiple risks)	<100 mg/dL	>60 mg/dL	<130 mg/dL

CAD, Coronary artery disease.

PHARMACOLOGY

TABLE 12-4   Medications for Lowering Cholesterol and Triglycerides

Antilipemic Agents (HMG-CoA Reductase Inhibitors)

Indications: used to lower total and LDL cholesterol and to help reduce the risk of acute myocardial infarction and stroke

Mechanism of action: competitively inhibit HMG-CoA reductase, the enzyme that catalyzes the rate-limiting step in cholesterol biosynthesis, resulting in lower total and LDL cholesterol levels with increased HDL cholesterol

Generic Name (Brand Name)	Dosage	Side Effects and Nursing Considerations
Lovastatin (Altocor, Mevacor)	10-80 mg PO once daily (in the evening) or in two divided doses	Headache, dizziness, constipation, weakness, and increased creatine phosphokinase levels Instruct patient to take with evening meal. Report severe muscle pain, weakness, or abdominal tenderness. Patient should have baseline liver function and lipid profile tests before starting therapy, then at 6 and 12 months. Do not give in pregnancy. Patient should be instructed in a low-cholesterol diet
Atorvastatin (Lipitor)	10-80 mg PO daily	Headache, peripheral edema, weakness, constipation Medicine can be taken with any meal during the day Instruct patient to maintain fluid status every day (2 L/day) unless on fluid restriction. Do not give in pregnancy. Patient should be instructed to consume a low-cholesterol diet. Patient should have baseline liver function and lipid profile tests before starting therapy, then at 6 and 12 months
Fluvastatin (Lescol)	20-80 mg daily PO at bedtime	Same
Pravastatin (Pravachol)	10-80 mg daily PO at bedtime	Same
Rosuvastatin (Crestor)	5-40 mg daily PO at bedtime	Same
Simvastatin (Apo-Simvastatin, Zocor)	5-80 mg daily PO at bedtime	Same

Antilipemic Agents (Bile Acid Sequestrants)

Indications: used to manage hypercholesterolemia

Mechanism of action: form a nonabsorbable complex with bile acids in the intestine, inhibiting enterohepatic reuptake of intestinal bile salts, which increases the fecal loss of bile salt–bound LDL cholesterol

Generic Name (Brand Name)	Dosage	Side Effects and Nursing Considerations
Cholestyramine (Novo-Cholamine, Prevalite, Questran, Questran-Lite)	Powder: 4-24 g 1-2 times a day Tablet: 4-16 g 1-2 times a day	Constipation, heartburn, nausea, flatulence, vomiting, abdominal pain, and headache Instruct patient to mix powder with fluid, pudding, or applesauce. Patient should take other medications at least 1 hour before taking this medication. Patient should report any stomach cramping, pain, blood in stool, and unresolved nausea or vomiting. Monitor cholesterol and triglyceride levels before and during therapy. Use during pregnancy must be cautious, weighing benefits of use against the possible risks involved

Continued

PHARMACOLOGY

TABLE 12-4 Medications for Lowering Cholesterol and Triglycerides—cont'd

Generic Name (Brand Name)	Dosage	Side Effects and Nursing Considerations
Colesevelam (Welchol)	4-6 tablets	Same
Colestipol (Colestid)	5-30 g in divided doses 2-4 times a day	Same

Antilipemic Agent (Miscellaneous, Niacin)
Indications: adjunctive treatment of hyperlipidemia
Mechanism of action: inhibits VLDL synthesis

Generic Name (Brand Name)	Dosage	Side Effects and Nursing Considerations
Nicotinic acid (Niacin)	1.5-6 g daily in 3 divided doses	Headache, bloating, flatulence, and nausea. Instruct patient to take it as directed and not to exceed recommended dosage. Should be taken after meals. Patient should report persistent gastrointestinal disturbances or changes in color of urine or stool

Antilipemic Agent (Fibric Acid)
Indications: treatment of hypertriglyceridemia in patients who have not responded to dietary intervention
Mechanism of action: inhibits lipolysis and decreases subsequent hepatic fatty acid uptake and hepatic VLDL secretion and thus reduces serum VLDL and increases HDL

Gemfibrozil (Lopid)	600 mg BID PO	Stomach upset, fatigue, headache, diarrhea, and nausea. Instruct patient to take before breakfast and dinner. May take with milk or meals if gastrointestinal upset occurs. Patient should report severe abdominal pain, nausea, or vomiting. Use during pregnancy must be weighed against the possible risks
Fenofibrate (Tricor)	67-200 mg PO	Diarrhea, nausea, constipation, abdominal pain, back pain, headaches

BID, Twice daily; *HDL,* high-density lipoprotein; *HMG-CoA,* 3-hydroxy-3-methylglutaryl-coenzyme A; *LDL,* low-density lipoprotein; *PO,* orally; *VLDL,* very low density lipoprotein.
From Hodgson B. B., & Kizior R. J. (2007). *Saunders nursing drug handbook.* Philadelphia: Saunders.

One disadvantage of the drugs is their high cost. Another disadvantage is that they can cause liver damage; therefore, it is important to ensure that the patient has liver enzymes drawn periodically to assess liver function.

The bile acid resins combine with cholesterol-containing bile acids in the intestines to form an insoluble complex that is eliminated through feces. These drugs lower LDL levels by 10% to 20%. Bile acid resins include cholestyramine and colestipol. The drugs are mixed in liquid and are taken twice daily. They are associated with side effects such as nausea and flatulence. The drugs interfere with absorption of many medications. It is recommended that other medications be given 1 hour before or 4 hours after administration of the resins to promote absorption.[14]

Nicotinic acid, or niacin, reduces total cholesterol, LDL, and triglyceride levels if it is given in high doses. The drug is available over-the-counter; however, its use in lowering cholesterol must be under the supervision of a health care provider. The drug is given three times daily; doses range from 500 mg to 2 g daily, according to the desired LDL effect. The drug should be gradually increased to the maximum effective daily dose. Common side effects include a metallic taste in mouth, flushing, and increased feelings of warmth. Major side effects include hepatic dysfunction, gout, and hyperglycemia. Because nicotinic acid affects the absorption of other drugs, the nurse must give the patient information about common drug-drug interactions.[14]

If triglyceride levels are elevated, patients may be prescribed agents that specifically lower triglyceride levels. One agent is gemfibrozil, a fibric acid derivative. This drug is associated with many gastrointestinal side effects.

If a patient does not respond adequately to single-drug therapy, combined-drug therapy is considered to lower LDL levels further. For example, statins may be combined with bile acid resins. Patients must be carefully monitored when two or more lipid-lowering agents are given simultaneously.

Medications to Prevent Platelet Adhesion and Aggregation. Drugs are often prescribed for the patient with CAD to reduce platelet adhesion and aggregation. They are used to provide long-term therapy for angina. A single dose of 81 to 325 mg of an enteric-coated aspirin per day is commonly prescribed. To prevent platelet aggregation, other agents that may be prescribed such as dipyridamole (Persantine), ticlopidine (Ticlid), and clopidogrel (Plavix). Dipyridamole or clopidogrel may be given with aspirin.[14]

Patient Outcomes

Several outcomes are expected after treatment. These include relief of pain, less anxiety related to the disease, adherence to health behavior modification to reduce cardiovascular risks, and the ability to describe the disease process, causes, and factors contributing to the symptoms, and the procedures for disease or symptom control.

ANGINA

Angina is chest pain or discomfort caused by myocardial ischemia that result from an imbalance between myocardial oxygen supply and demand. CAD and coronary artery spasms are common causes of angina.

Pathophysiology

Angina (from the Latin word meaning *squeezing*) is the chest pain associated with myocardial ischemia; it is transient and does not cause cell death, but it

may be a precursor to cell death from MI. The neural pain receptors are stimulated by accelerated metabolism, chemical changes and imbalances, and/or local mechanical stress resulting from abnormal myocardial contractions. The oxygen circulating via the vascular system to the myocardial cells decreases, causing ischemia to the tissue, resulting in pain.

Angina occurs when oxygen demand is higher than oxygen supply. Box 12-5 shows factors influencing oxygen supply and demand that may result in angina.

Types of Angina

Different types of angina exist: stable, unstable, and variant. *Stable angina* occurs with exertion and is relieved by rest. It is sometimes called chronic exertional angina. *Unstable angina* (along with AMI) is classified as an acute coronary syndrome (ACS). The common pathophysiology of these syndromes is a thrombus resulting from disruption of an atherosclerotic plaque. In unstable angina, some blood continues to flow through the affected coronary artery; however, flow is diminished. The pain in unstable angina is more severe, may occur at rest, and requires more frequent nitrate therapy. It is sometimes described as crescendo (increasing) in nature. During an unstable attack, the ECG may show ST-segment depression. The patient has an increased risk of MI within 18 months of onset of unstable angina; therefore, medical or surgical interventions, or both, are

---

BOX 12-5 Factors That Influence Oxygen Demand and Supply

Increased Oxygen Demand
- Increased heart rate: exercise, tachydysrhythmias, anemia, fever, anxiety, pain, thyrotoxicosis, medications, ingestion of heavy meals, adapting to extremes in temperature
- Increased preload: volume overload, medications
- Increased afterload: hypertension, aortic stenosis, vasopressors
- Increased contractility: exercise, medications, anxiety

Reduced Oxygen Supply
- Coronary artery disease
- Coronary artery spasms
- Medications
- Anemia
- Hypoxemia

warranted. Patients are often hospitalized for diagnostic workup and treatment.

Variant, or *Prinzmetal's*, *angina* is caused by coronary artery spasms. It often occurs at rest and without other precipitating factors. The ECG shows a marked ST elevation (usually seen only in AMI) during the episode. The ST segment returns to normal after the spasm subsides. AMI can occur with prolonged coronary artery spasm, even in the absence of CAD.

Assessment

Assessment of the patient with actual or suspected angina involves continual observation of the patient and monitoring of signs, symptoms, and diagnostic findings. The patient must be monitored for the type and degree of pain (see Clinical Alert: Symptoms of Angina).

CLINICAL ALERT
Symptoms of Angina

Pain is frequently retrosternal, left pectoral, or epigastric. It may radiate to the jaw, left shoulder, or left arm.

Pain can be described as burning, squeezing, heavy, or smothering.

Pain usually lasts 1 to 5 minutes.

Classic placing of clenched fist against the chest (sternum) may be seen, or may be absent if the sensation is confused with indigestion.

Pain usually begins with exertion and subsides with rest.

The precipitating factors that can be identified as bringing on an episode of anginal pain include physical or emotional stress, exposure to temperature extremes, and ingestion of a heavy meal. It is important to know what factors alleviate the anginal pain, including stopping activity or exercise and taking NTG sublingual tablets or spray.

Diagnostic Studies

Diagnostic studies for angina include the following: history and physical examination, in which patterns of pain and precipitating risk factors are sought; laboratory data, including blood studies for anemia (hemoglobin and hematocrit values), cardiac enzymes (CK_2-MB, cardiac troponin I, cardiac troponin T levels), and cholesterol and triglyceride levels; ECGs during resting periods, precipitating events (exercise), and anginal pain episodes; exercise tolerance or stress testing; cardiac scanning; and coronary arte-

riography. Complications of untreated or unstable angina include MI, HF, presence of dysrhythmias, psychological depression, and sudden death.[6]

Nursing Diagnoses

Several nursing diagnoses and interventions are identified for patients with angina. These include the following:[12]

- Acute chest pain related to myocardial ischemia
- Knowledge deficit related to unfamiliarity with disease process and treatment
- Activity intolerance related to chest pain; side effects of prescribed medications; imbalance between oxygen supply and demand

Interventions

Nursing Interventions

Nursing interventions for the patient with angina are aimed at assessing the patient's description of pain, noting exacerbating factors and measures used to relieve the pain; evaluating whether this is a chronic problem (stable angina) or a new presentation; assessing for appropriateness of performing an ECG to evaluate ST-segment and T-wave changes; monitoring vital signs during chest pain and after nitrate administration; and monitoring the effectiveness of interventions. The patient should be instructed to relax and rest at the first sign of pain or discomfort, and to notify the nurse at the onset of any type of chest pain so that nitrates and oxygen can be administered. The nurse should also offer assurance and emotional support by explaining all treatments and procedures and by encouraging questions. The nurse begins to assess the patient's knowledge base regarding the causes of angina, diagnostic procedures, the treatment plan, and risk factors for CAD. Patients who wish to stop smoking can be referred to the American Heart Association, American Lung Association, or American Cancer Society for support groups and interventions.

Medical Interventions

Unstable angina can be treated by conservative management, early intervention with percutaneous intervention, or surgical revascularization. Conservative intervention for the patient experiencing angina includes the administration of nitrates, beta-adrenergic blocking agents, and/or calcium channel blocking agents (Table 12-5). Angioplasty, stenting, and bypass surgery are approaches to revascularization.

Nitrates are the most common medications for angina. They are direct-acting smooth muscle

Text continued on p. 328

PHARMACOLOGY

TABLE 12-5   Drugs for Acute Coronary Syndromes

Nitrates
Indications: angina
Mechanism of action: directly relaxes smooth muscle, which causes vasodilation of the systemic vascular bed; decrease
myocardial oxygen demands

Generic Name (Brand Name)	Dosage	Side Effects and Nursing Considerations
Nitroglycerin (Tridil, Nitro-Bid, Nitro-Dur, Nitrostat)	SL: 0.4 mg SL every 5 minutes for 3 doses Topical: 0.5-2 inches every 6 hours IV: continuous infusion started at 5 mcg/min and titrated up to 200 mcg/min maximum	Headache, flushing, tachycardia, dizziness, and orthostatic hypotension Instruct patient to call 911 if chest pain does not subside after the third SL dose. For topical and oral doses, patient may need a nitrate-free interval (10-12 hours/day) to avoid development of tolerance. Instruct patient not to combine nitrate use with medications used for treatment of erectile dysfunction (e.g., Viagra)
Isosorbide dinitrate (Isordil)	5-40 mg TID PO, every 6 hours except at bedtime	Same
Isosorbide mononitrate (Imdur)	30-60 mg every day PO Maximum 240 mg every day PO	Same

Beta-Blockers
Indications: used to treat angina, acute myocardial infarction, and heart failure
Mechanism of action: block beta-adrenergic receptors, which results in decreased sympathetic nervous system response
such as decreased heart rate, blood pressure, and cardiac contractility

Generic Name (Brand Name)	Dosage	Side Effects and Nursing Considerations
Metoprolol (Lopressor, Toprol XL)	50-100 mg BID PO; 5 mg IV Toprol XL: 100-200 mg daily PO	Bradycardia, hypotension, atrioventricular blocks, asthma attacks, fatigue, impotence, may mask hypoglycemic episodes Teach patient to take pulse and blood pressure on regular basis. Patient should not abruptly stop taking beta-blockers. Close glucose monitoring is needed if diabetic. Patient should have ECG monitoring in place for IV administration
Propranolol (Inderal)	80-320 mg in divided doses 2-4 times a day IV: 1-3 mg SLOW IVP	Same
Labetalol (Trandate, Normodyne)	200-400 mg BID PO IV: 2 mg over 2 minutes at 10-minute intervals; slow IVP	Same Acts on both alpha and beta$_1$ and beta$_2$ receptors Monitor blood pressure continuously, maximum effect occurs within 5 minutes
Carvedilol (Coreg)	3.125-25 mg BID PO	Same

Continued

PHARMACOLOGY

TABLE 12-5   Drugs for Acute Coronary Syndromes—cont'd

Calcium Channel Blockers

Indications: used to treat hypertension, tachydysrhythmias, vasospasms, and angina
Mechanism of action: inhibit the flow of calcium ions across cellular membranes, with resulting increased coronary blood
  flow and myocardial perfusion and decreased myocardial oxygen requirements

Generic Name (Brand Name)	Dosage	Side Effects and Nursing Considerations
Verapamil (Calan, Isoptin)	80-120 mg TID PO	Dizziness, flushing, headaches, bradycardia, atrioventricular blocks, and hypotension Teach patient to monitor pulse and blood pressure, especially if taking nitrates and/or beta-blockers. Tablets cannot be crushed or chewed. Instruct patient to make position changes slowly
Nifedipine (Procardia)	10 mg TID PO	Same
Diltiazem (Cardizem, Cardizem CD)	30 mg QID PO, sustained release 120-180 mg daily	Same

Anticoagulants

Indications: unstable angina, acute myocardial infarction, and coronary interventions
Mechanism of action: inhibit clotting mechanisms within the clotting cascade or prevent platelet aggregation

Generic Name (Brand Name)	Dosage	Side Effects and Nursing Considerations
Aspirin	81-325 mg daily PO	Bleeding, epigastric discomfort, bruising, and gastric ulceration Instruct patient to take medication with food. Do not crush or chew the enteric-coated forms. Instruct patient to be aware of additive effects with OTC drugs containing aspirin or salicylate or other NSAIDs. Instruct patient to avoid high-risk activities that can cause injury
Clopidogrel (Plavix)	300 mg loading dose then 75 mg daily PO (in combination with aspirin)	Same
Dipyridamole (Persantine)	75-100 mg QID PO in divided doses	May worsen angina, dizziness, headache, and hypotension; increased risk of bleeding with aspirin use Medication should be taken 1 hour before meals with a full glass of water.
Ticlopidine (Ticlid)	250 mg BID PO	Bleeding, bruising, gastrointestinal upset, and diarrhea Instruct patient to take with food to reduce gastrointestinal upset. Instruct patient to report any unusual bleeding. Monitor CBC during therapy

PHARMACOLOGY

TABLE 12-5 Drugs for Acute Coronary Syndromes—cont'd

Glycoprotein IIb/IIIa Inhibitors

Indications: acute coronary syndromes and coronary intervention patients

Mechanism of action: antiplatelet agent and glycoprotein IIb/IIIa inhibitor; act by binding to the glycoprotein IIb/IIIa receptor site on the surface of the platelet

Generic Name (Brand Name)	Dosage	Side Effects and Nursing Considerations
Abciximab (ReoPro)	0.25 mg/kg IV bolus followed by a continuous infusion at 10 mcg/min for 18-24 hours after procedure	Bleeding, bruising, hemorrhage, thrombocytopenia, and hypotension Avoid IM injections. Avoid venipunctures. Observe and teach patient bleeding precautions and activities to avoid that may cause injury. Assess infusion insertion site for bleeding or hematoma formation. Assess femoral puncture site frequently. Abciximab is not reversible because of its binding to the platelet. For hemorrhage, give fresh frozen plasma and platelets. Monitor CBC and PTT daily
Tirofiban (Aggrastat)	0.4 mcg/kg/min for 30 minutes, then continued at 0.1 mcg/kg/min for 12-24 hours	Same Tirofiban stops working when the infusion is discontinued. Platelet function is restored 4 hours after stopping the infusion
Eptifibatide (Integrilin)	180 mcg/kg IV loading dose over 2 minutes, followed by continuous infusion of 2 mcg/kg/min until hospital discharge or for up to 18-24 hours. Concurrent aspirin and heparin therapy is recommended	Same Eptifibatide stops working when the infusion is discontinued. Platelet function is restored 4 hours after stopping the infusion

Antithrombin Agents

Indications: prevention of or delay in thrombus formation

Mechanism of action: accelerates formation of antithrombin III–thrombin complex and deactivates thrombin, preventing conversion of fibrinogen to fibrin

Generic Name (Brand Name)	Dosage	Side Effects and Nursing Considerations
Heparin	80 units/kg IV bolus, followed by initial infusion of 18 units/kg/hr, titrated to PTT (range, 10-30 units/kg/hr)	Bleeding, bruising, thrombocytopenia Monitor PTT. Monitor for signs of bleeding and hematoma formation. Avoid IM injections. Do not rub the site after giving the injection
Enoxaparin (Lovenox)	1 mg/kg subcutaneous every 12 hours, in conjunction with aspirin	Bleeding, bruising, local site hematomas, and hemorrhage Instruct patient to report persistent chest pain, unusual bleeding or bruising. Do not rub the site after giving the injection

Continued

PHARMACOLOGY

TABLE 12-5　Drugs for Acute Coronary Syndromes—cont'd

Analgesic

Indications: pain relief and anxiety reduction during acute myocardial infarction

Mechanism of action: binds to opioid receptors in the central nervous system and causes inhibition of ascending pain pathways, altering perception and response to pain

Generic Name (Brand Name)	Dosage	Side Effects and Nursing Considerations
Morphine	2-4 mg IVP every 5-10 minutes	Hypotension, respiratory depression, apnea, bradycardia, nausea, and restlessness titrated for chest pain Monitor level of consciousness, blood pressure, respiratory rate, and oxygen saturation during therapy. Effects are reversed with naloxone (Narcan)

Angiotensin-Converting Enzyme Inhibitors

Indications: used to treat hypertension, heart failure, and patients after myocardial infarction

Mechanism of action: prevent the conversion of angiotensin I to angiotensin II resulting in lower levels of angiotensin II, which causes an increase in plasma renin activity and a reduction of aldosterone secretion; also inhibit the remodeling process after myocardial injury

Generic Name (Brand Name)	Dosage	Side Effects and Nursing Considerations
Enalapril (Vasotec)	2.5-10 mg BID PO	Hypotension, bradycardia, renal impairment, cough, and orthostatic hypotension Do not give IV enalapril to patients with unstable heart failure or in those patients having an acute myocardial infarction. Monitor urine output. Monitor potassium levels. Avoid use of NSAIDs. Instruct patient to avoid rapid change in position such as from lying to standing. Angiotensin-converting enzyme inhibitors are contraindicated in pregnancy
Fosinopril (Monopril)	20-40 mg daily PO	Same
Captopril (Capoten)	6.25 mg once per day, increasing slowly to 50 mg TID	Same

BID, Twice daily; *CBC*, complete blood count; *ECG*, electrocardiogram; *IVP*, intravenous push; *NSAIDs*, nonsteroidal antiinflammatory drugs; *OTC*, over-the-counter; *PO*, orally; *PTT*, partial thromboplastin time; *QID*, four times daily; *SL*, sublingual; *TID*, three times daily.

From Hodgson B. B., & Kizior R. J. (2007). *Saunders nursing drug handbook*. Philadelphia: Saunders.

relaxants that cause vasodilation of the peripheral or systemic vascular bed.[14] Nitrate therapy is beneficial because it decreases myocardial oxygen demand. The vasodilating effect causes relief of pain and lowering of blood pressure. Forms or preparations of nitrates include sublingual, intravenous (IV), transdermal, spray, and ointment NTG, and sublingual and oral isosorbide (Isordil). Side effects of these vasodilators include headache, flushing, tachycardia, dizziness, and orthostatic hypotension. Instructions for NTG therapy are detailed in Box 12-6.

Beta-adrenergic blocking agents may also be used to treat angina. They block adrenergic receptors, thereby decreasing heart rate, blood pressure, and cardiac

BOX 12-6　Instructions Regarding Nitroglycerin

If the client is discharged on sublingual or buccal nitroglycerin, instruct client to:
- Avoid drinking alcoholic beverages.
- Have tablets readily available.
- Take a tablet before strenuous activity and in stressful situations.
- Take one tablet when chest pain occurs and another every 5 minutes up to a total of three times if necessary; obtain emergency medical assistance if pain persists.
- Place the tablet under the tongue or in the buccal pouch and allow it to dissolve thoroughly.
- Store tablets in a tightly capped, original container away from heat and moisture.
- Replace tablets every 6 months or sooner if they do not relieve discomfort.
- Avoid rising to a standing position quickly after taking nitroglycerin.
- Recognize that dizziness, flushing, and mild headache are common side effects.
- Report fainting, persistent or severe headache, blurred vision, or dry mouth.
- Caution use of drugs for erectile dysfunction (e.g., Viagra, Levitra) when taking nitrates because hypotensive effects are exaggerated.

If nitroglycerin skin patches are prescribed:
- Provide instructions about correct application, skin care, the need to rotate sites and to remove the old patch, and frequency of change.
- The patch may be ordered to be left off for a period each day to prevent development of nitrate tolerance.
- Caution the client that activities that increase blood flow to the skin (e.g., hot bath or shower, sauna) can cause a sudden reduction in blood pressure.

From Gulanick, M., & Myers, J. L. (2007). *Nursing care plans: Nursing diagnosis and intervention* (6th ed.). St. Louis: Mosby.

contractility.[14] Examples include metoprolol, propranolol, labetalol, carvedilol, nadolol, timolol, and pindolol. The side effects of these agents include bradycardia, AV block, asthma attacks, depression, hypotension, memory loss, and masking of hypoglycemic episodes. The patient is taught to take these agents as prescribed, not to stop taking them abruptly, and to monitor heart rate and blood pressure at regular intervals.

Calcium channel blockers inhibit the flow of calcium ions across cellular membranes, an effect that causes direct increases in coronary blood flow and myocardial perfusion, as well as decreases in myocardial oxygen requirements.[14] These drugs are used for treating tachydysrhythmias, vasospasms, and hypertension, as well as for treating angina. Examples of calcium channel blockers include verapamil (Calan, Isoptin), nifedipine (Procardia), and diltiazem (Cardizem). The side effects of calcium channel blockers include dizziness, flushing, headaches, decreased heart rate, and hypotension. The patient is taught to monitor blood pressure for hypotension, and heart rate for bradycardia, especially if the agents are taken in combination with nitrates and beta-blockers.

Conservative treatment also includes the administration of aspirin and heparin. In addition, Gp IIb/IIIa inhibitors (abciximab, tirofiban, and eptifibatide) are used in the management of ACSs.

Outcomes

The outcomes for patients with angina are that they will verbalize relief of chest discomfort; appear relaxed and comfortable; verbalize an understanding of angina pectoris and its management; describe their own cardiac risk factors and strategies to reduce them; and perform activities within limits of their ischemic disease, as evidenced by absence of chest pain or discomfort and no ECG changes reflecting ischemia.[12]

ACUTE MYOCARDIAL INFARCTION

AMI is ischemia with death of the myocardium that is caused by lack of blood supply from the occlusion of a coronary artery or its branches. AMI results when there is prolonged ischemia causing irreversible damage to the heart muscle.[6]

Pathophysiology

AMI is caused by an imbalance between myocardial oxygen supply and demand. This imbalance is the result of decreased coronary artery perfusion. Most cases of AMI are secondary to atherosclerosis. Other causes (<5%) include coronary artery spasm, coronary embolism, and blunt trauma. Reduced blood flow to an area of the myocardium causes significant and sustained oxygen deprivation to myocardial cells. Normal functioning is disrupted as ischemia and injury lead to eventual cellular death. Myocardial dysfunction occurs as more cells become involved.

EVIDENCE-BASED PRACTICE

PROBLEM

Treatment of acute coronary syndromes (ACS) presents a major health challenge. With new clinical trials being conducted, knowledge of latest therapies for ACS continually evolves.

QUESTION

What are the currently available pharmacological therapies and evidence-based rationale for the treatment of ACS?

REFERENCE

Ramanath, V. S., Kim A., & Eagle, K. A. (2007). Evidence-based medical therapy of patients with acute coronary syndromes. *American Journal of Cardiovascular Drugs,* 7(2), 95-116.

EVIDENCE

The authors reviewed currently available medical therapies and provided evidence-based rationale for current pharmacological therapies. Antiplatelet therapies (aspirin, clopidogrel, and glycoprotein IIb/IIIa inhibitors) demonstrated significant efficacy in reducing morbidity and mortality. Anticoagulants (unfractionated heparin and low–molecular weight heparin) remain the hallmarks of therapy. Fibrinolysis is an acceptable modality for reperfusion. Antiischemic therapy, beta-adrenoceptor antagonists, and nitrates remain critical. Inhibitors of the renin-angiotensin-aldosterone system have also reduced in the morbidity and mortality. Angiotensin-converting enzyme (ACE) inhibitors and lipid-lowering therapies (statins, specifically 3-hydroxy-3-methylglutaryl-coenzyme A [HMG-CoA] reductase inhibitors) are documented as being the most well-tolerated and most efficacious therapies. Finally, combination therapy including antiplatelet drugs, beta-adrenoceptor antagonists, ACE inhibitors, and lipid-lowering agents show a clear benefit.

IMPLICATIONS FOR NURSING

The acute phase of ACS care encompasses the time in which the risk of progression to myocardial infarction or development of a recurrent episode is the highest, and is generally complete within 2 months. As advocated in the American College of Cardiology/American Heart Association guidelines, direct patient instruction is imperative and must be reinforced with written instructions. After hospital discharge, in addition to follow-up with the cardiologist, primary care physician, or both, enrollment in a cardiac rehabilitation program enhances patient education and compliance with the newly prescribed or updated medication and lifestyle regimens.

Prolonged ischemia from cessation in blood flow is called infarction and evolves over time. Cardiac cells can withstand ischemic conditions for 20 minutes; after that period, cellular death begins. After only 30 to 60 seconds of lack of oxygen, ECG changes are noted. If blood flow is reestablished within 20 minutes, cells remain viable.[6]

Irreversible cellular damage and muscle death is shown in Figure 12-9. Contractility in the infarcted area becomes impaired. A nonfunctional zone and a zone of mild ischemia with potentially viable tissue surround the infarct. The ultimate size of the infarct depends on the fate of this ischemic zone. Early interventions, such as the administration of thrombolytics, can restore perfusion to the ischemic zone and can reduce the area of myocardial damage.

AMI is classified as a Q-wave or a non–Q-wave MI. Previously, non–Q-wave MI was believed to be associated with damage to only a portion (subendocardial) of the cardiac muscle, whereas Q-wave MI was believed to cause damage to the entire thickness of the cardiac muscle.[5] Currently, both types of MI are considered to cause damage throughout the muscular layers of the ventricle. A Q-wave MI occurs as a result of total occlusion of a coronary artery secondary to a thrombus or ruptured atherosclerotic plaque. Emergency treatment with thrombolytics is recommended. ST-segment elevation and elevated cardiac enzymes are seen in a Q-wave MI. The non–Q-wave MI usually results from a partially occluded coronary vessel, and it is associated

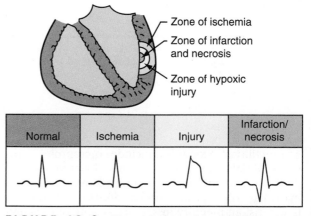

FIGURE 12-9. Electrocardiographic alterations associated with the three zones of myocardial infarction. *(From McCance, K. L., & Huether, S. E. [Eds.]. [2006]. Pathophysiology: The biologic basis for disease in adults and children [5th ed., p. 1114]. St. Louis: Mosby.)*

with ST-segment depression in two or more leads along with elevated cardiac enzymes.[5] Most infarcts occur in the left ventricle; however, right ventricular infarction occurs in more than half of the inferior wall MIs. The treatment for RV infarcts is usually fluid therapy.

The severity of the MI is determined by the success or lack of success of the treatment and by the degree of collateral circulation present at that particular part of the heart muscle. The collateral circulation consists of the alternative routes, or channels, that can develop in the myocardium in response to chronic ischemia or regional hypoperfusion. Through this small network of *extra* vessels, blood flow can be improved to the threatened myocardium.

Assessment

Patient Assessment

Patient assessment includes close observation to identify the classic signs and symptoms of AMI. Chest pain is the paramount symptom. It may be severe, crushing, tight, squeezing, or simply a feeling of pressure. It can be precordial, substernal, or in the back, radiating to the arms, neck, or jaw, and/or unrelated to exertion and respirations. It does not cease with rest or nitrate administration and thus can be distinguished from the pain of an angina attack. The longer the duration and the more severe the pain, the greater the likelihood that an MI is occurring.[5] The skin may be cool, clammy, pale, and diaphoretic; the patient's color may be dusky or ashen; and slight hyperthermia may be present. The patient may be short of breath, dyspneic, and tachypneic, and may feel faint or have intermittent loss of sensorium. Nausea and vomiting commonly occur. Hypotension may be present and is often accompanied by dysrhythmias, particularly ventricular ectopy, bradycardia, tachycardia, or heart block. The type of dysrhythmia present depends on the area of the MI. The patient may be anxious or restless, or may exhibit certain behavioral responses including denial, depression, and a sense of impending doom. Women are more likely to have atypical signs and symptoms, such as shortness of breath, nausea and vomiting, and back or jaw pain.

Some individuals have ischemic episodes without knowing it, thereby having a *silent* infarction. These occur with no presenting signs or symptoms. Asymptomatic or nontraditional symptoms are more common in elderly persons, in women, and in diabetic patients.[6]

Assessment of a patient experiencing an MI takes all the foregoing signs and symptoms into account during the history and physical examination. Risk factors for an MI are also considered.

Diagnosis

Diagnosis of AMI is based on symptoms, analysis of a 12-lead ECG, and cardiac enzyme values. A high index of suspicion is needed for anyone older than 35 years who has chest pain lasting more than 20 minutes.[5] The patient is assessed for other signs and symptoms indicating an AMI that were previously described. The ECG is inspected for ST-segment elevation (>1 mm) in two or more contiguous leads. ST-segment depression (≥ 0.5 mm) and new onset left bundle branch block also suggest an AMI. The type of AMI can be determined by the particular coronary artery involved and the blood supply to that area (Table 12-6).

Serum cardiac enzymes are used to confirm the diagnosis of AMI. As previously described, serum levels of total CK_2, CK-MB, troponin I and T, and myoglobin increase after AMI. These tests are ordered immediately when a diagnosis of AMI is suspected and periodically (usually every 8 hours) during the first 24 hours to assess for increasing levels.[5] Emergency cardiac arteriography may be performed in institutions with interventional cardiology services. Criteria for the diagnosis of ACS are summarized in Table 12-7.

Nursing Diagnoses

Nursing diagnoses and collaborative problems for the patient with AMI are described in the Nursing Care Plan for the Patient with Acute Myocardial Infarction.

Complications

Complications of AMI include cardiac dysrhythmias, HF, thromboembolism, rupture of a portion of the heart (e.g., ventricular wall, interventricular septum, or papillary muscle), pericarditis, infarct extension or recurrence, and cardiogenic shock (see Chapter 11).[15] Dysrhythmias, HF, and pericarditis are discussed later in this chapter.

Medical Interventions

Treatment goals for AMI are to establish reperfusion, to reduce infarct size, to prevent and treat complications, and to provide emotional support and education.[12] Medical treatment of AMI is aimed at relieving pain, providing adequate oxygenation to the myocardium, preventing platelet aggregation, and restoring blood flow to the myocardium through thrombolytic therapy or acute interventional therapy

TABLE 12-6   Myocardial Infarction by Site, Electrocardiographic Changes, and Complications

Location of MI	Primary Site of Occlusion	Primary ECG Changes	Complications
Inferior MI	RCA (80%-90%) LCX (10%-20%)	Leads: II, III, aV$_F$	First- and second-degree heart block, right ventricular infarct
Inferolateral MI	LCX	II, III, aV$_F$, V$_5$, V$_6$	Third-degree heart block, left HF, cardiomyopathy, left ventricular rupture
Posterior MI	RCA or LCX	No lead truly looks at posterior surface. Look for reciprocal changes in V$_1$ and V$_2$—tall, broad R waves; ST depression and tall T waves. Posterior leads V$_7$, V$_8$, and V$_9$ may be recorded and evaluated	First-, second-, and third-degree heart blocks, HF, bradydysrhythmias
Anterior MI	LAD	V$_2$-V$_4$	Third-degree heart block, HF, left bundle branch block
Anterior-septal MI	LAD	V$_1$-V$_3$	Second- and third-degree heart block
Lateral MI	LAD or LCX	V$_5$, V$_6$, I, aVL	HF
Right ventricular	RCA	V$_4$R. Right precordial leads V$_1$R-V$_6$R may be recorded and evaluated	Increased RAP, decreased cardiac output, bradydysrhythmias, heart blocks, hypotension, cardiogenic shock

AV, Atrioventricular; *ECG,* electrocardiographic; *HF,* heart failure; *LAD,* left anterior descending; *LCX,* circumflex; *MI,* myocardial infarction; *RAP,* right atrial pressure; *RCA,* right coronary artery.

such as angioplasty. Hemodynamic monitoring is also used to assess cardiac function and to monitor fluid balance in some patients.

Pain Relief. The initial pain of AMI is treated with morphine sulfate administered by the IV route. The dose is 2 to 4 mg IV push over 5 minutes. Patients must be observed for hypotension and respiratory depression (see Table 12-5).

NTG may be given to reduce the ischemic pain of AMI. NTG increases coronary perfusion because of its vasodilatory effects. It is usually started at doses of 5 to 10 mcg/min and titrated to a total dose of 50 to 200 mcg/min until chest pain is absent, pulmonary artery occlusion pressure decreases, and/or systolic blood pressure decreases. Caution should be used in administering NTG to patients with inferior or right ventricular infarcts.

Oxygen. Oxygen administration is important for assisting the myocardial tissue to continue its pumping activity and for repairing the damaged tissue around the site of the infarct. Treatment with oxygen via nasal cannula at 4 to 6 L/min assists in maintaining oxygenation. Rest also helps to improve

oxygenation. The goal is to maintain oxygen saturation above 90%.

Antidysrhythmics. Antidysrhythmic agents are used when the heart's natural pacemaker develops an abnormal rate or rhythm (see Chapter 7).

Prevention of Platelet Aggregation. Alterations in platelet function contribute to occlusion of the coronary arteries. Aspirin (162.5 mg) is given immediately to all patients with suspected AMI. Aspirin blocks synthesis of thromboxane A$_2$, thus inhibiting aggregation of platelets.

Thrombolytic Therapy. One common treatment for AMI is thrombolytic therapy. Research has shown that occlusion of the coronary vessel does not cause immediate myocardial cell death. Injury begins within minutes of the vessel occlusion. Within a period of hours, irreversible damage begins at the endocardial surface and progresses to the epicardium. The extent and the progression of the injury are determined by the completeness of the occlusion and the presence of collateral circulation.[5] The goals are to dissolve the lesion that is occluding the coronary artery and to increase blood flow to the myo-

TABLE 12-7   Criteria for Diagnosis of Acute Coronary Syndrome

Major Criteria	Minor Criteria	
A diagnosis of an ACS can be made if one or more of the following major criteria are present:	In the absence of a major criterion, a diagnosis of ACS requires the presence of at least one item from both columns I and II.	
	I	**II**
• ST-elevation or left bundle branch block (LBBB) in the setting of recent (<24 hours) or ongoing angina • New, or presumably new, ST-segment depression (≥0.05 mV) or T-wave inversion (≥0.2 mV) with rest symptoms • Elevated serum markers of myocardial damage (i.e., troponin I, troponin T, and CK_2-MB)	• Prolonged (i.e., >20 minutes) chest, arm/shoulder, neck, or epigastric discomfort • New onset chest, arm/shoulder, neck, or epigastric discomfort at rest, minimal exertion or ordinary activity • Previously documented chest, arm/shoulder, neck, or epigastric discomfort which has become distinctly more frequent or longer in duration	• Typical or atypical angina • Male age >40 or female age >60 • Known CAD • Heart failure, hypotension, or transient mitral regurgitation by examination • Diabetes • Documented extracardiac vascular disease • Pathologic Q-waves on ECG • Abnormal ST-segment or T-wave abnormalities not known to be new

ACS, Acute coronary syndrome; *CAD*, coronary artery disease; *CK₂-MB*, creatine kinase MB band; *ECG*, electrocardiogram. From Veterans Health Administration, Department of Defense. (2003) *VA/DoD clinical practice guideline for management of ischemic heart disease*. Washington, D.C.: Veterans Health Administration, Department of Defense.

cardium. The patient must be symptomatic for less than 6 hours, have pain for 20 minutes that was unrelieved by NTG, and have an ECG with an ST-segment elevation of 1 mm or greater in two or more contiguous ECG leads or an ST-segment depression of 0.5 mm or greater. Table 12-8 lists some of the common thrombolytics currently available. A summary of the use of thrombolytics includes the following:

- Fibrinolysis reduces mortality and salvages myocardium in anterior and inferior Q-wave MI.
- Fibrinolysis is not effective in the treatment of unstable angina or non–Q-wave MI.
- The sooner treatment is initiated, the better the outcome. Thrombolysis should be instituted within 30 to 60 minutes of arrival.[16]
- The worst possible complication of fibrinolysis is intracranial hemorrhage. Bleeding from puncture sites commonly occurs.

More investigation is being conducted to develop effective reperfusion therapy by combining thrombolytic therapy with antiplatelet therapy. Many patients do not achieve reperfusion sufficient to maintain adequate perfusion of the heart. However, with the current advances in percutaneous coronary intervention (PCI) and other new technologies, the rates of restenosis will decrease.

Nursing care of the patient includes rapid identification of whether the patient is a suitable candidate for IV thrombolytics, thus ensuring as little delay as possible before the therapy and screening for contraindications are initiated. Next, the nurse secures three vascular access lines and obtains necessary laboratory data. Initial ECG monitoring is documented before starting the infusion, at various times throughout the infusion, and at the end of the infusion. Finally, the patient is monitored for complications, including reperfusion dysrhythmias (premature ventricular contractions, sinus bradycardia, accelerated idioventricular rhythm, or ventricular tachycardia), oozing at venipuncture sites and gingival bleeding, reocclusion or reinfarction, and symptoms of hemorrhagic stroke.

Percutaneous Coronary Intervention. Emergency PCI is being used in the management of AMI with improved outcomes over thrombolytic therapy. PCI should be performed within 90 minutes of arrival with a target of less than 60 minutes.[16] Primary PCI has been demonstrated to be more effective than thrombolysis in opening acutely occluded arteries in settings where it can be rapidly performed by experienced interventional cardiologists.[16]

Text continued on p. 338

NURSING CARE PLAN for the Patient with Acute Myocardial Infarction

NURSING DIAGNOSIS

Acute Chest Pain

PATIENT OUTCOMES

- Verbalizes relief of pain
- Appears comfortable

NURSING INTERVENTIONS

- Assess for characteristics of AMI pain:
  Occurs suddenly
  More intense
  Quality varies
  Not relieved with rest of nitrates
  Atypical symptoms in older patients, women,
      diabetic patients, and patients with heart failure
- Note time since onset of first episode of chest pain;
  if less than 6 hours, patient may be a candidate
  for thrombolytic therapy
- Assess prior treatments for pain; patient may have
  taken sublingual nitroglycerin and a single dose
  of aspirin before arriving to hospital
- Monitor heart rate and blood pressure during pain
  episodes and during medication administration
- Assess baseline ECG for signs of MI: T- and
  ST changes and development of Q waves
- Monitor serial cardiac markers
- Continually reassess chest pain and response to
  medication; ongoing pain signifies prolonged
  myocardial ischemia and warrants immediate
  intervention
- Assess for contraindications to thrombolytic agents;
  absolute contraindications include active internal
  bleeding, bleeding diathesis, or history of
  hemorrhagic stroke or intracranial hemorrhage
- Assess for relative contraindications or warning
  conditions
- Maintain bed rest during periods of pain
- Administer oxygen therapy at 4-6 L/min; maintain
  oxygen saturation above 90%
- Initiate IV nitrates according to protocol

- Administer morphine sulfate according to unit
  protocol
- Administer IV beta-blockers according to protocol
- Administer oral aspirin

- Administer angiotensin-converting enzyme
  inhibitors

RATIONALES

- Assist in identification of AMI to provide early
  treatment

- Provide timely intervention

- Assess response to prior treatment; assess need
  for aspirin as part of treatment protocol

- Assess nonverbal indicators of pain and
  response to treatment
- Identify ischemia, injury, evolving AMI

- Assist in diagnosis and confirmation of AMI
- Assess response to treatment; ensure that pain
  is controlled

- Ensure that medication is administered safely
  when warranted. Prevent complications
  associated with the medication

- Risks of thrombolytic agents are weighed
  against benefits
- Reduce oxygen demand of the heart
- Ensure adequate oxygenation to the
  myocardium to prevent further damage
- Nitrates are both coronary dilators and
  peripheral vasodilators causing hypotension
- Reduce the workload on the heart through
  venodilation
- Reduce mortality in acute-phase MI
- Decrease platelet aggregation to improve
  mortality
- Reduce progression to heart failure and death
  in patients with large transmural MIs with LV
  dysfunction and in diabetics patients having
  an MI

NURSING CARE PLAN for the Patient with Acute Myocardial Infarction—cont'd

NURSING INTERVENTIONS	RATIONALES
• Administer thrombolytic agents according to unit protocol	• Restore perfusion
• Monitor for signs of bleeding: puncture sites, gingival bleeding, and prior cuts; observe for presence of occult or frank blood in urine, stool, emesis, and sputum	• Assess for complications of thrombolytic therapy (bleeding) so that treatment can be initiated as needed
• Assess for intracranial bleeding by frequent monitoring of neurological status; changes in mental status, visual disturbances, and headaches are frequent signs of intracranial bleeding	• Assess for complication of intracranial bleeding associated with thrombolytic therapy
• Administer IV heparin according to unit protocol, adjusting aPTT dose to 1.5 to 2 times normal	• Maintain vessel patency after thrombolysis
• Prepare for possible cardiac catheterization, percutaneous transluminal coronary angioplasty, or coronary artery bypass graft surgery if signs of reperfusion are not evident and infarction evolves	• Facilitate rapid intervention to restore coronary artery perfusion

NURSING DIAGNOSIS

Risk for decreased cardiac output

PATIENT OUTCOMES
Maintains normal cardiac rhythm with adequate cardiac output

• Strong peripheral pulses	• Good capillary refill
• Normal blood pressure	• Adequate urine output
• Clear breath sounds	• Clear mentation

NURSING INTERVENTIONS	RATIONALES
• Monitor heart rate and rhythm continuously; observe and/or anticipate common dysrhythmias —PVCs, ventricular tachycardia, atrial flutter, and atrial fibrillation	• Detect and treat dysrhythmias
• Assess for signs of decreased cardiac output	• Assist in identifying complications to ensure timely treatment
• Monitor PR, QRS, and QT intervals	• Detect abnormal conduction of impulses early
• Monitor continuous ECG in appropriate leads	• See Chapter 7 for details on best practice for monitoring
• Institute treatment according to advanced cardiac life support guidelines or unit protocol	• Surveillance may prevent lethal dysrhythmias
• Assess peripheral and central pulses	• Detect reduced stroke volume and cardiac output
• Assess for mental status changes—restlessness and anxiety	• Detect early signs of hypoxemia
• Assess respiratory rate, rhythm, and breath sounds; rapid, shallow respirations and presence of crackles and wheezes are signs of reduced cardiac output	• Assess respiratory symptoms associated with low cardiac output
• Assess urine output via Foley catheter	• Assess inadequate renal perfusion from reduced cardiac output

Continued

NURSING CARE PLAN for the Patient with Acute Myocardial Infarction—cont'd

NURSING INTERVENTIONS	RATIONALES
• Auscultate for presence of S_3, S_4, or systolic murmur	• S_3 denotes LV dysfunction; S_4 indicates a noncompliant ventricle after an ischemic event; a systolic murmur may be caused by papillary muscle rupture
• Assess pulse oximetry and arterial blood gases; maintain oxygen saturation of at least 90%	• Ensure adequate oxygenation
• If patient had a inferior wall MI, evaluate the right–sided 12—lead ECG; assess for signs of a right ventricular MI and right ventricular failure—increased RAP, absence of crackles, and decreased blood pressure	• Identify right ventricular MI and potential complication of right-sided heart failure
• Anticipate insertion of hemodynamic monitoring catheter	• Guide management of fluids and medications
• Administer IV fluids	• Maintain fluid balance
• Monitor for signs of left and right ventricular failure	• For left-sided failure anticipate diuretics, vasodilators, inotropics, and oxygen as indicated
	• For right-sided failure anticipate fluid resuscitation and possible inotropic and peripheral vasodilator therapy
• Carefully administer nitrates and morphine sulfate for pain	• Reduced preload and filling pressures may compromise cardiac output

NURSING DIAGNOSIS

Fear

PATIENT OUTCOMES

• Patient verbalizes reduced fear
• Patient demonstrates positive coping mechanisms

NURSING INTERVENTIONS	RATIONALES
• Assess level of fear noting nonverbal communication	• Identify fear and anxiety
• Assess coping factors	• Coping patterns are highly individualized
• Acknowledge awareness of patient's fears	• Validate feelings and communicate acceptance of those feelings
• Allow patient to verbalize fears of dying	• May reduce anxiety
• Offer realistic assurances of recovery	• Reduce anxiety by providing accurate information
• Maintain confident, assured manner	• Staff anxiety may be perceived by the patient
• Explain care provided and rationale so it is understandable for the patient	• Allay anxiety; lack of understanding can add to fear
• Assure the patient that continuous monitoring will ensure prompt intervention	• Provide a measure of safety
• Reduce unnecessary external stimuli	• Anxiety may escalate with excessive noise
• Provide diversional materials	• Decrease anxiety and prevent feelings of isolation
• Establish rest periods	• Ensure dedicate periods to facilitate physical and mental rest
• Refer to other support persons as appropriate	• Additional specialty expertise may be required
• Administer mild sedative as prescribed	• Medication may be required to reduce anxiety

NURSING CARE PLAN for the Patient with Acute Myocardial Infarction—cont'd

NURSING DIAGNOSIS

Risk for activity intolerance

PATIENT OUTCOMES
Tolerates progressive activity

- Heart rate and blood pressure within expected range and no complaints of dyspnea or fatigue
- Verbalizes realistic expectations for progressive activity

NURSING INTERVENTIONS	RATIONALES
• Assess respiratory and cardiac status before initiating activity	• Physical deconditioning may occur with prolonged bed rest
• Observe and document response to activity	• Assess response to activity progression
• Encourage adequate rest	• Provide time for energy conservation and recovery
• Provide small, frequent meals	• Facilitate digestion and reduce energy needs
• Instruct patient not to hold breath while exercising or moving about in bed and not to strain for bowel movements	• Valsalva maneuver affects endocardial repolarization
• Maintain progression of activity per cardiac rehabilitation protocol	• Provide gradual increase in activity as tolerated by the patient
• Provide emotional support when increasing activity	• Reduce anxiety about overexertion of the heart

AMI, Acute myocardial infarction; *aPTT*, activated partial thromboplastin time; *ECG*, electrocardiogram; *IV*, intravenous; *LV*, left ventricular; *PVCs*, premature ventricular contractions; *RAP*, right atrial pressure.

PHARMACOLOGY

TABLE 12-8   Thrombolytics

Name	Dose	Half-Life
Alteplase (tissue plasminogen activator; t-PA)	For adult patients weighing >67 kg, dose of 100 mg over 90 minutes, starting with 15-mg bolus intravenous over 1-2 minutes, then 50 mg over 30 minutes, then 35 mg over 60 minutes OR	4-5 minutes
Accelerated infusion	3-hour infusion, giving 60 mg over the first hour (6-10 mg as bolus over 1-2 minutes), 20 mg over second hour, and 20 mg over third hour For adult patients weighing ≤67 kg, maximum dose of 100 mg over 90 minutes, starting with 15-mg bolus IV, followed by 0.75 mg/kg over 30 minutes (not to exceed 50 mg), then 0.50 mg/kg over 60 minutes (not to exceed 35 mg)	
Reteplase (r-PA)	10 units IV bolus, repeat in 30 minutes; administer over 2 minutes Give through a dedicated line Do not give repeat bolus if serious bleeding occurs after first IV bolus is given	13-16 minutes
Tenecteplase (TNK)	Total dose 50 mg, based on weight (see package insert) given over 5 seconds	20-24 minutes
Streptokinase (SK)	1.5 million units IV infusion over 60 minutes	23 minutes

IV, Intravenous.
From Hodgson B. B., & Kizior R. J. (2007). *Saunders nursing drug handbook*. Philadelphia: Saunders.

Facilitated Percutaneous Coronary Intervention. Facilitated PCI is the use of additional agents—fibrinolysis, Gp IIb/IIIa inhibitors, or both—to pretreat the patient awaiting primary PCI.[16] It was thought that facilitated PCI would improve outcomes; however, administration of these agents before PCI is associated with higher rates of death, reinfarction, and bleeding complications. Therefore, primary PCI is the preferred treatment. Additional research is needed to test if fibrinolytic therapy is preferable to delayed PCI in facilities without an interventional cardiology service. Current American College of Cardiology guidelines recommend treating the affected vessel when feasible and deferring surgical or PCI-based revascularization of other vessels until the patient's condition has stabilized and the clinically most appropriate treatment strategy has been determined.

Medications. Several other medications may be ordered for the patient with AMI. Patients whose chest pain symptoms are suggestive of serious illness need immediate assessment in a monitored unit and early therapy to include an IV line, oxygen, aspirin, NTG, and morphine. Early therapy may consist of aspirin, heparin or low–molecular weight heparin, nitrates, beta-blockers, and clopidogrel.[16]

Nitrates. Nitrates are vasodilators that reduce pain, increase venous capacitance, and reduce platelet adhesion and aggregation. Sublingual NTG is often given in the emergency department. IV NTG is effective for relieving ischemia (see Table 12-5).

Beta-Blockers. Beta-blockers are used to decrease heart rate, blood pressure, and myocardial oxygen consumption. Morbidity and mortality after AMI have been reduced by the use of beta-blockers. Commonly used drugs include metoprolol, atenolol, and carvedilol. The patient is carefully assessed for hypotension and bradycardia.

Angiotensin-Converting Enzyme Inhibitors. After an AMI (Q-wave type), the area of ventricular damage changes shape or remodels. The ventricle becomes thinner and balloons out, thus reducing contractility. Cardiac tissue surrounding the area of infarction undergoes changes that can be categorized as (1) myocardial stunning (a temporary loss of contractile function that persists for hours to days after perfusion has been restored); (2) hibernating myocardium (tissue that is persistently ischemic and undergoes metabolic adaptation to prolong myocyte survival until perfusion can be restored); and (3) myocardial remodeling (a process mediated by angiotensin II, aldosterone, catecholamines, adenosine, and inflammatory cytokines that causes myocyte hypertrophy and loss of contractile function in the areas of the heart distant from the site of infarctions).[16] Angiotensin-converting enzyme (ACE) inhibitors should be started within 24 hours to reduce the incidence of ventricular remodeling. The drugs can be discontinued if the patient exhibits no signs of ventricular dysfunction (see Table 12-5).

Outcomes

Patient outcomes are generalized to encompass the wide spectrum of patients who have experienced an MI, uncomplicated or complicated, that requires medical or surgical intervention. Outcomes include verbalization of relief of pain and fear, adequate cardiac output, ability to tolerate progressive activity, and demonstration of positive coping mechanisms.

INTERVENTIONAL CARDIOLOGY

Several interventions are done to treat ACS. The goal is to treat the patient to prevent AMI. Intervention is also used after AMI to prevent further damage of the myocardium. PCIs consist of percutaneous transluminal coronary angioplasty (PTCA), percutaneous transluminal coronary rotational atherectomy, directional coronary atherectomy, laser atherectomy, and intracoronary stenting. An early, invasive PCI strategy is indicated for patients with unstable angina/non–ST-segment elevation MI and without serious comorbidity who have coronary lesions amenable to PCI.[19] For the purposes of this book, only PTCA and stenting are discussed. The postprocedure care for all patients who undergo PCI consists of the same interventions.

Percutaneous Transluminal Coronary Angioplasty

The purpose of PTCA is to compress intracoronary plaque to increase blood flow to the myocardium. It is usually the treatment of choice for patients with uncompromised collateral flow, noncalcified lesions, and lesions not present at bifurcations of vessels. In addition, the patient must be a candidate for coronary artery bypass graft (CABG) surgery. PTCA is performed in the cardiac catheterization laboratory with the operating room on standby. A balloon catheter is inserted in the manner of coronary arteriography, but it is threaded into the occluded coronary artery and is advanced with the use of a guidewire across the lesion. The balloon is inflated under pressure one or several times to compress the lesion (Figure 12-10).

Single-vessel disease remains the classic indication for PTCA. This procedure best treats fixed, noncalcified lesions in the proximal two thirds of the coronary circulation that are accessible for dilation. Stenosis of the left mainstem artery is considered

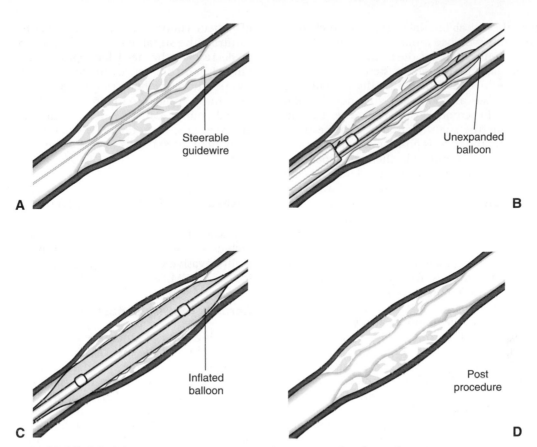

FIGURE 12-10. Coronary angioplasty procedure. **A-D,** Order of procedure. *(From Moser, D. K., & Riegel, B. [2008]. Cardiac nursing. St. Louis: Mosby.)*

unacceptable for dilation. The optimal goal after PTCA is open coronary arteries (Figure 12-11).

Complications

The major complication of PTCA is coronary artery dissection. It is reported in approximately 1% to 3% of patients who need emergency bypass surgery. In addition, myocardial ischemia may occur from coronary artery spasm, coronary embolization, or intimal trauma. Associated complications include bradycardia, ventricular fibrillation, hypotension, and vascular complications.[2]

Intracoronary Stent

Intracoronary stents are tubes that are implanted at the site of stenosis to widen the arterial lumen by squeezing atherosclerotic plaque against the artery's walls (as does PTCA). However, the stent also keeps the lumen open by providing structural support. Stent designs differ, but most are springs or slotted or mesh tubes about 15 mm in length, with some

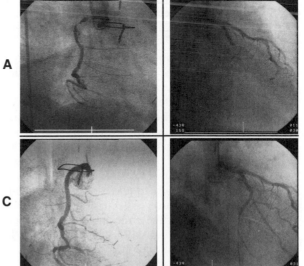

FIGURE 12-11. Radiographs of patients with triple-vessel disease with images before (**A** and **B**) and after (**C** and **D**) angioplasty. *(Courtesy of University Hospital, Cardiac Catheterization Laboratory, San Antonio, TX.)*

resembling the spiral bindings used in notebooks. These are tightly wrapped around a balloon catheter, which is inflated to implant the stent.

The procedure for placing a stent is similar to the procedure in PTCA, in which the patient first undergoes cardiac arteriography for identification of occlusions in coronary arteries. The balloon catheter bearing the stent is inserted into the coronary artery, and the stent is positioned at the desired site. The balloon is inflated, thereby expanding the stent, which squeezes the atherosclerotic plaque and intimal flaps against the vessel wall. After the balloon is deflated and removed, the stent remains, holding the plaque and other matter in place and providing structural support to keep the artery from collapsing.[2]

Aggressive anticoagulation therapy before, during, and after the procedure is necessary for the prevention of coagulation. Before sheath removal, peripheral perfusion is monitored because the sheath may cause occlusion of the femoral artery. Peripheral pulses, skin color, and temperature are monitored. The insertion site is inspected for any oozing or bleeding. After sheath removal, hemostasis is maintained with manual pressure, a femoral compression device, or an arterial puncture sealing device. Pain management and proper hydration aid in recovery. Retroperitoneal bleeding or impaired perfusion may occur after sheath removal. Restenosis can occur as a result of neointimal growth because of the body's natural defense when the inner intimal lining is injured, even slightly, as happens with stent placement. Restenosis occurs in 30% to 40% of patients who undergo this procedure.[2] The Gp IIb/IIIa inhibitors are being used after stent placement to prevent acute reocclusion through prevention of platelet aggregation.

After a stent procedure, a patient must take one or more antiplatelet or anticoagulant agents such as aspirin, ticlopidine, clopidogrel, and warfarin.[2] Aspirin is also used indefinitely at dose ranges of 81 to 325 mg,[19] whereas the other drugs are prescribed for 4 to 6 weeks. Oral clopidogrel, 75 mg/day, should be added to aspirin in patients with ST-elevation MI regardless of whether reperfusion with fibrinolytic therapy was done.[3] For 4 to 6 weeks after a stent procedure, it is necessary to take antibiotics for any minor surgical procedure (e.g., dental cleaning) to reduce the risk of infective endocarditis. In addition, for the next 4 weeks, an MRI scan should not be done without a cardiologist's approval.[2] However, metal detectors do not affect the stent.

Therapies in intracoronary stenting are advancing using both bare metal stents and drug-eluted stents. Drug-eluted stents are being evaluated for their outcomes in reducing restenosis rates. Follow-up study of patient cohorts of 4 years after revascularization confirms the sustained benefit of drug-eluted stents in decreasing the need for repeat revascularization but without differences in death or MI.[19] Normal reaction from the body to vascular injury is neointimal (new intimal cell) growth. When a stent is placed, minor damage to the inner lining of the artery occurs; thus, the body's natural defense is to grow new intimal cells to repair the damage, hence in-stent restenosis.

SURGICAL REVASCULARIZATION

Surgical approaches used for revascularization include coronary revascularization by CABG, minimally invasive CABG, and transmyocardial revascularization (TMR).

Coronary Artery Bypass Graft

CABG is a surgical procedure in which the ischemic area or areas of the myocardium are revascularized by implantation of the internal mammary artery or bypassing of the coronary occlusion with a saphenous vein graft or radial artery graft. The indications for CABG are chronic stable angina that is refractory to other therapies, significant left main coronary occlusion (>50%), triple-vessel CAD, unstable angina pectoris, AMI, intractable ventricular irritability, left ventricular failure, and failure of PTCA.[9,10]

CABG is performed in the operating room while the patient receives general anesthesia and is intubated. One approach is to make a midsternal, longitudinal incision into the chest cavity. Surgery is done either with cardiopulmonary bypass or without (off-pump). During cardiopulmonary bypass, blood is pumped through an oxygenator, or heart-lung machine, to receive oxygen. Cardioplegia solution is used to stop the heart so surgery can be performed.

The coronary arteries are visualized, and a segment of the saphenous vein is grafted or anastomosed to the distal end of the vessel, with the proximal end of the graft vessel anastomosed to the aorta (Figure 12-12). The internal mammary artery is often used for creating an artery-to-artery graft. Internal mammary revascularization has better long-term patency than saphenous vein grafts. It is the preferred graft for lesions of the left anterior descending coronary artery.

Once grafting is done, the cardiopulmonary bypass (if used) is progressively discontinued, chest and mediastinal tubes are inserted, and the chest is closed. Box 12-7 gives information related to chest and mediastinal tubes.[20]

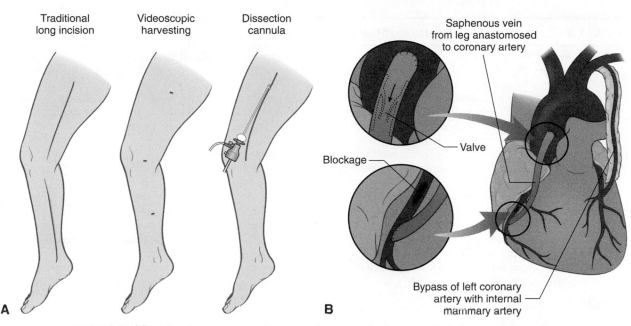

FIGURE 12-12. Coronary artery bypass graft surgery. Saphenous vein is harvested from the leg using either a traditional long incision or less-invasive videoscopic harvesting **(A)**. The vein is then anastomosed to the coronary artery **(B)**.

Minimally Invasive Coronary Artery Surgery

Minimally invasive coronary artery surgery is also called limited-access coronary artery surgery.[10] It has been evaluated as an alternative to the standard methods for CABG. Two commonly used approaches include port-access coronary artery bypass (PACAB or PortCAB) and minimally invasive coronary artery bypass (MIDCAB).

In PACAB, the heart is stopped, and the patient undergoes cardiopulmonary bypass. Small incisions (ports) are made in the patient's chest. The surgical team passes instruments through the ports to perform the bypasses using the internal mammary artery, saphenous vein, or radial artery. Procedures to replace damaged valves through limited-access ports are also being done.

The goal of MIDCAB is to avoid using cardiopulmonary bypass. It is performed while the patient's heart is still beating and is intended for use when only one or two arteries will be bypassed. MIDCAB uses a combination of small holes or ports in the chest and a small incision made directly over the coronary artery to be bypassed. The internal mammary artery is commonly used for the graft. The surgeon views and performs the attachment directly, so the artery to be bypassed must be right under the incision.

The American Heart Association's Council on Cardiothoracic and Vascular Surgery has been carefully monitoring these two procedures. MIDCAB appears to be easier on the patient and less expensive than CABG. However, complications may require an open-chest procedure.[10] As these surgical procedures are refined so that they are no more invasive than angioplasty, they will become more common.

Transmyocardial Revascularization

In TMR, a high-energy laser creates channels from the epicardial surface into the left ventricular chamber.[2] This procedure is also called laser revascularization. The purpose of TMR is to increase perfusion directly to the heart muscle. It is performed on patients who are poor candidates for CABG and whose symptoms are refractory to medical treatment. To do this procedure, a surgeon makes an incision on the left side of the chest and inserts a laser into the chest cavity. With the laser, the surgeon makes channels (1 mm) through the heart's left ventricle in between heartbeats. (The laser is fired when the chamber is full of blood so the blood can protect the inside of the heart.) Ten to 50 channels are created.[2] Then the surgeon applies pressure on the outside of the heart. This seals the outer openings but lets the inner channels stay open, to allow oxygen-rich blood to flow through the heart muscle.

TMR has received Food and Drug Administration approval for use in patients with severe angina who

BOX 12-7   Key Points for Maintaining Chest and Mediastinal Tubes

Definitions
- Chest tube: The tube is inserted into the pleural space to maintain the normal negative pressure and to facilitate respiration. It is inserted after cardiac surgery if the pleural space is opened. It is also inserted as treatment for pneumothorax or hemothorax.
- Mediastinal tube: The tube is inserted into the mediastinal space to provide drainage after cardiac surgery.
- Drainage system: A water-seal system assists in maintaining negative pressures (chest tube). Some devices are designed to function without water. Suction (up to 20 cm H_2O) is often applied to facilitate drainage.
- Autotransfusion: Reinfusion of autologous drainage from the system back to the patient.

Baseline Assessment
- Make sure that all connections are tight: insertion site to the chest drainage system, suction control chamber to the suction unit.
- Assess that the dressing over insertion site is dry and intact.
- Palpate for subcutaneous crepitus around the insertion site and chest wall.
- Auscultate breath sounds bilaterally.
- Observe the color and consistency of fluid in the collecting tubing (more accurate assessment than fluid in the drainage system); mark the fluid level on the drainage system.
- Assess the drainage system for proper functioning (read instructions for the device being used).
- Check the water in the water-seal level; the water level should fluctuate with respirations in chest tubes (not in mediastinal tubes).
- Check suction control and be sure that suction is on, if ordered.
- Check for intermittent bubbling in the water-seal chamber; it indicates an air leak from the pleural space (pleural tube).

Maintaining the Chest Drainage System
- Keep the tubing coiled on the bed near the patient.
- Record drainage on the flow sheet per unit protocol; notify the physician of excessive drainage (obtain written parameters; the normal amount varies depending on the purpose of the tube and the time since insertion).
- Change the dressing according to unit protocol.
- Splint the insertion site to facilitate coughing and deep breathing.
- Ensure that drainage flows into the drainage system by facilitating gravity drainage; *milking* and *stripping* the tubes are not recommended because these procedures generate high negative pressures in the system.
- If the patient must be transported (or ambulated) with the system, disconnect from suction and keep the drainage system upright below the level of the chest. Do not clamp the tube.
- Chest x-ray studies are done immediately after insertion and usually daily thereafter.

Assisting with Removal
- Chest and mediastinal tubes are usually removed by the physician.
- Ensure adequate pain medication before removal.
- Apply an occlusive dressing to the insertion site after removal.
- A chest x-ray study is usually done after removal.

Autotransfusion
- An autotransfusion collection system is attached to the chest drainage device.
- Anticoagulants may be ordered to be added to the autotransfusion system (citrate-phosphate-dextrose, acid-phosphate-dextrose, or heparin); these are not usually necessary with mediastinal drainage.
- Reinfuse drainage within the time frame specified by unit policy. It is recommended that reinfusion begin within 6 hours of initiating the collection and that drainage be reinfused to the patient within a 4-hour period.
- Evacuate air from the autotransfusion bag; air embolism may occur unless all air is removed.
- Attach a microaggregate filter and infuse via gravity or a pressure bag.

have no other treatment options. It has produced early promising results in that the angina of 80% to 90% of patients who have had this procedure has significantly improved (at least 50%) through 1 year after surgery. There are still limited follow-up data as to how long the benefits of this procedure might last, however.[2] Improvement in symptoms usually occurs over time, not immediately. TMR will not replace CABG or angioplasty as a common method of treating CAD. TMR may be used for patients who are high-risk candidates for a second bypass or angioplasty, for example, patients whose blockages are too diffuse to be treated with bypass alone, or some patients with heart transplants who develop atherosclerosis.

Management after Cardiac Surgery

Patients are usually admitted directly to the critical care unit after cardiac surgery. The patient often has a pulmonary artery catheter, arterial catheter, peripheral IV lines, chest tubes, mediastinal tube, and an indwelling urinary catheter. The patient is usually mechanically ventilated in the immediate postoperative period. The nurse assesses the patient often and provides rapid interventions to help the patient recover from anesthesia and to prevent complications. The nurse-to-patient ratio is often 1:1 during the first few hours after surgery or until the patient is extubated. Nursing care for these patients is summarized in Box 12-8.

Complications of Cardiac Surgery

Patients who have had cardiac surgery should be closely monitored for complications such as dysrhythmias (atrial fibrillation, atrial flutter, ventricular tachycardia, ventricular fibrillation), mediastinal bleeding and cardiac tamponade, and mediastinitis and sternal dehiscence.[10] The critical care nurse taking care of a patient who has just undergone CABG must have quick critical thinking skills and the ability to assess the whole picture, while prioritizing interventions that need to be performed.

CARDIAC DYSRHYTHMIAS

Cardiac dysrhythmias have many causes such as CAD, AMI, electrolyte imbalances, and HF. The various dysrhythmias and patient assessment are discussed in Chapter 7. Emergency treatments of dysrhythmias, such as medications, transcutaneous pacemakers, and cardioversion and defibrillation, are also discussed in Chapter 7. Other drugs that may be used to manage dysrhythmias are shown in Table 12-9. Additional surgical and electrical treatments are discussed in the following sections.

BOX 12-8   Nursing Interventions after Cardiac Surgery

- Monitor for hypotension; administer fluids and vasopressors as ordered or based on protocol.
- Assess for hypovolemia; monitor and trend output from the chest and mediastinal tubes and urine output.
- Monitor hemodynamic pressures, SvO_2, stroke index, cardiac index, PAOP, and RAP; treat the patient per protocol.
- Rewarm the patient gradually (if applicable).
- Monitor and treat fluid and electrolytes, hemoglobin, hematocrit, renal function, and coagulation studies.
- Provide pain relief.
- Monitor for complications: intraoperative acute myocardial infarction, dysrhythmias, heart failure, cardiac tamponade, thromboembolism, impaired renal function, pneumonia, pneumothorax, pleural effusion, cerebral ischemia, or stroke.
- Wean from mechanical ventilation per protocol; extubate; promote pulmonary hygiene every 1 to 2 hours while the patient is awake.
- Assess wounds and provide incisional care per hospital protocol.
- Gradually increase the patient's activity.
- Provide emotional support to the patient and family.

SvO_2, Mixed venous oxygen saturation; *PAOP*, pulmonary artery occlusion pressure; *RAP*, right atrial pressure.

Radiofrequency Catheter Ablation

Radiofrequency catheter ablation is a method of interrupting a supraventricular tachycardia, a dysrhythmia caused by a reentry circuit, an abnormal conduction pathway. The objective of catheter ablation is to interrupt electrical conduction or activity permanently in a region of dysrhythmogenic cardiac tissue.[2] Indications for radiofrequency catheter ablation include the presence of two conducting pathways that are in competition with each other, causing reentrant tachycardia.

Radiofrequency ablation is performed percutaneously. The procedure begins with a diagnostic electrophysiology study. A catheter with an electrode is positioned at the accessory (abnormal) pathway, and mild, painless radiofrequency energy (similar to microwave heat) is transmitted to the pathway, causing coagulation and necrosis in the conduction fibers without destroying the surrounding tissue. This stops the area from conducting the extra

PHARMACOLOGY

TABLE 12-9   Medications Used to Treat Dysrhythmias

Drug	Indications	Mechanism of Action	Dosage and Route	Side Effects	Nursing Implications
Diltiazem (Cardizem)	Atrial fibrillation/flutter SVT	Inhibits calcium ion influx into vascular smooth muscle and myocardium	IV: 0.25 mg/kg actual body weight over 2 minutes May repeat in 15 minutes at dose of 0.35 mg/kg actual body weight Infusion: 5-15 mg/hour × 24 hours	Hypotension, edema, dizziness, bradycardia	Often used in conjunction with digoxin for rate control Not used in heart failure Observe for dysrhythmias
Amiodarone (Cordarone)	Atrial fibrillation/flutter SVT Ventricular dysrhythmias	Prolongs action potential phase 3	PO: 200-600 mg/day IV: 150-mg bolus in 10 minutes, then 360 mg over 6 hours, then 540 mg over 18 hours May continue at 0.5 mg/min for up to 2-3 weeks regardless of age, renal status, or left ventricular function (ventricular dysrhythmias)	Bradycardia, complete atrioventricular block, hypotension Multiple side effects (thyroid, pulmonary, hepatic, neurological, dermatological)	Long half-life Monitor rhythm closely Obtain baseline pulmonary and liver function tests
Flecainide (Tambocor)	Ventricular dysrhythmias	Decreases conduction in all parts of the heart; stabilizes cardiac membrane	PO: 50-100 mg every 12 hours; increase as needed, not to exceed 400 mg/day	Hypotension, bradycardia, heart block, blurred vision, respiratory depression	Interacts with many other drugs; check drug guide Monitor cardiac rhythm Monitor intake and output Assess electrolytes Assess for central nervous system symptoms

Drug	Indication	Action	Dose	Adverse Effects	Nursing Considerations
Sotalol (Betapace)	Ventricular dysrhythmias	Nonselective beta-blocker	PO: 80 mg BID Increase to 160-640 mg/day	Hematological disorders, bronchospasm	Monitor blood pressure and pulse rate Check baseline liver and renal function before beginning therapy Monitor hydration Watch for QT prolongation Teach patient not to decrease drug abruptly
Ibutilide (Corvert)	Atrial fibrillation/flutter	Prolongs duration of action potential and refractory period	IV: 1 mg IV push over 10 minutes; may repeat after 10 minutes	Hypotension, bradycardia, sinus arrest	Continuous ECG monitoring to assess effectiveness Assess for central nervous system symptoms Use usually restricted to electrophysiology personnel
Propafenone (Rythmol)	Ventricular dysrhythmias	Stabilizes membranes; depresses action potential phase 0	PO: 150 mg every 8 hours; 450-900 mg/day	Ventricular dysrhythmias, congestive heart failure, dizziness, nausea/vomiting, altered taste	Monitor rhythm Use in patients without structural heart disease

BID, Twice daily; *ECG*, electrocardiogram; *IV*, intravenous; *PO*, orally; *SVT*, supraventricular tachycardia.
From Hodgson B. B., & Kizior R. J. (2007). *Saunders nursing drug handbook.* Philadelphia: Saunders.

impulses that caused the tachycardia. After each ablation attempt, the patient is retested until there is no recurrence of the tachycardiac rhythm.[2]

A radiofrequency ablation technique called circumferential radiofrequency ablation is used to treat atrial fibrillation. The lines of electrical conduction that may contribute to atrial fibrillation are located where the pulmonary veins connect to the left atrium. Radiofrequency ablation is done in a circular pattern around each pulmonary vein opening. This procedure has been found to be effective in treating and curing both episodic and chronic atrial fibrillation.

Permanent Pacemakers

Temporary pacemakers are used on an emergency basis to treat symptomatic bradycardia or to override tachydysrhythmias. Bradycardia often results from heart block associated with AMI, digoxin toxicity, or other cardiac abnormalities. If symptomatic bradycardia continues despite treatment and resolution of the cause, a permanent pacemaker is usually indicated. Permanent pacemakers may also be used to treat recurrent tachydysrhythmias unresponsive to pharmacological treatment. Biventricular pacemakers are discussed in the HF section of this chapter.

In the United States, most pacemakers are multiprogrammable for rate, voltage, sensitivity, stimulus duration, and refractory period. Most implanted pacemakers are of the ventricular demand type and have the ability to coincide with the patient's changing needs. Most permanent pacemakers use lithium batteries as their power source. These models have longevity of approximately 10 years.

Pacemaker functions are described in a code developed by the Intersociety Commission for Heart Disease (ICHD) which is a Modified Generic Code. The North American Society for Pacing and Electrophysiology (NASPE) uses a more specific code that may also be seen in the clinical setting. The code is used to denote the capabilities of the pacemaker as programmed for an individual patient. The code originally had three letters, was updated to five, but is more commonly seen with the original three letters denoting the chambers paced, the chamber sensed, and the mode of response to sensing (Table 12-10).

Programmable pacing devices have the ability to sense as well as trigger an output; they are classified as *atrial* or *ventricular* pacemakers and are coded as such, depending on their placement and inhibiting or triggering activity. A permanent pacemaker can be inserted in a transvenous mode by use of local anesthesia, with the lead wires traversing through the subclavian vein into the right atrium and ventricle. The battery or generator is implanted into the subcutaneous tissue, usually on the left side of the chest. This procedure may be performed in the operating room, but it is commonly performed in the cardiac catheterization laboratory or special procedures area of the radiology department.

Implantable Cardioverter-Defibrillator

Implantable cardioverter-defibrillators (ICDs) have become the dominant therapeutic modality for patients with life-threatening ventricular dysrhythmias. ICDs were initially used for patients with one or more sudden cardiac arrests or drug-refractory sustained ventricular tachycardia or ventricular fibrillation.[2]

Current indications for ICD therapy are listed in Box 12-9. Recent indications include patients awaiting cardiac transplantation who sustain life-threatening dysrhythmias, and prophylactic implantation in the following high-risk patient groups: patients with extensive MI and low ejection fraction, those with a history of MI with recurrent episodes of unexplained syncope, and children with congenital long-QT syndrome.[11]

An implantable atrial defibrillator has been introduced. In selected patients with recurrent atrial fibrillation with and without structural heart disease,

TABLE 12-10	Modified Generic Code for Pacemakers			
I Chamber Paced	**II** Chamber Sensed	**III** Response to Sensing	**IV** Programmable Functions/ Rate Modulation	**V** Antitachycardia Function(s)
V: Ventricle	V: Ventricle	T: Triggered	P: Programmable	P: Pace
A: Atrium	A: Atrium	I: Inhibited	M: Multiprogrammable	S: Shock
D: Dual (A + V)	D: Dual (A + V)	D: Dual (T + I)	C: Communicating	D: Dual (P + S)
O: None	O: None	O: None	R: Rate modulating	O: None
			O: None	

From Medtronic. (1998). *CorePace. PowerPoint presentation package.* Minneapolis, MN: Author.

a stand-alone atrial defibrillator was able to restore sinus rhythm promptly with low amounts of energy. In patients with no structural heart disease, the frequency of atrial fibrillation episodes decreased.[13]

ICDs provide high-energy shocks for ventricular fibrillation and rapid ventricular tachycardia, antitachycardia pacing for ventricular tachycardia, and pacing for bradycardia. Newer devices, incorporating an atrial lead, allow dual-chamber pacing with better discrimination between ventricular tachycardia and supraventricular tachycardia. ICDs can also provide resynchronization therapy for patients with HF.[4,7,13]

Just like the leads of a pacemaker, ICD leads are placed transvenously through the subclavian or cephalic vein and are positioned inside the heart. The defibrillator or pulse generator is placed in the pectoral region. Specific measurements are obtained at the time of the ICD implantation. Complications associated with ICD therapy include infection, lead failure, and unnecessary shocks for supraventricular tachycardia. Before hospital discharge, the device is programmed to determine thresholds and adequate safety margins along with rate-adaptive response rates determined through formal testing.[13]

Patients and family members must be educated about the device. Teaching is highlighted in Box 12-10. Quarterly clinic visits are important for the monitoring of ICD function and events.

The ICD comes with an identification card that specifies the heart rate at which shocks occur, the

---

BOX 12-9 Indications for an Implantable Cardioverter-Defibrillator

- Cardiac arrest resulting from ventricular fibrillation (VF) or ventricular tachycardia (VT) not produced by a transient or reversible cause
- Spontaneous sustained VT in association with structural heart disease
- Syncope of undetermined origin with clinically relevant, hemodynamically significant sustained VT or VF induced during electrophysiological study
- Nonsustained VT in patients with coronary artery disease, prior myocardial infarction, left ventricular dysfunction, and inducible VF or sustained VT during electrophysiological study
- Spontaneous sustained VT in patients who do not have structural heart disease that is not amenable to other treatments
- Patients with left ventricular ejection fraction of 30% or less, at least 1 month after myocardial infarction and 3 months after coronary artery bypass surgery

From Gregoratos, G., Abrams, J., Epstein, A., Freedman, R., Hayes, D., Hlatky, M., et al. (2002). ACC/AHA/NASPE 2002 guideline update for implantation of cardiac pacemakers and antiarrhythmia devices. Summary article: A report of the American College of Cardiology/American Heart Association Task Force on Practice Guidelines (ACC/AHA/NASPE Committee to Update the 1998 Pacemaker Guidelines). *Circulation, 106,* 2145-2161.

BOX 12-10 Patient and Family Teaching for an Implantable Cardioverter-Defibrillator

Preprocedural Teaching
- Device and how it works
- Lead and generator placement
- Implantation procedure
- Videos and materials from the manufacturer

Postprocedural Teaching
- Site care and symptoms of complications
- Hematoma at the site is most common when anticoagulant therapy is initiated
- Restricting activity of the arm on the side of the implant
- Identification (Medic Alert jewelry and ICD card)
- Diary of an event if the device fires
- Response if the device fires (varies from falling, tingling, or discomfort to no awareness of the shock); family members need to help in assessment
- Safety measures:
  - Avoid strong magnetic fields (no magnetic resonance imaging)
  - Avoid sources of high-power electricity
  - Keep cellular phones at least 6 inches from the ICD
  - Inform airline security personnel about the device; avoid the metal detector; the security wand may be used but should not be left over the device
  - The defibrillator must be turned off for surgical procedures using electrocautery
- Everyday activities:
  - Hairdryers, microwaves, and razors are safe
  - Sexual activity can be resumed; tachycardia associated with sexual activity may cause the device to fire; rate adjustments may be needed
  - If shock occurs during sexual activity, it will not harm the patient's partner
  - Avoid driving for 6 months if the patient has a history of sudden cardiac arrest
  - Testing of the device requiring additional electrophysiological studies
  - Replacement of the device
  - Instruction of family members in cardiopulmonary resuscitation and in how to contact emergency personnel
  - Support groups in the local community

ICD, Implantable cardioverter-defibrillator.

manufacturer and model number of the ICD, and the telephone numbers of the manufacturer and the primary physician. This card is carried with the patient.

Standard emergency procedures are to be followed with patients who have these devices and experience cardiovascular collapse. Cardiopulmonary resuscitation must not be delayed because the patient has an implanted device. Placement of paddles for external defibrillation is usually anteroposterior rather than sternum-apex.

HEART FAILURE

HF is a complex clinical syndrome that results from many disorders and can be exacerbated or worsened by comorbid conditions, lifestyle choices, psychological state, and the quality and quantity of care people receive once HF is diagnosed.[1] HF can result from any structural or functional cardiac disorder that impairs the ability of the ventricle to fill or eject blood. CAD is the primary underlying cause of HF; however, several nonischemic causes have been identified. These include hypertension, valvular disease, exposure to myocardial toxins, myocarditis, or unidentifiable causes such as idiopathic dilated cardiomyopathy.

Clinically, HF is defined as the heart's inability to pump a sufficient amount of blood to meet the needs of the body's tissues. The cardinal manifestations of HF are dyspnea, fatigue, exercise intolerance, and fluid retention, which may lead to pulmonary and peripheral edema.[1] Signs and symptoms of HF consist of progressive exertional dyspnea, paroxysmal nocturnal dyspnea, orthopnea, fatigability, loss of appetite, abdominal bloating, nausea or vomiting, and eventual organ system dysfunction, particularly the renal system as the failure advances.

The American Heart Association and American College of Cardiology developed a new classification system for HF. A patient is classified from stage A to D, based on results of physical examination and diagnostic tests, and clinical symptoms. This terminology helps in understanding that HF is often a progressive condition and worsens over time (Table 12-11). HF can be asymptomatic (stages A and B pre-HF) or symptomatic (stages C and D). The current goal of HF therapy is to cause regression and prevent progression.[1]

Pathophysiology

HF is impaired cardiac function of one or both ventricles. HF is also classified as systolic or diastolic. Systolic HF results from impaired pumping of the ventricles. Diastolic HF results from impaired filling

TABLE 12-11   Heart Failure Stages and Descriptions

Stages	Description of Stage
A	Those at high risk for developing heart failure: Hypertension Diabetes mellitus Coronary artery disease (including heart attack) History of cardiotoxic drug therapy History of alcohol abuse History of rheumatic fever Family history of cardiomyopathy
B	Those diagnosed with systolic heart failure but have never had symptoms of heart failure (ejection fraction less than 40% on echocardiogram)
C	Patients with known heart failure with current or prior symptoms: Shortness of breath Fatigue Reduced exercise intolerance
D	Presence of advanced symptoms, in the presence of optimized care

Heart and Vascular Institute Cleveland Clinic. *Understanding Heart Failure.* Retrieved January 2, 2008, from www.clevelandclinic.org/heartcenter/pub/guide/disease/heartfailure/understanding_hf.htm.

or relaxation of the ventricles. The most common type of HF is left-sided systolic dysfunction. Right-sided dysfunction is usually a consequence of left-sided HF; however, it can be a primary cause of HF after a right ventricular MI, or secondary to pulmonary pathology. Selected causes of HF are noted in Box 12-11.[17]

In left-sided HF, the left ventricle cannot pump efficiently. The ineffective pumping action causes a decrease in cardiac output, leading to poor perfusion. The volume of blood remaining in the left ventricle increases after each beat. As this volume builds, it backs up into the left atrium and pulmonary veins and into the lungs, causing congestion. Eventually, fluid accumulates in the lungs and pleural spaces, causing increased pressure in the lungs. Gas exchange (oxygen and carbon dioxide) in the pulmonary system is impaired. The backflow can continue into the right ventricle and right atrium and into the systemic circulation (right-sided HF).

When gas exchange is impaired and carbon dioxide increases, the respiratory rate increases to help eliminate the excess carbon dioxide. This phenomenon causes the heart rate to increase,

BOX 12-11   Causes of Heart Failure

Left Heart Systolic Failure
- Myocardial infarction
- Coronary artery disease
- Cardiomyopathy
- Hypertension
- Valvular heart disease
- Tachyarrhythmias
- Toxins: cocaine, ethanol, chemotherapy agents
- Myocarditis
- Pregnancy postpartum cardiomyopathy

Left Heart Diastolic Failure
- Myocardial infarction
- Coronary artery disease
- Hypertrophic heart disease
- Pericarditis
- Infiltrative disease: amyloid sarcoid
- Radiation therapy to the chest
- Age
- Hypertension

Right Heart Systolic Failure
- Right ventricular infarction
- Left-sided heart failure
- Pulmonary embolus
- Pulmonary hypertension
- Chronic obstructive pulmonary disease
- Septal defects

Right Heart Diastolic Failure
- Right ventricular hypertrophy
- Infiltrative disease: amyloid, sarcoid
- Radiation therapy to the chest

BOX 12-12   Signs and Symptoms of Heart Failure

Left-Sided Heart Failure: Poor Pump
- Dyspnea/orthopnea
- Paroxysmal nocturnal dyspnea
- Cough (orthopnea equivalent)
- Fatigue or activity intolerance
- Diaphoresis
- Slow capillary refill/cyanosis
- Elevated pulmonary capillary wedge pressure
- S_3 and S_4 gallop
- Increased heart rate

Right Sided Hearty Failure: Excess Volume
- Elevated jugular venous pressure
- Liver engorgement (hepatomegaly)
- Edema
- Elevated right atrial pressure
- Loss of appetite, nausea, vomiting
- Enlarged spleen

pumping more blood to the lungs for gas exchange. The increased heart rate results in the pumping of more blood from the systemic circulation into the cardiopulmonary circulation, which is already dangerously overloaded, thus a vicious cycle ensues.

As the heart begins to fail to meet the body's metabolic demands, several compensatory mechanisms are activated to improve cardiac output and tissue perfusion. The most noteworthy of these neurohormonal systems are the renin-angiotensin-aldosterone system and the sympathetic nervous system. These interrelated systems act in concert to redistribute blood to critical organs in the body by increasing peripheral vascular tone, heart rate, and contractility.[25] The activation of these diverse systems may account for many of the symptoms of HF and may contribute to the progression of the syndrome. Although these responses may be initially viewed as compensatory, many of them are or become counterregulatory and lead to adverse effects.

The renin-angiotensin-aldosterone system plays a major role in the pathogenesis and progression of HF. Angiotensin II is a potent vasoconstrictor and promotes salt and water retention by stimulation of aldosterone release. Sodium reabsorption increases, and this, in turn, increases blood volume. In patients with impaired function, the heart is unable to handle the extra volume effectively, resulting in edema (peripheral, visceral, and hepatic).

The sympathetic nervous system is activated. Although this is initially beneficial in preserving cardiac output and systemic blood pressure, chronic activation is deleterious. Activation (1) produces tachycardia, thereby decreasing preload and contributing to a further decrease in stroke index; (2) causes vasoconstriction, which increases afterload, further decreasing stroke index; and (3) increases contractility, which increases myocardial oxygen demand, thereby decreasing contractility and possibly decreasing stroke index. These changes are progressive. In time, the ventricle dilates, hypertrophies, and becomes more spherical. This process of cardiac remodeling generally precedes symptoms by months or even years.[25]

Assessment

Patient assessment includes the identification of the cause of both right-sided and left-sided HF, the signs and symptoms, and precipitating factors as well as diagnostic studies. Signs and symptoms of HF are presented in Box 12-12.[17]

In diagnosing HF, it is important to identify the etiology or precipitating factors. It is also important to determine whether ventricular dysfunction is systolic or diastolic because therapies are quite different. For example, some therapies for systolic dysfunction may be harmful if used to treat a patient with preserved systolic function. Ischemia is responsible for most cases of HF. Identifying ischemia as a cause of HF is important because a majority of these patients may benefit from revascularization.

Diagnosis of the patient with suspected HF includes the following:

- A complete history including precipitating factors
- Physical examination, including assessment of:
  Intravascular volume, with examination of neck veins and presence of hepatojugular reflux
  Presence or absence of edema
  Perfusion status, which includes blood pressure, quality of peripheral pulses, capillary refill, and temperature of extremities
  Lung sounds, which may not be helpful. In many cases, the lung fields are clear when the patient is obviously *congested*, a reflection of chronicity of the disease and adaptation.
- Chest x-ray study to view heart size and configuration and to check the lung fields to determine whether they are clear or opaque (fluid filled)
- Hemodynamic monitoring with pulmonary artery catheter. Mixed venous oxygen saturation, stroke index, cardiac index, cardiac output, and pulmonary artery pressures are important parameters to assess in the most critically ill patients, especially those who do not respond to conventional therapy. Noninvasive methods of determining hemodynamic parameters also helpful (see Chapter 8).
- Noninvasive imaging of cardiac structures. The single most useful test in evaluating patients with HF is the echocardiogram, which can evaluate ventricular enlargement, wall motion abnormalities, and valvular structures.
- Arterial blood gases to assess oxygenation and acid-base status
- Diagnostic studies
  Serum electrolytes. Many electrolyte imbalances are seen in patients with HF. Trending of electrolyte levels (sodium, potassium, chloride, calcium, and magnesium) is routinely done.[17] A low serum sodium level is a sign of advanced or end-stage disease; a low potassium level is associated with diuresis; a high potassium level is seen in renal impairment; blood urea nitrogen and creatinine levels are elevated in low perfusion states or with overdiuresis.
  Complete blood count to assess for anemia
  B (brain)-type natriuretic peptide (BNP). BNP is a cardiac hormone secreted by ventricular myocytes in response to wall stretch. BNP and ProBNP assays are useful in the diagnosis of patients with dyspnea of unknown etiology.[17] BNP is a good marker for differentiating between pulmonary and cardiac causes of dyspnea.[8] Plasma concentrations of BNP reflect the severity of HF. In decompensated HF, the BNP concentration increases as a response to wall stress or stretch. As the HF is treated, BNP is used to assess the response to therapy. The normal BNP concentration is less than 100 pg/mL. Patients are at risk of 30-day readmission if the BNP concentration is higher than 400 pg/mL at the time of discharge.
  Liver function studies. The liver often becomes enlarged with tenderness because of hepatic congestion. Serum transaminase and bilirubin levels are elevated with diminished liver function. Function usually returns once the patient is treated and euvolemic.
  ECG. Intraventricular conduction delays are common. Left bundle branch blocks are often associated with structural abnormalities. Patients frequently have premature ventricular contractions, premature atrial contractions, and atrial dysrhythmias such as atrial fibrillation or flutter. Resting sinus tachycardia implies substantive cardiac decompensation, and detection of this occurrence is essential.

Nursing Diagnoses

Many nursing diagnoses are associated with heart failure, such as decreased cardiac output, fluid volume excess, and activity intolerance. See the Nursing Care Plan for the Patient with Heart Failure for nursing diagnoses, outcomes, interventions, and rationale.

Interventions

Medical and nursing interventions for the patient with HF consist of a threefold approach: (1) treatment of the existing symptoms of the crisis situation, (2) prevention of further or expanding complications, and (3) treatment of the underlying cause. For example, some patients with HF can be treated by controlling hypertension or by repairing or replacing abnormal heart valves.

Text continued on p. 354

NURSING CARE PLAN for the Patient with Heart Failure

NURSING DIAGNOSIS

Decreased Cardiac Output

PATIENT OUTCOMES

Maintains optimally compensated cardiac output

- Clear lung sounds
- No shortness of breath
- Absence of or reduced edema

NURSING INTERVENTIONS	RATIONALES
• Assess rate and quality of apical and peripheral pulses	• Assess for compensatory tachycardia
• Assess BP for orthostatic changes	• Low CO as well as vasodilating medications may alter adequate perfusion
• Assess S_3 and S_4 heart sounds	• Assess left ventricular ejection or reduced compliance
• Assess lung sounds	• Crackles reflect fluid accumulation
• Assess for complaints of fatigue or altered activity tolerance	• Common in low CO states
• Assess urine output	• Assess renal perfusion
• Determine mental status changes, restlessness, irritability	• Assess for alteration in cerebral perfusion
• Assess oxygen saturation; administer supplemental oxygen to maintain saturation above 90%	• Ensure adequate oxygenation
• Monitor serum electrolytes	• Assess risk factors for dysrhythmias
• Assess BNP	• Elevated with increased left ventricular filling pressures
• Monitor for signs/symptoms of digitalis toxicity	• Therapeutic and toxic margin is narrow
• Weigh and evaluate trends	• Assess for fluid volume status
• Administer medications	• Many medications needed to improve CO; assess response
• Optimize preload Increased preload—restrict fluids and sodium Decreased preload—increase fluids and monitor response	• Promote adequate CO
• Consider invasive hemodynamic monitoring	• Provide data to guide treatment

NURSING DIAGNOSIS

Excess Fluid Volume

PATIENT OUTCOMES

Maintains optimal fluid balance

- Stable weight
- Absence of or reduction in edema
- Clear lung sounds

Continued

NURSING CARE PLAN for the Patient with Heart Failure—cont'd

NURSING INTERVENTIONS	RATIONALES
• Monitor and trend daily weight	• Weight gain of 2-3 lb indicates excess fluid volume
• Assess for presence of edema over ankles, feet, sacrum, and dependent areas	• Symmetrical dependent edema is characteristic in HF
• Auscultate for labored lung sounds	• Elevation of pulmonary pressure shifts fluid to interstitial and alveolar spaces
• Assess for JVD, ascites, nausea, and vomiting	• Right-sided HF increases venous pressure and fluid congestion backing up from the right side of the heart: hepatic and abdominal areas
• Monitor for side effects of diuretics	• Assess electrolyte imbalances—low potassium, low sodium, low magnesium, and elevated creatinine levels
• Consider hemofiltration or ultrafiltration for excess fluid volume	• Remove excess fluid volume

NURSING DIAGNOSIS

Risk for Alteration in Electrolyte Balance

PATIENT OUTCOMES

• Patient maintains electrolytes within normal range
• Patient receives medication adjustments as needed if electrolyte imbalance is noted

NURSING INTERVENTIONS	RATIONALES
• Monitor serum electrolyte levels Hyponatremia Hypokalemia Hypomagnesemia Hypernatremia Hyperkalemia	• Hyponatremia may be dilutional • Require higher safety range for normal potassium • Dysrhythmias increase risk of sudden death • Hypernatremia is caused by large loss of water • Coadministration of ACE inhibitors, ARBs, or aldosterone blockers can cause potassium retention
• Administer diuretics • Administer electrolyte supplements; provide appropriate diet with foods that contain supplements; if replacement is needed, administer by mouth or intravenously	• Restore water and sodium balance • Prevent electrolyte imbalances via medication and/or diet
• Place on ECG monitor	• Assess for dysrhythmias associated with electrolyte imbalances

NURSING DIAGNOSIS

Activity Intolerance

PATIENT OUTCOMES

• Reports improved activity tolerance and ability to perform required activities of daily living
• Verbalizes and uses energy conservation techniques

NURSING CARE PLAN for the Patient with Heart Failure—cont'd

NURSING INTERVENTIONS	RATIONALES
• Assess patient's current level of activity	• Assess baseline activity; intolerance is common
• Observe and document response to activity	• HR increases >20 beats/min; BP drop of >20 mm Hg, dyspnea, lightheadedness, and fatigue signify abnormal responses to activity
• Monitor sleep pattern and amount of sleep during night and day	• Provide adequate rest to facilitate progression of activity
• Evaluate need for oxygen with activity	• Supplemental oxygen compensates for increased oxygen demand
• Teach energy conservation techniques Sit for tasks Push rather than pull Slide rather than lift Store frequently used items within reach Organize a work-rest-work schedule	• Techniques reduce oxygen consumption
• Provide emotional support and encouragement	• Promote positive reinforcement to guide activity progression

NURSING DIAGNOSIS

Disturbed Sleep Pattern

PATIENT OUTCOMES

- Verbalizes improvement in hours and quality of sleep
- Appears rested and more alert
- Need for daytime napping decreases

NURSING INTERVENTIONS	RATIONALES
• Assess current sleep patterns	• Provide baseline assessment
• Assess for nocturia, dyspnea, orthopnea, PND, and fear of PND	• Assess for common issues associated with sleep disturbances
• Plan medication schedules; facilitate medication administration that will not cause patient to have to wake up to use the bathroom	• Promote periods of uninterrupted sleep
• Avoid caffeine and smoking	• Promote relaxation and sleep
• Encourage patient to elevate HOB	• Reduce pulmonary congestion and nighttime dyspnea
• Review how to summon for help during the night	• Reduce anxiety and fear that may disrupt sleep patterns

NURSING DIAGNOSIS

Deficient Knowledge

PATIENT OUTCOME

- Patient or significant others understand and verbalize causes, treatment, and care related to HF

Continued

NURSING CARE PLAN for the Patient with Heart Failure—cont'd

NURSING INTERVENTIONS	RATIONALE
• Assess knowledge of causes, treatment, and care related to HF	• Provide a base for educational planning
• Identify misconceptions regarding care	• Identify baseline knowledge and misperceptions that need to be corrected
• Educate about normal heart and circulation, HF disease process, symptoms, dietary modifications, activity guidelines, medications, psychological aspects of illness, goals of therapy, and community resources	• Reduce symptoms and readmission for exacerbation
• Encourage questions	• Verify understanding of information

ACE, Angiotensin-converting enzyme; *ARBs*, angiotensin II receptor blockers; *BNP*, B (brain)-type natriuretic peptide; *BP*, blood pressure; *CO*, cardiac output; *ECG*, electrocardiogram; *HF*, heart failure; *HOB*, head of bed; *HR*, heart rate; *JVD*, jugular venous distention; *PND*, paroxysmal nocturnal dyspnea.

Treatment of existing symptoms includes the following:

1. Improvement of pump function, fluid removal, and enhanced tissue perfusion (Tables 12-12 and 12-13)[14,17]
   a. First-line medications include ACE inhibitors and diuretics. Once symptoms and volume status are stable, a beta-blocker (metoprolol, carvedilol, bisoprolol) should be added. An ACE inhibitor and beta-blocker form the cornerstone of the treatment for HF.[22] When only one drug can be initiated, beta-blockers are preferred.[17] Additional drug therapies include digoxin, spironolactone, hydralazine, and nitrates.
   b. Inotropes—dobutamine, dopamine, and milrinone—have failed to demonstrate improved mortality in the treatment of severe decompensated HF. A review of the literature has shown an increase in mortality associated with administration of these agents.[17]
   c. Nesiritide (Natrecor) is administered IV to patients with acutely decompensated HF who have dyspnea at rest or with minimal activity. The best candidates for therapy are patients with decompensated HF who have clinical evidence of fluid overload, increased central venous pressure, or both.[17]
2. Reduction of cardiac workload and oxygen consumption
   a. The intraaortic balloon pump is an invasive strategy to preserve coronary flow in the presence of severe, acute decompensated

Text continued on p. 358

TABLE 12-12 Medication Subsets for Heart Failure

Medication	Management of Heart Failure
ACE inhibitors	Slow disease progression, improve exercise capacity, and decrease hospitalization and mortality
Angiotensin II receptor antagonists	Reduce afterload and improve cardiac output. Can be used for patients with ACE inhibitor cough
Hydralazine/ Isosorbide dinitrate	Vasodilator effect; useful in patients intolerant to ACE inhibitors
Diuretics	Manage fluid overload
Aldosterone antagonists	Manage HF associated with LV systolic dysfunction (<35%) while receiving standard therapy, including diuretics
Digoxin	Improve symptoms, exercise tolerance, and quality of life; no effect on mortality
Beta-blockers	Manage HF associated with LV systolic dysfunction (<40%); well tolerated in most patients, including those with comorbidities such as diabetes mellitus, chronic obstructive lung disease, and peripheral vascular disease

ACE, Angiotensin-converting enzyme.

PHARMACOLOGY

TABLE 12-13   Specific Medications for Heart Failure

Angiotensin-Converting Enzyme Inhibitors (ACE-Is)

Indications: used to treat hypertension, heart failure, and patients after myocardial infarction
Mechanism of action: prevent the conversion of angiotensin I to angiotensin II resulting in lower levels of angiotensin II, thus causing an increase in plasma renin activity and a reduction of aldosterone secretion; also inhibit the remodeling process after myocardial injury

Generic Name (Brand Name)	Dosage	Side Effects and Nursing Considerations
Enalapril (Vasotec)	2.5-20 mg BID PO	Hypotension, bradycardia, renal impairment, cough, and orthostatic hypotension Do not give IV enalapril to patients with unstable heart failure or patients having an acute myocardial infarction. Monitor urine output Monitor potassium levels. Avoid use of NSAIDs Instruct patient to avoid rapid change in position such as from lying to standing ACE-Is are contraindicated in pregnancy
Fosinopril (Monopril)	10-40 mg daily PO	Same
Captopril (Capoten)	12.5-100 mg TID PO	Same

Diuretics

Indication: for the management of edema or fluid volume overload associated with heart failure and hepatic or renal disease
Mechanism of action: inhibit reabsorption of sodium and chloride in the ascending loop of Henle and distal renal tubule, interfering with the chloride-binding cotransport system, causing increased excretion of water, sodium, chloride, magnesium, and calcium

Generic Name (Brand Name)	Dosage	Side Effects and Nursing Considerations
Furosemide (Lasix)	20-600 mg BID PO/IV	Orthostatic hypotension, vertigo, dizziness, gout, hypokalemia, cramping, diarrhea or constipation, hearing impairment, tinnitus (rapid IV administration) Monitor laboratory results, especially potassium levels. Monitor cardiovascular and hydration status regularly. In decompensated patients, use IV route until euvolemic status is reached Administer first dose early in the day and second dose late in afternoon, to avoid sleep disturbance
Bumetanide (Bumex)	0.5-4 mg daily PO/IV/IM	Same
Torsemide (Demadex)	10-200 mg daily PO/IV Maximum 200 mg daily	Same
Metolazone (Zaroxolyn)	5-10 mg daily PO	Increased diuretic effect occurs when it is given with furosemide and other loop diuretics
Ethacrynic acid (Edecrin)	50-200 mg daily PO	Same Used when patient has a sulfa allergy

Continued

PHARMACOLOGY

TABLE 12-13   Specific Medications for Heart Failure—cont'd

Beta-Blockers

Indications: used to treat angina, acute myocardial infarction, and heart failure
Mechanism of action: block beta-adrenergic receptors, with resulting decreased sympathetic nervous system responses such as decreases in heart rate, blood pressure, and cardiac contractility in heart failure may improve systolic function over time

Generic Name (Brand Name)	Dosage	Side Effects and Nursing Considerations
Metoprolol (Lopressor)	50-450 mg daily PO, 5 mg IV	Bradycardia, hypotension, atrioventricular blocks, asthma attacks, fatigue, impotence, may mask hypoglycemic episodes
Toprol XL	25-200 mg daily PO	Teach patient to take pulse and blood pressure on regular basis Patient should not abruptly stop taking these drugs Close glucose monitoring if the patient is diabetic Patients should be started on the lowest dose and slowly titrated to the maximum dose over 4-6 weeks as tolerated
Carvedilol (Coreg)	12.5-50 mg daily PO	Same This is better tolerated on a full stomach
Bisoprolol (Concor)	2.5-20 mg daily PO	Same

Aldosterone Receptor Antagonist

Indication: management of edema associated with excessive aldosterone secretion
Mechanism of action: competes with aldosterone for receptor sites in distal renal tubules, increasing sodium chloride and water excretion while conserving potassium and hydrogen ions; may block the effect of aldosterone on arterial smooth muscle

Generic Name (Brand Name)	Dosage	Side Effects and Nursing Considerations
Spironolactone (Aldactone)	25-200 mg daily PO	Monitor serum potassium and renal function. This is potassium sparing
Eplerenone (Inspra)	50 mg daily PO, may be increased to 50 mg BID if inadequate response after 4 weeks	Monitor blood pressure closely, especially at 2 weeks Monitor potassium and sodium levels

Inotropes

Indication: treatment of cardiac decompensation from heart failure, shock, or renal failure
Mechanism of action: augment cardiac output by increasing contractility and enhancing tissue perfusion; agents listed use different mechanisms

Generic Name (Brand Name)	Dosage	Side Effects and Nursing Considerations
Digoxin (Lanoxin)	0.125-0.5 mg daily PO/IV	Heart block, asystole, visual disturbances (blurred or yellow vision), confusion/mental disturbances, nausea, vomiting, diarrhea Monitor serum concentrations; digoxin possesses a narrow therapeutic range. Digoxin toxicity can be life-threatening. Maintain adequate serum potassium levels; hypokalemia increases risk of digoxin toxicity. Monitor heart rate and notify prescriber if heart rate is <50/min

PHARMACOLOGY

TABLE 12-13 Specific Medications for Heart Failure—cont'd

Generic Name (Brand Name)	Dosage	Side Effects and Nursing Considerations
Dopamine (Intropin)	1-50 mcg/kg/min IV infusion titrated to desired response Always administer via infusion device; administer into large vein	Frequent ventricular ectopy, tachycardia, anginal pain, vasoconstriction, headache, nausea, or vomiting. Extravasation into surrounding tissue can cause tissue necrosis and sloughing Monitor heart rate/rhythm and blood pressure closely Dopamine is most frequently used for treatment of hypotension because of its peripheral vasoconstrictor action. It is often used together with dobutamine to minimize hypotension. Thus, pressure is maintained by increased cardiac output (from dobutamine) and vasoconstriction (by dopamine) Monitor the IV site frequently
Dobutamine (Dobutrex)	2.5-20 mcg/kg/min continuous IV infusion titrated to desired response Always administer via infusion device; administer into large vein	Increased heart rate, ventricular ectopy, hypotension, angina, headache, nausea, and local inflammatory changes It has been used in outpatient settings (continuous at home or intermittent infusions in office) in patients with end-stage heart failure to stabilize symptoms, but it does increase mortality Monitor heart rate/rhythm and blood pressure closely
Milrinone (Primacor)	Loading dose of 50 mcg/kg administered over 10 minutes, followed by continuous infusion 0.375-0.75 mcg/kg/min Always administer via infusion device; administer into large vein	Same as dobutamine
Inamrinone (Inocor)	Initially, 0.75 mg/kg IV bolus over 2 to 3 minutes. Then begin maintenance infusion of 5 to 10 mcg/kg/min May give additional bolus of 0.75 mcg/kg/min 30 minutes after starting therapy Do not exceed total daily dose of 10 mg/kg	Same as dobutamine Because of confusion with amiodarone, the generic name amrinone was changed to inamrinone Do not administer furosemide and inamrinone through the same IV line because precipitation occurs

Brain Natriuretic Peptide
Indication: decompensated congestive heart failure
Mechanism of action: exogenous form of hormone produced by myocardial myocytes as a result of myocardial stress and stretching; vasodilates both veins and arteries and has a positive neurohormonal effect by decreasing aldosterone, and positive renal effects by increasing diuresis and natriuresis

Continued

PHARMACOLOGY

TABLE 12-13   Specific Medications for Heart Failure—cont'd

Generic Name (Brand Name)	Dosage	Side Effects and Nursing Considerations
Nesiritide (Natrecor)	Continuous infusion: 0.01 mcg/kg/min after bolus of 2 mcg/kg	Hypotension, enhanced diuresis, electrolyte imbalances (hypokalemia) Patients will usually respond quickly to therapy. Infusions generally run for 24 hours but can continue for days in the severely decompensated patient

Nitrates

Indications: to reduce afterload, elevated systemic vascular resistance
Mechanism of action: directly relax smooth muscle, which causes vasodilation of the peripheral vascular bed; decrease myocardial oxygen demands

Generic Name (Brand Name)	Dosage	Side Effects and Nursing Considerations
Nitroglycerin (Tridil)	IV: continuous infusion started at 5 mcg/min and titrated up to a maximum of 200 mcg/min	Headache, dizziness, flushing, orthostatic hypotension Monitor blood pressure closely. Titrate to effect

Angiotensin Receptor Blockers

Indications: hypertension, heart failure; used in patients who cannot tolerate use of ACE-Is
Mechanism of action: selective and competitive angiotensin II receptor antagonists; block the vasoconstrictor and aldosterone-secreting effects of angiotensin II

Generic Name (Brand Name)	Dosage	Side Effects and Nursing Considerations
Valsartan (Diovan)	80 mg daily BID PO up to 320 mg total daily dose	Hypotension, diarrhea, dyspepsia, upper respiratory infection Avoid use of NSAIDs, such as indomethacin or naproxen, which may cause renal impairment. Same as ACE-Is
Candesartan (Atacand)	4-32 mg PO daily	Same

BID, Twice daily; *IM*, intramuscular; *IV*, intravenous; *NSAIDs*, nonsteroidal antiinflammatory drugs; *PO*, orally; *TID*, three times daily.

HF. It is used to stabilize patients with marked hemodynamic instability to allow time for insertion of a ventricular assist device (VAD).[25]

b. VADs are capable of partial to complete circulatory support for short- to long-term use. They assist the failing heart and maintain adequate circulatory pressure. VADs attach to the patient's own heart and leave the patient's heart intact, and they have the potential for removal. At present, the left VAD is therapy for patients with terminal HF and has been used in patients who are not eligible for heart transplant.[25]

c. Biventricular pacing. Patients with chronic HF may exhibit dyssynchronous contraction of the left ventricle, resulting from abnormal electrical conduction pathways.[25] This results in contraction of the septum before contraction of the free wall of the left ventricle. The result is a significant alteration in the circulation of blood flow forward out of the left ventricle. Cardiac resynchronization therapy through biventricular pacing involves placing a ventricular lead in the right ventricle and another lead down the coronary sinus to the left ventricle.[25] Both ventricles are stimulated simultaneously, resulting in a synchronized contraction that improves cardiac performance, decreases wall stress, and reduces mitral regurgitation. Patients are showing improved exercise and activity tolerance and improved quality-of-life scores.

   d. Nursing measures that can reduce cardiac workload and oxygen consumption are to schedule rest periods and to encourage patients to modify their activities of daily living. Activity is advanced as tolerated. Many patients with HF derive tremendous benefit from formal cardiac rehabilitation to improve activity tolerance and endurance.

3. Optimization of gas exchange through supplemental oxygen and diuresis

   a. Evaluate the airway, the degree of respiratory distress, and the need for supplemental oxygenation by pulse oximetry, arterial blood gas measurement, or both. Patients are more comfortable in semi-Fowler's position. Adjust oxygen delivery. Consider noninvasive ventilatory support such as continuous positive airway pressure (CPAP) or bilevel positive airway pressure (BiPAP). CPAP and BiPAP have demonstrated effectiveness in the management of HF and often reduce the need for intubation.[17]

   b. Diurese aggressively. Administer IV diuretics; furosemide and bumetanide are the preferred diuretics. Ethacrynic acid is useful if the patient has a serious sulfa allergy. These agents are characterized by quick onset; diuresis is expected 10 to 15 minutes after administration. The goal is to achieve euvolemia, which may take days. When the patient is euvolemic, oral medications are reinstated because they are better absorbed, and the patient is less likely to be readmitted to the acute care setting.

   c. Patients with severe HF often have limited mobility; therefore, they are at high risk for venous thromboembolism.[25] Thromboprophylaxis is considered if the patient has limited or complete restriction of activity.

   d. Control of sodium and fluid retention involves fluid restriction of 2 L/day and sodium restriction of 2 g/day. Sodium restriction alone may provide substantial benefits for patients with HF.[17] Dietary counseling includes a discussion about fluid balance management and the importance of avoiding excess sodium or water intake, or both. Referral to a dietitian should be considered for patients with comorbid conditions or repeat episodes of HF.

   e. Daily weights are a priority in these patients.

Nurses make a tremendous impact by teaching and enforcing these concepts throughout the hospital stay. Patients may find it easier to continue these habits at discharge if their importance is stressed throughout hospitalization.

Cardiac transplantation is a therapeutic option of last resort for patients with end-stage HF. Patients who have severe cardiac disability refractory to expert management and who have a poor prognosis for 6-month survival are optimal candidates. For many patients with symptomatic HF and ominous objective findings (ejection fraction <20%, stroke volume <40 mL, severe ventricular dysrhythmias), timing of the surgery is difficult. A further consideration may be the quality of life, which is a judgment made by the patient and the patient's physicians.

Once the crisis stage has passed and the patient is stabilized, the precipitating factors for the complications must be addressed and treated. Treatment consists of surgical or catheter-based interventions as addressed for a patient with an MI, such as CABG, PTCA or stent, and pharmacological therapy (ACE inhibitors, beta-blocker); valve replacement or repair for valvular heart disease; restoration of sinus rhythm if atrial fibrillation or flutter and tachydysrhythmias are present; and management of risk factors such as hypertension, hyperlipidemia, diabetes, and obesity.[17,25] Compliance with medications and sodium restriction is continually and vigilantly readdressed.

Complications

Complications of HF can be devastating. Interventions must be provided to avoid extending the existing conditions or allowing the development of new, life-threatening complications. Two specific complications for which the patients are monitored are pulmonary edema and cardiogenic shock.

Pulmonary Edema

The failing heart is sensitive to increases in afterload. In some patients with HF, when systolic blood pressure is ≥150 mm Hg, pulmonary edema will ensue. The pulmonary vascular system becomes full and engorged. The results are increasing volume and pressure of blood in pulmonary vessels, increasing pressure in pulmonary capillaries, and leaking of fluid into the interstitial spaces of lung tissue.

Pulmonary edema greatly reduces the amount of lung tissue space available for gas exchange and results in clinical symptoms of extreme dyspnea, cyanosis, severe anxiety, diaphoresis, pallor, and blood-tinged, frothy sputum. Arterial blood gas results indicate severe respiratory acidosis and hypoxemia.

Patients with persistent volume overload may be candidates for continuous IV diuretics, ultrafiltra-

TRANSPLANTATION Cardiac

INDICATIONS

Cardiac transplantation is the primary therapeutic choice for patients younger than 65 years who have advanced heart failure and who remain symptomatic despite maximal medical therapy. In the United States, approximately 2000 new recipients receive cardiac transplants annually. These recipients have an 85% probability of surviving the first year with an excellent quality of life, and a 50% probability of surviving to 10 years.[3]

CRITERIA FOR TRANSPLANT RECIPIENT

Because of the huge discrepancy between the number of patients who meet the criteria for transplantation and the number of available donors, considerable efforts have focused on optimal pharmacological management (neurohormonal antagonists, vasodilators, inotropes, diuretics, and anticoagulants), cardiac resynchronization therapy with biventricular pacing, ventricular assist devices, and surgery.[1] Older age has often eliminated potential recipients; however, during the past 20 years, the percentage of recipients older than 65 years has increased steadily.[3]

CRITERIA FOR DONOR

Donor heart criteria have expanded to include older hearts (>55 years), donor hearts with an ischemic time greater than 4 hours, and the creation of an alternative list to match excluded potential recipients with donor hearts that otherwise would not be used.[2]

PATIENT MANAGEMENT

The immune system is programmed to recognize a transplanted organ as foreign, and therefore the immune system must be inhibited after organ transplantation (see Chapter 16). Immunosuppressive therapy targets different processes in the rejection process: induction, maintenance, and rejection. Induction therapy (antithymocyte agents and interleukin-2 receptor blockers) is initiated in the immediate posttransplant period when the risk for rejection is greatest and renal dysfunction, infection, and later malignancy can occur as a result of immunosuppressive therapy. Maintenance therapy consists of medications that inhibit T-cell proliferation and differentiation, deplete lymphocytes, and inhibit macrophages. These medications include a calcineurin inhibitor (cyclosporine [Neoral] or tacrolimus [Prograf]), a steroid (methylprednisolone), and an antiproliferative agent (mycophenolate mofetil [CellCept], azathioprine [Imuran], or sirolimus). Complications associated with immunosuppressive therapy include nephrotoxicity, hypertension, hyperlipidemia, bone loss, and infection.

COMPLICATIONS

Infection is the leading cause of death in the first year after transplantation. In the early postoperative period, nosocomial infections predominate including pneumonia, wound and urinary tract infections, and sepsis. Protective isolation has not been to be beneficial over standard universal precautions. Opportunistic infections predominate 1 to 6 months after cardiac transplantation. Causative organisms include cytomegalovirus, herpes simplex virus, varicella zoster (shingles), *Pneumocystis carinii*, *Aspergillus*, and *Candida*.

Cytomegalovirus has been a significant cause of morbidity and mortality after cardiac transplantation, as it is associated with acute and chronic rejection, allograft vasculopathy, and opportunistic superinfections. After 6 months, most infections are community acquired, and patients are instructed to avoid contact with anyone who is ill, avoid environments high in dust or mold, and to use good hand-washing practices. A high index of suspicion must be maintained, as fever can be masked by the effects of the immunosuppressive medications.

PREVENTING REJECTION

Cardiac transplant rejection is the result of the patient's immune system response to a donor heart and is the leading cause of death in the first year after transplantation.[3] Compliance with immunosuppressive medication is essential to reduce the risk of rejection. Hyperacute rejection occurs within minutes or hours of transplantation, is caused by preformed antibodies, and rarely occurs. Acute cellular rejection occurs 3 to 6 months after transplantation and involves the activation and proliferation of T lymphocytes with destruction of cardiac tissue. Humoral or antibody-mediated rejection involves B-cell–mediated production of immunoglobulin G antibody against the transplanted organ. Significant hemodynamic compromise and shock can occur, resulting in death.

Rejection is diagnosed by endomyocardial biopsy, initially weekly for 4 to 6 weeks and then at increasingly longer periods based on the recipient's clinical presentation and cardiac function. Biopsy specimens are graded according to the severity of the interstitial infiltration of lymphocytes by using a standard grading system (0, no rejection, to 4, severe rejection). Symptoms of rejection may be subtle and include weight gain, shortness of breath, fatigue, abdominal bloating, or fever. Management may include high-dose meth-

TRANSPLANTATION   Cardiac—cont'd

ylprednisolone; augmenting current maintenance immunosuppression with tacrolimus, mycophenolate mofetil, rapamycin, or orthoclone (OKT3); and/or plasmapheresis.

Cardiac allograft vasculopathy, also known in the past as chronic rejection, is an accelerated form of diffuse arteriosclerosis that remains one of the principal limiting factors to long-term survival in cardiac transplant recipients. It can result in myocardial ischemia, infarction, heart failure, ventricular arrhythmias, and death. Immunological mechanisms play a role in the development of cardiac allograft vasculopathy; however, smoking, obesity, diabetes, hyperlipidemia, hypertension, older recipient, and older donor are also considered risk factors.

REFERENCES

1. Jessup, M., Banner, N., Brozena, S., Campana, C., Costard-Jäckle, A., Dengler, T., et al. (2006). Optimal pharmacologic and non-pharmacologic management of cardiac transplant candidates: Approaches to be considered before transplant evaluation: International Society for Heart and Lung Transplantation guidelines for the care of cardiac transplant candidates—2006. *Journal of Heart and Lung Transplantation, 25*(9), 1003-1023.
2. Klein, D. G. (2007). Current trends in cardiac transplantation. *Critical Care Nursing Clinics of North America, 19*(4), 445-460.
3. Taylor, D. O., Edwards, L. B., Boucek, M. M., Trulock, E. P., Aurora, P., Christie, J., et al. (2007). Registry of the International Society for Heart and Lung Transplantation: Twenty-fourth official adult heart transplant report 2007. *Journal of Heart and Lung Transplantation, 26*(8), 769-781.

tion, or hemodialysis.[17] Loop diuretics given as an IV bolus are considered along with an IV infusion. Furosemide is the most commonly used loop diuretic, with the dose adjusted upward if the patient is currently on oral doses. The diuretic effect occurs in 30 minutes, with the peak effect in 1 to 2 hours.[14] IV torsemide or bumetanide are alternative loop diuretics.

The pharmacological characteristics of loop diuretics are similar. Therefore, a lack of response to adequate doses of one loop diuretic alleviates the need for administration of another loop diuretic. In patients who have poor responses to intermittent doses of a loop diuretic, a continuous IV infusion can be tried. If an effective amount of the diuretic is maintained at the site of action at all times, a small but clinically important increase in the response may occur. In addition, combinations of diuretics with different mechanisms of action are considered. Monitoring hourly urinary output assists in determining the effectiveness of the diuretic therapy.

Although diuretic therapy is important, it is also critical to lower the blood pressure and cardiac filling pressures. IV NTG is administered and titrated until the blood pressure is controlled, resulting in a reduction in both preload and afterload.[17] Patients who do not demonstrate improvement in symptoms require more aggressive treatment. A NTG infusion is initiated at 5 mcg/min, and initial titration is in increments of 5 mcg/min at intervals of 3 to 5 minutes, guided by patient response. If no response is seen at 20 mcg/min, incremental increases of 10 and 20 mcg/min may be used. The maximum dose is 200 mcg/min. Other care requirements for the administration of NTG include the use of non–polyvinyl chloride tubing. If this tubing is not available and traditional polyvinyl chloride tubing must be used, then the initial dose for NTG starts at 25 mcg/min IV.

Cardiogenic Shock

Cardiogenic shock is the most acute and ominous form of pump failure. Cardiogenic shock can be seen after a severe MI, with dysrhythmias, decompensated HF, pulmonary embolus, cardiac tamponade, and ruptured abdominal aortic aneurysm. Often, the outcome of cardiogenic shock is death. Cardiogenic shock and its treatment are discussed in depth in Chapter 11. Outcomes for the patient with HF are included in the nursing care plan.

PERICARDIAL DISEASE

Pericarditis

Pericarditis is acute or chronic inflammation of the pericardium. It may occur as a consequence of AMI or secondary to other diseases such as renal failure (uremic pericarditis), infection, and cancer. The pericardium has an inner and outer layer with a small amount of lubricating fluid between the layers. When the pericardium becomes inflamed, the amount of fluid between the two layers increases (pericardial effusion). This squeezes the heart and restricts its action and may result in cardiac tamponade. Chronic inflammation can result in constrictive pericarditis, which leads to scarring. The epicardium may thicken and calcify.

The patient with pericarditis usually has precordial pain; this pain frequently radiates to the shoulder, neck, back, and arm and is intensified during deep inspiration, movement, coughing, and even swallowing. Other signs and symptoms may include a pericardial friction rub, dyspnea, weakness, fatigue, a persistent temperature elevation, an increased white blood cell count and sedimentation rate, and an increased anxiety level.[21] Pulsus paradoxus may be noted while auscultating the blood pressure. Precordial pain must be distinguished from the pain of an AMI.

Detection of a pericardial friction rub is the most common method of diagnosing pericarditis. The friction rub is usually heard best on inspiration with the diaphragm of the stethoscope placed over the second, third, or fourth intercostal space at the sternal border. Friction rubs have been described as grating, scraping, squeaking, or scratching sounds. This rubbing sound results from an increase in fibrous exudate between the two irritated pericardial layers.

Other findings of pericarditis include ECG changes. There are anterior and inferior concave ST-segment elevation and PR-segment deviations opposite to P-wave polarity. T waves progressively flatten and invert, with generalized T-wave inversions present in most or all leads.[21] In addition, an echocardiogram is also useful in diagnosis to visualize the effusion.

The treatment of patients with pericarditis involves relief of pain (analgesic agents or antiinflammatory agents, such as indomethacin and ibuprofen), antibiotics if the causative agent is bacterial, and treatment of other systemic symptoms.[21] If excess fluid is seriously affecting the heart's action, a needle can be inserted into the pericardial space to remove the fluid (pericardiocentesis). In extreme cases, surgery may be required to remove part of the pericardium (pericardial window).

ENDOCARDITIS

Infective endocarditis is an infection of microorganisms circulating in the bloodstream that attach onto an endocardial surface. Endocarditis is classified as one of three types: left-sided native valve, right-sided native valve, and prosthetic valve.[26] It is caused by various microbes and frequently involves the heart valves. Bacteria of the genus *Streptococcus* are the organisms most commonly responsible for subacute infective endocarditis. Endocarditis can also be caused by staphylococci, gram-negative bacilli (e.g., *Escherichia coli* and *Klebsiella* species), and fungi (e.g., *Candida* and *Histoplasma* species).

Infectious lesions or vegetations form on the heart valves. These lesions have irregular edges and have been known to have a cauliflower-like appearance. The mitral valve is the most common area to be affected, followed by the aortic valve. The vegetative process can grow to involve the chordae tendineae, papillary muscles, and conduction system. Therefore, the patient may have dysrhythmias or acute HF.

Endocarditis rarely occurs in people with normal hearts. Certain preexisting heart conditions increase the risk of developing endocarditis: implantation of an artificial (prosthetic) heart valve and a history of previous endocarditis or damaged or abnormal heart valves by conditions such as rheumatic fever or congenital heart or valve defects.

The clinical presentation of patients with acute infectious endocarditis includes signs and symptoms of cardiogenic or septic shock.[26] Clinical manifestations include fever, chills, night sweats, cough, weight loss, general malaise, weakness, fatigue, headache, musculoskeletal complaints, new murmurs, right- or left-sided HF, positive blood cultures, and anemia. The presenting symptoms are determined by the valve involved, the organism present, and the length of time and extent of growth of the vegetative process. Treatment involves diagnosing the infective agent, treating with the appropriate antibiotics or antifungal agents, and performing valve replacement surgery in the most serious cases.[26]

VASCULAR ALTERATIONS

The aorta is the largest blood vessel in the body both in length and diameter. Shaped like a walking cane, the aorta is an artery that carries blood from the heart. Its many branches then feed all other areas of the body. The aorta is divided into the thoracic and abdominal aorta (Figure 12-13).

The thoracic aorta is divided into the ascending aorta, the aortic arch, and the descending aorta. The thoracic aorta begins at the left ventricle just beyond the aortic valve of the heart. The round segment, or cane handle, is the ascending aorta and the aortic arch. Branches of the ascending aorta include the right and left coronary arteries, which feed the myocardium. The arch vessels include the innominate artery, which branches into the right subclavian artery and right common carotid artery, and the left common carotid and subclavian arteries. These branches send blood to the head and the upper extremities.

The descending thoracic aorta, the long segment of the cane, is to the left of the midline of the chest. Branches of the descending aorta are the intercostal arteries. These arteries are the major blood supply to the distal spinal cord, feeding the artery of Adamkiewicz, and they arise anywhere along the spinal cord from T8 to L2.

The abdominal aorta begins at the level of the diaphragm. At the umbilicus, it bifurcates into the

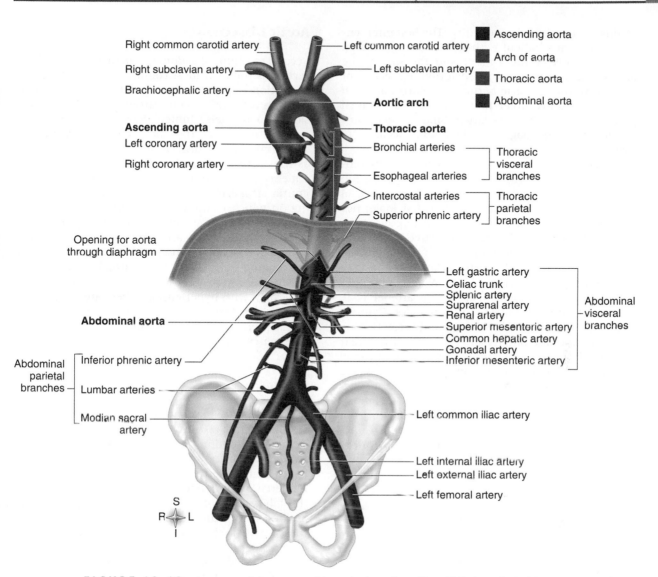

FIGURE 12-13. Anatomy of the aorta and its major branches. *(From Thibodeau, G. A. & Patton, K. T. [2007]. Anatomy and physiology [6th ed.]. St. Louis: Mosby.)*

iliac arteries. Abdominal branches include the celiac artery, the superior and inferior mesenteric arteries, and the renal arteries.

Aortic Aneurysms

The word *aneurysm* comes from the Greek *aneurysma*, which means *widening*. An aneurysm is a diseased area of an artery causing dilatation and thinning of the wall. Pathological examination often shows layered clot and mural thrombi at the aneurysm site.[24] Atherosclerosis and degeneration of elastin and collagen are the underlying causes in most cases.

Aneurysms are frequently hereditary and are associated with hypertension, with a predominance in males. The ratio of aneurysms in men compared with women is 2:1.[24] In the critical care arena, abdominal aortic aneurysms are the most common. Other artery locations for aneurysms include the iliac, femoral, popliteal, intracranial, splenic, subclavian, and hepatic. Anastomotic aneurysms are false aneurysms found at any graft-host artery anastomosis.

Aneurysms of the aorta are generally divided into thoracic aortic, thoracoabdominal aortic, and abdominal aortic. Most aneurysms are asymptomatic and are found on routine physical examination or when testing for another disease entity. The best intervention is to treat a patient with an aneurysm based on the symptoms of the patient and the size of the aneurysm. Size is the usual determining factor for surgical repair: thoracic aortic or thoracoabdominal aortic aneurysms larger than 6 cm and abdominal aortic aneurysms 5 cm or larger. Smaller aneurysms are followed up diagnostically for any change in size.

Patients with aortic aneurysms who are symptomatic will die within the first 24 to 48 hours if left untreated.[24] The goal of treatment is avoidance of rupture, which is dramatic and often fatal. Major risk factors for rupture include the coexisting diagnosis of hypertension or chronic obstructive pulmonary disease and larger aneurysm size.[24]

An aneurysm may be further classified as a false or true aneurysm (Figure 12-14). A false aneurysm results from a complete tear in the arterial wall. Blood leaks from the artery to form a clot. Connective tissue is then laid down around this cavity. One example of a false aneurysm is an arterial wall tear resulting from an arterial puncture in the groin area. This type of aneurysm is one of the more stable aneurysms. True aneurysms include fusiform, saccular, and dissecting aneurysms. Fusiform or spindle-shaped aneurysms are generally found in the abdominal aorta and are the most common. A saccular aneurysm is a bulbous pouching of the artery usually found in the thoracic aorta.

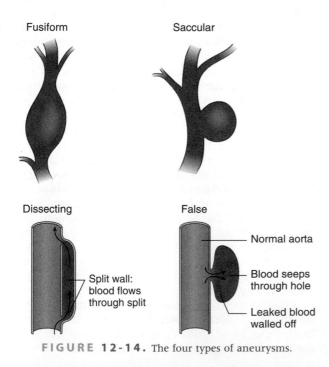

FIGURE 12-14. The four types of aneurysms.

Aortic Dissection

Second to ruptured abdominal aneurysms, aortic dissection is the next most common aortic emergency. Dissection is a tear in the intimal layer of the vessel creating a "false" lumen, causing blood flow diversion into the false lumen. Severe chest pain of a sudden nature is the most common presenting symptom of aortic dissection.[24] The pain is described as the "three Ss": sudden, sharp, and shifting pain. Patients may also have ischemic symptoms (i.e., anuria, stroke, or lower extremity ischemia), depending on which of the branch arteries are blocked by the dissection. Dissection can occur in any age group. Ascending dissections are more common in younger patients, especially those with Marfan syndrome. Descending dissections are usually seen with advanced atherosclerotic disease and are highly associated with hypertension. These are often misdiagnosed because of the copycat pain of MI or pulmonary embolism.[24] Aortic dissection is a surgical emergency.

Nursing Assessment

Knowledge of anatomy is the key factor in the treatment and care of patients with aortic aneurysms. Presentation of symptoms, intraoperative risk, and postoperative care are often location dependent. Blood flow to aortic branches may be hindered by the aneurysm itself, or embolization of thrombus may cause signs and symptoms such as chest pain, transient ischemic attacks, arm paresthesia with arch location, transient paralysis with descending aorta involvement, or abdominal or flank pain with abdominal aortic aneurysm. In the presence of atherosclerosis, lower extremity pain, buttock pain, or both, or loss of peripheral pulses may occur.[24]

Diagnostic Studies

1. Physical examination. Disparity in blood pressure measurements may be noted between the right and left arms or between the arms and legs, or a diminished pulse may be found in one of the limbs. Palpation reveals decreased or absent peripheral pulses. The patient may have a history of paresthesia, transient ischemic attacks, lower extremity or buttock claudication, and/or back or abdominal pain.
2. Imaging studies. Improved computed tomography, angiography, TEE, and MRI techniques are as accurate as aortic angiography and are usually far more rapidly obtained.

GENETICS

MARFAN SYNDROME

Many cardiovascular diseases have a genetic component. One of the more common disorders associated with a single gene variant is Marfan syndrome (MFS). MFS affects connective tissue in the blood vessels, bones, eyes, skin, lungs, and dura surrounding the brain and spinal cord.[1] This disorder demonstrates an autosomal dominant pattern of inheritance, which means that each child of an affected parent has a 50% chance of receiving a disease-causing gene variant. Most cases of MFS are caused by a mutation in the *FBN1* gene, located on chromosome 15.[2] This gene codes for a glycoprotein that is an extracellular component of connective tissue microfibrils.[4] Penetrance, or the probability that disease will occur when the gene is present, is high. About 75% of MFS is inherited, but another 25% of individuals develop the disease from de novo mutations, meaning that the mutation occurred in the egg or sperm or in the early embryo.[2] Whether inherited or a new alteration, variation exists in the number and severity of symptoms, despite inheriting a similarly altered gene. Thus, despite high penetrance, the presence of a *FBN1* MFS variant gene does not predict the onset or severity of disease.[1] Because the *FBN1* gene is not a sensitive or specific diagnostic test for disorders from altered fibrillin, the diagnosis of MFS is based on the presence of a positive family history and the number of organ systems with MFS-related defects.

The phenotypes—clinical manifestations—that are most commonly associated with MFS are aortic aneurysm (especially thoracic); dilation of the root of the aorta where it is connected to the left ventricle; tall stature with especially long arms, legs, fingers, and toes; a protruding or indented sternum; enlargement of the dural membrane surrounding the lower spine or brainstem (i.e., dural ectasia); and discoloration of the lens of the eye.[4] Individuals can also present with blebs or emphysema-like changes in the lung with possible spontaneous pneumothorax, inguinal or incisional hernias, skin stretch marks (i.e., striae), joint hypermobility, and visual disorders such as myopia or early cataracts.[2,4] Testing for the *FBN1* gene is commercially available; genetic testing is reserved for those with a positive family history or when the constellation of symptoms suggests a new mutation resulting in MFS.[3]

Management of MFS is tailored to each individual's manifestation of the disease. For persons who have cardiovascular manifestations of MFS, interventions typically include beta-blockers to slow the progression of widening for the aorta, restriction of contact sports and weight lifting, and surgical intervention when the aortic root enlargement meets specific criteria. Patients with MFS are at risk for aortic dissection and sudden death. Therefore, patients with MFS and their family members should be referred for genetic counseling, including psychosocial support and risk assessment.[2]

REFERENCES

1. Ades, L. (2007). Members of the CSANZ Cardiovascular Genetics Working Group. Guidelines for the diagnosis and management of Marfan syndrome. *Heart, Lung & Circulation, 16*, 28-30.
2. Grimes, S. J., Acheson, L. S., Matthews, A. L., & Wiesner, G. L. (2004). Clinical consult: Marfan syndrome. *Primary Care: Clinics in Office Practice 31*, 739-742.
3. National Marfan Foundation, Inc. Marfan Syndrome Foundation. (2005). *Molecular Testing for Marfan Syndrome.* Retrieved April 2, 2008, from www.marfan.org.
4. Pyeritz, R. E. (2005). Genetics and cardiovascular disease. In E. Braunwald, D. P. Zipes, P. Libby, et al. (Eds.), *Braunwald's heart disease: A textbook of cardiovascular medicine* (pp. 1977-2018). Philadelphia: Saunders.

Treatment

Surgical repair is the treatment for aortic aneurysms. Thoracic aneurysm repair is electively done in tertiary care centers. Surgery of the ascending aorta and arch requires a mediastinal open surgical approach and cardiopulmonary bypass. Endovascular repair is not an option because of possible occlusion of major arteries leading from the aorta.

Surgery of the descending aorta and the abdominal aorta may be done as an open repair or endovascularly. Both method and approach depend on the surgeon's preference and the patient's anatomy. The primary goal of surgical treatment of aortic dissection is to replace the aorta to prevent aortic rupture or proximal extension of the process.[24]

The open or conventional repair of aortic aneurysm is the endoaneurysmal repair (Figure 12-15). This requires a midline or transverse anterior approach or a retroperitoneal approach. Endovascular or aortic stent grafting is less invasive. Through a small opening in the exposed femoral artery, an intraluminal sheathed stent is introduced, placed, and deployed with fluoroscopic guidance. Once this is in place, the device excludes the aneurysm sac and significantly decreases the risk of rupture.[24] Patients and their families are informed during the preoperative teaching phase that a chance of an intraoperative event exists and may require open repair of the aneurysm. Care of the vascular surgery patient is detailed in Box 12-13.

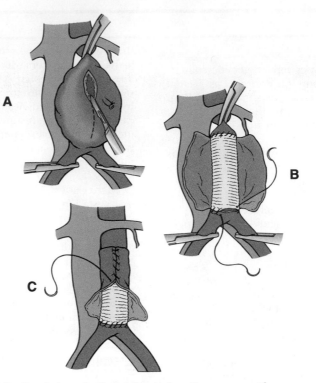

FIGURE 12-15. Surgical repair of an abdominal aortic aneurysm. The aneuysmal sac is incised **(A)**. The synthetic graft is inserted **(B)**, and the native aortic wall is sutured over the synthetic graft **(C)**. *(From O'Brien, P. G., & Bucher, L. [2007]. Medical-surgical nursing: Assessment and management of clinical problems, 7th ed. St. Louis: Mosby.)*

BOX 12-13   Nursing Interventions after Aortic Surgery

- Monitor vital signs every 1 hour: pulse; assess for tachycardia and irregular rhythms.
- Blood pressure: keep the patient normotensive; hypertension causes bleeding; give vasodilators per protocol. Hypotension causes organ ischemia; give fluids and vasoconstrictors.
- Monitor hemodynamic pressures: SvO₂, stroke index, cardiac index; PAOP and RAP; and treat per protocols.
- Assess for hypovolemia: monitor output from chest tubes, drains, and urine output every 1 hour.
- Assess for hypothermia: rewarm the patient per protocol.
- Monitor fluid and electrolytes, hemoglobin, hematocrit, renal function, and coagulation studies.
- Monitor the radial, dorsalis pedis, and posterior tibial pulses every 1 hour; use Doppler studies as needed. Assess the ankle-brachial index every 2 hours or as ordered.

- Monitor for complications: intraoperative acute myocardial infarction, dysrhythmias, heart failure, cardiac tamponade, thromboembolism, impaired renal function, pneumonia, pneumothorax, pleural effusion, cerebral ischemia, or stroke.
- Implement ventilator bundle of care (see Chapter 9), wean from mechanical ventilation and extubate as soon as possible; promote pulmonary hygiene.
- Assess wounds and provide incisional care per protocol.
- Organize nursing care; control environmental stimuli.
- Gradually increase the patient's activity.
- Provide emotional support to the patient and family; assess the family's level of understanding; discuss the postoperative course.

SvO₂, Mixed venous oxygen saturation; *PAOP,* pulmonary artery occlusion pressure; *RAP,* right atrial pressure.

CASE STUDY

Mr. Smith was admitted to the emergency department by the emergency medical service with a complaint of sudden onset of substernal chest pain while he was mowing his lawn. The paramedics have placed Mr. Smith on oxygen at 2 L/min by nasal cannula. They have started an 18-gauge intravenous line in his left antecubital area with normal saline to be kept open. They have given Mr. Smith aspirin and three sublingual nitroglycerin tablets en route. Mr. Smith states that his pain has gone from a 7, on a scale from 0 to 10, to a 3.

Jane, the emergency department nurse, places Mr. Smith on the heart monitor and notes that he is in sinus rhythm with frequent premature ventricular contractions. The paramedic states that Mr. Smith was diaphoretic, cool, and clammy on arrival of the emergency medical service at the scene. Mr. Smith is now warm and less clammy, although he still appears quite pale. Mr. Smith's blood pressure is 154/88 mm Hg, his pulse is 95 beats/min, and respiration rate is 24 breaths/min and nonlabored.

While awaiting the arrival of the emergency department physician to examine Mr. Smith, Jane starts a second IV line, gives Mr. Smith another nitroglycerin tablet, and then proceeds to obtain a brief history from Mr. Smith.

Mr. Smith is a 63-year-old white man, 220 lb, and he has been married for 41 years. He is hypertensive and diabetic, and he continues to smoke 1½ packs of cigarettes per day. He is allergic to penicillin.

While Jane is obtaining the history from Mr. Smith, she looks at the monitor and notices ventricular fibrillation. She begins cardiopulmonary resuscitation. The code team arrives, and Mr. Smith is defibrillated with 200 J using the biphasic defibrillator. His rhythm is now regular sinus with frequent premature ventricular contractions. His blood pressure is 92/56 mm Hg, his pulse is thready, and he is diaphoretic. His pupils are 4 mm, equal and reactive. His respiration rate is 16 breaths/min and shallow, and his oxygen saturation is 92%. He has developed crackles in his lower and middle lung fields bilaterally. He is not fully awake at this time, but he is moving all his extremities. A 150-mg bolus of amiodarone is given over 10 minutes, and a drip is started at 1 mg/min. Emergency laboratory tests and arterial blood gases are ordered, along with a 12-lead electrocardiogram. A request for an emergency consultation is placed to the cardiologist on call.

Mr. Smith's cardiac enzyme results return: creatine kinase, 456 units/L; creatine kinase–myocardial band, 52% of creatine phosphokinase; troponin I.5 ng/mL; and troponin T, 151 mcg/L. Electrolyte values are sodium, 143 mEq/L; potassium, 3.4 mEq/L; chloride, 109 mEq/L; carbon dioxide, 34 mEq/L; glucose, 354 mg/dL; and magnesium, 1.5 mEq/L.

Arterial blood gas values are pH, 7.32; $PaCO_2$, 49 mm Hg; PaO_2, 77 mm Hg; and bicarbonate, 24 mEq/L. His hemoglobin level is 16.9 g/dL, and his hematocrit is 47.2%.

A 12-lead electrocardiogram shows ST elevation in leads V_2, V_3, and V_4. Mr. Smith is diagnosed with an acute anterior myocardial infarction. Mr. Smith's oxygen is increased to 6 L/min by nasal cannula. Based on these study results, tissue plasminogen activator (t-PA) is administered.

QUESTIONS

1. What do Mr. Smith's cardiac enzyme values indicate about the time and extent of his myocardial infarction?
2. What would you expect his repeat troponin levels to be at the following times after his heart attack?
   a. 8 hours
   b. 12 hours
3. What complications may be anticipated for Mr. Smith related to the infusion of t-PA? What parameters would the nurse need to monitor?
4. What assessments would indicate that the t-PA was effective?

SUMMARY

This chapter focuses on the care of the patient with alterations in cardiovascular status. Geriatric patients are increasingly having medical and surgical interventions. They have even greater needs associated with the aging process (see Geriatric Considerations). The purpose of this chapter is to acquaint the critical care nurse with the problems and pathological conditions most commonly seen in the cardiovascular patient. This chapter is intended to provide a basic understanding of the cardiovascular patient that will facilitate sound clinical judgment in the planning of care that is holistic and incorporates a cooperative, interdisciplinary approach.

GERIATRIC CONSIDERATIONS

The geriatric cardiac patient needs special considerations when planning and implementing care. Many older patients react differently and with more sensitivity to medications, procedures, and other modes of treatment. Some areas of special consideration include the following:

MEDICATIONS

Great caution must be exercised when administering any medication to a geriatric patient, especially cardiac medications. Elderly persons may have greater sensitivity to these medications, they may not require the usual recommended dosage, or they may require more if they have been taking the medication in question for a long period of time. Monitor the patient closely for signs of drug effectiveness, adverse reactions, and possible interactions with other medications.

PROCEDURES

The geriatric patient may need more information, support, and attendance during diagnostic or treatment procedures. Always having someone in attendance is a major consideration. It is also necessary to answer any and all questions to the extent needed for understanding and compliance. Frequent repetition and intentionality to reassessment in the elderly patient will emphasize the importance of teaching.

SURGERY

Cardiac surgery is a major stress factor for anyone. The geriatric patient needs special attention to answer questions at the appropriate level of understanding and to provide the support for a very stressful, life-threatening procedure. Information and education are important, but be cautious of overwhelming the patient and causing greater stress.

POSTOPERATIVE

The geriatric patient has special needs in the postoperative period. The aging patient has a natural physiological process of gradually diminished circulation. Anesthesia and a major surgical procedure add to this problem area and warrant careful monitoring and continuous assessment.

FAMILY

It is imperative to have the involvement of family members or close friends. This can add a stabilizing factor that elderly patients need as they adjust to changes in treatment, activity, diet, medications, and ability to maintain activities of daily living.

REHABILITATION

Rehabilitation is a necessary part of the process for any cardiac patient, whether after a myocardial infarction or after surgery. The geriatric patient needs extra encouragement to adhere to the set regimen to progress to maximum cardiac and vascular function.

CRITICAL THINKING QUESTIONS   *evolve*

1. You are taking care of a 58-year-old post-MI patient readmitted to the unit because of recurrent chest pain, shortness of breath, and the need for IV NTG.
   a. Prioritize your actions at this time.
   b. What assessment findings regarding MI would concern you?
   c. What pertinent information from the patient's history would you want to obtain?
   d. What diagnostic tests do you anticipate?
2. Many patients now come into the hospital the same day that cardiac surgery is performed. Discuss methods for teaching patients effectively given this situation.
3. You are caring for a 63-year-old woman who has just returned to the cardiac care unit after PTCA and stent placement to the right coronary artery. Her proximal right coronary artery had a 90% occlusive lesion. She has her arterial sheath in place to the right femoral artery. She is receiving IV NTG and eptifibatide (Integrilin).
   a. What type of dysrhythmia would you anticipate if her right coronary artery were to reocclude?
   b. Prioritize your actions on her arrival.
   c. What type of assessment would you perform regarding the sheath?
4. A patient has been hospitalized three times in the past 2 months for chronic HF. What teaching and interventions can you implement to prevent rehospitalization after discharge?

> **evolve** Be sure to check out the bonus material, including free self-assessment exercises, on the Evolve Web site at http://evolve.elsevier.com/Sole.

REFERENCES

1. Albert, N. (2006). Evidence-based nursing care for patients with heart failure. *AACN Advanced Critical Care,* *17*(2), 170-185.
2. American Heart Association (AHA). (2007). *Percutaneous Coronary Interventions.* Retrieved October 12, 2007, from www.americanheart.org/presenter.jhtml?identifier=1200000.
3. Antman, E. M., Hand, M., & Armstrong, P. W. (2008). 2007 Focused update of the ACC/AHA 2004 guidelines for the management of patients with ST-elevation myocardial infarction. A report of the American College of Cardiology/American Heart Association Task Force on Practice Guidelines. *Circulation, 117,* 296-329.
4. Barnett, D., Phillips, S., & Longson, C. (2008). Cardiac resynchronisation therapy for the treatment of heart failure: NICE technology appraisal guidance. *Heart,* *93*(9), 1134-1135.
5. Brady, W. J., Ghaemmaghami, C. A., Baer, A., & Perron, A. D. (2005). Acute coronary syndromes: Pathophysiology and diagnosis. In M. P. Fink, E. Abraham, J. L. Vincent, & P. M. Kochanek (Eds.), *Textbook of critical care* (5th ed.). Philadelphia: Saunders.
6. Braslicis, V. J. (2006). Alterations of cardiovascular function. In K. L. McCance & S. E. Huether (Eds.), *Pathophysiology: The biologic basis for disease in adults and children* (5th ed., pp. 1081-1146). St. Louis: Mosby.
7. Cesario, D. A., & Dec, G. W. (2006). Implantable cardioverter-defibrillator therapy in clinical practice. *Journal of the American College of Cardiology, 47*(8), 1507-1517.
8. Chernecky, C. C., & Berger, B. J. (2008). *Laboratory tests and diagnostic procedures* (5th ed.). Philadelphia: Saunders.
9. Fleisher, L. A., Beckman, J. A., Brown, K. A., & ACC/AHA. (2007). 2007 Guidelines on perioperative cardiovascular evaluation and care for noncardiac surgery: A report of the American College of Cardiology/American Heart Association Task Force on Practice Guidelines (Writing Committee to Revise the 2002 Guidelines on Perioperative Cardiovascular Evaluation for Noncardiac Surgery). *Circulation, 16,* e418-e499. Retrieved December 30, 2007, from http://circ.ahajournals.org/cgi/content/full/116/17/e418.
10. Goldstein, J. P., & Wauthy, P. (2005). Cardiac surgery: Indications and complications. In M. P. Fink, E. Abraham, J. L. Vincent, & P. M. Kochanek (Eds.), *Textbook of critical care* (5th ed.). Philadelphia: Saunders.
11. Gregoratos, G., Abrams, J., Epstein, A., Freedman, R., Hayes, D., Hlatky, M., et al. (2002). ACC/AHA/NASPE 2002 guideline update for implantation of cardiac pacemakers and antiarrhythmia devices. Summary article: A report of the American College of Cardiology/American Heart Association Task Force on Practice Guidelines (ACC/AHA/NASPE Committee to Update the 1998 Pacemaker Guidelines). *Circulation, 106,* 2145-2161.
12. Gulanick, M., & Myers, J. L. (2007). *Nursing care plans: Nursing diagnosis and intervention* (6th ed.). St. Louis: Mosby.
13. Hayes, D. L., & Zips, D. P. (2005). Cardiac pacemakers and cardioverter-defibrillators. In M. P. Fink, E. Abraham, J. L. Vincent, & P. M. Kochanek (Eds.), *Textbook of critical care* (5th ed.). Philadelphia: Saunders.
14. Hodgson, B. B., & Kizior, R. J. (2007). *Saunders nursing drug handbook.* Philadelphia: Saunders.
15. Hollenberg, S. M. (2005). Acute coronary syndromes: Management and complications. In M. P. Fink, E. Abraham, J. L. Vincent, & P. M. Kochanek (Eds.), *Textbook of critical care* (5th ed.). Philadelphia: Saunders.
16. Institute for Clinical Systems Improvement (ICSI). (2006). *Diagnosis and treatment of chest pain and acute coronary syndrome (ACS).* Retrieved December 29, 2007, from www.ngc.gov/summary/summary.aspx?doc_id=10227&nbr=005390&string=Acute+AND+Coronary+AND+Syndrome.
17. Institute for Clinical Systems Improvement (ICSI). (2007). *Heart failure in adults.* Retrieved January 2, 2008, from www.guideline.gov/summary/summary.aspx?view_id=1&doc_id=11531.
18. Kern, M. J. (2005). Coronary blood flow and myocardial ischemia. In D. P. Zipes, P. Libby, R. O. Bonow, & E. Braunwald (Eds.), *Braunwald's heart disease: A textbook of cardiovascular medicine* (7th ed., pp. 1103-1127). Philadelphia: Saunders.
19. King, S. B., Smith, S. C., Hirshfeld, J. W., Jacobs, A. K., Morrison, D. A., Williams, D. O., et al. (2008). 2007 Focused update of the ACC/AHA/SCAI 2005 guideline update for percutaneous coronary intervention. A report of the American College of Cardiology/American Heart Association Task Force on Practice Guidelines. *Circulation, 117,* 261-295.
20. McHale, L., Wiegand, D. J., & Carlson, K. K. (2005). *AACN procedure manual for critical care* (pp. 121-169). Philadelphia: Saunders.
21. Maisch, B., & Ristic, A. D. (2005). Pericardial diseases. In M. P. Fink, E. Abraham, J. L. Vincent, & P. M. Kochanek (Eds.), *Textbook of critical care* (5th ed.). Philadelphia: Saunders.
22. McMurray, J., & Swedberg, K. (2006). Treatment of chronic heart failure: A comparison between the major guidelines. *European Heart Journal, 27*(15), 1773-1777.
23. National Heart Blood and Lung Institute. (n.d.). *Heart and valvular diseases.* Retrieved December 29, 2007, from www.nhlbi.nih.gov/health/public/web/index.htm.

24. Sellke, F. W. (2005). Aortic dissection. In M. P. Fink, E. Abraham, J. L. Vincent, & P. M. Kochanek (Eds.), *Textbook of critical care* (5th ed.). Philadelphia: Saunders.

25. Sosin, M. D., & Gregory, Y. H. (2005). Severe heart failure. In M. P. Fink, E. Abraham, J. L. Vincent, & P. M. Kochanek (Eds.), *Textbook of critical care* (5th ed.). Philadelphia: Saunders.

26. Wolff, M., & Timsit, J. F. (2005). Infectious endocarditis. In M. P. Fink, E. Abraham, J. L. Vincent, & P. M. Kochanek (Eds.), *Textbook of critical care* (5th ed.). Philadelphia: Saunders.

CHAPTER 13

Nervous System Alterations

Deborah G. Klein, MSN, RN, CCRN, CS
Christina Amidei, MSN, RN, CNRN, CCRN, CS
Joseph Haymore, MS, RN, CNRN, CCRN, ACNP

INTRODUCTION

Impaired neurological functioning, due to either disease or injury, has a profound effect on individuals and their families. In addition to being a potentially life-threatening event, neurological dysfunction alters an individual's independence and ability to care for one's self.

The brain is important in all aspects of our lives—consciousness, thinking, problem solving, judgment, memory, language, perception, emotion, movement, and autonomic function. The spinal cord is important because most sensory pathways go through the spinal cord on the way to the brain. Most motor pathways pass through the spinal cord to the rest of the body, and most reflex activity is accomplished at the spinal cord level. When these structures are damaged, a person's activities are greatly altered. In this chapter, the pathophysiology, assessment, and nursing and medical management related to increased intracranial pressure (ICP), head and traumatic brain injury (TBI), meningitis, status epilepticus (SE), cerebrovascular diseases, and spinal cord injury (SCI) are discussed.

ANATOMY AND PHYSIOLOGY OF THE NERVOUS SYSTEM

Cells of the Nervous System

The nervous system is composed of two types of cells, neurons and neuroglia. The *neuron*, or nerve cell, is the basic functioning unit of the nervous system and serves as the transmitter of nerve impulses (Figure 13-1). Of the billions of neurons in the central nervous system (CNS), three fourths are located in the cerebral cortex. Each neuron is unique in character, and its features are determined by its specific function.

One function of a neuron is to receive input from other neurons via dendrites and axons. *Axons* carry nervous impulses *away* from the cell body of the neuron while *dendrites* conduct impulses *toward* the cell body. Axons and dendrites are collectively referred to as *nerve fibers*. Each neuron possesses one axon, although it may have numerous dendrites. Some axons are surrounded by a white, protein-lipid complex *(myelin)* that is formed by Schwann cells in the peripheral nervous system (PNS) and by oligodendrocytes in the CNS. Along the axons are periodic constrictions that are nonmyelinated. These areas are known as nodes of Ranvier, and they facilitate faster and more efficient impulse conduction (see Figure 13-1).

Neuroglial cells (glia) constitute the supportive tissue and form the supporting structures for the CNS. These cells are approximately 5 to 10 times as numerous as neurons. Because neuroglial cells are capable of division, most primary CNS tumors originate from this cell type. Four types of neuroglial cells exist, each with specific functions. *Microglia* act as phagocytic scavenger cells when nervous tissue is damaged. *Astrocytes*, which means "star shaped," play a critical role in the basic structure of the blood-brain barrier. They provide nutrients for neurons and respond to brain trauma by forming scar tissue. Astrocytes also play a role in the transport of nutrients, gases, and waste products among neurons, the vascular system, and cerebrospinal fluid (CSF). *Oligodendrocytes* are responsible for myelin formation. *Ependymal* cells produce specialized glial tissue that forms the lining of the ventricles of the brain and the central canal of the spinal cord and play a role in production of CSF.

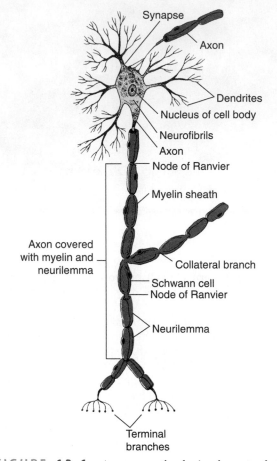

Synapse

Axon

Dendrites

Nucleus of cell body

Neurofibrils

Axon

Node of Ranvier

Myelin sheath

Axon covered
with myelin and
neurilemma

Collateral branch

Schwann cell
Node of Ranvier

Neurilemma

Terminal
branches

FIGURE 13-1. A neuron, the basic element of the nervous system. *(From Black, J. M., & Hawks, J. A. [2005]. Medical-surgical nursing: Clinical management for positive outcomes [7th ed.]. Philadelphia: Saunders.)*

Transmission of Nerve Impulses

The same principles of depolarization and repolarization that occur in the cardiac cycle apply in the conduction of a nerve impulse. An action potential alters the permeability of the cell membrane to certain ions, resulting in changes in the membrane potential. Sodium rapidly enters the cell and potassium exits the cell, creating an *action potential*. This positive ionic change is transmitted along the length of the neuron and is termed a *wave of depolarization*; the impulse is then conducted from one neuron to the next. The cell returns to a resting state in a process termed *repolarization*.

In myelinated neurons, the myelin sheath is non-insulated at the nodes of Ranvier. This noninsulated feature facilitates conduction of impulses along the neuron because the action potential hops from one node to the next. This is called *saltatory conduction*, which causes a rapid velocity of conduction and con-

serves energy. The speed of the impulse depends on both the thickness of the myelin and the distance between nodes.

Synapses

A *synapse* is the junction where one neuron transmits an impulse to another neuron or muscle cell. The three structures necessary for impulse transmission at the synapse are the presynaptic terminals (affector cell/neuron), the synaptic cleft, and the postsynaptic membrane (effector cell/neuron).

Presynaptic terminals are either predominantly inhibitory or excitatory. The neurotransmitter secretions from these terminals arise from the synaptic vesicles of the axon. Mitochondria within the axon supply the adenosine triphosphate (ATP) to form new transmitter secretions. The microscopic space between the presynaptic terminal and the receptor area of the effector cells is the synaptic cleft. The part of the effector membrane that is closest to the presynaptic terminals is the postsynaptic membrane.

As an action potential spreads through the presynaptic terminal, the membrane depolarizes, allowing contents from the synaptic vesicles to be emptied into the cleft. The neurotransmitter that is released binds to the effector membrane and changes the permeability of the postsynaptic membrane, resulting in either excitation or inhibition of the neuron, depending on the type of chemical transmitter released.

Neurotransmitters

Neurotransmitters are chemical substances that, when released from the synaptic vesicle, excite, inhibit, or modify the response of an effector cell. It is generally believed that each neuron releases the same neurotransmitter at all its separate terminals. Table 13-1 provides a summary of common neurotransmitters and their actions.

Cerebral Circulation

The cerebral circulation must provide sufficient blood to supply oxygen, glucose, and nutrients to the cerebral tissues. The brain does not have any effective energy stores; therefore, even a brief interruption in blood supply may result in significant ischemic tissue damage. The brain receives approximately 750 mL of blood per minute, or 15% to 20% of the total resting cardiac output.[9]

The blood supply of the brain arises from two major sets of arteries, the carotid arteries (anterior circulation) and the vertebral arteries (posterior circulation).

TABLE 13-1 Common Neurotransmitters and Their Actions

Neurotransmitter	Action
Acetylcholine	Generally excitation; inhibitory effect on some of parasympathetic nervous system
Dopamine	Inhibitory effect
Norepinephrine	Generally excitation; inhibitory effect on postsynaptic neurons
Serotonin	Inhibitory effect
Glutamate	Generally excitation
Gamma-aminobutyric acid (GABA)	Inhibitory effect
Substance P	Excitation
Endorphin	Excitation to systems that inhibit pain

Specifically, the left common carotid artery originates from the aortic arch, and the right common carotid artery originates from the innominate artery. The common carotid arteries then branch to form the external and internal carotid arteries. The external carotid artery supplies the face, scalp, and other extracranial structures. Each internal carotid artery terminates by dividing into anterior cerebral and middle cerebral arteries. The anterior cerebral artery and its branches supply the medial aspects of the motor cortex and the frontal lobes. The middle cerebral artery comprises the principal blood supply of the frontal, temporal, and parietal lobes. Almost 90% of all strokes involve this artery.

The paired vertebral arteries originate from the subclavian arteries and enter the skull through the foramen magnum. The vertebral arteries and their branches supply the upper spinal cord, medulla, and cerebellum before joining at the pons to form the basilar artery. The basilar artery sends branches to the cerebellum, medulla, pons, and internal ear. Then the basilar artery bifurcates and terminates as the posterior cerebral arteries, which serve the medial portions of the occipital and inferior temporal lobes.

These two arterial systems interconnect at the base of the brain via communicating arteries. The posterior communicating artery connects the internal carotid artery to the posterior cerebral artery, and the anterior communicating artery connects the two anterior cerebral arteries. This interconnection is known as the cerebral arterial circle (*circle of Willis*) (Figure 13-2).

Cerebral veins, which do not have a muscle layer or valves, empty blood into venous sinuses located throughout the cranium. Since the venous sinuses play a role in absorption of CSF, they parallel the ventricular system rather than the arterial system, as in most other organs. The venous blood is emptied into the internal jugular vein and, ultimately, the superior vena cava, which returns the blood to the heart.

Brain Metabolism

The continuous activity of the brain results in large metabolic energy needs. Glucose is the brain's sole source of energy for cellular function. Because the brain is unable to store glucose, it requires a continuous supply of glucose to maintain normal brain metabolism. If the cerebral glucose level drops below 70 mg/dL, confusion may develop. Seizures may occur if the glucose level continues to decrease. Cellular damage develops when the brain glucose level drops to less than 20 mg/dL.

Cerebral glucose metabolism is divided into aerobic and anaerobic metabolism. Because anaerobic metabolism produces only a minimal amount of ATP, aerobic metabolism is used to meet the high cerebral energy demands. If the brain is deprived of oxygen, even for a few minutes, metabolism changes from aerobic to the less efficient anaerobic cellular metabolism.

Maintaining a constant *cerebral blood flow (CBF)* is essential to sustain normal cerebral metabolism. In the absence of adequate blood flow, cell membrane integrity is lost, allowing extracellular fluid to flow into the cell, causing edema. The extracellular environment becomes acidotic as a result of lactic acid production from anaerobic metabolism, and cellular damage ensues. Neurological manifestations occur owing to slowing of electrical activity. If an anoxic state lasts for 5 minutes or longer at normal body temperature, cerebral neurons are destroyed and cannot regenerate.[9]

A process called autoregulation ensures continuous CBF regardless of the mean arterial pressure (MAP). *Autoregulation* is defined as the ability of cerebral blood vessels to adjust their diameter to arterial pressure changes within the brain. If a rapid increase in MAP occurs, the cerebral vessels constrict to prevent excessive distention of the cerebral arteries. Conversely, if the MAP drops, the cerebral blood vessels dilate to maintain normal CBF and to prevent cerebral ischemia.

The cerebral vessels are also sensitive to the chemical regulators to maintain CBF: the partial pressure of arterial carbon dioxide ($PaCO_2$) or oxygen (PaO_2),

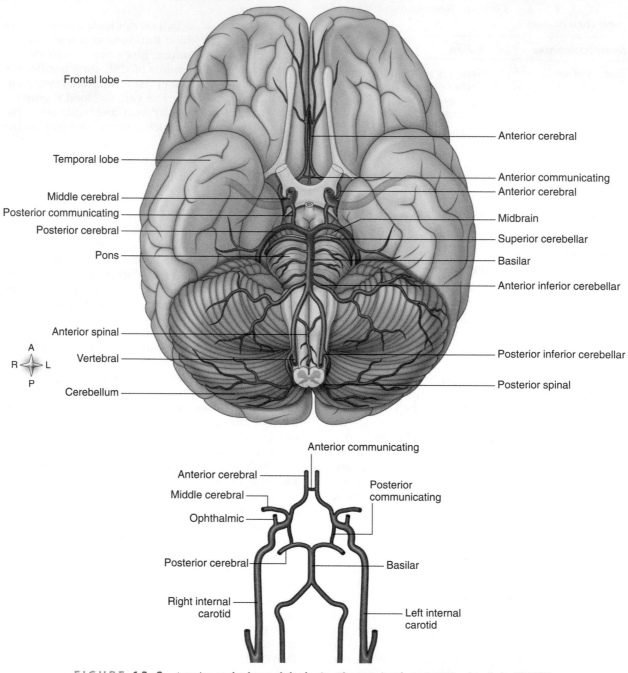

Frontal lobe

Temporal lobe

Middle cerebral

Posterior communicating

Posterior cerebral

Pons

Anterior spinal

Vertebral

Cerebellum

Anterior cerebral

Anterior communicating

Anterior cerebral

Midbrain

Superior cerebellar

Basilar

Anterior inferior cerebellar

Posterior inferior cerebellar

Posterior spinal

A
R L
P

Anterior communicating

Anterior cerebral

Middle cerebral

Ophthalmic

Posterior communicating

Posterior cerebral

Basilar

Right internal carotid

Left internal carotid

FIGURE 13-2. Arteries at the base of the brain. The arteries that compose the circle of Willis are the two anterior cerebral arteries, joined to each other by the anterior communicating two short segments of the internal carotids, off of which the posterior communicating arteries connect to the posterior cerebral arteries. *(From Thibodeau, G. A., & Patton, K. T. [2007]. Anatomy and physiology [6th ed.]. St. Louis: Mosby.)*

and the hydrogen ion concentration (*chemical auto-regulation*). Carbon dioxide is the most potent agent influencing CBF. When the $PaCO_2$ is greater than 45 mm Hg, cerebral blood vessels respond by vasodilating, which increases CBF. A low $PaCO_2$ causes the cerebral arteries to constrict, leading to decreased CBF and decreased tissue perfusion. Cerebral arteries are less sensitive to changes in PaO_2. The CBF is not affected until the PaO_2 is 50 mm Hg or less. This low PaO_2 causes cerebral hypoxia, resulting in vasodilation of the cerebral vessels to increase CBF and oxygen delivery. If the PaO_2 is not raised, anaerobic metabolism begins and results in lactic acid accumulation. The increased hydrogen ion concentration causes more vasodilation to facilitate the removal of acidic end products from cerebral tissue.[9]

Cerebral perfusion pressure (CPP) is the pressure required to perfuse the brain. CPP is calculated as the difference between the MAP and the ICP (normal, 0 to 15 mm Hg): CPP = MAP − ICP. The normal CPP in an adult is between 60 and 100 mm Hg and must be maintained at 70 mm Hg or greater in those with brain pathology. Any factor that decreases MAP and/or increases ICP decreases CPP. CPP determines CBF; therefore, ischemia or infarction can occur if the CPP is inadequate. Measures to promote adequate CPP include lowering of increased ICP or, if this is not possible, increasing MAP to offset the effects of ICP on CPP. Often MAP will rise in the presence of increased ICP; lowering MAP in this circumstance may actually decrease CPP and should be avoided.[9]

Brain Barrier System

The *blood-brain barrier system* protects the brain from toxic elements and disease-causing organisms that may circulate in the blood. The blood-brain barrier operates on the concept of tight junctions between adjacent cells and selective permeability that prevents the free movement of materials from the vascular bed into the brain. Typically, large molecules do not cross the blood-brain barrier, whereas small molecules cross easily. Water, carbon dioxide, oxygen, and glucose freely cross the cerebral capillaries. The movement of other substances into the brain is dependent on the chemical dissociation, lipid solubility, and protein-binding potential. Infections, tumors, and certain other disease states may also alter the blood-brain barrier.

Ventricular System and Cerebrospinal Fluid

The four *ventricles* of the adult brain are hollow spaces lined by ependyma. Specialized epithelium in the ventricular wall, called the *choroid plexus*, produce CSF. A smaller amount of CSF is secreted from the ependymal cells that line the ventricles, and the blood vessels of the meninges and the brain. CSF is continually secreted from these surfaces at about 500 mL per day, or 18 to 24 mL per hour.[9] On average, 150 mL of CSF is in the ventricles and subarachnoid space at any given time. The CSF provides a cushioning effect during rapid movements of the head and exerts a considerable buoyant effect on the brain. It also plays a role in metabolic function of the brain.

CSF flows from the two lateral ventricles into the third ventricle through the foramen of Monro. From the third ventricle, CSF flows through the aqueduct of Sylvius into the fourth ventricle. From there, the CSF flow is directed through the foramina of Luschka and Magendie into the cisterna and subarachnoid space (Figure 13-3). After circulating around the brain and spinal cord, CSF is reabsorbed into the venous sinuses of the brain through the arachnoid villi, which are dural projections from the arachnoid space.

FUNCTIONAL AND STRUCTURAL DIVISIONS OF THE CENTRAL NERVOUS SYSTEM

Meninges

Meninges cover the brain and spinal cord and consist of three layers: dura mater, arachnoid mater, and pia mater (Figure 13-4). The *dura mater* is the outermost covering and has two layers. The outer surface adheres to the skull, and the inner layer produces prominent folds (falx cerebri, tentorium cerebelli, falx cerebelli) that subdivide the interior cranial cavity to support and protect the brain. The inner dura mater also covers the spine. The *arachnoid mater* is located inside the dura mater. It is a delicate, avascular layer that loosely encloses the brain and spine. The *pia mater* closely adheres to the brain's outer surface and contains a network of blood vessels. The pia mater surrounding the spinal cord is less vascular.

Actual or potential spaces exist between the meningeal layers. The epidural space is a potential space between the skull and the outer dura mater. The subdural space is between the dura mater and the arachnoid mater and is filled with a small amount of lubricating fluid. The subarachnoid space, a considerable area between the arachnoid and pia mater, contains circulating CSF. In addition, the subarachnoid space has a vast network of arteries traveling through it.

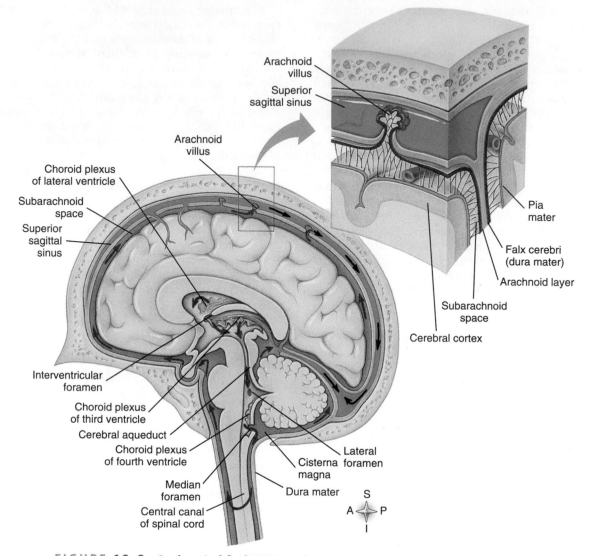

FIGURE 13-3. Cerebrospinal fluid (CSF) circulation. *Arrows* represent the route of CSF. CSF is produced in the ventricles and returns to the venous circulation in the superior sagittal sinus. *(From Thibodeau, G. A., & Patton, K. T. [2007]. Anatomy and physiology [6th ed.]. St. Louis: Mosby.)*

Brain (Encephalon)

The brain is approximately 2% of body weight. The average weight of a man's brain is approximately 1400 g, and the brain of a woman weighs less. Brain weight decreases with aging, primarily because of neuronal loss. The brain is divided into three major areas: the cerebrum, the brainstem, and the cerebellum (Figure 13-5).

Cerebrum

The *cerebrum* (Figure 13-6) is composed of the right and left cerebral hemispheres, which are separated by a deep longitudinal fissure. The cerebral hemi-spheres are joined by the *corpus callosum*, a thick area of nerve fibers. This provides a pathway for fibers to travel from one hemisphere to the other and thus makes the two hemispheres intricately connected.

Individuals have a dominant hemisphere. For example, 90% of the population are right-handed and the left side of the brain dominates. However, the right and left hemispheres specialize in different complex functions, regardless of handedness. This concept is known as *hemisphericity*. The left hemisphere specializes in language for most individuals and dominates skilled and gesturing hand movements. The right hemisphere specializes in the perception of certain nonspeech auditory stimuli such

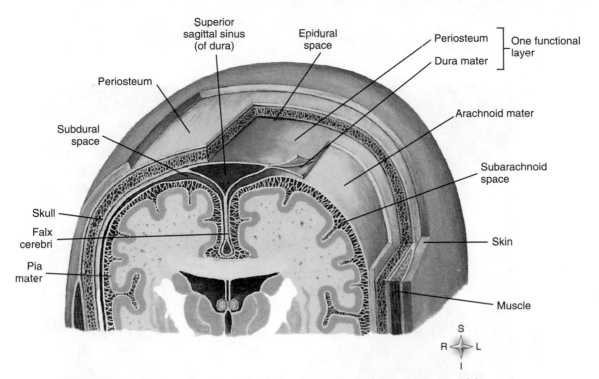

FIGURE 13-4. Frontal section of the skull and brain showing the relationships of the meninges. *(From Thibodeau, G. A., & Patton, K. T. [2007]. Anatomy and physiology [6th ed.]. St. Louis: Mosby.)*

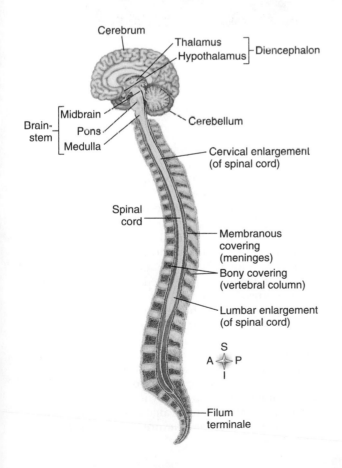

FIGURE 13-5. Major divisions of the central nervous system. *(From Thibodeau, G. A., & Patton, K. T. [2007]. Anatomy and physiology [6th ed.]. St. Louis: Mosby.)*

as melodies, crying, and laughing. The right hemisphere also specializes in the ability to perceive and visualize spatial relationships. Both sides of the brain communicate with each other to facilitate complex functions.

The surface of each hemisphere appears wrinkled because of the numerous raised areas, called *gyri* (Figure 13-7). Each gyrus folds into another, causing the convoluted appearance and substantially increasing the surface area of the brain. The surface of the cerebral hemisphere is approximately six cells deep and is called the *cerebral cortex*, or gray matter. Beneath the cortex is a layer of white matter consisting of mostly myelinated axons, which serve as association and projection pathways.

A *fissure*, or *sulcus*, is a separation in the cerebral hemisphere. The fissures serve as important divisions or landmarks (see Figure 13-7). The longitudinal fissure separates the cerebral hemispheres into left and right sections. The lateral, or Sylvian fissure, divides the frontal and temporal lobes. The central, or Rolandic, fissure separates the frontal and the parietal

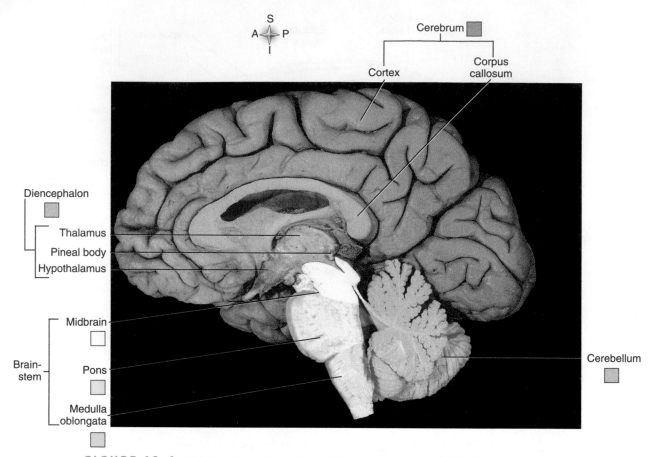

S
A — P
I

Cerebrum ▨

Cortex   Corpus
                callosum

Diencephalon
▨

Thalamus
Pineal body
Hypothalamus

Midbrain
Brain-
stem   Pons

Medulla
oblongata
▨

Cerebellum
▨

FIGURE 13-6. The structures of the brain (midsagittal section). *(From Thibodeau, G. A., & Patton, K. T. [2007]. Anatomy and physiology [6th ed.]. St. Louis: Mosby.)*

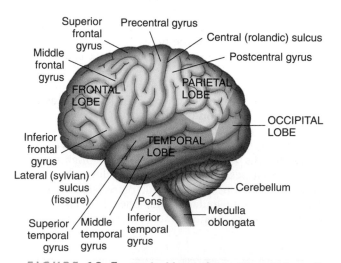

Superior   Precentral gyrus
frontal
gyrus   Central (rolandic) sulcus
Middle
frontal   Postcentral gyrus
gyrus
            PARIETAL
FRONTAL   LOBE
LOBE
                         OCCIPITAL
                         LOBE
Inferior   TEMPORAL
frontal   LOBE
gyrus
Lateral (sylvian)
sulcus   Cerebellum
(fissure)
            Pons
Superior Middle Inferior Medulla
temporal temporal temporal oblongata
gyrus   gyrus   gyrus

FIGURE 13-7. Cerebral hemispheres. *(From McCance, K. L., & Huether, S. E. [2006]. Pathophysiology: The biologic basis for disease in adults and children [5th ed.]. St. Louis: Mosby.)*

lobes. The parieto-occipital fissure separates the occipital lobe from the parietal and temporal lobes.

The cerebrum is divided into lobes (see Figure 13-7). Each lobe has a specific function. The *frontal lobes*, situated anterior to the central sulcus and above the lateral fissure, have as their major functions conscious thought, abstract thinking, judgment, and initiation of contralateral (opposite side of the body) voluntary motor activity. The motor expressive component of language is located in the left inferior frontal gyrus and is known as *Broca's area*. The prefrontal area of these lobes is concerned with affective reactions, memory, and concentration.

The *parietal lobes* extend from the central sulcus to the parieto-occipital fissure. The primary responsibilities of this lobe are sensory functioning, sensory perception, association, and processing of general sensory modalities at a higher level.

The *temporal lobes* are located in the middle cranial fossa under the Sylvian fissures. They serve as the primary auditory areas, which receive input from the auditory pathway and process auditory information. The auditory association area occupies a portion of the temporal gyrus and is known as *Wernicke's area*. The insula, considered the fifth cerebral hemisphere, are located medial to the temporal lobes and have memory and social behavior functions.

The *occipital lobes* are wedge shaped, extending posteriorly from the parieto-occipital fissures. They contain the primary cortex for visual reception and association.

The *basal ganglia* are masses of gray matter located deep within the cerebral hemisphere. Composed of several sections, these structures influence motor control of fine body movements, particularly of the hands and lower extremities.

Diencephalon

The *diencephalon* is the uppermost portion of the brainstem between the cerebrum and the midbrain. It is divided into four paired regions: thalamus, hypothalamus, subthalamus, and epithalamus. The *thalamus* is the largest structure within the diencephalon and integrates all bodily sensations except smell. The thalamus assists in recognizing pain, touch, and temperature, and relays sensory information to the cerebrum. It also plays a role in emotions, arousal and alertness, and complex reflexes.

The *hypothalamus* acts as the CNS regulatory centers for the autonomic nervous system (ANS). The general functions of the hypothalamus include temperature control, water balance, control of appetite and thirst, cardiovascular regulation, sleep-wakefulness cycle, circadian rhythms, and sexual activity. The hypothalamus also controls the release of hormones from the pituitary gland.

Brainstem

The *brainstem* is at the central core of the brain and controls vital functions. The major divisions of the brainstem are the midbrain, pons, and medulla (see Figure 13-6). The *midbrain*, also known as the mesencephalon, is a short segment of brainstem lying between the diencephalon and the pons. It contains nuclei of cranial nerves III (oculomotor) and IV (trochlear). The midbrain carries impulses down from the cerebrum and controls the wakefulness of the brain via the reticular activating system. It also serves as the center for auditory and visual reflexes.

The *pons* is seated between the midbrain and the medulla. It contains nuclei of cranial nerves V (trigeminal), VI (abducens), VII (facial), and VIII (vestibulocochlear). In conjunction with the medulla, the pons controls the rate and duration of respirations.

The *medulla oblongata* is situated between the pons and the spinal cord. It contains nuclei of cranial nerves IX (glossopharyngeal), X (vagus), XI (accessory), and XII (hypoglossal). The functions of the medulla include the regulation of the basic rhythm of respiration, rate and strength of the pulse, and vasomotor activity. In addition, neurons within the medulla regulate certain reflexes including sneezing, swallowing, coughing, and vomiting.

Cerebellum

The *cerebellum* is located in the posterior fossa of the cranium (see Figures 13-5 and 13-6). It is attached to the pons, medulla, and midbrain by three paired cerebellar peduncles. The peduncles receive input from the spinal cord and brainstem and send it to the cerebellar cortex. The functions of equilibrium, fine movement, muscle tone, and coordination are mediated by the cerebellum.

Specialized Systems within the Central Nervous System

The *limbic system* and the *reticular activating system* (RAS) are two important systems with the brain. These systems incorporate various structures within the brain to provide primitive control of emotional responses and arousal. The major structures of the limbic system include the amygdala (reward and fear stimuli), hippocampus (long-term memory), cingulate gyrus (attention and cognition), hypothalamus, and thalamus.

The RAS is a complex system involving the pons, midbrain, hypothalamus, and thalamus. The RAS also interacts with the cerebral hemispheres, especially the frontal lobes. If the RAS is intact, a person is capable of being aroused. When the RAS is impaired, the person experiences a decreased level of consciousness (LOC), the most extreme being coma.[19]

Spinal Cord

The *spinal cord* is located within and protected by the vertebral column and surrounded by the meninges. It is continuous with the medulla oblongata. The spinal cord usually measures 18 inches (46 cm) in the adult. The spinal canal is a continuation of the subarachnoid space and contains CSF.

The spinal cord has 31 segments, each of which gives off a pair of spinal nerves. The segments include 8 cervical, 12 thoracic, 5 lumbar, 5 sacral, and 1 coccygeal (Figure 13-8). The spinal nerves, part of the peripheral nervous system, transmit information from the periphery to the spinal cord, and from the spinal cord to the periphery. These nerves innervate the skin and musculature of most of the body. Each spinal nerve consists of a *dorsal root* (posterior) and

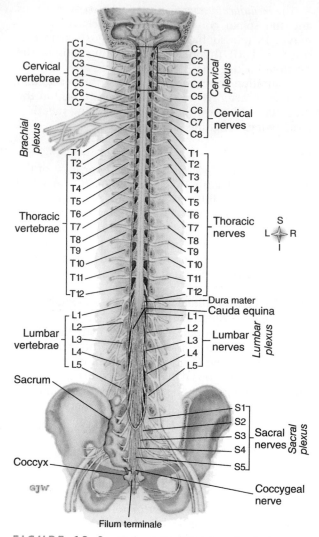

FIGURE 13-8. Each of the 31 pairs of spinal nerves exit the spinal cavity from the vertebrae. The names of the vertebrae are listed on the left, and the corresponding spinal nerves are listed on the right. *(From Thibodeau, G. A., & Patton, K. T. [2007]. Anatomy and physiology [6th ed.]. St. Louis: Mosby.)*

ventral root (anterior). The dorsal roots convey afferent impulses (sensory input) into the spinal cord from skin segments that represent specific areas of the body known as *dermatomes*. The ventral roots carry efferent impulses (muscle signals) from the spinal cord to the body. A dermatome chart traces the spinal nerves to their point of skin innervation and provides anatomical clues about the level of injury or dysfunction (Figure 13-9).

Four types of nerve fibers make up the spinal nerves. *Motor fibers*, which originate in the ventral horn of the spinal cord, have efferent fibers that relay motor impulses from the CNS to skeletal muscles. *Sensory fibers*, which begin in the dorsal horn of the spinal cord, have afferent fibers that convey sensory impulses from organs and muscles to the CNS. *Meningeal fibers* relay sensory and vasomotor innervation to the spinal meninges. *Autonomic fibers* are discussed in the section on the ANS.

Plexuses

Plexuses are networks of interlacing nerves. The spinal nerves interconnect in three areas: the cervical, brachial, and lumbosacral plexuses. These plexuses innervate specific areas of the body and form the major peripheral nerves. The *cervical plexus* includes spinal nerves C1 to C4 and innervates the muscles of the neck and shoulders. The phrenic nerve originates in this plexus and supplies the diaphragm. The *brachial plexus* comprises spinal nerves C4 to C8 and T1 and innervates the arms via the radial and ulnar nerves. The *lumbosacral plexus* is formed by spinal nerves L1 to L5 and S1 to S3. The femoral nerve arises from the lumbar plexus and the sciatic nerve from the sacral plexus, and both innervate the legs (see Figure 13-8).

Peripheral Nervous System

The PNS is the portion of the nervous system that is situated outside the CNS. It includes 12 paired cranial nerves and 31 paired spinal nerves, along with the ANS.

The 12 pairs of *cranial nerves* originate in the brain and brainstem and exit from the cranial cavity. Cranial nerves have sensory or motor functions, or both. These nerves are primarily responsible for the innervation of structures in the head and neck. A summary of the functions of the cranial nerves and their assessment in the critically ill patient is provided in Table 13-2.

Autonomic Nervous System

The ANS comprises motor nerves to visceral effectors: cardiac muscle, smooth muscle, adrenal medulla, and various glands, including salivary, gastric, and sweat glands. The ANS controls visceral activities at an unconscious level. The ANS consists of the *sympathetic nervous system* and the *parasympathetic nervous system*. These parallel systems act to regulate visceral organs in opposing ways—one system stimulates effects while the other inhibits—to maintain homeostasis.

The *sympathetic nervous system* is known as the thoracolumbar system because the nerve fibers originate in the thoracic and lumbar regions of the spinal cord.

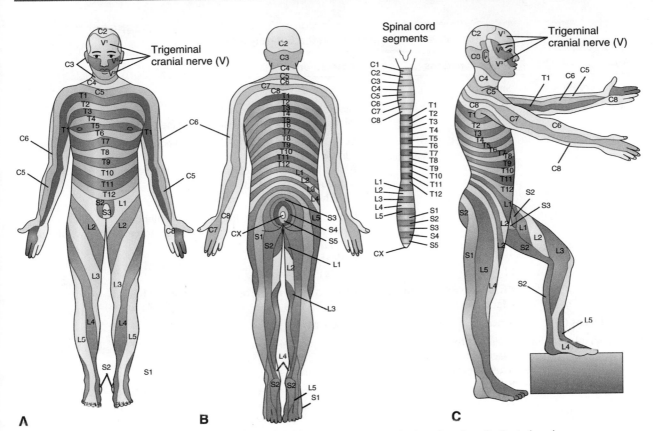

FIGURE 13-9. Dermatome distribution of spinal nerves. **A,** Anterior view. **B,** Posterior view. **C,** Side view. *(From Thibodeau, G. A., & Patton, K. T. [2007]. Anatomy and physiology [6th ed.]. St. Louis: Mosby.)*

This system contains a chain of ganglia located on both sides of the vertebrae. The sympathetic nervous system is sometimes called the *fight-or-flight* system because it is activated and dominates during stressful periods. Most sympathetic neurons release the neurotransmitter *norepinephrine* at the visceral effector. Sympathetic impulses cause vasoconstriction in the skin and viscera, vasodilation in the skeletal muscles, an increase in the heart rate and force of contraction, an increase in blood pressure (BP), dilation of the bronchioles, an increase in sweat gland activity, dilation of the pupils, a decrease in peristalsis, and contraction of the pilomotor muscles (gooseflesh).

The *parasympathetic nervous system* is known as the craniosacral system because the preganglionic fibers originate at certain cranial nerves and in the sacral spinal cord. The axons are long, and ganglia are situated adjacent to or within specific organs. The parasympathetic system is dominant in nonstressful situations. It stimulates visceral activities associated with maintenance of normal functions. The effects of parasympathetic nervous system stimulation induce a return of systems to a normal state of functioning. All neurons within the parasympathetic nervous system release the neurotransmitter *acetylcholine* at the visceral effector.

Effects of Aging

Aging affects the nervous system in a variety of ways (see Geriatric Considerations). Loss of myelin and altered conduction may result in a decrease in reaction time of specific nerves. Cellular degeneration and death of neurons may result in a decreased speed and intensity of reflexes with an increased risk of injury. Decreased sensation may reduce the ability to taste, smell, see, and feel pain. Proprioception (one's position in space) is altered, resulting in an increased risk for falling. Hardening of the pupil sphincter may result in a decreased responsiveness to light, especially when moving from one level of lighting to another. Increased rigidity of the iris may result in decreased pupil size, with the need for more light for visual clarity. Altered motor functioning may result in physiological tremors, decreased neuromuscular control, change in posture, a shuffling gait, and a short stride, resulting in an increased risk for falls. Muscle atrophy may also be present.

TABLE 13-2   The Cranial Nerves and Assessment in the Critically Ill Patient

Nerve	Major Functions	Assessment
I—Olfactory (S)	Smell	Not assessed.
II—Optic (S)	Vision	Assess gross ability to see. Evaluate pupillary response to light (see CN III).
III—Oculomotor (M)	Movement of eyes; pupillary constriction and accommodation	Evaluate pupil size (mm), shape, and equality with bright penlight in dimly lit room. Assess for direct and consensual reaction to light; rate as brisk, sluggish, or nonreactive. See CN IV for eye movement.
IV—Trochlear (M)	Movement of eyes	CNs III, IV, and VI test extraocular movements. If possible, assess whether eyes are able to move medial, lateral, and up and down. Evaluate if eyes move together. Assess for nystagmus.
V—Trigeminal (S/M)	Chewing; sensation of scalp, face, teeth	Assess corneal reflex; observe for bilateral blink.
VI—Abducens (M)	Movement of eyes	See CN IV.
VII—Facial (M)	Facial expression; lacrimation, salivation; taste anterior tongue	Assess for facial expressions and symmetry; if possible, ask patient to smile, frown, and puff cheeks. Assess corneal reflex.
VIII—Auditory (S)	Hearing (cochlear) Equilibrium (vestibular)	Assess response to verbalization (gross hearing ability). In unconscious patients with stable cervical spine, assess *oculocephalic reflex* (doll's eye): turn the patient's head quickly from side to side while holding the eyes open. Note movement of eyes. The doll's eye reflex is present if the eyes move bilaterally in the opposite direction of the head movement. In the unconscious patient, the caloric irrigation test is done to assess the *oculovestibular reflex* (may be more sensitive than the doll's eye): elevate the head of bed to 30 degrees, assess for intact tympanic membrane, irrigate the ear canal with cold water. Bilateral eye movement towards the irrigated ear indicates an intact reflex.
IX—Glossopharyngeal (S/M)	Swallowing; taste posterior tongue; general sensation pharynx	CNs IX and X evaluated together. Evaluate cough and gag reflex in response to suctioning the endotracheal tube and mouth. Assess ability to manage oral secretions by swallowing.
X—Vagus (S/M)	Swallowing and laryngeal control; parasympathetic function	See above.
XI—Spinal accessory (M)	Movement of head and shoulders	Assess ability to move/shrug shoulders and turn head.
XII—Hypoglossal (M)	Movement of tongue	Not usually assessed; if patient able to follow commands, assess ability to protrude and/or move tongue from side to side.

CN, Cranial nerve; *M,* motor; *S,* sensory; *S/M,* sensory and motor.

GERIATRIC CONSIDERATIONS

- Subdural hematomas are more common in the older population because of cerebral atrophy and subsequent increase in size of the subdural space. A large amount of blood can accumulate before the patient demonstrates overt signs and symptoms. Subtle changes in mental status may indicate a substantial intracranial hemorrhage.
- Assessment of admission Glasgow Coma Scale scores may underestimate the extent of brain injury in the older patient.
- The effects of certain medications used to decrease intracranial pressure (osmotic and loop diuretics, barbiturates) should be closely monitored because of the older patient's decreased ability to absorb, metabolize, and/or excrete these drugs.
- Assessment of preexisting renal insufficiency and use of diuretics is necessary because the use of these drugs may place older patients at risk of hypokalemia or hyponatremia when they receive medications to reduce intracranial pressure.
- In the older patient, elevating the head of the bed to decrease intracranial pressure may compromise an already diminished cerebral blood flow. Continuous assessment of neurological function and/or cerebral perfusion pressure is necessary to avoid decreasing brain blood flow.
- Central cord syndrome is more common in the older population and may result from hyperextension of an osteoarthritic spine.

Assessment

A thorough history provides information about the patient's condition. Ideally, the patient is the primary source of the historical data. If the patient is unable to give a history, family or friends should supply information related to symptoms, onset, progression, and chronology of the event. Comorbidities and contributing factors must also be considered. If pain is a presenting symptom, information must be obtained about the location, onset, type, duration, presence of other symptoms, and what makes the pain better or worse. If the patient is admitted secondary to nervous system trauma, specific information concerning the mechanism of injury, immediate posttrauma care, and emergency treatments is needed.

An initial baseline neurological assessment, along with ongoing assessments, assists in monitoring the patient's condition and response to treatments and nursing interventions. When performing a neurological assessment, the critical care nurse focuses on mental status, LOC, cranial nerve functioning, motor status, and sensory function. In addition to using tools such as the Glasgow Coma Scale (GCS), a narrative assessment may be written to document findings. It is also beneficial for nurses to review specific assessment findings with each other at the patient's bedside during the hand-off communication at change-of-shift report. Because many neurological changes represent life-threatening conditions that require emergent treatment, it is important for the nurse to immediately report adverse changes in assessment findings to the physician.

CLINICAL ALERT
Neurological Assessment

Perform the neurological assessment with the nurse who just cared for the patient. This ensures complete understanding of the prior documented assessment by the receiving nurse and quick recognition of neurological changes.

Mental Status. When assessing a patient's mental status, the critical care nurse tests arousal (consciousness), expressive and receptive language, and memory.

The GCS is a standardized tool to assess neurological status. It scores two aspects of the patient's LOC: arousal (awareness of the environment) and cognition (demonstrates an understanding of what the observer says through an ability to follow commands). The components of the GCS are *eye opening, best verbal response,* and *best motor response* (Figure 13-10). To assess arousal and cognition, the patient is asked to follow a verbal command. If the patient does not respond to the command, a noxious stimulus is used to elicit a response. A painful stimulus is applied by either a firm pressure to the patient's nailbed (use a pencil or pen), a trapezium squeeze (using thumb and two fingers, pinch the trapezius muscle where the head meets the shoulder), supraorbital pressure (place pressure on the notch felt along the bony ridge above the top of the eye), or sternal pressure (rub the center of sternum using knuckles of clenched fist). It is important not to apply noxious stimuli that results in injury, such as bruising, to the patient.

Glasgow Coma Scale			
Eyes	Open	Spontaneously	4
		To verbal command	3
		To pain	2
		No response	1
Best motor response	To verbal command	Obeys	6
	To painful stimulus	Localizes pain	5
		Flexion-withdrawal	4
		Flexion-abnormal (Decorticate rigidity)	3
		Extension (Decerebrate rigidity)	2
		No response	1
Best verbal response		Oriented and converses	5
		Disoriented and converses	4
		Inappropriate words	3
		Incomprehensible sounds	2
		No response	1
Total			3-15

FIGURE 13-10. The Glasgow Coma Scale is based on eye opening, movement, and verbal responses. Each response is given a number, and the three scores are summed. Scores range from 3 to 15.

A numeric rating is given to each of the three components of the GCS, and a total score is calculated. The GCS score ranges from 3 (deep coma), to 15 (normal functioning). A GCS of 8 or less is consistent with coma. Several conditions can limit application of the GCS, including medications and concurrent traumatic injuries, such as spinal cord injury (SCI). The GCS does not replace neurological assessment of specific brain functions. However, the GCS provides a universal, standardized approach to monitor trends in consciousness.

Language Skills. If the patient is not intubated, it is important to assess the ability to talk, fluency of speech, word-finding difficulty, comprehension, and whether the speech is spontaneous. Deficits are common in neurological disorders.

Expressive dysphasia is a deficit in language output or speech production from a dysfunction in the dominant frontal lobe. It varies from mild word-finding difficulty to complete loss of both verbal and written communication skills. If the patient is intubated, the ability to express thoughts in writing can be assessed.

The inability to comprehend language and follow commands is called *receptive dysphasia*. Receptive dysphasia indicates dysfunction in the dominant temporal lobe. The patient is asked to perform simple verbal commands such as pointing to the clock, blinking the eyes, or raising the right arm. If able to follow simple commands, the patient may be presented with a complex command such as raising the right arm and folding a piece of paper. A nonintubated patient with receptive problems can speak spontaneously, but the verbal response does not follow the context of the conversation. An intubated patient may appear to be responsive, but is unable to follow simple commands.

Memory. Both short- and long-term memory are evaluated. *Short-term memory* is assessed by asking the patient to recall the names of three common words or objects (e.g., chair, clock, blue) after a 3-minute interval. This simple test can be used with an intubated patient by having the patient write the words on a piece of paper. *Long-term memory* is tested by asking questions about the patient's distant past (e.g., birth place, year of birth, year of graduation from school, year of marriage). If intubated, the patient can write the answers.

Cranial Nerve Functioning. Knowledge of the function of each of the cranial nerves helps to identify problems related to cranial nerve deficits. On the initial baseline neurological assessment, all cranial nerves are assessed. Comprehensive testing of cranial nerve function is discussed in all health assessment texts. Table 13-2 focuses on assessments that can be done in patients who are critically ill, who often have a decreased LOC.

Examination of the pupils is an essential part of cranial nerve assessment. Pupils are often assessed hourly for size, shape, equality, and response to light. Normal pupil size ranges from 1.5 to 6 mm in diameter. Exact measurement with a millimeter scale is the most reliable method of determining size and equality. Unequal pupils (*anisocoria*) occurs in approximately 10% of the general population. Otherwise, inequality of pupils (>1 mm) is a sign of a pathological process. Direct and consensual responses of pupils to light are assessed. A change in pupil reaction to light is an important sign that may indicate increasing ICP or a deterioration in neurological status. A difference in response to light between pupils is also a significant finding. For example, pressure on the pathway of the oculomotor nerve may cause the *ipsilateral* pupil (same side as pressure) to be dilated and sluggish, or nonreactive to light, whereas the *contralateral* pupil (opposite side of pressure) remains normal in size and reactivity. Hypoxia and medications may also influence pupillary size and reactivity to light.

Motor Status. The nurse assesses spontaneous movement of all extremities, muscle strength, muscle tone, deep tendon reflexes, Babinski's reflex, coordination, and abnormal posturing. Muscle groups are assessed for symmetry. A more comprehensive assessment can be done if the patient is able to follow commands. If the patient is unable to follow commands, the nurse relies on neurological testing and observation skills.

Spontaneous Movement. Spontaneous movement is assessed by asking the patient to move the extremities on command, or by observing while the patient moves around in bed.

Muscle Strength. Muscle strength of the arms and legs is assessed and graded on a 5-point scale. The grading is based on the ability to move muscle groups, hold a position against gravity, and maintain that position against resistance. Ratings are as follows:

- 0/5—unable to lift the arm or leg to command, or in response to painful stimuli
- 1/5—flicker of movement is felt or seen in the muscle(s) of the limb
- 2/5—moves the limb, but unable to raise the extremity off the bed
- 3/5—able to lift the extremity off the bed briefly, but does not have the strength to maintain the lift
- 4/5—able to lift the extremity off the bed, but has difficulty resisting the examiner ("I am going to push your right arm/leg down, so try to prevent me from doing that")
- 5/5—able to lift the extremity off the bed and maintain the position against resistance

Lower extremity strength can also be tested by asking the patient to push the feet against the nurse's hands. It is important to assess each limb, as differences between the right and left sides can occur. *Hemiplegia* exists when one side of the patient's body stops moving spontaneously. This state indicates a cortical lesion that affects the fibers in the motor strip in the frontal lobe.

Testing generalized muscle strength in a conscious patient is also done with the *drift test*. The patient is asked to close the eyes and stretch out the arms with palms up for 20 to 30 seconds. A downward drift of the arm or pronation of the palm on one side indicates mild paresis of the involved extremity. This test is very sensitive to subtle changes. If the arm strength is normal but drift is demonstrated, the patient is displaying dysfunction in the contralateral frontal or parietal lobe of the brain.

Muscle Tone. Muscle tone is assessed by taking each extremity through passive range of motion. Normal muscle tone shows slight resistance to range of motion. Flaccid muscles have decreased or loss of muscle tone, so there is no resistance to movement.

Increased muscle tone is characterized by spasticity and rigidity.

Deep Tendon Reflexes. Deep tendon reflexes (DTRs) are obtained by a brisk tapping of a reflex hammer on the tendons of a muscle group (Figure 13-11). The biceps reflex assesses spinal nerve roots C5-C6; brachioradialis, C5-C6; triceps, C7-C8; patellar, L2-L4; and Achilles tendon, S1-S2. DTRs are graded according to the response elicited: 0, no reflex; 1+, hypoactive; 2+, normal; 3+, increased but normal; 4+, very brisk, hyperreflexive, clonus. Some references include a rating of 5+ for sustained clonus. Assessment of DTRs is useful in evaluating SCI. DTRs are absent below the level of injury initially, secondary to spinal shock; return of DTRs signals resolution of spinal shock. Alterations in DTRs may indicate subtle damage of the spinal cord or in the brain. Aging and metabolic factors, such as thyroid dysfunction or electrolyte abnormalities, may also affect DTRs.

Babinski's Reflex. Babinski's reflex is a pathological reflex (Figure 13-12). When the sole of the patient's foot is lightly stroked, the normal response is plantar flexion of the toes. Babinski's reflex is present when dorsiflexion of the great toe with fanning of the other toes is noted upon stimulation. In an adult, the presence of a Babinski's reflex is a sign of an upper motor neuron lesion and damage to the corticospinal tract.

Coordination. Coordination of movement is under cerebellar control. It is assessed by asking the patient to perform rapid alternating movements, such as touching the finger to the nose or running the heel down the shin bilaterally. These tests require the patient to be able to follow verbal commands.

Abnormal Posture. Abnormal posturing may be observed in unconscious patients with brain damage. These include flexion or extensor posturing (Figure 13-13). *Flexion posturing* (previously known as decorticate posturing) involves rigid flexion of the arms, wrist flexion with clenched fists, and extension and internal rotation of the legs. It usually occurs secondary to damage of the corticospinal tract. *Extensor posturing* (previously known as decerebrate posturing) is the result of a midbrain or pons lesion. In this posture, the patient's jaw is clenched, the arms and legs are rigidly extended, and the feet are in plantar extension. The forearms may be pronated, and the wrists and fingers are flexed. Abnormal posturing can occur in response to noxious stimuli, such as suctioning or pain, or may be spontaneous. Different posturing may be noted on each side of the body.

Sensory Assessment. Sensory assessment is performed to determine superficial response to pinprick (sharp, dull, hyperesthesia, absent), position sense, and temperature. The areas of sensation on the skin are supplied by one spinal segment, or sensory dermatome

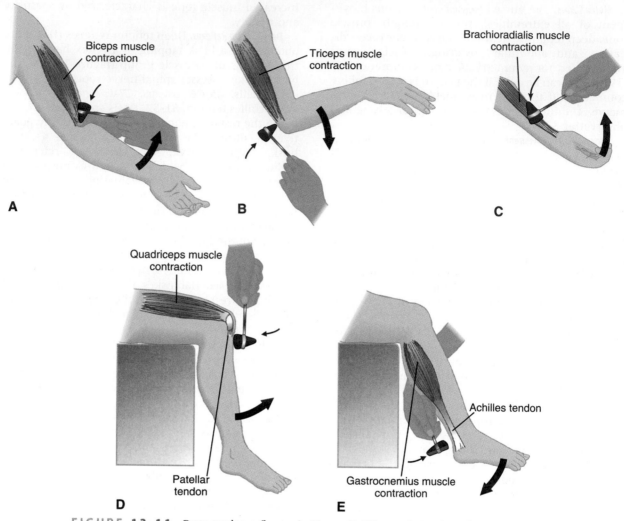

FIGURE 13-11. Deep tendon reflexes. **A**, Biceps. **B**, Triceps. **C**, Brachioradialis. **D**, Patellar. **E**, Achilles. *(From Black, J. M., & Hawks, J. H. [2005]. Medical-surgical nursing: Clinical management for positive outcomes [7th ed.]. Philadelphia: Saunders.)*

(see Figure 13-9; Table 13-3). For example, the ability to sense a superficial pinprick on the lateral forearm, thumb, and index finger tests the innervation of the C6 dermatome. To assess position sense, the patient is instructed to close the eyes. The nurse grasps the patient's thumb or big toe and moves the digit up or down, or leaves it in a neutral position. The patient is asked to identify the pattern of movement. The ability to differentiate between hot and cold is also tested. Temperature is assessed by filling up one container with hot water and another with cold water. The patient is asked to identify the sensation of hot or cold when the container is touched to the skin. Sensation cannot be assessed in coma but is implied if the patient responds to painful stimulation.

Respiratory Assessment. Assessing respiratory pattern and rate is performed as part of the neurological assessment. Changes in the respiratory pattern can indicate neurological deterioration. Table 13-4 describes abnormal respiratory patterns related to neurological dysfunction. However, these patterns are obscured in intubated and mechanically ventilated patients.

Hourly Assessment. The nurse assesses the neurological parameters based on ordered frequency (often hourly) and severity of the patient's condition. Reassessment is also done if changes are noted. Table 13-5 contains the components of an hourly neurological assessment for patients with increased ICP, head injury, or acute stroke. All findings are documented per unit protocol, and abnormal findings are immediately reported to the physician.

INCREASED INTRACRANIAL PRESSURE

A commonly encountered problem in the critical care setting is increased ICP. Many neurological disorders and injuries are associated with increased ICP,
such as brain injury and stroke. Along with MAP, the ICP determines the CPP. Therefore, it is important to assess and maintain ICP within normal limits to maintain an adequate CPP to promote optimal patient outcomes.

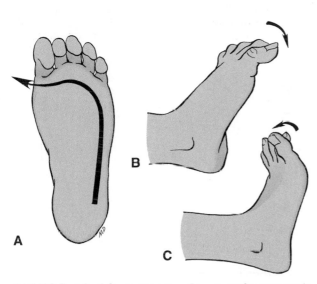

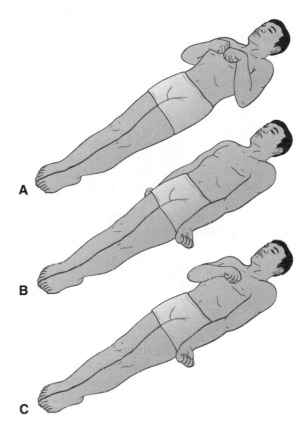

FIGURE 13-12. Babinski's reflex. A, Light pressure is applied with a hard object to the lateral surface of the sole, starting at the heel and going over the ball of the foot ending beneath the great toe. B, Normal response is flexion of all toes. C, Positive Babinski's response is dorsiflexion of the great toe and fanning of the other toes. (From Black, J. M., & Hawks, J. A. [2005]. Medical-surgical nursing: Clinical management for positive outcomes [7th ed., p. 2036]. Philadelphia: Saunders.)

FIGURE 13-13. Abnormal motor responses. A, Flexion posturing. B, Extensor posturing. C, Flexion posturing on right side and extensor posturing on left side.

TABLE 13-3	Spinal Nerve Innervation of Major Muscle Groups	
Spinal Nerve	**Muscle Group Movement**	**Assessment Technique**
C4-C5	Shoulder abduction	Shrug shoulders against downward pressure of examiner's hands
C5	Elbow flexion (biceps)	Arm pulled up from resting position against resistance
C7	Elbow extension (triceps)	From the flexed position, arm straightened out against resistance
	Thumb-index pinch	Index finger held firmly to thumb against resistance to pull apart
C8	Hand grasp	Hand grasp strength evaluated
L2	Hip flexion	Leg lifted from bed against resistance
L3	Knee extension	From flexed position, knee extended against resistance
L4	Foot dorsiflexion	Foot pulled up toward nose against resistance
S1	Foot plantar flexion	Foot pushed down (stepping on the gas) against resistance

Pathophysiology

The rigid cranial vault contains three types of noncompressible contents: the brain, arterial and venous blood supply, and CSF. This can be depicted by the following formula: Intracranial Volume $(Vol_{Intracranial}) = Vol_{Brain} + Vol_{Blood} + Vol_{CSF}$. The pressure exerted by the combined volumes of these three components is ICP. If the volume of any one of these three components increases, the volume of one or both of the other compartments must decrease proportionally, or an increase in ICP occurs (Monro-Kellie doctrine). This compensation is termed *compliance* (Figure 13-14). With adequate compliance, an increase in intracranial volume is compensated by displacement of CSF into the spinal subarachnoid space, displacement of blood into the venous sinuses, or both. The ICP remains normal despite increases in volume (flat part of curve). When compensatory mechanisms are exhausted, small increases in volume lead to large increases in ICP (steep part of curve).

As compliance decreases, ICP increases and CBF decreases. When CBF decreases, the brain becomes hypoxic, carbon dioxide levels increase, and acidosis occurs. In response to these changes, the cerebral blood vessels dilate to increase CBF. This compensatory response further increases intracranial volume, creating a vicious cycle that can be life-threatening (Figure 13-15).

Normal ICP ranges from 0 to 15 mm Hg. Increased ICP is defined as a pressure of 20 mm Hg or greater persisting for 5 minutes or longer, and is a life-threatening event. Sustained increases in ICP can lead to herniation syndromes. Herniation occurs from shifting of brain tissue from an area of high pressure

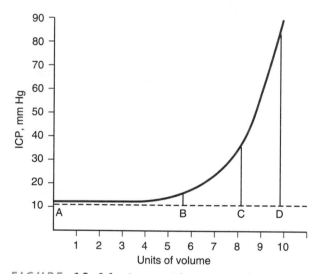

FIGURE 13-14. Intracranial pressure–volume curve. Between points *A* and *B*, intracranial compliance is present. Intracranial pressure (ICP) is normal, and increases in intracranial volume are tolerated without large increases in ICP. As compliance is lost, small increases in volume result in large and dangerous increases in ICP (points *C* and *D*).

TABLE 13-4 Respiratory Patterns in Neurological Disorders

Abnormal Pattern	Disorder
Cheyne-Stokes	Bilateral deep cerebral lesion or some cerebellar lesions
Central neurogenic hyperventilation	Lesions of the midbrain and upper pons
Apneustic	Lesions of the mid to lower pons
Cluster breathing	Lesions of the lower pons or upper medulla
Ataxic respirations	Lesions of the medulla

TABLE 13-5 Components of the Hourly Neurological Assessment for Patients with Increased Intracranial Pressure, Head Injury, or Acute Stroke

Mental Status	Focal Motor	Pupils	Brainstem/Cranial Nerves
Glasgow Coma Scale Assesses level of consciousness, expressive language, ability to follow commands	Move all extremities Strength of all extremities (compare right and left sides) Motor response	Size Shape Reaction to light (direct and consensual) Extraocular movements	Corneal reflex Present: immediate blinking bilaterally Diminished: blinking asymmetrically Absent: no blinking Cough, gag, swallow reflex Observe for excessive drooling Observe for cough/swallow reflex

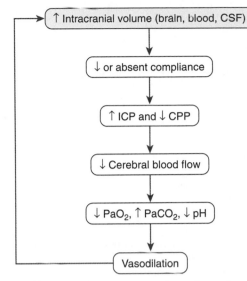

FIGURE 13-15. Pathophysiology flow diagram for increased intracranial pressure.

to one of lower pressure. Herniation syndromes are classified as supratentorial (cingulate, central, and uncal herniation) or infratentorial (cerebellar tonsil herniation). These herniation syndromes are described in Table 13-6 and shown in Figure 13-16.

Causes of Increased Intracranial Pressure

Factors that increase ICP are associated with increased brain volume, increased cerebral blood volume, and increased CSF (Box 13-1).

Increased Brain Volume

A common cause of increased brain volume is cerebral edema. Intracerebral masses such as tumors, abscesses, or hematomas also increase the brain volume.

Cerebral edema is an increase in the water content of the brain tissue; uncorrected, it may lead to increase in ICP and decrease in CBF. Cytotoxic edema and vasogenic edema are two categories of cerebral edema; they may occur independently or together. *Cytotoxic cerebral edema* is characterized by intracellular swelling of neurons, most often the result of hypoxia and hypo-osmolality. Hypoxia causes decreased ATP production; leads to the failure of the sodium-potassium pump; and causes sodium, chloride, and water to enter the cell while potassium exits. This failure leads to hypo-osmolality within the cell, which causes the cells to swell and to stop functioning. Cytotoxic edema is associated with brain ischemia or hypoxic events such as stroke or cardiac arrest. It is also seen with hypo-osmolar conditions including water intoxication and hyponatremia.

Vasogenic cerebral edema occurs as a result of a breakdown in the blood-brain barrier, leading to an increase in the extracellular fluid space. Normally, the highly selective blood-brain barrier closely regulates the internal brain environment. When this barrier is disrupted, osmotically active substances (proteins) leak into the brain interstitium and draw water from the vascular system. This results in an increase in extracellular fluid and consequently an increase in ICP. Brain injuries, brain tumors, meningitis, and abscesses are common causes of vasogenic cerebral edema.

Increased Cerebral Blood Volume

Several mechanisms can increase cerebral blood volume. These include loss of autoregulation, physiological responses to decreased cerebral oxygenation, increased oxygen demand and delivery, and obstruction of venous outflow.

Loss of Autoregulation. Within normal limits, the cerebral vasculature exhibits pressure and chemical autoregulation. Autoregulation provides a constant blood volume and CPP over a wide range of MAPs. Pathological states such as head injury or hypertension often lead to a loss of autoregulation.

Decreased Cerebral Oxygenation. A reduction in cerebral oxygenation leads to cerebral vasodilation in an attempt to increase oxygen delivery. Hypercapnia

TABLE 13-6   Herniation Syndromes

Syndrome	Definition	Symptoms
Cingulate	Shift of brain tissue from one cerebral hemisphere under the falx cerebri to the other hemisphere	No specific symptoms; may compromise cerebral blood flow
Central	Downward shift of cerebral hemispheres, basal ganglia, and diencephalon through the tentorial notch that compresses the brainstem	**Early** Decrease in LOC Motor weakness Cheyne-Stokes respiration Small, reactive pupils **Late** Coma Pupils dilated and fixed Abnormal flexion posturing, progressing to abnormal extensor posturing Unstable vital signs progressing to cardiopulmonary arrest
Uncal	Unilateral lesion forces uncus of temporal lobe to displace through the tentorial notch, compressing the midbrain Symptoms can progress rapidly	**Early** Decreased LOC Increased muscle tone Positive Babinski's reflex Cheyne-Stokes respiration, progressing to central neurogenic hyperventilation Ipsilateral dilated pupil Weakness **Late** Pupils dilated and fixed Paralyzed eye movements Contralateral hemiplegia Decerebrate posturing Unstable vital signs progressing to cardiopulmonary arrest
Cerebellar tonsil	Displacement of cerebellar tonsils through foramen magnum, compressing the pons and medulla	Alterations in respiratory and cardiopulmonary function, rapidly progressing to cardiopulmonary arrest

LOC, Level of consciousness.

also causes vasodilation and contributes to increased ICP. Any factor that results in hypoxemia or hypercapnia, such as ineffective airway, airway obstruction, or endotracheal suctioning, can contribute to increased ICP.

Increased Metabolic Demands. CBF increases to augment oxygen supply in response to increased metabolic demands. Several factors increase oxygen demands including fever, physical activity, pain, stimulation, and seizures. When several nursing activities are done together (e.g., bathing, suctioning, turning), metabolic demands are often increased. Although sleep and rest are important, oxygen demands are higher during rapid eye movement (REM) sleep. Increases in ICP may be noted during any of these situations.

Obstructed Venous Outflow. Several mechanisms can cause venous outflow obstruction that results in increased cerebral blood volume. Different neck positions (hyperflexion, hyperextension, rotation) or a tightly applied tracheostomy or endotracheal ties compress the jugular vein, inhibit venous return, and cause central venous engorgement. A tumor or abscess can compress the venous structures, causing an outflow obstruction. Mechanisms that increase intrathoracic or intraabdominal pressure also impair

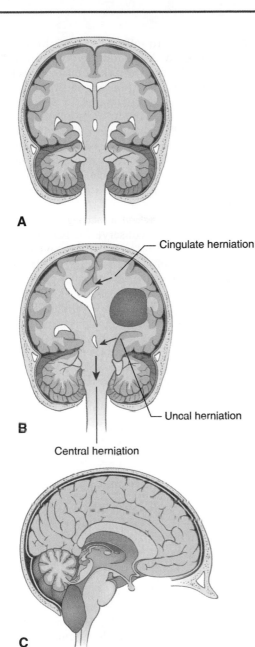

A

Cingulate herniation

Uncal herniation

B

Central herniation

C

FIGURE 13-16. Herniation syndromes. A, Normal intracranial structures. B, Supratentorial herniation syndromes. C, Cerebellar tonsil herniation. *(From McCance, K. L., & Huether, S. E. [2006]. Pathophysiology: The biologic basis for disease in adults and children [5th ed., p. 523]. St. Louis: Mosby.)*

CLINICAL ALERT
Optimal Positioning

Optimal head position to avoid complications related to increased intracranial pressure should be established on an individual basis rather than by placing all patients in a head-raised position.[33]

---

venous return (e.g., coughing, vomiting, posturing, isometric exercise, Valsalva's maneuver, positive end-expiratory pressure, hip flexion). Therefore, the patient at risk for increased ICP should be positioned to ensure unobstructed venous outflow as a compensatory mechanism.

Increased Cerebrospinal Fluid

Increased CSF can result in increased ICP. Hydrocephalus is a primary etiology of increased CSF. Hydrocephalus may occur after in any circumstance where CSF flow or absorption is blocked, such as subarachnoid hemorrhage or infection (meningitis, encephalitis).

Assessment

A thorough neurological examination is performed with an emphasis placed on LOC, motor function, and cranial nerve testing (pupillary response; extraocular movements; and corneal, cough, gag, and swallow reflexes).Vital signs are part of the routine assessment. Hypertension is common in increased ICP and represents a compensatory mechanism to augment CPP. Other changes related to increased ICP appear late in the course of neurological dysfunction and signify severe irreversible damage. Cushing's triad is a late sign of increased ICP and consists of systolic hypertension with a widening pulse pressure, bradycardia, and irregular respirations.

Monitoring Techniques

Other assessment parameters for a patient with increased ICP include ICP, hemodynamic, and cerebral oxygenation monitoring.

Intracranial Pressure Monitoring. ICP monitoring is used to correlate objective data with the clinical picture and to determine cerebral perfusion. Monitoring is indicated for patients with severe brain injury or other neurological disorders who have a GCS between 3 and 8. It may also be used to treat increased ICP by draining CSF, or to assess response to therapy, such as after administering mannitol.[3] A ventriculostomy allows for both ICP monitoring and draining of excessive CSF to relieve increased ICP.

ICP monitoring systems are classified by location of device or type of transducer system. Devices can be placed in the ventricle or in the parenchymal, subarachnoid, or epidural spaces (Figure 13-17). Local anesthesia is used during the insertion procedure. Each site has advantages and disadvantages (Table 13-7).

The transducer system may be a microchip sensor device, fiberoptic catheter, or fluid-filled system.[3] A fluid-filled system is often used for ICP monitoring.

This system is similar to that used for hemodynamic monitoring with a few exceptions. The pressure tubing is flushed with sterile normal saline *without* preservatives since preservatives may damage brain tissue, and no pressurized fluid or flush system is used. The device is zero referenced, and the air-fluid interface is leveled with the foramen of Munro. The ICP waveform is observed on a channel on the bedside monitor. The mean ICP pressure is recorded.

Catheters with internal microchip sensors and fiberoptic catheters have the transducer built into the tip of the catheter. These devices only need to be zero referenced before insertion. They are connected via a cable to a stand-alone monitor provided by the manufacturer. Some monitors can be connected to the bedside monitor for an additional display of ICP and waveforms.[3]

Intracranial Pressure Waveform Monitoring. Monitoring systems allow nurses to observe an ICP waveform pattern. The normal intracranial pulse waveform has three defined peaks of decreasing height that correlate with the arterial pulse waveform and are identified as P_1, P_2, and P_3 (Figure 13-18). P_1 (percussion wave) is fairly consistent in shape and amplitude; it represents the blood being ejected from the heart and correlates with cardiac systole. Extreme hypotension or hypertension produces changes in P_1. P_2 (tidal wave) represents intracranial brain bulk. It is variable in shape and is related to the state

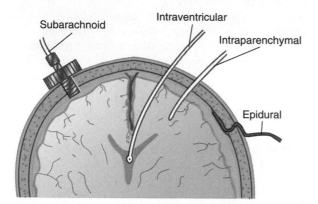

FIGURE 13-17. Intracranial pressure monitoring sites. *(From Kee, K. R., & Hoff, J. T. [1996]. Youman's neurological surgery [4th ed.]. Philadelphia: Saunders.)*

TABLE 13-7 Intracranial Pressure Monitoring Devices[3]

Device	Location	Advantages	Disadvantages
Intraventricular catheter (ventriculostomy) or fiberoptic transducer	Lateral ventricle of nondominant hemisphere; may be tunneled or bolted	Therapeutic or diagnostic removal of CSF to control ↑ ICP Good ICP waveform quality Accurate and reliable	Highest risk for infection; infection rate, 2%-5% Risk for hemorrhage Longer insertion time Rapid CSF drainage may result in collapsed ventricle CSF leakage around insertion site
Subarachnoid bolt or screw	Subarachnoid space	Inserted quickly Does not penetrate brain	Bolt can become occluded with clots or tissue, causing a dampened waveform CSF leakage may occur CSF drainage not possible
Epidural sensor or transducer	Between the skull and the dura	Least invasive Low risk of infection Low risk of hemorrhage Recommended in patients at risk for meningitis or other CNS infections	Indirect measure of ICP Less accurate and reliable CSF drainage not possible
Parenchymal fiberoptic catheter	1 cm into brain tissue	Inserted quickly Accurate and reliable Good ICP waveform quality	CSF drainage not possible Catheter relatively fragile Expensive

CNS, Central nervous system; *CSF,* cerebrospinal fluid; *ICP,* intracranial pressure.

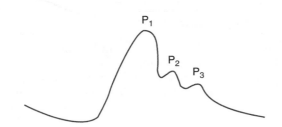

Normal intracranial waveform

A

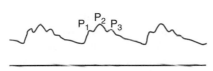

Abnormal ICP wave form

B

FIGURE 13-18. Intracranial pressure (ICP) waveforms. **A,** Normal ICP waveform. **B,** Abnormal waveform. *(From Barker, E. [2008]. Neuroscience nursing: A spectrum of care. [3rd ed.]. St. Louis: Mosby.)*

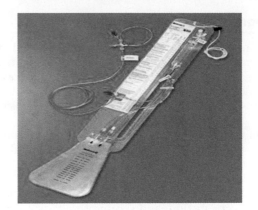

FIGURE 13-19. Becker external drainage and monitoring system. *(Courtesy of Medtronic, Minneapolis, MN.)*

of compliance. Decreased compliance exists when P_2 is equal to or higher than P_1. It also is helpful in predicting the risk for increases in ICP. P_3 (dicrotic wave) follows the dicrotic notch and represents closure of the aortic valve, correlating with cardiac diastole. Smaller peaks that follow the three main peaks vary among individual patients.[9]

Ventriculostomy. Some patients have a ventriculostomy placed for management of ICP. These devices allow concurrent monitoring of ICP as well as a drainage system (Figure 13-19). The decision to drain CSF is based on the ICP exceeding an individually established ICP and the patient's neurological condition.

Hemodynamic Monitoring. Hemodynamic monitoring may be used to monitor fluid management to assist in maintaining adequate cerebral perfusion (see Chapter 8).

Cerebral Oxygenation Monitoring. One technique for monitoring CBF and brain oxygen utilization is *jugular bulb oxygen saturation* (S_jO_2). The technology is similar to mixed venous oxygen saturation (SvO_2) measured in the pulmonary artery. S_jO_2 is monitored via a fiberoptic catheter inserted retrograde through the internal jugular vein into the jugular venous bulb. Placement of the catheter is verified by a neck x-ray study. Oxygen saturation of venous blood is measured as it leaves the brain and provides a global measure of cerebral oxygenation. The normal value is 60% to 70%. Values less than 50% suggest cerebral ischemia. However, normal values do not ensure adequate perfusion to all brain areas.[25]

Another type of device measures the *partial pressure of oxygen within brain tissue* ($PbtO_2$) through a monitoring probe placed directly into the brain white matter and attached to a stand-alone monitor. The probe may be inserted into the damaged portion of the brain to measure regional oxygenation, or inserted into an undamaged portion of the brain to measure global oxygenation. In a patient with traumatic brain injury, the goal of therapy is to maintain an adequate $PbtO_2$. Current studies recommend a $PbtO_2$ greater than 20 mm Hg. However, the science of brain tissue oxygenation is evolving, and target values may change. Values may also be device specific; therefore, it is important to review the manufacturer's literature. Management of low $PbtO_2$ is directed at treating the underlying cause.[6,8,24,26]

Respiratory Monitoring. Continuous monitoring of oxygen saturation via pulse oximetry (SpO_2), and of end-tidal carbon dioxide levels is useful to ensure adequate gas exchange in the neurological patient. Periodic arterial blood gas samples may also be obtained.

Bedside Electroencephalographic Monitoring. Continuous bedside electroencephalographic (EEG) monitoring provides a recording of electrical activity in the brain. The continuous EEG allows for recording, trending, and using evoked potentials to correlate with ICP monitoring. In some cases, EEG monitoring is used to assess the effects of sedation and paralytic agents. Bispectral index monitoring is rapidly becoming available in patients with neurological injury (see Chapter 5).

Diagnostic Testing

The initial baseline laboratory tests obtained in a patient with increased ICP include the following:

- Arterial blood gases, SpO_2, end-tidal carbon dioxide
- Complete blood count, with an emphasis on hematocrit, hemoglobin, and platelets
- Coagulation profile including prothrombin time, international normalized ratio, and activated partial thromboplastin time, as brain injury may induce a coagulopathy
- Electrolytes, blood urea nitrogen, creatinine, liver function, and serum osmolality
- Urinalysis and urine osmolality

The ongoing laboratory tests obtained in a patient with increased ICP include arterial blood gases, SpO_2, hemoglobin and hematocrit, electrolytes, blood urea nitrogen, creatinine, and serum osmolality.

A variety of x-ray studies and other diagnostic tests may be performed on a patient with increased ICP. These include the following:

- Computed tomography (CT) scan (usually noncontrast) to assess the potential for a worsening intracranial mass effect
- Magnetic resonance imaging (MRI) to provide anatomical detail of mass effects or the status of stroke patients
- Cerebral blood flow monitoring, in which a transcutaneous Doppler device (a noninvasive technology) measures the velocity of arterial flow and allows for the indirect monitoring of CBF at the bedside. Transcutaneous Doppler measurements are correlated with ICP values to assess patient response to treatment and nursing interventions. Monitoring is particularly useful to detect vasospasm in patients with a cerebral aneurysm. Vasospasm is noted by an increase in velocity.
- Evoked potential monitoring, which is a noninvasive procedure of applying sensory stimuli and recording the electrical potentials created. Each potential is recorded and stored in a computer, and an average curve is calculated. Brainstem auditory evoked potentials evaluate brainstem function and can be conducted on a conscious or unconscious patient, or even during surgery. Somatosensory evoked potentials measure peripheral nerve responses and are helpful in evaluating spinal cord function.
- EEG
- Xenon CT or CT angiography to measure CBF

Nursing Diagnoses

Refer to the Nursing Care Plan for the Patient with Traumatic Brain Injury, Increased Intracranial Pressure, or Acute Stroke for a detailed description of nursing diagnoses, specific nursing interventions, and selected rationales.

Management

Medical and Nursing Interventions (Nonsurgical)

The goal of management is to maintain an ICP of less than 20 mm Hg while maintaining the CPP above 70 mm Hg. The first task is to prevent an increase in ICP. If the ICP is elevated, therapy is instituted to decrease ICP and then identify the cause of increased ICP. Once the cause is discovered, management is centered on permanently decreasing the high ICP, maintaining CPP, maintaining the airway, providing ventilation and oxygenation, and decreasing the metabolic demands placed on the injured brain.

Nursing Actions to Manage Intracranial Pressure. Several nursing activities are associated with increases in ICP. These include turning, repositioning, and hygiene measures. Elevated ICP resulting from nursing care is usually temporary, and the ICP should return to the resting baseline value within a few minutes. Sustained increases in ICP lasting longer than 5 minutes should be avoided. This is accomplished by spacing nursing care activities to allow for rest between activities. If ICP pressure monitoring is available, the nurse directly monitors the ICP in response to care and other interventions.

The patient is positioned to minimize ICP and maximize CPP. Elevating the head of the bed up to 30 degrees and keeping the head in a neutral midline position in relation to the body facilitates venous drainage and decreases the risk of venous obstruction. However, care must be taken to evaluate blood pressure response to head elevation. Raising the head of the bed may decrease MAP, thereby decreasing CPP. Hemodynamically unstable patients may need to be cared for in a flat position. Patients with increased ICP can be turned from side to side. However, during any position change or change in elevation of the head of bed, it is imperative to monitor and document the patient's individualized cerebral and hemodynamic response. If the CPP does not return to the baseline value within 5 minutes after the position change, the patient must return to the position that maximized CPP.[33]

Since endotracheal suctioning is associated with hypoxemia, the patient is preoxygenated with 100% oxygen before and between suction attempts, and for 1 minute after the procedure. Each suction attempt is limited to less than 10 seconds, with no more than

Text continued on p. 399

NURSING CARE PLAN for the Patient with Traumatic Brain Injury, Increased Intracranial Pressure, or Acute Stroke

NURSING DIAGNOSIS

Decreased intracranial adaptive capacity related to trauma/neurological illness

PATIENT OUTCOMES
Optimal cerebral perfusion

- GCS >13
- CPP >70 mm Hg
- Absence of secondary neurological deficit
- PERLA
- Vital signs within normal limits

NURSING INTERVENTIONS	RATIONALES
• Assess neurological status hourly	• Detect changes in LOC and other signs of increased ICP; change in pupil size or reaction, decrease in motor function, and CN impairment indicate worsening condition
• Monitor ICP and CPP; notify physician if CPP <70 mm Hg	• Ensure adequate cerebral perfusion
• Maintain airway; monitor SpO_2 and $EtCO_2$ or ABGs for evidence of hypoxemia/hypercapnia	• Ensure adequate cerebral perfusion; prevent cerebral vasodilation
• Monitor VS. Be alert to changes in respiratory pattern, fluctuations in BP, bradycardia, widening pulse pressure	• Detect increased ICP; however, these signs occur very late
• Maintain patient's head in a neutral position; maintain head-of-bed elevation that keeps ICP <20 mm Hg and CPP >70 mm Hg	• Facilitate cerebral venous drainage and prevent increased ICP
• Monitor fluid volume status; ensure precise delivery of IV fluids	• Prevent fluid volume excess or deficit, both of which can affect ICP
• Evaluate patient's response to nursing interventions (ICP, CPP). Space activities to avoid increases in ICP	• Prevent sustained elevations in ICP. ICP should return to normal values within 5 minutes of completion of activities
• Prevent increases in intrathoracic and intraabdominal pressure through proper positioning, avoiding coughing and Valsalva's maneuver	• Facilitate cerebral venous drainage and prevent increased ICP
• If hyperthermic, administer treatments to reduce temperature to normal (or mild hypothermia) values	• Reduce cerebral metabolic demands
• Assess the need for medications (sedatives, analgesics, paralytics, anticonvulsants)	• Decrease cerebral metabolic demands and control ICP

NURSING DIAGNOSIS

Ineffective tissue perfusion related to increased ICP and decreased cerebral blood flow

Continued

NURSING CARE PLAN for the Patient with Traumatic Brain Injury, Increased Intracranial Pressure, or Acute Stroke—cont'd

PATIENT OUTCOMES
Improved cerebral tissue perfusion

- VS WNL
- Adequate hemodynamic values
- NSR

- Improved LOC
- Sensory/motor function
- Adequate urine output

NURSING INTERVENTIONS	RATIONALES
• Assess neurological status hourly; monitor VS, assess ECG	• Assess for alterations in ICP
• Perform interventions to prevent and treat increased ICP	• Ensure adequate cerebral tissue perfusion
• Implement measures to improve cerebral tissue perfusion by administering prescribed medications (e.g., diuretics) and maintaining IV fluid therapy	• Improve cerebral tissue perfusion
• Monitor hemodynamic values to achieve and maintain prescribed parameters	• Provide objective assessment of fluid volume needs
• Administer calcium channel blockers (nimodipine), if ordered	• Reduce cerebral vasospasm

NURSING DIAGNOSIS

Impaired gas exchange related to decreased oxygen supply and increased carbon dioxide production secondary to decreased ventilatory drive

PATIENT OUTCOMES
Optimal gas exchange

- $PaCO_2$ 35-40 mm Hg
- PaO_2 >80 mm Hg
- RR 12-20 breaths/min with normal depth/pattern
- Adventitious breath sounds absent
- LOC improved

NURSING INTERVENTIONS	RATIONALES
• Assess patient's RR, depth, and rhythm	• Assess adequacy of respiration; assess abnormal patterns
• Auscultate breath sounds every 1-4 hours	• Detect adventitious lung sounds
• Assess for signs of hypoxemia (confusion, agitation, restlessness, irritability)	• Identify need for oxygenation to prevent cerebral hypoxia
• Ensure a patent airway and assess the need for suctioning. Hyperoxygenate the patient before and after suctioning	• Prevent cerebral hypoxia
• Monitor ABGs, SpO_2, and $EtCO_2$	• Assess adequate oxygenation and ventilation
• Turn every 2 hours, within the limits of patient's status	• Promote lung drainage and alveolar expansion
• Monitor I&O	• Prevent fluid volume excess
• Weigh daily	• Monitor fluid volume status; prevent fluid volume excess

NURSING CARE PLAN for the Patient with Traumatic Brain Injury, Increased Intracranial Pressure, or Acute Stroke—cont'd

NURSING DIAGNOSIS

Risk for imbalanced fluid volume related to fluids/medications administered; development of complications (diabetes insipidus; SIADH); and gastrointestinal suction

PATIENT OUTCOMES
Optimal fluid balance

- Adequate VS, hemodynamic values, and I&O
- Appropriate weight
- Moist mucous membranes

NURSING INTERVENTIONS	RATIONALES
- Weigh daily - Monitor I&O hourly - Monitor laboratory results (electrolytes, serum and urine osmolality) - Assess skin and mucous membranes - Monitor VS and hemodynamic values	- Monitor fluid volume status (all interventions)

NURSING DIAGNOSIS

Imbalanced nutrition: less than body requirements related to hypermetabolic state

PATIENT OUTCOMES
Optimal nutrition

- Weight within normal range for patient
- Serum proteins and albumin within normal range
- Positive nitrogen balance

NURSING INTERVENTIONS	RATIONALES
- Implement early nutritional support - Auscultate bowel sounds and monitor for abdominal distention - Weigh daily - Assess gastric tube feeding residual as ordered - Monitor I&O	- Improve patient outcomes; reduce infection; promote healing - Monitor bowel function; assess tolerance to nutritional support - Monitor fluid volume and nutritional status - Prevent aspiration; neurological patients at increased risk - Monitor fluid volume status

NURSING DIAGNOSES

Risk of infection related to invasive techniques and devices; compromised immune system; and bacterial invasion caused by traumatic brain injury, pneumonia, or iatrogenic causes

Continued

NURSING CARE PLAN   for the Patient with Traumatic Brain Injury, Increased Intracranial Pressure, or Acute Stroke—cont'd

PATIENT OUTCOMES
Free of infection

- Normal WBCs
- Negative culture results
- VS WNL
- Absence of purulent drainage and other clinical indicators of infection
- Normothermia

NURSING INTERVENTIONS	RATIONALES
• Employ proper hand-washing technique before and after patient contact	• Hand washing is best strategy to prevent infection
• Use aseptic technique when performing invasive procedures and caring for catheters, tubes, and lines	• Prevent infection
• Assess VS, drainage, and skin for signs and symptoms of infection	• Detect signs of infection for early intervention
• Inspect cranial wounds for presence of erythema, tenderness, swelling, and drainage	• Detect signs of infection for early intervention
• Maintain a closed system for hemodynamic/ICP monitoring devices	• Prevent bacteria from entering systems and devices
• Monitor the results of CBC and cultures	• Assess for infection; guide treatment
• Assess and maintain adequate nutritional status	• Reduce risk for infection
• Administer antibiotics as ordered	• Treat infection

NURSING DIAGNOSIS

Disturbed thought processes related to impaired cerebral functioning

PATIENT OUTCOMES
Optimal thought processes

- Improved attention, memory, and judgment
- Appropriate response with an improved level of orientation

NURSING INTERVENTIONS	RATIONALES
• Reorient frequently; place a clock or calendar within patient's view	• Provide reorientation to place and time
• Explain activities clearly and simply in a calm manner; allow adequate time for response	• Provide information; prevent anxiety
• Instruct the family in methods to deal with patient's altered thought processes	• Provide ongoing reorientation by all who interact with patient
• Maintain a consistent and fairly structured routine	• Facilitates reorientation
• Allow for frequent rest periods for the patient	

NURSING DIAGNOSIS

Impaired family processes related to situational crisis (patient's illness)

NURSING CARE PLAN for the Patient with Traumatic Brain Injury, Increased Intracranial Pressure, or Acute Stroke—cont'd

PATIENT OUTCOME
Family demonstrates effective adaptation to the situation

- Seeking support
- Sharing concerns.

NURSING INTERVENTIONS	RATIONALES
• Assess family structure; assess social, environmental, ethnic, and cultural relationships, role, and communication patterns	• Establish family structure as a baseline for determining interventions
• Establish open, honest communication and provide information	• Facilitate communication; meet family needs
• Assess knowledge regarding the patient's status and therapies; allow sufficient time for questions	• Identify knowledge deficits
• Acknowledge the family/significant other's involvement in patient care	• Promote family involvement; reduce family stress
• Provide opportunities to talk and share concerns in a private setting	• Assist the family to develop realistic expectations
• Offer and support realistic hope	
• Assess for ineffective coping (depression, substance abuse, withdrawal)	• Identify need for intervention and/or referral
• Encourage the family/significant other to schedule periods of rest or activity	• Provide support for family

ABG, Arterial blood gas; *BP,* blood pressure; *CBC,* complete blood count; *CN,* cranial nerves; *CPP,* cerebral perfusion pressure; *ECG,* electrocardiogram; *EtCO₂,* end-tidal carbon dioxide concentration; *GCS,* Glasgow Coma Scale; *ICP,* intracranial pressure; *I&O,* intake & output; *IV,* intravenous; *LOC,* level of consciousness; *NSR,* normal sinus rhythm; *PaCO₂,* partial pressure of arterial carbon dioxide; *PaO₂,* partial pressure of arterial oxygen; *PERLA,* pupils equal and reactive to light and accommodation; *RR,* respiratory rate; *SIADH,* syndrome of inappropriate antidiuretic hormone secretion; *SpO₂,* oxygen saturation via pulse oximetry; *VS,* vital signs; *WBC,* white blood cell count; *WNL,* within normal limits.
Data from Baird, M. S., Keen, J. H., & Swearingen, P. L. (2005). *Manual of critical care nursing* (5th ed.). St. Louis: Mosby; and Gulanick, M., & Myers, J. L. (2007). *Nursing care plans: Nursing diagnosis and intervention* (6th ed.). St. Louis: Mosby.

two suction passes. The head is maintained in a neutral position during the suctioning procedure.

Although many nurses believe that visitors should be limited for the patient with neurological pathology, family presence has been shown to decrease ICP. However, family members need to be cautioned to avoid excess stimulation of the patient or unpleasant conversations that may emotionally stimulate the patient (e.g., discussing prognosis, condition, deficits, restraints), as this can cause an elevation in ICP.[9] Assessing the patient's physiological response to visitors is an important nursing function.

Medical Management. Medical management of increased ICP includes the following: adequate oxygenation and ventilation; cautious, limited use of hyperventilation; osmotic and loop diuretics; euvolemic fluid administration; maintenance of BP; and reducing metabolic demands. Administration of corticosteroids for reducing ICP in patients with head injury is not recommended. Corticosteroids reduce cerebral edema associated with brain tumors and meningitis, but recent studies do not support administration of corticosteroids to reduce ICP associated with other intracranial conditions.[12]

Adequate Oxygenation. The goal is to maintain a PaO₂ above 80 mm Hg and to ensure that oxygen delivery to the brain exceeds oxygen consumption. A PaO₂ below 50 mm Hg can precipitate increased ICP. For many patients with increased ICP, short-term management of the airway is accomplished by an endotracheal tube and mechanical ventilation. Positive end-expiratory pressure may be added to facilitate oxygenation; however, it must be used with extreme caution since it may prevent venous outflow and further increase ICP. A tracheostomy tube may be required for long-term ventilatory management. In addition, adequate hematocrit and hemoglobin levels are maintained to promote oxygenation.

Management of Carbon Dioxide. Hyperventilation decreases $PaCO_2$, which causes vasoconstriction of the cerebral arteries and a reduction of CBF. In the past, hyperventilation was commonly used to manage ICP. However, hyperventilation may cause neurological damage by decreasing cerebral perfusion, and it is no longer recommended as a first-line treatment to reduce ICP. It is recommended that the $PaCO_2$ be kept within a normal range, 35 to 45 mm Hg. Hyperventilation should also be avoided when providing manual ventilation via a bag-valve device.

Hyperventilation is only used to decrease ICP for short periods when acute neurological deterioration is occurring (i.e., herniation) and other methods to reduce ICP have failed. If the $PaCO_2$ level is purposefully lowered to less than 35 mm Hg for an extended period, oxygen delivery at the cellular level should be evaluated using a jugular bulb or cerebral tissue oxygen monitor.[9,12]

Diuretics. Osmotic and loop diuretics are administered to reduce cerebral brain volume by removing fluid from the brain's extracellular compartment. *Osmotic diuretics* (mannitol 20%) draw water from the extracellular space to the plasma by creating an osmotic gradient, thereby decreasing ICP. The effects of decreasing ICP and increasing CPP occur within 20 minutes of infusion. Side effects of osmotic diuretics include hypotension, electrolyte disturbances, and rebound increased ICP. If mannitol is used, the patient must have adequate intravascular volume to prevent hypotension and secondary brain injury. Osmotic diuretics are contraindicated in patients with renal failure because they are not metabolized and are excreted unchanged in the urine. Hypertonic saline solutions (in solutions ranging from 1.5% to 24% normal saline) also act as an osmotic and may be given to expand intravascular volume, extract water from intracellular spaces, decrease ICP, and increase cardiac contractility. *Loop diuretics* (furosemide, ethacrynic acid) decrease ICP by removing sodium and water from injured brain cells. These agents also decrease CSF formation (Table 13-8).

Optimal Fluid Administration. Fluid administration is provided to optimize MAP, maintain intravascular volume, and normalize CPP. Normal saline solution (0.9%), an isotonic solution, is recommended for volume resuscitation. Hypotonic solutions are avoided to prevent an increase in cerebral edema. Strict measurement of intake and output while monitoring serum sodium, potassium, and osmolarity is required. The goal is to keep serum osmolarity between 310 and 320 mOsm/L.[12] If needed, colloids or blood products are administered to restore volume and maintain adequate hematocrit and hemoglobin levels. Hemodynamic monitoring may be used to optimize fluid administration.

Blood Pressure Management. BP must be carefully controlled in a patient with increased ICP. Usually the MAP is kept between 70 and 90 mm Hg. However, it is critical to monitor the ICP and MAP collectively to sustain an adequate CPP of at least 70 mm Hg.[9] Hypotension decreases CBF, which leads to cerebral ischemia. When hypotension occurs, manipulating the systolic BP with vasopressor drugs and fluids may be needed to achieve an adequate CPP.

Hypertension (>160 mm Hg systolic) can worsen cerebral edema by increasing microvascular pressure. However, hypertension may be necessary for adequate cerebral perfusion. If necessary, systolic BP is lowered with antihypertensive drugs such as labetalol. This beta-blocker decreases the sympathetic response and catecholamine release associated with neurological injury. Some antihypertensive agents (nitroprusside, nitroglycerin) and some calcium channel blockers (verapamil, nifedipine) cause cerebral vasodilation. This vasodilation increases CBF and causes increased ICP. Administration of these agents is avoided in patients with poor intracranial compliance. Nicardipine is a calcium channel blocker that does not affect cerebral vasculature and is very effective in providing quicker and tighter control of BP than other antihypertensive agents.

Reducing Metabolic Demands. Several therapies may be required to reduce metabolic demands. These include temperature control, sedation, seizure prophylaxis, neuromuscular blockade, and barbiturate therapy.

Temperature Control. Aggressive management of hyperthermia is critical. Lowering body temperature to a normal or subnormal temperature decreases intracranial metabolism, decreases cerebral blood flow and volume, and decreases ICP.

Sedation. Patients are often sedated to lower increased ICP related to agitation, restlessness, and resistance to mechanical ventilation. Benzodiazepines are given for sedation and do not affect CBF or ICP. Propofol is a sedative-hypnotic agent that reduces cerebral metabolism and ICP. It is a short-acting drug with a rapid onset that is given by continuous infusion. Morphine can be administered for analgesia and sedation as a low-dose continuous infusion

Text continued on p. 405

PHARMACOLOGY

TABLE 13-8 Frequently Used Drugs in Nervous System Alterations

Drug	Actions/Uses	Adult Dosage/Route	Side Effects	Nursing Implications
Mannitol	Draws water from normal brain cells into plasma; treat ↑ ICP	0.5 to 1 g/kg IV over 5-10 minutes, then 0.25-2 g/kg IVP q4-6h as needed depending on ICP, CPP, serum osmolarity	Hypotension, dehydration, electrolyte disturbances, tachycardia Rebound edema	Neurological assessment q1h; monitor ICP, CPP, serum osmolarity, electrolytes, ABGs, VS, hourly I&O, daily weights; warm ampule or bottle in hot water and shake to dissolve crystals; use an in-line filter needle to administer
Furosemide (Lasix)	Reduces cerebral edema by drawing sodium and water out of injured neurons	Edema/HF: 20-40 mg IV over 1-2 minutes; may repeat in 1-2 hours; if necessary, increase dosage by 20 mg increments until desired diuresis; IV dose should not exceed 1 g/day Postcardiac arrest cerebral edema: 40 mg IV over 1-2 minutes; if no response in 1 hour, increase to 80 mg or 0.5-1 mg/kg IV over 1-2 minutes; if no response, increase dose to 2 mg/kg	Ototoxicity, polyuria, electrolyte disturbances, gastric irritation, muscle cramps, hypotension, dehydration, embolism, vascular thrombosis	Monitor hourly I&O, daily weights, electrolytes, ABGs, VS
Dexamethasone (Decadron)	Steroid that has a stabilizing effect on cell membrane; prevents destructive effect of oxygen-free radicals; ↓ inflammation by suppressing white blood cells	Cerebral edema: 10-mg IV loading dose over 1 minute; 4 mg every 6 hours; reduce dose after 2-4 days; discontinue gradually over 5-7 days Cerebral edema in recurrent or inoperable brain tumor: 2 mg every 8-12 hours (usually IM); adjust dose based on patient response	Flushing, sweating, hypertension, tachycardia, thrombocytopenia, weakness, nausea, diarrhea, GI irritation/hemorrhage, fluid retention, poor wound healing, weight gain, hyperglycemia, muscle wasting, hypokalemia	↑ or ↓ effects of anticoagulants; ↓ effects of anticonvulsants; adjust dose of antidiabetic agents; ↑ effects of digitalis; monitor glucose, potassium, daily weights, VS; masks signs of infection; taper drug before discontinuing

Continued

PHARMACOLOGY

TABLE 13-8   Frequently Used Drugs in Nervous System Alterations—cont'd

Drug	Actions/Uses	Adult Dosage/Route	Side Effects	Nursing Implications
Methylprednisolone (Solu-Medrol)	An adjunct to SCI management; improves blood flow to injury site facilitating tissue repair	30 mg/kg over 15 minutes; in 45 minutes, begin maintenance dose of 5.4 mg/kg/hr for 23 hours	Same as dexamethasone	Same as dexamethasone
Labetalol (Normodyne; Trandate)	Nonselective beta-blocker to decrease BP	10-20 mg IVP over 2 minutes; may repeat with 40-80 mg IVP at 10 minute intervals until desired BP is achieved; do not exceed total dose of 300 mg After bolus, can give as continuous infusion at 2-8 mg/min	Hypotension; bradycardia; HF; bronchospasm; ventricular dysrhythmias; diaphoresis; flushing; somnolence; weakness/fatigue	Monitor BP, HR; I&O, daily weight; may ↓ glucose; may cause further hypotension with nitroglycerin; may potentiate with calcium channel blockers; adjust dosage of antidiabetic drugs
Phenytoin (Dilantin)	Depresses seizure activity	For status epilepticus, 10-20 mg/kg in 0.9% NS only; follow with maintenance dose of 100 mg IV over 2 minutes q6-8h; do not exceed a total dose of 1.5 g; if seizure not terminated, consider other anticonvulsants, barbiturates, or anesthesia	Bradycardia, hypotension, nystagmus/ataxia; gingival hyperplasia; agranulocytosis; rash; Stevens-Johnson syndrome; lymphadenopathy; nausea; cardiac arrest; heart block	Slow rate if bradycardia, hypotension, or cardiac dysrhythmias occur; monitor ECG, BP, pulse, and respiratory function; dilute with 0.9% NS only; assess oral hygiene; assess for rash; monitor renal, hepatic, and hematological status; interacts with many drugs

Drug	Action/Use	Dosage	Side Effects	Nursing Considerations
Fosphenytoin (Cerebyx)	Anticonvulsant; depresses seizure activity	Status epilepticus loading dose 15-20 mg PE/kg IV [PE = phenytoin equivalent]; each 100-150 mg PE over a minimum of 1 minute; if full effect is not immediate, may be necessary to use with benzodiazepine to control status epilepticus; maintenance dose 4-6 mg PE/kg/24 hr Nonemergency loading dose: 10-20 mg PE/kg; maintenance dose 4-6 mg PE/kg/24 hr	Transient ataxia, dizziness, headache, nystagmus, paresthesia, pruritus, somnolence, hypotension, bradycardia, heart block, respiratory arrest, ventricular fibrillation, tonic seizures, nausea/vomiting, lethargy, hypocalcemia, metabolic acidosis, rash	Slow infusion rate or temporarily stop infusion for bradycardia, hypotension, burning, itching, numbness, or pain along injection site; assess neurological, respiratory, and cardiovascular status; assess seizure activity; monitor renal, hepatic, and hematological status; interacts with many drugs
Diazepam (Valium)	Depresses subcortical areas of CNS; anticonvulsant; sedative-hypnotic; antianxiety	For status epilepticus, 5-10 mg IV; give 5 mg over 1 minute. May be repeated every 10-15 minutes for a total dose of 30 mg; may repeat in 2-4 hours; or 0.2-0.5 mg/kg every 15-30 minutes for 2-3 doses; some specialists suggest 20 mg and titrate total dose over 10 minutes or until seizures stop; maximum dose in 24 hours is 100 mg	Respiratory depression; hypotension; drowsiness; lethargy; bradycardia; cardiac arrest	Monitor respiratory status, BP, HR; assess IV site for phlebitis and venous thrombosis
Lorazepam (Ativan)	Depresses subcortical areas of CNS; anticonvulsant; sedative-hypnotic; antianxiety	Status epilepticus: 4 mg IV over 1 minute as initial dose. may repeat once in 10-15 minutes if seizure continues; or 0.05 mg/kg to a total of 4 mg; may repeat once in 10-15 minutes; do not exceed 8 mg in 12 hours	Airway obstruction; apnea; blurred vision; confusion; excessive drowsiness; hypotension; bradycardia; respiratory depression; somnolence	Same as diazepam

Continued

PHARMACOLOGY

TABLE 13-8   Frequently Used Drugs in Nervous System Alterations—cont'd

Drug	Actions/Uses	Adult Dosage/Route	Side Effects	Nursing Implications
Pentobarbital sodium (Nembutal sodium)	Barbiturate; sedative; hypnotic agent; anticonvulsant	100 mg IV initially; give over 2 minutes; additional doses in increments of 25-50 mg IV; give 50 mg over 1 minute; maximum dose 200-500 mg IV	Hypotension; myocardial or respiratory depression; thrombocytopenia purpura	Monitor ICP, CPP, VS, and hemodynamic responses; monitor levels; response of each patient is variable
		Barbiturate coma: loading dose 3-10 mg/kg over 3 minutes to 3 hours	Overdose: apnea, coma, cough reflex depression, flat EEG, hypotension, sluggish or absent reflexes, pulmonary edema	
		Maintenance dose: 1.5-2 mg/kg IV every 2 hours or an infusion of 0.5-3 mg/kg/hr; adjust to maintain pentobarbital blood level between 110 and 177 mmol/L (25-40 mg/dL) or ICP below 25 mm Hg		
Nimodipine (Nimotop)	Calcium channel blocker; reduces neurological deficits after SAH; reduces vasospasm associated with SAH	60 mg PO every 4 hours for 21 days; start within 96 hours of SAH	Hypotension, peripheral edema, ECG abnormalities, nausea/vomiting, diarrhea, altered liver function, HF, cough, dyspnea	Assess neurological status; monitor VS, I&O, daily weights; watch for signs of HF

↑, Increase; ↓, decrease; *ABGs*, arterial blood gases; *BP*, blood pressure; *CNS*, central nervous system; *CPP*, cerebral perfusion pressure; *ECG*, electrocardiogram; *EEG*, electroencephalogram; *GI*, gastrointestinal; *HF*, heart failure; *HR*, heart rate; *I&O*, intake & output; *ICP*, intracranial pressure; *IM*, intramuscular; *IV*, intravenous; *IVP*, intravenous push; *IVPB*, intravenous piggyback; *LOC*, level of consciousness; *NS*, normal saline; *PO*, orally; *PT*, prothrombin time; *SAH*, subarachnoid hemorrhage; *SCI*, spinal cord injury; *VS*, vital signs.

Data from Gahart, B., & Nazareno, A. (2007). *2007 Intravenous medications* (23rd ed.). St. Louis: Mosby; and Hodgson, B. B. & Kisior, R. J. (2007). *Saunders nursing drug handbook 2007*. Philadelphia: Saunders.

EVIDENCE-BASED PRACTICE

PROBLEM

In the neurocritical care setting, seizures can occur in association with a variety of clinical problems, including traumatic brain injury, ischemic stroke, and hemorrhagic stroke. Since seizures can cause adverse events and worsen outcome, antiepileptic drug (AED) prophylaxis is often considered. However, prophylaxis itself carries risks. Therefore, clarification of situations where risk is warranted is necessary.

QUESTION

In what clinical paradigms in neurocritical care should prophylactic antiepileptic drugs be considered?

REFERENCE

Liu, K. C., & Bhardwaj, A. (2007). Use of prophylactic anticonvulsants in neurologic critical care: A critical appraisal. *Neurocritical Care* 7:175-184.

EVIDENCE

The authors performed a comprehensive search of the literature from 1973 through 2006 for all randomized trials in any language that included early seizure prophylaxis for children or adults with traumatic brain injury or stroke. Phenytoin was the dominant drug in investigations of seizure prophylaxis, but most studies were done before the advent of new AEDs. Class I evidence was found to recommend that AEDs be used for 7 days in critically ill traumatic brain patients to decrease the incidence of post-traumatic seizures. In patients with subarachnoid hemorrhage, a randomized, placebo-controlled study to assess effect of prophylaxis on seizure prevalence is recommended because contemporary information is contradictory. Similarly, there is a paucity of research in seizure prophylaxis following intracerebral hemorrhage. There are no data to suggest benefit of seizure prophylaxis after ischemic stroke, and, in fact, AED use in this population can adversely affect outcome.

IMPLICATIONS FOR NURSING

Nurses caring for critically ill patients with traumatic brain injury can anticipate the administration of prophylactic AEDs for the first 7 days after injury. For other neurocritical care populations, it is important for nurses to observe for seizure activity and institute seizure precautions, particularly during the acute phase of an illness. Since controversy exists about use in ischemic and hemorrhagic stroke, nurses must be astutely observant for adverse effects when prophylactic AEDs are used in these scenarios. Nurses must also remain apprised of current literature on prophylactic AED use, especially with the use of the newer generation of AEDs that may have fewer adverse effects.

(2-8 mg/hr) or in small frequent intravenous (IV) boluses.

Seizure Prophylaxis. Patients with brain disorders or injury are prone to seizures. Seizure activity is associated with high metabolic demands. Seizure prophylaxis is often initiated in high-risk situations, since adverse effects can occur from prophylactic agents.

Neuromuscular Blockade and Barbiturate Therapy. Neuromuscular blockade is considered for patients unresponsive to other treatments. Barbiturates are given selectively to reduce ICP refractory to other treatments. Pentobarbital is the most common agent used. Patients receiving neuromuscular blockade or barbiturate therapy require hemodynamic monitoring, mechanical ventilation, and intensive nursing management. Table 13-8 outlines drug therapy for patients with increased ICP.

Surgical Interventions

Surgical intervention may be required to remove the source of a mass or lesion causing the increased ICP. Surgery may involve the removal of infarcted areas and hematomas (epidural, subdural, or intracerebral). Decompressive hemicraniotomy is occasionally performed for severe brain injury or large volume stroke. The cranial bone is removed and the dura is opened to create more space for edematous tissue. The nurse must be aware of the missing flap and protect the patient's brain from trauma.[34]

Psychosocial Support

Neurological injury usually occurs without warning and may be severe. This places the family in a state of shock and disbelief. In addition, the patient has suffered an insult to the nervous system and may respond inappropriately or uncharacteristically, or may not be able to respond at all to the family. Neurological insults cause uncertainty in the patient's physical and mental outcomes. The personality and mental changes associated with brain insults can be devastating to the family. Nurses support the family by providing information and psychosocial support to families to reduce their anxiety.

TRAUMATIC BRAIN INJURY

TBI is a common occurrence in the United States and is the leading cause of trauma-related deaths in persons younger than 45 years. Each year, 1.4 million TBIs occur, resulting in 50,000 immediate deaths and hospitalization of 200,000 individuals. Males are 1.5 times as likely as females to sustain a TBI. The highest incidences of TBI occur in children younger than 4 years and in persons aged 15 to 19 years. Survival of TBI is dependent on prompt emergency treatment and focused management of primary and secondary injuries.[22]

Pathophysiology

Traumatic injury can result in damage to the scalp, skull, meninges, and brain, including neuronal pathways, cranial nerves, and intracranial vessels. The extent of TBI can range from mild to severe (Figure 13-20). Mechanisms of closed TBI, along with associated signs and symptoms, are listed in Table 13-9.

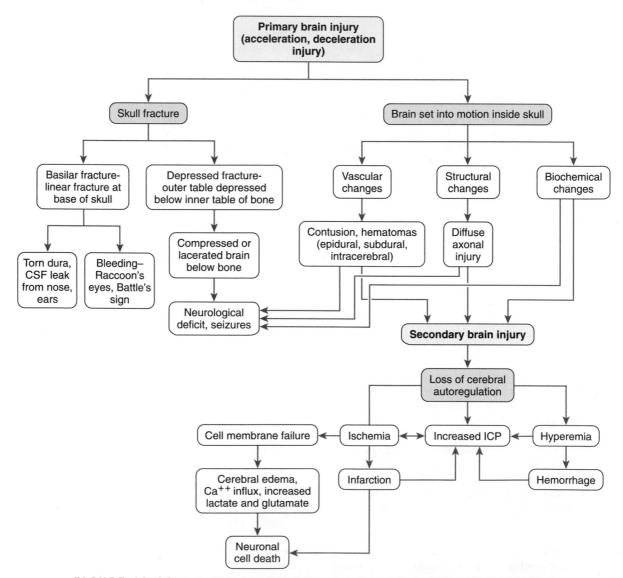

FIGURE 13-20. Pathophysiology flow diagram for traumatic brain injury. *CSF*, Cerebrospinal fluid; *Ca*++, calcium; *ICP*, intracranial pressure.

TABLE 13-9   Types of Traumatic Injury with Associated Signs and Symptoms

Injury	Signs and Symptoms
Skull Fractures	
Linear: Starts at out-bent area, moves toward point of impact and to base of skull	Swelling, redness, bruising, tenderness on scalp, scalp laceration
Depressed: Outer table depressed below the inner table, associated with torn dura, and brain beneath depressed bone is bruised	Depressed area in contour of skull is palpable; CSF leak from nose, ear, postnasal; scalp bruising, tenderness, laceration
Basilar: Fracture in the anterior, middle, and/or posterior fossa along the floor of the cranial vault; dura is torn	
Anterior fossa	"Raccoon" or "panda" eyes, periorbital edema, CSF leak from nose, nasal congestion, cranial nerve deficits
Middle fossa	CSF leak from ear, hemotympanum, Battle's sign, decreased hearing, cranial nerve deficits
Posterior fossa	Bruising at base of neck, cranial nerve deficits
Primary Brain Injuries	
Concussion: Temporary failure of impulse conduction	Altered LOC, confusion, disorientation, retrograde amnesia
Contusion: Injury can be to the area directly beneath impact (coup) or injury can be to the brain's poles (contrecoup)	Altered LOC, retrograde amnesia, motor deficits (weakness to paralysis), restlessness, combativeness, confusion, speech disturbances, cranial nerve dysfunction, decorticate and decerebrate posturing, abnormal breathing patterns, coma
Diffuse axonal injury: Tearing of axons and myelin sheaths, secondary to generalized movement of brain from impact	Prolonged coma, cranial nerve deficits, motor deficits, abnormal posturing, increased ICP, hypertension, elevated temperature
Penetrating injuries: Injury is caused by deep laceration of brain tissue, damage to the ventricular system	Symptoms depend on location of injury and amount of tissue damage
Hematomas	
Epidural: Tearing of an artery from a skull fracture; brisk bleeding and rapid accumulation in the epidural space	Short period of loss of consciousness then lucid, then confusion, irritability, headache, deterioration in LOC, motor, cranial nerve dysfunction
Subdural: Tearing of bridging cortical veins: blood accumulates in the space between the dura and arachnoid	Acute and subacute: Depressed LOC, pupil and extraocular movement changes, motor changes, headache Chronic: personality changes, gait problems
Subarachnoid: Bleeding into the subarachnoid space	Altered LOC, headache, nuchal rigidity, photophobia
Intraventricular: Bleeding into the ventricles	Altered LOC, cranial nerve dysfunction, motor changes
Intracerebral: Bleeding into brain tissue	Similar to focal injuries

CSF, Cerebrospinal fluid; *ICP,* intracranial pressure; *LOC,* level of consciousness.

Injuries may be open or closed. With an open injury, the scalp is torn or a fracture extends into the sinuses or middle ear. The meninges can also be penetrated. A closed TBI occurs when there is no break in the scalp. Acceleration-deceleration is a common mechanism for TBI. With this injury, the movement of the head follows a straight line, and the moving head (acceleration) hits a stationary object (deceleration). Rotation or a twisting of the brain within the cranial vault adds to the insult (Figure 13-21).

Scalp Lacerations
Scalp lacerations are common in traumatic injury and are often associated with skull fracture. The scalp offers some resistance to compression and absorbs

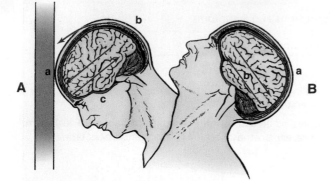

FIGURE 13-21. Coup and contrecoup head injury after blunt trauma. **A,** Coup injury: impact against object. *a,* Site of impact and direct trauma to the brain. *b,* Shearing of the subdural veins. *c,* Trauma to the base of the brain. **B,** Contrecoup injury: impact within skull. *a,* Site of impact from brain hitting opposite side of skull. *b,* Shearing forces throughout the brain. These injuries occur in one continuous motion—the head strikes the wall (coup), then rebounds (contrecoup). *(From Barker, E. [2008]. Neuroscience nursing: A spectrum of care [3rd ed.]. St. Louis: Mosby.)*

mild blows by distributing forces over the entire area of the scalp. The scalp is very vascular and can be the source of significant blood loss. The wound is cleansed, debrided, and inspected for a depressed skull fracture, then sutured closed. Inattention to these details can lead to infection.

Skull Fractures

The skull has high compressive strength and is somewhat elastic. After impact, there is an in-bending of the skull at the point of impact and an out-bending at the vertex. The area of out-bending of tensile stresses creates a fracture line that moves toward the base of the skull. There are several types of skull fractures—linear, depressed, and comminuted—and various locations of the fractures (Figure 13-22).

Linear Skull Fracture. A linear fracture is the most common type of skull fracture. This fracture usually does not lead to significant complications unless there is an extension of the fracture to the orbit, sinus, or across a vessel. When there is extension of the fracture, the patient is admitted for observation of signs of intracranial bleeding and epidural hematoma.

Linear fractures at the skull base are termed *basilar fractures.* This type of fracture is difficult to confirm on a skull x-ray study and is diagnosed by clinical presentation of the patient (see Table 13-9). Battle's sign (bruising behind the ear) and the presence of "raccoon's eyes" (bilateral periorbital edema and bruising) may be indicative of a basilar skull fracture (Figure 13-23). Dural tears are very common with a basilar skull fracture and may lead

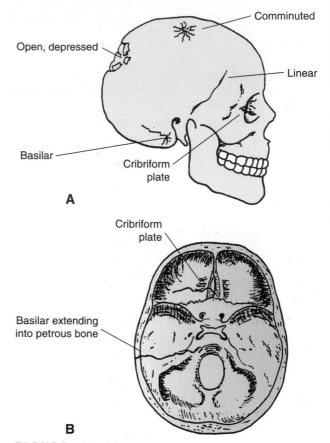

FIGURE 13-22. Skull fractures. **A,** Linear; open, depressed; basilar and comminuted fractures. **B,** View of base of skull with fractures. *(From Barker, E. [2008]. Neuroscience nursing: A spectrum of care [3rd ed.]. St. Louis: Mosby.)*

to meningitis. Drainage of CSF from the nose (rhinorrhea), postnasal drainage, or drainage of CSF from the ear (otorrhea) may indicate a dural tear. When blood encircled by a yellowish stain is seen on a dressing or bed linen, it is called the *halo sign* and usually indicates CSF (see Figure 13-23). If CSF is suspected in the drainage, a sample of the drainage is sent to the laboratory for analysis. In the event of a CSF leak, it is important to allow the CSF to flow freely. Nothing should be placed in the nose or ear, although small bandages under the nose or around the ear can be used to collect the drainage. The patient is instructed not to blow the nose. To avoid penetrating the brain as a result of the dural tear, tubes (e.g., gastric, suction catheters, endotracheal tubes) should be inserted through the mouth rather than through the nose.

Depressed Skull Fracture. A depressed skull fracture occurs when the outer table of the skull is depressed below the inner table of the surrounding intact skull.

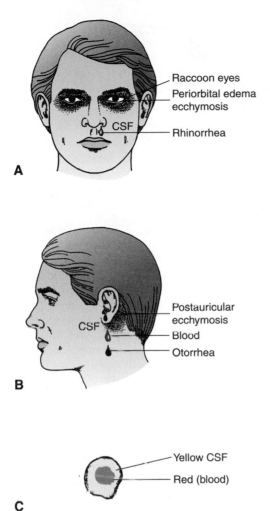

FIGURE 13-23. **A,** Raccoon eyes, rhinorrhea. **B,** Battle's sign with otorrhea. **C,** Halo or ring sign. *(From Barker, E. [2008]. Neuroscience nursing: A spectrum of care [3rd ed.]. St. Louis: Mosby.)*

The dura may be intact, bruised, or torn. If the dura is torn, there is direct communication between the brain and the environment, and meningitis can occur. In addition, the compressed and bruised brain beneath the depressed bone or bone lodged in brain parenchyma is the source of focal neurological deficit and may become a seizure focus.

Comminuted Skull Fracture. A comminuted skull fracture occurs from multiple linear fractures with a depressed area at the site of impact. The fracture originates and radiates toward the impact site and base of the skull. Comminuted skull fracture is referred to as an "eggshell fracture" because of the appearance of the skull. Risks are similar to those occurring with a depressed fracture.

Brain Injury

TBI is classified as primary and secondary. Primary brain injury can be further divided into focal (contusions, hematomas, penetrating injuries) and diffuse lesions (diffuse axonal injury). Figure 13-20 summarizes physiological changes.

Primary Brain Injury. Primary brain injury is a direct injury that occurs to the brain from an impact. With impact, the semisolid brain moves around inside the skull. The area under the direct impact is injured (coup injury). Injury to adjacent poles occurs from the movement of the brain inside the skull (contrecoup injury). The stretching, shearing, rotational, and tearing forces that result from impact interrupt normal neuronal pathways. The initial insult causes biomechanical damage to the axonal membrane. The damaged cells trigger secondary brain injury (see Figure 13-20). Concussion, contusion, penetrating injuries, hematomas, and intracerebral hemorrhage are all types of primary brain injury (see Table 13-9). Concussion represents a mild form of TBI, whereas contusion, penetrating injuries, hematomas, and hemorrhage constitute severe head injuries.

Concussion. Concussion occurs when a mechanical force of short duration is applied to the skull. This injury results in the temporary failure of impulse conduction. The neurological deficits are reversible and are generally mild. Patients may lose consciousness for a few seconds at the time of injury, but lasting effects are not common.

Contusion. Contusion is the result of coup and contrecoup injuries, accompanied by bruising and generalized hemorrhage into brain tissue. Lacerations of the cortical surface associated with contrecoup injuries may be greater than those seen directly under the point of impact. Signs and symptoms are variable, depending on location and extent of bleeding.

Diffuse Axonal Injury. A more global brain injury is diffuse axonal injury. With this injury, widespread white matter axonal damage occurs secondary to rotational and shearing forces. This type of injury is associated with disruption of axons in the cerebral hemispheres, diencephalon, and brainstem. This injury results in vasodilation and increased cerebral blood volume that precipitates increased ICP. Signs and symptoms are variable, and prognosis is poor.

Penetrating Injury. Penetrating injuries are the result of low- or high-velocity forces such as gunshots, knives, or sharp objects. With this type of injury, there is a deep laceration of brain tissue and possible damage to the ventricular system. A low-velocity (stabbing) injury is limited to the tract of entry, and the greatest concern is bleeding and infection.

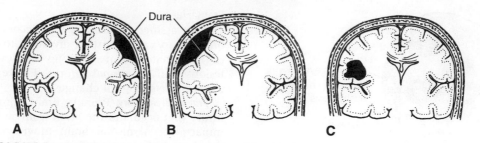

FIGURE 13-24. Types of hematomas. **A,** Subdural (takes on contour of brain). **B,** Epidural. **C,** Intracerebral. *(From Barker, E. [2008]. Neuroscience nursing: A spectrum of care [3rd ed.]. St. Louis: Mosby.)*

A high-velocity (gunshot) injury causes extensive damage because of the entry of bone fragments at the site. In addition, because bullets spin irregularly, they create many paths and shock waves that cause extensive brain damage.

Hematoma. Acute hematomas can be life-threatening. There are three types of hematomas: epidural, subdural, and intracerebral (Figure 13-24).

Epidural Hematoma. Collection of blood in the potential space between the inner table of the skull and the dura causes an *epidural hematoma.* This hematoma is typically associated with a linear fracture of the temporal bone and results from the tearing of the middle meningeal artery. Arterial blood accumulates rapidly in this space. The patient typically experiences a brief loss of consciousness followed by a lucid period before neurological deterioration. The lucid period can last for a few hours to 48 hours. As the patient's condition deteriorates, the LOC decreases, contralateral deficits appear, and the pupil on the side of the lesion *(ipsilateral)* becomes fixed and dilated.

Subdural Hematoma. Collection of blood in the subdural space causes a *subdural hematoma.* It occurs when a surface vein is torn around the cerebral cortex. There are three kinds of subdural hematomas: acute, subacute, and chronic. *Acute subdural hematoma* occurs within 48 hours of an injury. It is nearly always seen with cortical or brainstem injury and represents a mass lesion. The risk of death is high because of injury to brain tissue and the mass effect caused by an expanding hematoma. Surgical intervention occurring within 4 hours of injury improves mortality.[9] Symptoms of a *subacute subdural hematoma* occur anywhere from 48 hours to 2 weeks after an injury. The onset of symptoms is later because the normal compensatory mechanisms promote CBF as the hematoma grows slowly. A *chronic subdural hematoma* occurs as a result of a low-velocity impact. Symptoms occur from 2 weeks to several months after an injury. A higher incidence of chronic subdural hematomas is seen in the elderly, chronic alcohol abusers, or those taking anticoagulants including warfarin, clop-idogrel (Plavix), or aspirin.[7] Because symptoms are often subtle, the diagnosis of chronic subdural hematoma is often missed.

Intracerebral Hematoma. An intracerebral hematoma is a hemorrhage into brain tissue that creates a mass lesion. This lesion can occur anywhere in the brain. It can be caused by penetrating injuries, gunshot wounds, deep depressed skull fractures, stab wounds, or extension of a contusion. Signs and symptoms vary according to the location of the lesion.

Secondary Brain Injury. Secondary brain injury occurs as a consequence of the initial trauma and is characterized by an inflammatory response and release of cytokines from macrophages that cause increased vascular permeability of the blood vessel wall, leading to vasogenic cerebral edema. A series of biochemical events also contributes to the overproduction of free oxygen radicals that disrupt the cellular membrane, impair cellular metabolism, and cause neuronal deterioration. Decreased cerebral perfusion from numerous causes, hypoxia, infection, and/or fluid and electrolyte imbalances all contribute to secondary brain injury. These insults add to the degree and extent of cellular dysfunction after TBI, increase the extent of brain damage, and affect functional recovery. Proper management minimizes the effects of secondary brain injury.

Assessment

The GCS is used as a guide in assessing a patient with a TBI. The assessment is supplemented with a thorough neurological examination, including pupillary changes. Assessment should be specific to the area of the brain involved. Assessment of airway and oxygenation status is essential to ensure adequate oxygenation and CBF. Abnormal respiratory patterns must be reported and documented because pattern changes usually indicate deterioration in neurological status. Additional assessment data include ICP, CPP, and hemodynamic monitoring. A patient with a TBI requires the same laboratory and diagnostic studies as a patient with increased ICP.

Nursing Diagnoses

The same nursing diagnoses are applicable for a TBI patient as for a patient with increased ICP (see Nursing Care Plan for the Patient with Increased Intracranial Pressure, Traumatic Brain Injury, or Acute Stroke). These diagnoses cover both primary and secondary head injuries. Additional nursing diagnoses include Impaired Swallowing, Disturbed Sensory Perception, Hyperthermia, Acute Pain, Decreased Cardiac Output, Risk for Constipation, Risk for Imbalanced Fluid Volume, Risk for Infection, Imbalanced Nutrition, Impaired Physical Mobility, Risk for Impaired Skin Integrity, and Impaired Verbal Communication.

Management

Medical (Nonsurgical) Interventions

The nonsurgical treatment of a patient with a TBI is the same as for a patient with increased ICP. The emphasis is on reducing ICP, maintaining the airway, providing oxygenation, maintaining cerebral perfusion, and preventing secondary TBI. Because the injured brain is sensitive to changes in body temperature, therapeutic hypothermia may be implemented to protect the injured brain.[27] Hypothermia decreases the cerebral metabolic rate and oxygen consumption, lowers levels of glutamate and interleukin-1β, decreases ICP, and increases CPP. Protecting the brain by using hypothermia may improve outcomes in persons with TBI.[30] Several strategies are available to induce hypothermia including external cooling systems, hypothermia blankets, endovascular or endonasal cooling devices, antipyretics, sponging with cold water, and applying ice packs. If available, monitoring the brain temperature to thermoregulate the patient is an optimal choice because the actual brain temperature is higher than the blood temperature. The nurse should assess for adverse effects of hypothermia including dysrhythmias (atrial fibrillation), acidosis, shivering, and coagulopathies.

Nutritional support after TBI is essential. Hypermetabolism, accelerated catabolism, and excess nitrogen losses are responses to TBI. These responses result in depletion of energy stores, loss of lean muscle mass, reduced protein synthesis, loss of gastrointestinal mucosal integrity, and immune compromise. Nutritional support decreases susceptibility to infections, promotes wound healing, and facilitates weaning from mechanical ventilation.[12]

Surgical Interventions

Various surgical procedures exist to treat TBI. A depressed skull fracture may require surgery to elevate and repair or remove bone fragments. Acute subdural hematomas are usually evacuated via burr holes and epidural hematomas via craniotomy to prevent herniation. Penetrating wounds to the skull and brain may necessitate a craniotomy to explore the pathway of the missile, repair lacerations of intracranial vessels and brain tissue, remove bone fragments, or retrieve a foreign body such as a bullet.

Postoperative care is directed at the several interventions. Maintaining normal ICP and CPP; maintaining the airway and ventilation; preventing fluid and electrolyte imbalances; preventing complications of immobility; avoiding nutritional deficits; and reducing the incidence of infection are important.

The craniotomy dressing is assessed for drainage including color, odor, and amount. Once the dressing is removed, the incision is assessed for swelling, redness, drainage, and tenderness. Persistent CSF drainage from the wound after surgery may indicate a dural tear and may require a lumbar drain or ventriculostomy for several days to decrease pressure at the fistula site and to aid in healing. A craniotomy may be necessary to repair the dura if leakage persists. Patients with penetrating wounds to the brain are at high risk for the development of not only infections, but also brain abscesses.

ACUTE STROKE

Stroke is a major public health problem. It is the third leading cause of death in the United States, the most frequent cause of adult disability, and the leading cause of long-term care. Although most strokes are preventable by controlling major risk factors such as hypertension, more than 700,000 new strokes occur each year in the United States. More than 4 million people are stroke survivors.[4] Persons who have a stroke have a 10- to 20-fold increased risk of having another stroke. The cost of hospitalization, rehabilitation, long-term care, and lost wages from stroke is estimated at $57 billion annually. Stroke, also known as "brain attack," results in infarction of a focal area of the brain. Early recognition of the signs and symptoms is essential in order to reperfuse the brain. A stroke should be assessed and treated as a life-threatening emergency because optimal early treatment improves long-term outcome.[1]

The hallmark of stroke is the sudden onset of focal neurological symptoms associated with changes in blood flow to the brain resulting from either a blockage of flow or hemorrhage. Stroke can present with maximal focal neurological deficits, or as stroke in evolution in which symptoms evolve over several hours. The definition of stroke includes neurological deficits lasting 24 hours or longer. Although symptoms may completely resolve, CT or MRI will show evidence of permanent cerebral tissue damage.

GENETICS

APOLIPOPROTEIN E AND COGNITIVE RECOVERY AFTER BRAIN INJURY

A genetic variation that influences recovery from central nervous system (CNS) injury is found on chromosome 19, which contains the genetic codes for apolipoprotein E (APOE). APOE is one of a family of compounds that transport lipids and lipid-soluble vitamins through the bloodstream. The role of APOE in the CNS is not as well defined, but it appears to contribute to cognition by promoting normal neuronal function. It has also been implicated in neuronal repair after ischemia and injury. A variation in the chemical structure of APOE may have a role in the development and progression of both cardiac and neurological disease.

The gene that codes for APOE is polymorphic, with three variations or alleles: *ApoE2*, *ApoE3*, and *ApoE4*. Each allele contains 3597 base pairs and produces three APOE versions or isoforms: APOE-ε2, APOE-ε3, and APOE-ε4. Each isoform differs by only one amino acid substitution (at positions 112 and 158 in a string of 299 amino acids).[4] *ApoE3* is the most common allele, present in more than half of the U.S. population. Patients with the *ApoE4* gene produce the APOE-ε4 version of the lipoprotein. It is this version of the gene that contributes to derangements in CNS and cardiovascular health. Inheriting two copies of the *ApoE4* gene increases risk over inheritance of a single allele.

APOE was originally investigated for its role in lipoprotein metabolism and cardiovascular disease. In the liver and peripheral circulation, apolipoproteins bind lipids for transportation and also serve as enzyme cofactors and intermediaries on cell receptors that regulate lipid uptake into tissues. Patients who are homozygous (carrying two copies of the gene) for *ApoE4* have significantly more risk for cardiovascular disorders and familial hypercholesterolemia than other combinations of APOE inheritance.[3]

APOE is recognized as a contributor to impaired cognition. In the CNS, nonneuronal cells like astroglial and microglia cells produce APOE, while neurons have APOE receptors. APOE is associated with the transportation of lipids within the brain, maintains the structural integrity of microtubules within neurons, and assists with the transmission of neural impulses. It may have a role in inflammation and in influencing the synthesis of excitatory neurotransmitters that contribute to adverse changes in neurons after brain injury.[7] When a gene codes for APOE-ε4, the neurons in the CNS appear to be more vulnerable to stress from injury or ischemia. The presence of APOE-ε4 is also associated with an increased risk for developing neurodegenerative conditions such as Alzheimer disease.[9]

Among critically ill patients, APOE appears to play an important role in the ability of the brain to recover from serious injury. Inheritance of two copies of the *ApoE4* gene (homozygosity), or even single copies of the gene (heterozygosity), is associated with a poorer outcome after brain trauma, hemorrhagic stroke, and subarachnoid hemorrhage.[8] For example, lower Glasgow Coma Scale scores on admission have been demonstrated after moderate and severe traumatic brain injury among patients with one or two copies of *ApoE4*.[2] Long-term consequences among brain-injured patients homozygous for *ApoE4* include poorer retention, deficits in episodic memory, difficulties in learning and verbal comprehension, and impaired executive functioning as well as global cognitive dysfunction for as long as three decades after traumatic brain injury.[1,5,6]

Clinical outcomes after brain injury are variable. Genetic influences are only one factor associated with unfavorable outcomes. Examining genetic influences may help uncover the key mechanisms underlying the response to different patterns of brain injury, resulting in better treatments as well as the ability to predict outcomes. Results from genetic studies suggest that *ApoE4* is a susceptibility gene but not a causative factor in poor recovery after acute brain injury. Genetic testing for APOE profiles is not routinely performed. Nurses caring for patients tested for an APOE genetic profile should realize that the results will have implications for both cardiovascular and neurodegenerative disease as well as recovery from some types of brain injury.

REFERENCES

1. Ariza, M., Pueyo, R., Matarin Mdel, M., Junque, C., Mataro, M., Clemente, I., et al. (2006). Influence of APOE polymorphism on cognitive and behavioural outcome in moderate and severe traumatic brain injury. *Journal of Neurology, Neurosurgery and Psychiatry, 77*(10), 1191-1193.
2. Chiang, M. F., Chang, H. G., & Hu, C. J. (2003). Association between apolipoprotein E genotype and outcome of traumatic brain injury. *Acta Neurochirurgica, 145*(8), 649-653.
3. Foley, S. M. (2005). Update on risk factors for atherosclerosis: The role of inflammation and apolipoprotein E. *Medical-Surgical Nursing, 14*(1), 43-50.
4. Helbecque, N., & Amouyel, P. (2004). Commonalities between genetics of cardiovascular disease and neurodegenerative disorders. *Current Opinion in Lipidology, 15*(2), 121-127.
5. Isoniemi, H., Tenovuo, O., Portin, R., Himanen, L., & Kairisto, V. (2006). Outcome after traumatic brain injury after three decades—Relationship to ApoE genotype. *Journal of Neurotrauma, 23*(11), 1600-1608.

GENETICS—cont'd

6. Jiang, Y., Sun, X., Xia, Y., Tang, W., Cao, Y., & Gu, Y. (2006). Effect of APOE polymorphisms on early responses to traumatic brain injury. *Neuroscience Letter, 408*(2), 155-158.
7. Kerr, M. E., Ilyas Kamboh, M., Yookyung, K., Kraus, M. F., Puccio, A. M., DeKosky, S. T., et al. (2003). Relationship between apoE4 allele and excitatory amino acid levels after traumatic brain injury. *Critical Care Medicine, 31*(9), 2371-2379.
8. Waters, R. J., & Nicoll, J. A. (2005). Genetic influences on outcome following acute neurological insults. *Current Opinion in Critical Care, 11*(2), 105-110.
9. Wolozin, B., & Bednar, M. M. (2006). Interventions for heart disease and their effects on Alzheimer's disease. *Neurological Research, 28*(6), 630-636.

Pathophysiology

Stroke occurs when the blood supply to the brain is disturbed by occlusion (ischemic) or hemorrhage. Brain cells survive only about 3 to 4 minutes when deprived of blood and oxygen. Normal CBF is 50 mL/100 g of brain tissue/min. When CBF drops to 25 mL/100 g/min, neurons become electrically silent but remain potentially viable for several hours. This region of brain is known as the ischemic penumbra (Figure 13-25). If CBF falls to less than the critical level of 10 mL/100 g/min, irreversible damage occurs. A cascade of metabolic disturbances follows, including lactic acidosis production, glutamate release, depletion of ATP, and the entry of sodium and calcium into the cells, leading to cytotoxic cerebral edema and mitochondrial failure.

Ischemic Stroke

Ischemic strokes are caused by large artery atherosclerosis, cardioembolic events, or small artery occlusive disease (lacunar stroke), or the cause is unknown (cryptogenic stroke) (Figure 13-26). Approximately 85% of all strokes in the United States are ischemic.

Large Artery Atherosclerosis. *Large artery atherosclerosis* is the result of stenosis in the large arteries of the head and neck, caused by a cholesterol plaque or a thrombus superimposed on the plaque. Blood flow may be greatly reduced (stenosis), causing ischemia, or occluded completely, causing a stroke. Hypertension, diabetes, smoking, obesity, and hyperlipidemia are risk factors for this type of stroke.

Cardioembolic Stroke. Low-flow states or stasis of blood within the cardiac chambers may result in blood clot formation. An embolism occurs when a blood clot or plaque fractures, breaks off, and travels to the brain. The most common causes of *cardioembolic stroke* are atrial fibrillation, rheumatic heart disease, acute myocardial infarction, endocarditis, mitral valve stenosis, and prosthetic heart valves. Because a cardiac abnormality is the source of the cerebral emboli, it is important to treat the underlying cardiac problem as well as the neurological problem.

Lacunar Stroke. *Lacunar strokes* (small vessel occlusive disease) are caused by chronic hypertension, hyperlipidemia, obesity, and diabetes. These disease states

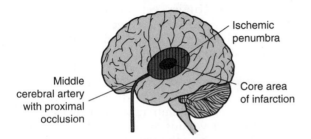

FIGURE 13-25. Proximal occlusion of left middle cerebral artery with infarction. Ischemic penumbra represents regional blood flow at about 25 mL/100 g/min. Ischemic penumbra is the area where acute therapies for stroke are targeted.

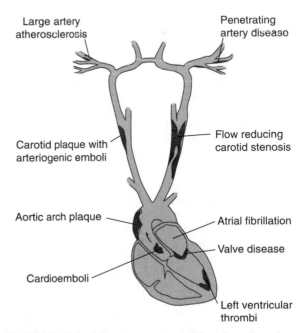

FIGURE 13-26. Common arterial and cardiac abnormalities causing ischemic stroke. *(From Albers, G. W., Easton, J. D., Sacco, R. L., & Teal P. [1998]. Antithrombotic and thrombolytic therapy for ischemic stroke. Chest, 114[Suppl. 5], 683S-698S.*

cause lipid material to coat the small cerebral arteries within deep structures of the brain. This process leads to a thickening of the arterial walls, decreased blood flow, and ultimately a stroke. The characteristic locations of lacunar infarcts are the basal ganglia, subcortical white matter, thalamus, cerebellum, and brainstem. The recurrence rate of these strokes is about 10- to 12-fold compared with other types of stroke. This type of stroke causes not only physical impairment, but also cognitive impairment such as vascular dementia. Patients can have pure motor, pure sensory, or both motor and sensory features of stroke.

Cryptogenic Stroke. The *cryptogenic* subtype refers to a stroke of unknown origin.

Hemorrhagic Stroke

Hemorrhagic strokes account for approximately 15% of all strokes in the United States. The most common causes of hemorrhagic stroke are primary intraparenchymal hemorrhage and ruptured vascular malformations, such as cerebral aneurysm or arteriovenous malformations (AVMs). Secondary causes include overanticoagulation (warfarin, heparin, or recombinant tissue plasminogen activator [rt-PA]), vasopressor drugs, drug abuse (cocaine abuse), and coagulopathies.

Intraparenchymal Hemorrhage. About 10% of strokes in the United States are intraparencymal hemorrhages, with bleeding into the brain substance. These hemorrhages are usually caused by uncontrolled hypertension. Another cause of intraparenchymal hemorrhage is cerebral amyloid angiopathy. This condition is the result of abnormal amyloid protein deposits in the cerebral blood vessels. As a result, the cerebral blood vessels become friable and therefore prone to spontaneous rupture, even in patients without hypertension.[5] When a blood vessel ruptures within the brain parenchyma, the escaped blood forms a mass that displaces and compresses brain tissue. The severity of the symptoms is dependent on the location of the hemorrhage. If the hemorrhage is large enough, herniation may result.

Ruptured Cerebral Aneurysm with Subarachnoid Hemorrhage. *Cerebral aneurysm* is a localized dilation of the cerebral artery wall that causes the artery to weaken and become susceptible to rupture. The aneurysm usually occurs at the bifurcation of large arteries at the base of the brain (circle of Willis). Most patients with cerebral aneurysms are asymptomatic before the rupture unless they experience a warning "leak" or sentinel bleeding. The aneurysm commonly ruptures into the subarachnoid space of the basal cisterns and causes a *subarachnoid hemorrhage* (SAH). Bleeding into the subarachnoid space causes increased ICP, impaired cerebral autoregulation, reduced CBF,

and irritation of the meninges. The bleeding generally stops through the formation of a fibrin plug and platelet aggregation within the artery.

After an aneurysm rupture, the patient can develop cardiac dysrhythmias, rebleeding, hydrocephalus, seizures, and cerebral vasospasm. Cardiac dysrhythmias occur as a result of sympathetic nervous system stimulation. Increased sympathetic tone can cause elevated T waves, prolonged QT intervals, and ST abnormalities. Rebleeding after the initial aneurysm rupture may occur before the aneurysm is secured. The mechanism causing the rebleeding is increased tension on the artery from hypertension, or normal breakdown of the clot, which occurs 7 to 10 days after the initial hemorrhage. Early endovascular or surgical intervention is recommended to prevent rebleeding.

Hydrocephalus can occur after SAH through two mechanisms. Bleeding into the intraventricular space can block flow of CSF and cause acute obstructive hydrocephalus. As blood enters the subarachnoid space, an inflammatory response is triggered that causes fibrosis and thickening of the arachnoid villi, thereby preventing reabsorption of CSF and producing hydrocephalus.

Seizures occurring within the first 12 hours after rupture are attributed to increased ICP or rebleeding of the aneurysm. Seizures occurring later are more likely due to ischemic damage secondary to vasospasm. Because of the adverse effects of medications, seizure prophylaxis is not recommended unless seizures occur beyond the first 12 hours after hemorrhage.

Cerebral vasospasm is a narrowing of arteries adjacent to the aneurysm that results in ischemia and infarction of brain tissue if it progresses. It is the leading cause of death after aneurysmal SAH. The usual period for vasospasm to occur can be anywhere between 3 and 14 days after the rupture. The exact mechanism for vasospasm is unknown, but some factors that contribute to vasospasm are structural changes in the adjacent cerebral arteries, denervation of adjacent arteries, generation of oxygen-free radicals, and release of vasoactive substances (serotonin, catecholamines, prostaglandins) that initiate vasospasm, the inflammatory response, and calcium influx.

Arteriovenous Malformation. An AVM is a congenital abnormality resulting in tangled, dilated vessels that form an abnormal communication network between the arterial and venous systems. Arterial blood is directly shunted into the venous system without a capillary network. This predisposes the vessels to rupture and hemorrhage into the ventricular system or subarachnoid system, causing SAH, or into the brain parenchyma, causing ICH. Impaired perfusion of the cerebral tissue adjacent to the AVM also occurs. The size and location of AVMs differ. Some AVMs do not hemorrhage, but rather cause varying degrees of ischemia, scarring of brain tissue, abnormal tissue development, compression, or hydrocephalus. AVMs are more prevalent in males and are commonly diagnosed after a patient has had a seizure. Headache is another common manifestation of AVM.

Assessment

Early identification of a stroke is imperative so rapid treatment can be initiated. The public must be educated on the symptoms of a brain attack because early intervention can minimize stroke deficit. Patients at high risk of stroke are taught risk reduction, the signs and symptoms of stroke, and to seek medical attention immediately (Box 13-2). Specialized stroke centers improve patient outcomes. The stroke center concept is designed to expedite evaluation and management of patients with suspected ischemic stroke, transient ischemic attack, or intracerebral hemorrhage. A stroke center is equipped with an emergency department (ED); a stroke team of physicians, nurses, and allied professionals with stroke-specific training; treatment protocols; emergent neuroradiology services; and access to neurosurgical services. Assessment in the ED includes an eyewitness description of symptoms, identification of the exact time symptoms started, and a neurological assessment.

The neurological examination includes evaluating mental status (LOC, arousal, orientation), cranial nerve function, motor strength, sensory function, neglect, coordination, and deep tendon reflexes. The National Institutes of Health Stroke Scale (Table 13-10) is used to assess the severity of the presenting signs and symptoms, especially if the patient is a candidate for thrombolytic therapy.

BOX 13-2   Signs and Symptoms of Stroke

- Weakness or numbness of one side of the body (face, arm, leg, or any combination of these)
- Slurred speech
- Inability to comprehend what is being said
- Visual disturbance (transient loss of vision in one or both eyes [transient monocular blindness] or a visual field deficit)
- Dizziness, incoordination or ataxia, double vision, vertigo
- Nausea or vomiting
- Severe headache ("worst headache of my life")

Assessment and stabilization of the airway, breathing, and circulation are a priority. Vital signs are monitored, generally every 15 minutes for the first 6 hours. BP elevations are common in these patients. Because reducing the BP can decrease blood flow and oxygenation to the ischemic brain tissue, a gradual 20% lowering of the BP is recommended to prevent enlargement of the infarcted area and worsening of the neurological deficit. The goal for ischemic stroke is to keep the systolic BP less than 220 mm Hg and the diastolic BP less than 120 mm Hg.[1] In hemorrhagic stroke, the goal is a MAP less than 130 mm Hg.[11] Monitoring the respiratory pattern is important because changes can indicate that the stroke is extending and more neurological damage is occurring. Hypoxemia after a stroke is common as a result of concurrent medical conditions such as aspiration, pneumonia, hypoventilation, atelectasis, and pulmonary embolism.[20] A baseline SpO_2 is obtained while the patient is breathing room air, and supplemental oxygen is provided when the SpO_2 is less than 95%. Cardiac assessment, including the presence of cardiac dysrhythmias, is important to determine whether the stroke was potentially caused by a cardioembolic event. IV access is obtained, and normal saline infusions are started; hypertonic solutions are avoided. Laboratory studies include electrolytes, cardiac enzymes, complete blood count, urinalysis, and coagulation studies. A serum glucose level is obtained because many patients who present with stroke are hyperglycemic. In addition, up to 20% of patients with stroke are diabetic.[10] Several studies indicate that individuals with hyperglycemia have poorer outcomes after stroke as compared with normoglycemic patients, even without a history of diabetes. The hyperglycemia seems to increase neuronal injury.[32]

Once the patient is transferred to the critical care unit, assessments are compared with the baseline assessments performed in the ED. Hemodynamic instability is common in an acute stroke because of cardiac disorders and the sympathetic response; therefore, assessment of the airway, vital signs, and fluid and electrolyte status continues to be a priority. Elderly patients with stroke often are dehydrated. Dehydration is caused by inadequate water intake, drowsiness, dysphagia, possible infection, diuretic use, and uncontrolled diabetes.[10,23] Dehydration after a stroke can cause an increased hematocrit and a reduced BP that can worsen the ischemic process. In a patient with an acute stroke, neurological status, hemodynamic status, laboratory values, and cardiac function are monitored. Ongoing assessments are similar to those in patients with increased ICP. Patients with subarachnoid hemorrhage present differently than those with ischemic stroke. When

TABLE 13-10   National Institutes of Health Stroke Scale

Instructions	Scale Definition
1a. Level of Consciousness: The investigator must choose a response if a full evaluation is prevented by such obstacles as an endotracheal tube, language barrier, orotracheal trauma/bandages.	0 = **Alert;** keenly responsive. 1 = **Not alert;** but arousable by minor stimulation. 2 = **Not alert;** requires repeated stimulation to attend. 3 = **Responds** only with reflex motor or autonomic effects or totally unresponsive, flaccid, and areflexic.
1b. LOC Questions: The patient is asked the month and his/her age. The answer must be correct—there is no partial credit for being close.	0 = **Answers** both questions correctly. 1 = **Answers** one question correctly. 2 = **Answers** neither question correctly.
1c. LOC Commands: The patient is asked to open and close the eyes and then to grip and release the nonparetic hand. Substitute another one-step command if the hands cannot be used.	0 = **Performs** both tasks correctly. 1 = **Performs** one task correctly. 2 = **Performs** neither task correctly.
2. Best Gaze: Only horizontal eye movements will be tested. Voluntary or reflexive (oculocephalic) eye movements will be scored, but caloric testing is not done.	0 = **Normal.** 1 = **Partial gaze palsy;** gaze is abnormal in one or both eyes. 2 = **Forced deviation,** or total gaze paresis not overcome by the oculocephalic maneuver.
3. Visual: Visual fields (upper and lower quadrants) are tested by confrontation, using finger counting or visual threat, as appropriate.	0 = **No visual loss.** 1 = **Partial hemianopia.** 2 = **Complete hemianopia.** 3 = **Bilateral hemianopia** (blind).
4. Facial Palsy: Ask—or use pantomime to encourage—the patient to show teeth or raise eyebrows and close eyes.	0 = **Normal** symmetrical movements. 1 = **Minor paralysis** (asymmetry on smiling). 2 = **Partial paralysis** (total or near-total paralysis of lower face). 3 = **Complete paralysis** of one or both sides.
5. Motor Arm: The limb is placed in the appropriate position: extend the arms (palms down) 90 degrees (if sitting) or 45 degrees (if supine). Drift is scored if the arm falls before 10 seconds. **5a.** Left arm **5b.** Right arm	0 = **No drift;** limb holds position for 10 seconds. 1 = **Drift;** limb holds position, but drifts down before full 10 seconds. 2 = **Some effort against gravity;** limb cannot get to or maintain position, drifts down to bed, some effort against gravity. 3 = **No effort against gravity; limb falls.** 4 = **No movement.** UN = **Amputation** or joint fusion.
6. Motor Leg: The limb is placed in the appropriate position: hold the leg at 30 degrees (always tested supine). Drift is scored if the leg falls before 5 seconds. **6a.** Left leg **6b.** Right leg	0 = **No drift;** leg holds position for full 5 seconds. 1 = **Drift;** leg falls by the end of the 5-second period but does not hit bed. 2 = **Some effort against gravity;** leg falls to bed. By 5 seconds, has some effort against gravity. 3 = **No effort against gravity;** leg falls to bed immediately. 4 = **No movement.** UN = **Amputation** or joint fusion
7. Limb Ataxia: The finger-nose-finger and heel-shin tests are performed on both sides with eyes open.	0 = **Absent.** 1 = **Present in one limb.** 2 = **Present in two limbs.** UN = **Amputation** or joint fusion.

TABLE 13-10	National Institutes of Health Stroke Scale—cont'd

Instructions	Scale Definition
8. **Sensory:** Sensation or grimace to pinprick when tested, or withdrawal from noxious stimulus in the obtunded or aphasic patient.	0 = **Normal;** no sensory loss. 1 = **Mild-to-moderate sensory loss;** feels pinprick is less sharp or is dull on the affected side; or there is a loss of superficial pain with pinprick, but aware of being touched. 2 = **Severe to total sensory loss;** patient is not aware of being touched in the face, arm, and leg.
9. **Best Language:** Patient is asked to describe what is happening in the attached picture, to name the items on the attached naming sheet, and to read from the attached list of sentences. Comprehension is judged from responses here, as well as to all of the commands in the preceding general neurological exam.	0 = **No aphasia;** normal. 1 = **Mild-to-moderate aphasia;** some obvious loss of fluency or facility of comprehension, without significant limitation on ideas. 2 = **Severe aphasia;** all communication is through fragmentary expression; great need for inference, questioning, and guessing by the listener. 3 = **Mute, global aphasia;** no usable speech or auditory comprehension.
10. **Dysarthria:** An adequate sample of speech must be obtained by asking patient to read or repeat words from the attached list.	0 = **Normal.** 1 = **Mild-to-moderate dysarthria;** patient slurs some words; can be understood with some difficulty. 2 = **Severe dysarthria;** patient's speech is so slurred as to be unintelligible; or is mute/anarthric. UN = **Intubated** or other physical barrier.
11. **Extinction and Inattention (formerly Neglect):** Sufficient information to identify neglect may be obtained during prior testing. If the patient has a severe visual loss preventing visual double simultaneous stimulation, and the cutaneous stimuli are normal, the score is normal.	0 = **No abnormality.** 1 = **Visual, tactile, auditory, spatial, or personal inattention** or extinction to bilateral simultaneous stimulation in one of the sensory modalities. 2 = **Profound hemi-inattention or extinction to more than one modality;** does not recognize own hand or orients to only one side of space.

From National Institute of Neurological Disorders and Stroke at the National Institutes of Health. (2003). *NIH stroke scale.* Retrieved January 27, 2008 from www.ninds.nih.gov.

arterial blood enters the subarachnoid space, its presence is irritating to the meninges. The patient may complain of a localized headache, stiff neck *(nuchal rigidity)*, pain above and behind the eye, and photophobia. Patients with SAH are often anxious and agitated as a result of pain, altered LOC, and cognitive changes. If conscious, the patient may complain of "the worst headache of my life." Vomiting and decreased LOC are commonly seen. Neurological assessment includes LOC, motor and sensory deficits, and pupillary response. Assessment findings may include mental status changes and subtle focal deficits to coma or severe neurological deficits.

Diagnostic Tests

Diagnostic tests are performed to differentiate ischemic from hemorrhagic stroke and to establish base-line parameters to monitor the effects of treatment.[1] A summary of common diagnostic tests is listed in Box 13-3.

Management

Nursing Diagnoses
A patient with stroke has similar nursing diagnoses as a patient with increased ICP and TBI. Refer to the Nursing Care Plan for the Patient with Traumatic Brain Injury, Increased Intracranial Pressure, or Acute Stroke.

Ischemic Stroke
Thrombolytic Candidates. Early intervention for ischemic stroke is recommended. rt-PA is the only approved therapy for acute ischemic stroke and must be given within 3 hours of the onset of symptoms;

BOX 13-3   Diagnostic Testing for Stroke

Initial Diagnostic Testing
- Emergency CT scan without contrast
- 12-lead electrocardiogram
- Chest x-ray study
- Review of time of onset and inclusion criteria for patients eligible for rt-PA, including NIHSS assessment
- Complete blood count (red blood cells, hemoglobin, hematocrit, platelet count)
- Coagulation studies: prothrombin time, activated partial thromboplastin time, INR
- Serum electrolytes and glucose
- Urinalysis
- Troponin and cardiac enzymes, to rule out myocardial infarction

Additional Diagnostic Testing[1]
- MRI with diffusion and perfusion images: detects ischemia, altered CBF, and cerebral blood volume
- Arteriography: detects shallow ulcerated plaques, thrombus, aneurysms, dissections, multiple lesions, AVMs, and collateral blood flow
- MRA images: detects carotid occlusion, intracranial stenoses or occlusions
- CT perfusion images: detects altered CBF and cerebral blood volume
- CT angiography images: detects carotid occlusion and intracranial stenoses or occlusions
- Digital subtraction angiography: detects carotid occlusion, and intracranial stenoses or occlusions
- Doppler carotid ultrasound: detects stenoses or occlusions of the carotid arteries
- Transcranial Doppler ultrasound: detects stenoses and occlusions of the circle of Willis, vertebral arteries, and basilar artery
- Transthoracic echocardiogram: detects cardioembolic abnormalities
- Transesophageal echocardiogram: detects cardioembolic abnormalities; more sensitive than transthoracic echocardiogram

AVMs, Arteriovenous malformations; *CBF*, cerebral blood flow; *CT*, computerized tomography; *INR*, international normalized ratio; *MRA*, magnetic resonance angiography; *MRI*, magnetic resonance imaging; *NIHSS*, National Institutes of Health Stroke Scale; *rt-PA*, recombinant tissue plasminogen activator.

unfortunately, only about 5% of eligible patients actually receive the treatment.[29] Administration after 3 hours has not shown to be beneficial. The medication lyses the clot and restores blood flow to the ischemic penumbra, limiting secondary brain damage and improving overall neurological function. rt-PA does not affect the infarcted area but revitalizes the ischemic penumbra. Careful assessment of patients potentially eligible for thrombolytic therapy must be made (Box 13-4).

Before the administration of rt-PA, two peripheral IV lines are inserted—one for the administration of rt-PA and one for fluids. Any catheters that are needed (e.g., urinary catheters, nasogastric tubes) are ideally placed before the administration of rt-PA to reduce the risk for bleeding. After the administration of rt-PA, invasive procedures may be performed; however, the risk of bleeding is higher. Antithrombotics such as heparin, warfarin, and aspirin are withheld for 24 hours after administration of rt-PA to prevent bleeding complications.

Symptomatic hemorrhage is the most common complication after rt-PA administration, with an incidence of 6.4%.[1] The highest risk for hemorrhage is within the first 36 hours. Intracerebral hemorrhage usually occurs as a result of secondary bleeding into the area of infarct, also known as hemorrhagic transformation. The incidence of hemorrhage may be reduced by detecting neurological changes early and maintaining the systolic BP at less than 185 mm Hg and the diastolic BP at less than 110 mm Hg. Antihypertensive agents are administered as needed to control the BP.

Signs and symptoms of intracerebral hemorrhage manifest as neurological deterioration, increased ICP, or cerebral herniation. If intracerebral hemorrhage is suspected, the rt-PA infusion is stopped, an emergency noncontrast CT scan of the head is obtained, and fresh frozen plasma or platelets are administered. Systemic bleeding can also occur. Signs and symptoms include hypotension, tachycardia, pallor, restlessness, or low back pain. Stool, urine, and gastric secretions are monitored for the presence of blood. IV sites and gums are monitored for signs of external bleeding. Baseline coagulation studies are compared with current studies.

Neurological assessment (LOC, language, motor and sensory testing, pupillary response) and vital signs are performed every 15 minutes for the first 2 hours, every 30 minutes for the next 6 hours, and every hour for 16 hours. Accurate intake and output are maintained. Continuous cardiac monitoring is done throughout the hyperacute phase (first 24 to 72 hours). Oxygen is given to maintain the SpO_2 at 95%. Pneumonia is a common complication after stroke; therefore, frequent patient repositioning and nebulizer therapy may be indicated.[20]

Nonthrombolytic Candidates. For a patient with stroke who is a not a candidate for thrombolytic therapy, interventions include neurological, respiratory, and

BOX 13-4 Administration of Tissue Plasminogen Activator for Acute Ischemic Stroke

Inclusion Criteria
- Onset of stroke symptoms <3 hours
- Clinical diagnosis of ischemic stroke with a measurable deficit using the NIHSS
- Age >18 years
- CT scan consistent with ischemic stroke

Exclusion Criteria
- Stroke symptoms >3 hours of symptoms onset
- Rapidly improving minor or major stroke (i.e., transient ischemic attack)
- Evidence of intracerebral bleed including intraparenchymal subarachnoid hemorrhage or other pathological condition (neoplasm, AVM, or aneurysm on CT scan)
- Systolic BP >185 mm Hg or diastolic BP >110 mm Hg
- Glucose <50 mg/dL or >400 mg/dL
- Rapidly improving or deteriorating neurological signs or minor symptoms
- Recent myocardial infarction
- Seizure at the onset of stroke
- Active internal bleeding (e.g., urinary) within 21 days
- Arterial puncture at noncompressible site
- Known bleeding diathesis, including but not limited to:
  a. Current use of oral anticoagulants (e.g., warfarin, sodium) with prothrombin time of >15 seconds
  b. Administration of heparin within 48 hours preceding the onset of stroke and have an elevated aPTT at presentation
  c. Platelet count <100,000/μl
- Lumbar puncture within 7 days, major surgery within 14 days

Administration
- rt-PA dosing: 0.9 mg/kg intravenously up to maximum of 90 mg
- Give bolus of 10% of total calculated dose intravenously over 1 minute
- Administer the remaining 90% over the next 60 minutes

aPTT, Activated partial thromboplastin time; *AVM,* arteriovenous malformation; *BP,* blood pressure; *CT,* computed tomography; *NIHSS,* National Institutes of Health Stroke Scale; *rt-PA,* recombinant tissue plasminogen activator. Modified from the National Institute of Neurological Disorders and Stroke (NINDS) t-PA Stroke Study Group. (1995). Tissue plasminogen activator for acute ischemic stroke. *New England Journal of Medicine,* 333, 1581-1587; and the Activase (alteplase), Genentech, Inc., South San Francisco, CA package insert.

cardiac assessments. These assessments and vital signs are performed every 1 to 2 hours during the first 24 hours after stroke. BP is controlled to prevent bleeding while maintaining an adequate CPP. For patients with uncontrolled hypertension, BP is managed carefully with IV medications including labetalol or nicardipine. Rapid drops in BP can cause further neurological deterioration by decreasing cerebral perfusion and extending the area of cerebral ischemia. Laboratory tests (complete blood count, chemistries, urinalysis, coagulations studies, cardiac enzymes) are performed, and a urinary catheter may be indicated.

Other interventions include the administration of medications to decrease ICP and maintenance of hemodynamic stability. The incidence of cerebral herniation peaks at about 72 hours after the stroke (refer to Table 13-6). Since hyperglycemia may exacerbate the extent of neurological injury, glycemic control is advocated (see Chapter 18). Hyponatremia due to cerebral salt wasting may occur; sodium and fluid replacement are necessary to maintain a normal sodium level.

Antithrombotics such as warfarin, aspirin, combination aspirin/dipyridamole (Aggrenox), and clopidogrel (Plavix) may be given for prevention of secondary stroke. Some patients require antihypertensive agents or antiepileptic medications. Maintaining adequate fluid balance is crucial to ensure proper hydration. Maintaining normothermia is important to reduce the metabolic needs of the brain. Hyperthermia may be the result of direct injury or bleeding into the hypothalamus, systemic infection, or drug-induced fever from anticonvulsant medications. Aspiration precautions are implemented including elevating the head of the bed and maintaining nothing-by-mouth status until a swallow screening or formal study rules out dysphagia.

Other Ischemic Events

Transient Ischemic Attacks. A *transient ischemic attack* (TIA) is defined as the sudden onset of a temporary focal neurological deficit caused by a vascular event. During a TIA, a transient decrease in CBF occurs, but the patient does not experience any permanent deficits.

A TIA is commonly caused by stenosis of the carotid arteries. A common presentation of a TIA is amaurosis fugax (monocular blindness), a transient occlusion of the central retinal artery. Although symptoms of a TIA mimic those of stroke, by definition TIA symptoms last 24 hours or less.[23] Generally, patients with symptoms of TIA should receive a complete stroke workup to determine the cause of TIA. Patients may be managed with anticoagulants such as heparin if the symptoms wax and wane or with antiplatelet therapy such as aspirin if symptoms are stable and do not recur.

It is important that TIAs be diagnosed so that preventive measures to avoid stroke can be initiated. Unfortunately, persons experiencing a TIA often ignore the symptoms because the symptoms are painless and short-lived, usually about 5 to 10 minutes. Within a year of having a TIA, many persons have a stroke and sustain permanent neurological deficits.

Patients experiencing TIAs with carotid stenosis are evaluated for carotid endarterectomy or carotid angioplasty and stenting. If a patient has carotid stenosis greater than 69% on the symptomatic side, carotid endarterectomy is recommended. Carotid angioplasty with stenting is also an accepted method of treating carotid stenosis for selected patients.

Hemorrhagic Stroke

Intraparenchymal Stroke. Control of BP is important to prevent recurrent hemorrhage. The optimum threshold for BP is unknown. Elevations in BP are not usually treated unless the MAP is greater than 130 mm Hg, or the patient has a history of heart failure. If treatment is required, BP is lowered cautiously to prehemorrhage levels. Control of BP is important to prevent continued bleeding.

Medical assessment focuses on determining the size and location of the intracranial hemorrhage, and whether it is amenable to surgical intervention. Small clots usually resolve without surgery. In these instances, more aggressive BP management may be indicated. Surgery is considered in patients with hematomas larger than 3 cm or who are deteriorating neurologically, although the role of surgical intervention is controversial. Comatose patients with large lesions usually have poorer outcomes, regardless of treatment.[11]

Subarachnoid Hemorrhage

Early diagnosis of the cause of SAH helps to guide treatment. Although a CT scan helps differentiate an aneurysm from an AVM, definitive diagnosis of an aneurysm is determined by digital subtraction or CT angiography. Early surgical or endovascular intervention (within 24 hours of admission) is recommended for patients in good neurological condition whose aneurysm is surgically or endovascularly accessible. The goal is to operate when there is minimal neurological dysfunction and before any episodes of rebleeding or vasospasm occur.

Surgery for a cerebral aneurysm involves occluding the neck of the aneurysm with a ligature or metal clip, reinforcing the sac by wrapping the sac with muscle, fibrin foam, or solidifying polymer, or proximally ligating a feeding vessel. If the neck of the aneurysm is narrow and accessible, using a ligature or metal clip is desirable. When the neck of the aneurysm is too broad, reinforcing the aneurysmal sac is the goal of surgery. Proximal ligation may be preferred when the aneurysm is directly fed by the internal carotid artery. The disadvantage of this procedure is the potential for stroke should collateral circulation fail.

Interventional techniques such as endovascular therapy with coils or stents may be used to occlude the aneurysm. This therapy consists of navigating a microcatheter through the femoral artery to the aneurysm and placing platinum coils into the aneurysm sac or a stent to cover the opening. Thrombosis occurs, thus occluding the aneurysm from the feeder vessel. This technique can be done with ruptured or unruptured aneurysms.

Patients with severe neurological compromise after a ruptured aneurysm may benefit from emergency ventriculostomy. The ventriculostomy assists in treating the hydrocephalus associated with the bleeding. The ventriculostomy also allows the clinician to monitor ICP and remove CSF to lower ICP if needed. However, where possible, venticulostomy is not performed until after the aneurusym has been secured, as changing the ICP can contribute to rebleeding.

Management of BP is an important treatment of aneurysmal SAH. Medications are administered to reduce BP before the aneurysm is secured to prevent rebleeding. After securing the aneurysm, blood pressure is allowed to rise to prevent vasospasm. If vasospasm occurs, blood pressure may be purposely increased with fluids and medications to augment CBF. Neurological status is assessed frequently by using the GCS and monitoring for focal deficits and pupillary changes. Temperature monitoring is important because persons with SAH often have a fever, which is associated with worse neurological outcome.[16] Elevation of the head of the bed may reduce ICP. A feeding tube may be required for nutritional support. Measures for venous thromboembolism prevention are initiated. Other important interventions include providing an analgesia and bed rest.

Monitoring for signs of vasospasm is of paramount importance because early intervention results in better patient outcomes. Nimodipine, a neurospecific calcium channel blocker, reduces the incidence and severity of deficits associated with SAH. The recommended dosage is 60 mg every 4 hours for 21 days. Vasospasm is often treated with volume expansion to increase CPP. The modalities used are hypervolemia and hypertension. Hypervolemia refers to increasing the blood volume by using crystalloids, colloids, albumin, plasma protein fraction, or blood. Systolic BP is maintained between 150 and 160 mm Hg (and sometimes higher). The increase in volume and BP forces blood through the vasospastic area at higher pressures. If the patient's BP becomes lower than prehemorrhage levels, vasoactive infusions, such as dopamine, dobutamine, or phenylephrine (Neo-Synephrine), may be warranted.

Recent therapies for the treatment of symptomatic vasospasm include papaverine and angioplasty. Intraarterial papaverine application increases the diameter of the vasospastic blood vessel and lasts less than 24 hours. Intraarterial administration of nicardipine (Cardene) is another option for treating vasospasm. Nicardipine, a calcium channel blocker, has a vasodilatory effect. The clinical indications for intraarterial nicardipine are similar to those for papaverine; however, nicardipine is effective for 2 to 5 days. Cerebral angioplasty is indicated for vasospasm when pharmacological therapy has failed. Risks of angioplasty include perforation or rupture, cerebral artery thrombosis, recurrent vasospasm, and transient neurological deficits.

Arteriovenous Malformation

Spontaneous bleeding from an AVM can occur into the ventricular system, intraparenchymal tissue, or subarachnoid space. Hemorrhage from an AVM is usually low-pressure bleeding, and the mortality from such a hemorrhage is lower than that from a ruptured aneurysm. The rebleeding rate is also much lower than that of an aneurysm. AVMs may also cause symptoms due to ischemia or act as a space-occupying lesion, similar to a tumor.

Treatment interventions for an AVM include embolization, surgery, radiotherapy, or a combination of all three. Surgery for removal of an AVM is done either as a single step or in multiple stages. Postoperatively, the major problem is breakthrough bleeding from cauterized vessels. Rapid increases in BP during recovery from anesthesia are to be avoided, and blood pressure must be tightly controlled for the first 48 hours after resection to prevent bleeding. Embolization is not a curative approach to the majority of AVMs, but rather is used as preparation for surgery. Embolization may occur in a single setting or may be staged in several procedures over days to weeks. Radiotherapy may be performed alone or for residual AVM after surgery; results are manifest over years.

Postoperative Neurosurgical Care

The postoperative care of a patient who has undergone a neurosurgical procedure involves frequent and ongoing hemodynamic, respiratory, metabolic, and neurological assessments. Neurological assessments are done every 15 to 30 minutes for the first 2 to 12 hours postoperatively, then every hour while the patient is in the critical care unit. Oxygenation and tissue perfusion are monitored. Chest x-rays, CT scans, EEGs, and other diagnostic tests may be necessary to monitor progress.

The position of the head of the bed depends on the specific surgical procedure, patient condition, and physician preference. Unless the patient is intubated, unconscious patients are never positioned on their backs because the tongue can slip backward and obstruct the airway. However, unconscious patients may be positioned in a lateral position with the head of the bed flat. The neck must always be maintained in a neutral position.

The most common postoperative complications include infection, cerebral hemorrhage, increased ICP, hydrocephalus, and seizures.[9] Intracerebral hemorrhage is detected by a decline in neurological status, signs of increasing ICP, and new or worsened focal deficits (i.e., hemiparesis/hemiplegia, aphasia). It is confirmed by CT scan. Treatment depends on CT findings and may require emergency surgery.

Hydrocephalus can develop any time during the postoperative course as a result of edema or bleeding into the subarachnoid space. Treatment may include placement of a ventriculostomy to drain CSF temporarily. If the hydrocephalus does not resolve, a surgical shunting procedure may be indicated to relieve the brain of excessive CSF.

Seizures can occur at any time but are most common within the first 7 days after surgery. Focal seizures in the form of twitching of selected muscles, particularly of the face and hand, are often seen. Patients may receive postoperative antiepileptic drugs, most commonly phenytoin, if concern for seizures is high. Serum phenytoin levels are monitored to maintain a therapeutic range.

SEIZURES AND STATUS EPILEPTICUS

A seizure is an abnormal electrical discharge in the brain caused by a variety of neurological disorders, systemic diseases, and metabolic disorders. Seizures consist of repetitive depolarization of hyperactive, hypersensitive cells that cause an altered state of brain function. Abnormalities can occur in the motor system, sensory system, and/or ANS. Seizures are classified as either partial or generalized (Table 13-11). *Partial seizures* usually begin in one cerebral hemisphere and cause motor activity to be localized to one area of the body (e.g., arm, face). The seizure is classified as *simple partial* if consciousness remains

TABLE 13-11   Classification of Seizures

Type	Symptoms
I. Partial	
Simple (no loss of consciousness)	
Motor	"Jacksonian" march
	Movement of eye, head, and body to one side
	Stopping of movement or speech
Sensory or somatosensory	Tingling, numbness of body part
	Visual, auditory, olfactory, or taste sensations
	Dizzy spells
Autonomic	Pallor, sweating, flushing, piloerection, pupillary dilation
Psychic	Déjà vu ("already seen")
	Distortion of time sense
	Hallucinations
	Objects appearing small, large, or far away
Complex (alteration of consciousness); automatisms	Automatisms (lip smacking, picking with hands), wandering
II. Generalized	
Absence	
Simple	Staring spell lasting less than 15 seconds
Atypical	Staring spell with myoclonic jerks and automatisms
Myoclonic	Brief jerk of one or more muscle groups
Clonic	Repetitive jerking of muscle groups
Tonic	Stiffening of muscle groups
Tonic-clonic	Starts with the stiffening or tonic phase, followed by the jerking or clonic phase
	Unconsciousness
	Tongue biting
	Bowel and bladder incontinence
Atonic	Drop attack or abrupt loss of muscle tone

Modified from Barker, E. (2008). *Neuroscience nursing: A spectrum of care* (3rd ed., p. 691). St. Louis: Mosby.

intact, and *complex partial* if consciousness is impaired. *Generalized seizures* involve both cerebral hemispheres and cause altered consciousness and bilateral motor manifestations.

Pathophysiology of Status Epilepticus

When seizures occur in close proximity to each other, they have the potential to lead to a life-threatening medical emergency known as *status epilepticus* (SE). SE can occur with any type of seizure. By definition, SE is present when seizure activity lasts for 30 minutes or longer, or when two or more sequential seizures occur without full recovery of consciousness between seizures. SE is more likely to occur with tonic-clonic seizures that have a specific causative factor than with idiopathic seizures. The most frequent precipitating factors for SE are irregular intake of antiepileptic drugs, withdrawal from habitual use of alcohol or sedative drugs, electrolyte imbalance, azotemia, head trauma, infection, and brain tumor.

Physiological changes that occur during SE are divided into two phases. During phase 1, cerebral metabolism is increased and compensatory mechanisms (increased CBF and catecholamine release) prevent cerebral damage from hypoxia or metabolic injury. However, these changes can lead to other problems. Hyperglycemia occurs from release of epinephrine and activation of hepatic gluconeogenesis. Hypertension occurs to increase CBF. Hyperpyrexia results from excessive muscle activity and catecholamine release. Lactic acidosis occurs from anaerobic metabolism. Elevated epinephrine and norepinephrine levels and acidosis contribute to cardiac dysrhythmias. Autonomic dysfunction causes excessive sweating and vomiting, leading to dehydration and electrolyte loss.

Phase 2 begins 30 to 60 minutes after phase 1. Decompensation occurs because the increased metabolic demands cannot be met. This causes decreased CBF, systemic hypotension, increased ICP, and cerebral autoregulation failure. The patient develops metabolic and respiratory acidosis from hypoxemia, hypoglycemia from depleted energy stores, hyponatremia, and hypokalemia or hyperkalemia. The lack of oxygen and glucose results in cellular injury. Pulmonary edema is common, and pulmonary aspiration can occur from decreased laryngeal reflex sensitivity. Cardiac dysrhythmias and heart failure result from hypoxemia, hyperkalemia caused by increased muscle activity, and metabolic acidosis. Renal failure may result from rhabdomyolysis and acute myoglobinuria. Myoglobin is released secondary to excessive muscle activity from prolonged skeletal muscle contraction and traumatic injury during the seizure.

Death from SE is more likely to occur when an underlying disease is responsible for the seizure, or from the acute illness that precipitated the seizure. Generalized seizures that last for 30 to 45 minutes can result in neuronal necrosis and permanent neurological deficits. Prompt diagnosis and treatment are important because seizure duration is an important prognostic factor.

Assessment

Assessment during SE incorporates the neurological, respiratory, and cardiovascular systems. Characteristics of the seizure and the neurological state before, between, and after seizures are important to monitor. Information to collect includes precipitating factors, preceding aura, type of movement observed, automatisms, changes in size of pupils or eye deviation, responsiveness to auditory or tactile stimuli, LOC throughout the seizure, urinary or bowel incontinence, patient's behavior after the seizure, weakness or paralysis of extremities after the seizure, injuries caused by the seizure, and duration of the seizure.[9] Assessment of respirations and monitoring of SpO_2 are needed to ensure adequate oxygenation. Because autonomic changes can result in pulmonary edema, it is imperative to observe for the onset of fine basilar crackles. Suction equipment and oxygen should be readily available. Cardiac monitoring is necessary to assess for dysrhythmias.

Diagnostic Tests

Laboratory studies for a patient with SE include serum electrolytes, liver function studies, serum medication levels, and blood and urine toxicology screens. Cardiac enzymes and arterial blood gases assist in assessing the effect of the seizure on other body systems. Patient monitoring includes ECG, EEG, noninvasive BP, and pulse oximetry.

Radiological studies are performed to rule out a space-occupying lesion that may be responsible for the episode of SE. These may include CT or MRI with contrast, or both. Additional studies may be ordered to rule out injury.

Management

Nursing Diagnoses

Nursing diagnoses that are relevant to the patient experiencing SE are as follows: ineffective tissue perfusion (cerebral and cardiopulmonary) related to continuous seizure activity or vasodilating effects of antiepileptic medications; ineffective breathing pattern or impaired gas exchange related to hypoventilation; ineffective airway clearance related to underlying neurological problem and seizure activity; risk for trauma (oral and musculoskeletal) related to seizure activity; disturbed thought processes related to the postictal state; and deficient knowledge related to disease process, treatment, and necessary lifestyle changes.

Nursing and Medical Interventions

Management during SE includes maintaining a patent airway, providing adequate oxygenation, maintaining vascular access for the administration of medications and fluids, administering appropriate medications, and maintaining seizure precautions. A patent airway is facilitated by positioning appropriately; use of an oral/nasal airway or endotracheal tube may be necessary. Padded tongue blades are not to be inserted between the clenched teeth of a patient undergoing a seizure. Patients have inadvertently been injured from aspirating teeth that were loosened during forceful attempts to insert a padded tongue blade between their teeth. Suctioning is often needed to remove secretions that collect in the oropharynx. Supplemental oxygen is administered to improve oxygenation. A nasogastric tube with intermittent suction may be needed to ensure that the airway is not compromised by aspiration.

Vascular access must be maintained to provide a route for the administration of medication. If unable to establish IV access, some antiseizure medications can be administered rectally. The specific medication given to arrest the seizure depends on the physician's preference and the type and duration of the seizure (see Table 13-8). It is essential to monitor BP and to administer volume replacement and vasoactive drugs if necessary. IV dextrose is administered unless the blood glucose level is known to be normal or high. Thiamine may also be given.

Seizure precautions are continued during SE. This includes padding the side rails on the patient's bed and making sure that the bed has full-length side rails. The bed is kept in a low position with side rails up, except when providing direct nursing care. If the patient is in a chair when a seizure begins, the patient is lowered to the floor and a soft object is placed under the patient's head. It is important to remove the patient's restrictive clothing and jewelry while always maintaining the patient's privacy. The patient should not be restrained because forceful tonic-clonic movements can traumatize the patient.

SE must be treated immediately. The nurse ensures a patent airway and maintains breathing and circulation. Medications are given using a sequential approach that progressively uses more potent medications to control the seizure. The first-line medication is a benzodiazepine, usually IV lorazepam (Ativan). If lorazepam fails to stop seizure activity within 10 minutes, or if intermittent seizures persist for longer than 20 minutes, phenytoin (Dilantin) or fosphenytoin (Cerebyx) may be administered. Phenytoin is mixed only with normal saline, and it is stable in solution for only 20 minutes, thus making it impractical for IV piggyback administration. It may be given slowly by IV push after clearing the line with saline. Phenobarbital may be used as the third-line agent to control SE, but its utility in SE is lessened by the length of time required to achieve a therapeutic effect.

If SE continues despite phenytoin administration, propofol (Diprivan) is given. Propofol is a general anesthetic and sedative-hypnotic agent. Patients may require intubation and mechanical ventilation because inefficient ventilation may result. Pentobarbital may also be considered. Patients must be assessed for hypotension. Refer to Table 13-8 for specifics regarding medication therapy for SE.

CENTRAL NERVOUS SYSTEM INFECTIONS

The brain and spinal cord are relatively well protected from infective agents by the bones of the skull and veterbral column, the meninges, and the blood-brain barrier. However, infective agents can enter the CNS through the air sinuses, middle ear, or blood. Penetrating injuries that disrupt the dura (e.g., basilar skull fractures, missile injuries, neurosurgical procedures) also increase the risk for infection. *Meningitis* (infection of the meninges) may be caused by bacteria, viruses, fungi, parasites, or other toxins. These infections are classified as acute, subacute, or chronic. The pathophysiology, clinical presentation, and management differ for each type of microorganism. Box 13-5 lists common organisms that cause meningitis.

Bacterial Meningitis

Bacterial meningitis is a neurological emergency and can lead to substantial morbidity and mortality.[36,37] Approximately 3000 cases occur in the United States each year, and more than 300 people die, with a significant fatality rate in adolescents.[13] Meningitis affects the very young, the very old, and immunosuppressed individuals. Because of its high mortality, vaccination against bacterial meningitis is recommended.

Pathophysiology
Bacterial meningitis is an infection of the pia mater and arachnoid layers of the meninges, and the CSF in the subarachnoid space. Bacteria gain access in one of three ways: (1) via the blood or through the

---

BOX 13-5   Causes of Meningitis

Bacterial
- *Streptococcus pneumoniae* (pneumococcus)
- *Neisseria meningitidis* (meningococcus)
- *Haemophilus influenzae* (Hib)
- Staphylococci *(Staphylococcus aureus)*
- Gram-negative bacilli *(Escherichia coli, Enterobacter, Serratia)*

Viruses
- Echovirus
- Coxsackievirus
- Mumps
- Herpes simplex types 1 and 2
- St. Louis encephalitis
- Colorado tick fever
- Epstein-Barr
- West Nile
- Influenza types A and B

Fungal
- Histoplasmosis
- Candidiasis
- Aspergillosis

---

spread of nearby infection, such as sinusitis; (2) CSF contamination through surgical procedures or catheters; or (3) through the skull. Airborne droplets passed from infected individuals through sneezing, coughing, or kissing, or droplets passed along through saliva and transmitted via drinks, cigarettes, or utensils, can occur. Bacteria enter through the choroid plexuses, multiply in the subarachnoid space, and irritate the meninges. An exudate forms that thickens the CSF and alters CSF flow through and around the brain and spinal cord, resulting in obstruction, interstitial edema, and further inflammation.

Assessment
The clinical assessment of adults with bacterial meningitis requires a thorough history and neurological assessment. Patients often are seen in the ED with an acute onset of symptoms (e.g., headache, fever, stiff neck, vomiting) that developed over 1 to 2 days. There may be a recent history of infection (ear, sinus, or upper respiratory), foreign travel, or illicit drug use. The clinical presentation often reveals signs of systemic infection including fever (temperature as high as 39.5° C), tachycardia, chills, and petechial rash. Initially the rash may be macular, but it progresses to petechiae and purpura, mainly on the trunk and extremities. Meningeal irritation produces a throbbing headache, photophobia, vomiting, and

nuchal rigidity. A positive *Kernig's sign* (pain in the neck when the thigh is flexed on the abdomen and the leg extended at the knee) and a positive *Brudzinski's sign* (involuntary flexion of the hips when the neck is flexed toward the chest) may be present. The patient's condition can quickly deteriorate to hypotension, shock, and sepsis.

Assessment of the patient's LOC, motor response, and cranial nerves is performed. Confusion and decreasing LOC are evidence of cortical involvement. Focal neurological deficits may be seen including hemiparesis, hemiplegia, and ataxia as well as seizure activity and projectile vomiting. Irritation and damage to cranial nerves occur as a result of inflamed sheaths (Table 13-12). As ICP increases, unconsciousness may occur.

Diagnostic Tests

The gold standard for the diagnosis of meningitis is examination of CSF via lumbar puncture, or aspiration of CSF from a ventricular catheter. Diagnosis is also based on a nasopharyngeal smear and antigen tests. Blood and urine cultures are obtained before starting antibiotics. A CT scan, MRI, or both, may be beneficial in diagnosing bacterial meningitis to exclude other neurological pathological conditions such as cerebral edema, hydrocephalus, fractures, inner ear infection, or mastoiditis. However, scanning should not delay the lumbar puncture procedure if the patient has significant neurological deficits.[17,37]

Management

Nursing Diagnoses. The following nursing diagnoses may be applicable to a patient with a CNS infection including bacterial meningitis: infection related to presence of bacteria, virus, or fungus within the CNS; risk for injury (seizures) related to cerebral irritation, focal edema, and/or inflammation; risk for ineffective cerebral tissue perfusion related to cerebral edema, increased ICP, and/or hydrocephalus; and acute pain related to meningeal irritation, increased ICP, or both.

Nursing and Medical Management. Antibiotics are started as soon as possible once the diagnosis is suspected because of the rapid progression of the disease process.[17] After administration of antibiotic therapy, the search begins for the offending organism based on patient history, physical examination, CSF cultures, and blood cultures. Droplet isolation is maintained for 24 hours after the initiation of antibiotic therapy. Unusual bacteria or other microorganisms are increasingly responsible for meningitis. Identification of the offending organism(s) may take time; final culture results may redirect treatment.

During the acute phase of bacterial meningitis, the patient requires close monitoring. Increased ICP may occur, requiring administration of mannitol, placement of a ventriculostomy catheter to drain CSF, or both. Patients are maintained on bedrest with the head of the bed elevated 30 to 40 degrees. IV antibiotic therapy is continued to treat the specific organism identified. IV corticosteroids may reduce mortality, hearing loss, and neurological sequelae in adults with bacterial meningitis by decreasing meningeal inflammation.[14] Current practice guidelines recommend that dexamethasone (Decadron) 10 mg be initiated before or with the first dose of antibiotics, and then every 6 hours for 4 days in adult patients with suspected bacterial meningitis.[35,36]

Patients are placed in a private room, and the lighting is dimmed. Seizure precautions are implemented. Fever is managed with antipyretics and cooling devices.

As the acute inflammatory period subsides, the patient continues to require close monitoring to prevent secondary complications. These include seizures, increased ICP, syndrome of inappropriate antidiuretic hormone secretion, cerebral infarction, gastric bleeding, venous thromboembolism, pneumonia, and sepsis.

TABLE 13-12 Manifestations of Cranial Nerve Inflammation in Bacterial Meningitis

Cranial Nerve	Manifestations
II (Optic)	Papilledema, blindness
III, IV, VI (Oculomotor, trochlear, abducens)	Ptosis, visual field deficits, diplopia
V (Trigeminal)	Photophobia
VII (Facial)	Facial paresis
VIII (Auditory)	Deafness, tinnitus, vertigo

SPINAL CORD INJURY

Approximately 200,000 people in the United States are living with SCI. Each year, about 11,000 additional individuals sustain SCI. Most SCIs occur in individuals between the ages of 16 and 30 years. The most common causes of SCI are motor vehicle crashes, falls, acts of violence (primarily gunshot wounds), sports injuries, and diving accidents. TBI often occurs with SCI; therefore, SCI should be considered a possibility in all unconscious patients.[28] Providing emergency intervention at the scene by skilled providers, decreasing transport time to the hospital, and implementing evidence-based SCI guidelines improve a patient's outcome.

Pathophysiology

SCI occurs when force is exerted on the vertebral column, resulting in damage to the spinal cord. A series of complex and multifaceted responses results from this injury, known as *neurogenic shock* or *spinal shock*. Neurogenic shock is the result of the concussive effect of the primary SCI on the nervous system with the loss of facilitory input from the brain and inhibitory input below the level of the injury. It results in temporary and complete loss of autonomic, sensory, motor, and reflex functions below the level of the lesion. Altered autonomic function leads to cardiovascular instability (Figure 13-27). Specifically, sympathetic input is lost, causing decreased vascular resistance and vascular dilation, resulting in bradycardia, hypotension, and hypothermia. The duration of spinal shock is variable and may last days to months. A sign of the termination of spinal shock is the return of reflex activity below the level of the lesion.

Another response to SCI is an inflammatory reaction that creates spinal cord edema. Cord edema compresses spinal cord tissue as well as cord blood vessels. Cord edema can ascend or descend from the level of injury.

The SCI results in a series of biochemical changes. These changes lead to vasoconstriction of blood vessels, decrease in tissue oxygen, lactic acidosis, and ischemia. If the ischemia is not reversed, axonal degeneration and conduction failure of the neurons occur. Eventually, cell death occurs with permanent loss of function (see Figure 13-27).

Vascular changes also occur in SCI. After injury, microscopic hemorrhages occur in the central gray matter of the spinal cord. Hemorrhages may invade the surrounding white matter, cause edema and decreased blood flow, resulting in ischemia. If the ischemia is not reversed, neuronal cell death occurs.

SCI can result in a complete or incomplete lesion (Figure 13-28). A *complete lesion* causes total, permanent loss of motor and sensory function below the level of injury. An incomplete lesion results in the sparing of some motor and sensory function below the level of injury. The three types of *incomplete lesions* are *central cord, anterior cord,* and *Brown-Séquard* syndromes. The clinical presentation of each syndrome is based on damage to spinal cord organization and crossing of tracts. Most patients with an incomplete lesion show a mixed pattern of motor and sensory function and have a potential for partial or full recovery.

Assessment

Airway and Respiratory Assessment

Assessment of the airway, respiratory status, and neurological status is the first assessment priority. The higher the level of SCI, the greater the functional impairment. Respiratory problems are common with cervical and thoracic SCI. Ineffective breathing patterns are caused by paralysis of the diaphragm or intercostal muscles, or both. Baseline arterial blood gases are obtained on admission. Ongoing assessment of the adequacy of the airway and ventilation, including continuous monitoring of SpO_2, is essential. Emergent treatment, including endotracheal intubation and mechanical ventilation, may be needed.

Respiratory impairment varies with the level and type of injury (complete or incomplete). Complete lesions are associated with the following:

- C1-C3—ventilator dependency;
- C4-C5—phrenic nerve impairment that may be treated with a phrenic nerve pacemaker;
- Cervical injury below C5—intact diaphragmatic breathing, without intercostal and abdominal muscle function, and varying amounts of intercostal and abdominal muscle loss.

Those with incomplete spinal cord lesions present with varying degrees of respiratory impairment, depending on the level of the lesion and whether the motor system is impaired.

Neurological Assessment

All components of the neurological examination are performed on the patient with an SCI, with an emphasis on the motor, reflex, and sensory responses. In addition, an assessment of the spinal nerve innervation of major muscle groups is completed to determine the level of injury to the motor system (see Table 13-3). Components of the hourly assessment for an SCI patient are reviewed in Table 13-13.

A patient with a high-level SCI (above C5) is unable to regulate body temperature. The level of injury interrupts the pathway between the hypothalamus and the blood vessels and causes body temperature to rise and fall according to the environmental temperature. The inability to adequately autoregulate body temperature is called *poikilothermia*. Attention to the temperature of the patient's room is imperative to avoid hypothermia and hyperthermia.

Hemodynamic Assessment

Patients with an SCI are managed in a critical care unit for the first 7 to 14 days after injury to allow early detection and management of hemodynamic instability.[2] Spinal shock is common in complete

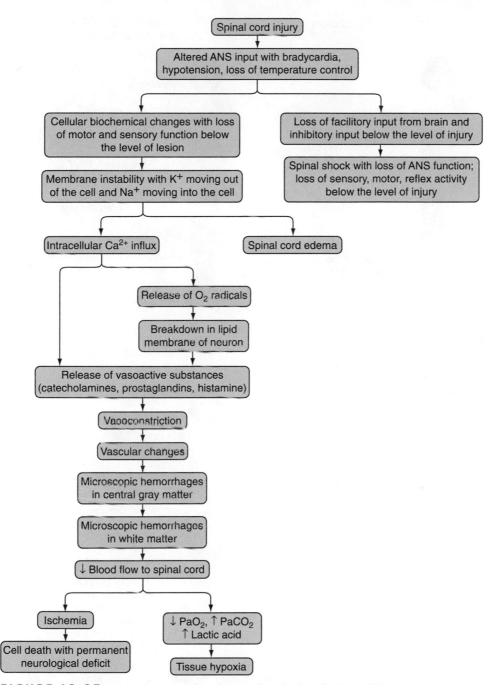

FIGURE 13-27. Pathophysiology flow diagram for spinal cord injury. *ANS,* Autonomic nervous system; K^+, potassium; Na^+, sodium; Ca^{2+}, calcium; O_2, oxygen; PaO_2, partial pressure of oxygen in arterial blood; $PaCO_2$, partial pressure of carbon dioxide in arterial blood.

injuries above the C5 level; therefore, the patient is assessed for hypotension and bradycardia. Decreases in heart rate may also be associated with hypothermia and hypoxemia. Venous stasis occurs as a result of loss of vasomotor tone and paralysis. This stasis increases the risk of venous thromboembolism.

Bowel and Bladder Function

Spinal shock results in atony of the bowel and bladder. The bladder does not contract, and the detrusor muscle does not open. Urinary retention is a common problem, and an indwelling urinary catheter is required. Loss of peristaltic movement

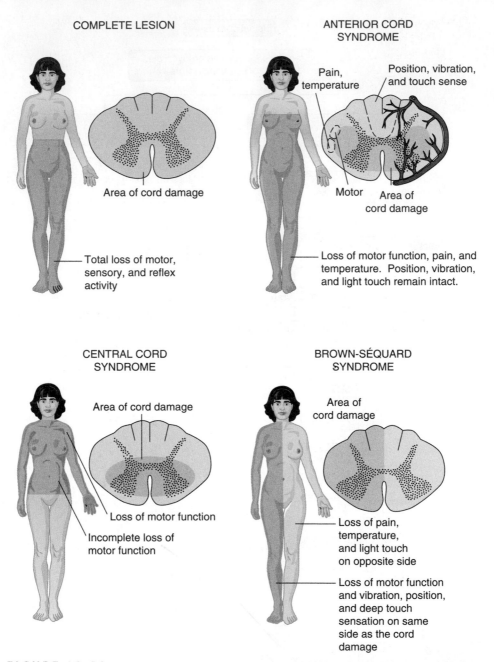

COMPLETE LESION

Area of cord damage

Total loss of motor, sensory, and reflex activity

ANTERIOR CORD SYNDROME

Pain, temperature

Position, vibration, and touch sense

Motor   Area of cord damage

Loss of motor function, pain, and temperature. Position, vibration, and light touch remain intact.

CENTRAL CORD SYNDROME

Area of cord damage

Loss of motor function

Incomplete loss of motor function

BROWN-SÉQUARD SYNDROME

Area of cord damage

Loss of pain, temperature, and light touch on opposite side

Loss of motor function and vibration, position, and deep touch sensation on same side as the cord damage

FIGURE 13-28. Common spinal cord syndromes. *(Modified from Ignatavicius, D. D., & Workman, M. L. [2002]. Medical-surgical nursing: Critical thinking for collaborative care [4th ed.]. Philadelphia: Saunders.)*

increases the risk of paralytic ileus. The patient is assessed for return of bowel sounds, flatus, and bowel movement.

Skin Assessment
Because of impaired circulation and immobility, the patient with SCI is at risk of skin breakdown. A complete assessment of all skin surfaces is done every 8 to 12 hours. If halo traction or cervical tongs is used to stabilize a cervical fracture, the skin around pin sites and under traction devices is carefully inspected. Assessment includes observing the site for redness, swelling, drainage, and pain. If a cervical collar is in place, skin integrity is assessed with an emphasis on pressure points (occipital, chin, and sternal region).

TABLE 13-13 Components of the Hourly Neurological Assessment for Patients with Spinal Cord Injury*

Motor	Sensation
Respirations—rate, rhythm, effort	Pinprick (sharp, dull) all surfaces of body
Movement/strength bilaterally	Position sense
Shrug shoulders	Temperature all surfaces of body
Elbow flexion	
Elbow extension	
Bending wrists	
Touch thumb to index finger	
Hand grasp	
Lift leg off the bed	
Bend knee	
Extend knee	
Pull feet up	
Push feet down	

*If patient has a suspected traumatic brain injury, see Table 13-5 for additional assessments.

Psychological Assessment

A psychological assessment is important during the acute phase of SCI. Initially, the patient is concerned with surviving the injury and does not realize the extent of injury or disability. The patient's perceptions are also impaired by medications and the physiological effects of injury. Patients often experience denial, anger, and depression. As the patient gains insight into the situation, it is important for the nurse to include the patient in care planning and to give the patient choices, because feelings of powerlessness are common.

Family members also go through a similar experience. First they experience shock related to the injury itself and the seriousness of the patient's condition. During this time, family members need support and answers to their questions.[21,31] Consultation with a psychiatric or mental health nurse or a psychiatrist may be indicated.[15,18] Early involvement of the patient and family in plans for rehabilitation is also important.

Diagnostic Studies

Baseline laboratory studies include electrolytes, complete blood count, prothrombin time, partial thromboplastin time, platelet count, and arterial blood gases. Common diagnostic studies to confirm the extent of vertebral and cord injury include anteroposterior and lateral spine x-ray studies, chest

BOX 13-6 Autonomic Dysreflexia

Medical Emergency; Can Result in Stroke, Seizures, or Other Complications
- Common in lesions above T6; occurs after spinal shock has resolved
- Characterized by exaggerated response of the sympathetic nervous system

Triggered by a Variety of Stimuli
- Bladder—kinked indwelling catheter, distention, infection, calculi, cystoscopy
- Bowel—fecal impaction, rectal examination, insertion of suppository
- Skin—tight clothing, irritation from bed linens, temperature extremes

Common Signs and Symptoms
- Sudden, severe, pounding headache
- Elevated, uncontrolled blood pressure
- Bradycardia
- Nasal congestion
- Blurred vision
- Profuse diaphoresis above the level of the lesion
- Flushing of the face and neck
- Pallor, chills, and pilomotor erection below the level of the injury
- Anxiety

Treatment
- Find and remove the cause of stimulation
- Elevate the head of bed
- Remain calm and supportive
- If symptoms persist, give vasodilators to decrease blood pressure
- Teach patients to recognize and report symptoms

x-ray studies, CT scan, MRI, and myelography. Somatosensory-cortical evoked potentials may be performed to see whether sensory pathways between the site of stimulation and the site of recording are intact.

Management

Nursing Interventions

Nursing interventions are focused on maintaining stabilization of the spinal alignment, preserving the airway and respiratory status, and preventing complications associated with immobility and the SCI (see Nursing Care Plan for the Patient with Spinal Cord Injury). Once spinal shock has resolved, the patient with a complete SCI above T6 must be observed for autonomic dysreflexia (Box 13-6).

Text continued on p. 435

NURSING CARE PLAN for the Patient with Spinal Cord Injury

NURSING DIAGNOSIS

Risk for injury related to displacement of fracture; spinal shock; and ascending cord edema

PATIENT OUTCOMES
Risk for injury minimized

- Maintenance of vertebral alignment
- Absence of progressive neurological dysfunction
- Improved sensory, motor, and reflex function

NURSING INTERVENTIONS	RATIONALES
• Perform neurological assessments (motor, reflex, and sensory)	• Assess subtle changes indicating neurological deterioration or improvement
• Report progression of deficits from baseline (↑ difficulty with swallowing or coughing, respiratory stridor, sternal retraction, bradycardia, fluctuating BP, and ↑ motor and sensory loss at a higher level than the initial findings)	• Detect worsening of symptoms that indicate need for interventions (e.g., airway management and ventilation)
• Maintain halo or tong traction for immobilization	• Maintain alignment and prevent complications
• Perform pin care every 8 hours	• Prevent infection at the pin site
• If skeletal traction slips or is accidentally removed, maintain the patient's head in a neutral position	• Maintain alignment and prevent further damage
• Turn, lift, and transfer the patient with at least three people, with one at head to stabilize neck and to coordinate the move	• Proper turning keeps the spinal cord in alignment and prevents further trauma to the spinal cord

NURSING DIAGNOSIS

Impaired gas exchange related to hypoventilation secondary to paresis or paralysis of respiratory muscles

PATIENT OUTCOMES
Adequate gas exchange

- Orientation
- PaO_2 ≥80 mm Hg
- $PaCO_2$ >35-45 mm Hg
- RR 12-20 breaths/min with normal depth and pattern
- HR 60-100 beats/min
- BP stable

NURSING INTERVENTIONS	RATIONALES
• Assess for signs of respiratory distress	• Indicates the need for assisted ventilation
• Monitor ABG studies and pulse oximetry values	• Assess oxygenation status
• Monitor chest x-ray studies	• Assess worsening or improvement of status
• Monitor respiratory status, especially in a patient with cranial tongs or traction with a halo vest	• Ensure that the vest is not restricting diaphragmatic movement
• Assess for absent or adventitious breath sounds and inspect chest movement	• Assess adequacy of ventilation

NURSING CARE PLAN for the Patient with Spinal Cord Injury—cont'd

NURSING DIAGNOSIS

Ineffective airway clearance related to decreased or absent cough reflex secondary to injury or depressant effect of some medications

PATIENT OUTCOME
Within 24-48 hours, airway clear

- Absence of adventitious breath sounds

NURSING INTERVENTIONS	RATIONALES
• Monitor lung sounds every 1-4 hours	• Identify need for coughing and/or suctioning
• Suction airway as needed; provide oxygenation before and between suction attempts	• Clear airway of secretions; improve gas exchange
• Assess ability to cough	• Identify need for assistance in removing secretions
• Perform incentive spirometry every hour patient is able	• Promote expansion of lungs and facilitate secretion removal
• Turn and reposition patient every 2 hours; consider need for therapeutic bed (e.g., RotoRest)	• Mobilize secretions; reduce risk for pneumonia

NURSING DIAGNOSIS

Ineffective thermoregulation related to inability of body to adapt to environmental temperature changes secondary to loss of sympathetic innervation

PATIENT OUTCOME

- Within 2-4 hours of diagnosis, patient normothermic

NURSING INTERVENTIONS	RATIONALES
• Monitor temperature at least every 4 hours	• Assess need for intervention
• Assess for signs of ineffective thermoregulation (diaphoresis, skin warm above level of injury or cool below; complaints of being too cold or warm, pilomotor erection)	• Identify need for intervention to maintain normothermia
• Implement measures to attain normothermia (warmth or cooling as indicated; adjust ambient room temperature)	• Maintain normothermia; prevent complications

NURSING DIAGNOSIS

Risk for decreased CO related to relative hypovolemia secondary to neurogenic/spinal shock

PATIENT OUTCOMES
Adequate CO

- Orientation to name, place, time
- SBP >90 mm Hg
- Urine output ≥0.5 mL/kg/hr

- ECG NSR
- HR 60-100 beats/min
- Normal peripheral pulses

Continued

NURSING CARE PLAN for the Patient with Spinal Cord Injury—cont'd

NURSING INTERVENTIONS	RATIONALES
• Monitor symptoms of low CO: hypotension, increased HR, lightheadedness, confusion, diminished peripheral pulses	• Identify low CO to provide prompt interventions
• Monitor hemodynamic measurements; administer fluids and/or vasopressors	• Provide objective data to guide and monitor treatment
• Continuously assess the ECG	• Identify dysrhythmias associated with low CO
• Implement measures to prevent orthostatic hypotension: change position slowly; antiembolic hose	• Prevent orthostatic hypotension

NURSING DIAGNOSIS

Imbalanced nutrition: less than body requirements related to hypermetabolic state; decreased oral intake secondary; difficulty eating in prone position; fear of choking and aspiration; inability to feed self; and decreased gastrointestinal motility

PATIENT OUTCOMES
Adequate nutrition

• Balanced nitrogen state
• Serum albumin 3.5-5.5 g/dL

NURSING INTERVENTIONS	RATIONALES
• Weigh the patient daily	• Assess fluid volume and nutritional status
• Attach NGT on low suction to prevent abdominal distention or aspiration	• Decompress the stomach; reduce risk of aspiration
• Maintain NPO until bowel sounds	• Prevent complications associated with spinal shock
• Assess readiness for oral intake (bowel sounds present, passing flatus, or bowel movement)	• Assess resolution of spinal shock and return of GI function
• Perform a nutrition assessment	• Assess nutritional needs
• Give parenteral or enteral nutrition if ordered	• Maintain adequate nutrition
• Progress slowly from liquids to solids	• Assess tolerance to change in diet
• Give small, frequent feedings	• Prevent abdominal distention and also less tiring

NURSING DIAGNOSIS

Ineffective tissue perfusion related to venous stasis; vascular intimal injury; and hypercoagulability from decreased vasomotor tone and immobility (see Chapter 14 for interventions)

PATIENT OUTCOME

• Absence of venous thromboembolism

NURSING CARE PLAN for the Patient with Spinal Cord Injury—cont'd

NURSING DIAGNOSIS

Risk for infection related to inadequate primary defenses (broken skin) secondary to immobilization and presence of invasive devices

PATIENT OUTCOMES
Free of infection

- No infection at insertion site for tongs, IV, urinary catheter, pneumonia
- Negative culture results
- Absence of erythema, swelling, warmth, purulent drainage, tenderness
- Normal WBCs

NURSING INTERVENTIONS	RATIONALES
• Perform pin, IV, and urinary catheter care	• Prevent infection
• Monitor WBCs	• Assess for infection
• Use sterile technique to change all dressing	• Prevent infection
• Use proper hand-washing techniques	• Prevent infection

NURSING DIAGNOSIS

Risk for impaired skin integrity related to prolonged immobility

PATIENT OUTCOME

- Skin remains intact

NURSING INTERVENTIONS	RATIONALES
• Assess the patient's skin every 4 hours; include area under the halo vest or cervical collar	• Assess potential for skin breakdown early
• Ensure that the patient's skin is clean and dry	• Prevent skin breakdown
• Pad the halo vest to decrease irritation and friction	• Prevent skin breakdown
• Turn the patient every 2 hours	• Increase circulation to prevent skin breakdown
• Consider need for therapeutic bed or other protective devices	• Prevent skin breakdown

NURSING DIAGNOSIS

Constipation related to neuromuscular impairment secondary to spinal shock, SCI

PATIENT OUTCOME

- Soft, formed bowel movement within 48 hours of admission

Continued

NURSING CARE PLAN for the Patient with Spinal Cord Injury—cont'd

NURSING INTERVENTIONS	RATIONALES
• Monitor for nausea, vomiting, abdominal distention, malaise, and the presence of a hard fecal mass on digital examination	• Assess constipation and fecal impaction
• Monitor the patient's bowel sounds	• Assess bowel function
• Administer stool softeners	• Promote adequate bowel movement
• Document the patient's bowel movements	• Assess effectiveness of bowel management program

NURSING DIAGNOSIS

Fear/anxiety related to loss of motor and sensory function; immobilizing device to stabilize and align spine; lack of understanding of diagnostic tests and treatment; unfamiliar environment; financial concerns; and anticipated effect of SCI on lifestyle and roles

PATIENT OUTCOMES
Reduced fear and anxiety

• Verbalization of feeling less anxious
• Usual sleep pattern
• Relaxed facial expression
• Healthy interaction with others

NURSING INTERVENTIONS	RATIONALES
• Assess for signs and symptoms of fear and anxiety (tense, insomnia)	• Assess need for intervention
• Implement measures to reduce fear and anxiety	• Assist in coping with changes and reduce anxiety
• Explain the need for frequent neurological checks	• Provide information to reduce anxiety
• Provide information concerning all nursing care	• Promote successful resolution of the crisis and establish a positive coping mechanism
• Assure the patient that staff members are nearby; provide a call signal that is adapted to meet the patient's needs. Answer the call signal as soon as possible	• Assure that needs will be met; reduce anxiety
• Include the patient in planning care	• Provide a sense of control
• Encourage expressions of fear or questions	• Identify concerns; provide information to reduce anxiety

NURSING DIAGNOSIS

Powerlessness related to SCI

PATIENT OUTCOME

• Verbalizing of increased control over activities

NURSING CARE PLAN for the Patient with Spinal Cord Injury—cont'd

NURSING INTERVENTIONS	RATIONALES
• Encourage talking • Include the patient in planning • Allow the patient to make choices • Display sensitivity toward events that could cause powerlessness • Encourage asking questions	• All facilitate communication and promote sense of control

↑, Increase; ↓, decrease; *ABG*, arterial blood gas; *BP*, blood pressure; *CO*, cardiac output; *ECG*, electrocardiogram; *GI*, gastrointestinal; *HR*, heart rate; *IV*, intravenous; *NGT*, nasogastric tube; *NPO*, nothing by mouth; *NSR*, normal sinus rhythm; *PaCO$_2$*, partial pressure of arterial carbon dioxide; *PaO$_2$*, partial pressure of arterial oxygen; *RR*, respiratory rate; *SBP*, systolic blood pressure; *SCI*, spinal cord injury; *WBC*, white blood cell count.
Data from Baird, M. S., Keen, J. H., & Swearingen, P. L. (2005). *Manual of critical care nursing* (5th ed.). St. Louis: Mosby; and Gulanick, M., Myers, J. L. (2007). *Nursing care plans: Nursing diagnosis and intervention* (6th ed.). St. Louis: Mosby.

Nursing and Medical Interventions

Maintaining a patent airway and respiratory function is a priority. Endotracheal intubation and mechanical ventilation are often required, especially in high cervical spine injuries. Care must be taken to prevent neck hyperextension during endotracheal intubation. Patients with complete cervical injury may be placed on a rotational bed (e.g., Roto-Rest, KCI) to optimize pulmonary function; however, patients must be assessed for the risk of skin breakdown.

Immobilization of the spinal cord must occur at the scene. A rigid cervical collar with supporting blocks on a rigid backboard is recommended.[2] Once the patient is hospitalized, external stabilization of the fracture or dislocation is often accomplished by cervical collar, skeletal traction (cervical tongs), a halo vest, or brace (Figure 13-29). The halo vest offers many advantages, such as easy access to the neck for diagnostic procedures and surgery, early mobilization, and ambulation. Surgical stabilization may be required.

Maintaining perfusion to the spinal cord is crucial. The MAP should be maintained at 85 to 90 mm Hg for the first 7 days after the SCI. A systolic BP less than 90 mm Hg must be avoided, as hypotension contributes to secondary injury by decreasing spinal cord blood flow and perfusion, leading to ischemia and neurological deficit. Fluid volume administration and vasopressor drugs may be needed to sustain the BP.[2] A pulmonary artery catheter may be used to determine the need for fluids accurately.

Acute management of SCI often includes administration of glucocorticoids. Guidelines for the management of acute cervical spine and spinal cord injuries recommend treatment with high-dose methylprednisolone (Solu-Medrol) within the first 8 hours of injury as an option for the patient with SCI. The dosing regimen is initiated with a bolus of 30 mg/kg over 15 minutes, followed in 45 minutes by a continuous IV infusion of 5.4 mg/kg/hr for 23 hours.[2] Continuation of therapy for up to 48 hours is being tested to assess improvement in function. Potential adverse effects of glucocorticoids include hyperglycemia, infection, gastrointestinal hemorrhage, poor wound healing, edema, and thrombocytopenia.[2]

During the first 72 hours after SCI, a nasogastric tube is inserted for gastric decompression until bowel sounds return. This also helps to prevent vomiting and possible aspiration and to improve pulmonary function. Stress ulcers can occur as a result of vagus-stimulated gastric acid production. Administration of steroids also increases the risk of gastric irritation. Histamine (H$_2$)-antagonists or proton pump inhibitors are given to prevent stress ulcers. A bowel care program should be instituted within 72 hours after injury.

The skin must be kept clean and dry at all times. Various skin protection devices may be required including therapeutic beds, mattress overlays, boots, and skin barrier creams. An indwelling urinary catheter is inserted immediately on admission to prevent bladder distention; an intermittent catherization program is instituted upon resolution of spinal shock.

Because of the limited mobility of patients with SCIs, measures to prevent venous thromboembolism are started immediately on admission.[9] Intermittent pneumatic compression devices are commonly ordered. Heparin prophylaxis may be

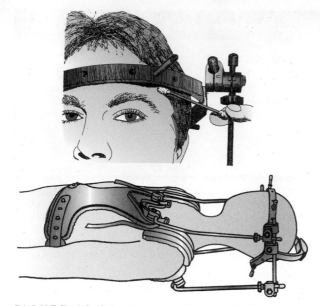

FIGURE 13-29. Halo vest. *(Courtesy of DePuy Acromed, Raynham, MA.)*

initiated if the risk of intramedullary or epidural hemorrhage into the spine is low. If the patient is not a candidate for anticoagulation, a vena cava filter may be considered; however, the effectiveness of its use is controversial. Since metabolic demands are initially increased, adequate nutrition must also be provided.

Surgical Intervention

SCIs may require surgical intervention to achieve greater neurological recovery and restore spinal stability. Surgery is indicated for neurological deterioration, unstable fractures, cord compression in the presence of an incomplete injury, and gross spinal misalignment. Surgery may involve the placement of plates or rods, and a bone graft to fuse the spine. Depending on the injury, bone fragments may be removed, or the spine may need to be realigned. The issue of when surgery should be performed is controversial.[9] External immobilzation devices, such as cervical traction or halo vest, may also be used.

CASE STUDY   *evolve*

Ms. Jones is a 45-year-old patient who had a subarachnoid hemorrhage followed by clipping of an aneurysm 5 days ago. At present, she is receiving mechanical ventilation and has a pulmonary artery catheter, arterial line, and ventriculostomy in place. Cerebral angiography performed today indicates that she is experiencing cerebral vasospasm. To reverse the vasospasm, she is started on hypervolemic hypertensive therapy.

QUESTIONS
1. When is a patient at greatest risk for developing vasospasm?
2. What effects does vasospasm have on cerebral function?
3. Discuss the benefits of administering hypervolemic hypertensive therapy.
4. Explain the purpose of a ventriculostomy in this patient.

SUMMARY

Care of the patient with a neurological problem is challenging and complex. Knowledge of normal structure and function of the nervous system is essential to understand common disorders and injuries. Nurses must carefully consider how interventions affect patients. Skills in neurological assessment are important to learn because changes are often subtle. Nursing assessments and interventions that are tailored to each patient are essential to promote positive patient outcomes. In addition,

many nervous system disorders result in a prolonged recovery period. It is important for the nurse to provide comprehensive care that prevents the complications that can result from bedrest and immobility. Other disciplines need to be involved in the patient's care as soon as possible to assist in promoting rehabilitation, including physical therapists, occupational therapists, and speech therapists. The nurse is instrumental in getting consults for these services and coordinating the multidisciplinary plan of care that improves outcomes for this patient population.

CRITICAL THINKING QUESTIONS

evolve

1. You are caring for Tim Smith, who has sustained a traumatic brain injury from a motor vehicle crash. He has an intraventricular catheter for continuous measurement of intracranial pressure (ICP). His ICP has been stable at 13 mm Hg for the past 4 hours. The alarm on the monitor sounds because his ICP is now 20 mm Hg. What are your priority assessments and interventions at this time?

2. Many nurses believe that visiting should be restricted for neurological patients, especially those with brain injuries. What assessments can you make to determine whether family visits are helpful or harmful to your patient?

3. What interventions can you teach families to assist in the care and rehabilitation of patients with prolonged unconsciousness after a traumatic brain injury or cranial surgery?

4. Barry Brown is an 18-year-old patient who was admitted in generalized convulsive status epilepticus. Describe the appropriate nursing and medical interventions.

evolve Be sure to check out the bonus material, including free self-assessment exercises, on the Evolve Web site at http://evolve.elsevier.com/Sole.

REFERENCES

1. Adams, H., del Zoppo, G., Alberts, M., Bhatt D. L., Brass L., Furlan A., et al. (2007). Guidelines for the early management of adults with ischemic stroke: A guideline from the American Heart Association/American Stroke Association Stroke Council, Clinical Cardiology Council, Cardiovascular Radiology and Intervention Council, and the Atherosclerotic Peripheral Vascular Disease and Quality of Care Outcomes in Research Interdisciplinary Working Groups. *Stroke, 38,* 1655-1711.

2. American Association of Neurological Surgeons & Congress of Neurological Surgeons. (2002). Guidelines for the management of acute cervical spine and spinal cord injuries. *Neurosurgery, 50*(3 Suppl).

3. American Association of Neuroscience Nurses (AANN). (2005). *Guide to the care of the patient with intracranial pressure monitoring.* Glenville, IL: Author.

4. American Stroke Association/American Heart Association. (2005). *Heart disease & stroke statistics—2005.* Dallas: Author.

5. Auer, R., & Sutherland, G. (2005). Primary intracerebral hemorrhage: Pathophysiology. *Canadian Journal of Neurological Sciences, 32*(Suppl. 2), S3-S12.

6. Bader, M. K. (2006). Recognizing and treating ischemic insults to the brain: The role of brain tissue oxygen monitoring. *Critical Care Nursing Clinics, 18*(2), 243-256.

7. Bader, M. K., & Littlejohns, L. (2004). AANN *core curriculum for neuroscience nursing* (4th ed.). St. Louis: Saunders.

8. Bader, M. K., Littlejohns, L., & March, K. (2003). Brain tissue oxygen monitoring in severe brain injury. II. Implications for critical care teams and case study. *Critical Care Nurse, 23*(4), 29-44.

9. Barker, E. (2008). *Neuroscience nursing: A spectrum of care* (3rd ed.). St. Louis: Mosby.

10. Bhalla, A., Wolfe, C. D. A., & Rudd, A. G. (2001). Management of acute physiological parameters after stroke. *QJM, 94,* 167-172.

11. Broderick, J., Connolly, S., Feldmann, E., Hanley, D., Kase, C., Krieger, D., et al. (2007). Guidelines for the management of spontaneous intracerebral hemorrhage in adults: 2007 update a guideline from the American Heart Association/American Stroke Association Stroke Council, High Blood Pressure Research Council, and the Quality of Care and Outcomes in Research Interdisciplinary Working Group. *Stroke, 38,* 2001-2023.

12. Bullock, R., Chestnut, R. M., Clifton, G., Ghajar, J., Marion, D. W., Narayan, R. K., et al. (2000). *Management and prognosis of severe traumatic brain injury.* New York: Brain Trauma Foundation and American Association of Neurological Surgeons.

13. Center for Disease Control and Prevention. *Bacterial meningitis statistics 2006.* Retrieved March 31, 2008 from www.cdc.gov.

14. de Gans, J., & van de Beek, D. (2002). Dexamethasone in adults with bacterial meningitis. *New England Journal of Medicine, 347,* 1549-1556.

15. Elliott, T. R. (2004). Treatment of depression following spinal cord injury: An evidence-based review. *Rehabilitation Psychology, 49*(2), 134-139.

16. Fernandez, A., Schmidt, J. M., Claassen, J., Pavlicova, M., Huddleston, K., Kreiter, T, et al. (2007). Fever after subarachnoid hemorrhage: Risk factors and impact on outcome. *Neurology, 68,* 1013-1019.

17. Fitch, M. T., & von de Beek, D. (2007). Emergency diagnosis and treatment of adult meningitis. *The Lancet Infectious Diseases, 7*(3), 191-200.

18. Fitchenbaum, J., & Kirshblum, S. (2002). Psychological adaptation to spinal cord injury. In S. Kirshblum, D. I. Campagnolo, & J. A. DeLisa, (Eds.), *Spinal cord medicine*. Philadelphia: Lippincott Williams & Wilkins.

19. Haymore, J. (2004). A neuron in a haystack: Advanced neurologic assessment. *AACN Clinical Issues, 15*(4), 568-581.

20. Hilker, R., Poetter, C., Findeisen, N., Sobesky, J., Jacobs, A., Neveling, M., et al. (2003). Nosocomial pneumonia after acute stroke: Implications for neurological intensive care medicine. *Stroke, 34*, 975-981.

21. Kosco, M., & Warren, N. A. (2000). Critical care nurses' perspective of family needs as met. *Critical Care Nursing Quarterly, 23*(2), 60-72.

22. Langlois, J. A., Rutland-Brown, W., & Thomas, K. E. (2006). *Traumatic brain injury in the United States: Emergency department visits, hospitalizations, and deaths.* Atlanta, GA: Centers for Disease Control and Prevention, National Center for Injury Prevention and Control.

23. Leonard, A. (2002). *Acute stroke principles of modern management: General care after stroke, including stroke units and prevention and treatment of complications of stroke.* St. Paul, MN: American Academy of Neurology.

24. Littlejohns, L., & Bader, M. K. (2001). Guidelines for the management of severe head injury: Clinical application and changes in practice. *Critical Care Nurse, 21*(6), 48-65.

25. Littlejohns, L., & Bader, M. K. (2005). Prevention of secondary brain injury: Targeting technology. *AACN Clinical Issues: Advanced Practice in Acute and Critical Care, 15*(4), 501-514.

26. Littlejohns, L., Bader, M. K., & March, K. (2003). Brain tissue oxygen monitoring in severe brain injury. I. *Critical Care Nurse, 23*(4), 17-25.

27. Marik, P., Varon, J., & Trask, T. (2002). Management of head trauma. *Chest, 122*, 699-711.

28. National Spinal Cord Injury Statistical Center. *Spinal cord injury: Facts and figures, 2006.* Retrieved December 8, 2007, from www.spinalcord.uab.edu.

29. National Institute of Neurological Disorders and Stroke t-PA Stroke Study Group. (1995). Tissue plasminogen activator for acute ischemic stroke. *New England Journal of Medicine, 333*, 1581-1587.

30. Qui, W. S., Liu, W. G., Shen, H., Wang, W. M., Hang, Z. L., Zhang, Y., et al. (2005). Therapeutic effect of mild hypothermia on severe traumatic head injury. *China Journal of Trauma, 8*(1), 27-32.

31. Roland, R., Russell, J., Richards, K. C., & Sullivan, S.C. (2001). Visitation in critical care: Processes and outcomes of a performance improvement initiative. *Journal of Nursing Care Quality, 15*(2), 18-26.

32. Sabin-Alverez, J., Molina, C. A., Montaner, J., Arenillas, J. F., Huertas, R., Ribo, M., et al. (2003). Effects of admission hyperglycemia on stroke outcome in reperfused tissue plasminogen activator treated patients. *Stroke, 34*, 1235.

33. Sullivan, J. (2000). Positioning of patients with severe traumatic brain injury: Research-based practice. *Journal of Neuroscience Nursing, 32*(4), 204-209.

34. Tazbir, J., Marthaler, M. T., Moredich, C., & Keresztes, P. (2005). Decompressive hemicraniectomy with duraplasty: A treatment for large-volume ischemic stroke. *Journal of Neuroscience Nursing, 37*(4), 194-199.

35. Tunkel, A. R., Hartman, B. J., Kaplan, S. L., Kaufman, B. A., Roos, K. L., Scheld, W. M., et al. (2004). Practice guidelines for the management of bacterial meningitis. *Clinical Infectious Diseases, 39*, 1267-1284.

36. van de Beek, D., de Gans, T., Tunkel, A. R., & Wijdicks, E.F. (2006). Community acquired bacterial meningitis in adults. *New England Journal of Medicine, 354*, 44-53.

37. Ziai, W. C., & Lewin, J. J. (2006). Advances in the management of central nervous system infections in the ICU. *Critical Care Clinics, 22*(4), 661-694.

CHAPTER 14

Acute Respiratory Failure

Carolyn D. Hix, DNP, RN, CNAA
Linda M. Tamburri, MSN, RN, CCRN, CS

INTRODUCTION

Acute respiratory failure (ARF) occurs in many disease states. It may be the patient's primary problem or a complicating factor in other conditions. This chapter reviews the pathophysiology of ARF, several common causes, and the nursing care involved in the treatment of these patients.

ACUTE RESPIRATORY FAILURE

Definition

ARF is defined as a state of altered gas exchange resulting in the following abnormal arterial blood gas (ABG) values obtained with the patient breathing room air: a partial pressure of oxygen (O_2) in arterial blood (PaO_2) of less than 60 mm Hg, and a partial pressure of carbon dioxide (CO_2) in arterial blood ($PaCO_2$) of greater than 45 mm Hg with a pH of less than 7.30.[55] Causes of ARF are classified into one of three categories: failure of respiration or oxygenation, failure of ventilation, or a combination of respiratory and ventilatory failure. ARF differs from chronic respiratory failure in the length of time necessary for it to develop. ARF occurs rapidly, with little time for physiologic compensation. Chronic respiratory failure develops over time and allows the body's compensatory mechanisms to activate. ARF and chronic respiratory failure are not mutually exclusive. ARF may occur when a person who has chronic respiratory failure develops a sudden respiratory infection or is exposed to other types of stressors. This is referred to as acute-on-chronic respiratory failure.

Pathophysiology

Failure of Oxygenation

Failure of oxygenation is present when the PaO_2 cannot be adequately maintained. Five generally accepted mechanisms that reduce PaO_2 and create a state of hypoxemia are (1) hypoventilation, (2) intrapulmonary shunting, (3) ventilation-perfusion mismatching, (4) diffusion defects, and (5) decreased barometric pressure (Figure 14-1). Decreased barometric pressure, which occurs at high altitudes, is not addressed in this text. Nonpulmonary conditions such as decreased cardiac output and low hemoglobin level may also result in tissue hypoxia.

Hypoventilation. In the normal lung, the partial pressure of alveolar O_2 (PAO_2) is approximately equal to the PaO_2. Alveolar ventilation refers to the amount of gas that enters the alveoli per minute. If the alveolar ventilation is reduced because of hypoventilation, the PAO_2 and the PaO_2 are reduced. Factors that may lead to hypoventilation include a drug overdose that causes central nervous system depression, neurological disorders that cause a decrease in the rate or depth of respirations, and abdominal or thoracic surgery leading to shallow breathing patterns secondary to pain on inspiration. Hypoventilation also produces an increase in the alveolar CO_2 level because the CO_2 that is produced in the tissues is delivered to the lungs but is not released from the body.

Intrapulmonary Shunting. In normally functioning lungs, a small amount of blood returns to the left side of the heart without engaging in alveolar gas exchange. This is referred to as the physiological shunt. If, however, a larger amount of blood returns to the left side of the heart without participating in gas exchange, the shunt becomes pathological and a decrease in the PaO_2 occurs.[55] The condition exists

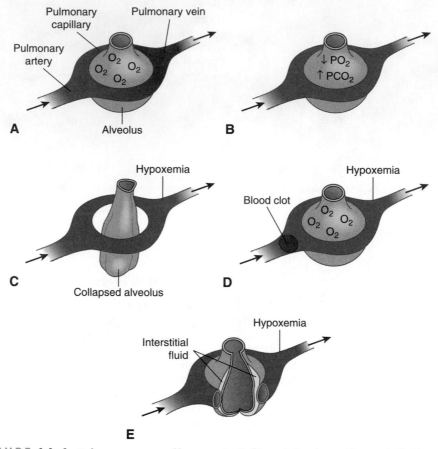

FIGURE 14-1. Pulmonary causes of hypoxemia. **A,** Normal alveolar-capillary unit. **B,** Hypoventilation causes an increased $PaCO_2$ and decreased PaO_2. **C,** Shunt. **D,** Ventilation-perfusion mismatch resulting from pulmonary embolus. **E,** Diffusion defect due to increased interstitial fluid.

when areas of the lung that are inadequately ventilated are adequately perfused (see Figure 14-1). The blood, therefore, is shunted past the lung and returns unoxygenated to the left side of the heart. Causes of shunting include atrial or ventricular septal defects, atelectasis, pneumonia, and pulmonary edema.[60]

As the shunt worsens, the PaO_2 continues to decrease. This cause of hypoxemia cannot be effectively treated by increasing the fraction of inspired O_2 (FiO_2) because the unventilated alveolar units do not receive any of the enriched air.

Ventilation-Perfusion Mismatch. Gas exchange in the lungs is dependent upon ventilation (the movement of gas) and perfusion (blood flow). The rate of ventilation ($\dot{V}$) usually equals the rate of perfusion ($\dot{Q}$), resulting in a ventilation-perfusion ($\dot{V}/\dot{Q}$) ratio of 1. If ventilation exceeds blood flow, the $\dot{V}/\dot{Q}$ ratio is greater than 1; if ventilation is less than blood flow, the $\dot{V}/\dot{Q}$ ratio is less than 1. Both of these conditions are examples of $\dot{V}/\dot{Q}$ mismatch. In respiratory failure, $\dot{V}/\dot{Q}$ mismatch is the most common cause of hypox-

emia and can often be corrected by increasing the FiO_2.[60] $\dot{V}/\dot{Q}$ mismatch can occur in conditions such as pneumonia or pulmonary edema when obstructed airways inhibit ventilation (and perfusion is normal), or in the case of pulmonary embolism when a clot in the pulmonary circulation obstructs perfusion.[60]

Diffusion Defects. Diffusion is the movement of gas from an area of high concentration to an area of low concentration. In the lungs, O_2 and CO_2 move between the alveoli and the blood by diffusing across the alveolar-capillary membrane. The alveolar-capillary membrane has six barriers to the diffusion of O_2 and CO_2: surfactant, alveolar epithelium, interstitial fluid, capillary endothelium, plasma, and red blood cell membrane. Under normal circumstances, O_2 and CO_2 diffuse across the alveolar-capillary membrane in 0.25 seconds. The distance between an alveolus and a pulmonary capillary is usually only one or two cells thick. This narrowness of space facilitates efficient diffusion of O_2 and CO_2 across the cell membrane.

In respiratory failure, the distance between the alveoli and the capillaries may be increased by the accumulation of fluid in the interstitial space (see Figure 14-1). Changes in capillary perfusion pressure, leakage of plasma proteins into the interstitial space, and destruction of the capillary membrane contribute to the buildup of fluids around the alveolus. Fibrotic changes in the lung tissue itself, such as those seen in chronic obstructive pulmonary disease (COPD), may also contribute to a reduction in the diffusion capacity of the lung. As this capacity is reduced, PaO_2 is the first parameter affected and hypoxemia results. Because CO_2 is more readily diffusible than O_2, hypercapnia is a late sign of diffusion defects.

Low Cardiac Output. Adequate tissue oxygenation depends on a balance between O_2 supply and demand. The mechanism for delivering O_2 to the tissues is cardiac output. A normal cardiac output results in the delivery of 600 to 1000 mL/min of O_2, which generally exceeds the normal amount of O_2 needed by the tissues. If the cardiac output decreases, less oxygenated blood is delivered. To maintain normal aerobic metabolism in low cardiac output states, the tissues must extract increasing amounts of O_2 from the blood. When this increase in extraction can no longer compensate for the decreased cardiac output, the cells convert to anaerobic metabolism. This results in the production of lactic acid, which depresses the function of the myocardium and further lowers cardiac output.

Low Hemoglobin Level. Approximately 95% of the body's O_2 is transported to the tissues bound to hemoglobin. Each gram of hemoglobin can carry 1.34 mL of O_2 when all of its O_2 binding sites are completely filled. Oxygen saturation (SaO_2) refers to the percentage of O_2 binding sites on each hemoglobin molecule that are filled with O_2. The hemoglobin of a healthy person breathing room air is about 95% saturated. If a patient's hemoglobin level is less than normal, the O_2 supply to the tissues may be impaired and tissue hypoxia can occur. An alteration in hemoglobin function (i.e., carbon monoxide poisoning or sickle cell disease) can also decrease O_2 delivery to the tissues.

Tissue Hypoxia. The final step in oxygenation is the use of O_2 by the tissues. Anaerobic metabolism occurs when the tissues cannot obtain adequate O_2 to meet metabolic needs. In addition, some conditions such as cyanide poisoning may leave the tissues unable to use O_2 despite normal O_2 delivery.[55] Anaerobic metabolism is inefficient and results in the accumulation of lactic acid. The point at which anaerobic metabolism begins to occur is not known and may vary with different organ systems. The effects of tissue hypoxia vary with the severity of the hypoxia

but may result in cellular death and subsequent organ failure.

Failure of Ventilation

$PaCO_2$ is the index used to evaluate ventilation. When ventilation is reduced, $PaCO_2$ is increased (hypercapnia). When ventilation is increased, $PaCO_2$ is reduced (hypocapnia). Hypoventilation and $\dot{V}/\dot{Q}$ mismatching are the two mechanisms responsible for hypercapnia. Hypercapnia greatly increases cerebral blood flow. The patient may appear restless and anxious, and may demonstrate slurred speech and a decreased level of consciousness.

Hypoventilation. Hypoventilation is the cause of respiratory failure that occurs in patients with neuromuscular disorders, drug overdoses, and chest wall abnormalities (see Figure 14-1). In hypoventilation, CO_2 accumulates in the alveoli and is not blown off. Respiratory acidosis occurs rapidly before renal compensation can occur. Mechanical ventilation may be necessary to support the patient until the initial cause of the hypoventilation can be corrected.

Ventilation-Perfusion Mismatch. Because the upper and lower airways do not play a part in gas exchange, the volume of inspired gas that fills these structures is referred to as physiologic dead space. This dead space is normally 25% to 30% of the inspired volume. A major mechanism for the elevation of $PaCO_2$ is an increase in the volume of dead space in relation to the entire tidal volume. Dead space increases when an area that is well ventilated has reduced perfusion and no longer participates in gas exchange.

Assessment

Respiratory assessment and evaluation of gas exchange are discussed in depth in Chapter 9. Assessment of the patient with ARF begins with the neurological system. Changes in mental status resulting from hypoxia and hypercapnia begin with anxiety, restlessness, and confusion and may progress to lethargy, severe somnolence, and coma.

The respiratory assessment continues with observing the rate, depth, and pattern of respiration. In response to hypoxemia, compensatory mechanisms produce tachypnea and an increase in tidal volume. As these compensatory mechanisms fail, respirations become shallow. A decrease in respiratory rate is an ominous sign. Use of accessory muscles and sternal retractions are a cause for concern as they indicate respiratory muscle fatigue. By auscultation, the nurse assesses the adequacy of airflow and the presence of adventitious breath sounds. The presence of a cough and the amount and characteristics of any sputum production should be noted.

A thorough cardiac assessment provides information about the heart's ability to deliver O_2 to the tissues. The patient must be closely monitored for changes in blood pressure, heart rate, and cardiac rhythm. ARF initially causes tachycardia and increased blood pressure. As ARF progresses, it may lead to dysrhythmias, angina, bradycardia, hypotension, and cardiac arrest. The nurse should evaluate peripheral perfusion by assessing pulses for strength and bilateral equality. The skin is assessed for a decrease in temperature and the presence of cyanosis or pallor, which are additional indicators of poor perfusion.

The patient's nutritional status must be evaluated because this is an important factor in maintaining respiratory muscle strength. The nurse looks for recent weight loss, muscle wasting, nausea, vomiting, abdominal distention, and skin turgor quality.

It is important to assess the patient's psychosocial status. This includes identifying the patient's significant others and their role in the family structure. An understanding of the patient's educational level, socioeconomic background, spiritual beliefs, and cultural or ethnic practices is important in determining an educational plan for discharge and future self-care.

Serial chest x-rays and pulmonary function tests provide important assessment information. Laboratory studies that are essential for the patient with respiratory failure include the following: electrolytes, which determine adequate muscle function; hemoglobin and hematocrit to evaluate the blood's O_2 carrying capacity; and ABG measurements to assess gas exchange and acid-base balance. Noninvasive monitoring such as pulse oximetry (SpO_2) and end-tidal CO_2 provides continuous information about the patient's oxygenation and ventilation.

Effects of Aging

Many age-related factors increase the older adult's risk for developing ARF (see Geriatric Considerations). Physiological changes may make identifying the signs and symptoms of ARF more difficult in the elderly. The most common early sign of hypoxemia in the elderly is a change in mental status, such as confusion or agitation. These changes are often mistaken for dementia or a normal sign of advancing age.[24]

Because of age-related decreases in chemoreceptor and central nervous system function, older adults have a lower ventilatory response to hypoxia and hypercapnia, and they may be less likely to perceive the sensation of dyspnea.[82] In addition, hypoxia in the elderly may not produce the same compensatory increases in heart rate, stroke volume, and cardiac output that are seen in younger adults. This may be due to preexisting cardiac disease or the effects of cardiac medications such as digoxin or beta-blockers. Increasing age can also lead to a slower response to O_2 therapy, making early identification and treatment of hypoxia essential in this population. Finally, normal PaO_2 levels decrease with age, but aging does not produce alterations in $PaCO_2$. For this reason hypercapnia and a falling pH are causes for concern.

GERIATRIC CONSIDERATIONS

PHYSIOLOGICAL CHANGES	NURSING IMPLICATIONS
Calcification of costal and sternal cartilage	Decreased chest wall mobility
Osteoporosis	Increased functional residual capacity and residual volume
Spinal degeneration	Decreased tidal volume, vital capacity, and forced expiratory
Kyphosis	volume
Flattening of diaphragm	Increased work of breathing
Decline in muscle mass	Respiratory muscle fatigue
Diminished cough reflex	Ventilation/perfusion mismatch
Decreased mucociliary clearance	Early airway collapse
Decline in surfactant production	Increased risk of atelectasis and pneumonia
Decreased effectiveness of immune system	
Thickening of alveolar-capillary membrane	Ventilation-perfusion mismatch
Decreased pulmonary blood flow	

Data from El Sohl, A. A., & Ramadan, F. H. (2006). Overview of respiratory failure in older adults. *Journal of Intensive Care Medicine, 21*(6), 345-351; and Zeleznik, J. (2003). Normative aging of the respiratory system. *Clinics in Geriatric Medicine, 19*(1), 1-18.

Interventions

The goals of treating patients with ARF are fivefold and include (1) maintaining a patent airway, (2) optimizing O_2 delivery, (3) minimizing O_2 demand, (4) treating the cause of ARF, and (5) preventing complications.

If a patient is unable to maintain a patent airway, it is the responsibility of the critical care team to protect the airway. This usually involves insertion of an endotracheal tube (ETT) or tracheostomy tube. Preventing inadvertent extubation is an important aspect of maintaining the airway. (Refer to Chapter 9 for nursing care interventions for the patient with an artificial airway.)

Optimizing O_2 delivery can be achieved in many ways, depending on the needs of the patient. The first is to provide supplemental O_2 via nasal cannula or face mask to maintain the PaO_2 above 60 mm Hg or the SaO_2 above 90%.[55] Higher PaO_2 values are indicated in cases of severe tissue hypoxia, low flow states, or deficiencies in O_2 carrying capacity.[55] If supplemental O_2 is ineffective in raising PaO_2 levels, noninvasive or invasive mechanical ventilation is indicated (see Clinical Alert: Acute Respiratory Failure). Patients are positioned for comfort and to enhance $\dot{V}/\dot{Q}$ matching. Some patients who are alert and are dyspneic oxygenate more effectively in the semi-Fowler to high-Fowler's position. Patients with unilateral lung disease should be positioned on their side with the better-functioning lung down. This allows gravity to perfuse the lung that has the best ventilation. Other methods to optimize O_2 delivery include red blood cell transfusion to ensure adequate hemoglobin levels to transport O_2, and enhancing cardiac output to deliver sufficient O_2 to the tissues.

Decreasing the patient's O_2 demand begins with providing adequate rest. Unnecessary physical activity is avoided in the patient with ARF. Agitation, restlessness, fever, sepsis, and patient-ventilator dyssynchrony must be addressed because they all contribute to increased O_2 demand and consumption.

While the patient's hypoxia is being treated, efforts must be made to identify and reverse the cause of the ARF. Specific interventions for acute respiratory distress syndrome (ARDS), COPD, asthma, pneumonia, and pulmonary embolism are detailed later in this chapter.

Finally, the critical care nurse must be alert to the potential complications that the patient with ARF may encounter. Preventive measures must be taken to avoid the complications of immobility, adverse effects from medications, fluid and electrolyte imbalances, development of gastric ulcers, and the hazards of mechanical ventilation (see Chapter 9).

CLINICAL ALERT
Acute Respiratory Failure

Concern	Symptoms	Nursing Actions

Respiratory muscle fatigue	Diaphoresis
	Nasal flaring
	Tachycardia
	Abdominal paradox
	Muscle retractions
	   Intercostal
	   Suprasternal
	   Supraclavicular
	Tachycardia
	Central cyanosis
		Improve O_2 delivery:
		   Administer O_2
		   Ensure adequate cardiac output
		   Correct low hemoglobin
		   Administer bronchodilators
		Decrease O_2 demand:
		   Provide rest
		   Reduce fever
		   Relieve pain and anxiety
		Decrease work of breathing
		Position patient for optimum gas exchange and perfusion

Cerebral hypoxia and carbon dioxide narcosis from increased CO_2 retention	Lethargy Somnolence Coma Respiratory acidosis	Maintain airway patency Prepare for intubation and mechanical ventilation

Nursing Diagnoses

Several nursing diagnoses must be considered in the care of a patient with ARF and are discussed in the Nursing Care Plan for a Patient with Acute Respiratory Failure. Expected outcomes include adequate organ and tissue oxygenation, and effective breathing and adequate gas exchange.

RESPIRATORY FAILURE IN ACUTE RESPIRATORY DISTRESS SYNDROME

Definition

ARDS was originally described in 1967 as an acute illness manifested by dyspnea, tachypnea, decreased

NURSING CARE PLAN for a Patient with Acute Respiratory Failure*

NURSING DIAGNOSIS

Impaired spontaneous ventilation related to hypoventilation, respiratory muscle fatigue, bronchospasm, infection, inflammation, central nervous system depression

PATIENT OUTCOMES

- Ventilatory demand decreased
- Respiratory distress absent
- Respirations unlabored at a rate of 12-16 breaths/min
- Arterial blood gases WNL

NURSING INTERVENTIONS	RATIONALES
• Assess and document respiratory status every 1 to 2 hours, including breath sounds, breathing pattern, rate, depth, and rhythm respirations	• Assess for respiratory distress. Changes in breath sounds may indicate fluid in the airways (crackles), accumulation of mucus (rhonchi), or airway obstruction (wheezes)
• Monitor for dyspnea and signs of increasing respiratory distress	• Indicate worsening of condition
• Assess for restlessness or change in the level of consciousness	• Assess for signs of hypoxemia
• Position patient in semi-Fowler's position (45 degrees) or position in which breathing pattern is most comfortable	• Promote maximal air exchange and lung expansion
• If patient has lung pathology, position for maximal gas exchange; place the "good" lung down	• Increase perfusion to the good lung and facilitate gas exchange
• Assist with activities. Provide patient with adequate periods of rest	• Reduce oxygen consumption and demands
• Administer medications to increase airflow as prescribed; evaluate their effectiveness	• Decrease airway resistance secondary to bronchoconstriction
• Give oxygen therapy or maintain mechanical ventilation as indicated	• Correct hypoxemia
• Monitor ABGs	• Assess for worsening hypoxemia and/or increasing $PaCO_2$; assess response to treatments
• If patient is mechanically ventilated, sedate according to goals for patient. Avoid oversedation	• Facilitate gas exchange and mechanical ventilation. Oversedation prolongs time on mechanical ventilation and its associated risks

NURSING DIAGNOSIS

Risk for ineffective airway clearance related to inability to cough, presence of endotracheal tube, thick secretions, fatigue.

PATIENT OUTCOMES

- Airway clear of secretions
- Lung sounds clear

*Please see Chapter 9 for Nursing Care Plan for the Mechanically Ventilated Patient.

NURSING CARE PLAN for a Patient with Acute Respiratory Failure—cont'd

NURSING INTERVENTIONS	RATIONALES
• Assess lung sounds	• Rhonchi may be audible with accumulation of secretions
• Change patient's position every 2 hours	• Mobilize secretions
• Encourage patient to cough and deep breathe	• Improve lung capacity and facilitate gas exchange
• Suction (nasotracheal or endotracheal) as determined by patient assessment	• "As needed" suctioning prevents damage to the airway from the suctioning procedure
• Provide adequate humidification with supplemental oxygen or mechanical ventilation	• Prevent drying of secretions and facilitate secretion removal
• Assess amount, color, consistency of secretions	• Indicate need for humidification and/or signs of infection

NURSING DIAGNOSIS

Risk for infection related to underlying illness/disease process, endotracheal intubation

PATIENT OUTCOMES
Absence of infection

- Normal temperature
- White blood cell count WNL
- Chest x-ray normal
- Negative cultures of sputum and bronchial aspirates

NURSING INTERVENTIONS	RATIONALES
• Monitor temperature every 4 hours, more frequently if elevated	• Fever may be first sign of infection
• Monitor white blood cell count	• Rising count indicates body's response to combat pathogens
• Assess amount, color, consistency of secretions	• Assess for infection
• Monitor results of cultures of sputum and/or bronchial specimens	• Assess need for antibiotic and appropriate antibiotic coverage
• Elevate the head of bed to at least 30 degrees	• Reduce the risk of aspiration and ventilator-associated pneumonia
• Provide oral care every 2 to 4 hours and as needed; brush teeth every 12 hours	• Reduce bacterial growth and colonization of oropharyngeal secretions; promotes patient comfort

NURSING DIAGNOSIS

Anxiety related to inability to speak, situational crises, uncertainty, fear of death, and lack of control

PATIENT OUTCOMES
Anxiety decreased or absent

- Vital signs WNL
- Relaxed facial expression and body movements, and normal sleep patterns
- Usual perceptual ability and interactions with others

Continued

NURSING CARE PLAN | for a Patient with Acute Respiratory Failure—cont'd

NURSING INTERVENTIONS	RATIONALES
• Monitor for signs of anxiety: increased heart rate, blood pressure, respiratory rate, muscle tension, inappropriate behaviors	• Anxiety is highly individualized response to life events. Signs must be recognized to provide interventions
• Develop trusting relationship by using calm, consistent, and reliable behaviors	• Encourage communication and enhance feelings of safety
• Always introduce yourself and all unfamiliar persons to the patient and explain why they are there	• Uncertainty and lack of predictability contribute to feelings of anxiety
• Provide nurturing environment. Allow the patient some control over decision making	• Increase sense of independence and normality
• Provide a means of communication (e.g., nonverbal, yes/no, picture charts, pencil/paper)	• Assist in meeting patient's needs and reduce anxiety
• Teach relaxation techniques (e.g., the use of slow rhythmic breathing during stressful periods)	• Enhance coping and improve physiological response
• Reassure patient of staff member's presence and prompt interventions as needed	• Assist in meeting needs and reducing anxiety
• Allow family member to remain at bedside to decrease isolation	• Provide a sense of security and familiarity; facilitate communication

NURSING DIAGNOSIS

Risk for impaired skin integrity related to bed rest and altered metabolic state

PATIENT OUTCOMES

• Skin intact
• Perfusion to all areas of the body maximized

NURSING INTERVENTIONS	RATIONALES
• Assess skin every shift for areas of breakdown	• Identify problems and promote preventive interventions
• Keep patient's skin clean and dry	• Decrease the risk of skin breakdown
• Reposition every 2 hours. If unable to turn patient because of hemodynamic instability, consider continuous lateral rotation or kinetic therapy with pressure relief mattress	• Reduce pressure on bony prominences

NURSING DIAGNOSIS

• Risk for ineffective family coping related to knowledge deficits of family members

PATIENT OUTCOMES
Family integrity maintained

• Family members verbalize educational needs and fears
• Family members feel comfortable asking questions related to patient's prognosis

NURSING CARE PLAN	for a Patient with Acute Respiratory Failure—cont'd

NURSING INTERVENTIONS	RATIONALES
• Assess family unit and coping behaviors	• Allow for anticipatory care and guidance to help family unit maintain support and coping strategies
• Assist family to identify roles to maintain family integrity	• Positive feedback from one family member can reinforce a behavior of another member
• Assist family members to verbalize fears and distress	• Promote effective communication
• Answer questions. Explain procedures, equipment, changes in patient's condition, and outcomes to family members in a sensitive manner	• Establish a trusting relationship; reduce anxiety
• Inform family of resources available to them such as chaplain and psychiatric liaison	• Enhance the use of services that may assist family
• Initiate multidisciplinary conferences with family to provide information and make decisions regarding ongoing treatment	• Establish trust with all health care team and encourages compliance with treatments

ABGs, Arterial blood gases; *HOB,* head of bed; *PaCO₂,* partial pressure of carbon dioxide in arterial blood; *WNL,* within normal limits.

lung compliance, and diffuse alveolar infiltrates on chest x-ray studies. The syndrome was observed in young adult patients after trauma who developed shock, required excessive fluid administration, or both. Autopsy results revealed that pathological heart and lung findings were similar to those described in infant respiratory distress syndrome.

The definition of ARDS has been expanded and refined over the years. In 1994, the American-European Consensus Conference recommended a definition of ARDS as a subset of acute lung injury. The definition included three criteria: PaO_2/FiO_2 ratio less than 200, bilateral infiltrates on chest x-ray, and pulmonary artery occlusion pressure less than 18 mm Hg or no clinical evidence of left atrial hypertension.[7] A lung injury score is often computed to assist in identifying ARDS.[7,26,74] The lung injury score is based on the amount of infiltrates on chest x-ray, the degree of hypoxemia, the amount of positive end-expiratory pressure (PEEP) that is required, and the static lung compliance (Table 14-1).

Etiology

Several possible causes of ARDS are listed in Box 14-1, and are categorized into direct and indirect factors. However, certain risk factors have a higher associated frequency of ARDS, and the presence of two or more factors increases the risk. The most common risk factors or disease processes associated with ARDS are sepsis, pneumonia, trauma, and aspiration of gastric contents. These four risk factors are believed to account for approximately 85% of all ARDS cases, with sepsis being the most common at a rate of about 50%. Approximately one third of hospitalized patients who aspirate gastric contents develop ARDS. In addition, critically ill patients with a history of chronic alcoholism are at an increased risk of developing ARDS.[74] Other causes with significant incidences are multiple transfusions including fresh frozen plasma and platelets, fat embolism, ischemia reperfusion, and pancreatitis.[7] Acute lung injury is the most common cause of mortality related to transfusions with an incidence of about 1 for every 5000 transfusions, and a mortality of 6% to 23%. The syndrome has been named TRALI (transfusion-related acute lung injury) with defined criteria.[62]

The mortality rate for patients with diagnosed ARDS has been improving over the last decade. The 28-day mortality rate is reported to be 25% to 30%.[7] As more individuals survive ARDS, prevention of long-term disabilities associated with a decrease in quality of life must be a priority of care. A recent study of patients who survived ARDS revealed that although lung volume and pulmonary function were normal by 6 months, functional disability persisted 1 year after discharge.[36] Another study reported that nearly half of ARDS survivors had significant neurocognitive impairment and a decrease in quality of life that persisted for at least 2 years.[38]

TABLE 14-1 Mechanical Ventilation Protocol for Acute Respiratory Distress Syndrome (NHLBI, NIH)

Definition of ALI/ARDS:

1. Acute onset

2. $PaO_2/FiO_2 \leq 300$, ALI; $PaO_2/FiO_2 \leq 200$, ARDS (referred to as P/F ratio)

3. Bilateral (patchy, diffuse, or homogeneous) infiltrates consistent with pulmonary edema

4. No clinical evidence of left atrial hypertension

Ventilator Setup and Adjustment:

1. Calculate predicted body weight (PBW)

  Males = 50.0 + 2.3 (height [inches] − 60)

  Females = 45.5 + 2.3 (height [inches] − 60)

2. Select Assist-Control mode

3. Set initial V_T to 8 mL/kg PBW

4. Reduce V_T by 1 mL/kg at intervals ≤ 2 hours until V_T = 6 mL/kg PBW

5. Set initial rate to approximate baseline VE (not >35 breaths/min)

6. Adjust V_T and RR to achieve pH and plateau pressure goals.

7. Set inspiratory flow rate above patient demand (usually >80 L/min)

Oxygenation Goal: PaO_2 55-80 mm Hg or SpO_2 88%-95%

FiO_2	0.3	0.4	0.4	0.5	0.5	0.6	0.7	0.7
PEEP cm H_2O	5	5	8	8	10	10	10	12
FiO_2	0.7	0.8	0.9	0.9	0.9	1.0	1.0	1.0
PEEP cm H_2O	14	14	14	16	18	20	22	24

Plateau Pressure Goal: ≤ 30 cm H_2O

Check Pplat, SaO_2, Total RR, V_T, and pH at least every 4 hours and after each change in PEEP or V_T

  1. If Pplat >30 cm H_2O: decrease V_T by 1-mL/kg steps (minimum, 4 mL/kg)

  2. If Pplat <25 cm H_2O: V_T <6 mL/kg, increase V_T by 1 mL/kg until Pplat >25 cm H_2O or V_T = 6 mL/kg

  3. If Pplat <30 cm H_2O and breath stacking occurs: may increase V_T in 1-mL/kg increments (maximum, 8 mL/kg)

pH Goal: 7.30-7.45

Acidosis Management: (pH < 7.30)

1. If pH 7.15-7.30: Increase RR until pH >7.30 or $PaCO_2$ <25 mm Hg (maximum RR, 35 breaths/min)

2. If RR = 35 breaths/min and $PaCO_2$ <25 mm Hg: may give $NaHCO_3$

3. If pH < 7.15: Increase RR to 35 breaths/min, if pH remains 7.15 and $NaHCO_3$ considered or infused, V_T may be increased in 1-mL/kg steps until pH >7.15 (Pplat target may be exceeded).

Alkalosis Management: (pH >7.45)

1. Decrease ventilator breaths/min rate if possible

I:E Ratio Goal: 1:10 to 1:3

1. Adjust flow rate to achieve goal

2. If FiO_2 = 1.0 and PEEP >24 cm H_2O, may adjust I:E to 1:1

ALI, Acute lung injury; *ARDS*, acute respiratory distress syndrome; *FiO2*, fraction of inspired oxygen; *H2O*, water; *I:E*, inspiration-to-expiration ratio; *NaHCO3*, sodium bicarbonate; *NHLBI*, National Heart, Lung, and Blood Institute; *NIH*, National Institutes of Health; *PaO2*, partial pressure of oxygen in arterial blood; *PaCO2*, partial pressure of carbon dioxide in arterial blood; *Pplat*, peak plateau pressure; *PEEP*, positive end-expiratory pressure; *P/F*, PaO_2/FiO_2 (oxygenation index); *RR*, respiratory rate; *SaO2*, arterial oxygen saturation; *SpO2*, arterial oxygen saturation via pulse oximeter; *VT*, tidal volume; *VE*, minute ventilation.
Adapted from the NIH NHLBI ARDS Clinical Network Mechanical Ventilation Protocol Summary Retrieved on June 10, 2007, from www.ardsnet.org.

BOX 14-1 Possible Causes for Acute Respiratory Distress Syndrome

Direct Causes
- Aspiration of gastric contents
- Diffuse pneumonia
- Fat embolism
- Near-drowning
- Neurogenic pulmonary edema
- Oxygen toxicity
- Prolonged mechanical ventilation
- Pulmonary contusion
- Multisystem trauma (chest and/or lung injury)
- Radiation (chest)

Indirect Causes
- Sepsis
- Multisystem trauma (without chest and/or lung injury)
- Cardiopulmonary bypass
- Anaphylaxis
- Disseminated intravascular coagulation
- Drug overdose
- Eclampsia
- Fractures, especially of the pelvis or long bones
- Increased intracranial pressure
- Leukemia
- Multiple transfusions
- Pancreatitis
- Thrombotic thrombocytopenic purpura
- Hypotension
- Radiation

Pathophysiology

ARDS is characterized by acute and diffuse injury to the lungs, leading to respiratory failure. It is a two-phase condition including the acute exudation response phase and the late phase of fibroproliferation. The acute response is a systemic inflammatory reaction secondary to direct or indirect lung injury. Initial injury causes damage to the pulmonary capillary endothelium, which activates massive aggregation of platelets and formation of intravascular thrombi. The platelets release serotonin and a substance that activates neutrophils. Other inflammatory factors such as endotoxin, tumor necrosis factor, and interleukin-1 are also activated. Neutrophil activation causes release of inflammatory mediators such as proteolytic enzymes, toxic O_2 products, arachidonic acid metabolites, and platelet-activating factors. The release of these mediators damages the alveolar-capillary membrane, which leads to increased capillary membrane permeability. Fluids, protein, and blood cells leak from the capillary beds into the alveoli, resulting in pulmonary edema. Pulmonary

hypertension occurs secondary to vasoconstriction caused by the inflammatory mediators. The pulmonary hypertension and pulmonary edema lead to $\dot{V}/\dot{Q}$ mismatching. The production of surfactant is stopped, and the surfactant present is inactivated.[40,65]

During the acute phase of ARDS, damage to the alveolar epithelium and vascular endothelium occurs. The damaged cells become susceptible to bacterial infection and pneumonia. The lungs become less compliant, resulting in decreased ventilation. A right-to-left shunt of pulmonary blood develops, and hypoxemia refractory to O_2 supplementation becomes profound. The work of breathing increases.[40]

The late phase of ARDS is the fibroproliferation stage. As ARDS proceeds over time (greater than 24 to 48 hours), a fibrin matrix (hyaline membrane) forms. After approximately 7 days, fibrosis obliterates the alveoli, bronchioles, and interstitium. The lungs become fibrotic with decreased functional residual capacity and severe right-to-left shunting. The inflammation and edema become worse with narrowing of the airways. Resistance to airflow and atelectasis increase.[40,65]

The inflammatory mediators responsible for lung damage also cause harm to other organs in the body, often resulting in multiple organ dysfunction syndrome.[40,65] The pathophysiology of ARDS is outlined in Figure 14-2.

Assessment

Assessment of a patient with ARDS is collaborative. A key clinical finding that is often diagnostic of ARDS is a lung insult (direct or indirect) followed by respiratory distress with dyspnea, tachypnea, and hypoxemia that does not respond to O_2 therapy. Initial signs of ARDS include restlessness, disorientation, and change in the level of consciousness. Pulse and temperature may be increased. Chest x-ray studies are usually normal in the initial stage.

As the process progresses and the PaO_2 decreases, dyspnea becomes severe and the patient may grunt with respirations. The grunting is an unconscious self-regulated response that increases intrathoracic pressures, causing positive expiratory pressure.[65] Intercostal and suprasternal retractions are often present. Other signs may include tachycardia and central cyanosis. The $PaCO_2$ continues to decrease, resulting in respiratory alkalosis. Hypocapnia and hypoxemia do not respond to increasing levels of supplemental O_2. Patients developing ARDS frequently need their noninvasive supplemental O_2 increased until it is at the maximum level, with little effect on the PaO_2. Metabolic acidosis caused by lactic acid buildup often results, and is confirmed by serum lactate level determinations. The metabolic imbal-

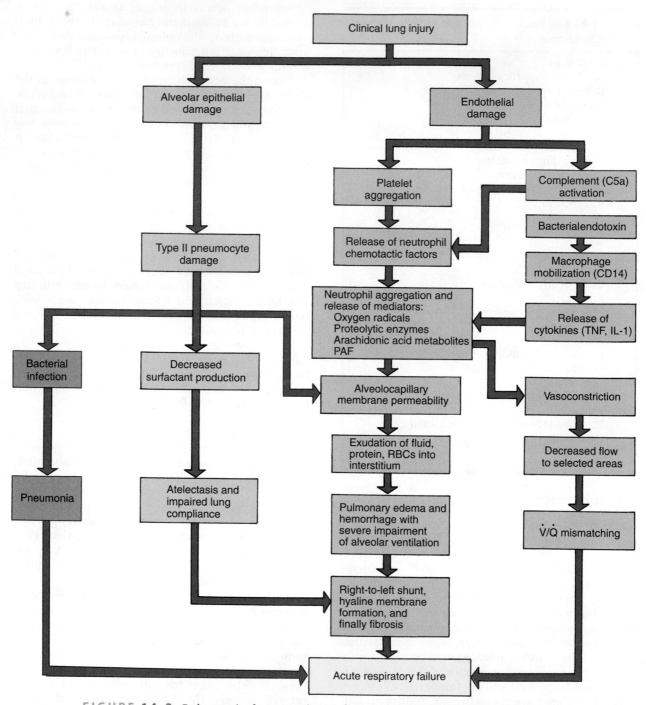

FIGURE 14-2. Pathogenesis of acute respiratory distress syndrome (ARDS). *TNF,* Tumor necrosis factor; *IL-1,* interleukin-1; *PAF,* platelet-activating factor; *RBCs,* red blood cells. *(From Huether, S. E., & McCance, K. L. [2004].* Understanding pathophysiology *[3rd ed., p. 765]. St. Louis: Mosby.)*

ances are a result of a low $\dot{V}/\dot{Q}$ ratio and a deteriorating PaO_2/FiO_2 ratio. As the ARDS progresses, crackles, rhonchi, and bronchial breath sounds are audible as fluid moves into the airways. Initially, the chest x-ray shows bilateral patchy infiltrates that have a "ground glass appearance." As ARDS worsens, the chest x-ray shows complete opacity, sometimes referred to as a "whiteout." The cardiac silhouette is normal.[49] (See Clinical Alert: Acute Respiratory Failure.)

Pulmonary mechanics show a decrease in lung volume, especially functional residual capacity, and a decrease in static and dynamic compliance. Peak inspiratory pressures rise, indicating a decrease in compliance.

Once ARDS is diagnosed, important assessment data that are used to guide treatment include hemodynamic measurements, ABGs, mixed venous blood gases, breath sounds, serial chest x-ray studies, computerized tomography (CT), complete blood cell count with differential, blood and sputum cultures, and fluid and electrolyte values. Metabolic and nutritional needs, and psychosocial needs of the patient and family, must also be assessed.

Interventions

Achieving adequate oxygenation is the primary goal in the treatment of ARDS. Other treatments are primarily supportive.

Oxygenation

Patients with ARDS generally require intubation and mechanical ventilation (see Chapter 9). Selection of ventilator settings is based on lung-protective strategies that attempt to achieve adequate oxygenation while minimizing the risks of ventilator-associated complications. Lung-protective strategies consist of low tidal volume (V_T), low end-inspiratory plateau pressure, FiO_2 at nontoxic levels (<0.60), and PEEP (see Table 14-1). Recent large clinical studies have shown reduced mortality and complications with the use of low V_T. The target V_T recommended is 6 mL/kg of predicted body weight (calculated from sex and height) (see Table 14-1). Actual body weight should not be used. The body weight may change secondary to accumulation of body fluid, but the size of the lungs does not change. The V_T may be reduced to 4 to 5 mL/kg to maintain the end-inspiratory plateau pressure at 30 cm H_2O or less. These lower volumes and plateau pressures prevent the alveoli from overdistending and minimize shearing. The respiratory acidosis that occurs secondary to the low V_Ts can be controlled by increasing the ventilator respiratory rate in a stepwise manner generally to an upper limit of 35 breaths per minute. The $PaCO_2$ should be kept within a permissive hypercapnia range of 50 to 70 mm Hg, and the pH maintained between 7.30 and 7.45.[7,8,29,74] (See Evidence-Based Practice feature.)

Patients with ARDS require significant support to achieve and maintain arterial oxygenation. High levels of FiO_2 may be required for short periods while aggressively working to reduce the FiO_2 to the lowest level that maintains the PaO_2 above 60 mm Hg. To prevent O_2 toxicity, the goal is to maintain the PaO_2 with levels of FiO_2 at 0.60 or below.

Ventilatory support typically includes PEEP to restore functional residual capacity, open collapsed alveoli, prevent collapse of unstable alveoli, and improve arterial oxygenation.[65] The National Heart, Lung, and Blood Institute ARDS network developed a protocol for PEEP application based on amount of FiO_2 requirements (see Table 14-1). A recent study found that higher PEEP resulted in improved PaO_2/FiO_2 ratios and lung compliance; however, no difference was noted in survival or length of time on

EVIDENCE-BASED PRACTICE

PROBLEM

Patients with acute respiratory distress syndrome (ARDS) require mechanical ventilation and other support to ensure adequate oxygenation and ventilation.

QUESTION

What are the best practices for mechanical ventilation for patients with ARDS?

REFERENCE

Girard, T. D., & Bernard, G. R. (2007). Mechanical ventilation in ARDS: A state-of-the-art review. *Chest, 131*, 921-929.

EVIDENCE

The authors reviewed 12 clinical trials that evaluated mechanical ventilation and other strategies as part of the treatment for patients with ARDS. They concluded that mechanical ventilation with low tidal volumes (<6 mL/kg of predicted body weight) significantly improved survival in patients with ARDS. Studies testing high positive end-expiratory pressures, maneuvers to increase alveolar recruitment, and prone positioning were useful as rescue therapies but did not affect patient mortality.

IMPLICATIONS FOR NURSING

Nurses must collaborate with respiratory therapists and the intensivists in determining the best management of patients with ARDS. Protocols for ventilator management that include low tidal volumes may assist in implementation of practices that improve patient outcomes. Some providers are concerned that ventilation with low tidal volumes is associated with patient discomfort, tachypnea, and hypercapnia. The nurse can assist by assessing the patient regularly for these potential outcomes of low–tidal volume ventilation and provide appropriate sedation.

mechanical ventilation.[7] Most experts in the field recommend using the National Heart, Lung, and Blood Institutes ARDS network protocol as a guideline and reserve the use of high levels of PEEP for patients with complex cases such as chest wall abnormalities or life-threatening hypoxemia.[7,26,29,48]

When using high levels of PEEP, the nurse must assess for potential adverse effects. PEEP increases intrathoracic pressure, potentially leading to decreased cardiac output. Excessive pressure in stiff lungs increases peak inspiratory and plateau pressures, which may result in barotrauma and pneumothorax. Treatment of a pneumothorax requires prompt insertion of a chest tube. A patient receiving high levels of PEEP therapy should be monitored every 2 to 4 hours, and after every adjustment in the PEEP setting, for changes in respiratory status such as increased respiratory rate, worsening adventitious breath sounds, decreased or absent breath sounds, decreased SpO_2, and increasing dyspnea.

A few unconventional modes of mechanical ventilation are used to treat ARDS when patients are unable to be oxygenated with standard modes of ventilation. These modes include high-frequency oscillatory ventilation; pressure-controlled, inverse-ratio ventilation; and airway pressure release ventilation. These modes often improve alveolar ventilation and arterial oxygenation while decreasing the risk of lung injury. None have been successful enough to be considered standard therapy. (See Chapter 9.)

Sedation/Comfort

Patients with ARDS routinely receive continuous sedation to promote comfort and sleep/rest, alleviate anxiety, prevent self-extubation or harm, and ensure adequate ventilation. A major adverse effect of undersedation is breathing dyssynchrony between the patient and ventilator. Ventilator dyssynchrony causes inadequate gas exchange and increases the patient's risk for ventilator-induced lung injury.[20,67]

The amount of sedation used must be monitored carefully to achieve predetermined end points or goals (see Chapter 5). Sedation goals are based on the patient's response to therapy and are determined through a collaborative effort between the physician, clinical pharmacist, and the critical care nurse. Regular assessment and documentation of response to therapy with a validated sedation assessment scale are essential.[44,67]

Therapeutic paralysis with a neuromuscular blocking agent may be required to completely control ventilation and promote adequate oxygenation. Patients who require unconventional modes of mechanical ventilation often need neuromuscular blockade because these modes are uncomfortable for

the patient and provide an unnatural means of respiration.[10] (See Chapter 5.)

Prone Positioning

Patients with ARDS who do not respond to standard treatment may benefit from prone positioning. Turning the patient to the prone position (proning) alters the $\dot{V}/\dot{Q}$ ratio by shifting blood from the posterior bases of the lung to the anterior portion. Proning also removes the weight of the heart and abdomen from the lungs, facilitates removal of secretions, improves oxygenation, and enhances recruitment of airways.[67,75] Proning should be considered when the PaO_2/FiO_2 ratio falls below 100, other lung recruitment strategies have been maximized, and/or the pulmonary status continues to deteriorate.[1] Once turned to the prone position, the optimal duration of therapy is 18 to 23 hours daily, with therapy continuing until the improvement in oxygenation is maximized.[75]

Turning the patient to the prone position is a cumbersome procedure requiring involvement of several health care professionals to ensure the patient's safety. Care must be taken to prevent dislodging the ETT and other tubes and lines. Several commercial devices are available to assist in turning the patient such as the Vollman Prone Positioner (Hill-Rom Services Corp.) and specialized proning beds.

Potential complications from the prone position are gastric aspiration, peripheral nerve injury, skin necrosis, corneal ulceration, and facial edema. Tube feedings are turned off for 1 hour before turning the patient to reduce the risk of aspiration. Proper body alignment must be maintained while the patient is in the prone position to decrease the risk of nerve damage. Pillows and foam support equipment are used to prevent overextension or flexion of the spine and reduce weight-bearing on bony prominences. Protective pads are used at the shoulders, iliac crest, and knees to decrease alterations in skin integrity and peripheral nerve damage. To avoid peripheral nerve injury and contractures of the shoulders, the arms are positioned carefully and repositioned often. A moisture barrier is applied to the patient's entire face to protect the skin from the massive amount of drainage from the mouth and nose. Absorbent pads, an emesis basin, or both, can be placed to capture the excessive oral and nasal drainage. The eyes must be protected to prevent direct ocular pressure caused by facial edema. The eyes are lubricated and taped shut to prevent corneal drying and abrasions.[75]

Fluid and Electrolytes

The National Heart, Lung, and Blood Institute ARDS network recently completed a large multicenter clinical trial to determine optimal fluid management for patients with ARDS. Patients who received a conservative fluid management protocol had reduced mortality, improved lung function, shorter length of mechanical ventilation, and fewer intensive care unit (ICU) days.[35] This study in combination with others strongly supports the use of conservative fluid strategies during the early phase of ARDS unless the patient is in shock. If the patient is in shock, aggressive fluid resuscitation is required until the shock has been resolved.[35]

Nutrition

The goal of nutritional support is to provide adequate nutrition to meet the patient's level of metabolism and reduce morbidity.[22] (See Chapter 6.) Several studies have recently evaluated the effects of a specialized enteral nutritional formula enriched with eicosapentaenoic acid (EPA), gamma-linolenic acid (GLA), and elevated antioxidants (EPA/GLA) in the treatment of ARDS. The studies have demonstrated reduced mortality, improved oxygenation secondary to reduced pulmonary inflammation, and fewer days of mechanical ventilation.[28,61,65]

Pharmacological Treatment

Despite clinical studies of various medications, no pharmacological agents are considered standard therapy for ARDS. Furosemide with albumin is advocated when the patient's protein level is low. The combination has resulted in improved oxygenation and reduced time receiving mechanical ventilation. Corticosteroids administration in both early and late ARDS has been associated with mixed findings. Studies of surfactant, inhaled nitric oxide, antifungal drugs, and phosphodiesterase inhibitors have not shown significant improvement of ARDS. Several new and different drugs are being studied, including activated protein C, granulocyte-macrophage colony-stimulating factor, and inhaled beta-agonist.[11]

Psychosocial Support

The onset of ARDS and its long recovery phase result in stress and anxiety for both the patient and the family. The patient may also experience feelings of isolation and dependence because of the length of the recovery phase. Health care team members must always remember to provide a warm, nurturing environment in which the patient and family can feel safe. A therapeutic environment includes taking the time to explain procedures, equipment, changes in the patient's condition, and outcomes to the patient and family members. Allowing the patient to participate in the planning of care and to verbalize fears and questions may help reduce stress and anxiety. In the intubated patient, communication is impaired, which increases the patient's sense of isolation. The isolation and accompanying depression can be minimized by encouraging a family member to stay with the patient and displaying personal items from home, such as photographs of loved ones.

ACUTE RESPIRATORY FAILURE IN CHRONIC OBSTRUCTIVE PULMONARY DISEASE

Pathophysiology

COPD is a progressive disease characterized by airflow limitations that are not fully reversible. These airflow limitations are associated with an abnormal inflammatory response to noxious particles or gases.[58] COPD is a preventable and treatable disease. Its incidence and impact on chronic morbidity and mortality are increasing. COPD is the fourth leading cause of death in the United States after cardiac disease, cancer, and stroke. Whereas the mortality rates for heart disease and stroke have declined since 1970, the death rate for COPD has doubled.[45] The primary cause of COPD is tobacco smoke, and smoking cessation is the most effective intervention to reduce the risk of developing COPD and stop disease progression.[58] Other contributing factors to the development of COPD include air pollution, occupational exposure to dust or chemicals, and the genetic abnormality alpha$_1$-antitrypsin deficiency.[58]

The primary pathogenic mechanism in COPD is chronic inflammation. Exposure to inhaled particles leads to airway inflammation and injury. The body repairs this injury through the process of airway remodeling, which causes scarring, narrowing, and obstruction of the airways. Destruction of alveolar walls and connective tissue results in permanent enlargement of air spaces. Increased mucus production results from enlargement of mucus-secreting glands and an increase in the number of goblet cells. Areas of cilia are destroyed, contributing to the patient's inability to clear thick, tenacious mucus. Structural changes in the pulmonary capillaries thicken the vascular walls and inhibit gas exchange. Table 14-2 outlines the physiological changes that result from COPD.

ARF can occur at any time in the patient with COPD. These patients normally have little respiratory reserve, and any condition that increases the work of breathing worsens $\dot{V}/\dot{Q}$ mismatching. Common causes of ARF in patients with COPD are acute exacerbations, heart failure, dysrhythmias, pulmonary edema, pneumonia, dehydration, and electrolyte imbalances.

TABLE 14-2　　Pathological and Physiological Changes in Chronic Obstructive Pulmonary Disease

Pathological Changes	Physiological Changes
Mucus hypersecretion	Sputum production
Ciliary dysfunction	Retained secretions
	Chronic cough
Chronic airway inflammation	Expiratory airflow limitation
Airway remodeling	Terminal airway collapse
	Air trapping
	Lung hyperinflation
Thickening of pulmonary vessels	Poor gas exchange with hypoxemia and hypercapnia
	Pulmonary hypertension
	Cor pulmonale (right ventricular enlargement and heart failure)

From the National Heart, Lung, and Blood Institute, World Health Organization. (2007). *Global Initiative for Chronic Obstructive Lung Disease (GOLD) global strategy for the diagnosis, management and prevention of chronic obstructive pulmonary disease.* Retrieved on March 24, 2008, from www.goldcopd.org.

Assessment

The hallmark symptoms of COPD are dyspnea, chronic cough, and sputum production. The diagnosis is confirmed by postbronchodilator spirometry that documents irreversible airflow limitations.[58] These pulmonary function tests show an increase in total lung capacity and a reduction in forced expiratory volume over 1 second (FEV_1). Functional residual capacity is increased as a result of air trapping.

By the time the characteristic physical findings of COPD are evident on physical examination, a significant decline in lung function has occurred. The chest will be overexpanded, or barrel-shaped, because the anteroposterior diameter increases in size. Respiration may include the use of accessory muscles and pursed-lip breathing. Clubbing of the fingers indicates long-term hypoxemia. Lung auscultation usually reveals diminished breath sounds, prolonged exhalation, wheezing, and crackles. ABG results show mild hypoxemia in the early stages of the disease, and worsening hypoxemia and hypercapnia as the disease progresses. Over time, as a compensatory mechanism, the kidneys increase bicarbonate production and retention (metabolic alkalosis) in an attempt to keep the pH within normal limits.

Exacerbations of COPD often result in dyspnea and an increase in sputum volume. Changes in the character of the sputum may signal the development of a respiratory infection. Additional symptoms may include anxiety, chest tightness, weakness, malaise, weight loss, fever, and sleeping difficulties. Wheezing indicates narrowing of the airways. Retraction of intercostal muscles may occur with inspiration, and exhalation is prolonged through pursed lips. The

CLINICAL ALERT
Chronic Obstructive Pulmonary Disease

During an acute exacerbation of chronic obstructive pulmonary disease, the risk of death is highest in patients with a low PaO_2, respiratory acidosis, significant comorbidities, and the need for ventilatory support.

patient is generally more comfortable in the upright position. Tachycardia and hypotension may result from reduced cardiac output.

ABG monitoring is a sensitive indicator of the respiratory status of the patient with COPD. It is important to know the patient's baseline ABG values to detect changes that indicate ARF. The patient with COPD usually has baseline ABG results that show a normal pH, a moderately low PaO_2 in the range of 60 to 65 mm Hg, and an elevated $PaCO_2$ in the range of 50 to 60 mm Hg (compensated respiratory acidosis). When ARF ensues, the $PaCO_2$ increases and the PaO_2 often decreases, resulting in respiratory acidosis and tissue hypoxia (see Clinical Alert: Chronic Obstructive Pulmonary Disease).

Interventions

Box 14-2 outlines the care of patients with stable COPD. These interventions should be individualized to reduce risk factors, manage symptoms, limit complications, and enhance the patient's quality of life. When a patient has an acute exacerbation, the goals of therapy are to provide support during the episode of acute failure, to treat the triggering event, and to return the patient to the previous level of functioning.

Oxygen

The most important intervention for acute exacerbation is to correct hypoxemia. O_2 should be administered to achieve a PaO_2 greater than 60 mm Hg or an SaO_2 greater than 90%.[12,58] Delivering high concentrations of O_2 in an attempt to raise the PaO_2 above 60 mm Hg will not significantly raise the SaO_2. Administering high concentrations of O_2 may also blunt the patient's hypoxic drive, which can diminish respiratory efforts and increase the risk of CO_2 retention.

Bronchodilator Therapy

Table 14-3 lists commonly administered bronchodilator agents. Short-acting, inhaled beta$_2$-agonists cause bronchial smooth muscle relaxation that reverses bronchoconstriction. They are primarily administered via a nebulizer or a metered-dose inhaler with a spacer. The dosage and frequency vary, depending on the delivery method and the severity of bronchoconstriction. Adverse effects are dose related and are more common with oral or intravenous administration compared with inhalation.[6] Adverse effects include tachycardia, dysrhythmias, tremors, hypokalemia, anxiety, bronchospasm, and dyspnea. Beta$_2$-agonists should be administered cautiously in patients with cardiac disease. Long-acting beta$_2$-agonists are effective in controlling stable COPD, but their onset of action is too long to be useful in the rapid treatment of acute exacerbations. They are administered by inhalation using a metered-dose inhaler or dry powder inhaler.

Anticholinergics may also be administered to treat bronchoconstriction. They are indicated for patients who cannot tolerate beta$_2$-agonists, or they may be

---

BOX 14-2 Treatment of Stable Chronic Obstructive Pulmonary Disease

- Reduce exposure to airway irritants
- Counseling/treatment for smoking cessation
- Remain in air-conditioned environment during times of high air pollution
- Influenza and pneumococcal vaccinations
- Inhaled bronchodilators (short-acting, long-acting, or combination)
- Inhaled glucocorticosteroids (for severe disease and repeated exacerbations)
- Pulmonary rehabilitation program with exercise training
- Long-term administration of oxygen more than 15 hours/day (for severe disease)

National Heart, Lung, and Blood Institute, World Health Organization. (2007). *Global Initiative for Chronic Obstructive Lung Disease (GOLD) global strategy for the diagnosis, management and prevention of chronic obstructive pulmonary disease.* Retrieved on March 24, 2008, from www.goldcopd.org.

TABLE 14-3 Bronchodilators

Medication	Mechanism of Action	Adverse Effects/Nursing Implications
Beta$_2$-agonists (short-acting) Albuterol Bitolterol Fenoterol Pirbuterol Terbutaline	Bronchial smooth muscle relaxation; relief of acute symptoms	Tremor, anxiety, bronchospasm, dyspnea, tachycardia, dysrhythmias, palpitations, hypertension, hypokalemia, throat irritation
Beta$_2$-agonists (long-acting) Salmeterol Formoterol	Bronchial smooth muscle relaxation; long-term prevention of symptoms	Same as above; do not use to treat acute exacerbations
Anticholinergics Ipratropium bromide Oxitropium bromide Tiotropium bromide	Inhibit action of acetylcholine, causing bronchial smooth muscle relaxation	Dry mouth, bitter taste, dizziness, bronchoconstriction, palpitations; lower incidence of tachycardia than beta$_2$-agonists; avoid contact with eyes.
Methylxanthines Theophylline Aminophylline	Phosphodiesterase inhibitor	Tremor, tachycardia, dysrhythmias, CNS stimulation (headache, seizures, restlessness), nausea, vomiting; do not crush sustained-release capsules; monitor trough levels.

CNS, Central nervous system.

used in combination with beta$_2$-agonists. The use of methylxanthines for acute exacerbation is controversial and requires the monitoring of trough blood levels to maintain therapeutic concentrations.[58] Cardiac side effects may be seen in addition to central nervous system stimulation that may lead to headache, restlessness, and seizures. The use of expectorants, mucolytic agents, and chest physical therapy has not been found to be effective in the management of COPD exacerbations.

Corticosteroids

Administration of systemic corticosteroids for a period of 7 to 10 days to decrease airway inflammation has been shown to be beneficial in the management of an acute exacerbation of COPD.[58] Studies show a reduction in hospital length of stay and an improved FEV$_1$ and PaO$_2$, with no significant difference seen between oral and parenteral steroids.[71] Common adverse effects of steroid therapy include hyperglycemia and an increased risk of infection. There may also be an unexplained association between steroid use in the critically ill and the development of skeletal muscle neuromyopathy.[46]

Antibiotics

Antibiotic therapy is recommended when dyspnea is accompanied by increased sputum volume and purulence, or if mechanical ventilation is needed.[58] Infections are commonly caused by *Haemophilus influenzae*, *Streptococcus pneumoniae*, and *Moraxella catarrhalis*.[58] Multiple drug-resistant bacterial infections are common in COPD exacerbations, and antibiotic selection should be based on local bacterial resistance patterns and on sensitivity reports from sputum cultures.[12,59]

Ventilatory Assistance

Patients with ARF from a COPD exacerbation benefit from early treatment with noninvasive positive pressure ventilation (NPPV) (see Chapter 9). Unlike invasive mechanical ventilation that requires insertion of an ETT or a tracheostomy, NPPV assists the patient's respiratory efforts by delivering positive airway pressure through a nasal, oronasal, or full face mask. Contraindications to NPPV include hemodynamic instability, thick or copious secretions, a change in mental status, and head or facial trauma/surgery.[18] Studies on the use of NPPV in COPD exacerbations have shown a decrease in the need for intubation, lower mortality rates, a decreased ICU length of stay, and a decrease in the occurrence of health care–acquired pneumonia.[18,23,54]

Intubation and invasive mechanical ventilation are indicated in those patients who, despite aggressive therapy, develop significant mental status changes, severe dyspnea and respiratory muscle fatigue, respiratory acidosis, significant hypoxemia, or hypercapnia.

In the late stages of severe COPD, patients often report that their quality of life deteriorates because of severe activity limitations and comorbid conditions. Decisions regarding the use or avoidance of intubation, mechanical ventilation, cardiopulmonary resuscitation, and other forms of life support should be made by the patient in conjunction with the patient's family and physician before ARF occurs. Critical care nurses are in an ideal position to facilitate discussions about advance directives and to answer questions for the patient and significant others.

ACUTE RESPIRATORY FAILURE IN ASTHMA

Pathophysiology

Asthma is a chronic inflammatory disorder of the airways. The inflammation causes the airways to become hyperresponsive when the patient inhales allergens, viruses, or other irritants (Box 14-3). Episodic airflow obstruction results because these irritants cause bronchoconstriction, airway edema, mucus plugging, and airway remodeling[57a] (Figure 14-3). Air trapping, prolonged exhalation, and $\dot{V}/\dot{Q}$ mismatching with an increased intrapulmonary shunt occur. The airflow limitations in asthma are largely reversible. When asthma is controlled, symptoms and exacerbations should be infrequent.

Assessment

Symptoms of asthma exacerbation are wheezing, dyspnea, chest tightness, and cough, especially at night or in the morning. The patient initially hyperventilates, producing respiratory alkalosis. As the airways continue to narrow, it becomes more difficult for the patient to exhale. Peak expiratory flow readings will be less than 50% of the patient's normal values. The lungs become overinflated and stiff, which further increases the work of breathing. Nursing assessment will reveal tachypnea, tachycardia, pulsus paradoxus greater than 25 mm Hg, agitation, possible use of accessory muscles, and suprasternal retractions. A severe asthma exacerbation, previously referred to as status asthmaticus, occurs when the bronchoconstriction does not respond to bronchodilator therapy, and ARF ensues. The patient experiences fatigue from the severe dyspnea, cough, and increased work of breathing. Hypercapnia, hypoxia, and respiratory acidosis develop, and cardiac output decreases as a result of a

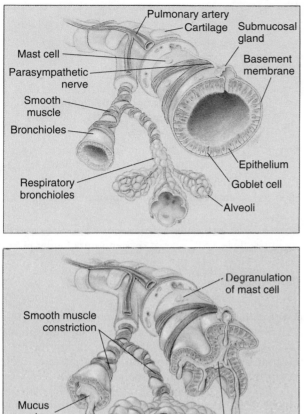

FIGURE 14-3. Airway obstruction caused by asthma. **A,** Normal lung. **B,** Bronchial asthma: thick mucus, mucosal edema, and smooth muscle spasm causing obstruction of small airways. *(From Huether, S. E., & McCance, K. L. [2004]. Understanding pathophysiology [3rd ed., p. 1121]. St. Louis: Mosby.)*

decreased venous return that is related to increased intrathoracic pressures (see Clinical Alert: Asthma).

Interventions

Mild exacerbations of asthma can be managed by the patient at home with the use of short-acting beta$_2$-agonists to treat bronchoconstriction (see Table 14-3). Treatment of acute, severe exacerbations of asthma requires O_2 therapy, repeated administration of rapid-acting inhaled bronchodilators, and systemic steroid administration (Table 14-4). Most patients respond well to treatment, but some may need intubation and mechanical ventilation. Because of severe airflow obstruction, these patients are at risk for developing dynamic lung hyperinflation (auto-

---

BOX 14-3   Asthma Triggers

Inhalant Allergens
- Animals
- House-dust mites
- Cockroaches
- Indoor fungi
- Outdoor allergens

Occupational Exposure
- Organic and inorganic dusts
- Chemical agents
- Fumes

Irritants
- Tobacco smoke
- Indoor/outdoor pollution
- Fumes: perfumes, cleaning agents, sprays

Other Factors Influencing Asthma Severity
- Viral respiratory infections
- Rhinitis/sinusitis
- Gastroesophageal reflux disease
- Exercise
- Sensitivity: aspirin, other nonsteroidal anti-inflammatory drugs, sulfites
- Topical and systemic beta-blockers

National Heart, Lung, and Blood Institute. (2007). *Global Initiative for Asthma (GINA) global strategy for asthma management and prevention* Retrieved March 24, 2008, from www.ginasthma.org.

CLINICAL ALERT
Asthma

Signs of impending acute respiratory failure in a patient with severe asthma may include:
- Breathlessness at rest and the need to sit upright
- Speaking in single words; unable to speak in sentences or phrases
- Lethargy or confusion
- Paradoxical thoracoabdominal movement
- Absence of wheezing ("silent chest") indicating no air movement and respiratory muscle fatigue
- Bradycardia
- Respiratory acidosis and hypoxemia with $PaCO_2$ > 45 mm Hg and PaO_2 < 60 mm Hg

National Heart, Lung, and Blood Institute. (2007). *Global Initiative for Asthma (GINA) global strategy for asthma management and prevention.* Retrieved March 24, 2008, from www.ginasthma.org.

TABLE 14-4 Emergency Treatment of Severe Asthma

Therapy	Purpose	Goals
Oxygen via nasal cannula or face mask	Correct hypoxemia	Maintain SpO_2 ≥90%
Inhaled rapid-acting beta$_2$-agonists via nebulizer (continuous); followed by intermittent on-demand therapy	Relieve airway obstruction caused by bronchoconstriction	Achieve PEF >70% of predicted or personal best; normalizing/improving ABGs; respiratory rate <30 bpm without use of accessory muscles
Inhaled anticholinergics (added to beta$_2$-agonist therapy)	Relieve bronchoconstriction	Relieve sensation of dyspnea; patient able to complete full sentences without breathlessness
Systemic corticosteroids (orally or intravenous)	Reverse airway inflammation	Improve lung sounds; prevent intubation

ABGs, Arterial blood gases; *bpm*, breaths per minute; *PEF*, peak expiratory flow; *SpO₂*, arterial oxygen saturation by pulse oximetry.
National Heart, Lung, and Blood Institute. (2007). *Global Initiative for Asthma (GINA) global strategy for asthma management and prevention.* Retrieved March 24, 2008, from www.ginasthma.org.

PEEP), lung injury from barotrauma, and hemodynamic compromise.[9] Precise management of mechanical ventilation is required to enhance outcomes and prevent complications. In cases that are refractory to standard treatment, oxygenation may be improved by delivering a mixture of helium and O_2 (heliox) to the lungs. Because helium is less dense than O_2, enhances gas flow through the constricted airways and may improve oxygenation.[9]

During a patient's recovery from a severe asthmatic event, the critical care nurse should focus efforts on teaching the patient asthma management techniques because patient and family education is essential for achieving asthma control. Persons with asthma are taught how to implement environmental controls to prevent symptoms, understand the differences between medications that relieve and control symptoms, properly use inhaler devices, and monitor their level of asthma control.[57a] A written action plan and goals of treatment mutually determined by the patient and the health care provider helps patients to achieve asthma control and assists with early identification and treatment of exacerbations.

ACUTE RESPIRATORY FAILURE RESULTING FROM VENTILATOR-ASSOCIATED PNEUMONIA

Definition and Etiology

Pneumonia is a common consequence of illness and hospitalization, and may include hospital-acquired pneumonia (HAP), ventilator-associated pneumonia (VAP), or health care-associated pneumonia (HCAP). HAP is defined as pneumonia occurring more than 48 hours after hospital admission excluding any infection incubating at the time of admission. HAP accounts for 25% of nosocomial infections in the ICU and 50% of the antibiotics administered. The patient with HAP may be treated in a medical/surgical unit or in a critical care unit depending upon the severity of the illness. Critically ill patients who receive mechanical ventilation are especially vulnerable to the development of VAP, defined as pneumonia that develops 48 hours or more after intubation (Figure 14-4). HCAP is defined as pneumonia that develops in any patient who (1) was hospitalized in an acute care hospital for 2 or more days within 90 days of the infection; (2) resides in a long-term care facility; (3) received intravenous antibiotic therapy, chemotherapy, or wound care within the past 30 days; or (4) had hemodialysis at a hospital or clinic.[4,51] Most of the information in this chapter focuses on VAP, but it is important to have an understanding of all categories of nosocomial pneumonia because the treatments are the same if the patient requires ventilatory support.

Epidemiological investigations have shown the incidence of VAP to be 10% to 25%. Crude mortality varies from 10% to 40% and reaches as high as 76% if the disease is caused by high-risk pathogens.[4] Ventilated patients who develop VAP are more likely to die.[42] VAP also increases the length of stay and hospital cost; up to $57,000 in mean hospital charges per patient has been reported.[17] The risk for developing VAP is highest during the first 5 days of ventilation.[51,53] Recently reported VAP rates ranged from 2.7 cases per 1000 ventilator days

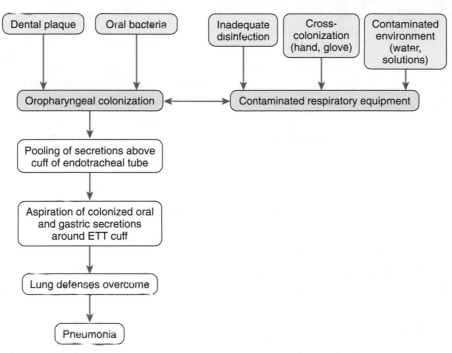

FIGURE 14-4. Role of airway management in the pathogenesis of ventilator-associated pneumonia.

in medical units to 12.3 cases per 1000 ventilator days in burn units.[23a]

Pathophysiology

For VAP to occur, enough organisms must accumulate in the lower respiratory tract to overwhelm the patient's natural defense mechanism, or the patient must be immunocompromised. The pathogens responsible for VAP may be inherent in the patient's endogenous flora or in the hospital environment. Endogenous sources of pathogens include aspiration of colonized oropharyngeal secretions around the ETT cuff, sinusitis, aspiration of gastric contents, and inhalation of infected organisms. Patients with an ETT are at increased risk for aspiration secondary to the natural anatomical barrier of the glottis being violated. The ETT is inserted into the trachea past the vocal cords, thereby holding the glottis in the open position and compromising its ability to prevent aspiration.[4,64] Sources of exogenous pathogens include contamination from health care personnel, ventilator equipment, nebulizers, and the biofilm coating on the ETT. The patient's underlying condition may contribute to the development of VAP. Preexisting pulmonary disease such as COPD, recent neurosurgical illness, severe trauma, ARDS, and age greater than 70 years increase the risk for developing VAP.[4,64]

VAP is categorized into two stages based on the time of onset from intubation. Early-onset VAP occurs within the first 4 days of intubation and is commonly associated with community-acquired organisms, such as *S. pneumoniae*, methicillin-susceptible *Staphylococcus aureus*, *H. influenzae*, or *Enterobacteriaceae*. Late-onset VAP occurs 5 or more days after intubation and is associated with enteric gram-negative rods, multidrug-resistant (MDR) organisms, or both. The pathogens associated with late-onset VAP include *Pseudomonas aeruginosa*, *Acinetobacter* species, methicillin-resistant *S. aureus*, and other MDR gram-negative bacilli. HCAP is associated with a high incidence of infection with MDR organisms.[4,53]

Assessment

The diagnosis of VAP is complicated by a lack of sensitive and specific criteria; there is no "gold standard." Many conditions can produce new lung infiltrates in critically ill patients. Cultures obtained by bronchoscopic and nonbronchoscopic methods are useful in diagnosis. A protected-specimen brush culture with at least 10^3 cfu/mL or a bronchoalveolar lavage culture with at least 10^4 cfu/mL is considered specific for diagnosing VAP. Some clinicians use clinical criteria to diagnose VAP. The presence of a new or persistent lung density seen on chest x-rays with two or more of the following is considered

---

TABLE 14-5 Modified Clinical Pulmonary Infection Score

CPIS Points	0	1	2
Tracheal secretions	Rare	Abundant	Abundant and purulent
Chest x-ray infiltrates	No infiltrate	Diffuse	Localized
Temperature (°C)	≥36.5 and ≤38.4	≥38.5 and ≤38.9	≥39 or ≤36
Leukocyte count (per microliter)	≥4000 and ≤11,000	<4000 or >11,000	<4000 or >11,000 + band forms ≥500
PaO₂/FiO₂ ratio (mm Hg)	>240 or ARDS		≤240 and no evidence of ARDS
Microbiology	Negative		Positive

Score each section and determine total points. A score of more than 6 at baseline or after incorporating the Gram stains or culture results is suggestive of pneumonia.

ARDS, Acute respiratory distress syndrome; *CPIS,* clinical pulmonary infection score; *FiO₂,* fraction of inspired oxygen; *PaO₂,* partial pressure of oxygen in arterial blood.

From Fartoukh, M., Maitre, B., Honore, S., Cerf, C., Zahar, J. R., & Brun-Buisson, C. (2003). Diagnosing pneumonia during mechanical ventilation: The clinical pulmonary infection score revisited. *American Journal of Respiratory and Critical Care Medicine, 168,* 173-179.

diagnostic: temperature of more than 38.5°C or less than 36.5°C, leukocyte count of more than 11,000 cells/microliter or less than 5000 cells/microliter, and the presence of purulent endotracheal secretions.[4,14,53] The clinical pulmonary infection score may also aid in diagnosis. This score combines clinical, radiographic, physiological (PaO₂/FiO₂ ratio), and microbiological information into a numerical value that predicts the presence or absence of VAP (Table 14-5).[4,27,53]

Interventions

The interventions for VAP are aimed at prevention and treatment. The prevention of VAP is a major focus of many recent safety initiatives and focuses on modification of risk factors. The Institute for Healthcare Improvement proposed a "bundle of care" for mechanically ventilated patients. Bundles are evidence-based interventions grouped together to improve outcomes. Four strategies are included in the ventilator bundle: elevation of head of bed (HOB) to at least 30 degrees, daily awakening ("sedation vacation") with assessment of the need for mechanical ventilation, prophylaxis for stress ulcers, and prophylaxis for deep venous thrombosis.[5,42] Strategies for prevention of VAP are summarized in Box 14-4.

Prevention

Hand Hygiene and Universal Precautions. The most effective method to prevent VAP caused by the hospital environment is hand hygiene and following universal precautions.[5,13,76] Hand hygiene includes washing hands before and after touching any patient's respiratory equipment or anything else in the patient's environment.[14] Gloves are required when suctioning the patient both orally and through the ETT tube, including the closed suction technique.

Respiratory Equipment. The first step to preventing VAP is to avoid endotracheal intubation when possible. Noninvasive mechanical ventilation is an option to consider before intubation. Use of NPPV for acute exacerbations of COPD and cardiac-related pulmonary edema is associated with lower rates of VAP and reduced mortality[30] (see Chapter 9). If the patient requires endotracheal intubation, oral intubation is the preferred site. Nasal intubation has been linked to an increased risk of sinusitis with potential aspiration of infected nasal secretions into the lungs.[14,53]

The ETT itself increases the risk for VAP by several mechanisms. The ETT results in injury to the tracheal mucosa, which reduces mucociliary function. Gag and cough reflexes are impaired. The ETT prevents the upper respiratory system from heating and humidifying inspired air, leading to thickening of secretions. The ETT can create binding sites for bacteria in the bronchial tree and increase mucus secretion. It serves as a reservoir where bacteria remain inaccessible to antibiotics. Bacteria that colonize the ETT form a bacterial biofilm.[66,69] Suctioning, coughing, or movement of the tube may dislodge this biofilm. No significant differences in VAP are noted between closed and open suctioning procedures.[77] Instillation of normal saline during suctioning may facilitate inoculation of bacteria into the respiratory tract by dislodging the bacteria adhered to the ETT and should be avoided. If the patient has thick secretions, the key strategies to facilitate secretion removal are adequate hydration, increased mobility, and humidification of the airway.[14,76]

BOX 14-4 Prevention of Ventilator-Associated Pneumonia

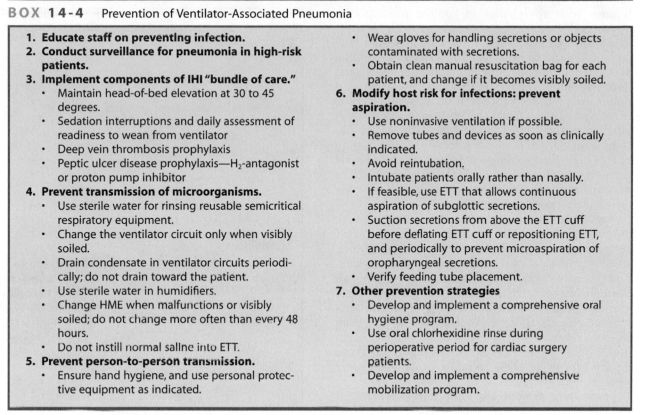

1. **Educate staff on preventing infection.**
2. **Conduct surveillance for pneumonia in high-risk patients.**
3. **Implement components of IHI "bundle of care."**
   - Maintain head-of-bed elevation at 30 to 45 degrees.
   - Sedation interruptions and daily assessment of readiness to wean from ventilator
   - Deep vein thrombosis prophylaxis
   - Peptic ulcer disease prophylaxis—H$_2$-antagonist or proton pump inhibitor
4. **Prevent transmission of microorganisms.**
   - Use sterile water for rinsing reusable semicritical respiratory equipment.
   - Change the ventilator circuit only when visibly soiled.
   - Drain condensate in ventilator circuits periodically; do not drain toward the patient.
   - Use sterile water in humidifiers.
   - Change HME when malfunctions or visibly soiled; do not change more often than every 48 hours.
   - Do not instill normal saline into ETT.
5. **Prevent person-to-person transmission.**
   - Ensure hand hygiene, and use personal protective equipment as indicated.
   - Wear gloves for handling secretions or objects contaminated with secretions.
   - Obtain clean manual resuscitation bag for each patient, and change if it becomes visibly soiled.
6. **Modify host risk for infections: prevent aspiration.**
   - Use noninvasive ventilation if possible.
   - Remove tubes and devices as soon as clinically indicated.
   - Avoid reintubation.
   - Intubate patients orally rather than nasally.
   - If feasible, use ETT that allows continuous aspiration of subglottic secretions.
   - Suction secretions from above the ETT cuff before deflating ETT cuff or repositioning ETT, and periodically to prevent microaspiration of oropharyngeal secretions.
   - Verify feeding tube placement.
7. **Other prevention strategies**
   - Develop and implement a comprehensive oral hygiene program.
   - Use oral chlorhexidine rinse during perioperative period for cardiac surgery patients.
   - Develop and implement a comprehensive mobilization program.

ETT, Endotracheal tube; *HME,* heat moisture exchanger; *IHI,* Institute for Healthcare Improvement.
Modified from Centers for Disease Control and Prevention. (2004). Guidelines for prevention of healthcare associated pneumonia, 2003. *MMWR. Morbidity and Mortality Weekly Report, 53*(RR03), 1-36.

Maintaining aseptic technique during ETT suctioning and meticulous care of the respiratory equipment decrease the incidence of VAP. The condensate in the ventilator tubing is periodically drained away from the patient to prevent aspiration (or lavage). When turning a patient, meticulous care must be taken to prevent accidental lavage of the condensate. The ventilator circuit is changed only if it is visibly soiled or mechanically malfunctioning, as reducing the number of times the circuit is opened is associated with a reduction in VAP. A clean manual resuscitation bag is used for each patient and changed if it becomes visibly soiled.[4,13]

Prevention of aspiration of oropharyngeal secretions is an important nursing intervention. An initial step to prevent aspiration of oropharyngeal secretions is to thoroughly suction the patient's oropharynx before intubation. After intubation, oropharyngeal secretions accumulate above the ETT cuff and may result in microaspiration. Regular suctioning of oral secretions and keeping the ETT cuff pressure between 20 and 30 cm H$_2$O may assist in preventing aspiration.[2] ETT cuff pressure is routinely checked and adjusted, usually by a respiratory therapist. The mouth and the area above the ETT cuff need to be suctioned periodically because coughing or movement of the ETT (including tube repositioning) can cause these secretions to enter the lungs. A special dual-lumen ETT that has a suction port in the subglottic area above the cuff is commercially available (see Chapter 9). These specialized ETTs are associated with a reduction in VAP and a delay in onset of VAP, and are recommended in clinical practice guidelines.[4,5,14] Newer ETTs are being tested in clinical trials, including tubes with redesigned cuffs to prevent aspiration[81] and silver-coated tubes to reduce biofilm and bacterial growth.[53]

Patient Position and Mobility. The supine position places mechanically ventilated patients at an increased risk for aspiration and VAP. Semirecumbency or HOB elevation to at least 30 degrees with a goal of 45 degrees is recommended to reduce VAP.[42] HOB elevation also facilitates ventilation and minimizes atelectasis.[5,34,57,64,76] Keeping the HOB elevated is challenging, as nurses often underestimate the degree of elevation.[34] Other barriers to HOB elevation include hemodynamic instability, increased risk of pressure ulcers, reduced patient comfort, and interference with completion of routine nursing care activities.[64,76]

A protocol for progressive mobility for critically ill patients should be established to assist in preventing atelectasis, pulmonary infection, pressure ulcers, and deconditioning. The protocol should include decision points to progress patients from turning every 2 hours, to sitting (chair or dangling), to weight-bearing, to transferring to a bedside chair, to ambulation. If the patient does not tolerate manual turning or is at high risk for complications, continuous lateral rotation or kinetic therapy needs to be initiated. In patients with severe refractory hypoxemia, turning to the prone position is considered.[5,34,57,76]

Oral Care. Implementing a comprehensive oral care program that includes brushing the teeth and oral suctioning is an effective intervention for preventing VAP.[5,14,34,64,76] Oral care reduces oropharyngeal colonization and dental plaque. Box 14-5 describes an example of a comprehensive oral care protocol. Some oral care protocols include swabbing with chlorhexidine gluconate. Chlorhexidine gluconate has been shown to reduce VAP in the cardiac surgery population.[39] The effectiveness of chlorhexidine gluconate in oral care protocols is being investigated in other patient populations.[5]

Gastric Tubes, Nutrition, and Peptic Ulcer Prophylaxis. A nasogastric or orogastric tube impairs swallowing, produces stagnation of oropharyngeal secretions, increases reflux, and acts as a conduit for bacteria to migrate from the stomach to the oropharynx. A nasogastric tube also increases the risk of maxillary sinusitis. When possible, insertion of an orogastric tube is preferred.[4,14]

Early initiation of nutritional support is a standard of care.[15,53] Enteral nutrition is the preferred method of support; however, enteral feedings may increase the risk of VAP by promoting overgrowth of gram-negative organisms secondary to an increased pH of stomach contents, an increased gastric volume, and an increased reflux. Starting early enteral feedings helps to maintain the gut mucosa, which prevents microbial translocation and minimizes the effect of malnutrition on the immune system.[4] Tube placement must be verified radiographically before initiating enteral feeding. Placement and gastric residual volumes are reassessed every 4 hours and before medications are instilled. Several issues related to enteral feeding and VAP remain unresolved, such as gastric versus postpyloric feeding.

Mechanical ventilation for longer than 24 hours is a major risk factor for gastrointestinal bleeding. Gastrointestinal bleeding that requires treatment with blood transfusions places the patient at risk for VAP and ARDS.[53,73] Peptic ulcer disease prophylaxis is part of the ventilator bundle, and administration

---

BOX 14-5   Example of a Comprehensive Oral Care Protocol

Interventions
1. Assess the oral cavity on admission and every 12 hours.
2. Administer oral care to unconscious or intubated patients every 2-4 hours and as needed.
3. Brush teeth every 12 hours as part of oral care protocol.
4. Assess intubated patients every 2 hours, before repositioning or deflating the endotracheal tube, and as needed to determine the need for removal of oropharyngeal secretions. Suction as the need is identified.

Equipment
1. Soft-tipped, covered Yankauer for nontraumatic suctioning
2. Soft-suction toothbrush with a compact head that can maneuver around the endotracheal tube
3. Suction oral swab for stimulation of mucosal tissue
4. 1.5% Hydrogen peroxide mouth rinse for oral cleansing and reduction of respiratory pathogens
5. Water-based mouth moisturizer with vitamin E to improve the healing of lesions
6. Deep suction catheters for suctioning secretions above the endotracheal tube cuff
7. Dedicated tubing for oral suctioning equipment for infection control
8. Oral chlorhexidine rinse during perioperative period for cardiac surgery patients or other patients as prescribed

---

of H_2-receptor inhibitors or proton pump inhibitors is recommended.[21,73]

Sedation Interruption and Daily Assessment of Readiness to Extubate. Daily interruption of sedation infusions to assess the readiness to extubate is associated with a reduction in the number of days that mechanical ventilation is required and a reduction in the length of stay in the ICU.[50] Fewer days of mechanical ventilation will result in a decreased incidence of VAP. Protocols for sedation interruption have been published, including assessment for complications.[42,64]

Treatment

VAP is associated with a high risk of mortality if an appropriate antibiotic regimen is not started in a timely manner.[43] The guidelines for antibiotic use have two major goals: to provide therapy with an appropriate and adequate empirical antibiotic regimen, and to achieve the first goal without over-using and abusing antibiotics.[4,15] The initial anti-biotic therapy algorithm includes two groups of patients: patients with early-onset VAP without any risk factors for MDR pathogens, and patients with late-onset VAP or risk factors for MDR pathogens. Patients with early-onset VAP without any risk factors for MDR may be placed on narrow-spectrum monotherapy based on knowledge of local micro-biological data. Patients at risk for MDR pathogens require broad-spectrum therapy based on knowl-edge of the local hospital antibiogram. When the patient is at high risk for MDR, three antibiotics are prescribed: two drugs of different classes active against *P. aeruginosa* and a third drug to treat methicillin-resistant *S. aureus*. The antibiotic regi-mens for both classifications of patients should be narrowed once the results of the quantitative cul-tures are known (deescalation therapy). Clinical improvement takes about 3 days. If clinical improve-ment does not occur within 72 hours, the patient should be evaluated for noninfectious causes of the symptoms or extrapulmonary infections. If a patient receives an appropriate antibiotic regimen, the dura-tion of therapy can be reduced to 7 to 8 days versus the traditional 14 to 21 days.[4,15,63]

ACUTE RESPIRATORY FAILURE RESULTING FROM PULMONARY EMBOLISM

Definition/Classification

An embolus is a clot or plug of material that travels from one blood vessel to another smaller vessel. The clot lodges in the smaller vessel and obstructs blood flow. An embolus in the pulmonary vasculature is called a pulmonary embolism (PE). The embolus may be a clot that has broken off from a deep vein thrombosis (DVT), a globule of fat from a long bone fracture, septic vegetation, or an iatrogenic catheter fragment. In pregnancy, amniotic fluid can be the cause of a PE. Most PEs originate from DVT of the lower extremities.[52,70] PE and DVT are the two com-ponents of the disease process known as venous thromboembolism (VTE).

PE is classified in several different ways. An initial classification may be acute or chronic. An acute PE occurs quickly and either responds to treatment, or death occurs. A chronic PE initially responds to treat-ment but then reoccurs. In chronic PE, small clots continue to develop and travel to the pulmonary vascular bed after treatment. Chronic PE is typically caused by a coagulopathy. A PE is also classified based on the amount of pulmonary vascular occlusion:

massive, submassive, or nonmassive. A massive PE obstructs 50% or more of the pulmonary vasculature or two or more lobar arteries. From a clinical presen-tation, a massive PE is defined as an embolus causing hypotension (systolic blood pressure <90 mm Hg or a decrease in systolic blood pressure >40 mm Hg for 15 minutes or longer if the hypotension is not caused by a new-onset dysrhythmia, hypovolemia, or shock).[25,79] A *submassive* PE is usually noted on an echocardio-gram as right ventricular dysfunction without hemo-dynamic instability. A *nonmassive* PE is not associated with right ventricular dysfunction. Repeated small, nonmassive or submassive pulmonary emboli can precede a massive PE.[25,79] *Major* is another term used to define a PE. The PE is considered to be major if the patient becomes hemodynamically unstable second-ary to its size, location, or the patient's underlying cardiovascular status. A major PE is considered a medical emergency. Patients who are initially seen with hemodynamic instability and shock frequently die within the first hour and require rapid, accurate assessment and treatment.[25,70]

Etiology

The three main mechanisms that favor the develop-ment of VTE, often referred to as Virchow's triad, are (1) venous stasis, or a reduction in blood flow; (2) altered coagulability of blood; and (3) damage to the vessel walls. Specific causes of VTE are listed in Box 14-6.

Acute PE remains a cardiovascular emergency and has a high mortality rate. PE is considered to be the most preventable cause of hospital deaths in the United States, with autopsy results showing that approximately 60% of patients dying in a hospital have had a PE, with the diagnosis missed about 70% of the time.[16,25,28,32] Critically ill patients are at high risk for VTE, and DVT prophylaxis is a part of the ventilator bundle. PE is also the leading cause of maternal death after delivery. It occurs in 2 of every 100,000 live births.[70]

Pathophysiology

When an embolus completely or partially occludes the pulmonary artery or one of its branches, a mechanical obstruction impedes forward flow of blood. The pulmonary circulation has an enormous capacity to compensate for a PE. This compensatory mechanism results from the lung vasculature that is necessary to accommodate increased blood flow during exercise, and is the reason many patients do not initially decompensate from a massive PE. After an embolus lodges in the pulmonary vasculature, blood flow to the alveoli beyond the occlusion is

BOX 14-6 Risk Factors for Venous Thromboembolism

Venous Stasis
- Heart disease
  - Heart failure
  - Myocardial infarction
  - Cardiomyopathy
  - Constrictive pericarditis
- Dehydration
- Immobility (bed rest >72 hours)
- Paralysis
- Incompetent venous valves
- Obesity (>20% ideal body weight)
- Pregnancy
- Surgery lasting more than 45 minutes
- Age >40 years

Vessel Wall Injury
- Trauma
  - Fracture
  - Extensive burns
- Infection
- Venipuncture
- Central venous catheter
- Intravenous infusion of irritant solutions
- Previous history of deep venous thrombosis
- History of previous major surgery

Hypercoagulability
- Alterations in hemostatic mechanisms
- Protein C resistance or deficiency
- Antithrombin III deficiency or resistance
- Protein S deficiency
- Leiden mutation
- Polycythemia vera
- Anemia
- Trauma/surgery
- Malignancy
- Hormone replacement therapy
- Oral contraceptive use
- Systemic infection

eliminated. The result is a lack of perfusion to ventilated alveoli, an increase in dead space, a $\dot{V}/\dot{Q}$ mismatch, and a decrease in CO_2 tension in the embolized lung zone. Gas exchange cannot occur. Reaction to the mechanical obstruction causes the release of a number of inflammatory mediators such as prostaglandin, serotonin, and histamine. The ensuing inflammation causes constriction of bronchi and surrounding blood vessels.[78]

Constriction in the terminal airways of the non-perfused lung zones results in alveolar shrinking and an increase in the work of breathing. The reduction in blood flow to the alveoli also results in hypoxia for the type II pneumocytes, which are responsible for the production of surfactant. Although the effects are not seen for 24 to 48 hours, the decrease in surfactant results in an unequal gas distribution, an increase in the work of breathing, and a stiffening and collapse of the alveoli. Ventilation is then shifted away from these units, thus worsening the $\dot{V}/\dot{Q}$ mismatch. Atelectasis and shunting transpire as a result of the release of serotonin from the platelets that surround the clot. The result is peripheral airway constriction, which often involves functioning alveoli. In this situation, perfusion with inadequate ventilation occurs.[33,52,78]

The entire process may lead to an increase in pulmonary arterial pressure and an increase in right ventricular workload to maintain pulmonary blood flow. The right ventricle increases in size, causing a leftward shift of the septum. As the process continues, it can lead to decreased left ventricular filling and output. The patient may develop right and left ventricular failure, leading to decreased cardiac output and shock.[33,78]

The overall prognosis after a PE depends on two main factors. The first is whether any underlying cardiopulmonary problem preceded the PE, and the second is the extent of the pulmonary vascular circulation that is occluded by the thrombus. The PE is considered major if circulatory shock occurs.[33,52,78]

Assessment

Dyspnea, hemoptysis, and chest pain have been called the "classic" signs and symptoms for a PE, but the three signs and symptoms actually occur in less than 20% of cases.[25] A PE should be suspected in any patient who has unexplained cardiorespiratory complaints and has any risk factors for VTE. A relatively common symptom of PE is the sudden onset of dyspnea. The patient may also be especially apprehensive or anxious, with a feeling of impending doom. Syncope, defined as a loss of consciousness lasting at least 2 minutes, is the presenting symptom in 10% to 15% of patients with a PE. Other common signs and symptoms of PE are chest wall tenderness, chest pain aggravated by deep inspiration, tachypnea, decreased SpO_2, tachycardia, cough, crackles, wheezing, and hemoptysis. Additional signs and symptoms that may occur are an accentuated pulmonic component of the second heart sound, new-onset atrial fibrillation, fever, new-onset reactive airway disease (adult onset asthma), cyanosis, and diaphoresis.[25,28] Patients should also be assessed for the presence of a DVT, which may include calf tenderness, redness, or a positive Homan's sign (only 50% of cases).

Diagnosis

Arterial Blood Gases. The PaO_2 on initial ABGs may be normal even in situations where the patient has had a massive PE. ABGs cannot be used to determine whether a patient has a PE.[28,70]

Electrocardiogram. Tachycardia and nonspecific ST-segment and T-wave changes are the most common abnormalities found on the electrocardiogram. Other findings are peaked P waves in leads II, III, and aVF, or a right bundle branch block.[31] The pattern of anterior T-wave inversions in the precordial leads correlates best with PE severity.[28,70]

Chest X-ray. The initial chest x-ray is frequently normal. Serial chest x-rays over time often show atelectasis or a pulmonary parenchymal abnormality. A small pleural effusion is present in about half of the cases. Other changes that correlate with increased pulmonary artery pressure are pulmonary edema, cardiomegaly, and a prominent central pulmonary artery. A triangular wedge-shaped pleural infiltrate (Hampton hump) indicative of pulmonary infarction and dilatation of the pulmonary vasculature near the embolus (Westermark sign) are two other findings that may be present.[28,70]

D-dimer Assay. D-dimers are fibrin degradation products or fragments produced during fibrinolysis. The D-dimer assay is a sensitive but nonspecific test to diagnose a PE. A negative D-dimer assay has about a 90% sensitivity for ruling out a PE. A positive D-dimer assay can occur in a number of other conditions such as infection, cancer, surgery, pregnancy, heart failure, or kidney failure.[28,32,70]

Ventilation-Perfusion Scan. A $\dot{V}/\dot{Q}$ scan is a noninvasive scintigraphic lung scan that calculates pulmonary airflow and blood flow. A $\dot{V}/\dot{Q}$ scan may detect dead space from impaired perfusion of ventilated alveoli. Results of $\dot{V}/\dot{Q}$ scans are reported as low, medium, or high probability.[28]

Duplex Ultrasonography. Duplex ultrasonography is a noninvasive imaging study useful in detecting lower extremity DVT. It has a high sensitivity and specificity for DVT in the leg above the knee, but is not accurate in detecting DVT in pelvic vessels or small vessels in the calf.[52,70]

Echocardiogram. The echocardiogram may show signs of enlarged right-sided chambers or tricuspid regurgitation. Right ventricular dilatation is reported in 50% to 100% of patients with a PE. Transthoracic echocardiography may visualize intracardiac thrombi. Transesophageal echocardiography may detect emboli in transit and thrombi within the central pulmonary artery.[70]

High-Resolution Multidetector Computed Tomography Angiography. High-resolution multidetector CT angiography (MDCTA; spiral CT) has become the preferred tool for detecting a PE. It is highly accurate for direct visualization of large emboli in the main and lobar pulmonary arteries. MDCTA does not always visualize small emboli in distal vessels, but a pulmonary angiogram has the same limitation.[28]

Magnetic Resonance Imaging. Magnetic resonance imaging has a sensitivity and specificity comparable to that of spiral CT, but it is rarely used to diagnose PE in critically ill patients.[28]

Pulmonary Angiogram. A pulmonary angiogram is considered the gold standard for detecting a PE. It provides direct anatomical visualization of the pulmonary vasculature. Pulmonary angiography is an invasive procedure consisting of catheterization of the right side of the heart with contrast medium injected through the catheter into the pulmonary vascular system. MDCTA is replacing pulmonary angiography as the standard because it is noninvasive and has a high level of sensitivity and specificity.[28]

Prevention

The best therapy for VTE is prevention. Evidence-based strategies for prevention of VTE include the following: (1) Assess patients on admission and routinely throughout their ICU stay for risk of DVT/VTE.[37] The nurse, physician, and other members of the multidisciplinary team need to review daily the current DVT risk and the current status of DVT prophylaxis including the patient's response and the need for a central venous catheter. It is recommended that all ICU patients receive some type of prophylaxis treatment. (2) It is recommended that patients at high risk for bleeding use mechanical prophylaxis with graduated compression stockings, intermittent pneumatic compression devices, or both, until the risk for bleeding has been resolved.[37] When using these devices, it is imperative to ensure that they are applied correctly and removed for only short periods each day. (3) Patients at moderate risk for developing VTE should receive either low-dose unfractionated heparin or low–molecular weight heparin.[37] (4) Low–molecular weight heparin is recommended for patients at high risk for VTE.[37] (5) The nurse should implement a mobilization regimen for the patient, with the goal of maximizing the patient's mobility.[3] Other nursing interventions that may reduce the risk of VTE include not adjusting the knee section of the patient's bed and avoiding the use of pillows below the knees. Box 14-7 outlines some nursing interventions to prevent VTE.

Treatment

Fibrinolytic therapy is the standard of care for a patient with a PE who is in shock or hemodynamically unstable. Unless absolute contraindications are present, fibrinolytic therapy needs to be considered for a patient who is hemodynamically stable but has signs and symptoms of reduced right ventricular function.[56] Fibrinolytic regimens with short infusion times are recommended. Of the four fibrinolytic drugs available—streptokinase, urokinase, t-PA

BOX 14-7   Nursing Measures to Prevent Venous Thromboembolism

---

Assess Patient on Admission to Unit and Daily to Determine Risk for VTE

Discuss with Other Health Care Professionals Strategies to Reduce Risk Based on Assessment (Initially and Daily)

Implement Prescribed Prophylactic Regimen
- Nonpharmacological (mechanical) (patient at high risk for bleeding)
  - Graduated compression stockings
  - Intermittent pneumatic compression
  - Venous foot pump
  - Ensure applied correctly
  - Remove only for short periods
- Pharmacological (according to risk level)
  - Subcutaneous low-dose unfractionated heparin (moderate risk)
  - Subcutaneous low–molecular weight heparin (moderate or high risk)
  - Oral anticoagulants (documented DVT or other medical condition requiring)

Document Implementation Tolerance, and Complications, of Prophylaxis

Assess Extremities on a Regular Basis
- Pain/tenderness
- Unilateral edema
- Erythema
- Warmth

Implement a Comprehensive Mobility Program

Monitor for Low-Grade Fever

Encourage Fluids to Prevent Dehydration; Administer IV Fluids as Prescribed; Maintain Accurate Intake and Output Records

Avoid Adjusting the Knee Section of the Bed or Using Pillows Under Knees

Provide Patient Education Regarding Prevention

DVT, Deep vein thrombosis; *IV*, intravenous; *VTE*, venous thromboembolism.

(alteplase), and r-PA (reteplase)—alteplase and reteplase have the shortest infusion times. Alteplase can be administered as an intravenous infusion over 90 minutes, and reteplase can be given as one or two intravenous boluses. Reteplase is not approved for VTE but is under investigation for use in PE, with promising results.[28]

Heparin remains the mainstay of treatment of a PE. Heparin does not dissolve the existing clot, but it prevents the clot from enlarging and prevents more thrombi from forming by inhibiting the conversion of prothrombin to thrombin. Heparin may also stimulate the intrinsic fibrinolytic system, thereby enhancing the degradation of the PE. Heparin is the initial treatment of choice for a patient with a PE who is hemodynamically stable and has normal right ventricular function. Patients presenting with a PE who receive fibrinolytic therapy will also receive heparin. An initial bolus is given followed by a continuous infusion to achieve an activated partial thromboplastin time that is 1.5 to 2.5 times greater than the control value. Studies have demonstrated that using a dose-adjusted nomogram based on weight is more likely to achieve the desired effect within the first 24 hours. The heparin infusion is continued for 5 to 7 days. Oral anticoagulation with warfarin overlaps with the heparin for at least 4 days.[28,56] It is essential that the critical care nurse regularly monitor the laboratory values to titrate the heparin to a therapeutic level and to monitor the patient for any signs or symptoms of bleeding or heparin-induced thrombocytopenia. The nurse must be attuned to major bleeding, such as intracranial or retroperitoneal hemorrhage, and minor bleeding. Heparin-induced thrombocytopenia is a well-known complication of heparin therapy. It is caused by antibodies that activate platelets and leads to thrombocytopenia.[70] Fondaparinux, a synthetic antithrombotic agent, is an alternative to heparin infusion for patients with a PE who are hemodynamically stable and have no signs of right ventricular dysfunction.[68]

Catheter embolectomy is reserved for patients who have contraindications to fibrinolytic therapy. Catheter embolectomy is performed during pulmonary angiography by either suction aspiration or mechanical fragmentation of the embolus. Mechanical fragmentation has about an 80% success rate but is associated with greater risk.[70] Surgical embolectomy is rarely used and involves manual removal of the thrombus from the pulmonary artery. The patient must be placed on a cardiopulmonary support system during the procedure.

Inferior vena cava filters are placed in the inferior vena cava to prevent recurrence of PE by preventing clots from migrating from the lower extremities. Two types of filters are available: permanent and temporary retrievable. Permanent vena cava filters are rarely used and have a number of associated complications. Temporary vena cava filters are used to prevent PE in patients who have contraindications for anticoagulation therapy, have recurring PE, or have severe cardiac or pulmonary disease. Many of these devices can be placed in the vena cava by a minimally invasive technique under fluoroscopy.[56]

Other treatments are focused on maintaining the airway, breathing, and circulation. Supplemental O_2 may be administered to maintain SaO_2 at more than 90%. If the location of the PE is known, positioning the patient with the "good" lung in the dependent position is warranted. Analgesics are given to allevi-

CYSTIC FIBROSIS: A HERITABLE DISORDER WITH PULMONARY AND GASTROINTESTINAL COMPLICATIONS

Cystic fibrosis (CF) is a lifelong disorder that may lead to critical illness. The basic pathologic abnormality in this disease is a defect in a protein that forms part of the ion channel that transports chloride across epithelial cell membranes on mucosal surfaces. The defective protein is a result of a variation in the *CFTR* gene on chromosome 7.[6] There are more than 1300 variations in this gene. All of them cause some degree of alteration in the chloride ion channel; most of these alterations result in reduced chloride transport across cell membranes.[7]

Organs and tissues most profoundly affected by the defective chloride ion channels are in the pancreas, intestines, lungs, sweat glands, and vas deferens. As a result of this chloride ion channel defect, there is a decrease in the secretion of chloride and increased reabsorption of sodium and water across epithelial cells. This leads to mucus-producing cells that synthesize thick mucus. Thick mucus in the respiratory and gastrointestinal tracts, the pancreas, the sweat glands, and other tissues is difficult to clear. The thick mucus interferes with normal organ function. For example, mucus production in the lungs interferes with gas exchange, leading to chronic hypoxemia. Mucus production in the gastrointestinal tract can block intestinal fluids, resulting in gastrointestinal obstruction.[3] Thick mucus is also more likely to colonize microorganisms, resulting in infection and inflammation and contributing to adverse and irreversible changes in these organs.[4]

The degree of impairment in the chloride ion channel as a result of differences in the CFTR protein components varies. Abnormalities are typically not seen unless CFTR function is less than 10%.[5] Those patients with the most severe symptoms have less than 1% CFTR activity and manifest the full spectrum of disease involvement including pancreatic insufficiency, recurrent, severe pulmonary infections, gastrointestinal obstruction, and congenital absence of the vas deferens.[5]

CF is the most common lethal disease inherited by the Caucasian population. One in 22 people of European heritage carry one gene for CF. CF is an autosomal recessive disease, which means that both parents must be a carrier of variant *CFTR* genes or have the disease in order for their children to inherit the gene variation that causes CF. Because so many individuals in the United States are symptomless carriers of CF (estimated at more than 10 million people), the American College of Obstetricians and Gynecologists suggests genetic testing for all couples who are at high risk for being a carrier because of their ethnicity or family history.[1] In general, testing is performed on just one future parent initially; if that person is a carrier, then the other future parent is tested to calculate the risk that their children will have CF. It is not possible to test for all 1300 variations of the *CFTR* gene in a single genetic test. Testing typically looks for 32 to 70 common mutations.[5] Therefore, a negative screen does not guarantee that a child will not have CF. A child with CF usually has the same mutation as the carrier parent. If a family has a known uncommon variant, then specific testing for that polymorphism can be performed.

Symptoms of CF are most often manifested in infancy and early childhood by a persistent cough with mucus production that is frequently colonized with bacteria; by loose, bulky stools; and by failure to thrive. Those with milder disease may not have CF diagnosed until adolescence or early adulthood. The presence of aspermia or male infertility is an indication to the clinician to include CF as a diagnostic possibility. In addition to genotyping, tests of pancreatic function and nasal potential-difference measurements are used to diagnose CF. Diagnosis by sweat testing is also used since the defect in chloride ion channels leads to salty secretions. About 1000 new cases of CF are diagnosed in the United States annually.[2]

There is no cure for CF. If CF genetic testing shows both parents are carriers, genetic counseling is strongly recommended by health care providers. When both parents have a *CFTR* variant, as with any autosomal disorder, there is a 1-in-4 chance with each pregnancy that the child will have CF.[1,7] Remember, many variants of CF are not included in the typical genetic test, manifestations of CF can be mild, and not all parents will perceive the diagnosis of CF as a serious disorder. In addition, genetic testing and counseling may not be covered by insurance companies. Thus, the health care provider needs to individualize the approach to advising persons seeking CF genetic testing. The Cystic Fibrosis Foundation has links to information as well as support groups when CF is a potential or actual condition in a family.[2] Because of improved treatments over the past four decades, the average lifespan of a child with diagnosed CF has increased from 10 to 36 years. Active research programs in several academic centers continue to pursue a cure.

REFERENCES

1. American College of Obstetricians and Gynecologists. (2001). *Cystic fibrosis carrier testing: The decision is yours.* Washington, D.C.: ACOG.
2. Cystic Fibrosis Foundation. (2007). About cystic fibrosis. Retrieved March 28, 2008, from www.cff.org.
3. Jenkins, J. F., & Lea, D. H. (2005). *Nursing care in the genomic era.* Boston: Jones and Bartlett.
4. Lashley, F. R. (2005). *Clinical genetics in nursing practice* (3rd ed.). New York: Springer.
5. Lashley, F. R. (2007). *Essentials of clinical genetics in nursing practice.* New York: Springer.
6. National Institutes of Health. (2007). *Learning about cystic fibrosis.* Retrieved March 28, 2008 from www.genome.gov/10001213.
7. Sharma, G. (2006). Cystic fibrosis. *eMedicine.* Retrieved March 28, 2008 from www.emedicine.com.

INTRODUCTION

Lung transplantation has become the treatment of choice for patients with end-stage lung disease when no other medical and surgical options are available. The most common indications are chronic obstructive pulmonary disease, idiopathic pulmonary fibrosis, pulmonary hypertension, and cystic fibrosis. Because of significant advances in surgical techniques and pharmacological management, lung transplantation offers many patients an improved quality of life and an increased likelihood of survival.[5] Currently, there are 2337 patients on the national waiting list for lung transplantation. In 2007, 1210 lung transplants were performed, with a projected 1-year survival of 85%, 3-year survival of 66%, and 5-year survival of 51%.[3]

CRITERIA FOR TRANSPLANT RECIPIENTS

Criteria for placement on the waiting list include a life expectancy of less than 24 to 36 months, significant impact of the lung disease on other organ systems, and the effects of the disease process on quality of life. Because of the significant shortage of organs, the waiting time must also be considered, as allocation of donor lungs is based on the length of time on the waiting list. This system is different than that used for the allocation of donor hearts and livers, in which priority status is based on severity of illness.

Contraindications for lung transplantation include current steroid use of greater than 20 mg daily, significant coronary artery disease, cachexia or obesity, alcohol or drug abuse, cigarette smoking, active infection, previous cardiothoracic surgery, ventilation dependency, and a positive test for hepatitis B virus antigen.

CRITERIA FOR DONORS

The lack of organ donors is a significant problem. Many factors influence the low procurement rate including acute lung injury after brain death, pneumonia, aspiration, and atelectasis.[1]

Characteristics of optimal lung donors include being younger than 55 years and having no history of smoking or pulmonary disease; having a clear chest x-ray; having a PaO_2 of greater than 300 mm Hg on 100% oxygen and 5 cm H_2O positive end-expiratory pressure for 5 minutes; having no previous surgery, pulmonary contusions, or trauma; and having an airway clear of purulent or aspirated material. Donor and recipient size are also considered.

Efforts to increase the number of liver transplant recipients have resulted in a variety of lung transplantation options including heart-lung transplantation, single lung transplantation, double lung en bloc, and living donor lobar transplantation. Considerations in selecting the type of lung transplantation include the specific disease process, the need for cardiac transplantation, and donor availability.

PATIENT MANAGEMENT

The immune system is programmed to recognize a transplanted organ as foreign, and therefore the immune system must be inhibited after organ transplantation (see Chapter 16). Maintenance therapy consists of medications that inhibit T-cell proliferation and differentiation, deplete lymphocytes, and inhibit macrophages. Immunosuppressive medications consist of triple therapy—a calcineurin inhibitor (tacrolimus [Prograf] or cyclosporine [Neoral]), a corticosteroid (prednisone), and mycophenolate mofetil (CellCept). Complications associated with immunosuppressive therapy include nephrotoxicity, hypertension, hyperlipidemia, bone loss, new-onset diabetes mellitus, and infection.

COMPLICATIONS

Primary graft dysfunction is a major cause of morbidity and mortality and is comparable to acute respiratory distress syndrome. Possible causes include increased capillary permeability of the transplanted lung tissue, edema from extended ischemic time, and changes in compliance and vascular resistance in the donor and recipient. Patients present with malaise, increased work of breathing, activity intolerance, and oxygen desaturation. Management includes supplemental oxygen, positive pressure ventilation, and aggressive pulmonary toilet. Mechanical ventilation, nitric oxide inhalation, and extracorporeal membranous oxygenation may be indicated.

Infection is one of the major complications of immunosuppression therapy after transplantation. The lung is the most common site and is the leading cause of death after lung transplantation. Bacterial and fungal infections occur most frequently in the first months; viral infections, especially cytomegalovirus, are more prevalent in the following months after transplantation. Other complications include inadequate bronchial anastomosis, pneumothorax, pleural effusions, and gastroesophageal reflux disease.

PREVENTING REJECTION

Rejection after lung transplantation is the result of the patient's immune system response to the donor lung. Compliance with immunosuppressive medication is essential to avoid or decrease the incidence of rejection episodes. Hyperacute rejection occurs within minutes or hours of transplantation and is caused by humoral or antibody-mediated B-cell production against the transplanted organ. It may present as acute desaturation and tissue hypoxia or by radiographic changes. Acute or cellular-mediated rejection occurs within the first 12 weeks after transplant in 60% to 70% of recipients.[2] Symptoms may include fatigue, dyspnea, fever, hypoxemia, pulmonary infiltrates, pleural effusions, and chest pressure. Because these signs of rejection are similar to the signs of a pulmonary infection, a biopsy may be indicated. Manage-

TRANSPLANTATION   Lung—cont'd

ment includes high-dose corticosteroids and optimizing maintenance immunosuppression.

Recurrent acute rejection has been associated with the development of chronic rejection, or obliterative bronchiolitis, in which inflammation and fibrosis of the small airways occur. More than 40% of lung transplant recipients develop obliterative bronchiolitis by 2 years after transplant.[4] Other risk factors include inadequate immunosuppression and pulmonary infection. Symptoms include progressive shortness of breath, decreased exercise tolerance, airflow limitation, and progressive decline in forced expiratory volume in 1 second. Management is individualized and includes aggressively managing acute rejection and infection and optimizing the immunosuppression regimen.

REFERENCES

1. Angel, L. F., Levine, D. J., Restrepo, M. I., et al. (2006). Impact of lung transplantation donor-management protocol on lung donation and recipient outcomes. *American Journal of Respiratory and Critical Care Medicine, 174*(6), 710-716.
2. Myers, B., de la Morena, M., Sweet, S., et al. (2005). Primary graft dysfunction and other selected complications of lung transplantation: A single center experience of 983 patients. *Journal of Thoracic and Cardiovascular Surgery, 129*(6), 1421-1429.
3. United Network for Organ Sharing (UNOS). Retrieved, from www.unos.org.
4. White-Williams, C., Kugler, C., & Widmar, B. (2008). Lung and heart-lung transplantation. In L. Ohler, & S. Cupples (Eds.), *Core curriculum for transplant nurses*. St. Louis: Mosby.
5. Wilkes, D. S., Egan, T. M., & Reynolds, H. Y. (2005). Lung transplantation: Opportunities for research and clinical advancement. *American Journal of Respiratory and Critical Care Medicine, 172*(8), 944-955.

ate pain and anxiety. If the patient is hemodynamically unstable, inotropic support may be required.

ACUTE RESPIRATORY FAILURE IN ADULT PATIENTS WITH CYSTIC FIBROSIS

Definition

Cystic fibrosis (CF) is a genetic disorder (see Genetics feature) resulting from defective chloride ion transport. The mutation in chloride transport causes the formation of mucus with little water. The thick, sticky mucus obstructs the glands of the lungs, pancreas, liver, salivary glands, and testes causing organ dysfunction. While CF is a multisystem disease, it has the greatest effect on the lungs. The thick mucus narrows the airways and reduces airflow. The constant presence of thick mucus provides an excellent breeding ground for bacteria, leading to chronic lower respiratory tract bacterial infection, chronic bronchitis, and dilatation of the bronchioles. The mucus-producing cells in the lungs increase in number and size over time. Respiratory complications of CF include pneumothorax, arterial erosion, hemorrhage, chronic bacterial infection, and respiratory failure.[40,41]

Etiology

CF affects primarily Caucasians but is occasionally seen in other races. For many years, CF was considered a disease of children. Because of significant improvements in care, most people with CF are now living into the third decade of life or longer, and 40% of CF patients are older than 18 years.[19] The mean age of death from CF is 36.5 years.[19] The diagnosis of CF is typically made early in life (70% by age 1 year), but a few patients receive a diagnosis of CF as adults. A sweat test is the typical diagnostics tool for CF in children. Patients who do not receive a diagnosis until adulthood generally present with respiratory problems and have fewer other systems involved. Many of these patients have a normal or borderline sweat test result. They generally have a better prognosis.[19]

Interventions

Respiratory failure is the cause of death for more than 90% of patients with CF. As the disease process progresses, patients develop increased ventilator requirements, air trapping, and respiratory muscle weakness. All of these conditions are complicated by chronic bacterial infections that can quickly become overwhelming. In the past, mechanical ventilation was not considered a treatment option because patient outcomes were poor. During the last 20 years, the standard of care for ARF in CF has been revisited because of improved ventilator modalities, more aggressive pharmacological therapy, and the option of lung transplantation. Lung transplantation provides the opportunity for a tremendous improvement in the quality of life, but acute exacerbations of respiratory failure must be overcome during the long wait for a transplant.[71]

The three cornerstones of care for a patient with CF are antibiotic therapy, airway clearance, and nutritional support. Any patient with CF who is admitted to a critical care unit in ARF must have these three issues addressed immediately. A frequent cause of respiratory failure is pneumonia. Antibiotic selection is based on the patient's most recent sputum bacterial isolates. *Pseudomonas aeruginosa* is the most common pathogen found in adult patients with CF. Patients with CF are at high risk to have MDR bacterial isolates. They require higher doses of antibiotics and shorter dosing intervals than other patients because of differences in the volume of drug distribution and the rate of elimination. Mucolytic agents are routinely administered to facilitate clearance of mucus. Recombinant human DNase (Pulmozyme) is the drug of choice. It decreases the viscosity of sputum by catalyzing extracellular DNA into smaller fragments. Chest physiotherapy is used to increase airway clearance. Bronchodilators are routinely prescribed and administered before chest physiotherapy to increase airway clearance. Enteral nutrition with pancreatic enzyme supplements, if needed, is started early in the course of treatment.[72,80] If ventilator support is necessary, noninvasive mechanical ventilation is the first line of therapy. Endotracheal intubation with mechanical ventilation is the next step. The goal of mechanical ventilation is the same as with any patient with ARF. Adult patients with CF are at high risk for pneumothorax and massive hemoptysis. The critical care nurse must be aware of these life-threatening complications, constantly monitoring for them, and respond quickly.[72,80]

CASE STUDY

Mrs. P. is a 57-year-old woman admitted to the trauma intensive care unit after a motor vehicle crash. She sustained multiple long bone fractures and a chest contusion, and experienced an episode of hypotension in the emergency department. She received 3 units of blood and 2 L of intravenous fluid in the emergency department. Within 12 hours she became short of breath with an increase in respiratory rate requiring high levels of supplemental oxygen. She was electively intubated and placed on volume-control mechanical ventilation with a positive end-expiratory pressure (PEEP) of 5 cm H_2O. A continuous intravenous sedation infusion was started. The decision was made to titrate the infusion to keep her not fully alert but able to open her eyes to voice stimuli. During the next 8 hours, her oxygen saturation by pulse oximetry (SpO_2) steadily deteriorated, and the high-pressure alarms on the ventilator activated frequently. The nurse noted steadily rising peak airway pressures. The fraction of inspired oxygen (FiO_2) had to be increased to 0.80 and the PEEP increased to 14 cm H_2O to maintain her partial pressure of oxygen in arterial blood (PaO_2) at 60 mm Hg. Her chest x-ray study showed bilateral infiltrates with normal heart size. A pulmonary artery catheter was inserted with an initial pulmonary artery occlusion pressure of 14 mm Hg. The sedation infusion required frequent upward titrations to maintain the desired goal of sedation. The diagnosis of acute respiratory distress syndrome (ARDS) was made.

During the next 6 hours, Mrs. P. steadily became more hypoxemic. She was changed to pressure-controlled ventilation with a PEEP of 20 cm H_2O. The FiO_2 had to be increased to 1.0 (100%) to maintain a PaO_2 of greater than 60 mm Hg. She was extremely restless, with tachycardia, diaphoresis, and a labile SaO_2. The decision was made to start a neuromuscular blocking agent with sedation. During the next few hours her general condition continued to deteriorate. Her SaO_2 ranged from 85% to 87%. Her chest x-ray findings were worse. The nurses and physicians decided to turn her to the prone position in an effort to improve oxygenation. An hour after turning her to the prone position, her SpO_2 began to slowly rise. After 2 hours in the prone position, her SpO_2 stabilized at 93%. Slowly, the FiO_2 was decreased to 0.50, with a stable SpO_2 of 92%. After 18 hours she was returned to the supine position. Her SpO_2 decreased to 90% and it remained stable. She was weaned off the neuromuscular blocking agent, and the sedation level was reduced to reach a goal of alert and calm.

Mrs. P. slowly improved over the next week. Her ventilator settings were changed from pressure-control to assist-control then to synchronized intermittent mandatory ventilation (SIMV). The PEEP level was decreased to a physiological level. The sedation was interrupted on a daily basis to allow assessment for the ability to wean from the ventilator. On the seventh day, she was extubated and the following day transferred to the general orthopedic nursing unit.

QUESTIONS
1. Identify the risk factors Mrs. P. had for developing ARDS.
2. The American-European Consensus Conference recommended three criteria for diagnosing ARDS in the presence of a risk factor. List the criteria.
3. Explain the use of the high PEEP and the nursing monitoring responsibilities.
4. Explain the rationale for the use of sedation and neuromuscular blocking agents and what nursing interventions should occur when using these agents.
5. Explain the rationale for placing the patient in the prone position and what nursing interventions should occur before and after turning a patient to the prone position.

SUMMARY

ARF is a disorder that can affect all segments of the population, from young trauma patients to elderly persons with long-standing pulmonary disease. Patients in the critical care areas are at high risk of ARF. The critical care nurse must be constantly alert to signs of impending respiratory failure. Changes in respiratory rate and character, breath sounds, and blood gas values must be closely evaluated. Frequent position changes, good pulmonary hygiene, and careful attention to nutritional status all contribute to maintaining a patient's respiratory system and preventing ARF.

CRITICAL THINKING QUESTIONS   *evolve*

1. Mr. R. is a 66-year-old man who has smoked 1.5 packs of cigarettes a day for 40 years (60 pack-years). He is admitted with an acute exacerbation of COPD. His baseline ABGs drawn in the clinic 2 weeks ago showed: pH, 7.36; $PaCO_2$, 55 mm Hg; PaO_2, 69 mm Hg; bicarbonate, 30 mEq/L; SaO_2, 92%. In the critical care unit, Mr. R. has coarse crackles in his left lower lung base and a mild expiratory wheeze bilaterally. His cough is productive of thick yellow sputum. His skin turgor is poor; he is febrile, tachycardic, and tachypneic. Currently, Mr. R's ABGs while receiving O_2 at 2 L/min via a nasal cannula are: pH, 7.32; $PaCO_2$, 64 mm Hg; PaO_2, 50 mm Hg; bicarbonate, 30 mEq/L; SaO_2, 86%.
   a. What is your interpretation of Mr. R's baseline ABGs from the clinic?
   b. What is the probable cause of Mr. R's COPD exacerbation, and what treatment is indicated at this time?
   c. What ABG changes would indicate that Mr. R's respiratory status is deteriorating?
2. Ms. T. is a 41-year-old woman admitted to the critical care unit and mechanically ventilated for acute asthma. She was extubated yesterday and will be transferred out of the critical care unit tomorrow. What are the important points you must cover in your teaching with Ms. T.?
3. Mr. B. has just been intubated for ARF. Currently, he is agitated and very restless. What risks are associated with Mr. B's agitation? What nursing actions are indicated in this situation?
4. Mr. C., age 27 years, was hospitalized 3 days ago after fracturing his femur in a snow-skiing accident. He has just been admitted to the critical care unit with a PE and is orally intubated and receiving mechanical ventilation. What actions would you take to decrease Mr. C's risk of developing VAP?

evolve Be sure to check out the bonus material, including free self-assessment exercises, on the Evolve Web site at http://evolve.elsevier.com/Sole.

REFERENCES

1. Ahrens, T., Burns, S., Phillips, J., Vollman, K. M., & Whitman, J. (2005). Progressive mobility algorithm for critically ill patients, mobility. *Advancing Nursing Consultant*, Retrieved June 25, 2007, from www.vollman.com.
2. Akca, O. (2007). Endotracheal tube cuff leak: Can optimum management of cuff pressure prevent pneumonia? *Critical Care Medicine, 35*(6), 60374-60375.
3. American Association of Critical-Care Nurses. (2005). *American Association of Critical-Care Nurses practice alert. Deep vein thrombosis prevention.* Retrieved July 27, 2007, from www.aacn.org.
4. American Thoracic Society. (2005). Guidelines for the management of adults with hospital-acquired, ventilator-acquired pneumonia, and healthcare-associated pneumonia. *American Journal of Respiratory and Critical Care Medicine, 171*, 388-416.
5. Aragon, D., & Sole, M. L. (2006). Implementing best practice strategies to prevent infection in the ICU. *Critical Care Nursing Clinics of North America, 18*(4), 441-452.
6. Barnes, P. J. (2004). β-Agonists, anticholinergics, and other nonsteroidal drugs. In R. K. Albert, S. G. Spiro, & J. R. Jett (Eds.), *Clinical respiratory medicine* (2nd ed.). St. Louis: Mosby.
7. Bernard, G. R. (2005). Acute respiratory distress syndrome. *American Journal of Respiratory and Critical Care Medicine, 172*, 798-806.
8. Burns, S. M. (2005). Mechanical ventilation of patients with acute respiratory distress syndrome and patients requiring weaning. *Critical Care Nurse, 25*(4), 14-24.
9. Burns, S. M. (2006). Ventilating patients with acute severe asthma: What do we really know? *AACN Advanced Critical Care, 17*(2) 186-193.
10. Burton, S., & Alexander, E. (2006). Avoiding the pitfalls of ensuring the safety of sustained neuromuscular blockade. *AACN Advanced Critical Care, 17*(3), 239-243.
11. Cafee, C. S., & Matthay, M. A. (2007). Nonventilatory treatments for acute lung injury and ARDS. *Chest, 131*, 913-920.
12. Celli, B. R., MacNee, W., Agusti, A., Anzueto, A., Berg, B., Buist, A. S., et al. (2004). Standards for the diagnosis and treatment of patients with COPD: A summary of the ATS/ERS position paper. *European Respiratory Journal, 23*(6), 932-946.

13. Centers for Disease Control and Prevention. (2003). *Hand hygiene guidelines fact sheet*. Retrieved June 10, 2007, from www.cdc.gov.

14. Centers for Disease Control and Prevention. (2004). Guidelines for preventing health-care associated pneumonia, 2003. Recommendation of CDC and the healthcare infection control practices advisory committee. *MMWR Morbidity and Mortality Weekly Report*, 53(RR03), 1-36.

15. Chastre, J. (2006). Ventilator-associated pneumonia: What is new? *Surgical Infection*, 7(Suppl. 2), S81-S85.

16. Coalition to Prevent Deep Vein Thrombosis. (2007). *Why is there an urgent need to make DVT a major health priority?* Retrieved June 17, 2007, from www.clotcare.com/clotcare/deepveinthrombosisdvtcoalition.aspx.

17. Cocanour, C. S., Ostrosky-Zeichner, L., Peninger, M., Garbade, D., Tideman, T., Domonsoske, B. D., et al. (2005). Cost of a ventilator-associated pneumonia in a shock trauma intensive care unit. *Surgical Infection*, 6(1), 65-72.

18. Crummy, F., & Naughton, N. T. (2007). Non-invasive positive pressure ventilation for acute respiratory failure: Justified or just hot air? *Internal Medicine Journal*, 37(2), 112-118.

19. Cystic Fibrosis Foundation. (2005). *Cystic Fibrosis Foundation annual data report*. Retrieved June 26, 2007, from www.cff.org/LivingwithCF/QualityImprovement/PatientRegistryReport.

20. De Jong, M. M., Burns, S. M., Campbell, M. L., Chulay, M., Grap, M. J., Pierce, L. N. B., et al. (2005). Development of the American Association of Critical-Care Nurses' sedation assessment scale for critically ill patients. *American Journal of Critical Care*, 14(6), 531-544.

21. Dellinger, P. R. (2004). Surviving Sepsis Campaign: Guidelines for management of severe sepsis and septic shock. *Critical Care Medicine*, 32(3), 858-873.

22. DeMichele, S. J., Wood, S. M., & Wennberg, A. K. (2006). A nutritional strategy to improve oxygenation and decrease morbidity in patients who have acute respiratory distress syndrome. *Respiratory Care Clinics of North America*, 12(4), 547-566.

23. Demoule, A., Girou, E., Richard, J., Taille, S., & Brochard, L. (2006). Benefits and risks of success or failure of noninvasive ventilation. *Intensive Care Medicine*, 32(11), 1756-1765.

23a. Edwards, J. R., Peterson, K. D., Andrus, M. L., Tolson J. S., Goulding, J. S., Dudeck, M. A., et al. (2007). National Healthcare Safety Network (NHSN) Report, data summary for 2006, issued June 2007. *American Journal Infection Control*, 35(5), 290-301.

24. El Sohl, A. A., & Ramadan, F. H. (2006). Overview of respiratory failure in older adults. *Journal of Intensive Care Medicine*, 21(6), 345-351.

25. English, J. B. (2006). Prodromal signs and symptoms of a venous pulmonary embolism. *Medical-Surgical Nursing: The Journal of Adult Health*, 15(6), 352-356.

26. Fan, E., Needham, D. M., & Stewart, T. E. (2005). Ventilatory management of acute lung injury and acute respiratory distress syndrome. *Journal of the American Medical Association*, 294(22), 2889-2896.

27. Fartoukh, M., Maitre, B., Honore, S., Cerf, C., Zahar, J. R., & Brun-Buisson, C. (2003). Diagnosing pneumonia during mechanical ventilation: The clinical pulmonary infection score revisited. *American Journal of Respiratory and Critical Care Medicine*, 168, 173-179.

28. Feied, C., & Handler, J. A. (2006). Pulmonary embolism. In M. S. Beeson, F. Talavera, G. Selnik, et al. (Eds.), *eMedicine* (from WebMD). Retrieved on June 27, 2007 from www.emedicine.com/EMERG/topic490.htm.

29. Girard, T. D., & Bernard, G. R. (2007). Mechanical ventilation in ARDS: A state-of-art review. *Chest*, 131, 921-929.

30. Girou, E., Brun-Buisson, C., Taille, S., Lemaire, F., & Brochard, L. (2003). Secular trends in nosocomial infections and mortality associated with noninvasive ventilation in patients with exacerbation of COPD and pulmonary edema. *Journal of American Medical Association*, 290(22), 2985-2989.

31. Goldhaber, S. Z. (2008). Assessing the prognosis of acute pulmonary embolism: tricks of the trade. *Chest*, 133(2), 334-336.

32. Goldhaber, S. Z. (2007). Venous thromboembolism risk among hospitalized patients: magnitude of the risk is staggering. *American Journal of Hematology*, 82(9), 775-776.

33. Goldhaber, S. Z., & Elliot, C. E. (2003). Acute pulmonary embolism: Part 1. Epidemiology, pathophysiology, and diagnosis. *Circulation*, 108, 2726-2734.

34. Grap, M. J., & Munro, C. L. (2004). Preventing ventilator-associated pneumonia: Evidence-based care. *Critical Care Nursing Clinics of North America*, 16(3), 334-358.

35. Heresi, G. A., Arroliga, A. C., Weidemann, H. P., & Matthay, M. A. (2006). Pulmonary artery catheter and fluid management in acute lung injury and the acute respiratory distress syndrome. *Clinics of Chest Medicine*, 27(4), 627-635.

36. Herridge, M. S., Cheung, A. M., Taney, M. S., et al. (2003). One-year outcomes in survivors of the acute respiratory distress syndrome. *New England Journal of Medicine*, 348(8), 683-693.

37. Hirsch, J., Guyatt, G., Albers, G. W., Harrington, R., & Schunemann, H. J. (2008). Executive summary. American College of Chest Physicians Evidence-Based Clinical Practice Guidelines (8th ed.). *Chest*, 133(6 suppl.), 71S-105S.

38. Hopkins, R. O., Weaver, l. K., Collingridge, D., Parkinson, R. B., Chan K. J., & Orme, J. F. (2005). Two-year cognitive, emotional, and quality-of-life outcomes in acute respiratory distress syndrome. *American Journal of Respiratory and Critical Care Medicine*, 171, 340-347.

39. Houston, S., Hougland, P., Anderson, J. J., LaRocco, M., Kennedy, V., & Gentry, L. O. (2002). Effectiveness of 0.12% chlorhexidine gluconate oral rinse in reducing prevalence of nosocomial pneumonia in patients undergoing heart surgery. *American Journal of Critical Care*, 11(6), 567-570.

40. Huether, S. E., & McCance, K. L. (2004). *Understanding pathophysiology* (3rd ed., pp. 762-803), St. Louis: Mosby.

41. Ignatavicius, D. D., & Workman, M. L. (2005). *Medical surgical nursing: Critical thinking for collaborative care* (5th ed., pp. 591-594). St. Louis: Mosby.

42. Institute of Healthcare Improvement. (2007). *Protecting 5 million lives. Getting started kit: Prevent ventilator-associated pneumonia how-to guide.* Retrieved June 5, 2007, from www.ihi.org/IHI/Programs/Campaign.

43. Iregui, M., Ward, S., Sherman, G., Fraser, V. J., & Kollef, M. H. (2002). Clinical importance of delays in the initiation of appropriate antibiotic treatment for ventilator-associated pneumonia. *Chest, 122*(1), 262-268.

44. Jacobi, J., Fraser, G. L., Coursin, D. B., Riker, R. R., Fontaine, D., Wittbrodt, E. T., et al. (2002). Clinical practice guidelines for the sustained use of sedatives and analgesics in the critically ill patient. *Critical Care Medicine, 30*(1), 119-141.

45. Jemal, A., Ward, E., Hao, Y., & Thun, M. (2005). Trends in the leading causes of death in the United States, 1970-2002. *Journal of the American Medical Association, 294*(10), 1255-1259.

46. Johnson, K. L. (2007). Neuromuscular complications in the intensive care unit: Critical illness polyneuromyopathy. *AACN Advanced Critical Care, 18*(2), 167-182.

47. Reference deleted in proof.

48. Kallet, R. H., & Branson, R. D. (2007). Do the NIH ARDS Clinical Trials Network PEEP/FiO$_2$ tables provide the best evidence-based guide to balancing PEEP and FiO$_2$ setting in adults? *Respiratory Care, 52*(4), 461-475.

49. Kane, C., & Galanes, S. (2004). Adult respiratory distress syndrome. *Critical Care Nursing Quarterly, 27*(4), 325-335.

50. Kess, J. P., Pohlman, A. S., O'Connor, M. F., & Hall, J. B. (2000). Daily interruption of sedative infusions in critically ill patients undergoing mechanical ventilation. *New England Journal of Medicine, 342*, 1471-1477.

51. Kollef, M. H. (2005). What is ventilator-associated pneumonia and why is it important? *Respiratory Care, 50*(6), 714-721.

52. Koschel, M. J. (2004). Pulmonary embolism: Quick diagnosis can save a patient's life. *American Journal of Nursing, 104*(6), 46-50.

53. Leong, J. R., & Huang D. T. (2006). Ventilator-associated pneumonia. *Surgical Clinics of North America, 86*(6), 1409-1429.

54. Majid, A., & Hill, N. S. (2005). Noninvasive ventilation for acute respiratory failure. *Current Opinion in Critical Care, 11*(1), 77-81.

55. Markou, N. K., Myrianthefs, P. M., & Baltopoulos, G. J. (2004). Respiratory failure: An overview. *Critical Care Nursing Quarterly, 27*(4), 353-379.

56. Motsch, J., Walther, A., Bock, M., & Bottiger, B. W. (2006). *Current Opinion in Anaesthesiology, 19*(1), 52-58.

57. Murray, T., & Goodyear-Bruch, C. (2007). Ventilator-associated pneumonia improvement program. *AACN Advanced Critical Care, 18*(2), 190-199.

57a. National Heart, Lung, and Blood Institute. (2007). *Global Initiative for Asthma (GINA) global strategy for asthma management and prevention.* Retrieved March 24, 2008, from www.ginasthma.org.

58. National Heart, Lung, and Blood Institute, World Health Organization. (2007). *Global Initiative for Chronic Obstructive Lung Disease (GOLD) global strategy for the diagnosis, management and prevention of chronic obstructive pulmonary disease.* Retrieved on March 24, 2008, from www.goldcopd.org.

59. Nseir, S., Pompeo, C., Calvestri, B., Jozefowicz, E., Nyunga, M., Soubrier, S., et al. (2006). Multiple-drug-resistant bacteria in patients with severe acute exacerbation of chronic obstructive pulmonary disease: Prevalence, risk factors and outcome. *Critical Care Medicine, 34*(12), 2959-2966.

60. Peters, J., & Chalaby, M. A. (2004). Acute respiratory failure, part 1: Establishing the diagnosis. *Journal of Respiratory Diseases, 25*(7), 294-297.

61. Pontes-Arruda, A., Aragao, A. M. A., & Albuquerque, J. D. (2006). Effects of enteral feeding with eicosapentaenoic acid, γ-linolenic acid, and antioxidants in mechanically ventilated patients with severe sepsis and septic shock. *Critical Care Medicine, 34*(9), 2325-2333.

62. Popovsky, M. A. (2005). Acute lung injury, transfusion and the anesthesiologist. *Journal Clinical Anesthesia, 17*(5), 331-333.

63. Porzecanski, I., & Bowton, D. L. (2006). Diagnosis and treatment of ventilator-associated pneumonia. *Chest, 130*, 597-604.

64. Powers, J. (2006). Managing VAP effectively to optimize outcomes and costs. *Nursing Management, 37*(11), 48B-48F.

65. Pruitt, B. (2007). Take an evidence based approach to treating acute lung injury. *Critical Care Insider*, Spring, 14-18.

66. Pruitt, B., & Jacobs, M. (2006). Best-practice interventions: How can you prevent ventilator-associated pneumonia?, *Nursing, 36*(2), 36-41.

67. Pun, B., & Dunn, J. (2007). The sedation of critically ill adults: Part 1: Assessment. *American Journal of Nursing, 107*(7), 40-48.

68. Robinson, D. M., & Wellington, K. (2005). Fondaparinux sodium, a review of its use in the treatment of acute venous thromboembolism. *American Journal Cardiovascular Drugs, 5*(5), 335-346.

69. Safdar, N., Crnich, C., & Maki, D. G. (2005). The pathogenesis of ventilator-associated pneumonia: Its relevance to developing effective strategies for prevention. *Respiratory Care, 50*(6), 725-739.

70. Shaughnessy, K. (2007). Massive pulmonary embolism. *Critical Care Nurse, 27*(1), 39-50.

71. Singh, J. M., Palda, V. A., Stanbrook, M. B., & Chapman, K. R. (2002). Corticosteroid therapy for patients with acute exacerbations of chronic obstructive pulmonary disease: A systematic review. *Archives of Internal Medicine, 162*(22), 2527-2536.

72. Sood, N., Paradowski, L. J., & Yankaskas, J. R. (2001). Outcomes of intensive care unit care in adults with cystic fibrosis. *American Journal of Respiratory and Critical Care Medicine, 163*(2), 335-338.

73. Spirt, M. J., & Stanley, S. (2006). Update on stress ulcer prophylaxis in critically ill patients. *Critical Care Nurse, 26*(1), 18-28.

74. Taylor, M. M. (2005). ARDS diagnosis and management implications for critical care nurses. *Dimensions of Critical Care Nursing, 24*(5), 197-207.

75. Vollman, K. M. (2004). Prone positioning in the patient with acute respiratory distress syndrome: The art and science. *Critical Care Nursing Clinic of North America, 16,* 319-336.

76. Vollman, K. M. (2006). Ventilator associated pneumonia and pressure ulcer prevention as targets for quality improvement in the ICU. *Critical Care Nursing Clinics of North America, 18*(4), 453-467.

77. Vonberg, R. P., Eckmanns, T., Welte, T., & Gastmeier, P. (2006). Impact of the suctioning system (open vs. closed) on the incidence of ventilation-associated pneumonia: Meta-analysis of randomized controlled trials. *Intensive Care Medicine, 32,* 1329-1335.

78. Wood, K. E. (2002). Major pulmonary embolism: Review of a pathophysiology approach to the golden hour of hemodynamically significant pulmonary embolism. *Chest, 121,* 877-905.

79. Yamamoto, T., Sato, N., Tajima, H., Takagi, H., Morita, N., Akutsu, K., et al. (2004). Differences in the clinical course of acute massive and submassive pulmonary embolism in-hospital onset vs. out-of-hospital onset. *Circulation Journal, 68,* 988-992.

80. Yankaskas, J. R., Marshall, B. C., Sufian, B., Simon, R. H., & Rodman, D. (2004). Cystic fibrosis adult care consensus conference report. *Chest, 125*(Suppl. 1), 1S-39S.

81. Young, P. J., Pakeerathan, S., Blunt, M. C., & Subramanya, S. (2006). A low-volume, low-pressure tracheal tube cuff reduces pulmonary aspiration. *Critical Care Medicine, 34*(3), 632-639.

82. Zeleznik, J. (2003). Normative aging of the respiratory system. *Clinics in Geriatric Medicine, 19*(1), 1-18.

CHAPTER 15

Acute Renal Failure

Janet Goshorn, MSN, ARNP, BC

INTRODUCTION

The renal system is the primary regulator of the body's internal environment. With sudden cessation of renal function, all body systems are disrupted. The incidence of acute renal failure varies depending on how it is defined and the patient population studied, but ranges from 1% to 13% in hospitalized patients, and up to 25% in critically ill patients.[10]

Despite advances in renal replacement therapies and critical care management, acute renal failure is associated with significant morbidity and mortality, ranging between 30% and 70%. Mortality rates have not improved much since the mid-1970s, thus making prevention of acute renal failure a high priority for all health care professionals.[30,53]

Nurses play a pivotal role in promoting positive outcomes in patients with acute renal failure. Recognition of high-risk patients, preventive measures, sharp assessment skills, and supportive nursing care are fundamental to ensure delivery of high-quality care to these challenging and complex patients. In this chapter, the pathophysiology, assessment, and collaborative management of acute renal failure are discussed.

REVIEW OF ANATOMY AND PHYSIOLOGY

The kidneys are a pair of highly vascularized, bean-shaped organs that are located retroperitoneally on each side of the vertebral column, adjacent to the first and second lumbar vertebrae. The right kidney sits slightly lower than the left kidney because the liver lies above it. An adrenal gland sits on top of each kidney and is responsible for the production of aldosterone, a hormone that influences sodium and water balance. Each kidney is divided into two regions: an outer region, called the *cortex*, and an inner region, called the *medulla*.

The *nephron* is the basic functional unit of the kidney. A nephron is composed of a renal corpuscle (glomerulus and Bowman's capsule) and a tubular structure, as depicted in Figure 15-1. Approximately 1 to 3 million nephrons exist in each kidney. About 85% of these nephrons are found in the cortex of the kidney and have short loops of Henle. The remaining 15% of nephrons are called *juxtamedullary nephrons* because of their location just outside the medulla. Juxtamedullary nephrons have long loops of Henle and, along with the vasa recta (long capillary loops), are primarily responsible for concentration of urine.

The kidneys receive approximately 20% to 25% of the cardiac output, which computes to 1200 mL of blood per minute. Blood enters the kidneys through the renal artery, travels through a series of arterial branches, and reaches the glomerulus by way of the afferent arteriole (*afferent* meaning to carry toward). Blood leaves the glomerulus through the efferent arteriole (*efferent* meaning to carry away from), which then divides into two extensive capillary networks called the *peritubular capillaries* and the *vasa recta*. The capillaries then rejoin to form venous branches by which blood eventually exits the kidney via the renal vein. The glomerulus is a cluster of minute blood vessels that filter blood. The glomerular walls are composed of three layers: the endothelium, the basement membrane, and the epithelium. The epithelium of the glomerulus is continuous with the inner layer of Bowman's capsule, the sac that surrounds the glomerulus. Bowman's capsule is the entry site for filtrate leaving the glomerulus.[4]

The kidneys perform numerous functions that are essential for the maintenance of a stable internal environment. The following text provides a brief overview of key roles the kidneys perform in

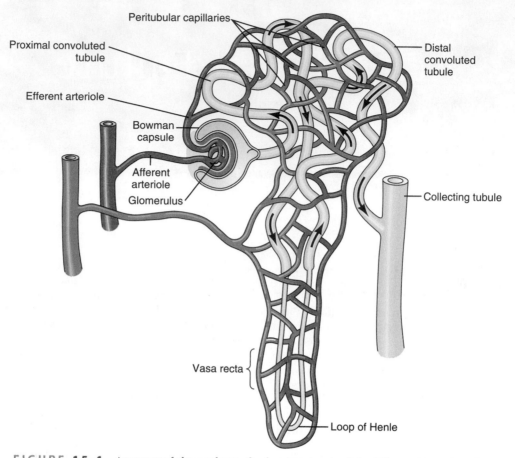

FIGURE 15-1. Anatomy of the nephron, the functional unit of the kidney. *(From Banasik, J.* *[2005]. Renal function. In L. Copstead, & J. Banasik [Eds.],* Pathophysiology *[3rd ed., pp. 684-709]. Philadelphia: Saunders.)*

BOX 15-1 Functions of the Kidney

- Regulation of fluid volume
- Regulation of electrolyte balance
- Regulation of acid-base balance
- Regulation of blood pressure
- Excretion of nitrogenous waste products
- Regulation of erythropoiesis
- Metabolism of vitamin D
- Synthesis of prostaglandin

maintaining homeostasis. Box 15-1 provides a listing of kidney functions.

Regulation of Fluid and Electrolytes and Excretion of Waste Products

As blood flows through each glomerulus, water, electrolytes, and waste products are filtered out of the blood across the glomerular membrane and into Bowman's capsule, to form what is known as *filtrate*. The glomerular capillary membrane is approximately 100 times more permeable than other capillaries. It acts as a high-efficiency sieve and normally allows only substances with a certain molecular weight to cross. Normal glomerular filtrate is basically protein free and contains electrolytes, including sodium, chloride, and phosphate, and nitrogenous waste products, such as creatinine, urea, and uric acid, in amounts similar to those in plasma.[23] Red blood cells, albumin, and globulin are too large to pass through the healthy glomerular membrane.

Glomerular filtration occurs as a result of a pressure gradient, which is the difference between the forces that favor filtration and the pressures that oppose filtration. Generally, the capillary hydrostatic pressure favors glomerular filtration, whereas the colloid osmotic pressure and the hydrostatic pressure in Bowman's capsule oppose filtration (Figure 15-2). Under normal conditions, the capillary hydrostatic pressure is greater than the two opposing forces, and glomerular filtration occurs.

At a normal glomerular filtration rate (GFR) of 80 to 125 mL/min, the kidneys produce 180 L/day of filtrate. As the filtrate passes through the various components of the nephron's tubules, 99% is reabsorbed into the peritubular capillaries or vasa recta. Reabsorption is the movement of substances from the filtrate back into the capillaries. A second process that occurs in the tubules is secretion, or the movement of substances from the peritubular capillaries into the tubular network. Various electrolytes are reabsorbed or secreted at numerous points along the tubules, thus helping to regulate the electrolyte composition of the internal environment.

Aldosterone and antidiuretic hormone (ADH) play a role in water reabsorption in the distal convoluted tubule and collecting duct. Aldosterone also plays a role in sodium reabsorption and promotes the excretion of potassium. Eventually, the remaining filtrate (1% of the original 180 L/day) is excreted as urine, for an average urine output of 1 to 2 L/day.

Regulation of Acid-Base Balance

The kidneys help to maintain acid-base equilibrium in three ways: by reabsorbing filtered bicarbonate, producing new bicarbonate, and excreting small amounts of hydrogen ions (acid) buffered by phosphates and ammonia.[4] The tubular cells are capable of generating ammonia to help with excretion of hydrogen ions. This ability of the kidney to assist with ammonia production and excretion of hydrogen ions (in exchange for sodium) is the predominant adaptive response by the kidney when the patient is acidotic. When alkalosis is present, increased amounts of bicarbonate are excreted in the urine and cause the serum pH to return toward normal.

Regulation of Blood Pressure

Specialized cells in the afferent and efferent arterioles and the distal tubule are collectively known as the *juxtaglomerular apparatus*. These cells are responsible for the production of a hormone called *renin*, which plays a role in blood pressure regulation. Renin is released whenever blood flow through the afferent and efferent arterioles decreases. A decrease in the sodium ion concentration of the blood flowing past the specialized cells (e.g., in hypovolemia) also stimulates the release of renin. Renin activates the renin-angiotensin-aldosterone cascade, as depicted in Figure 15-3, which ultimately results in

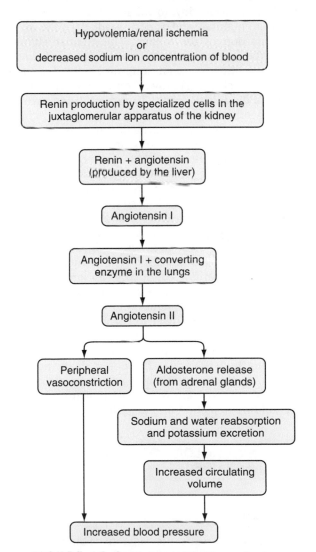

FIGURE 15-3. Renin-angiotensin mechanism.

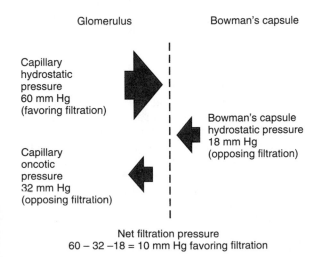

FIGURE 15-2. Average pressures involved in filtration from the glomerular capillaries.

angiotensin II production. Angiotensin II causes vasoconstriction and release of aldosterone from the adrenal glands, thereby raising blood pressure and flow and increasing sodium and water reabsorption in the distal tubule and collecting ducts.

Effects of Aging

The most important renal physiological change that occurs with aging is a decrease in the GFR. After age 40, there is a decline of approximately 8 to 10 mL/min per decade. This decrease occurs because of a reduction in renal mass, number of glomeruli, and blood flow. Serum creatinine levels may remain the same in the elderly patient even with a declining GFR because of decreased muscle mass and hence decreased creatinine production.

The ability to concentrate and dilute urine is impaired as well, due to an inability of the renal tubules to maintain the osmotic gradient in the medullary portion of the kidney. This tubular change affects the countercurrent mechanism, significantly altering sodium conservation, especially if a salt-restricted diet is being followed. Other tubular changes include a diminished ability to excrete drugs, including radiocontrast dyes used in diagnostic testing, which necessitates a decrease in drug dosing to avoid nephrotoxicity. Many medications, including antibiotics require dose adjustments as kidney function declines. Drug databases are available for appropriate dosing.

Age-related changes in renin and aldosterone levels also occur that can lead to fluid and electrolyte abnormalities. Renin levels are decreased by 30% to 50% in the elderly, resulting in less angiotensin II production and lower aldosterone levels. Together these can cause an increased risk of hyperkalemia (with possible cardiac conduction abnormalities), a decreased ability to conserve sodium, and a tendency to develop volume depletion and dehydration. The aging kidney is also slower to correct an increase in acids, causing a prolonged metabolic acidosis and the subsequent shifting of potassium out of cells and worsening hyperkalemia. There is a slight increase in ADH production with aging, but an associated decreased responsiveness to ADH that may exacerbate volume depletion and dehydration.[51,54]

PATHOPHYSIOLOGY OF ACUTE RENAL FAILURE

Definition

Acute renal failure is the sudden decline in GFR, resulting in retention of nitrogenous waste products (*azotemia*). It is usually accompanied by *oliguria* (urine output <400 mL in 24 hours), although many patients are nonoliguric and have a urine output of greater than 400 mL in 24 hours.[10,19] Patients with nonoliguric acute renal failure may excrete 2 to 4 L of fluid in 24 hours, but the fluid is deficient in the solutes and waste products that compose normal urine. Anuria (urine output <100 mL in 24 hours) is less commonly seen in acute renal failure.

Etiology

Numerous conditions can precipitate acute renal failure. The causes of acute renal failure are classified into three categories: prerenal, postrenal, and intrarenal. Classification depends on where the precipitating factor exerts its pathophysiological effect on the kidney.

Prerenal Causes of Acute Renal Failure

Conditions that produce acute renal failure by interfering with renal perfusion are classified as *prerenal*. Most prerenal causes of renal failure are fluid volume loss, extracellular fluid volume sequestration (third spacing), inadequate cardiac output, or vasoconstriction of the renal blood vessels (see Box 15-2). All these conditions reduce the glomerular perfusion and the GFR, and hypoperfuse the kidney. For example, major abdominal surgery can cause hypoperfusion of the kidney as a result of blood loss during surgery, or as a result of excess vomiting or nasogastric suction during the postoperative period. The body attempts to normalize renal perfusion by reabsorbing sodium and water. If adequate blood flow is restored to the kidney, normal renal function resumes. However, if the prerenal situation is prolonged or severe, it can progress to intrarenal damage, acute tubular necrosis (ATN), or acute cortical necrosis.[28] Implementation of preventive measures, recognition of the condition, and prompt treatment of prerenal conditions are extremely important.

Postrenal Causes of Acute Renal Failure

Acute renal failure resulting from obstruction of the flow of urine is classified as *postrenal*, or obstructive renal failure. Obstruction can occur at any point along the urinary system (Box 15-3). With postrenal conditions, increased intratubular pressure results in a decrease in the GFR and abnormal nephron function. Acute renal failure caused by postrenal conditions usually reverses rapidly once the obstruction is removed.[28]

Intrarenal Causes of Acute Renal Failure

Conditions that produce acute renal failure by directly acting on functioning kidney tissue (either the glomerulus or the renal tubules) are classified as

BOX 15-2   Prerenal Causes of Acute Renal Failure

Volume Depletion
- Hemorrhage
- Trauma
- Surgery
- Postpartum period
- Gastrointestinal loss
- Diarrhea
- Nasogastric suction
- Vomiting
- Renal loss
- Diuretics
- Osmotic diuresis
- Diabetes insipidus
- Volume shifts
- Burns
- Ileus
- Pancreatitis
- Peritonitis
- Hypoalbuminemia

Vasodilation
- Sepsis
- Anaphylaxis
- Medications
  - Antihypertensives
  - Afterload reducing agents
- Anesthesia

Impaired Cardiac Performance
- Heart failure
- Myocardial infarction
- Cardiogenic shock
- Dysrhythmias
- Pulmonary embolism
- Pulmonary hypertension
- Positive-pressure ventilation
- Pericardial tamponade

Miscellaneous
- Angiotensin-converting enzyme inhibitors in renal artery stenosis
- Inhibition of prostaglandins by nonsteroidal antiinflammatory drug use during renal hypoperfusion
- Renal vasoconstriction
- Norepinephrine
- Ergotamine
- Hypercalcemia

BOX 15-3   Postrenal Causes of Acute Renal Failure

- Benign prostatic hypertrophy
- Blood clots
- Renal stones or crystals
- Tumors
- Postoperative edema
- Drugs
  - Tricyclic antidepressants
  - Ganglionic blocking agents
- Foley catheter obstruction
- Ligation of ureter during surgery

autoregulatory defenses of the kidneys and thus initiates cell injury that may lead to cell death. Some patients have ATN after only several minutes of hypotension or hypovolemia, whereas others can tolerate hours of renal ischemia without having any apparent tubular damage. The most commonly injured portions of the renal tubule are the proximal tubule and the ascending limb of the loop of Henle.[15,28]

Nephrotoxic agents (particularly aminoglycosides and radiographic contrast materials) can also damage the tubular epithelium as a result of direct drug toxicity, intrarenal vasoconstriction, and intratubular obstruction. Acute renal failure does not occur in all patients who receive nephrotoxic agents; however, predisposing factors such as advanced age, diabetes mellitus, and dehydration enhance susceptibility to intrinsic damage. Patients with nephrotoxic ATN often have a good chance of complete recovery from renal failure.[10] Other intrarenal causes of acute renal failure are listed in Box 15-4.

Acute Tubular Necrosis. Dramatic advances have been made in our understanding of the pathophysiology of ATN. Multiple studies with renal biopsies have shown the following typical cellular findings in ATN:[10,39,42,54]

- Patchy loss of epithelial cells that causes gaps and exposed basement membrane
- Diffuse loss of brush cell border in the proximal tubule
- Patchy necrosis most often in the outer medulla region
- Dilatation of tubules with tubular cast formation and sloughing
- Evidence of cell regeneration along with freshly damaged cells that suggests multiple cycles of injury and repair

Multiple mechanisms are involved in the pathophysiology of ATN. Figure 15-4 is a detailed schematic of some of the mechanisms that play a role in the ATN cascade resulting in a reduced GFR. Mechanisms

intrarenal. The most common intrarenal condition is ATN. This condition may occur after prolonged ischemia (prerenal), exposure to nephrotoxic substances, or a combination of these. Ischemic ATN usually occurs when perfusion to the kidney is considerably reduced. The renal ischemia overwhelms the normal

BOX 15-4   Intrarenal Causes of Acute Renal Failure

Glomerular, Vascular, or Hematological Problems
- Glomerulonephritis (poststreptococcal)
- Vasculitis
- Malignant hypertension
- Systemic lupus erythematosus
- Hemolytic uremic syndrome
- Disseminated intravascular coagulation
- Scleroderma
- Bacterial endocarditis
- Hypertension of pregnancy
- Thrombosis of renal artery or vein

Tubular Problem (Acute Tubular Necrosis or Acute Interstitial Nephritis)
- Ischemia
- Causes of prerenal azotemia (see Box 15-2)
- Hypotension from any cause
- Hypovolemia from any cause
- Obstetric complications (hemorrhage, abruptio placentae, placenta previa)
- Medications (see Box 15-5)
- Radiocontrast dyes (large volume; multiple procedures)
- Transfusion reaction causing hemoglobinuria
- Tumor lysis syndrome
- Rhabdomyolysis
- Miscellaneous: heavy metals (mercury, arsenic), paraquat, snake bites, organic solvents (ethylene glycol, toluene, carbon tetrachloride), pesticides, fungicides
- Preexisting renal impairment
- Diabetes mellitus
- Hypertension
- Volume depletion
- Severe heart failure
- Advanced age

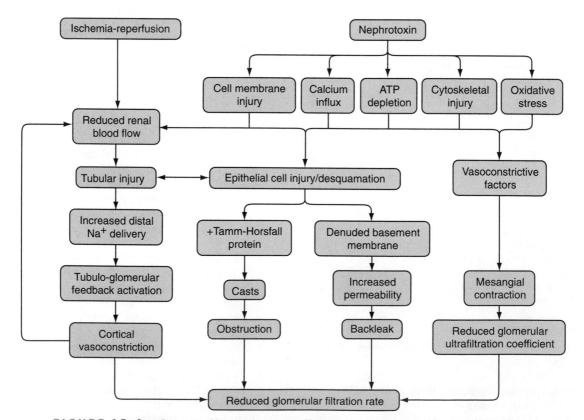

FIGURE 15-4. Schematic of loss of glomerular filtration seen in ischemic and nephrotoxic acute tubular necrosis. *(From Woolfson, R., & Hillman, K. [2003]. Causes of acute renal failure. In R. Johnson, & J. Feehally [Eds.],* Comprehensive clinical nephrology *[pp. 16.1-16.16]. London: Mosby.)*

include alterations in renal hemodynamics, tubular function, and tubular cellular metabolism.

Decreases in cardiac output, intravascular volume, or renal blood flow activate the renin-angiotensin system. Angiotensin II causes further renal vasoconstriction and decreased glomerular capillary pressure, resulting in a decreased GFR. The decreased GFR and renal blood flow lead to tubular dysfunction. In addition, administration of medications that cause vasoconstriction of the renal vessels can precipitate ATN, including nonsteroidal antiinflammatory drugs, angiotensin-converting enzyme inhibitors, angiotensin receptor blockers, cyclosporine, and tacrolimus. Endogenous substances that have been implicated in both causing and maintaining renal vessel vasoconstriction include endothelium 1, prostaglandins, adenosine, angiotensin II, and nitric oxide. A deficiency of renal vasodilators (prostaglandins, atrial natriuretic peptide, and endothelium-derived nitric oxide) has also been implicated.[10,41]

The renal tubules in the medulla are very susceptible to ischemia (the medulla receives only 20% of the renal blood flow and is very sensitive to any reduction in blood flow). When the tubules are damaged, necrotic endothelial cells and other cellular debris accumulate and can obstruct the lumen of the tubule. This intratubular obstruction increases the intratubular pressure, which decreases the GFR and leads to tubular dysfunction. In addition, the tubular damage often produces alterations in the tubular structure that permit the glomerular filtrate to leak out of the tubular lumen and back into the plasma, resulting in oliguria.[10,39]

Ischemic episodes cause decreased energy supplies, such as adenosine triphosphate (ATP). Oxygen deprivation results in a rapid breakdown of ATP. The proximal tubule is very dependent on ATP, a feature that explains why it is often the most commonly injured portion of the renal tubule. Without ATP, the sodium-potassium ATPase of the cell membrane can no longer effectively transport electrolytes across the membrane. This leads to an increase of intracellular calcium, free radical formation (which produces toxic effects), and a breakdown of phospholipids. Cellular edema occurs and further decreases renal blood flow, damages the tubules, and ultimately leads to tubular dysfunction and oliguria.[10,24,39]

Contrast-Induced Nephropathy. A leading cause of acute renal failure is contrast-induced nephropathy, accounting for about one third of all hospital-acquired cases of renal failure (see Evidence-Based Practices feature). More than a million procedures are done yearly using radiocontrast, with about 150,000 cases resulting in acute renal failure. Approximately 1% of these patients require renal replacement thera-

pies, prolonging hospitalization by 17 days and costing about $32 million annually. Patients with a milder renal failure not needing renal replacement therapies have an average extra 2 days of hospitalization costing about $148 million annually.[9,33] *Contrast-induced nephropathy* is defined as an increase in the serum creatinine level within the first 24 hours after administration of radiocontrast; however, levels may rise up to 5 days after the procedure. The most commonly used definition in clinical trials is an increase in the serum creatinine level of 0.5 mg/dL, or a 25% increase above the patient's baseline serum creatinine level, assessed at 48 hours after the procedure.[32]

The pathophysiology of contrast-induced nephropathy is not well understood. Radiocontrast is thought to initially cause a vasodilation of renal blood vessels, followed by an intense and persistent vasoconstriction. It is unclear why vasoconstriction occurs, but it is thought to be due to reduced production of prostaglandins (causing vasodilation), increased endothelin and adenosine release (causing vasoconstriction), or changes in intracellular calcium.[7] Blood flow to the renal medulla is markedly reduced with decreased oxygen delivery. The renal medulla is very susceptible to ischemic injury because of its high metabolic rate, and this medullary hypoxia may play a role. In addition, radiocontrast agents stimulate the influx of extracellular calcium, which may lead to a loss of medullary autoregulation as well as a direct toxic effect on the renal tubules.[50]

Patients usually have an increase in serum creatinine levels within 24 hours after receiving the radiocontrast, with levels peaking at about 7 days. Urine output usually remains normal; however, in severe cases oliguria may be seen. The most important risk factor is a preexisting reduction in renal function. Approximately 10% to 12% of patients with preexisting renal impairment who receive radiocontrast will develop worsening renal function requiring renal replacement therapies. Contrast-induced nephropathy rarely develops in patients with normal renal function.[7,9] Patients with diabetes mellitus have a fivefold greater risk for contrast-induced nephropathy than do nondiabetic patients.[33]

Cholesterol embolism or atheromatous emboli are a common cause of acute renal failure after a radiocontrast procedure and must be considered when a patient has what is thought to be contrast-induced nephropathy. Any arterial angiographic procedure such as cardiac catheterization can dislodge atheromatous emboli, which can lodge in small renal arteries producing an occlusion of the vessel, ischemia, and tubular dysfunction. A decline in renal function typically occurs over a period of 3 to 8 weeks, rather than the rapid decline seen with contrast-induced

EVIDENCE-BASED PRACTICE
Acute Renal Failure

PROBLEM

With more than one million radiocontrast procedures performed in the United States annually, contrast-induced nephropathy is a common and potentially serious complication in hospitalized patients, resulting in approximately 150,000 cases of acute renal failure per year.[33] It is the third leading cause of acute renal failure in hospitalized patients and is associated with significant patient morbidity, prolongation of hospital stays, and increased health care costs.[43] Preventive measures are needed to reduce the risk of contrast-induced nephropathy.

QUESTION

What are the most effective interventions for preventing contrast-induced renal failure?

REFERENCE

Stacul, F., On behalf of the CIN Consensus Working Panel. (2006). Strategies to reduce the risk of contrast-induced nephropathy. *American Journal of Cardiology, 98*(6A), 59-77.

EVIDENCE

Many studies have been conducted to evaluate interventions to reduce the risk of contrast-induced nephropathy; however, results have been inconsistent. The CIN Consensus Working Panel of experts studying the issue conducted an extensive review of clinical trials looking at clinical approaches to reduce risk. Studies conducted in both animal and human subjects suggest that intravascular volume expansion with fluids reduces the risk of contrast-induced nephropathy. Data are controversial on which intravenous fluid is superior. A variety of protocols have been studied in multiple clinical trials including normal saline (0.9%), half-normal (0.45%) saline, isotonic sodium bicarbonate (154 mEq/L in 5% dextrose), albumin, or oral fluids for hydration. The CIN Consensus Working Panel considered that isotonic saline was the most appropriate intravenous fluid for use at the present time. No clear evidence is available to guide the choice of an optimal rate or duration of intravenous infusions. The panel reported that although recent studies of isotonic sodium bicarbonate at 3 mL/kg/hr for 6 hours appear promising, further studies are needed.

The following consensus statement has been released by the CIN Consensus Working Panel:

> Adequate intravenous volume expansion with isotonic crystalloid (normal saline [0.9%], 1.0-1.5 mL/kg/hr) for 3 to 12 hours before the procedure and continued for 6 to 24 hours afterward can lessen the probability of contrast-induced nephropathy in patients at risk.

IMPLICATIONS FOR NURSING

This recommendation appears reasonable in both hospitalized patients and outpatients. High-risk hospitalized patients can begin intravenous hydration 12 hours before the procedure, and the infusion can be continued for at least 6 hours afterwards. For outpatients, especially those with risk factors for contrast-induced nephropathy, intravenous hydration can be started 3 hours before the procedure and continued for 6 or more hours afterwards. Ongoing clinical trials will determine additional preventive strategies in hopes of reducing the incidence of contrast-induced nephropathy. Nurses must assist in identifying patients at risk for contrast-induced nephropathy and advocating for early and adequate hydration.

---

nephropathy. Patients also typically have evidence of embolization to other areas of the body, including the skin (digital necrosis and gangrene), central nervous system (stroke, blindness), or gastrointestinal involvement (pancreatitis).

Course of Acute Renal Failure

The patient with acute renal failure progresses through three phases of the disease process: the initiation phase, the maintenance phase, and the recovery phase.[39]

Initiation (Onset) Phase. The initiation phase is the period that elapses from the occurrence of the precipitating event to the beginning of the change in urine output. This phase usually spans several hours to 2 days, during which time the normal renal processes begin to deteriorate, but actual intrinsic renal damage is not yet established. The patient cannot compensate for the diminished renal function and exhibits substantial clinical signs and symptoms that reflect the chemical imbalances in the internal environment. Acute renal failure is potentially reversible during the initiation phase.

Maintenance (Oliguric/Anuric) Phase. During the maintenance phase, intrinsic renal damage is well established, and the GFR stabilizes at approximately 5 to 10 mL/min. Urine volume is usually at its lowest point during the maintenance phase; however, patients may be nonoliguric, with urine outputs greater than 400 mL in 24 hours. This phase usually lasts 8 to 14 days, but it may last as long as 1 to 11 months. The longer a patient remains in this stage, the slower the recovery will be and the greater the chance of permanent renal damage is. Complications resulting from uremia, including hyperkalemia and infection, usually arise during this phase.

Recovery (Diuretic) Phase. This phase is the period during which the renal tissue recovers and repairs itself. A gradual increase in urine output and an improvement in laboratory values occur. Some patients may have a large diuresis during this phase that is caused by (1) salt and water accumulation in extracellular spaces that results from the inability of the renal tubules to regulate sodium and water, (2) osmotic diuresis that results from retained waste products, or (3) diuretics given to speed up salt and water excretion. However, with early and aggressive use of dialytic therapy, many patients are maintained in a relatively "dry" or volume-depleted state and do not have a large post-ATN diuresis. Recovery may take as long as 4 to 6 months.

ASSESSMENT

Patient History

Several aspects of the patient's history are important to remember in discussions of the renal system. Many patients do not volunteer essential parts of the history unless they are asked specific questions. Renal-related symptoms provide valuable clues to assist the clinician in focusing the assessment to obtain essential data. For example, dysuria, frequency, incontinence, nocturia, pyuria, and hematuria can be indicative of urinary tract infection. The history provides clues about medical conditions that predispose the patient to acute renal failure, including diabetes mellitus, hypertension, immunological diseases, and any hereditary disorders, such as polycystic disease. The medical record should be carefully examined to elicit additional risk factors, such as hypotensive episodes or any surgical or radiographic procedures performed. Information regarding exposure to potential nephrotoxins is extremely important. Common nephrotoxins include antibiotics such as aminoglycosides. Nephrotoxicity occurs in 7% to 36% of patients receiving aminoglycosides. Risk factors for development of aminoglycoside nephrotoxicity include volume depletion, prolonged use of the drug (>10 days), hypokalemia, sepsis, preexisting renal disease, high trough concentrations, concurrent use of other nephrotoxic drugs, and older age. Symptoms of acute renal failure are usually seen about 1 to 2 weeks after

BOX 15-5 Common Nephrotoxic Medications

- Aminoglycosides
- Amphotericin B
- Penicillins
- Acyclovir
- Vancomycin
- Pentamidine
- Rifampin
- Cephalosporins
- Cyclosporine
- Tacrolimus
- Methotrexate
- Cisplatin
- Fluorouracil (5-FU)
- Nonsteroidal antiinflammatory drugs (NSAIDs)
- Angiotensin-converting enzyme (ACE) inhibitors
- Angiotensin receptor blockers (ARBs)
- Interferon
- Indinavir
- Ritonavir
- Adefovir

exposure. Because of this delay, the patient must be questioned about any recent medical therapy (clinic or emergency department visits) for which an aminoglycoside may have been prescribed. In addition, a history of over-the-counter medication use, including nonsteroidal antiinflammatory medications, is important. Box 15-5 lists medications that have been associated with acute renal failure.

Vital Signs

Changes in blood pressure are common in acute renal failure. Patients with renal failure from prerenal causes may be hypotensive and tachycardic as a result of volume deficits. ATN, particularly if associated with oliguria, often causes hypertension. Patients may hyperventilate as the lungs attempt to compensate for the metabolic acidosis often seen in acute renal failure. Body temperature may be decreased (as a result of the antipyretic effect of the uremic toxins), normal, or increased (as a result of infection).[20]

Physical Assessment

The patient's general appearance is assessed for signs of *uremia* (retention of nitrogenous substances normally excreted by the kidneys) such as malaise, fatigue, disorientation, and drowsiness. The skin is assessed for color, texture, bruising, petechiae, and edema. The patient's hydration status is also carefully assessed. Current and admission body weight and intake and output information are evaluated. Skin turgor, mucous membranes, breath sounds, presence of edema, neck vein distention, and vital signs (blood pressure and heart rate) are all key indicators of fluid balance. An oliguric patient with weight loss, tachycardia, hypotension, dry mucous membranes, flat neck veins, and poor skin turgor may be volume depleted (prerenal cause). Weight gain, edema, distended neck veins, and hypertension in the presence of oliguria suggest an intrarenal cause. Table 15-1 summarizes the systemic manifestations of acute renal failure according to body system and also lists the pathophysiological mechanisms involved.

TABLE 15-1 Systemic Manifestations of Acute Renal Failure

System	Manifestation	Pathophysiological Mechanism
Cardiovascular	Heart failure	Fluid overload and hypertension
	Pulmonary edema	↑ Pulmonary capillary permeability Fluid overload Left ventricular dysfunction
	Dysrhythmias	Electrolyte imbalances (especially hyperkalemia and hypocalcemia)
	Peripheral edema	Fluid overload Right ventricular dysfunction
	Hypertension	Fluid overload ↑ Sodium retention
Hematological	Anemia	↓ Erythropoietin secretion Loss of RBCs through GI tract, mucous membranes, or dialysis ↓ RBC survival time Uremic toxins' interference with folic acid secretion
	Alterations in coagulation	Platelet dysfunction
	↑ Susceptibility to infection	↓ Neutrophil phagocytosis
Electrolyte imbalances	Metabolic acidosis	↓ Hydrogen ion excretion ↓ Bicarbonate ion reabsorption and generation ↓ Excretion of phosphate salts or titratable acids ↓ Ammonia synthesis and ammonium excretion
Respiratory	Pneumonia	Thick tenacious sputum from ↓ oral intake Depressed cough reflex ↓ Pulmonary macrophage activity
	Pulmonary edema	Fluid overload Left ventricular dysfunction ↑ Pulmonary capillary permeability
Gastrointestinal	Anorexia, nausea, vomiting	Uremic toxins Decomposition of urea releasing ammonia that irritates mucosa
	Stomatitis and uremic halitosis	Uremic toxins Decomposition of urea releasing ammonia that irritates oral mucosa
	Gastritis and bleeding	Uremic toxins Decomposition of urea releasing ammonia that irritates mucosa, causing ulcerations and increased capillary fragility
Neuromuscular	Drowsiness, confusion, irritability, and coma	Uremic toxins produce encephalopathy Metabolic acidosis Electrolyte imbalances
	Tremors, twitching, and convulsions	Uremic toxins produce encephalopathy ↓ Nerve conduction from uremic toxins

TABLE 15-1 Systemic Manifestations of Acute Renal Failure—cont'd

System	Manifestation	Pathophysiological Mechanism
Psychosocial	Decreased mentation, decreased concentration, and altered perceptions (even to the point of psychosis)	Uremic toxins produce encephalopathy Electrolyte imbalances Metabolic acidosis Tendency to develop cerebral edema
Integumentary	Pallor	Anemia
	Yellowness	Retained urochrome pigment
	Dryness	↓ Secretions from oil and sweat glands
	Pruritus	Dry skin Calcium and/or phosphate deposits in skin Uremic toxins' effect on nerve endings
	Purpura	↑ Capillary fragility Platelet dysfunction
	Uremic frost (rarely seen)	Urea or urate crystal excretion
Endocrine	Glucose intolerance (usually not clinically significant)	Peripheral insensitivity to insulin Prolonged insulin half-life from ↓ renal metabolism
Skeletal	Hypocalcemia	Hyperphosphatemia from ↓ excretion of phosphates ↓ GI absorption of vitamin D Deposition of calcium phosphate crystals in soft tissues

↑ Increased; ↓ decreased; *GI*, gastrointestinal; *RBC*, red blood cell.

Evaluation of Laboratory Values

Because the renal system is the primary regulator of the internal environment of the body, any alteration in its function can be rapidly noted in serum and urine laboratory values. In daily practice, the serum creatinine level is often used to evaluate renal function. Creatinine is a byproduct of muscle metabolism and is produced at a relatively constant rate, then cleared by the kidneys. With stable kidney function, creatinine production and excretion are fairly equal, and serum creatinine levels remain constant. When kidney function decreases, creatinine levels rapidly rise, indicating a decline in renal function or a decrease in the GFR. The serum creatinine level should not be the only measure used to assess renal function (see Clinical Alert: Serum Creatinine). When evaluating the serum creatinine level, it is helpful if past levels are available to determine whether the elevated creatinine level is due to an acute insult or a progressive loss of renal function. If past creatinine levels are not available, it is often difficult to distinguish acute from chronic renal failure.

The serum blood urea nitrogen (BUN) level is also used to evaluate renal function. The BUN level is not a reliable indicator of renal function because the rate of protein metabolism (urea is a byproduct of protein

> **CLINICAL ALERT**
> **Serum Creatinine**
>
> The same serum creatinine level can reflect very different glomerular filtration rates in patients because of differences in muscle mass. For example, a 25-year-old man weighing 220 lbs with a serum creatinine level of 1.2 mg/dL has an estimated glomerular filtration rate of 133 mL/hr (normal), whereas a 75-year-old woman weighing 121 lb with the same serum creatinine level of 1.2 mg/dL has an estimated glomerular filtration rate of 35 mL/hr (markedly decreased).

metabolism) is not constant. Extrarenal factors including dehydration, a high-protein diet, starvation, blood in the gastrointestinal tract, corticosteroids, and fever all can elevate the BUN level. For example, when a patient has gastrointestinal bleeding, the blood in the gut breaks down and results in an increased protein load and hence an elevated BUN level.

The relationship between the BUN and creatinine levels, known as the BUN/creatinine ratio, provides useful information. The normal BUN/creatinine ratio is 10:1 to 20:1 (e.g., BUN level, 20 mg/dL, and creatinine level, 1.0 mg/dL). If this ratio is greater than 20:1 (e.g., BUN level, 60 mg/dL, and creatinine level, 1.0 mg/dL), problems other than renal failure should be suspected. In prerenal conditions, an increased BUN/creatinine ratio is typically noted. There is a decrease in the GFR and hence a drop in urine flow through the renal tubules. This allows more time for urea to be reabsorbed from the renal tubules back into the blood. Creatinine is not readily reabsorbed; therefore, the serum BUN level rises out of proportion to the serum creatinine level. A normal BUN/creatinine ratio is present in ATN. In ATN, there is actual injury to the renal tubules and a rapid decline in the GFR; hence, urea and creatinine levels both rise proportionally as a result of increased reabsorption and decreased clearance.[35]

Assessment of the urine is extremely valuable in the evaluation of acute renal failure. Historically, timed 24-hour urine collections have been used to evaluate GFR or creatinine clearance. Timed urine collections are cumbersome and time-consuming, and are susceptible to multiple errors in collection. To measure creatinine clearance accurately, the nurse and patient must rigidly adhere to the following procedure:

1. The patient empties his or her bladder, the exact time is recorded, and the specimen is discarded.
2. All urine for the next 24 hours is saved in a container and stored in a refrigerator.
3. Exactly 24 hours after the start of the procedure, the patient voids again, and the specimen is saved.
4. The serum creatinine level is assessed at the end of 24 hours.
5. All the urine that was saved is sent to the laboratory for testing. (Urine can also be obtained from an indwelling urinary catheter.)

Urinary *creatinine clearance* is calculated with the following formula:

$$U_c \times V/P_c = C_{cr}$$

U_c = concentration of creatinine in the urine
V = volume of urine per unit of time
P_c = concentration of creatinine in the plasma
C_{cr} = creatinine clearance.

Creatinine clearance is an estimate of GFR and is measured in mL/min. Thus, given the following set of patient data,

U_c = 175 mg/100 mL
V = 288 mL/1440 min (24 hours = 1440 min)
P_c = 17.5 mg/100 mL

the patient's creatinine clearance would be calculated as follows:

$$\frac{175\,mg/100\,mL \times 288\,mL/1440\,min}{17.5\,mg/100\,mL} = 2\,mL/min$$

Because a normal creatinine clearance is about 84 to 138 mL/min, the clinician would recognize this patient's creatinine clearance as being consistent with severe renal dysfunction.

If a reliable 24-hour urine collection is not possible, the Cockcroft and Guault formula[44] may be used to determine the creatinine clearance from a serum creatinine value:

$$C_{cr} = \frac{(140 - Age[yr]) \times (Lean\ body\ weight\ [kg])}{72 \times Serum\ creatinine\ (mg/dL)}$$

For women, the calculated result is multiplied by 0.85 to account for the smaller muscle mass as compared to men.

Analysis of urinary sediment and electrolyte levels is extremely helpful in distinguishing among the various causes of acute renal failure. Urine should be inspected for the presence of cells, casts, and crystals. In prerenal conditions, the urine typically has no cells but may contain hyaline casts.[13,41] Casts are cylindrical bodies that form when proteins precipitate in the distal tubules and collecting ducts. Postrenal conditions may present with stones, crystals, sediment, bacteria, and clots from the obstruction. Coarse, muddy brown granular casts are classic findings in ATN.[1] Microscopic hematuria and a small amount of protein (<1 g/dL) may also be seen.

Urine electrolyte levels help in discriminating between prerenal causes and ATN. The nurse must obtain urine samples (often called spot urine levels) for electrolyte determinations before diuretics are administered because these drugs alter the urine results for up to 24 hours. Urinary sodium concentrations of less than 10 mEq/L are seen in prerenal conditions, as the kidneys attempt to conserve sodium and water to compensate for the hypoperfusion state. Urine sodium concentrations are greater than 40 mEq/L in ATN as a result of impaired reabsorption in the diseased tubules.[41]

The fractional excretion of sodium (FE_{Na}) is a useful test for assessing how well the kidney can concentrate urine and conserve sodium. To determine the FE_{Na} the following formula is used:

$$FE_{Na} = \frac{(Urine\ sodium)(Serum\ creatinine) \times 100}{(Urine\ creatinine)(Serum\ sodium)}$$

In prerenal conditions, the FE_{Na} is less than 1%, whereas ATN presents with an FE_{Na} of greater than

TABLE 15-2   Laboratory Findings Useful in Differentiating Causes of Acute Renal Failure

Type of Acute Renal Failure	Specific Gravity	Urine Osmolality	Urine Sodium	Microscopic Examination	BUN/CR Ratio	FE$_{Na}$
Prerenal	>1.020	>500 mOsm/L	<10 mEq/L	Few hyaline casts possible	Elevated	<1%
Intrarenal	1.010	<350 mOsm/L	>20 mEq/L	Epithelial casts, red blood cell casts, pigmented granular casts	Normal	>1%
Postrenal	Normal to 1.010	Variable	Normal to 40 mEq/L	May have stones, crystals, sediment, clots, or bacteria	Normal	>1%

BUN, Blood urea nitrogen; *CR*, creatinine; *FE$_{Na}$*, fractional excretion of sodium.

1%.[21] Table 15-2 summarizes laboratory data useful in differentiating among the three categories of acute renal failure.

Urine specific gravity and osmolality have a limited role in the diagnosis of acute renal failure, especially in older adults, because the body's ability to concentrate urine decreases with age.[54] In general, prerenal conditions cause concentrated urine (high specific gravity and osmolality), whereas intrinsic azotemia causes dilute urine (low specific gravity and osmolality) The volume of urine output is also not a good indicator of renal function. Patients with nonoliguric acute renal failure excrete large volumes of fluid with little solute. These patients still have renal dysfunction and azotemia even though they excrete large volumes of fluid. In an older adult, assessment parameters are modified when assessing for acute renal failure (see Geriatric Considerations).

Diagnostic Procedures

Various diagnostic procedures are used to evaluate renal function. Noninvasive diagnostic procedures are often performed before any invasive diagnostic procedures are conducted. Noninvasive diagnostic procedures that assess the renal system are radiography of the kidneys, ureters, and bladder (KUB) and renal ultrasonography. A KUB x-ray delineates the size, shape, and position of the kidneys. It may also detect abnormalities such as calculi, hydronephrosis (dilatation of the renal pelvis), cysts, or tumors. Renal ultrasound is helpful in evaluating the urinary collecting system for obstruction, which is manifest by hydronephrosis or hydroureter (dilatation of the ureters). Ultrasound can also document the size of the kidneys, which may be helpful in differentiating acute from chronic renal failure. The kidneys are often small (<10 cm) in chronic kidney disease. Real-time ultrasound is used during renal biopsy and during placement of percutaneous nephrostomy tubes (often placed for hydronephrosis).

Invasive diagnostic procedures for assessing the renal system include intravenous pyelography, computed tomography, renal angiography, renal scanning, and renal biopsy.[14] These procedures are summarized in Table 15-3.

For all diagnostic procedures, the nurse implements the following general interventions:

- Explain the procedure to the patient, reinforce previous explanations provided by other health care personnel, and emphasize the patient's responsibilities during the procedure.
- Notify the physician if the patient has any allergies to contrast media.
- Carry out any preparatory activities for the procedure, such as administration of a special diet, bowel preparations, laboratory testing, placement of intravenous line, and completion of consent forms.
- Provide appropriate fluids to the patient to maintain adequate hydration before and after the procedure.
- Provide emotional support to the patient before, during, and after the procedure.
- Assist with the procedure as necessary.
- Monitor the patient for any complications after the procedure, particularly for signs of infection after any invasive diagnostic procedure.
- Document the patient's response to the procedure.

GERIATRIC CONSIDERATIONS

MANAGEMENT OF ACUTE RENAL FAILURE

- Older adults are at increased risk for acute renal failure related to multiple comorbidities such as diabetes mellitus and hypertension, and from the multiple medications they may take. Two commonly prescribed classes of medications are nonsteroidal antiinflammatory drugs and angiotensin-converting enzyme inhibitors, both of which have adverse effects on renal blood flow.[48]
- The aging kidney is more susceptible to nephrotoxic and ischemic injury. Monitor drug dosages carefully, adjust drug dosages for underlying renal insufficiency, and use nephrotoxic agents judiciously.
- The primary risk factor for contrast-induced nephropathy is a preexisting decline in renal function, which places the elderly patient at risk, based on normal age-related changes. Monitor radiographic contrast media usage closely, using only as necessary. Maintain adequate hydration if radiographic contrast media must be used.
- Older adults are more prone to develop volume depletion (prerenal conditions) because of a decreased ability to concentrate urine and conserve sodium. Volume status is difficult to assess because of altered skin turgor and decreased skin elasticity, decreased baroreceptor reflexes, and mouth dryness caused by mouth breathing. Be sure fluids are easily within reach of older adults not on fluid restriction. Offer fluids frequently if not on fluid restriction (diminished thirst response and may not feel thirsty). Provide intravenous fluids to maintain adequate hydration as prescribed.
- Urinary indices are of limited value in assessment of older adults because of impaired ability to concentrate urine.

- Older patients tend to exhibit uremic symptoms at lower levels of serum blood urea nitrogen and creatinine than do younger patients. The typical signs and symptoms of acute renal failure may be attributed to other disorders associated with aging, thus delaying prompt diagnosis and treatment.
- Atypical signs and symptoms of uremia may be seen, such as an unexplained exacerbation of well-controlled heart failure, unexplained mental status changes, or personality changes.
- Older adults often have poor nutritional status before acute renal failure and require early and adequate nutrition.
- Older adults have special needs in regard to renal replacement therapies: they may need dialysis or continuous renal replacement therapy earlier than younger patients, because they tend to become symptomatic with lower serum creatinine and blood urea nitrogen levels than younger patients. Monitor for increased vascular access problems from comorbidities such as diabetes mellitus and peripheral vascular disease. Keep ultrafiltration rate less than 1 L per hour because decreased cardiac reserve and autonomic dysfunction make ultrafiltration difficult.
- Supply supplemental oxygen if needed to offset the hypoxemia that often develops at the start of dialysis. Monitor for increased risk of complications associated with systemic heparinization, including subdural hematomas from falls and gastritis.
- Older adults are more prone to infection because of a compromised immune system. Use meticulous technique for all procedures. Avoid indwelling catheterization especially if the patient is anuric; use intermittent catheterization as necessary.

NURSING DIAGNOSES

Nursing care of the patient with acute renal failure is complex. Multiple nursing diagnoses must be dealt with in these often critically ill patients. The Nursing Care Plan for the Patient with Acute Renal Failure addresses nursing diagnoses, patient outcomes, and interventions.

NURSING INTERVENTIONS

Measurement of intake and output, and determination of daily weights are two vital interventions performed by the nurse who is caring for patients with acute renal failure. Accuracy is extremely important. Appropriate measuring devices rather than clinician "guesstimations" must be used for the measurement of urine. For example, a urine meter or some other type of accurate measuring device is used if the patient has an indwelling catheter. Normal urine output is 0.5 to 1 mL/kg of body weight each hour. Oral fluid intake must also be carefully monitored. Fluid intake levels are often restricted to the amount of urine output in a 24-hour period plus insensible losses (approximately 600-1000 mL/day).[6] Administration of intravenous fluids as prescribed before procedures in which radiocontrast agents will be given is critical.[43]

Daily weights are one of the most useful noninvasive diagnostic tools available for clinicians. Daily

TABLE 15-3 Invasive Diagnostic Procedures for Assessing the Renal System

Procedure	Purpose	Potential Problems
Intravenous pyelography	To visualize the renal parenchyma, calyces, renal pelvis, ureters, and bladder to obtain information regarding size, shape, position, and function of the kidneys	Hypersensitivity reaction to contrast medium Acute renal failure
Computed tomography	To visualize the renal parenchyma to obtain data regarding the size, shape, and presence of lesions, cysts, masses, calculi, obstructions, congenital anomalies, and abnormal accumulations of fluid	Hypersensitivity reaction to contrast medium (if used)
Renal angiography	To visualize the arterial tree, capillaries, and venous drainage of the kidneys to obtain data regarding the presence of tumors, cysts, stenosis infarction, aneurysms, hematomas, lacerations, and abscesses	Hypersensitivity reaction to contrast medium Hemorrhage or hematoma at the catheter insertion site Acute renal failure
Renal scanning	To determine renal function by visualizing the appearance and disappearance of the radioisotopes within the kidney; also provides some anatomical information	Hypersensitivity reaction to contrast medium
Renal biopsy	To obtain data for making a histological diagnosis to determine the extent of the pathology, the appropriate therapy, and the possible prognosis	Hemorrhage Post-biopsy hematoma

NURSING CARE PLAN for the Patient with Acute Renal Failure

NURSING DIAGNOSIS

Excess fluid volume related to sodium and water retention and excess intake

PATIENT OUTCOMES
Stable fluid balance

- Body weight within 2 lb of dry weight
- Intake and output balanced; bilateral breath sounds clear; vital signs normal

NURSING INTERVENTIONS	RATIONALES
• Obtain daily weights	• Weight gain is best indicator of fluid gain
• Maintain accurate intake and output records	• Identify imbalances
• Monitor respiratory status, including respiratory rate and crackles	• Assess volume overload
• Assess heart rate, blood pressure, and respiratory rate	• Hypertension, tachycardia, and tachypnea indicate volume overload
• Administer all fluids and medications in the least amount of fluid possible	• Minimize intake

NURSING DIAGNOSIS

Risk for infection related to depressed immune response secondary to uremia and impaired skin integrity

Continued

NURSING CARE PLAN   for the Patient with Acute Renal Failure—cont'd

PATIENT OUTCOMES
Absence of infection

- Infection will be absent
- Patient will be afebrile
- WBC count and differential will be normal
- All cultures will be negative

NURSING INTERVENTIONS	RATIONALES
• Monitor WBC count and culture results	• Detect infection early
• Monitor temperature	• Fever may indicate infection
• Avoid invasive equipment whenever possible, such as indwelling urinary catheters and central lines	• Prevent infection
• Use good hand-washing technique	• Prevent infection
• Use aseptic technique for all procedures	• Prevent infection
• Perform pulmonary preventive techniques (turn, cough, deep breathing)	• Mobilize secretions to prevent pneumonia
• Assess potential sites of infection (urinary, pulmonary, wound, intravenous catheters)	• Detect early signs of infection

NURSING DIAGNOSIS

Imbalanced nutrition: less than body requirements related to uremia, altered oral mucous membranes, and dietary restrictions

PATIENT OUTCOMES
Adequate nutritional and caloric intake

- Body weight at patient's baseline
- Energy level appropriate
- Verbalizes comfort of oral cavity and ability to taste food normally

NURSING INTERVENTIONS	RATIONALES
• Monitor body weight and caloric intake daily	• Identify deficits in nutritional intake and response to nutritional therapy
• Collaborate with dietitian about nutritional needs	• Provide optimal nutritional support
• Provide diet with essential nutrients but within restrictions	• Prevent nutritional deficits; avoid electrolyte imbalances and fluid overload
• Provide oral hygiene every 2-4 hours	• Minimize dryness of oral mucosa and promote patient comfort
• Remove noxious stimuli from room	• Reduce nausea, vomiting, and anorexia

NURSING DIAGNOSIS

Anxiety related to diagnosis, treatment plan, prognosis, and unfamiliar environment

PATIENT OUTCOME
Anxiety levels reduced

- Effective coping mechanisms
- Participation in treatment plan

NURSING CARE PLAN for the Patient with Acute Renal Failure—cont'd

NURSING INTERVENTIONS	RATIONALES
• Monitor for signs of anxiety: tachycardia, muscle tension, inappropriate behaviors	• Recognize anxiety
• Explain all procedures; provide calm, relaxing environment	• Reduce anxiety by providing factual information
• Implement measures to reduce fear and anxiety	• Facilitate relaxation
• Allow patient to make choices	• Promote feelings of control to reduce anxiety
• Assess for ineffective coping (depression, withdrawal)	• Assess need for counseling and/or medications
• Administer antianxiety medications as prescribed	• Reduce anxiety

NURSING DIAGNOSIS

Deficient knowledge related to disease process and therapeutic regimen

PATIENT OUTCOME

• Patient and family have sufficient, accurate information related to condition to be informed participants in the care

NURSING INTERVENTIONS	RATIONALES
• Provide specific, factual information on acute renal failure, impact on the patient, and treatment plan	• Knowledge will enhance patient understanding
• Encourage patient and family to ask questions	• Promote increased knowledge
• Encourage patient and family members to participate in care	• Facilitate self-care management

WBC, White blood cell.

weights are used to validate intake and output measurements. A 1-kg gain in body weight is equal to a 1000-mL fluid gain. Weights should be obtained at the same time each day with the same scale. Many critical care beds have built-in scales, which simplify the procedure. When the patient is weighed, the nurse ensures that the scale is properly calibrated and that the same number of bed linens and pillows are weighed with the patient each time. The nurse must recognize signs and symptoms of fluid volume overload, which can lead to pulmonary edema and severe respiratory distress (see Clinical Alert: Fluid Volume Overload).

The nurse plays a key role in preventing infection in patients with acute renal failure. Infection accounts for about 70% of deaths in patients with acute renal

CLINICAL ALERT
Fluid Volume Overload

Signs and symptoms of fluid volume overload include hypertension, edema, crackles, neck vein distention, weight gain, increased pulmonary artery pressures, decreased urine output, decreased hematocrit, and presence of an S_3 heart sound.

failure.[42] Indwelling urinary catheters should not routinely be inserted because they increase the risk of infection, and many patients remain oliguric for 8 to 14 days. Strict aseptic technique with all intravenous lines (central and peripheral), including temporary access devices used for dialysis, is also of extreme importance, both at the time of insertion and during daily maintenance.

Another important role of the nurse in preventing acute renal failure, as well as delaying its progression, is monitoring peak and trough drug levels. Nurses are responsible for scheduling and obtaining the peak and trough blood levels at the appropriate times to ensure accurate results. Drug dosage adjustments must be made to avoid accumulation of the drug and toxic side effects. For example, aminoglycoside doses are based on drug levels and the patient's estimated creatinine clearance. If the drug level is too high, either the dose of the aminoglycoside can be kept constant and the interval between doses increased, or the interval can be kept constant and the dose is decreased. A peak level is usually drawn 1 to 2 hours after the drug is administered and reflects the highest level achieved after the drug has been rapidly distributed and before any substantial elimination has occurred. A trough level is drawn just before the next dose is given and is an indicator of how the body has cleared the drug.

MEDICAL MANAGEMENT OF ACUTE RENAL FAILURE

Prerenal Causes

Acute renal failure from prerenal conditions is usually reversible if renal perfusion is quickly restored; therefore, early recognition and prompt treatment are essential. However, prevention of prerenal conditions is just as important as early recognition and aggressive management. Prompt replacement of extracellular fluids and aggressive treatment of shock may help prevent acute renal failure. Hypovolemia is treated in various ways, depending on the cause. Blood loss necessitates blood transfusions, whereas patients with pancreatitis and peritonitis are usually treated with isotonic solutions such as normal saline. Hypovolemia resulting from large urine or gastrointestinal losses often requires the administration of a hypotonic solution, such as 0.45% saline. Patients with cardiac instability usually require positive inotropic agents, antidysrhythmic agents, preload or afterload reducers, or an intraaortic balloon pump. Hypovolemia from intense vasodilation may require vasoconstrictor medications, isotonic fluid replacement, and antibiotics (if the patient has sepsis) until the underlying problem has been resolved. Invasive hemodynamic monitoring with a pulmonary artery catheter is extremely valuable in the management of fluid balance.

Postrenal Causes

Postrenal obstruction should be suspected whenever a patient has an unexpected decrease in urine volume. Postrenal conditions are usually resolved with the insertion of an indwelling bladder catheter, either transurethral or suprapubic. Occasionally, a ureteral stent may have to be placed if the obstruction is caused by calculi or carcinoma.

Intrarenal Causes: Acute Tubular Necrosis

Common interventions for the patient with ATN include the following: drug therapy, dietary management such as protein and electrolyte restrictions, management of fluid and electrolyte imbalances, and dialysis or continuous renal replacement therapies (CRRTs).

Considering the detrimental impact of acute renal failure, nurses must focus on efforts aimed at prevention. The most important preventive strategies include identification of patients at risk and elimination of potential contributing factors. Aggressive treatment must begin at the earliest sign of renal dysfunction.

In general, maintenance of cardiovascular function and adequate intravascular volume are the two key goals in the prevention of ATN. Box 15-6 summarizes important measures for preventing acute renal failure. Primary measures include the following:

1. Maintaining an adequate hydration state for the patient, especially before surgery or invasive procedures in which radiocontrast material will be administered
2. Maintaining renal perfusion by administering vasoactive agents that may increase renal blood flow, such as low doses of dopamine, acetylcholine, isoproterenol, kinins, prostaglandins, and calcium antagonists
3. Monitoring the duration, dosage, and combinations of all nephrotoxic agents (radiocontrast agents, antibiotics, chemotherapy agents, nonsteroidal antiinflammatory drugs) administered to the patient, weighing the risk-to-benefit ratio carefully, and considering nontoxic alternatives.[7]

Pharmacological Management

Diuretics. Diuretic therapy in the treatment of patients with acute renal failure is controversial. In clinical practice, diuretics are commonly used to convert oliguria to a nonoliguric state (urine output

BOX 15-6   Measures to Prevent Acute Renal Failure

Avoid Nephrotoxins
- Use iso-osmolar radiocontrast agents (e.g., odixanol)
- Limit contrast volume to <100 mL
- Cautious use of antibiotics with appropriate dose modification
- Monitor drug levels (aminoglycosides)
- Stop certain medications (NSAIDs, ACE inhibitors, ARBs) before high-risk procedures

Optimize Volume Status Before Surgery or Invasive Procedures
- Aim for urinary output >40 mL/hr
- Keep mean arterial pressure >80 mm Hg
- Hydrate with normal saline before and after procedures requiring radiocontrast
- Hold diuretics day before and day of procedure

Reduce Incidence of Nosocomial Infections
- Judicious use of indwelling urinary catheters
- Remove of indwelling urinary catheters when no longer needed
- Strict aseptic technique with all intravenous lines

Implement Tight Glycemic Control in the Critically Ill

Aggressively Investigate and Treat Sepsis

ACE, Angiotensin-converting enzyme; *NSAIDs,* nonsteroidal antiinflammatory drugs; *ARBs,* angiotensin receptor blockers.

>400 mL/day). This conversion is thought to be beneficial for several reasons. In general, nonoliguric patients are easier to treat because they require less hemodialysis, have a shorter hospital stay, and have fewer complications and a lower mortality rate.[17] Although it is believed that diuretics increase renal blood flow, GFR (thereby increasing urine output), and reduce tubular dysfunction and obstruction, there is increasing evidence that they may cause excess diuresis and renal hypoperfusion, compromising an already insulted renal system.[8] Diuretics may increase the risk of acute renal failure (from volume depletion) when they are given before procedures requiring radiological contrast agents. Even though diuretics are commonly given, there is little evidence that they are of any benefit to patients with acute renal failure, and their widespread use should be discouraged.[45]

Hypovolemia should be corrected before any diuretics are administered. If diuretic therapy is implemented, a loop diuretic is commonly ordered. Furosemide has the dual effect of creating a solute diuresis (increased flow of tubular cellular debris) and augmenting renal blood flow.[19] Large doses of furosemide are often needed in acute renal failure to induce diuresis. This may lead to excessive diuresis and volume depletion. High doses of furosemide have been associated with deafness, which may become permanent. Patients who are also receiving aminoglycosides are at increased risk of ototoxicity.[15]

Mannitol, an osmotic diuretic often used in acute renal failure caused by rhabdomyolysis, increases plasma volume and is believed to protect the kidney by minimizing post-ischemic swelling. However, it may cause volume depletion and may inhibit oxygen perfusion and increase oxygen demand in the renal medulla.[27]

Dopamine. The role of dopamine is controversial in the treatment of acute renal failure. Low-dose dopamine has been used in acute renal failure despite numerous studies that have failed to show any benefit. Dopamine in low doses (1 to 3 mcg/kg/min) may increase renal blood flow and GFR by stimulating the dopaminergic receptors in the kidney. Sodium excretion is increased as a result of the enhanced blood flow. The administration of dopamine immediately at the onset of acute renal failure (particularly if the patient is hypotensive) is believed to avert further damage and to help maintain urine output. However, there has been growing concern regarding potential adverse effects of dopamine even at low doses. Dopamine causes a decrease in T-cell function and thereby increases the susceptibility to infection. It has been found to suppress circulating concentrations of most anterior pituitary–dependent hormones such as prolactin, growth hormone, and thyrotropin, which alters normal endocrine responses in critical illness. Dopamine has also been shown to reduce respiratory drive, increase intrapulmonary shunting, decrease splanchnic perfusion, and cause tachydysrhythmias. The routine administration of dopamine is diminishing because of growing evidence that it has no role in preventing acute renal failure and may actually be detrimental.[27,40]

Acetylcysteine. Multiple studies have been conducted using prophylactic acetylcysteine (Mucomyst) in patients at risk of contrast-induced acute renal failure. Acetylcysteine, an antioxidant, in conjunction with intravenous fluids has been thought to reduce the incidence of contrast-induced acute renal failure. The mechanism of action is unclear, but acetylcysteine is thought to act by scavenging oxygen-free radicals or enhancing the vasodilatory effects of nitric oxide.[37] Prophylactic administration of acetylcysteine (600 mg orally twice a day on the day before and on the day of the contrast), along with hydration (half-normal [0.45%] saline at 1 mL/kg/hr overnight before procedure) is hypothesized to reduce the amount of acute renal damage in high-risk patients undergoing procedures requiring contrast agents.[2,55] However, current data on the administration of acetylcysteine do not provide definitive conclusions about its use in preventing contrast-induced nephropathy.

Fenoldopam. Another agent that is postulated to protect against contrast-induced acute renal failure is fenoldopam, a dopamine A1 receptor agonist. Fenoldopam (Corlopam) acts predominately as a vasodilator of peripheral arteries (reducing blood pressure) and as a potent renal vasodilator (increasing renal blood flow). It is six times more potent than dopamine in increasing renal blood flow, especially to critical regions in the renal medulla. Fenoldopam is given via intravenous infusion several hours before the contrast agent is given and is continued for a minimum of 4 hours after the procedure.[3,34] Studies are ongoing with the use of fenoldopam in the prevention of contrast-induced nephropathy; however, no consistent outcome has been noted.

Theophylline. A potentially beneficial agent that may be considered for use in patients at risk for contrast-induced nephropathy is theophylline, a nonselective adenosine A1 and A2 receptor antagonist. Theophylline, usually given as a single 200 mg dose intravenously 30 minutes before the procedure, has had some positive results in preventing contrast-induced nephropathy. However, theophylline is associated with serious adverse effects including tachycardia, dysrhythmias, and seizures. Current studies are ongoing using theophylline in the prevention of contrast-induced nephropathy.[22,43]

Miscellaneous Agents. Multiple miscellaneous agents have been administered in an attempt to attenuate the course of acute renal failure and to hasten recovery. None, however, has consistently proved effective. Many of these drugs attempt to improve renal blood flow through vasodilation (atrial natriuretic peptide, endothelium-1 receptor antagonists, prostaglandin E_1), prevent accumulation of intracellular calcium as occurs in ischemic azotemia (calcium channel blockers), protect renal tubule cells during ischemia (glycine, magnesium adenosine triphosphate dichloride), or stimulate renal cell regeneration (epidermal growth factor, growth hormone, insulin-like growth factor). Many of these agents and numerous others have shown beneficial results in experimental models, but have had inconsistent results in the clinical setting.

Prostaglandin E_1 has a vasodilatory effect and has been shown in small studies to counteract the vasoconstriction from radiocontrast media that may cause acute renal failure in high-risk patients. Administra-tion of an intravenous sodium bicarbonate solution before and after the procedure is also thought to prevent contrast-induced nephropathy. It is speculated that alkalinizing the urine may reduce the nephrotoxic potential of the radiocontrast agent in the renal capillaries or tubules. Ongoing studies are being conducted on a variety of agents in the prevention and treatment of acute renal failure.[27,43]

Epoetin Alfa (Epogen). Patients with acute renal failure often develop anemia from a variety of causes (see Table 15-1). Epoetin alfa is an agent commonly given to treat the anemia of chronic renal failure, but it is occasionally administered in acute renal failure. Patients should have adequate iron stores (serum ferritin must be ≥300 ng/mL) before epoetin alfa is administered. If iron levels are low, oral or intravenous iron therapy is indicated. The most prominent side effect of epoetin alfa is hypertension. Blood pressure must be adequately controlled before starting epoetin alfa and closely monitored thereafter. Various dosing patterns may be used; however, starting doses in the range of 50 to 100 units/kg three times weekly are commonly used.

Pharmacological Management Considerations. Drug therapy for the patient with acute renal failure poses a challenge because two-thirds of all drugs or their metabolites are eliminated from the body by the kidneys. In acute renal failure, substantial alterations in drug dosages are often necessary to prevent toxic levels and adverse reactions. Assessment of renal function by creatinine clearance is often used to assist with drug dosing. The pharmacokinetic characteristics of the drug to be given, the route of elimination, and the extent of protein binding are also considered. Pharmacists often assist in determining optimum drug dosages for critically ill patients.

Many drugs are removed by dialysis, and extra doses are often required to avoid suboptimal drug levels. In general, drugs that are primarily water soluble, such as vitamins, cimetidine, and phenobarbital, are removed by dialysis and should be administered after dialysis. Drugs that are protein bound, lipid bound, or metabolized by the liver, such as phenytoin, lidocaine, and vancomycin, are not removed by dialysis and can be given at any time.[31] Box 15-7 is a partial list of drugs that are removed by dialysis.

Dietary Management

Dietary management in patients with acute renal failure is a major component of the therapeutic regimen. Energy expenditure in catabolic patients with acute renal failure is much higher than normal basal requirements. Dialysis also contributes to protein catabolism. The loss of amino acids and water-soluble vitamins in the dialysate solution constitutes another drain on the patient's nutritional stores. The overall goal of dietary management for acute renal failure is provision of adequate energy, protein, and micronutrients to maintain homeostasis in patients who may be extremely catabolic. Nutritional recommendations include the following:[26]

- Caloric intake of 25 to 35 kcal/kg of ideal body weight per day
- Protein intake of no less than 0.8 g/kg body weight. Patients who are extremely catabolic should receive 1.5 to 2 g/kg of ideal body weight per day—75% to 80% of which contains all the required essential amino acids.
- Sodium intake of 0.5 to 1.0 g/day
- Potassium intake of 20 to 50 mEq/day

- Calcium intake of 800 to 1200 mg/day
- Fluid intake equal to the volume of the patient's urine output plus an additional 600 to 1000 mL/day

In addition, patients undergoing dialysis usually receive multivitamins, folic acid, and occasionally an iron supplement to replace the water-soluble vitamins and other essential elements lost during dialysis. If the patient is unable to ingest or tolerate an adequate oral nutritional intake, enteral feedings or total parenteral nutrition are prescribed. Nutritional support must supply the patient with sufficient nonprotein glucose calories, essential amino acids, fluids, electrolytes, and essential vitamins to create a more stable internal environment. Such an internal environment not only prevents further catabolism, negative nitrogen balance, muscle wasting, and other uremic complications, but also enhances the patient's tubular regenerating capacity, resistance to infection, and ability to combat other multisystem dysfunctions. The physician may also prescribe early dialysis therapy to handle the increased fluid volume the patient receives from enteral or total parenteral nutrition.

BOX 15-7   Common Drugs Removed by Hemodialysis*

- Aminoglycosides (gentamicin, tobramycin)
- Cephalosporins (including cefoxitin and ceftazidime)
- Penicillins (piperacillin, penicillin G)
- Erythromycin
- Isoniazid
- Sulfonamides (sulfamethoxazole, sulfisoxazole)
- Trimethoprim-sulfamethoxazole
- Procainamide
- Quinidine
- Nitroprusside
- Lithium carbonate
- Water-soluble vitamins
- Folic acid
- Phenobarbital
- Cimetidine
- Ranitidine

*If possible, hold daily doses until after dialysis; supplemental doses may be required for many of these agents.

Management of Fluid, Electrolyte, and Acid-Base Imbalances

Fluid Imbalance. Volume overload is generally managed by dietary restriction of salt and water and administration of diuretics. In addition, dialysis or other renal replacement therapies may be indicated for fluid control. These modalities are discussed later in this chapter.

Electrolyte Imbalance. Common electrolyte imbalances in acute renal failure are listed in the Laboratory Alert, along with their "critical" values and the significance of the laboratory alert. The nurse immediately notifies the physician once a critical laboratory value is known. Hyperkalemia is common in acute

---

LABORATORY ALERT
Acute Renal Failure

Laboratory Test	Critical Value	Significance
Potassium (K+)	>6.6 mEq/L	Hyperkalemia: potential for heart blocks, asystole, ventricular fibrillation; may cause muscle weakness, diarrhea, and abdominal cramps
Sodium (Na+)	≤110 mEq/L	Hyponatremia: potential for lethargy, confusion, coma, or seizures; may cause nausea, vomiting, and headaches
Total calcium (Ca++)	<7 mg/dL	Hypocalcemia: potential for seizures, laryngospasm, stridor, tetany, heart blocks, and cardiac arrest; may see positive Chvostek's or Trousseau's sign
Magnesium (Mg+)	>3 mg/dL	Hypermagnesemia: potential for bradycardia and heart blocks, lethargy, coma, hypotension, hypoventilation, and weak-to-absent deep tendon reflexes

renal failure, especially if the patient is hypercatabolic. Hyperkalemia occurs when potassium excretion is reduced as a result of the decrease in GFR. Sudden changes in the serum potassium level can cause dysrhythmias, which may be fatal. Figure 15-5 shows the electrocardiographic changes commonly seen in hyperkalemia.

Three approaches are used in treating hyperkalemia: (1) reduce the body potassium content, (2) shift the potassium intracellularly, and (3) antagonize the membrane effect of the hyperkalemia. Only dialysis and administration of cation exchange resins (sodium polystyrene sulfonate [Kayexalate]) with sorbitol actually reduce plasma potassium levels and total body potassium content in a patient with acute renal failure. Other treatments only "protect" the patient for a short time until dialysis or cation exchange resins can be instituted. Table 15-4 summarizes medications used in the treatment of hyperkalemia. A commonly prescribed regimen for hyperkalemia consists of the following:[18]

- Calcium gluconate, 10 mL of a 10% solution given intravenously over 5 minutes
- Glucose (50 mL of 50% dextrose) given intravenously
- Regular insulin, 10 units given intravenously

- Sodium bicarbonate, 50 to 100 mEq/L given intravenously
- Sodium polystyrene sulfonate (Kayexalate), 15 g one to four times daily by mouth, or 30 to 50 g with 50 to 100 mL of a 20% sorbitol solution rectally every 6 hours as a retention enema.

Hyponatremia generally occurs from water overload. However, as nephrons are progressively damaged, the ability to conserve sodium is lost, and major salt-wasting states can develop, causing hyponatremia. Hyponatremia is usually treated with fluid restriction, specifically restriction of free water intake. Alterations in the serum calcium and phosphorus levels occur frequently in acute renal failure as a result of abnormalities in excretion, absorption, and metabolism of the electrolytes. Mild degrees of hypermagnesemia are common in acute renal failure as a result of decreased renal excretion.

Acid-Base Imbalance. Metabolic acidosis is the primary acid-base imbalance seen in acute renal failure. Box 15-8 summarizes the etiology and the signs and symptoms of metabolic acidosis in acute renal failure. Treatment of metabolic acidosis depends on its severity. In mild metabolic acidosis, the lungs are able to compensate by excreting carbon dioxide. Patients with a serum bicarbonate level of less than 15 mEq/L and a pH of less than 7.20 are usually treated with intravenous sodium bicarbonate. The goal of treatment is to raise the pH to a value greater than 7.20. Rapid correction of the

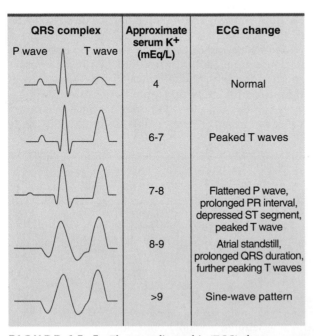

QRS complex	Approximate serum K+ (mEq/L)	ECG change
P wave ∧ T wave	4	Normal
	6-7	Peaked T waves
	7-8	Flattened P wave, prolonged PR interval, depressed ST segment, peaked T wave
	8-9	Atrial standstill, prolonged QRS duration, further peaking T waves
	>9	Sine-wave pattern

FIGURE 15-5. Electrocardiographic (ECG) changes seen in hyperkalemia. *(From Weiner, D., Linas, S., & Wingo, C. [2007]. Disorders of potassium metabolism. In J. Feehally, J. Floege, & R. Johnson [Eds], Comprehensive clinical nephrology [pp. 111-122]. Philadelphia: Mosby.)*

BOX 15-8   Metabolic Acidosis in Acute Renal Failure

Etiology
- Inability of kidney to excrete hydrogen ions; decreased production of ammonia by the kidney (normally assists with hydrogen ion excretion)
- Retention of acid end-products of metabolism, which use available buffers in the body; inability of kidney to synthesize bicarbonate

Signs and Symptoms
- Low pH of arterial blood (pH < 7.35)
- Low serum bicarbonate
- Increased rate and depth of respirations to excrete carbon dioxide from the lungs (compensatory mechanism); known as Kussmaul's respiration
- Low $PaCO_2$
- Lethargy and coma if severe

$PaCO_2$, Partial pressure of carbon dioxide in arterial blood.

PHARMACOLOGY

TABLE 15-4 Medications to Treat Hyperkalemia

Drug	Mechanism of Action	Dosage	Side Effects	Nursing Implications
Kayexalate (sodium polystyrene sulfonate)	↑ Fecal excretion of potassium by exchanging sodium ions for potassium ions	Oral: 15 g 1-4 times daily by mouth Rectal: 30-50 g via enema every 6 hours	Constipation, hypokalemia, hypernatremia, nausea and vomiting, fecal impaction in the elderly	Available as a powder or suspension Mix powder with full glass of liquid and chill to increase palatability Do not mix oral powder with orange juice May be mixed with sorbitol to facilitate movement through the intestinal tract
Sorbitol	Hyperosmotic laxative	20-100 mL rectally via enema every 6 hours	Hyperglycemia, diarrhea, edema, abdominal discomfort, hypokalemia	Administer as retention enema in combination with Kayexelate
Furosemide (Lasix)	↑ Renal excretion of potassium	Oral: 20-80 mg daily twice a day IV: 20-40 mg/dose every 6-12 hours Continuous infusion: 10-40 mg/hr	Orthostatic hypotension, hypokalemia, urinary frequency, dizziness, ototoxicity	Administer IV dose over several minutes; ototoxicity is associated with rapid administration Assess for allergy to sulfonylurea before giving Monitor for dehydration, hypokalemia, hypotension Diuretics only work if the patient is nonoliguric
Insulin/dextrose	Shifts potassium temporarily from the extracellular fluid (blood) into the intracellular fluid; the dextrose helps prevent hypoglycemia	10 Units regular insulin and 50 mL of 50% dextrose as a bolus IV	Hyperglycemia, hypoglycemia, hypokalemia	If the serum glucose is >300 mg/dL, the physician may order only the insulin
Sodium bicarbonate	Shifts potassium temporarily from the extracellular fluid (blood) to the intracellular fluid	50-100 mEq/L IV push	Hypernatremia, hypokalemia, pulmonary edema	Do not mix with any other medications to avoid precipitation Helpful if patient has a severe metabolic acidosis
Albuterol	Adrenergic agonist ↑ plasma insulin concentration; shifts potassium to intracellular space	Inhalation: 10-20 mg over 10 minutes IV: 0.5 mg over 15 min	Tachycardia, angina, palpitations, hypertension, nervousness, irritability	Note that the dose used is much higher than that used in treating pulmonary conditions Use concentrated form (5 mg/mL) so the volume to be inhaled is minimized
Calcium gluconate	Electrolyte replacement	10 mL IV over 5 minutes	Bradycardia, hypotension, syncope, necrosis if infiltrated	Has no effect on actually lowering serum potassium Will see almost immediate effect on ECG appearance Be sure IV is patent; avoid extravasation

ECG, Electrocardiogram; *IV,* Intravenous.

acidosis should be avoided, because tetany may occur as a result of hypocalcemia. The pH determines how much ionized calcium is present in the serum; the more acidic the serum; the more ionized calcium is present. If the metabolic acidosis is rapidly corrected, the serum ionized calcium level decreases as the calcium binds with albumin and other substances such as phosphate and sulfate. For this reason, intravenous calcium gluconate may be prescribed. Dialysis also corrects metabolic acidosis because it removes excess hydrogen ions and because bicarbonate is added to the dialysate solution.[46]

Renal Replacement Therapy

Renal replacement therapy is the primary treatment for the patient with acute renal failure. Without some form of renal replacement therapy, the patient is unable to sustain life during the acute renal failure episode. Therapy may include hemodialysis, CRRT, or peritoneal dialysis.

Definition. *Dialysis* is defined as the separation of solutes by differential diffusion through a porous or semipermeable membrane that is placed between two solutions. This general definition permits the clinician to distinguish among the various types of dialysis merely by identifying the semipermeable membrane and describing the two solutions that are involved.

Indications for Dialysis. The most common reasons for instituting dialysis in acute renal failure include fluid overload with pulmonary edema, hypertension, heart failure, electrolyte imbalances, and acid-base imbalances. Dialysis is usually initiated early in the course of the renal failure before uremic complications such as nausea and vomiting, pericarditis, and hematological abnormalities occur. In addition, dialysis is often started for fluid control when total parenteral nutrition is administered.[5,38] Prophylactic dialysis to prevent contrast-induced nephropathy has not been validated as an effective strategy and is not recommended.[33]

Principles and Mechanisms. Dialysis therapy is based on two physical principles that operate simultaneously: diffusion and ultrafiltration. *Diffusion* (or clearance) is the movement of solutes such as urea from the patient's blood to the dialysate cleansing fluid, across a semipermeable membrane (the artificial kidney). Substances such as bicarbonate may also cross in the opposite direction, from the dialysate across the semipermeable membrane into the patient's blood. Movement of solutes across the semipermeable membrane is dependent on the following:

- The amount of solutes on each side of the semipermeable membrane; typically, the patient's blood has larger amounts of solutes such as urea, creatinine, and potassium
- The surface area of the semipermeable membrane (the size of the artificial kidney)
- The permeability of the semipermeable membrane
- The size and charge of the solutes
- The rate of blood flowing through the artificial kidney
- The rate of dialysate cleansing fluid flowing through the artificial kidney

Ultrafiltration is the removal of plasma water and some low–molecular weight particles by using a pressure or osmotic gradient. Ultrafiltration is primarily aimed at controlling fluid volume, whereas dialysis is aimed at decreasing waste products and treating fluid and electrolyte imbalances.[49,52]

Vascular Access. An essential component of all the renal replacement therapies is adequate, easy access to the patient's bloodstream. Various types of vascular access devices (Figures 15-6 and 15-7) are used for hemodialysis: percutaneous venous catheters, arteriovenous fistulas, arteriovenous grafts, and external arteriovenous shunts. The terms fistula, graft, and shunt are often used interchangeably.

Temporary percutaneous catheters are commonly used in patients with acute renal failure because they can be used immediately. They are inserted into the subclavian, jugular, or femoral vein. The typical catheter has a single or double lumen and is designed only for short-term renal replacement therapy during acute situations. These catheters are replaced approximately every 7 days to decrease the risk of nosocomial infection. One example of such a device is the Vas-Cath catheter. Occasionally a percutaneous tunneled catheter is placed if the patient needs ongoing hemodialysis. These catheters are usually inserted in the operating room and do not need routine replacement unless they malfunction or become infected. Examples of tunneled hemodialysis catheters include the Permacath and Tesio twin catheters.

An *arteriovenous fistula* is an internal, surgically created communication between an artery and a vein. The most frequently created fistula is the Brescio-Cimino fistula, which involves anastomosing the radial artery and cephalic vein in a side-to-side or end-to-side manner. The anastomosis permits blood to bypass the capillaries and to flow directly from the artery into the vein. As a result, the vein is forced to dilate to accommodate the increased pressure that accompanies the arterial blood. This method produces a vessel that is easy to cannulate but requires 4 to 6 weeks before it is mature enough to use.

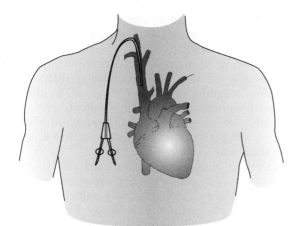

FIGURE 15-6. Central venous catheter used for hemodialysis.

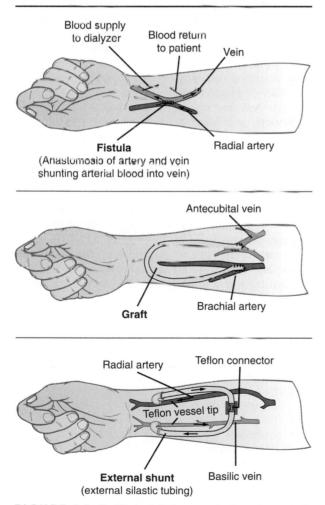

FIGURE 15-7. Hemodialysis access devices. *(From Lewis, S. L., Heitkemper, M. M., & Dirksen, S. R. [2004]. Medical-surgical nursing: Assessment and management of clinical problems (6th ed.). St. Louis: Mosby.)*

Arteriovenous grafts are created by using different types of prosthetic material, most commonly polytetrafluoroethylene and Gore-Tex.[16] Anastomoses are made with the graft ends connected to an artery and a vein.

An external *arteriovenous shunt* (Quinton-Scribner) consists of a surgically implanted extracorporeal apparatus that connects an artery and a vein. This type of device has become less popular since the advent of percutaneous catheters and is rarely used in the critical care unit. The external shunt poses a risk of infection and clotting problems.

Nursing Care of Arteriovenous Fistula or Graft. The nurse must protect the vascular access site. An arteriovenous fistula or graft should be auscultated for a bruit and palpated for the presence of a thrill or buzz every 8 hours. The extremity that has a fistula or graft must never be used for drawing blood specimens, obtaining blood pressure measurements, intravenous therapy, or intramuscular injections. Such activities produce pressure changes within the altered vessels that could result in clotting or rupture. The nurse must alert other health care personnel of the presence of the fistula or graft by posting a large sign at the head of the patient's bed that indicates which arm should be used. Constrictive clothing and jewelry must be avoided on the affected arm. Patients should be cautioned against sleeping on the affected arm. All these situations may decrease blood flow through the fistula or graft and may cause clotting. The presence and strength of the distal pulse past the fistula or graft are evaluated at least every 8 hours. Inadequate collateral circulation past the fistula or graft may result in loss of this pulse. The physician is notified immediately if no bruit is auscultated, no thrill is palpated, or the distal pulse is absent.[16]

Nursing Care of Percutaneous Catheters. Strict aseptic technique must be applied to any percutaneous catheter placed for dialysis. Exit sites should be inspected daily for signs of infection, such as redness, drainage, and swelling.[25] Dressing changes are performed using sterile technique. To avoid accidental dislodging, there is minimal manipulation of the catheter. The catheter is not used for the administration of fluids or medications or for the sampling of blood unless a specific order is obtained to do so. Dialysis personnel may instill heparin in the catheter to maintain patency, and clamp the catheter when not in use.

Hemodialysis. Hemodialysis is the most frequently used renal replacement therapy for treating acute renal failure. Hemodialysis consists of simply cleansing the patient's blood through an artificial kidney or dialyzer by the use of diffusion and ultrafiltration. Water and waste products of metabolism are easily removed. Hemodialysis is efficient and corrects biochemical disturbances quickly. Treatments are typically 3 to 4 hours long and are performed in the critical care unit at the patient's bedside. Patients with acute renal failure may be hemodynamically unstable and unable to tolerate conventional hemodialysis. In those instances, other methods of renal replacement therapy such as peritoneal dialysis or CRRT are considered.

Complications. Several complications are associated with hemodialysis. Hypotension occurs in approximately 10% to 50% of patients and is usually the result of preexisting hypovolemia, excessive amounts of fluid removal, or excessively rapid removal of fluid.[29] Other factors that contribute to hypotension include left ventricular dysfunction from preexisting heart disease or medications, autonomic dysfunction resulting from medication or diabetes, and inappropriate vasodilation resulting from sepsis or antihypertensive drug therapy. Dialyzer membrane incompatibility may also cause hypotension.

Dysrhythmias may occur during dialysis. Causes of dysrhythmias include a rapid shift in the serum potassium level, clearance of antidysrhythmic medications, preexisting coronary artery disease, hypoxemia, or hypercalcemia from rapid influx of calcium from the dialysate solution.

Muscle cramps may occur during dialysis, but they occur more commonly in chronic renal failure. Cramping is thought to be caused by ischemia of the skeletal muscles that results from aggressive fluid removal. The cramps typically involve the legs, feet, and hands and occur most often during the last half of the dialysis treatment.

A decrease in the arterial oxygen content of the blood can occur in patients undergoing hemodialysis. Usually, the decrease ranges from 5 to 35 mm Hg (mean, 15 mm Hg) and is not clinically significant except in the critically ill patient. Several theories have been offered to explain the hypoxemia, including leukocyte interactions with the artificial kidney and a decrease in carbon dioxide levels, resulting from either an acetate dialysate solution or a loss of carbon dioxide across the semipermeable membrane.

Dialysis disequilibrium syndrome often occurs after the first or second dialysis treatment or in patients who have had sudden, large decreases in BUN and creatinine levels as a result of the hemodialysis. Because of the blood-brain barrier, dialysis does not deplete the concentrations of BUN, creatinine, and other uremic toxins in the brain as rapidly as it does those substances in the extracellular fluid. An osmotic concentration gradient established in the brain allows fluid to enter until the concentration levels equal those of the extracellular fluid. The extra fluid in the brain tissue creates a state of cerebral edema for the patient, which results in severe headaches, nausea and vomiting, twitching, mental confusion, and occasionally seizures. The incidence of dialysis disequilibrium syndrome may be decreased by the use of shorter, more frequent, dialysis treatments. It is also safest to use a dialysis solution sodium value close to the patient's serum sodium value to avoid fluid shifts into the brain.[29]

Infectious complications associated with hemodialysis include vascular access infections and hepatitis C. Vascular access infections are usually caused by a break in sterile technique, whereas hepatitis C is usually acquired through transfusion.

Hemolysis, air embolism, and hyperthermia are rare complications of hemodialysis. Hemolysis can occur when the patient's blood is exposed to incorrectly mixed dialysate solution or hypotonic chemicals (formaldehyde and bleach). An air embolism can occur when air is introduced into the bloodstream through a break in the dialysis circuit. Hyperthermia may result if the temperature control devices on the dialysis machine malfunction. Complications of hemodialysis are summarized in Box 15-9.

Nursing Care of the Patient. The patient receiving hemodialysis requires specialized monitoring and interventions by the critical care nurse. Laboratory values are monitored and abnormal results reported to the nephrologist and dialysis staff. The patient is weighed daily to monitor fluid status. On the day of dialysis, dialyzable (water-soluble) medications are not given until after treatment. The dialysis nurse or pharmacist can be consulted to determine which medications to withhold or administer. Supplemental doses are administered as ordered after dialysis. Administration of antihypertensive agents is avoided

---

BOX 15-9   Complications of Dialysis

- Hypotension
- Cramps
- Bleeding/clotting
- Dialyzer reaction
- Hemolysis
- Dysrhythmias
- Infections
- Hypoxemia
- Pyrogen reactions
- Dialysis disequilibrium syndrome
- Vascular access dysfunction
- Technical mishaps (incorrect dialysate mixture, contaminated dialysate, or air embolism)

for 4 to 6 hours before treatment, if possible. Doses of other medications that lower blood pressure (narcotics, sedatives) are reduced, if possible. The percutaneous catheter, fistula, or graft is assessed frequently; unusual findings such as loss of bruit, redness, or drainage at the site must be reported. After dialysis, the patient is assessed for signs of bleeding, hypovolemia, and dialysis disequilibrium syndrome.

Continuous Renal Replacement Therapy. CRRT is frequently used in patients with acute renal failure because of its ability to provide continuous ultrafiltration of fluids and clearance of uremic toxins. CRRT is particularly useful for patients in the critical care unit whose cardiovascular status is too unstable to tolerate rapid fluid removal. Table 15-5 outlines the various CRRT modalities. The type of CRRT selected is based on clinical assessment, metabolic status,

TABLE 15-5 Continuous Renal Replacement Therapies

Abbreviation	Name	Purpose	Vascular Access Required	Brief Description
CAVH	Continuous arteriovenous hemofiltration	Fluid and some uremic waste product removal	Arterial and large venous catheter	Arterial blood is circulated through a hemofilter and returned to the patient through a venous catheter; ultrafiltrate (fluid removed) is collected in a drainage bag as it exits the hemofilter
CAVHD	Continuous arteriovenous hemodialysis	Fluid and uremic waste product removal	Arterial and large venous catheter	Arterial blood is circulated through a hemofilter (surrounded by a dialysate solution) and returned to the patient through a venous catheter; ultrafiltrate (fluid and waste products removed) is collected in a drainage bag as it exits the hemofilter
CVVH	Continuous venovenous hemofiltration	Fluid and some uremic waste product removal	Dual-lumen venous catheter or two large venous catheters	Venous blood is circulated through a hemofilter and returned to the patient through a venous catheter; replacement fluid is used to increase flow through the hemofilter; ultrafiltrate (fluid removed) is collected in a drainage bag as it exits the hemofilter
CVVHD	Continuous venovenous hemodialysis	Fluid and maximal uremic waste product removal	Dual-lumen venous catheter or two large venous catheters	Venous blood is circulated through a hemofilter (surrounded by a dialysate solution) and returned to the patient through a venous catheter; replacement solution may be used to improve convection; ultrafiltrate (fluid and waste products removed) is collected in a drainage bag as it exits the hemofilter
CVVHDF	Continuous venovenous hemodiafiltration	Maximal fluid and uremic waste product removal	Dual-lumen venous catheter or two large venous catheters	Venous blood is circulated through a hemofilter (surrounded by a dialysate solution) and returned to the patient through a venous catheter; replacement solution is used to maintain fluid balance; ultrafiltration (fluid and waste products removed) is collected in a drainage bag as it exits the hemofilter

severity of uremia, and whether the therapy is available.

Indications. The clinical indications for CRRT are similar to those for dialysis, such as hypervolemia, cardiac failure, and electrolyte and acid-base imbalances. CRRT modalities have also been thought to absorb specific proinflammatory substances such as tumor necrosis factor in patients with septic shock.[5]

CRRT is a continuous, 24-hour-a-day process with a more gradual solute removal than hemodialysis, with a decreased risk of hemodynamic instability. CRRT allows flexibility in fluid administration and requires minimal hyalinization.

Principles. CRRT is the extracorporeal circulation of blood through a hemofilter for the removal of fluid and small solutes via the process of hemofiltration. Hemofiltration occurs when blood under pressure passes down one side of a highly permeable membrane allowing both water and other substances to pass across the membrane. Several different types of hemofilters are available. All have highly porous membranes that permit the clearance of molecules less than 50,000 daltons, such as urea, creatinine, sodium, and potassium. Substances such as albumin and red blood cells are too large to pass through the hemofilter.[36] Solute clearance is enhanced with the addition of a dialysate solution, either a standard commercially prepared peritoneal solution (1.5% dextrose) or a solution formulated to meet the individual patient's electrolyte needs.

Depending on the method of CRRT, vascular access is gained via arterial or venous cannulation. In *continuous arteriovenous hemofiltration* (CAVH), an arterial and a venous catheter are inserted; the patient's own blood pressure pumps the blood through the hemofilter system and returns the blood via the venous catheter. However, because of complications associated with arterial vascular access, two venous accesses or a dual-lumen venous catheter are most often used. For example, in *continuous venovenous hemofiltration* (CVVH), venous blood from the patient is circulated through the hemofilter system by a blood pump and is then returned to the patient through the venous catheter (Figure 15-8). A continuous heparin infusion may be needed to keep the filter from clotting. Another option to continuous heparin therapy is sodium citrate, which anticoagulates blood by binding with calcium ions. Automated devices are currently marketed to facilitate the CRRT procedure (Figure 15-9).

In CAVH or *continuous arteriovenous hemodialysis* (CAVHD), *ultrafiltration* (rate of fluid removal) occurs as a result of the difference between the patient's hydrostatic pressure and oncotic pressure. In CVVH, a pressure gradient is established so water is pushed or pumped across the dialysis filter and carries the uremic waste products from the bloodstream with it (convection). Blood flow and ultrafiltration rates are controlled by adjusting the blood pump speed and ultrafiltration pump rate. Replacement solutions are occasionally used with CVVH, *continuous venovenous hemodialysis* (CVVHD), and *continuous venovenous hemodiafiltration* (CVVHDF) to achieve optimal fluid balance. The most commonly administered solutions are normal saline, lactated Ringer's, or a physiological solution prepared by the pharmacy containing a bicarbonate base. Replacement solutions can be administered before the hemofilter (predilution) or after the hemofilter (postdilution).[36]

Complications. Numerous complications are associated with CRRT including electrolyte and acid-base imbalances, fluid imbalances, hypotension, infection, bleeding from disruption of the catheter or system connections in the CRRT system, filter clotting, and air embolism. Some patients experience chills and hypothermia during the procedure. A blood warmer may be indicated to warm the dialysate or replacement fluid.

Nursing Care. The critical care nurse is responsible for monitoring the patient receiving CRRT. In many critical care units, the CRRT system is set up by the dialysis staff but is maintained by critical care nurses with additional training. The patient's hemodynamic status is monitored hourly, including fluid intake and output. Ultrafiltration volume is assessed hourly, and appropriate replacement fluid is administered. The hemofilter is assessed every 2 to 4 hours for clotting (as evidenced by dark fibers or a rapid decrease in the amount of ultrafiltration without a change in the patient's hemodynamic status). If clotting is suspected, the system is flushed with 50 mL of normal saline and observed for dark streaks or clots. If present, the system may have to be changed. Results of serum chemistries, clotting studies, and other tests are monitored. The CRRT system is frequently assessed to ensure filter and lines are visible at all times, kinks are avoided, and the blood tubing is warm to the touch. The ultrafiltrate is assessed for blood (pink-tinged to frank blood), which is indicative of membrane rupture. Sterile technique is performed during vascular access dressing changes.

Peritoneal Dialysis. Peritoneal dialysis is the removal of solutes and fluid by diffusion through a patient's own semipermeable membrane (the peritoneal membrane) with a dialysate solution that has been instilled into the peritoneal cavity. The peritoneal membrane surrounds the abdominal cavity and lines the organs inside the abdominal cavity. This renal replacement therapy is not commonly used

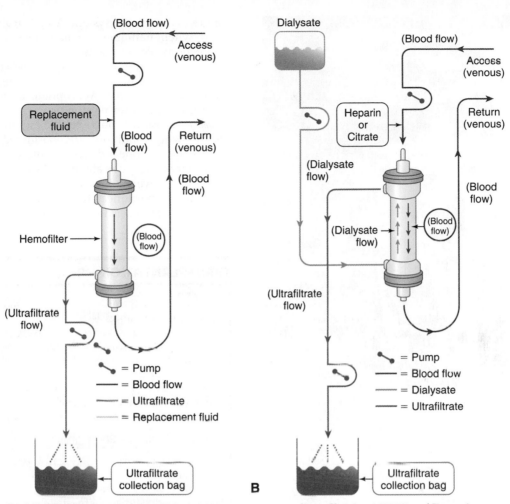

FIGURE 15-8. Schematic of **A,** continuous venovenous hemofiltration (CVVH) and **B,** continuous venovenous hemofiltration dialysis (CVVHD). *(In L. Urden, K. Stacy, & M. Lough [Eds]. [2005]. Thelan's critical care nursing: Diagnosis and management (5th ed.). St. Louis: Mosby.)*

for the treatment of acute renal failure because of its comparatively slow ability to alter biochemical imbalances.

Indications. Clinical indications for peritoneal dialysis include acute and chronic renal failure, severe water intoxication, electrolyte disorders, and drug overdose. Advantages of peritoneal dialysis include that the equipment is easily and rapidly assembled, the cost is relatively inexpensive, the danger of acute electrolyte imbalances or hemorrhage is minimal, and dialysate solutions can be individualized. In addition, automated peritoneal dialysis systems are available. Disadvantages of peritoneal dialysis include that it is time-intensive, requiring at least 36 hours for a therapeutic effect to be achieved; biochemical disturbances are corrected slowly; access to the peritoneal cavity is sometimes difficult; and the risk of peritonitis is high.

Complications. Although rare, many complications can result from peritoneal dialysis. Complications can be divided into three categories: mechanical problems, metabolic imbalances, and inflammatory reactions. Potential complications resulting from mechanical problems include perforation of the abdominal viscera during insertion of the catheter, poor drainage in or out of the abdominal cavity as a result of catheter blockage, patient discomfort from the pressure of the fluid within the peritoneal cavity, and pulmonary complications as a result of the pressure of the fluid in the peritoneal cavity. Metabolic imbalances include hypovolemia and hypernatremia from excessively rapid removal of fluid, hypervolemia from impaired drainage of fluid, hypokalemia from the use of potassium-free dialysate, alkalosis from the use of an alkaline dialysate, disequilibrium syndrome from excessively rapid removal of fluid and

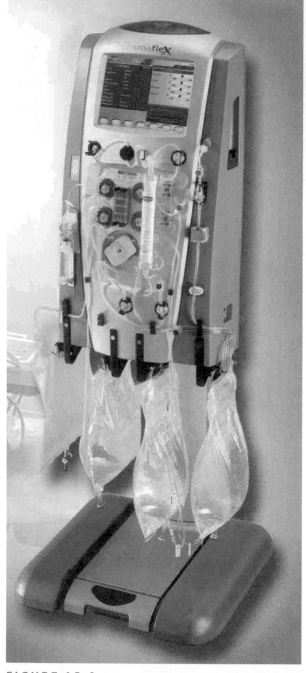

FIGURE 15-9. Prismaflex continuous renal replacement therapy system. *(Courtesy of Gambro, Lakewood, CO.)*

waste products, and hyperglycemia from the high glucose concentration of the dialysate. Inflammatory reactions include peritoneal irritation produced by the catheter and peritonitis from bacterial infection.

Peritonitis is the most common complication of peritoneal dialysis therapy and is usually caused by

contamination in the system. Aseptic technique must occur when handling the peritoneal catheter and connections. Peritonitis is manifested by abdominal pain, cloudy peritoneal fluid, fever and chills, nausea and vomiting, and difficulty in draining fluid from the peritoneal cavity. Appropriate antibiotic treatment is indicated for peritonitis.[11,47]

Contraindications. Although conflicting opinions exist, the following conditions are considered contraindications for peritoneal dialysis: acute active peritonitis, recent or extensive abdominal surgery, peritoneal adhesions, severe abdominal trauma or burns, massive intraperitoneal hematoma, and any major vascular anastomosis in the abdomen.[12]

TRANSPLANTATION   Renal

INDICATIONS

Renal transplantation is the therapeutic choice for patients with end-stage renal disease. After successful renal transplantation, the patient is free from the restrictions of dialysis and free from the manifestations of uremia. Survival at 5 years is approximately 85%. In 2007, 16,623 renal transplants were performed in the United States. However, 78,395 patients were on the UNOS Scientific Registry waiting list.[2]

CRITERIA FOR TRANSPLANT RECIPIENT

Selection of a transplant recipient is based on careful evaluation of medical, immunologic, and psychosocial status. Usually, the recipient is younger than 70 years, has an estimated life expectancy of 2 years or more, and is expected to have an improved quality of life after transplantation. Infection and active malignancy are the only two absolute contraindications to transplantation.

CRITERIA FOR DONORS

Attempts to increase the donor pool have resulted in two types of donation: living related donor and cadaver donor. The most desirable source is a living related donor who matches the recipient closely. Willing family members undergo physical and psychological evaluation and are screened for ABO blood group, tissue-specific antigen, and human leukocyte antigen histocompatibility. The number of living donors is slowly increasing because of the limited supply of cadaver donors. In 2007, 37% of renal transplants came from living donors and 63% came from deceased donors.[2]

PATIENT MANAGEMENT

The kidney from a living donor functions almost immediately after transplantation; however, a kidney

TRANSPLANTATION   Renal—cont'd

from a cadaver may not function immediately, and hemodialysis may be needed until it functions adequately. Careful monitoring of fluid and electrolyte balance is imperative. Patients with end-stage renal disease have chronic anemia; therefore hemoglobin and hematocrit levels are monitored for downward trends that could indicate bleeding.

The immune system is programmed to recognize a transplanted organ as foreign, and therefore the immune system must be inhibited after organ transplantation (see Chapter 16). Maintenance therapy consists of medications that inhibit T-cell proliferation and differentiation, deplete lymphocytes, and inhibit macrophages. Immunosuppressive medications consist of triple therapy—a calcineurin inhibitor (tacrolimus [Prograf] or cyclosporine [Neoral]), a corticosteroid (prednisone), and mycophenolate mofetil (CellCept).[3] Complications associated with immunosuppressive therapy include nephrotoxicity, hypertension, hyperlipidemia, bone loss, new-onset diabetes mellitus, and infection.

COMPLICATIONS

Postoperative complications include acute tubular necrosis, urine leaks, arterial or venous thrombosis, renal artery stenosis, and infection. Patients must be carefully monitored, and the patient and family must be knowledgeable of the signs and symptoms of infection. One of the most common infections seen is cytomegalovirus infection, which presents with a decrease in the white blood cell count, fatigue, and fever.

The most common cause of death after a renal transplant is cardiovascular disease (e.g., myocardial infarction, heart failure, or stroke) because of the presence of comorbid conditions including diabetes, hypertension, and older age. In addition, the immunosuppressants, especially corticosteroids, play a role in the development and progression of atherosclerosis and lipid disorders.

PREVENTING REJECTION

Rejection after renal transplantation is the result of the patient's immune system response to the donor kidney. Compliance with immunosuppressive medication is essential to avoid or decrease the incidence of rejection episodes. *Hyperacute rejection* occurs within minutes or hours of transplantation and is caused by humoral or antibody-mediated B-cell production against the transplanted organ. *Accelerated rejection* occurs 24 hours to 5 days after transplantation and is due to presensitization from prior exposure to one or more of the donor's antigens. *Acute rejection* occurs days to 3 months after transplantation and involves the activation and proliferation of T cells with destruction of renal tissue. Acute rejection accounts for about 90% of all rejection episodes.[1] *Chronic rejection* occurs months to years after transplantation and is caused by chronic renal allograft dysfunction in which there is a gradual deterioration in renal function. Risk factors include acute rejection episodes, hyperlipidemia, hypertension, hyperglycemia, and an increased risk of infection.

Acute rejection is diagnosed based on clinical presentation and biopsy findings. Biopsy specimens are graded according to the severity of tubulitis and arteritis by using the Banff 97 Grading System (borderline, 1A, 1B, 2A, 2B, and 3). Signs and symptoms of rejection include fever, edema, gross hematuria, pain over the graft site, increased BUN and creatinine levels, weight gain, increased blood pressure, and/or decreased urine output. Management includes administering methylprednisolone and augmenting current maintenance immunosuppression with thymoglobulin and muromonab-CD3.

REFERENCES

1. Holechek, M. J., & Armstrong, G. (2008). Kidney transplantation. In L. Ohler, & S. Cupples (Eds), *Core curriculum for transplant nurses*. St. Louis: Mosby.
2. United Network for Organ Sharing (UNOS). National Data Report. Retrieved March 23, 2008 from www.unos.org.
3. Yang, H. (2006). Maintenance immunosuppression regimens: Conversion, minimization, withdrawal, and avoidance. *American Journal of Kidney Diseases*, 47(4 Suppl. 2), S37-S51.

OUTCOMES

With appropriate nursing and medical interventions, expected outcomes for the patient with acute renal failure include the following:
- Fluid balance and hemodynamic status are stable.
- Body weight is within 2 lb of dry weight.
- Vital signs are stable and are consistent with baseline.
- Skin turgor is normal, and oral mucosa is intact and well hydrated.
- Serum laboratory values and arterial blood gas results are within normal limits.
- Infection is absent.
- Nutritional intake is adequate for the maintenance of the desired weight.
- The patient and family members are able to participate in the patient's care and are able to make informed decisions.

CASE STUDY

Mr. K. G. is a thin 60-year-old man admitted to the hospital for cardiac catheterization for recurrent angina. Past medical history includes hypertension, type 2 diabetes mellitus, and a previous myocardial infarction 2 years ago. Current medications are metformin (Glucophage), glipizide (Glucotrol), enteric-coated aspirin (Ecotrin), and lisinopril (Zestril). Laboratory tests on admission revealed the following: normal electrolyte levels; blood urea nitrogen (BUN), 40 mg/dL; and serum creatinine, 2.0 mg/dL. A complete blood cell count and urinalysis were unremarkable. Mr. K. G. receives intravenous fluids at (20 mL/hr) on the morning of the procedure. He successfully undergoes the catheterization and returns to the telemetry unit. The day after the procedure, Mr. K. G.'s urine output decreases to less than 10 mL/hr. Mr. K. G. is given a fluid bolus of normal saline without any increase in urine output. Furosemide is administered intravenously, with a slight increase in urine output to 15 mL/hr for several hours. Laboratory studies reveal the following: potassium, 5.9 mEq/L; BUN, 70 mg/dL; serum creatinine, 7.1 mg/dL, and carbon dioxide total content, 16 mEq/L. The next day Mr. K. G. has 2+ edema and basilar crackles, and he complains of feeling short of breath. A preliminary diagnosis of acute renal failure is made.

QUESTIONS

1. What are possible factors predisposing Mr. K. G. for acute renal failure?
2. What laboratory studies assist in the diagnosis of acute renal failure? Describe expected results for a patient with acute tubular necrosis.
3. What medical interventions do you anticipate for Mr. K. G.?
4. What interventions could have been taken before Mr. K. G.'s cardiac catheterization to possibly prevent his acute renal failure?
5. Discuss the advantages and disadvantages of using diuretic therapy in patients with acute renal failure.

SUMMARY

The patient with acute renal failure poses many clinical challenges for health care personnel. Many of these patients have multisystem failure and require intensive and aggressive care. In addition, the development of acute renal failure is an event that often catches the patient and family unprepared. Nurses play a pivotal role in promoting positive patient outcomes through prevention, sharp assessment skills, and supportive nursing care.

CRITICAL THINKING QUESTIONS

1. Identify two strategies that the critical care nurse can use to help prevent acute renal failure.
2. Describe physical examination and laboratory findings that may be seen in patients with prerenal acute renal failure.
3. Describe patients who are at high risk for contrast-induced nephropathy and discuss medical and nursing interventions that may be used to decrease their risk.
4. You are caring for a patient with acute renal failure postoperatively. The cardiac monitor demonstrates tall, tented T waves and a PR interval of 0.26 seconds.
   a. What electrolyte imbalance do you suspect?
   b. What medical interventions do you anticipate?
   c. Describe the mechanism of action for each medical intervention.
5. What are common indications for initiating dialysis in patients with acute renal failure?

evolve Be sure to check out the bonus material, including free self-assessment exercises, on the Evolve Web site at http://evolve.elsevier.com/Sole.

REFERENCES

1. Bagshaw, S., Langenberg, C., & Bellomo R. (2006). Urinary biochemistry and microscopy in septic acute renal failure: A systematic review. *American Journal of Kidney Diseases, 48*(5), 695-705.

2. Barrett, B., & Parfrey, P. (2006). Preventing nephropathy induced by contrast medium. *New England Journal of Medicine 354*(4), 379-386.

3. Brienza, N., Malcangi, V., Dalfino, L., Trerotoli, P., Guagliardi, C., Bortone, D., et al. (2006). A comparison between fenoldopam and low-dose dopamine in early renal dysfunction of critically ill patients. *Critical Care Medicine, 34*(3), 707-714.

4. Briggs, J., Kriz, W., & Schnermann, J. (2005). Overview of kidney function and structure. In A. Greenberg (Ed.), *Primer on kidney diseases* (4th ed., pp. 2-19). Philadelphia: Saunders.

5. Cheung, A. (2005). Hemodialysis and hemofiltration. In A. Greenberg (Ed.), *Primer on kidney diseases* (4th ed., pp. 464-476). Philadelphia: Saunders.

6. Cho, K., & Chertow, G. (2005). Management of acute renal failure. In A. Greenberg (Ed.), *Primer on kidney diseases* (4th ed., pp. 315-323). Philadelphia: Saunders.

7. Coffman, T. (2005). Kidney failure due to therapeutic agents. In A. Greenberg (Ed.), *Primer on kidney diseases* (4th ed., pp. 293-300). Philadelphia: Saunders.

8. Davis, A. (2006). The use of loop diuretics in acute renal failure in critically ill patients to reduce mortality, maintain renal function, or avoid the requirements for renal support. *Emergency Medicine Journal, 23*(7), 560-570.

9. Detrenis, S., Meschi, M., Bertolini, L., & Savazzi, G. (2007). Contrast medium administration in the elderly patient: Is advancing age an independent risk factor for contrast nephropathy after angiographic procedures? *Journal of Vascular Interventional Radiology, 18*(2), 177-185.

10. Duffield, J., & Bonventre, J. (2005). Acute renal failure: Bench to bedside. In B. Pereira, M. Sayegh, & P. Blake (Eds.), *Chronic kidney disease, dialysis & transplantation: A companion to Brenner & Rector's the kidney* (2nd ed., pp. 765-786). Philadelphia: Saunders.

11. Gabriel, P., Nascimento, G., Caramori, J., Martim, L., Barretti, P., & Balbi, A. (2006). Peritoneal dialysis in acute renal failure. *Renal Failure, 28*(6), 451-456.

12. Gokal, R., & Hutchison, A. (2005). Peritoneal dialysis. In A. Greenberg (Ed.), *Primer on kidney diseases* (4th ed., pp. 477-488). Philadelphia: Saunders.

13. Greenberg, A. (2005). Urinalysis. In A. Greenberg (Ed.), *Primer on kidney diseases* (4th ed., pp. 26-35). Philadelphia: Saunders.

14. Higgins, T., Mindell, H., & Fairbank, J. (2005). Kidney imaging techniques. In A. Greenberg (Ed.), *Primer on kidney diseases* (4th ed., pp. 47-57). Philadelphia: Saunders.

15. Hilton, R. (2006). Acute renal failure. *British Medical Journal, 333*(7572), 786-790.

16. Himmelfarb, J., Dember, L., & Dixon, B. (2005). Vascular access. In B. Pereira, M. Sayegh, & P. Blake (Eds.), *Chronic kidney disease, dialysis & transplantation: A companion to Brenner & Rector's the kidney* (2nd ed., pp. 341-362). Philadelphia: Saunders.

17. Ho, K., & Sheridan, D. (2006). Meta-analysis of furosemide to prevent or treat acute renal failure. *British Medical Journal, 333*(7565), 406-407.

18. Hollander-Rodriguez, J., & Calvert, J. (2006). Hyperkalemia. *American Family Physician, 73*(2), 283-290.

19. Holley, J. (2005). Clinical approach to the diagnosis of acute renal failure. In A. Greenberg (Ed.), *Primer on kidney diseases* (4th ed., pp. 287-292). Philadelphia: Saunders.

20. Hoste, E., & Waele, J. (2005). Physiological consequences of acute renal failure on the critically ill. *Critical Care Clinics, 21*(2), 251-260.

21. Hsu, C. (2005). Clinical evaluation of kidney function. In A. Greenberg (Ed.), *Primer on kidney diseases* (4th ed., pp. 20-25). Philadelphia: Saunders.

22. Huber, W., Eckel, F., Hennig, M., Rosenbrock, H., Wacker, A., Saur, D., et al. (2006). Prophylaxis of contrast material-induced nephropathy in patients in intensive care: Acetylcysteine, theophylline, or both? A randomized study. *Radiology, 239*(3), 793-804.

23. Ix, J., & Lingappa, V. (2006). Renal disease. In S. McPhee, & W. Ganong (Eds.), *Pathophysiology of disease: An introduction to clinical medicine* (5th ed., pp. 456-481). New York: Lange Medical Books/McGraw-Hill.

24. Klenzak, J., & Himmelfarb, J. (2005). Sepsis and the kidney. *Critical Care Clinics, 21*(2), 211-222.

25. Klouche, K., Amigues, L., Deleuse, S., Beraud, J., Canaud, B. (2007). Complications, effects on dialysis dose, and survival of tunneled femoral dialysis catheters in acute renal failure. *American Journal of Kidney Diseases, 49*(1), 99-108.

26. Kopple, J. (2007). Dietary considerations in patients with chronic renal failure, acute renal failure, and transplantation. In R. Schrier (Ed.), *Diseases of the kidney and urinary tract* (8th ed., pp. 2737-2746). Philadelphia: Lippincott Williams & Wilkins.

27. Lafayette, R., & Hladunewich, M. (2005). Pharmacologic interventions in acute renal failure. In B. Pereira, M. Sayegh, & P. Blake (Eds.), *Chronic kidney disease, dialysis & transplantation: A companion to Brenner & Rector's the kidney* (2nd ed., pp. 787-806). Philadelphia: Saunders.

28. Lameire, N. (2005). The pathophysiology of acute renal failure. *Critical Care Clinics, 21*(2), 197-210.

29. Liangos, O., Pereira, B., & Jaber, B. (2005). Acute complications associated with hemodialysis. In B. Pereira, M. Sayegh, & P. Blake (Eds.), *Chronic kidney disease, dialysis & transplantation: A companion to Brenner & Rector's the kidney* (2nd ed., pp. 451-471). Philadelphia: Saunders.

30. Liu, K., Matthay, M., & Chertow, G. (2006). Evolving practices in critical care and potential implications for management of acute kidney injury. *Clinical Journal of the American Society of Nephrology, 1*(4), 869-873.

31. Matzke, G. (2005). Principles of drug therapy in kidney failure. In A. Greenberg (Ed.), *Primer on kidney diseases* (4th ed., pp. 331-337). Philadelphia: Saunders.

32. McCullough, P., Adam, A., Becker, CR., Davidson, C., Lameire, N., Stacul, F., et al. (2006). Epidemiology and prognostic implications of contrast-induced nephropathy. *American Journal of Cardiology, 98*(6A), 5K-13K.

33. McCullough, P., & Soman, S. (2005). Contrast-induced nephropathy. *Critical Care Clinics, 21*(2), 261-280.

34. Morelli, A., Ricci, Z., Bellomo, R., Ronco, C., Rocco, M., Conti, G., et al. (2005). Prophylactic fenoldopam for renal protection in sepsis: A randomized, double-blind, placebo-controlled pilot trial. *Critical Care Medicine, 33*(11), 2451-2456.

35. Needham, E. (2005). Management of acute renal failure. *American Family Physician, 72*(9), 1739-1746.

36. O'Reilly, P., & Tolwani, A. (2005). Renal replacement therapy III: IHD, CRRT, SLED. *Critical Care Clinics, 21*(2), 367-378.

37. Pannu, N., Wiebe, N., & Tonelli, M. (2006). Prophylaxis strategies for contrast-induced nephropathy. *Journal of the American Medical Association, 295*(23), 2765-2779.

38. Pavelsky, P. (2005). Renal replacement therapy I: Indications and timing. *Critical Care Clinics, 21*(2), 347-356.

39. Safirstein, R. (2005). Pathophysiology of acute renal failure. In A. Greenberg (Ed.), *Primer on kidney diseases* (4th ed., pp. 280-286). Philadelphia: Saunders.

40. Schenarts, P., Sagraves, S., Bard, M., Toschlog E., Goettler, C., Newell, M., et al. (2006). Low-dose dopamine: A physiologically based review. *Current Surgery, 63*(3), 219-225.

41. Schrier, R. (2006). Urinary indices and microscopy in sepsis-related acute renal failure. *American Journal of Kidney Diseases, 48*(5), 838-841.

42. Schrier, R., & Wang, W. (2004). Acute renal failure and sepsis. *New England Journal of Medicine, 351*(2), 159-169.

43. Stacul, F., Adam, A., Becker, C., Davidson, C., Lameire, N., McCullough, R., et al. (2006). Strategies to reduce the risk of contrast-induced nephropathy. *American Journal of Cardiology, 98*(6A), 59K-77K.

44. Stevens, L., Coresh, J., Greene, T., & Levey, A. (2006). Assessing kidney function: Measured and estimated glomerular filtration rate. *New England Journal of Medicine, 354*(23), 2473-2483.

45. Subramanian, S., & Ziedalski, T. (2005). Oliguria, volume overload, Na$^+$ balance, and diuretics. *Critical Care Clinics, 21*(2), 291-303.

46. Szerlip, H. (2005). Metabolic acidosis. In A. Greenberg (Ed.), *Primer on kidney diseases* (4th ed., pp. 74-89). Philadelphia: Saunders.

47. Szeto, C., & Kam-Tao, P. (2005). Peritoneal dialysis-related infections. In B. Pereira, M. Sayegh, & P. Blake (Eds.), *Chronic kidney disease, dialysis & transplantation: A companion to Brenner & Rector's the kidney* (2nd ed., pp. 569-587). Philadelphia: Saunders.

48. Taber, S., & Mueller, B. (2006). Drug-associated renal dysfunction. *Critical Care Clinics, 22*(2), 357-384.

49. Teehan, G., Mehta, R., & Chertow, G. (2005). Dialytic management for acute renal failure. In B. Pereira, M. Sayegh, & P. Blake (Eds.), *Chronic kidney disease, dialysis & transplantation: A companion to Brenner & Rector's the kidney* (2nd ed., pp. 807-822). Philadelphia: Saunders.

50. Tumlin, J., Stacul, F., Adam, A., Becker, C., Davidson, C., Lameire, N., et al. (2006). Pathophysiology of contrast-induced nephropathy. *American Journal of Cardiology, 98*(6A), 14K-20K.

51. Watnick, S. (2007). Kidney. In S. McPhee., M. Papadakis., & L. Tierney (Eds.), *2007 Current Medical Diagnosis & Treatment* (46th ed., pp. 918-953). New York: McGraw Hill.

52. Yeun, J., & Depner, T. (2005). Principles of hemodialysis. In B. Pereira, M. Sayegh, & P. Blake (Eds.), *Chronic kidney disease, dialysis & transplantation: A companion to Brenner & Rector's the kidney* (2nd ed., pp. 307-340). Philadelphia: Saunders.

53. Ympa, Y., Sakr, Y., Reinhart, K., & Vincent, J. (2005). Has mortality from acute renal failure decreased? A systematic review of the literature. *The American Journal of Medicine, 118*(8), 827-832.

54. Yuan, F., & Anderson, S. (2005). The kidney in aging. In A. Greenberg (Ed.), *Primer on kidney diseases* (4th ed., pp. 436-443). Philadelphia: Saunders.

55. Zagler, A., Azadpour, M., Mercado, C., Hennekens, C. (2005). N-acetylcysteine and contrast-induced nephropathy: A meta-analysis of 13 randomized trials. *American Heart Journal, 151*(1), 140-145.

CHAPTER 16

Hematological and Immune Disorders

Patricia B. Wolff, MSN, APRN, BC, AOCNS

INTRODUCTION

Hematological and immunological functions are necessary for gas exchange, tissue perfusion, nutrition, acid-base balance, protection against infection, and hemostasis. These complex, integrated responses are easily disrupted, and most critically ill patients experience some abnormalities in hematological and immune function. This chapter provides a general overview of the pertinent anatomy and physiology of these organ systems and the typical alterations in red blood cells (RBCs), immune activity, and coagulation function. Table 16-1 defines key terms used in this chapter in describing hematological and immunological disorders. The text provides guidelines for assessment and nursing care strategies needed by beginning critical care nurses caring for patients at risk for these disorders.

REVIEW OF ANATOMY AND PHYSIOLOGY

Hematopoiesis

Hematopoiesis is defined as the formation and maturation of blood cells. The primary site of hematopoietic cell production is the bone marrow; however, secondary hematopoietic organs that participate in this process include the spleen, liver, thymus, lymphatic system, and lymphoid tissues. Negative feedback mechanisms within the body induce the bone marrow's pluripotent hematopoietic stem cells to differentiate into one of the three blood cells: erythrocytes (RBCs), leukocytes (white blood cells [WBCs]), or thrombocytes (platelets)[16] (Figure 16-1).

In infancy, most bones are filled with blood-forming red marrow; in adulthood, productive bone marrow is found in the vertebrae, skull, mandible, thoracic cage, shoulder, pelvis, femora, and humeri.[16] The hematopoietic and immunological organs and their key functions are summarized in Figure 16-2.

Effects of Aging

Aging affects several aspects of both hematological and immune systems. For example, elderly individuals have a greater risk of infection related to alterations in immunoglobulin levels. Changes in bone marrow reserve, immune function, lean body mass, hepatic function, and renal function contribute to the challenges of caring for this rapidly expanding, vulnerable population. These changes and implications are described in the Geriatric Considerations feature.

Components and Characteristics of Blood

Blood was recognized as being essential to life as early as the 1600s, but the specific composition and characteristics of blood were not defined until the twentieth century. Blood has four major components: (1) a fluid component called plasma, (2) circulating solutes such as ions, (3) serum proteins, and (4) cells. Plasma comprises about 55% of blood volume and is the transportation medium for important serum proteins such as albumin, globulin, fibrinogen, prothrombin, and plasminogen. The hematopoietic cells comprise the remaining 45% of blood volume. Characteristics of blood and potential alterations that may be encountered in critically ill patients are shown in Table 16-2.[16]

TABLE 16-1   Hematology-Immunology Key Terms

Term	Definition
Active immunity	A term used when the body actively produces cells and mediators that result in the destruction of the antigen
Anemia	A reduction in the number of circulating red blood cells or hemoglobin that leads to inadequate oxygenation of tissues. Subtypes named by etiology (e.g., aplastic anemia means "without cells") or by cell appearance (e.g., macrocytic anemia has large cells)
Antibody	Immune globulin, created by specific lymphocytes, and designed to immunologically destroy a specific foreign antigen
Anticoagulants	Factors inhibiting the clotting process
Antigen	Any substance that is capable of stimulating an immune response in the host
Autoimmunity	Situation in which the body abnormally sees self as nonself, and an immune response is activated against those tissues
Bone marrow	Replacement of a defective bone marrow with one that is functional; described in transplant terms of the source (e.g., autologous comes from self, and allogeneic comes from another person)
Cellular immunity	Production of cytokines in response to foreign antigen
Coagulation pathway	A predetermined cascade of coagulation proteins that are stimulated by production of the platelet plug, and occurs progressively, producing a fibrin clot; there are two pathways (intrinsic and extrinsic) triggered by different events that merge into a single list of events leading to a fibrin clot; clotting may be initiated by either or both pathways
Coagulopathy	Disorder of normal clotting mechanisms; usually used to describe inappropriate bleeding more often than excess clotting, but can refer to either one
Cytokines	Cell killer substances, or mediators secreted by white blood cells; when secreted by a lymphocyte, also called lymphokine, and secretions from monocytes are called monokines
Disseminated	Disorder of hemostasis characterized by exaggerated microvascular coagulation and intravascular depletion of clotting factors, with subsequent bleeding, also called consumption coagulation coagulopathy
Ecchymosis	Blue or purplish hemorrhagic spot on skin or mucous membrane, round or irregular, nonelevated
Epistaxis	Bleeding from the nose
Erythrocyte	Red blood cell
Fibrinolysis	Breakdown of fibrin clots that naturally occurs 1-3 days after clot development
Hemarthrosis	Blood in a joint cavity
Hematemesis	Bloody emesis
Hematochezia	Blood in stool; bright red
Hematoma	Raised, hardened mass indicative of blood vessel rupture and clotting beneath the skin surface; if subcutaneous, appears as a blue-purple or purple-black area; may occur in spaces such as pleural or retroperitoneal area
Hematopoiesis	Development of the early blood cells (erythrocytes, leukocytes, thrombocytes), encompassing their maturation in the bone marrow or lymphoreticular organs
Hematuria	Blood in the urine
Hemoglobinuria	Hemoglobin in the urine
Hemoptysis	Coughing up blood from the airways or lungs
Hemorrhage	Copious, active bleeding

TABLE 16-1   Hematology-Immunology Key Terms—cont'd

Term	Definition
Hemostasis	A physiological process involving hematological and nonhematological factors to form a platelet or fibrin clot to control the loss of blood
Human immunodeficiency virus	A retrovirus that transcribes its RNA-containing genetic material into DNA of the host cell nucleus; this virus has a propensity for the immune cells, replacing the RNA of lymphocytes and macrophages, causing an immunodeficient state
Humoral immunity	Production of antibodies in response to foreign proteins
Immunocompromised	Quantitative or qualitative defects in white blood cells or immune physiology; defect may be congenital or acquired and involve a single element or multiple processes; immune incompetence leads to lack of normal inflammatory, phagocytic, antibody, or cytokine responses
Immunoglobulin	A specific type of antibody named by its molecular structure (e.g., immunoglobulin A or immunoglobulin against cytomegalovirus)
Leukocyte	General word encompassing white blood cells; made up of three major subtypes: granulocytes (neutrophils, basophils, eosinophils), lymphocytes, and monocytes
Lymphoreticular system	Cells and organs containing immunologically active cells
Macrophage	Differentiated monocyte that migrates to lymphoreticular tissues of the body
Melena	Blood pigments in stool; dark or black
Menorrhagia	Excessive bleeding during menstruation
Neutropenia	Serum neutrophil count lower than normal; predisposes patients to infection
Passive immunity	A situation in which antibodies against a specific disease are transferred from another person
Petechiae	Small, red or purple, nonelevated dots indicative of capillary rupture, often located in areas of increased pressure (e.g., feet or back), or on the chest and trunk
Primary immunodeficiency	Congenital disorders in which some part of the immune system fails to develop
Procoagulants	Factors enhancing clotting mechanisms
Purpura	Large, mottled bruises
Reticulocytes	Slightly immature erythrocytes able to continue some essential functions of red blood cells
Secondary or acquired immunodeficiency	Immune disorder resulting from factors outside the immune system and involving the loss of a previously functional immune defense
Thrombocyte	Platelet
Thrombocytopenia	Serum platelet count less than normal. Predisposes individuals to bleeding as a result of inadequate platelet plugs
Thrombosis	Creation of clots; usually refers to excess clotting
Tissue anergy	Absence of a "wheal" tissue response to antigens and evidence of altered antibody capabilities
Tolerance	The body's ability to recognize self as self and therefore mount a rejection response against nonself, but not itself
Transfusion	Intravenous infusion of blood or blood products

Hematopoietic Cells

Erythrocytes

Erythrocytes (RBCs) are flexible biconcave disks without nuclei whose primary component is an oxygen-carrying molecule called hemoglobin. This physiological configuration permits RBCs to travel at high speeds and to perfuse small blood vessels, exposing more surface area for gas exchange. In each microliter of blood, there are approximately 5 million RBCs.[16]

RBCs are generated from precursor stem cells under the influence of a growth factor called *erythropoietin*.

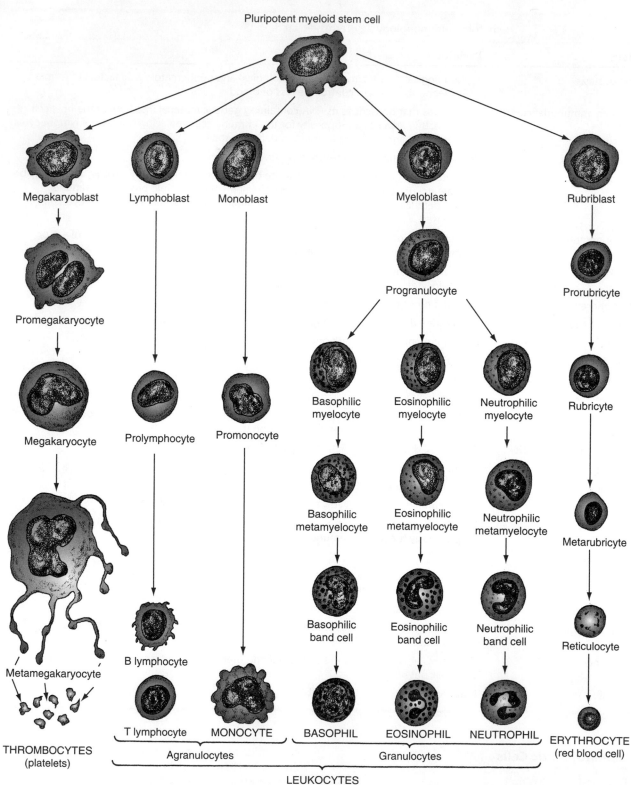

FIGURE 16-1. Hematopoietic stem cell and lineage.

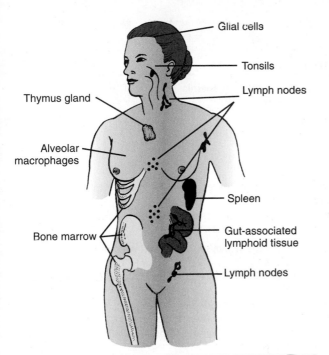

Organ	Key Functions
Spleen	The spleen is a highly vascular organ involved in the production of lymphocytes; the filtering and destruction of erythrocytes; the filtering and trapping of foreign matter, including bacteria and viruses; and the storage of blood. Although it is not necessary for survival, the spleen plays an important role in hemostasis and protection against infection.
Liver	The liver produces clotting factors, produces bile from RBC breakdown, and detoxifies many substances in the blood; its proper functioning is essential for normal hemostasis and metabolism. The liver filters and stores blood in addition to its many other metabolic functions.
Thymus gland	The thymus gland and lymph nodes are also part of the hematopoietic system; they are primarily involved in immunological functions.
Bone marrow	Site of production for all hematopoietic cells.
Tonsils, glial cells, alveolar macrophages, gut-associated lymphoid tissue	Lymphoid tissue responsive to antigens passing the initial barrier defenses, and possessing some inflammatory properties.
Lymph nodes	Storage site for lymphocytes. Part of the continuous lymphatic system that filters foreign matter.

FIGURE 16-1. Hematopoietic organs and their function. (Modified from Black, J. M., & Hawks, J. H. [Eds.] [2009], Medical-surgical nursing: Clinical management for positive outcomes [8th ed.]. Philadelphia: Saunders.)

GERIATRIC CONSIDERATIONS

AGE-RELATED CHANGES	IMPLICATIONS
Decreased percentage of marrow space occupied by hematopoietic tissue	Ineffective erythropoiesis, especially after blood loss
Decreased number of T cells produced	Delayed hypersensitivity
Decreased T-cell function	Increased incidence of infection
Appearance of autoimmune antibodies	Increased risk of autoimmune disorders
Increased IgA and decreased IgG levels	Increased prevalence of infection

IgA, Immunoglobulin A; *IgG*, immunoglobulin G.

Erythropoietin is secreted by the kidney in response to a perceived decrease in perfusion or tissue hypoxia. Maturation of RBCs takes 4 to 5 days, and their life span is about 120 days. *Reticulocytes* are immature RBCs that may be released when there is a demand for RBCs that exceeds the number of available mature cells. Reticulocytes are active but less effective than mature cells and circulate about 24 hours before maturing. The spleen and liver are important for removal and clearance of senescent RBCs.[16]

The RBC transports *hemoglobin*, whose function is the transport of oxygen and carbon dioxide. Hemoglobin binds with oxygen in the lungs and transports it to the tissues. The rate of erythrocyte production increases when oxygen transport to tissues is impaired, and it decreases when tissues are hypertransfused or exposed to high oxygen tension. The oxygen affinity for hemoglobin is modulated primarily by the concentration of 2,3-diphosphoglycerate (2,3-DPG) and depends on the blood pH and body temperature. Erythrocytes are also vital in the maintenance of acid-base balance because they transport carbon dioxide away from the tissues.[2]

Platelets

Platelets, or *thrombocytes*, are the smallest of the formed elements of the blood. A normal platelet count ranges from 150,000 to 400,000 per microliter of blood. Platelets are created by hematopoietic stem cells in response to hormonal stimulation. Platelets have a life span of 8 to 11 days, but they may be used more rapidly if there are many vascular injuries or clotting stimuli. Two thirds of the platelets circulate in the blood. The spleen stores the remaining third and may become enlarged if excess or rapid platelet removal

TABLE 16-2   Characteristics of Blood

Characteristic	Normal	Alterations
Color	Arterial: bright red Venous: dark red or crimson	Hypochromic (light color) in anemia Lighter color in dilution
pH	Arterial: 7.35-7.45	<7.35 acidosis >7.45 alkalosis
Specific gravity	Plasma: 1.026 Red blood cells: 1.093	— —
Viscosity	3.5-4.5 times that of water	Loss of plasma volume or increased cell production increases viscosity Abnormal immunoglobulin such as multiple myeloma increases viscosity
Volume	Plasma volume 45 mL/kg Cell volume 30 mL/kg Average male about 5000 mL	Fat tissue contains little water, so total blood volume best correlates to lean body mass Women have more fat, and therefore blood volume is usually lower than in men Plasma volume rises with progression of pregnancy Volume increases with immobility and decreases with prolonged standing. May be result of changes in pressure in glomerulus and glomerular filtration rate Blood volume highest in neonate and lowest in elderly Lack of nutrients causes decreased red blood cell and plasma formation Increased environmental temperature increases blood volume

occurs. In patients who have had a splenectomy, 100% of the platelets remain in circulation.[11,16]

Platelets are the first responders in the clotting response, and they form a platelet plug that temporarily repairs an injured vessel. During circulation they detect and adhere to roughened or sheared surfaces, such as blood vessel walls or indwelling catheters. Platelets also release mediators necessary for completion of clotting. Mediators include histamine and serotonin, which contribute to vasospasm; adenosine diphosphate, which assists platelet adhesion and aggregation; and calcium and phospholipids, which are necessary for clotting.[16,21]

Leukocytes

Leukocytes (WBCs) are larger and less numerous than RBCs and have nuclei. The average number of WBCs ranges from 5000 to 10,000 per microliter of blood in the adult. Leukocytes are derived from hematopoietic stem cells that are stimulated by a triggering mechanism within the immunological response. Cells vary in appearance, function, storage site, and life span. Specific characteristics of cell development and life cycle are shown in Table 16-3.

Leukocytes are released into the bloodstream for transport to the tissues, where they perform specific functions.[16] WBCs play a key role in the defense against infectious organisms and foreign antigens. They produce and transport factors such as antibodies that are vital in maintaining immunity. Although they possess a variety of unique and specialized functions, WBCs work in an integrated fashion to protect the body. Numbers of WBCs are increased in circumstances of inflammation, tissue injury, allergy, or invasion with pathogenic organisms. Their numbers are diminished in malnutrition, advancing age, and immune diseases.[12,15]

WBCs are classified according to their structure (granulocytes or agranulocytes), function (phagocytes or immunocytes), and affinity for certain dyes. The *granulocytes* (or *polymorphonuclear leukocytes*) include neutrophils, basophils, and eosinophils, and all function in phagocytosis. The *agranulocytes* consist of *monocytes* (phagocytes) and *lymphocytes* (immunocytes).[16]

Granular Leukocytes

Neutrophils. Neutrophils are the most numerous of the granulocytes, constituting 57% to 67% of the

TABLE 16-3   Overview of Leukocytes

Cell Type	Characteristics	Development and Migration	Life Span
Granulocytes			
Polymorphonuclear leukocytes (polys)	Large granules and horseshoe-shaped nuclei that differentiate and become multilobed	Mature in the bone marrow Maturing granulocytes that are no longer dividing, accumulate as a reserve in the bone marrow Normally about a 5-day supply in the bone marrow	Average of 12 hours in the circulation About 2 to 3 days in the tissues
Neutrophils	Have small, fine, light pink or lilac acidophilic granules stained and a segmented, irregularly lobed, purple nucleus		
Band neutrophils	Bands less well defined, because they are slightly immature forms of the same cell		
Eosinophils	Have large, round granules that contain red-staining basic mucopolysaccharides and multilobed purple-blue nuclei		
Basophils	Coarse blue granules conceal the segmented nucleus Granules contain histamine, heparin, and acid mucopolysaccharides		
Agranulocytes			
Lymphocytes	Small cell with a large, round, deep-staining, single-lobed nucleus and very little cytoplasm Cytoplasm slightly basophilic and stains pale blue	T lymphocytes constantly circulate, following a path from the blood to the lymphatic tissue, through the lymphatic channels, and back to the blood through the thoracic duct B lymphocytes largely noncirculating; remain mainly in the lymphoid tissue and may differentiate into plasma cells	Life span varies Small populations of memory lymphocytes survive for many years Most T lymphocytes of the peripheral lymphatic tissue recirculate about every 10 hours Mature plasma cells have a survival rate of about 2 to 3 days
Monocytes	Large cell with a prominent, multishaped nucleus that is sometimes kidney shaped Chromatin in the nucleus looks like lace, with small particles linked together like strands Blue-gray cytoplasm filled with many fine lysozymes that stain pink with Wright's stain	Monocytes spend less time in the bone marrow pool than granulocytes	Circulation about 36 hours After the monocyte is transformed into macrophage in the tissues, life span ranges from months to years

WBC differential count.[16] The differential count measures the percentage of each type of WBC present in the venous blood sample. These cells are further broken down into segmented neutrophils, in which filaments in the cell give the nuclei an appearance of having lobes, and band neutrophils, which are immature and have a thicker or U-shaped nucleus. Normally, segmented neutrophils make up the majority of WBCs, whereas band neutrophils constitute only about 5%.[4] The phrase *a shift to the left* refers to an increased number of "bands," or band neutrophils, compared with mature neutrophils on a complete blood count (CBC) report. This finding generally indicates an acute bacterial infectious process that draws on the WBC reserves in the bone marrow and causes less mature forms to be released. Likewise, a *shift to the right* indicates an increased number of circulating mature cells and may be associated with liver disease, Down syndrome, and megaloblastic and pernicious anemia.[4,15]

The survival time of neutrophils is short. Once released from the bone marrow, they circulate in the blood less than 24 hours before migrating to the tissues, where they live another few days. When serious infection is present, neutrophils may live only hours while they phagocytize infectious organisms.[16,21] Because of this short life span, drugs that affect rapidly multiplying cells (e.g., chemotherapeutic agents) quickly decrease the neutrophil count and alter the patient's ability to fight infection.

Eosinophils. Eosinophils are larger than neutrophils and make up 1% to 4% of the WBC count.[16] They are important in the defense against allergens and parasites, and are thought to be involved in the detoxification of foreign proteins. Eosinophils are found largely in the tissues of the skin, lung, and gastrointestinal tract. Eosinophils respond to chemotactic mechanisms triggering them to participate in phagocytosis, but they also contain bactericidal substances and lysosomal enzymes that aid in the destruction of invading organisms.[15,21]

Basophils. The third type of granulocyte is the basophil, which has large granules that contain heparin, serotonin, and histamine. Basophils participate in the body's inflammatory and allergic responses by releasing these substances. Basophils, which constitute up to 0.75% of the WBC differential, play an important role in acute systemic allergic reactions and inflammatory responses.[16]

Nongranular Leukocytes (Agranulocytes)

Monocytes. Monocytes are the largest of the leukocytes and constitute only 3% to 7% of the WBC differential.[4,16] Once they migrate from the bloodstream into the tissues, monocytes mature into tissue macrophages, which are powerful phagocytes. In the lung, these tissue macrophages are known as alveolar macrophages; in the liver, they are Kupffer's cells; in connective tissue, they are histiocytes. In addition to "eating" large foreign particles and cell fragments, macrophages are vital in the phagocytosis of necrotic tissue and debris. Like eosinophils, macrophages contain lysosomal enzymes and bactericidal substances. When activated by antigens, macrophages secrete substances called monokines that act as chemical communicators between the cells involved in the immune response. Although monocytes may circulate for only 36 hours, they can survive for months or even years as tissue macrophages.[16,21]

Lymphocytes. In the adult, approximately 25% to 33% of the total WBCs are lymphocytes.[4,16] Lymphocytes circulate in and out of tissues and may live days or years, depending on their type. They contribute to the body's defense against microorganisms, but they are also essential for tumor immunity (surveillance for abnormal cells), delayed hypersensitivity reactions, autoimmune diseases, and foreign tissue rejection. Lymphocytes are responsible for specific immune responses and participate in two types of immunity: *humoral immunity*, which is mediated by B lymphocytes; and *cellular immunity*, which is mediated by T lymphocytes. B lymphocytes, or B cells, originate in the bone marrow and are also thought to mature there. B cells perform in antibody production. T cells are produced in the bone marrow, but they migrate to the thymus for maturation; then most travel and reside in lymphoid tissues throughout the body. They live longer than B cells and participate in long-term immunity. The natural killer cell is a third type of lymphocyte thought to be a differentiated form of the T lymphocyte. It is responsible for surveillance and destruction of virus-infected and malignant cells. T-cell functions include delayed hypersensitivity, graft rejection, graft-versus-host reaction, defense against intracellular organisms, and defense against neoplasms.[20]

Immune Anatomy

Immune activity involves an integrated, multilevel response against invading pathogens. It requires both WBCs of the hematopoietic system and the secondary hematopoietic organs, also termed the *lymphoreticular system*. The lymphoreticular system consists of lymphoid tissue, lymphatic channels and nodes, and phagocytic cells, which engulf and process foreign materials (see Figure 16-2).

The body's ability to resist and fight infection is termed *immunity*. Our bodies are constantly exposed to normal and unusual microorganisms that are capable of causing disease. The healthy person's immune system recognizes potential pathogens and destroys them before tissue invasion can occur;

however, the person with a dysfunctional immune system is at risk of overwhelming, life-threatening infection.

Immune Physiology

The immune response protects the body from disease by recognizing, processing, and destroying foreign invaders. It aids in the removal of damaged cells and defends the body against the proliferation of abnormal or malignant cells. Key terms related to immune physiology are defined in Table 16-1.

The recognition and destruction of nonself molecules called *antigens* are the key triggering activities of the immune system. Microorganisms (e.g., bacteria, viruses, fungi, and parasites), abnormal or mutated cells, transplanted cells, nonself protein molecules (e.g., vaccines), and nonhuman molecules (e.g., penicillin) can act as antigens. These antigens are detected by the body as foreign, or nonself, and are destroyed by immunological processes. The body's response to an antigen is determined by factors such as genetics, amount of antigen, and route of exposure. In autoimmunity, the body abnormally sees self as nonself (i.e., it has no tolerance), and an immune response is activated against those tissues. Autoimmunity can result from injury to tissues, infection, or malignancy, although in many cases the cause is not known. An example of an autoimmune disease is systemic lupus erythematosus.[19,20]

An intact and healthy immune system consists of both natural (nonspecific) defenses and acquired (specific) defenses. The nonspecific defenses are the first line of protection and include the processes of inflammation and phagocytosis. When nonspecific mechanisms fail to protect the body from invasion, the specific defenses of humoral and cellular immunity are put into action. *Active immunity* is a term used when the body actively produces cells and mediators that result in the destruction of the antigen. *Passive immunity* is that which is transferred from another person (e.g., maternal antibodies transferred to the newborn through the placenta and breast milk).[21]

Nonspecific Defenses

The body's nonspecific defenses consist of the physical and chemical barriers to invasion, the protective and repairing processes of inflammation and phagocytosis, and other substances that stimulate the body to fight back. The body's first line of defense against infection consists of physical and chemical barriers.

Epithelial Surfaces. The epithelial surfaces are those that are exposed to the environment. Intact skin and mucous membranes provide a protective covering; they also secrete substances that have antimicrobial effects. For example, sweat glands produce an antimicrobial enzyme, lysozyme; and sebaceous glands secrete sebum, which has antimicrobial and antifungal properties. The skin constantly exfoliates, a process that sloughs off bacterial and chemical hazards. These same epithelial surfaces are colonized by "normal" bacterial flora. These normal flora help to protect the body from microorganisms by occupying space on the epithelium, which prevents pathogen attachment.

Epithelial surfaces also have unique physical and chemical properties protecting them from pathogen invasion. For example, mucus and cilia work together to trap and remove harmful substances in the respiratory tract. The motility of the intestines maintains an even distribution of bacterial flora, thereby preventing overgrowth or invasion of pathogens, and promotes evacuation of harmful microbes. Chemical barriers to pathogenic entry include the unique pH of the skin and mucosa of the gastrointestinal and urinary tracts. This pH inhibits the growth of many microorganisms. Immunoglobulin A (IgA, also called *secretory IgA*) and phagocytic cells are biological factors present in respiratory and gastrointestinal secretions. They are essential for destruction of particular pyogenic bacteria.[21]

Inflammation and Phagocytosis. The second line of defense involves the processes of inflammation and phagocytosis. Inflammation is initiated by cellular injury, is necessary for tissue repair, and is harmful when uncontrolled. When cellular injury occurs, a process called *chemotaxis* generates both a mediator and a neutrophil response. Mediator substances (histamine, serotonin, kinins, lysosomal enzymes, prostaglandin, platelet-activating factor, clotting factors, and complement proteins) are released at the site of injury. These mediators cause vasodilation, increase blood flow, induce capillary permeability, and promote chemotaxis and phagocytosis by neutrophils. Inflammatory symptoms such as redness, heat, pain, and swelling are sequelae of these responses. Complement proteins enhance the antibody activity, phagocytosis, and inflammation.[21]

Neutrophils are attracted to and migrate to areas of inflammation or bacterial invasion, where they ingest and kill invading microorganisms by phagocytosis. The inflammatory response is a rapid process initiated by granulocytes and macrophages, with granulocytes arriving within minutes of cellular injury. Once phagocytes have been attracted to an area by the release of mediators, a process called opsonization occurs, in which antibody and complement proteins attach to the target cell and enhance the phagocyte's ability to engulf the target cell. Once the bacteria have been engulfed, they are killed and digested within the cell by lysosomal enzymes.

Exudate formation at the inflammatory site has three functions: dilute toxins produced, deliver proteins and leukocytes to the site, and carry away toxins and debris.[21]

When infectious organisms escape the local phagocytic responses, they may be engulfed and destroyed in a similar fashion by the tissue macrophages within the lymphoreticular organs. The portal circulation of the spleen and liver filters the majority of blood, where infectious organisms can be removed before infecting the tissues. In the lymphatic system, pathogenic substances are filtered by the lymph nodes and are phagocytized by tissue macrophages. Here they may also stimulate immune responses by the lymphoid cells.

Other Nonspecific Defenses. Another nonspecific defensive activity is the release of cytokines and chemokines from WBCs, and are either proinflammatory, antiinflammatory, or both. These naturally occurring biological response modifiers, which include interleukins (ILs), tumor necrosis factor, colony-stimulating factors, monoclonal antibodies, and interferons (IFNs), mediate various interactions between immune system cells.[21,22] At least 30 human ILs have been identified. IL-1 is a proinflammatory cytokine that increases body temperature in infection (endogenous pyrogen), thereby inhibiting the growth of temperature-sensitive pathogens. IL-1 also activates phagocytes and lymphocytes, and acts as a growth factor for many cells. The IFNs have antitumor and antiviral activity and include 20 subtypes of IFN-alpha, two subtypes of IFN-beta, and IFN-gamma.[23] Through recombinant DNA technology, IFNs and other naturally occurring substances can be produced synthetically for the treatment of many disorders. IFNs, colony-stimulating factors, and monoclonal antibodies are some examples of biological therapies currently approved for the treatment of certain malignant disorders.[23]

Specific Defenses

Specificity refers to the finding that an immune response stimulates cells to develop immunity for a specific antigen. Two types of specific immune responses exist: humoral immunity and cell-mediated immunity. They are not mutually exclusive but act together to provide immunity.

Humoral Immunity. Humoral immunity is mediated by B lymphocytes and involves the formation of antibodies (immunoglobulins) in response to specific antigens that bind to their receptor sites. Antigen binding activates B-lymphocyte differentiation into plasma cells that produce specific antibodies in response to those antigens. Five classes of immunoglobulins exist: IgG, IgM, IgA, IgE, and IgD. The clinical features and abnormalities associated with these immunoglobulins are described in Table 16-4.[21]

Once antibodies have been synthesized and released, they bind to their specific antigen and form an antigen-antibody complex that activates phagocytosis and complement proteins. This humoral response is regulated by the activity of T lymphocytes. Helper T cells promote B-lymphocyte activity and the production of antibodies, whereas suppressor T cells downgrade the humoral response.

The body generates both primary and secondary humoral responses. In the *primary response*, antigens that have evaded the nonspecific defenses are engulfed and processed by macrophages. The macrophages then present the processed antigens to the lymphocytes, which proliferate, differentiate, and produce antibodies. In this first exposure, antibodies of the IgM subtype appear first and predominate, while IgG immunoglobulins appear later. During this primary response, the immunoglobulins develop an immunological memory for antigens that provides the basis for the secondary response on subsequent exposure.

When any subsequent exposure to the antigen occurs, a quicker, stronger, and longer-lasting IgG-mediated *secondary response* occurs. IgG antibodies predominate and may be detectable in the serum for decades.[20]

Cell-Mediated Immunity. Cellular immunity is mediated by the T lymphocyte. Cell-mediated immunity is a more delayed reaction than the humoral response and can occur only when in direct contact with sensitized lymphocytes. It is important in viral, fungal, and intracellular infections and is the mechanism involved in transplant rejection and recognition of neoplastic cells.

Cell-mediated immunity is initiated by macrophage recognition of nonself foreign materials. The macrophages trap, process, and present such materials to T lymphocytes, which then migrate to the site of the antigen, where they complete antigen destruction. Once contact is made with a specific antigen, the T lymphocyte differentiates into helper/inducer T cells, suppressor T cells, and cytotoxic killer cells. Although these T cells are microscopically identical, they can be distinguished by proteins present on the cell surface called cluster of differentiation (CD).[20] Helper T cells (also known as T4 cells because they carry a CD4 marker) enhance the humoral immune response by stimulating B cells to differentiate and produce antibodies. Suppressor T cells downgrade and suppress the humoral and cell-mediated responses. The ratio of helper to suppressor T cells is normally 2:1, and an alteration in this ratio may cause disease.[4] For example, a depressed ratio (a decrease of helper T cells in relation to suppressor T

TABLE 16-4   Immunoglobulins

Antibody	Description	Normal Value
IgG	Most abundant immunoglobulin Major influence with bacterial disease Crosses the placenta Coats microorganisms to enhance phagocytosis Activates complement	75% of total 500-1600 mg/dL
IgM	Primary Ig response to antigen, with levels increased within 7 days of exposure Present mostly in intravascular space Causes antigenic agglutination and cell lysis via complement activation	10% of total 60-280 mg/dL
IgA	Found on mucosal surfaces of respiratory, GI, and GU systems preventing antigen adherence Influential with bacteria and some viral organisms First antibody formed with exposure to antigen but rapidly diminishes as IgG increases Does not cross the placenta, but passes to newborn through colostrum and breast milk Deficiency caused by congenital autosomal dominant or recessive disease or related to anticonvulsant use Deficiency (<5 mg/dL) manifests as chronic sinopulmonary infection	15% of total 90-450 mg/dL
IgD	Activates B lymphocytes to plasma cells, which are the key immunoglobulin-producing cells	1% of total 0.5-3 mg/dL
IgE	Attaches to mast cells and basophils on epithelial surfaces and enhances release of histamine and other vasoactive mediators responsible for the "wheal flare" reaction Important for allergic responses, inflammatory reactions, and parasitic infections	0.002% of total 0.01-0.04 mg/dL

GI, Gastrointestinal; *GU*, genitourinary; *Ig*, immunoglobulin.

cells) is found in acquired immunodeficiency syndrome (AIDS), whereas a higher ratio (a decrease in suppressor T cells in relation to helper T cells) is a feature of an autoimmune disease. Cytotoxic or killer T cells (CD8 marker) participate directly in the destruction of antigens by binding to and altering the intracellular environment, which ultimately destroys the cell. Killer cells also release cytotoxic substances into the antigen cell that cause cell lysis. Killer T cells additionally provide the body with immunosurveillance capabilities that monitor for abnormal cells or tissue. This mechanism is responsible for the rejection of transplanted tissue and the destruction of single malignant cells.[20]

Hemostasis

Hemostasis is a physiological process involving platelets, blood proteins (clotting factors), and the vasculature. This process involves the formation of blood clots to stop bleeding from injured vessels, and natural anticoagulant and fibrinolytic systems to limit clot formation. Many substances are released during tissue destruction, including collagen, proteases, and bacterial endotoxins, that may activate the clotting system. The three physiological mechanisms

known to trigger clotting in the body are tissue injury, vessel injury, and the presence of a foreign body in the bloodstream. When one of these trigger factors is present, a series of physical events occurs that results in a fibrin clot.

Although the events of hemostasis are sequential, they require integration of components from the hematopoietic and coagulation systems. Within seconds after injury, platelets are attracted to the site and adhere to the site of injury. The activated platelets then undergo changes in shape to expose receptors on their surfaces. RBCs increase the rate of platelet adherence by facilitating migration of platelets to the site and by liberating adenosine diphosphate, which enables platelets to stick to the exposed tissue (collagen). The exposed receptors on the activated platelet surfaces are capable of binding fibrinogen, an essential component underlying platelet aggregation. Serotonin and histamine are released by the adhered platelets and cause immediate constriction of the injured vessel to lessen bleeding. Vasoconstriction is followed by vasodilation, bringing the necessary cellular products of the inflammatory response to the site. With minor vessel injury, *primary hemostasis* is temporarily achieved with platelet plugs, usually within seconds. During *secondary*

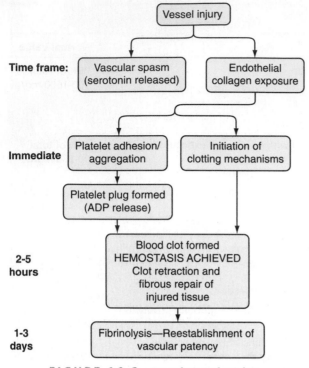

FIGURE 16-3. Coagulation physiology.

hemostasis, the platelet plug is solidified with fibrin, an end product of the coagulation pathway, and requires several minutes to reach completion (Figure 16-3).[10,16]

Coagulation Pathway

The classic theory of coagulation is viewed as occurring through two distinct pathways, *intrinsic* and *extrinsic*, which share a common "final" pathway, formation of insoluble fibrin (Figure 16-4). It is now known that the classic cascade theory of coagulation illustrates what occurs in vitro. In vivo, the primary activator of the coagulation cascade occurs via the extrinsic pathway. The intrinsic pathway serves to amplify the coagulation cascade.[13,16]

Both pathways begin with an initiating event and have a cascade sequence of clotting factor activation precipitated by a preceding reaction. The soluble clotting factors become insoluble fibrin. When blood is exposed to subendothelial collagen or is "injured," factor XII is activated, which initiates coagulation via the *intrinsic pathway*. In the *extrinsic pathway*, tissue injury precipitates release of a substance known as tissue factor, which activates factor VII. Factor VII is key in initiating blood coagulation, and the two pathways intersect at the activation of factor

X.[10,13,14] Both coagulation pathways illustrate a *final common pathway* of clot formation, retraction, and fibrinolysis.

The coagulation factors are plasma proteins that circulate as inactive enzymes, and most are synthesized in the liver. Vitamin K is necessary for synthesis of factors II, VII, IX, X, and protein C and protein S (anticoagulation factors). Thus, liver disease and vitamin K deficiency are commonly associated with impaired hemostasis.[15]

Coagulation Antagonists and Clot Lysis

Activation of the clotting factors, inhibition of these activated clotting factors, and production of circulating anticoagulant proteins maintain the balance of the coagulation processes. Normal vascular endothelium is smooth and intact, thereby preventing the collagen exposure that initiates the intrinsic clotting pathway. Rapid blood flow dilutes and disperses clotting factors. Clotting factors that are not contained within a formed clot are filtered and removed from circulation by the liver. Several plasma proteins, including antiplasmin and antithrombin III, are present to localize clotting at the site of injury. When coagulation protein levels are deficient, clotting may become inappropriately widespread, such as in disseminated intravascular coagulation (DIC). The most potent anticoagulant forces are the fibrin threads, which absorb 85% to 90% of thrombin during clot formation, and antithrombin III, which inactivates thrombin that is not contained within the clot. Heparin, which is produced in small quantities by basophils and tissue mast cells, acts as a potent anticoagulant. Heparin combines with antithrombin III to increase the effectiveness of the latter greatly. This complex removes several of the activated coagulation factors from the blood.[16]

Once blood vessel integrity has been restored via hemostasis, blood flow must be reestablished. This goal is accomplished by the fibrinolytic system, by which clots are broken down (lysed) and removed. *Fibrinolysis* occurs 1 to 3 days after clot formation and is mediated by plasmin, an enzyme that digests fibrinogen and fibrin (Figure 16-5). The plasma protein plasminogen is the inactive form of plasmin. It is incorporated into the blood clot as the clot forms, and it cannot initiate clot lysis until it is activated. Substances capable of activating plasminogen include tissue plasminogen activator, thrombin, fibrin, factor XII, lysosomal enzymes, and urokinase.[16] Thrombin and plasmin are key for the balance between coagulation and lysis. Fibrinolysis is active within the microcirculation, where it maintains the patency of the capillary beds. Larger vessels contain less plasminogen activator, a characteristic that may predispose them to clot formation.

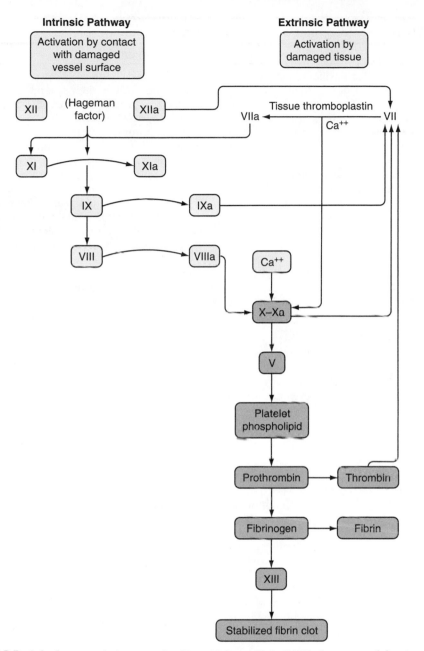

Intrinsic Pathway

Activation by contact with damaged vessel surface

Extrinsic Pathway

Activation by damaged tissue

FIGURE 16-4. Coagulation cascade. *(From McCance, K. L. [2002]. Structure and function of the hematological system. In K. L. McCance, & S. E. Huether [Eds.], Pathophysiology: The biologic basis for disease in adults and children [4th ed., p. 834]. St. Louis: Mosby.)*

When plasmin digests fibrinogen, fragments known as fibrin split products, or fibrin degradation products, are produced and function as potent anticoagulants. In cases of excessive clotting and clot lysis, these fibrin split products contribute to the coagulopathy. Fibrin split products are not normally present in the circulation but are seen in some hematological disorders as well as with thrombolytic therapy.

NURSING ASSESSMENT OF HEMATOLOGICAL AND IMMUNOLOGICAL FUNCTION

An understanding of both normal and disrupted hematological and immunological system activities is paramount to good assessment skills and use of therapeutic interventions. Nursing assessment involves

TRANSPLANTATION   Hematopoietic Stem Cell Transplantation

INDICATIONS

Hematopoietic stem cell transplantation (HSCT) includes multiple sources of donor stem cells: bone marrow transplantation (BMT), peripheral blood stem cell transplantation (PBSCT), and cord blood. The indications for HSCT may include a variety of hematological or immunological diseases caused by: abnormal RBC production (sickle cell disease), hematological malignancies (leukemia, lymphoma, myeloma, myelodysplastic syndrome), lack of normal blood cell production (aplastic anemia), immune system disorders (congenital neutropenia, severe combined immunodeficiency syndrome).

CATEGORIES

There are three types of transplants:

Autologous transplant: patient receives their own stem cells

Syngeneic transplants: patient receives stem cells from their identical twin (immunologically identical match)

Allogeneic transplants: patient receives stem cells from a sibling, parent, or unrelated donor (not immunologically identical)

TISSUE TYPING

Proteins on the surface of leukocytes, called human leukocyte antigens (HLA), are present on both donor and recipient cells. HLA-matching between donor and recipient is critically important for determining an appropriate donor. If the donor's cells are not an adequate match, they will recognize the patient's organs and tissues as foreign, and destroy them—known as graft-versus-host-disease (GVHD). Additionally, the patient's immune system could recognize the donor stem cells as foreign and destroy them—known as graft rejection. The higher the number of matching HLA antigens, the greater the chance the transplant will be successful.

COMPLICATIONS

Patients receiving HSCT are susceptible to severe infections, due to their severely immunocompromised state resulting from their disease; ablation of their bone marrow in preparation for transplant; or because of the immunosuppressive therapy used post transplant to prevent GVHD and graft rejection. Complications may occur at any time during the HSCT continuum: preengraftment (bone marrow ablation with high-dose chemotherapy and/or radiation) to day 30 post transplant; early after engraftment, usually from day 30-100; and late after transplantation, more than 100 days post transplant of donor stem cells.

Complications may include bacterial, fungal, protozoal, or viral infections; bleeding; sepsis; GVHD (acute or chronic); hepatic veno-occlusive disease (weight gain, painful hepatomegaly, and jaundice); and respiratory complications. Short-term side effects may include nausea, vomiting, fatigue, anorexia, mucositis, alopecia, and skin reactions. Potential long-term risks related to the pre-transplant chemotherapy and radiation includes: infertility, cataracts, new cancers, and damage to major organs.

REFERENCES

1. Applebaum, F. R. (2005). Hematopoietic cell transplantation. In D. L. Kasper, E. Braunwald, A. S. Fauci, S. L. Hauser, D. L. Longo, & J. L. Jameson (Eds.), *Harrison's principles of internal medicine.* (16th ed., pp. 668-673). New York: McGraw-Hill.
2. Bone Marrow Transplantation and Peripheral Blood Stem Cell Transplantation: Questions and Answers. Retrieved April 6, 2008, from www.cancer.gov/cancertopics/factsheet/therapy/bone-marrow-transplant.
3. Bone Marrow Transplant. Retrieved April 6, 2008, from www.nlm.nih.gov/medlineplus/ency/article/003009.htm.
4. Saria, M. G., & Gosselin-Acomb, T. K. (2007). Hematopoietic stem cell transplantation: Implications for critical care nurses. *Clinical Journal of Oncology Nursing, 11*(1), 53-63.
5. Stewart, S. K., & Sugar, J. (2006). Bone marrow and blood stem cell transplants: A guide for patients. Highland Park, Ill: Bone & Marrow Transplant Information Network.

evaluation of risk factors for hematological and immunological alterations, assessment of the patient's complaints, performance of a focused physical examination, and interpretation of pertinent laboratory tests.

Past Medical History

A complete health history includes a record of prior medical and surgical problems, allergies, medication or homeopathic remedy use, and family history. Conditions that may indicate hematological or immunological disorders are noted in Box 16-1.

Evaluation of Patient Complaints and Physical Examination

The nurse notes the patient's general appearance and assesses for signs of fatigue, acute illness, or chronic disease. The most common manifestations of either hematological or immunological disease include indicators of altered oxygenation, bleeding or clotting tendencies, and infection or accentuated immunological activity. The most important assessment

parameters for detection of anemia, bleeding, and infection are shown in Table 16-5.

Diagnostic Tests

Hematological or immunological abnormalities can usually be diagnosed by using the patient's clinical profile in conjunction with a few key laboratory tests. The most invasive microscopic examinations of the bone marrow or lymph nodes are reserved for circumstances when laboratory tests are inconclusive or when an abnormality in cellular maturation is suspected (e.g., aplastic anemia, leukemia, or lymphoma).

The first screening diagnostic tests performed to detect hematological or immunological dysfunction are a CBC with differential and a coagulation profile. The CBC reveals the total RBC count and RBC indices, hematocrit, hemoglobin, WBC count and differential,

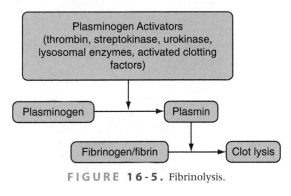

FIGURE 16-5. Fibrinolysis.

BOX 16-1 Conditions that may Indicate Hematological and Immunological Problems*

Hematological Disorders
- Alcohol consumption, excess
- Allergies
- Anemia of any kind
- Benzene exposure (gasoline, dry cleaning chemicals)
- Blood clots
- Delayed wound healing
- Excess bleeding
- Jaundice
- Liver disease
- Medications: allopurinol, antibiotics, anticoagulants, anticonvulsants, antidiabetics, antidysrhythmics, antiinflammatory agents, aspirin derivatives, chemotherapy, histamine blockers
- Neoplastic disease
- Pertinent surgical procedures: hepatic resection, partial or total gastric resection, splenectomy, tumor removal, valve replacement
- Pesticide exposure
- Previous transfusion of blood or blood products
- Poor nutrition
- Radiation: occupational, environmental
- Recurrent infection
- Renal disease
- Substance abuse

Immunological Disorders
- Alcohol consumption, excess
- Allergies
- Anorexia
- Bone tenderness
- Delayed wound healing
- Diabetes mellitus
- Diarrhea
- Fever
- Joint pain
- Liver disease
- Lymphadenopathy
- Medications: antibiotics, antiinflammatory agents, corticosteroids, chemotherapy, immunosuppressives
- Nausea and vomiting
- Neoplastic disease
- Night sweats
- Pertinent surgeries: hepatic resection, lung resection, small bowel resection, splenectomy, tumor removal
- Pesticide exposure
- Poor nutrition
- Previous transfusion of blood or blood products
- Radiation: occupational, environmental
- Recurrent infections
- Renal disease
- Sexual practices
- Substance abuse
- Weight loss

*A thorough history assessing for the foregoing clinical conditions may provide information suggesting predisposition to hematological or immunological disorders. This chart does not correlate specific risks with particular disease conditions, because many overlap or are not confirmed risk factors. History information should be supplemented with physical examination and laboratory test information.[5]

platelet count, and cell morphologies. Depending on these findings and the patient's clinical presentation, further studies may be performed. A summary of common hematological diagnostic laboratory tests with their normal values, and general implications of abnormal findings, is shown in Table 16-6 (RBCs and WBCs) and Table 16-7 (coagulation).

SELECTED ERYTHROCYTE DISORDERS

Many pathological conditions affect the erythrocytes, ranging from mild anemias to life-threatening RBC lysis. A decrease in functional RBCs with a resulting oxygenation deficit is termed *anemia* and is a common problem in critically ill patients. *Polycythemia*, a dis-

TABLE 16-5   Physical Assessment for Hemotological and Immune Disorders

Body System	Anemia	Bleeding	Infection*
Neurological	Difficulty concentrating Dizziness Fatigue Somnolence Vertigo	*Bleeding into brain (cerebrum, cerebellum):* alteration in level of consciousness, focal deficits such as unequal pupils or motor movement, headache *Bleeding into potential spaces*	*Encephalitis:* confusion, lethargy, difficulty arousing, headache, visual difficulty/photosensitivity, nausea, hypertension *Meningitis:* lethargy and somnolence, confusion, nuchal rigidity
Head/Neck	Headache Tinnitus	*Bleeding into eye:* visual disturbances, frank hemorrhagic conjunctiva, bloody tears *Bleeding into nasopharyngeal area:* nasal stuffiness, epistaxis *Oral bleeding:* petechiae of buccal mucosa or gums, hemorrhagic oral lesions *Bleeding into subcutaneous tissue of head or neck:* enlarged, bruised areas, raccoon's eyes, bruising	*Conjunctivitis:* reddened conjunctiva, excess tearing of eye, puslike exudates from eye, blurred vision, swelling of eyelid, eye itching *Otitis media:* earache, difficulty hearing, itching inner ear, ear drainage *Sinusitis:* discolored nasal mucus, nasal congestion, face pain, eye pain, blurred vision *Oropharyngeal:* oral ulcerations or plaques, halitosis, reddened gums, abnormal papillae of the tongue, sore throat, difficulty swallowing *Lymphadenitis:* swollen neck lymph glands, tender lymph glands, a lump left when patient swallows
Pulmonary	Air hunger Anxiety Dyspnea Tachypnea	*Alveolar bleeding:* crackles on breath sound assessment, alveolar fluid on x-ray, low oxygen saturation *Upper airway bleeding (e.g., trachea or bronchi):* hemoptysis *Pleural space bleeding:* decreased breath sounds, unequal chest excursion	*Bronchitis:* persistent cough, sputum production, gurgles in upper airways, wheezes in upper airways, hypoxemia and/or hypercapnia *Pneumonia:* chest discomfort pronounced with inspiration, persistent cough, sputum production, diminished breath sounds, crackles or gurgles, asymmetrical chest wall movement, labored breathing, nasal flaring with breathing, hypoxemia *Pleurisy:* chest discomfort pronounced with inspiration, sides of chest more painful, usually unilateral discomfort, splinting with deep breaths
Cardiovascular	Clubbing of digits Heart murmur Hypotension Nailbeds pale and slow capillary refill Peripheral pulses weak and thready Tachycardia	*Pericardial bleeding:* dyspnea, chest discomfort, hypotension, narrow pulse pressure, muffled heart sounds, increased jugular venous distention *Vascular bleeding:* visible blood, hematoma, or bruising of subcutaneous tissue	*Myocarditis:* dysrhythmias, murmurs or gallops, elevated jugular venous pulsations, weak thready pulses, hypotension, point of maximal impulse shifted laterally *Pericarditis:* constant aching discomfort in the chest unrelieved by rest or nitrates; pericardial rub; muffled heart sounds

TABLE 16-5   Physical Assessment for Hemo-Immune Disorders—cont'd

Body System	Anemia	Bleeding	Infection*
Gastrointestinal	Abdominal pain Constipation Splenic enlargement, tenderness	*Upper GI bleeding:* hematemesis, vomiting (coffee ground appearance) *Lower GI bleeding:* melena *Hepatic or splenic rupture:* acute abdominal pain; abdominal distention, rapid onset hypotension with ↓ hematocrit and hemoglobin *Hemorrhagic pancreatitis:* acute abdominal pain, abdominal distention, hypotension with ↓ hematocrit and hemoglobin	*Gastritis:* nausea, vomiting within 30 minutes of eating, heme-positive emesis, gastric pain that is initially improved by eating *Infectious diarrhea:* greater than six loose stools per day, clay-colored or foul-smelling stools, abdominal cramping or distention *Cholelithiasis/pancreatitis:* epigastric pain, intolerance to high-fat meal, clay-colored stools, nausea and vomiting, hyperglycemia, hypocalcemia, ↓ albumin, ↑ lipase and amylase *Hepatitis:* jaundice, right upper quadrant discomfort, hepatomegaly, elevated transaminases and bilirubin, fatty food intolerances, nausea and vomiting, diarrhea
Genitourinary		Bladder spasms with distended bladder Hematuria	*Urethritis:* painful urination, difficulty urinating, genitourinary itching *Cystitis:* small frequent urination, feeling of bladder fullness *Nephritis:* flank discomfort, oliguria, protein in urine *Vaginitis:* itching or vaginal discharge
Musculoskeletal	Muscle fatigue Muscle weakness	Altered joint mobility Painful or swollen joints Warm, painful, swollen muscles	*Arthritis:* joint discomfort, swollen and warm joints *Myositis:* aching muscles, weakness
Dermatological	Cyanosis Jaundice (hemolytic anemia) Pallor Poor skin turgor Skin cool to touch	Bleeding from line insertion sites, puncture wounds, skin tears Ecchymoses Petechiae	*Superficial skin infection:* rashes, itching, raised and/or discolored skin lesions, open-draining skin lesions; patterns are unique to specific microorganism *Cellulitis:* redness, warmth and swelling of subcutaneous tissue area, radiating pain from area toward middle of body
Hematological/ Immunological			*Bacteremia:* Positive blood culture

*Signs and symptoms presented in this chart are unique features of each process and do not include the common constitutional signs and symptoms seen with all infections such as fever, chills, malaise, leukocytosis, positive tissue culture for microorganisms, or increased erythrocyte sedimentation rate.
↑, Increased; ↓, decreased; *GI,* gastrointestinal.

order in which the number of circulating RBCs is increased, is seen less often but can affect hypoxic patients (e.g., chronic obstructive pulmonary disease). It leads to increased blood viscosity and thrombotic complications.

Anemia

Pathophysiology

The term *anemia* refers to a reduction in the number of circulating RBCs or hemoglobin, which leads to inadequate oxygenation of tissues. Although symptoms vary depending on the type, cause, or severity of anemia, the basic clinical findings are the same. As oxygenation delivery is decreased, tissues become hypoxic and 2,3-DPG increases to cause hemoglobin to release oxygen. Blood flow is redistributed to areas where oxygenation is most vital, such as the brain, heart, and lungs. Anemia is described as mild, moderate, or severe, based on symptoms, irrespective of actual RBC serum values. Patients are able to adjust and compensate to lower

TABLE 16-6   Functions and Normal Values of Blood Cells

Test	Reason Evaluated	Normal Value	Alterations
RBCs			
Erythrocyte (RBC)	Respiration Oxygen transport Acid-base balance	5 million/ microliter	↑ Polycythemia, dehydration ↓ Anemia, fluid overload, hemorrhage
Mean corpuscular volume (MCV)	Average size of each RBC reflects maturity	80-100/femtoliter	Nutrition deficiency cause ↑ ↓ Iron deficiency
Mean corpuscular hemoglobin (MCH)	Average amount of hemoglobin in each RBC	26-34 pg	↓ Disorders of hemoglobin production
Mean corpuscular hemoglobin concentration (MCHC)	Average concentration of hemoglobin within a single RBC	31%-38%	↓ Cell has hemoglobin deficiency
Reticulocyte count	Immature RBCs released when sudden ↑ demand	1%-2% of total RBC count	↑ Recent blood loss or with chronic hemolysis
Serum folate	Amount of available vitamin for RBC development	95-500 mcg/mL	↓ Malnutrition or folic acid deficiency
Serum iron level	Iron stores within the body	40-160 mcg/dL	↓ Inadequate iron intake or inadequate absorption (e.g., gastric resection)
Total iron binding capacity (TIBC)	Reflection of liver function and nutrition	250-400 mcg/dL	↓ Chronic illness (infection, neoplasia, cirrhosis)
Ferritin level	Precursor to iron reflective of body's ability to create new iron stores	15-200 ng/mL	↓ Levels demonstrate inability to regenerate iron stores and hemoglobin
Transferrin level	Protein that binds to iron for removal or recirculation after RBCs are hemolyzed	200-400 mg/dL	↓ Excess hemolysis
Haptoglobin level	Protein that binds with heme for removal or recirculation after RBCs are hemolyzed	40-240 mg/dL	↓ Excess hemolysis
WBCs			
Leukocytes (WBCs)	Inflammatory and immune responses Defend against infection, foreign tissue	4500-11,000/ microliter	↑ Inflammation, tissue necrosis, infection, hematologic malignancy ↓ Bone marrow depression (radiation, immune disorders), chronic disease
Granular Leukocytes			
Neutrophils	Polymorphonuclear neutrophils Phagocytosis of invading organisms	50%-70% of WBCs	↑ Inflammation, infection, surgery, myocardial infarction ↓ Aplastic anemia, hepatitis, some pharmacological agents
Eosinophils	Defend against parasites; detoxification of foreign proteins Phagocytosis	1%-5% of WBCs	↑ Allergic attacks, autoimmune diseases, parasitic infections, dermatological conditions ↓ Stress reactions, severe infection
Basophils	Release heparin, serotonin, and histamine in allergic reactions; inflammatory response	0%-1% of WBCs	↑ Postsplenectomy, hemolytic anemia, radiation, hypothyroidism, leukemia, chronic hypersensitivity ↓ Stress reactions

TABLE 16-6 Functions and Normal Values of Blood Cells—cont'd

Test	Reason Evaluated	Normal Value	Alterations
Nongranular Leukocytes			
Monocytes	Mature into macrophages; phagocytosis of necrotic tissue, debris, foreign particles	1%-8% of WBCs	↑ Bacterial, parasitic, and some viral infections, chronic inflammation ↓ Stress reactions
Lymphocytes	Defend against microorganisms	20%-40% of WBCs	↑ Bacterial and viral infections, lymphocytic leukemia ↓ Immunoglobulin deficiency
B lymphocytes	Humoral immunity and production of antibodies	270-640/microliter	↑ Bacterial and viral infections, lymphocytic leukemia ↓ Immunoglobulin deficiency, stress
T lymphocytes	Cell-mediated immunity	500-2400/microliter	↓ Chemotherapy, immunodeficiencies, HIV disease, end-stage renal disease, immunosuppressive drugs
Platelets			
Thrombocytes (platelets)	Blood clotting; hemostasis	150,000-400,000/ microliter	↑ Polycythemia vera, postsplenectomy, certain cancers ↓ Leukemia, bone marrow failure, disseminated intravascular coagulation, hemorrhage, hypersplenism, radiation exposure, large foreign bodies in blood (e.g., aortic balloon pump), hypothermia, hyperthermia, severe infection

↑, Increased; ↓, decreased; *HIV*, human immunodeficiency virus; *pg*, picograms; *RBCs*, red blood cells; *WBCs*, white blood cells.

RBC levels when the condition is chronic or slow in onset.

Anemia is classified by its origin or by the microscopic appearance of the RBCs. Hematologists generally use the microscopic classifications (e.g., microcytic, hypochromic), but critical care nurses can best plan their nursing care by using the etiological classifications. Causes of anemia include (1) blood loss (acute or chronic), (2) impaired production, (3) increased RBC destruction, or (4) a combination of these. Iron deficiency anemia is the most common type of anemia. The types of anemia are described in Table 16-8.

Assessment and Clinical Manifestations

Signs and symptoms of anemia begin gradually and initially may include fatigue, weakness, and shortness of breath.[14] Signs and symptoms are related to three physiological effects of reduced RBCs: (1) decreased circulating volume caused by loss of RBC mass, (2) decreased oxygenation of tissues resulting from reduced hemoglobin binding sites, and (3) compensatory mechanisms implemented by the body in its attempt to improve tissue oxygenation.

Decreased circulating volume is manifested by clinical findings reflective of low blood volume (e.g., low right atrial pressure) and the effects of gravity on the lack of volume (e.g., orthostasis). Tissue hypoxia from inadequate oxygen delivery results in compensatory activities, including an increased depth and rate of respiration to increase oxygen availability, tachycardia to increase oxygen delivery, and the shunting of blood away from nonvital organs to perfuse the vital organs.[14] Inadequate oxygenation of the tissues leads to organ dysfunction.

In addition to the general symptoms of anemia, unique disorders have their own classic clinical features. The patient with aplastic anemia may have bruising, nosebleeds, petechiae, and a decreased ability to fight infections. These effects result from thrombocytopenia and decreased WBC counts, which occur when the bone marrow fails to produce blood cells. Assessment of the patient with hemolytic anemia may reveal jaundice, abdominal pain, and enlargement of the spleen or liver. These findings result from the increased destruction of RBCs, their sequestration (abnormal distribution in the spleen and liver), and the accumulation of break-

TABLE 16-7   Coagulation Profile Studies

Test	Normal Value	Comments
Lee-White clotting time	6-12 minutes	Nonspecific for clotting abnormalities
Activated partial thromboplastin time (APTT)	<35 seconds	Used to monitor heparin therapy and detect bleeding tendencies, hemorrhagic disorders ↑ Anticoagulation therapy, liver disease, vitamin K deficiency, DIC
Prothrombin time (PT)	10-15 seconds 1-1.2 INR	Evaluates extrinsic pathway; used to monitor oral anticoagulant therapy ↑ Warfarin therapy, liver disease, vitamin K deficiency, obstructive jaundice
Thrombin time (TT)	9-13 seconds	Detect fibrinogen abnormalities, monitor heparin therapy ↑ Fibrinogen abnormalities, multiple myeloma, cirrhosis of liver, heparin therapy
Fibrinogen level	150-400 mg/dL	↓ DIC and fibrinogen disorders ↑ Acute infection, hepatitis, or with oral contraceptive use
Fibrin degradation products (FDPs)	<10 mcg/mL	Evaluates hematological disorders ↑ DIC, fibrinolysis, thrombolytic therapy
Fibrin D-dimer	0-0.5 mcg/mL	Presence diagnostic for DIC
Platelet count	150,000-400,000/microliter	Measures number of circulating platelets ↓ Thrombocytopenia
Platelet aggregation test	3-5 minutes	Measures platelet adherence ability Prolonged in von Willebrand's disease, acute leukemia, idiopathic thrombocytopenic purpura, liver cirrhosis, aspirin use
Bleeding time	1-4 minutes	Evaluates platelet function ↑ Thrombocytopenia and aspirin therapy
Calcium	9-11 mg/dL	↓ Massive transfusions of stored blood

↑, Increased; ↓, decreased; *DIC*, disseminated intravascular coagulation; *Hgb*, hemoglobin; *INR*, international normalized ratio.

down products. Patients with sickle cell anemia may have joint swelling or pain, and delayed physical and sexual development. In crisis, the sickle cell patient often has decreased urine output, peripheral edema, and signs of uremia because renal tissue perfusion is impaired as a result of sluggish blood flow.

Laboratory findings in anemia include a decreased RBC count and decreased hemoglobin and hematocrit values. The reticulocyte count is usually increased, indicating a compensatory increased RBC production with release of immature cells. Patients with hemolytic anemia also have an increased bilirubin level. In sickle cell disease, a stained blood smear reveals sickled cells. In aplastic anemia, the reticulocyte, platelet, RBC, and WBC counts are decreased because the marrow fails to produce any cells.

Nursing Diagnoses

Nursing diagnoses of the anemic patient may include the following:

- Decreased cardiac output related to decreased circulating blood volume
- Altered tissue perfusion, impaired gas exchange, or both, related to decreased or dysfunctional RBCs or hemoglobin
- Risk for fluid volume excess or deficit related to fluid replacement or hemorrhage
- Impaired skin integrity related to inadequate perfusion and tissue hypoxia
- Pain related to tissue ischemia and microvascular occlusion
- Risk for infection related to bone marrow failure and low WBC count
- Risk for injury related to transfusions

TABLE 16-8 Anemias

Marrow Failure to Produce RBCs	Aplastic Anemia	Hemolytic Anemia	Sickle Cell Anemia (Hemolytic Subtype)	Vitamin B$_{12}$ Deficiency	Folic Acid Deficiency	Iron Deficiency
			Pathophysiology			
Disorder or bone marrow toxin damages the erythrocyte precursors, leading to ↓ RBC production	Disorder or bone marrow toxin damages hematopoietic stem cells and results in ↓ production of RBCs, WBCs, and platelets	Stimulus causes extrasplenic destruction of the RBC, leading to hemolyzed RBC fragments in the circulating bloodstream; cell fragments ↑ blood viscosity and slow blood flow, leading to ischemia and/or infarction Extrasplenic hemolysis also leads to ↑ levels of circulating bilirubin and unbound iron	Presence of abnormal hemoglobin causes RBCs to assume a sickle or crescent shape Sickling alters the blood viscosity, leading to microvascular occlusion; sickling crisis leads to hypoxia, thrombosis, and infarction in tissues and organs	Pernicious anemia is caused by decreased gastric production of HCl and intrinsic factor that play a role in vitamin B$_{12}$ absorption	Malabsorption of dietary folic acid resulting from the lack of intake or absorption	Body's iron stores inadequate for RBC development; Hgb-deficient RBCs result

Continued

TABLE 16-8   Anemias—cont'd

	Marrow Failure to Produce RBCs	Aplastic Anemia	Hemolytic Anemia	Sickle Cell Anemia (Hemolytic Subtype)	Vitamin B$_{12}$ Deficiency	Folic Acid Deficiency	Iron Deficiency
Etiology							
	Disorders: Bone metastases *Drugs:* Chemotherapy agents Antiretroviral agents *Toxic exposures:* Radiation to long bones	*Disorders:* Immune suppression Postorthotopic liver transplant status Pregnancy Vitamin B$_{12}$ deficiency Viral infection: EBV, CMV *Drugs:* Anticonvulsants Antidysrhythmics Antiinflammatory agents Chloramphenicol Quinines *Toxic exposures:* Benzene Arsenic Herbicides/ Insecticides Lacquers Paint thinners Radiation exposure Toluene (glue)	*Abnormal RBC membrane or hemoglobin:* Anemia of liver or renal disease Hereditary RBC shape disorders Paroxysmal nocturnal hemoglobinuria Porphyria Sickle cell disease G6PD deficiency Thalassemias *Immune reaction:* Autoimmune hemolytic syndrome: BMT hemolytic transfusion reaction Autoimmune diseases *Physical damage to RBC:* Blunt trauma Extracorporeal circulation Prosthetic heart valves Thermal injury *Unknown:* Diabetes mellitus IgA deficiency Illicit drug stimulants: cocaine Ovarian cyst Snake or spider bite	Hereditary hemolytic anemia caused by abnormal amount of hemoglobin S in relation to hemoglobin A	Familial incidence related to autoimmune response with gastric mucosal atrophy Higher incidence in autoimmune disorders: SLE, myxedema, Graves' disease Common in Northern Europeans; rare in children, black and Asian populations Occurs postoperatively with gastric surgery	Common in infants, adolescents, pregnant and lactating women, alcoholic patients, older adults, cancer, intestinal disease (jejunitis, small bowel resection), prolonged anticonvulsants and estrogens, excessive cooking of foods	10%-30% of all American adults; primarily from dietary deficiency Also in pregnant and lactating women, infants, adolescents Malabsorption such as diarrhea, gastric resection, blood loss, or intravascular hemolysis

Clinical Presentation

Clinical Presentation	Diagnostic Tests
↓ Production of cells in the earliest phase: bone marrow resulting in low RBC count. Signs and symptoms are those common in profound anemia	CBC used as screening test. Bone marrow aspiration and biopsy confirm maturation failure
Symptoms of infection, bleeding, and anemia occur simultaneously; earliest symptoms usually the result of WBC dysfunction. Platelet production abnormalities lead to bleeding symptoms within 7-10 days followed by symptoms of anemia	CBC used as screening test. Bone marrow aspiration and biopsy reflect absence of precursor or stem cells
Rapid hemolysis of RBCs leads to spleen uptake with enlarged and tender spleen; metabolism of RBCs often leads to excess bilirubin with jaundice and itching	Reticulocytes usually ≥4% total RBC count. ↑ Total bilirubin. ↑ Direct bilirubin. ↓ Transferrin. ↓ Haptoglobin
Hyperviscosity and poor perfusion (e.g., altered mentation, hypoxemia, abdominal cramping); sickled cells removed from circulation, causing enlarged and tender spleen; long-term sickling and thrombosis causes ↓ joint mobility, gut dysfunction, cardiac failure, and risk for stroke	Hemoglobin electrophoresis abnormality
Inhibited growth of all cells: anemia, leukopenia, thrombocytopenia. Demyelination of peripheral nerves to spinal cord. Triad: weakness, sore tongue, paresthesias	Schilling test. ↓ Hgb and RBC. ↓ MCV. ↑ MCHC. ↓ WBC. ↓ Platelets. ↑ LDH
Similar to vitamin B_{12} deficiency but without neurological symptoms. Signs: poor oxygenation, dizziness, irritability, dyspnea, pallor, headache, oral ulcers, tachycardia	Macrocytosis. Serum folate <4 mg/dL. Abnormal platelet appearance. ↑ Reticulocyte count
Classic: "pica" (desire to eat nonfood items), ice or dirt cravings. Symptoms of cardiovascular/respiratory compromise: hypoxia, fatigue, headache, cracks in mouth corners, smooth tongue, paresthesias, neuralgias	↓ Hct and Hgb. ↓ Iron level with ↑ binding capacity. ↓ Ferritin level. ↓ RBC with hypochromia and microcytes. ↓ MCHC

Diagnostic Tests

Continued

TABLE 16-8 Anemias—cont'd

	Marrow Failure to Produce RBCs	Aplastic Anemia	Hemolytic Anemia	Sickle Cell Anemia (Hemolytic Subtype)	Vitamin B₁₂ Deficiency	Folic Acid Deficiency	Iron Deficiency
Management	Erythropoietin per dosing guidelines (Procrit, Aranesp)	Eliminate cause; Bone marrow stimulants may be tried early; Corticosteroids; Immunosuppressive agents if suspected autoimmune process; Chelating (iron binding) agents; Limit transfusions when possible to ↓ risk of rejection; Allogenic BMT	Staphylococcal protein A is capable of trapping IgG complexes that are thought to cause RBC autoantibodies; If autoantibodies are present, give immunosuppressive agents; Administer antiplatelet medications (e.g., salicylic acid)	Administer large volumes of IV fluids to dilute viscous blood; Oxygen therapy reduces sickling; Treat infections early with fluids and antibiotics; Sickling causes extreme pain (result of ischemia); narcotics may be required; Gene transplants used experimentally	Vitamin B₁₂ 30 mcg IM or deep SC for 5-10 days then 100-200 micrograms IM or deep SC every month	Folic acid 0.25-1 mg/day PO	Ferrous sulfate 325 mg PO TID and ascorbic acid to aid absorption; Iron replacement
Nursing Implications	Monitor diet and medications that interfere with marrow production of cells	High risk of infection and bleeding: implement bleeding precautions; Administer transfusions cautiously; ↑ exposure to antigens may enhance rejection if BMT is required later	Begin plasma reinfusion at a rate of 25 mL/hour for 15 minutes, then ↑ to 100 mL/hour; Assess for hypersensitivity; Assess for fluid shifts into the interstitial spaces during infusion or within 6-12 hours after infusion; Monitor for vomiting, pain at infusion site, diarrhea	Incurable, although severity remains consistent throughout lifetime; Children who do not have pain managed effectively can develop maladaptive coping; Life expectancy prolonged as a result of more effective supportive care; Common cause of death is intracranial thrombosis or hemorrhage	Lifetime treatment requires ongoing patient teaching; Heart failure prevention; Special oral hygiene; Monitor for persistent neurological deficits	Foods high in folic acid: beef, liver, peanut butter, red beans, oatmeal, asparagus, broccoli	Monitor for allergic reactions to iron; Give oral supplements with straw so not to stain teeth; causes skin irritation and iron deposits

↑, Increased; ↓, decreased; *BMT*, bone marrow transplant; *CMV*, cytomegalovirus; *2,3-DPG*, 2,3-, diphosphoglycerate; *EBV*, Epstein-Barr virus; *G6PD*, glucose-6-phosphate dehydrogenase; *Hct*, Hematocrit; *Hgb*, hemoglobin; *IM*, intramuscularly; *IV*, intravenous; *LDH*, lactate dehydrogenase; *MCHC*, mean corpuscular hemoglobin concentration; *MCV*, mean corpuscular volume; *PO*, orally; *RBC*, red blood cell; *SC*, subcutaneously; *SLE*, systemic lupus erythematosus; *TID*, three times a day; *WBC*, white blood cell.

Medical Interventions

Medical treatment of anemia includes identification and removal of causative agents or conditions, supplemental oxygen, blood component therapy, and cardiovascular system support. In anemia associated with blood loss, initial treatment is restoration of blood volume with intravenous administration of volume expanders (crystalloid or colloid) and/or transfusion of packed red blood cells. Erythropoietin products are given to stimulate RBC production. For certain types of anemia, cause-specific interventions may be indicated. Splenectomy may be performed for hemolytic anemia, and bone marrow transplantation may be preferred for refractory aplastic anemia. In sickle cell disease, oxygenation and correction of dehydration are important for the prevention or reversal of erythrocyte sickling.

Nursing Interventions

Nursing management of anemia is based on a continuous, thorough nursing assessment and the prescribed medical treatment. Physical assessment is vital; monitoring of vital signs, the electrocardiogram, hemodynamics, heart and lung sounds, and peripheral pulses assists the nurse in the assessment of tissue perfusion and gas exchange. Tachycardia and orthostatic hypotension are important signs that indicate that the patient's cardiovascular system is not adequately compensating for the anemia. Mental status, urine output, and skin color or temperature are important general indicators of tissue perfusion. Pain management and comfort measures are instituted as needed. Scrupulous skin care is given to prevent tissue breakdown, and the patient is monitored closely for signs of infection. For patients at risk of further blood loss, bleeding precautions are instituted. Interventions for patients at risk of bleeding or infection are listed later in this chapter.

Laboratory results, such as the CBC, are carefully monitored. Other vital nursing interventions include the following: promotion of rest and oxygen conservation; careful administration of blood components, drug therapy, and intravenous fluids; and monitoring of the patient's responses to the therapy. The desired goal of treatment and nursing intervention is optimal tissue perfusion, oxygenation, and gas exchange.

WHITE BLOOD CELL AND IMMUNE DISORDERS

Many pathological conditions can be classified as WBC or immune disorders. They may involve the WBCs themselves or other complementary immune processes. The immune system can fail to develop properly, lose its ability to react to invasion by pathogens, overreact to harmless antigens, or turn immune functions against self. Regardless of the cause, WBC and immune disorders or their treatments suppress the mechanisms needed for inflammation and combating infection. Because the clinical features and complications are similar among a variety of disorders, this first section addresses general causes, signs and symptoms, and management of immunological suppression. This is followed by in-depth descriptions of specific WBC and immune disorders.

The Immunocompromised Patient

Pathophysiology

The *immunocompromised* patient is one with defined quantitative or qualitative defects in WBCs or immune physiology. The defect may be congenital or acquired, and may involve a single element or multiple processes. Regardless of the cause, the physiological outcome is immune incompetence, with lack of normal inflammatory, phagocytic, antibody, or cytokine responses. Immune incompetence is often asymptomatic until pathogenic organisms invade the body and create infection. Infection is the leading cause of death in the immunocompromised patient.

Assessment and Clinical Manifestations

The nursing diagnosis *risk for infection* is frequently documented in critically ill patients and is the primary clinical problem for those with immune compromise. A detailed database containing the patient's history, physical examination findings, and laboratory studies is paramount for rapid detection of infection.

Immunocompromise in the critically ill is caused by many factors. In addition to existing immunodeficiency diseases and life-threatening illness, immune defenses are altered by invasive procedures, inadequate nutrition, and the presence of opportunistic pathogens. Many of the drugs and treatments administered in critical care can also depress the patient's immune system. The patient's medical and social history, current medications, and risk factors for infection are evaluated. Risk factors for immune compromise are described in Table 16-9. Immunosuppressed patients do not respond to infection with typical signs and symptoms of inflammation (see Clinical Alert: Infection in Immunocompromised Patients).

Laboratory results which reflect leukopenia, low CD4 counts, and decreased immunoglobulin levels may demonstrate disorders of immune components. A common test of the humoral (antibody) response to antigens is a skin test with intradermal injection of typical pathogens capable of initiating an antibody response. Absence of a "wheal" tissue response to the antigens (called tissue anergy) is evidence of altered antibody capabilities.

Nursing Diagnoses

The patient with compromised immune system function is most likely to have one of the following nursing diagnoses: risk for infection, altered protection, or hyperthermia.

Medical Interventions

Medical therapy is directed at reversing the cause of the immune dysfunction and preventing infectious complications. In *primary immunodeficiencies*, B-cell

---

CLINICAL ALERT

Infection in Immunocompromised Patients

Immunocompromised patients do not have typical signs and symptoms of infection.

- Erythema, swelling, and exudate formation are usually not evident.
- Symptoms of infection may be absent, masked, or present atypically.
- Fever is considered the cardinal and sometimes only symptom of infection.
- Patients are also more likely to describe pain at the site of infection, although physical inflammatory signs may be absent.

TABLE 16-9　Risk Factors for Infections in the Immunocompromised Patient

Patient Characteristics	Physiological Mechanism of Risk of Infection
Host Characteristics	
Alcoholism	↓ Neutrophil activity Hepatic/splenic congestion also slows phagocytic response
Abuse of intravenous drugs	Chronic altered barrier defense leads to reduced WBCs and slowed phagocytic responses Constant viral exposure may also alter T-cell function
Older adults	Slowed phagocytosis: ↑ bacterial infection, more rapid dissemination of infection Slowed macrophage activity—more fungal infection, more visceral infection Atrophy of thymus: ↑ risk of viral illness ↓ Antigen-specific immunoglobulins: diminished immune memory
Frequent hospitalizations	Frequent exposure to environmental organisms other than own normal flora Potential exposure to resistant organisms Potential exposure to other people's organisms via equipment, supplies, transport, person-to-person exposure
Malnutrition	Inadequate WBC count: infection ↓ Neutrophil activity: bacterial infection, at risk of infection dissemination Impaired phagocytic function: bacterial infection Impaired integumentary/mucosal barrier: general infection risk ↓ Macrophage mobilization: ↑ risk of fungal or rapidly disseminating infection ↓ Lymphocyte function: ↑ risk of viral and opportunistic infection Thymus and lymph node atrophy with iron deficiency
Stress	Induces ↑ release of adrenal hormones (cortisol), which causes ↓ circulating eosinophils and lymphocytes
Immune Defects and Disorders	
Lymphopenia	↓ Antibody response to previous exposed antigens ↓ Recognition and destruction of viral and opportunistic organisms
Macrophage dysfunction/ destruction	Altered response to fungi Inadequate antigen-antibody response Greater potential for visceral infection
Neutropenia	Inadequate neutrophils to combat pathogens (especially bacterial)
Splenectomy	Inability to recognize and remove encapsulated bacteria (e.g., streptococcus) Compromised reticuloendothelial system and ↓ antibodies lead to frequent and early bacteremia

TABLE 16-9   Risk Factors for Infections in the Immunocompromised Patient—cont'd

Patient Characteristics	Physiological Mechanism of Risk of Infection
Disease Processes	
Burns	Physiological stressor thought to ↓ phagocytic responses Altered barrier defenses allowing pathogen entry Protein loss through skin leads to malnutrition-related immunocompromise
Cancer	Structural disruption may lead to bone marrow or lymphatic abnormalities Certain cancers have specific immune defects (e.g., diminished phagocytic activity or T-cell defects) Radiation therapy destroys lymphocytes and causes shrinkage of lymphoid tissue Chemotherapy causes ↓ lymphocytes and alters the proliferation and differentiation of stem cells
Cardiovascular disease	Inadequate tissue perfusion slows WBC response to tissue with pathogenic organism
Diabetes mellitus	↓ Numbers of neutrophils Hyperglycemia causes ↓ phagocytic activity and immunoglobin defects Vascular insufficiency leads to slowed phagocytic response to pathogens Neuropathy and glycosuria predisposes person to ↓ bladder emptying and urinary tract infections
Gastrointestinal disease	↓ Bowel motility allows normal flora to translocate across the gastrointestinal wall to the bloodstream
Hepatic disease	↓ Neutrophil count
Infectious diseases	↓ Phagocytic activity Hypermetabolism with infection accelerates phagocytic cell use and death Certain viral and opportunistic infections ↓ bone marrow production of WBCs
Pulmonary disease	Inadequate oxygenation suppresses neutrophil activity
Renal disease	↓ Neutrophil activity caused by uremic toxins ↓ Immunoglobulin activity
Traumatic injuries	Altered barrier defenses allowing pathogen entry Type of infection dependent on source and severity of injury (e.g., soil contamination, water contamination, skin flora)
Medication/Treatment	
Antibiotics	Normal flora destroyed and enhanced resistant organism growth, fungal superinfection
Immunosuppressive agents and corticosteroids	↓ Phagocytic activity Altered T-cell recognition of pathogens, especially viral ↓ Interleukin-2 production leads to increased risk of malignancy ↓ IgG production Lack of immune memory to recall antibodies to previously encountered pathogens
Invasive devices	Altered barrier defenses allowing pathogen entry, especially skin organisms
Surgical procedures/wounds	Normal flora may be translocated by surgical procedure Altered barrier defenses caused by surgical entry Stress of surgery and anesthetic agents reduce neutrophil activity
Transfusion of blood products	Risk of transfusion-transmitted infections undetected by donor screening: cytomegalovirus, hepatitis, human immunodeficiency virus Exposure to foreign antigens in blood products causes T-lymphocytic immune suppression and increases risk of infection

↑, Increased; ↓, decreased; *IgG*, immunoglobulin G; *WBC*, white blood cell.

and T-cell defects are treated with specific replacement therapy or bone marrow transplantation. IgG blood levels of less than 300 mg/dL warrant immunoglobulin infusion. Gene replacement therapy may soon be a realistic curative treatment option for some disorders. In *secondary immunodeficiencies*, the underlying causative condition is treated. For example, malnutrition is corrected, or doses of immunosuppressive medications are adjusted.

Additional risk factors for infection are carefully monitored and avoided when possible. Invasive lines pose the most common risk for iatrogenic infection; lines should be kept to a minimum and managed with meticulous sterile technique.

Administration of prophylactic antimicrobial agents during the period of highest risk of infection is common. For example, patients receiving bone marrow–suppressing cancer chemotherapy receive broad-spectrum antimicrobials during the time of their lowest WBC count. Patients who have human immunodeficiency virus (HIV) infection or are recovering from organ transplantation have defined CD4 or immune suppression levels that place them at risk of specific infections. Depending on predetermined criteria, these patients can receive antimicrobial prophylaxis against infections with herpes simplex, *Candida albicans*, *Pneumocystis carinii*, Mycobacterium avium-intracellulare, *Mycobacterium tuberculosis*, and cytomegalovirus.

Nursing Interventions

Nursing interventions focus on protecting the patient from infection. It has been proposed that a protective environment could reduce the risk of infection. Research studies support the use of high-efficiency particulate air (HEPA) filtration of air and laminar air flow in single-patient rooms for prevention of infection with airborne microorganisms. Comparative studies of isolation precautions and careful infection control practices, such as hand washing with an antimicrobial soap, do not demonstrate any added advantage to isolation techniques.

Nurses should diligently ensure adequate hygiene measures that include general bathing with antimicrobial soaps, oral care, and perineal care. Hand washing is paramount for staff, patients, and visitors. Nursing staff members play an important role in limiting breaks in skin integrity and ensuring sterile technique when procedures are unavoidable.

General health promotion of adequate fluid, nutrition, and sleep are important in bolstering the patient's defenses against infection. Dietary restriction, such as prohibiting raw fruits and vegetables, is controversial and not standardized.[6,17] For a more comprehensive list of nursing interventions, consult the Nursing Care Plan for the Immunocompromised Patient.

Several patient outcomes are desired as a result of nursing interventions. These include absence of fever, negative cultures, and normal laboratory test results. Both family members and patients should be able to verbalize strategies to control infection risks.

Neutropenia

Pathophysiology

Neutropenia is defined as an absolute neutrophil count of less than 1500 cells/microliter of blood. Neutropenia may occur as a result of inadequate production or excess destruction. Patients with low neutrophil counts are predisposed to infections because of the body's reduced phagocytic ability.[15] Neutropenia is classified based on the patient's predicted risk for infection: mild (1000 to 1500 cells/microliter), moderate (500 to 1000 cells/microliter), and severe (<500 cells/microliter).

Assessment and Clinical Manifestations

The nurse must obtain a thorough medical and social history to identify risk factors for neutropenia. Common causes include acute or overwhelming infections, radiation, exposure to chemicals and drugs, or other disease states (Box 16-2).

There are no specific signs or symptoms of a low neutrophil count, although many patients describe fatigue or malaise that coincides with the drop in counts and precedes infectious signs and symptoms. This lack of a clear pattern of symptoms makes it essential to evaluate the patient carefully for risk factors for neutropenia. The patient is also monitored for clinical findings consistent with infection.

Every body system is examined for physical findings of infection. Typical signs may not be evident. Pain such as sore throat or urethral discomfort may be indicative of an infected site. Areas of heavy bacterial colonization (e.g., oral mucosa, perineal area, and venipuncture and catheter sites) have the highest risk of infection; however, the most common clinical infections are sepsis and pneumonia. Additional signs or symptoms of systemic infection include a rise in temperature from its normal set point, chills, and accompanying tachycardia.

The diagnostic test indicated when neutropenia is suspected is the WBC count with differential. The differential demonstrates the percentage of each type of WBC circulating in the bloodstream. The absolute neutrophil count is calculated by multiplying the total WBC count (without a decimal point) times the percentages (with decimal points) of polymorphonuclear leukocytes (polys; also called segs or neutrophils) and bands (immature neutrophils). This gives an actual number that is translated into the categories of mild, moderate, or severe neutropenia.

NURSING CARE PLAN for the Immunocompromised Patient

NURSING DIAGNOSIS

Risk for infection related to immunocompromise or immunosuppression; invasive procedures; and presence of opportunistic pathogens

PATIENT OUTCOMES
Patient will remain free of infection

- Absence of fever, redness, swelling, pain, and heat
- WBC and differential, urinalysis, and cultures within normal limits
- Chest x-ray study without infiltrates
- Absence of adventitious breath sounds

NURSING INTERVENTIONS	RATIONALES
• Establish baseline assessment with documented history, physical examination, and laboratory study results	• Establish trends to guide and monitor treatment
• Follow universal precautions, including hand hygiene	• Prevent infection
• Plan nurses' assignments to reduce the possibility of infection spread between patients	• Prevent spread of infection
• Be careful handling secretions/excretions that are known to be infected (e.g., use different washcloth for rectal and urinary areas)	• Prevent cross-contamination
• Monitor visitors for any recent history of communicable diseases	• Prevent infection
• Clean all multipurpose equipment (e.g., oximeter probes, noninvasive BP cuffs, bed scale slings, electronic thermometers) between patient use	• Prevent cross-contamination
• Assess patient for signs/symptoms of infection	• Accurate and timely interventions improve patient outcomes
• Monitor vital signs with temperature at least every 4 hours; any elevation in temperature is reported and investigated. Rectal temperatures are not recommended	• Assess for infection
• Monitor laboratory results: WBC and differential, blood, urine, sputum, wound, and throat cultures; report abnormal results	• Assess for infection
• Note the presence of chills, tachycardia, oliguria, or altered mentation that may indicate sepsis; report subtle changes to physician	• Assess for infection
• Encourage incentive spirometry, changes of position every 1-2 hours	• Prevent atelectasis
• Avoid breaks in the skin and mucous membranes; change position every 2 hours, avoid wetness, provide skin lubricants, provide meticulous oral and bathing hygiene	• Maintain intact skin—the first line of defense

Continued

NURSING CARE PLAN for the Immunocompromised Patient—cont'd

NURSING INTERVENTIONS	RATIONALES
• Use strict aseptic technique for dressing changes	• Prevent infection
• Avoid stopcocks in IV systems, use closed injection of site systems	• Stopcocks can harbor bacteria and are a source entry for any infectious agent
• Limit invasive devices/procedures when possible	• Decrease risk for infection
• Use private room, limit visitors, limit fresh flowers and standing water	• Fresh flowers have a potential to introduce pathogenic organisms
• Ensure that sleep needs are being met	• Enhance resistance to infection and aid in healing
• Control glucose levels	• Hyperglycemia compromises phagocytic activity
• Change oxygen setups with humidification (e.g., nasal cannula) every 24 hours	• Prevent bacterial growth

• For first fever (38.0°C two times 4 hours apart or any three consecutive times) or new fever (38.3°C after 72 hours on an antimicrobial regimen), obtain cultures:
  ▪ Blood cultures from two different sites
  ▪ Blood cultures from existing venous/arterial access devices
  ▪ Urine culture
  ▪ Sputum culture, if obtainable
  ▪ Stool culture, if obtainable
  ▪ Culture of open lesions or wounds
	• Determine site of infections and pathogens for proper antimicrobial treatment

• Administer antimicrobial therapy as ordered; perform antimicrobial peak and trough levels as ordered	• Treat infection and assess effectiveness of antibiotics
• Be alert to superinfection with fungal flora any time 7-10 days after initiation of antibiotics	• Assess complication of antibiotic therapy; oral or topical nystatin may be indicated

NURSING DIAGNOSIS

Risk for impaired skin integrity and altered oral mucous membranes related to immobility, invasive devices and procedures, dehydration, malnutrition, immunosuppression

PATIENT OUTCOMES
Skin and mucous membranes intact

• Absence of signs of pressure areas, breakdown, lesions, excoriation
• Skin turgor and moisture of mucous membranes adequate

NURSING CARE PLAN for the Immunocompromised Patient—cont'd

NURSING INTERVENTIONS	RATIONALES
• Assess skin and mucous membranes every shift for pressure, breakdown, lesions, and excoriation	• Assess for complications
• Monitor incisions, IV and venipuncture sites, axillae, perineal areas for redness, swelling, pain, heat	• Signs of infection may not be obvious
• Provide meticulous skin care; keep skin clean, dry, and lubricated	• Prevent infection
• Provide frequent mouth care with nonirritating solutions and soft-bristled brush	• Maintain moisture of mucous membranes
• Turn/reposition the patient at least every 2 hours; evaluate need for therapeutic beds/mattresses	• Prevent skin breakdown
• Treat any pressure ulcers or areas of breakdown promptly; consult with wound care specialist	• Prevent further complications; obtain advice from wound experts
• Maintain adequate hydration and optimal nutritional status	• Decrease risk for skin breakdown

NURSING DIAGNOSIS

Altered nutrition (less than body requirements) related to NPO status; anorexia, nausea/vomiting; and painful oral mucosa

PATIENT OUTCOMES
Optimal nutritional status maintained

• Adequate caloric and protein intake
• Ideal/stable body weight
• Laboratory values will remain within normal limits (total protein, serum albumin, electrolytes, hemoglobin, and hematocrit)

NURSING INTERVENTIONS	RATIONALES
• Assess baseline nutritional status: height and weight, laboratory values; presence of weakness, fatigue, infection, or other signs of malnutrition	• Obtain baseline assessment
• Obtain dietary consult to determine nutrients/intake required. Administer enteral/parenteral nutritional therapy as ordered and observe response	• Optimize nutritional therapy to reduce risks
• Establish food preferences. Encourage meals from home and provides relaxed atmosphere during meals	• Tailor nutritional support based on patient's preferences (see EBP box)
• Determine deterrents to adequate intake: fasting (NPO) status, presence of anorexia, nausea, vomiting, stomatitis	• Assess risks for decreased nutrition

Continued

NURSING CARE PLAN   for the Immunocompromised Patient—cont'd

NURSING INTERVENTIONS	RATIONALES
• Monitor daily weight, laboratory values, protein and caloric intake, I&O	• Monitor status
• Encourage small, frequent, high-calorie and high-protein meals	• Promote adequate intake
• Provide meticulous mouth care before and after meals	• Maintain oral mucosa and facilitate oral intake
• Administer antiemetics as needed, 30 minutes before meals	• Encourage adequate intake

BP, Blood pressure; *HEPA*, high-efficiency particulate air; *I&O*, intake and output; *IV*, intravenous; *NPO*, nothing by mouth; *WBC*, white blood cell.

EVIDENCE-BASED PRACTICE

PROBLEM

Neutropenia is an expected side effect associated with many chemotherapy agents. It becomes problematic, and can be life-threatening, when patients develop infections while neutropenic. A neutropenic diet is sometimes recommended as part of the treatment for patients with neutropenia. Dietary modifications are prescribed to help protect patients from bacteria and harmful organisms found in some food and drinks. The role of the neutropenic diet for patients with neutropenia is controversial, in both medicine and nursing.

QUESTION

What is the evidence that guides the teaching of neutropenic diet precautions to patients receiving outpatient chemotherapy?

REFERENCE

De Mille, D., Deming, P., Lupinacci, P., & Jacobs, L. A. (2006). The effect of the neutropenic diet in the outpatient setting: A pilot study. *Oncology Nursing Forum, 33*(2), 337-343.

EVIDENCE

The risk for infection is related to the severity and duration of the neutropenia. The literature review for this study was thorough and found that providers and patients make changes in the diet to prevent infections, even though no standard definition for what constitutes a neutropenic diet exists. It is well documented that many institutional practices advise dietary restrictions despite a lack of scientific evidence that it makes a difference in patient outcomes. In this pilot study, 16 of 28 subjects were compliant with the neutropenic diet. The rates of admissions for fever and positive blood cultures were not different between those compliant and noncompliant with the diet, although the study was limited by sample size.

IMPLICATIONS FOR NURSING

The majority of chemotherapy is provided in an outpatient setting. Neutropenic diet precautions are being recommended and taught to patients receiving chemotherapy, even though the definition is ambiguous and there is no evidence base supporting its use. This study was one of the first to test the outcomes of an intervention (diet) that has been advocated for years. Nurses should familiarize themselves with the literature regarding neutropenic diets, so that the teaching reflects the lack of scientific evidence. Evidence-based research studies are lacking for a commonly taught practice. Nurses have an opportunity to fill this gap in knowledge by designing studies that focus on patient outcomes; perhaps good hand washing and proper food-handling techniques are sufficient in providing best outcomes.

Nursing Diagnoses

The specific nursing diagnosis related to all patients with neutropenia is risk for infection.

Medical Interventions

Medical treatment of neutropenia is aimed at preventing and treating infection while reversing the cause of neutropenia. Patients with anticipated neutropenia, such as those receiving antineoplastic or antiretroviral therapy, may be administered bone marrow growth factors. Also known as colony-stimulating factors (CSF), these agents enhance bone marrow regeneration of the granulocyte (G-CSF), macrophage (M-CSF), or both cell lines (GM-CSF).[16]

Malnutrition
- Vitamin B deficiency
- Calorie deficiency
- Iron deficiency
- Protein deficiency

Health States
- Addison's disease
- Anaphylactic shock
- Anorexia nervosa
- Brucellosis
- Chronic fever
- Chronic illness
- Cirrhosis
- Diabetes mellitus
- Elderly status
- Hypothermia
- Infectious diseases (any severe bacterial or viral): mononucleosis, measles, mumps, influenza
- Renal trauma

Medications
- Alcohol
- Alkylating agents (antineoplastic and immunosuppressive; e.g., cyclophosphamide)
- Allopurinol (Zyloprim)
- Anticonvulsants (e.g., phenytoin)
- Antidysrhythmics (e.g., procainamide, quinidine)
- Antimicrobials (e.g., aminoglycosides, chloramphenicol, sulfonamides, trimethoprim-sulfamethoxazole)
- Antiretroviral agents (e.g., zidovudine)
- Antitumor antibiotics (e.g., bleomycin, doxorubicin [Adriamycin])
- Arsenic
- Phenothiazines (e.g., prochlorperazine)

Prophylactic antiinfective agents may be ordered to prevent infection, and potent broad-spectrum bactericidal antimicrobial agents are ordered when there is evidence of infection. In sepsis accompanying neutropenia, granulocyte transfusions are occasionally used to supplement phagocytosis.

Nursing Interventions

Nursing care of patients with neutropenia is the same as for all immunocompromised patients (see Nursing Care Plan for the Immunocompromised Patient). Desired patient outcomes related to medical and nursing interventions include absence of infection, negative cultures, and an absolute neutrophil count of 1500 cells/microliter or higher.

Malignant White Blood Cell Disorders: Leukemia, Lymphoma, and Multiple Myeloma

Pathophysiology

Malignant diseases involving WBCs are termed leukemia, lymphoma, and plasma cell neoplasm (multiple myeloma). They are differentiated by the cell affected and by the stage of cell development when malignancy occurs. Regardless of the specific neoplastic disorder, a deficiency of functional WBCs is a common problem. The unique pathophysiological and clinical characteristics of these disorders are described in Table 16-10. Despite normal serum cell counts, WBC activity is always impaired, and infection is the most common complication of all these disorders.

Assessment and Clinical Manifestations

Malignant hematological diseases have common risk factors such as genetic mutations, viral infection (especially retroviral), radiation, carcinogens, benzene derivatives, pesticides, and T-lymphocyte immune suppression (e.g., high-dose steroids, immunosuppressives after transplantation). Other risk factors that are unique to the specific malignancy are included in Table 16-10.

Assessment findings common to all malignant WBC disorders involve alterations in the immunological response to injury or microbes. As in other disorders affecting WBC function, minimized inflammatory reactions and response to pathogens are typical. Fever is particularly difficult to interpret because it may be a manifestation of the disease process or may accompany an infectious complication. General signs and symptoms such as fatigue, malaise, myalgias, activity intolerance, and night sweats are nonspecific indicators of immune disease. Each malignant WBC disorder is also associated with signs and symptoms representative of the cell line and location of the malignancy. For example, bone pain is common in multiple myeloma, while lymph node enlargement is more representative of lymphoma.[15] When symptoms overlap into more than one component of the immune system, it may be difficult to differentiate between these disorders.

The critical care nurse must be aware of unique oncological emergencies associated with these malignant diseases. Oncological emergencies may be the consequence of the cancer itself, a specific treatment plan, or tumor lysis. These complications are more likely to precipitate admission to the intensive care unit and are associated with significant morbidity and mortality. Information about complications are identified in Table 16-10.

TABLE 16-10　Malignant White Blood Cell Disorders

Leukemia	Lymphoma	Multiple Myeloma
Pathophysiology		
Cancer involving any of the WBCs during the early phase of maturation within the bone marrow	Cancer affects the lymphocytes after their bone marrow maturation, when they reside within the lymph node	Cancer involves the mature and differentiated immunoglobulin-producing macrophage called a plasma cell; the malignancy is primarily manifested by excess abnormal immunoglobulin
Classification		
Excess proliferation of immature cells is termed *acute* leukemia Excess proliferation of mature cells is termed *chronic* leukemia Leukemias are further classified according to whether they originate in the lymphocyte cell line or are nonlymphocytic	Hodgkin's and non-Hodgkin's subtypes have more subclassifications denoting the maturity of the cell involved and aggressiveness of the malignancy	Disease is classified as limited or extensive depending on the plasma viscosity, bone manifestations, presence of hypercalcemia, and renal involvement
Risk Factors		
Chromosomal abnormalities Viral infection Radiation Herbicides/pesticides Benzene/toluene Immunosuppressive therapy (e.g., high-dose steroids or posttransplant immunosuppressives) Alkylating agents	Chromosomal abnormalities Viral infection Radiation Herbicides/pesticides Benzene/toluene Immunosuppressive therapy (e.g., high-dose steroids or posttransplant immunosuppressives) Alkylating agents Autoimmune disease	Older age Male gender African American descent Chronic hypersensitivity reactions Autoimmune diseases
Clinical Manifestations		
Fever Constitutional symptoms: fatigue, malaise, weakness, night sweats Easy bruising and bleeding from mucous membranes such as gums Bone pain	Enlarged >2 cm, nontender lymph node Usually immovable, and irregularly shaped Masses in body cavities or other organs (e.g., peritoneal cavity, lungs)	Thrombotic events: deep vein thrombosis, pulmonary embolism, cerebral infarction Bone pain Renal failure
Acute Complications		
Leukostasis Disseminated intravascular coagulation Tumor lysis syndrome	Airway obstruction Superior vena cava syndrome Bowel obstruction Neoplastic tamponade Pleural effusion	Hyperviscosity Renal failure Hypercalcemia
Staging		
All patients are viewed as having systemic disease, or late-stage disease	Classified by the number of lymph nodes involved, the number of lymph node groups, whether involved nodes are only above the diaphragm or on both sides of the diaphragm, and how many extranodal sites are involved	Disease is classified as limited when there are only elevated abnormal immunoglobin levels; described as extensive when there are bone lesions, hypercalcemia, or renal dysfunction

TABLE 16-10 Malignant White Blood Cell Disorders—cont'd

Leukemia	Lymphoma	Multiple Myeloma
Diagnostic Tests		
CBC show either ↓ WBCs or large number of immature WBCs (blasts), ↓ RBCs, ↓ platelets Bone marrow aspiration and biopsy	Lymph node biopsy CT scans Chemistry: alkaline phosphatase	Bence Jones protein in urine Immunoglobulin electrophoresis Plasma viscosity
Medical Management		
Systemic chemotherapy BMT	Radiation therapy for single node or node group if above diaphragm for control or remission Radiation used if palliation of tumor is goal of therapy Systemic chemotherapy for multinode involvement, aggressive tumor subtypes Autologous BMT for patients with high risk of relapse Allogeneic BMT for patients with residual disease, especially involving bone marrow	Systemic chemotherapy only provides average of 14-36 months remission. BMT or "double" BMT may increase survival Radiation therapy used to palliatively treat bone lesions
Nursing Care Issues		
Infection control practices Bleeding precautions	Infection control practices Edema management Monitoring for lymphoma masses compressing body organs	Infection control practices Safe mobility Thrombosis precautions Aspiration precautions if hypercalcemic

↓, Decreased; *BMT*, bone marrow transplant; *CBC*, complete blood count; *CT*, computed tomography; *RBCs*, red blood cells; *WBCs*, white blood cells.

Nursing Diagnoses

The nursing diagnoses associated with hematological malignancies have some variation with each disorder. Common nursing diagnoses include risk for infection, altered tissue perfusion related to anemia, and risk for injury (bleeding).

Medical Interventions

Each major subtype of hematological malignancy denotes an additional list of further classification subdivisions, each with slightly differing presenting symptoms, prognostic variables, and treatment implications. The treatment plan is based on the stage of the definitive diagnosis established by accurate histopathology. The stage of disease dictates the choice of therapy in Hodgkin's lymphoma, multiple myeloma, and some non-Hodgkin's lymphomas.

Therapy commonly includes chemotherapy and biotherapy, and in selected cases, bone marrow transplantation. Surgery may be performed to establish a pathological diagnosis by excisional or incisional biopsy, but has no other significant role in the management of hematological malignancies. Radiation may be used to treat lymphoma when the disease is limited to single nodes or node groups.

The complexity of treatment is noted in the following examples. Leukemia is considered a *systemic* disease at diagnosis. Acute leukemias require complex chemotherapy treatment plans called *induction* chemotherapy at the time of diagnosis, and are associated with a period of severe cytopenias that require supportive care and transfusion therapy. The management of chronic myelogenous leukemia has been dramatically improved with the development of imatinib mesylate (Gleevec), an oral agent that results in high remission rates. The management of chronic lymphocytic leukemia has seen major changes with the availability of newer agents.

Multiple myeloma therapy involves careful staging and a choice of induction chemotherapy plans, leading to autologous stem cell transplantation for most patients. Radiation therapy is used palliatively to control the pain associated with bone lesions. Because of the rapid application of the advances in molecular biology, there has been a dramatic improvement in remission and cure rates for most hematological malignancies. Curing lymphomas and leukemias with the least chance for long-term treatment-related complications is now a realistic approach.[8]

Nursing Interventions

The care of patients with hematological malignancies is similar to that for all immunocompromised patients; however, specialized management of cancer therapies must be incorporated into the individual care plan. Oncology nursing references for chemotherapy administration guidelines, management of acute therapy–related nausea and vomiting, and oncological treatment modalities are available from the Oncology Nursing Society (ONS).

SELECTED IMMUNOLOGICAL DISORDERS

Primary Immunodeficiency

In primary immunodeficiency, the dysfunction exists in the immune system. Most primary immunodeficiencies are congenital disorders related to a single gene defect. The onset of symptoms may occur within the first 2 years of life, or in the second or third decade of life.[19] These defects of the immune system typically result in frequent or recurrent infections, and sometimes may predispose the affected individual to unusual or severe infections.[18] Disorders are grouped by their immunological disruption.

Secondary Immunodeficiency

In secondary, or acquired, immunodeficiency the immune disorder is the result of factors outside the immune system, not related to a genetic defect, and involves the loss of a previously functional immune defense. AIDS is the most notable secondary immunodeficiency disorder caused by an infection. AIDS-infected individuals are extremely susceptible to severe infections and malignancies. Risk factors for infections in immunocompromised patients are further described in Table 16-9. AIDS is discussed in more detail in the next section. Aging, dietary insufficiencies, malignancies, stressors (emotional, physi-

cal), immunosuppressive therapies, and certain diseases such as diabetes or sickle cell disease are additional examples of conditions that may be associated with acquired immunodeficiencies.

Acquired Immunodeficiency Syndrome

Pathophysiology. HIV is a retrovirus that transcribes its RNA-containing genetic material into the DNA of the host cell nucleus by using an enzyme called reverse transcriptase. HIV causes AIDS by depleting helper T cells, CD4 cells, and macrophages. Seroconversion is manifested by the presence of HIV antibodies and is likely to occur within 4 to 7 weeks after infection through blood products, or it may take several months when a patient is infected through sexual exposure.[19] This seroconversion is followed by a decrease in the HIV antibody titer as infected cells are sequestered in the lymph nodes. The earlier stages of HIV infection may last as long as 10 years and may produce few or no symptoms, although viral particles are actively replacing normal cells. This phenomenon is evident through the decreasing CD4 cell counts as the disease progresses.[19] As the CD4 cell count decreases, the patient becomes more susceptible to opportunistic infections, malignancies, and neurological disease. AIDS is the final stage of HIV infection. Figure 16-6 shows the progression of disease and common clinical manifestations. It is estimated that 99% of untreated HIV-infected individuals will progress to AIDS.[19] Treatment regimens with combined antiviral drug regimens are controlling the progression to AIDS; AIDS is now considered, for many infected individuals, a chronic disease.

HIV is transmitted through exposure to infected body fluids, blood, or blood products. Common modes of transmission include rectal or vaginal intercourse with an infected person, intravenous drug use with contaminated equipment, transfusion with contaminated blood or blood products, and accidental exposure through needle sticks, breaks in the skin, gestation, or childbirth (from mother to fetus). Risk of transmission is more likely when the infected person has advanced disease, although transmission of HIV can occur at any time or stage of infection. Since the 1980s, all blood products have been screened for HIV, hepatitis virus, and human T-cell lymphotrophic virus. The risk of HIV transmission to health care workers is small and is further diminished through consistent observance of universal precautions.

Assessment and Clinical Manifestations. The initial phase of HIV disease may be asymptomatic, or it may manifest as an acute seroconversion syndrome with symptoms similar to those of mononucleosis. This is followed by asymptomatic disease as HIV progressively destroys immune cells, which leads to

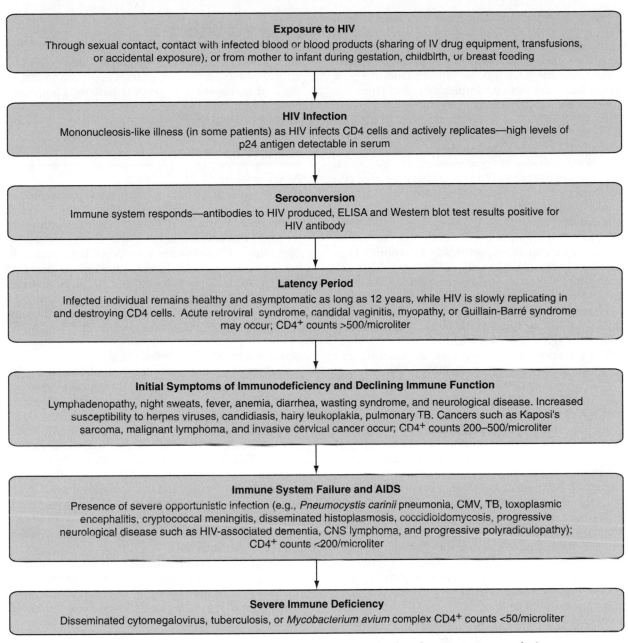

Exposure to HIV
Through sexual contact, contact with infected blood or blood products (sharing of IV drug equipment, transfusions, or accidental exposure), or from mother to infant during gestation, childbirth, or breast feeding

HIV Infection
Mononucleosis-like illness (in some patients) as HIV infects CD4 cells and actively replicates—high levels of p24 antigen detectable in serum

Seroconversion
Immune system responds—antibodies to HIV produced, ELISA and Western blot test results positive for HIV antibody

Latency Period
Infected individual remains healthy and asymptomatic as long as 12 years, while HIV is slowly replicating in and destroying CD4 cells. Acute retroviral syndrome, candidal vaginitis, myopathy, or Guillain-Barré syndrome may occur; CD4$^+$ counts >500/microliter

Initial Symptoms of Immunodeficiency and Declining Immune Function
Lymphadenopathy, night sweats, fever, anemia, diarrhea, wasting syndrome, and neurological disease. Increased susceptibility to herpes viruses, candidiasis, hairy leukoplakia, pulmonary TB. Cancers such as Kaposi's sarcoma, malignant lymphoma, and invasive cervical cancer occur; CD4$^+$ counts 200–500/microliter

Immune System Failure and AIDS
Presence of severe opportunistic infection (e.g., *Pneumocystis carinii* pneumonia, CMV, TB, toxoplasmic encephalitis, cryptococcal meningitis, disseminated histoplasmosis, coccidioidomycosis, progressive neurological disease such as HIV-associated dementia, CNS lymphoma, and progressive polyradiculopathy); CD4$^+$ counts <200/microliter

Severe Immune Deficiency
Disseminated cytomegalovirus, tuberculosis, or *Mycobacterium avium* complex CD4$^+$ counts <50/microliter

FIGURE 16-6. Human immunodeficiency virus (HIV) pathophysiology. *CMV*, Cytomegalovirus; *CNS*, central nervous system; *ELISA*, enzyme-linked immunosorbent assay; *TB*, tuberculosis.

AIDS. AIDS is defined by the presence of a CD4 count that is less than 200/microliter and the presence of an indicator condition[3] (see Figure 16-6). The signs and symptoms of AIDS vary with the CD4 count and the particular indicator disease manifested.

Diagnosis of HIV infection is made by the presence of one of the core antigens of HIV or the presence of antibodies to HIV. Core antigens are tested through protein electrophoresis. HIV antibodies are detected by enzyme-linked immunosorbent assay (ELISA) and are confirmed by the Western blot test and polymerase chain reaction (PCR).[4] Positive antibody test results are accurate for the presence of HIV infection, although a negative test result does not rule out HIV infection. Additional laboratory findings in AIDS may include an abnormal helper-to-suppressor ratio (<1.0), leukopenia, and thrombocytopenia.

Nursing Diagnoses. Nursing care of the patient with AIDS is complex, and nursing diagnoses depend on the particular clinical manifestations of the disease. Universal nursing diagnoses for these patients may include risk for infection, impaired tissue integrity, altered nutrition, activity intolerance, and pain.

Medical Interventions. Medical treatment consists of primary control of HIV invasion of CD4 cells through antiretroviral therapy. Antiretroviral medications are categorized as nucleoside reverse transcriptase inhibitors, nonnucleoside reverse transcriptase inhibitors, and protease inhibitors. The specific agents used and the strategies of combination therapy are a rapidly changing science that would be quickly outdated if included in this text.

Equally important to quality of life are prevention and management of opportunistic infections. Antimicrobials are administered to prevent high-risk opportunistic infections when predefined CD4 levels are reached. Additional treatment may include respiratory support, nutritional support, administration of blood products or intravenous fluids, administration of analgesics, and physical therapy.

Nursing Interventions. Nursing care of patients with HIV infection requires complex assessment and intervention skills. As with all immunosuppressed patients, those with HIV infection must be protected from infection. Precautions outlined in the Nursing Care Plan for the Immunocompromised Patient are followed. These patients provide additional clinical challenges because of their multisystemic clinical complications.

Nursing assessment must be comprehensive and include evaluation of the neurological status, mouth, respiratory status, abdominal symptoms, and peripheral sensation. For unclear reasons, persons with HIV infection have a higher propensity for adverse drug reactions than other patient groups and require careful monitoring of all medication regimens.

Staff members are encouraged to consult with support personnel and psychosocial health professionals to assist with the physical and emotional demands of caring for this population. The potential risk of exposure, although small, places an additional emotional stressor on nurses. Continuing education must be available to address prevention of HIV transmission, current research, and treatments.

Desired patient outcomes of medical treatment and nursing interventions include absence of infection, adequate oxygenation, adequate nutrition and hydration, skin integrity, and absence of pain. Complications such as diarrhea and seizures will be controlled. Lastly, the patient will understand disease transmission, the course of the disease, symptoms of opportunistic infections, treatments, and medications.

BLEEDING DISORDERS

Patients with abnormal hemostasis often require critical care treatment. A general approach to assessing and managing the bleeding patient is addressed before a more thorough discussion of thrombocytopenia and DIC.

The Bleeding Patient

Pathophysiology

Bleeding disorders, also referred to as *coagulopathies*, are caused by abnormalities in one of the stages of clotting: (1) vasoconstriction, (2) creation of a platelet plug, (3) development of the fibrin clot, or (4) fibrinolysis. Disorders are considered inherited (e.g., hemophilia, von Willebrand's disease) or acquired (e.g., vitamin K deficiency, DIC). Coagulopathies induce bleeding manifestations, and many care principles are universal. This section addresses the universal care of patients with disorders of coagulation.

Assessment and Clinical Manifestations

A patient with abnormal bleeding requires a careful medical and social history. It is important to assess for medical disorders and medications known to interfere with platelets, coagulation proteins, or fibrinolysis. Disruptions in hemostasis commonly occur in conjunction with renal disease, hepatic or gastrointestinal disorders, and malnutrition. Medications that may alter hemostasis include aminoglycosides, anticoagulants, antiplatelets, cephalosporins, histamine blockers, nitrates, sulfonamides, sympathomimetics, and vasodilators. Recognition of these risk factors, and modification when possible, may reduce the severity of bleeding.

The physical examination is extremely important. Although many patients with bleeding disorders demonstrate active bleeding from body orifices, mucous membranes, and open lesions or intravenous line sites, equal numbers of patients have less obvious bleeding. The most susceptible sites for bleeding are existing openings in the epithelial surfaces. Mucous membranes have a low threshold for bleeding because the capillaries lie close to the membrane surface, and minor injury may damage and expose vessels. A general overview of assessment findings that indicate bleeding is included in Table 16-5.

Substantial blood loss can occur in any coagulopathy. The physical consequences of blood loss are apparent in all body systems, most prominently the cardiac and pulmonary systems. Guidelines for assessment of bleeding and blood loss are described in the Nursing Care Plan for the Patient with a Bleeding Disorder.

Diagnostic tests are performed to evaluate the cause of the bleeding disorder and the extent of blood loss. The CBC provides quantitative values for RBCs and platelets. When the disorder arises from coagulation protein or clot lysis abnormalities, screening coagulation tests of fibrinogen level, prothrombin time, and partial thromboplastin time are usually ordered. Point-of-care tests for hemoglobin, hematocrit, and partial thromboplastin time are important resources to obtain immediate feedback regarding the patient's response to interventions in a bleeding disorder. In certain disease states, additional specialized tests such as bleeding time and levels of fibrin degradation products are monitored.

Nursing Diagnoses

The actively bleeding patient or one with a hemostatic disorder can have bleeding into any body system. The major diagnoses include risk for bleeding, altered protection, decreased tissue perfusion, fluid volume deficit, and pain.

Medical Interventions

Medical treatment for bleeding patients depends on the suspected cause. Component-specific replacement transfusions are preferred over whole blood because they provide more specific treatment of the bleeding disorder. Transfusion thresholds are established based on laboratory values and patient-specific variables. In general, a threshold for RBC transfusion is considered a hematocrit of 28% to 31%, based on the patient's cardiovascular tolerance. If angina or orthostasis is present, a higher threshold may be maintained. The platelet count may drop as low as 5000 to 10,000/microliter before spontaneous bleeding is likely to occur. This transfusion threshold may be too low for patients with preexisting conditions such as recent surgical procedures or

---

NURSING CARE PLAN for the Patient with a Bleeding Disorder

NURSING DIAGNOSIS

Altered tissue perfusion related to abnormal clotting, hypotension, and/or anemia

PATIENT OUTCOMES
Adequate perfusion maintained and damage to vital organs prevented

- Vital signs and hemodynamic stability, values within normal limits
- Normal mental status
- ABG results within normal limits
- Urine output >30 mL/hr; adequate peripheral pulses
- Skin warm with normal color

NURSING INTERVENTIONS	RATIONALES
• Monitor hemodynamics, vital signs, ABGs, I&O, and laboratory results	• Assess hemodynamic status to provide baseline
• Assess for and report signs of altered perfusion	• Assess for blood loss
• Provide good skin and oral care	• Promote circulation
• Evaluate vital signs for orthostatic changes	• Assess for blood loss
• Recognize signs and symptoms of subcutaneous bleeding (e.g., ecchymoses, hematomas)	• Assess for bleeding disorders
• Note increased girth of limbs or abdomen. Mark anatomical area for consistency of measurement	• Assess for bleeding into limbs and/or abdomen
• Elevate any limb that is bleeding	• Reduce blood flow to the area
• Administer blood components as ordered and monitor for adverse effects (see Table 16-11)	• Treat etiology of bleeding disorder
• Administer selective vasoconstrictor agents (e.g., vasopressin) as ordered	• Promote vasoconstriction and decrease bleeding
• Administer procoagulants (e.g., somatostatin, estrogen) as ordered	• Promote clotting and decrease bleeding

Continued

NURSING CARE PLAN   for the Patient with a Bleeding Disorder—cont'd

NURSING DIAGNOSIS

Fluid volume deficit related to hemorrhage

PATIENT OUTCOMES
Free of bleeding and normovolemic

- Absence of oozing/bleeding
- Laboratory study results within normal limits
- Vital signs and hemodynamics stable and within normal limits

NURSING INTERVENTIONS	RATIONALES
• Monitor hemodynamics, vital signs, I&O, and laboratory study results	• Assess for changes in volume status
• Weigh dressings/linens (urine, NG, stool)	• Estimate blood loss more accurately
• Assess body fluids for occult blood	• Assess for hidden sources of blood loss
• Assess and report signs of bleeding, such as oozing or bleeding from venipunctures, IV access sites, incisions, wounds, mucous membranes, and body orifices	• Assess sources of blood loss and provide early intervention
• Control bleeding using ice packs, pressure dressings, or direct pressure	• Reduce bleeding through vasoconstriction (cold) or pressure
• Leave existing clots undisturbed	• Prevent disruption of clot
• Administer topical hemostatic agents as ordered	• Promote clotting
• Severe bleeding requires administration of fluid to replenish volume even if blood components are administered (normal saline or Ringer's lactate)	• Maintain adequate volume; Ringer's lactate aids in maintaining the acid-base balance

ABGs, Arterial blood gases; *I&O*, intake and output; *NG*, nasogastric.

peptic ulcer disease. A more conservative platelet transfusion marker used in many critical care units is between 20,000 and 50,000/microliter. Cryoprecipitate is usually infused if the fibrinogen level is less than 100 mg/dL.[4] Fresh frozen plasma is used to correct a prolonged prothrombin time and partial thromboplastin time or a specific factor deficiency.[4] A summary of blood product components, clinical indications, and nursing implications is included in Table 16-11.

When the cause of bleeding is unknown or multifactorial, nonspecific interventions aimed at stopping bleeding are used. These include local and systemic procoagulant medications and therapies.

Local therapies to stop bleeding are used when systemic anticoagulation is necessary for treatment of another health condition (e.g., myocardial infarction, ischemic stroke, or pulmonary embolism). Local procoagulants usually act by direct tissue contact and initiation of a surface clot.

Systemic procoagulant medications may be used to enhance vasoconstriction (e.g., vasopressin), enhance clot formation (e.g., somatostatin), or prevent clot breakdown (e.g., aminocaproic acid). These agents are used judiciously in clinical situations when it is believed that inadequate clot formation and premature clot dissolution are the causes of excess bleeding. Each agent has significant adverse effects that must be considered before implementation. All may enhance clot production and induce thrombotic vascular or neurological events. They may be contraindicated when the patient has simultaneous procoagulant risk factors.

Nursing Interventions

Patients with bleeding disorders often have multisystemic manifestations. Administration of fluids and blood products is a priority nursing intervention that requires careful consideration of the patient's specific coagulation defect. When the patient's blood does

TABLE 16-11 Summary of Blood Products and Administration

Blood Component	Description	Actions	Indications	Administration	Complications
Whole blood	RBCs, plasma, and stable clotting factors	Restores oxygen-carrying capacity and intravascular volume	Symptomatic anemia with major circulating volume deficit Massive hemorrhage with shock	Donor and recipient must be ABO compatible and Rh compatible Use microaggregate filter Rate of infusion: usually 2-4 unit/hour but more rapid in cases of shock	Hemolytic reaction Allergic reaction Hypothermia Electrolyte disturbances Citrate intoxication Infectious diseases
RBCs	RBCs centrifuged from whole blood	Restores oxygen-carrying capacity and intravascular volume	Symptomatic anemia when patient is at risk for fluid overload Acute hemorrhage	Donor and recipient must be ABO and Rh compatible Use microaggregate filter Rate of infusion: 2-4 unit/hour but more rapid in cases of shock	Infectious diseases Hemolytic reaction Allergic reaction Hypothermia Electrolyte disturbances Citrate intoxication
Leukocyte-poor cells or washed RBCs	RBCs from which leukocytes and plasma proteins have been reduced	Restores oxygen-carrying capacity and intravascular volume	Symptomatic anemia with patient history of repeated, febrile, nonhemolytic transfusion reactions Acute hemorrhage	Donor and recipient must be ABO and Rh compatible Use microaggregate filter Rate of infusion: 2-4 unit/hour but more rapid in cases of shock	Allergic reaction Hemolytic reaction Hypothermia Electrolyte disturbances Citrate intoxication Infectious diseases
Fresh frozen plasma	Plasma rich in clotting factors with platelets removed	Replaces clotting factors	Deficit of coagulation factors as in DIC, liver disease, and massive transfusions Major trauma with signs/symptoms of hemorrhage	Donor and recipient must be ABO compatible, but not necessary to be Rh compatible Rate of Infusion: 10 mL/min	Allergic reaction Febrile reactions Circulatory overload Infectious diseases
Platelets	Removed from whole blood	Increases platelet count and improves hemostasis	Thrombocytopenia Platelet dysfunction (prophylactically for platelet counts 10,000-20,000/microliter), evidence of bleeding with platelet count <50,000/microliter	Do not use microaggregate filter; component filter obtained from blood bank ABO testing not necessary unless contaminated with RBCs but is usually done Usually give 6 units at one time	Infectious diseases Allergic reactions Febrile reactions

Continued

TABLE 16-11 Summary of Blood Products and Administration—cont'd

Blood Component	Description	Actions	Indications	Administration	Complications
Cryoprecipitate antihemophilic factor	Primarily coagulation factor VIII with 250 mg of fibrinogen and 20%-30% of factor XIII	Replaces selected clotting factors	Hemophilia A, von Willebrand's disease Hypofibrinogenemia Factor XIII deficiency Massive transfusions	Repeat doses may be necessary to attain satisfactory serum level Rate of infusion: approximately 10 mL of diluted component per minute	Allergic reactions Infectious diseases
Albumin	Prepared from plasma	Expands intravascular volume by increasing oncotic pressure	Hypovolemic shock Liver failure	Special administration set Rate of infusion: over 30-60 minutes	Circulatory overload Febrile reaction
Granulocytes	Prepared by centrifugation or filtration leukopheresis, which removes granulocytes from whole blood	Increases the leukocyte level	Decreased WBCs usually from chemotherapy or radiation	Must be ABO compatible and Rh compatible Rate of infusion: 1 unit over 2-4 hours; closely observe for reaction	Rash Febrile reaction Hepatitis
Plasma proteins	Pooled from human plasma	Expands intravascular volume by increasing oncotic pressure	Hypovolemic shock	ABO compatibility not necessary Rate of infusion: over 30-60 minutes	Circulatory overload Febrile reaction

DIC, Disseminated intravascular coagulation; *RBCs*, red blood cells; *WBCs*, white blood cells.

not clot because of thrombocytopenia, administration of RBCs before platelets will result in RBC loss from disrupted vascular structures.

Precautions such as limiting invasive procedures, including indwelling urinary catheters or rectal temperature measurement, are important. A comprehensive listing of bleeding precautions is included in the Nursing Care Plan for the Patient with a Bleeding Disorder.

Thrombocytopenia

Pathophysiology

A quantitative deficiency of platelets is termed *thrombocytopenia*. By definition, this is a platelet count of less than 100,000/microliter; however, levels greater than 50,000/microliter rarely cause significant complications. Thrombocytopenia can cause severe hemorrhage if it is not corrected. The pathophysiology may be related to decreased production of platelets by the bone marrow, increased destruction of platelets, or sequestration of platelets (abnormal distribution).[15]

Assessment and Clinical Manifestations

Many critical care therapies and medications interfere with platelet production or life span and cause thrombocytopenia. A thorough medical, social, and medication history can help to identify factors that may cause thrombocytopenia. A comprehensive listing of causes is included in Box 16-3. Thrombocytopenia is also a complication of heparin therapy. Box 16-4 describes heparin-induced thrombocytopenia (HIT).

Clinically, the patient with thrombocytopenia presents with petechiae, purpura, and ecchymoses,

BOX 16-3   Causes of Thrombocytopenia

Bone Marrow Suppression
- Aplastic anemia
- Burns
- Cancer chemotherapy
- Exposure to ionizing radiation
- Nutritional deficiency (vitamin B_{12}, folate)

Interference with Platelet Production (Other than Nonspecific Marrow Suppression)
- Alcohol
- Histamine$_2$-blocking agents
- Histoplasmosis
- Hormones
- Thiazide diuretics

Platelet Destruction Outside the Bone Marrow
- Artificial heart valves
- Cardiac bypass machine
- Heat stroke
- Heparin
- Infections: severe or sepsis
- Large-bore intravenous lines
- Intraaortic balloon pump
- Splenic sequestration of platelets
- Sulfonamides
- Transfusions
- Trimethoprim-sulfamethoxazole

Immune Response Against Platelets
- Idiopathic thrombocytopenic purpura
- Mononucleosis
- Thrombotic thrombocytopenic purpura
- Vaccinations
- Viral illness

Interference with Platelet Function
- Aminoglycosides
- Catecholamines: epinephrine, dopamine
- Cirrhosis
- Dextran
- Diabetes mellitus
- Diazepam
- Digitoxin
- Hypothermia
- Loop diuretics (e.g., furosemide)
- Malignant lymphomas
- Nonsteroidal antiinflammatory agents
- Phenothiazines
- Phenytoin
- Salicylate derivatives
- Sarcoidosis
- Scleroderma
- Systemic lupus erythematosus
- Thyrotoxicosis
- Tricyclic antidepressants
- Uremia
- Vitamin E

with oozing from mucous membranes. Laboratory findings reveal a platelet count of less than 150,000/microliter, predisposing the patient to an increased risk of bleeding. When the count drops to less than 20,000 to 30,000/microliter, spontaneous bleeding may occur. Fatal hemorrhage is a great risk when the count is less than 10,000/microliter.[15]

Nursing Diagnoses
Patients with thrombocytopenia have many of the nursing diagnoses listed in care of the bleeding patient. Additional diagnoses include potential for bleeding and altered body image related to petechiae and ecchymoses (see Clinical Alert: Bleeding Disorders).

Medical Interventions
Medical treatment of thrombocytopenia includes infusions of platelets. Patients who require multiple platelet transfusions should be evaluated for single-donor platelet products. A single-donor product

CLINICAL ALERT
Bleeding Disorders

All body surfaces should be inspected for overt bleeding such as bruising or petechiae that indicate subcutaneous bleeding. Internal bleeding is more difficult to recognize as bleeding may occur even without a known injury, and symptoms are often subtle.

permits administration of 6 to 10 units of platelets with exposure to the antigens of only one person. For every 1 unit of single-donor platelets, the platelet count should increase by 5000 to 10,000/microliter.[7] Patients who receive many platelet transfusions can become refractory, or alloimmunized, to the many different platelet antigens and may fail to obtain benefit from non–human leukocyte antigen (HLA)-matched platelets (tissue typed to match the patient).

BOX 16-4 Heparin-Induced Thrombocytopenia[11,15,22]

Definition

Two types of heparin-induced thrombocytopenia (HIT) have been identified. Type I HIT is a nonimmunologic response to heparin treatment. Type I HIT is thought to occur from an interaction between heparin and circulating platelets; heparin causes direct agglutination of platelets. It is usually self-limiting. Type II HIT is a severe immune-mediated drug reaction that can occur in any patient who has received heparin. Heparin binds to platelet factor 4 (PF4), forming an antigenic complex on the surface of the platelets. Some patients develop an antibody to this complex. The antibody stimulates removal of platelets by splenic macrophages, and thrombocytopenia develops. Thrombosis also occurs secondary to platelet activation and generation of procoagulants.

Risks

Up to 50% of patients who receive heparin will develop antibodies. About 0.5% to 5% will develop Type II HIT. All patients who have been exposed to heparin are at risk for Type II HIT.

Complications

Complications of Type I HIT are those associated with a low platelet count. Type II HIT is more severe, and its major complications are thromboembolic in nature. These include deep vein thrombosis, pulmonary embo-lism, myocardial infarction, thrombotic stroke, arterial occlusion in limbs, and disseminated intravascular coagulation.

Diagnosis

HIT usually develops 5 to 14 days after initiation of heparin therapy; however, rapid-onset HIT can occur within the first hours after heparin exposure. Type I HIT occurs in approximately 10% of patients receiving heparin, and the platelet count does not usually fall below 100,000/microliter; no laboratory tests are required. Type II HIT is suspected if the platelet count drops below 100,000/microliter or more than 50% from baseline values. Heparin-PF4 antibody testing assists in confirmation of Type II HIT. However, results may not be known rapidly, and treatment should start if HIT is suspected.

Treatment

Type I HIT is usually self-limiting. Type II HIT is treated by discontinuing all heparin products, including heparin flushes and heparin-coated infusion catheters. Treatment focuses on administration of drugs that inhibit thrombin formation or cause direct thrombin inhibition. These drugs include lepirudin (Refludan), bivalirudin (Angiomax), or argatroban (Novastan).

After multiple platelet transfusions, febrile and allergic transfusion reactions are common but can be reduced by administration of acetaminophen and diphenhydramine before transfusion.

Thrombopoietin, a platelet stimulating cytokine, is being investigated as an alternative to platelet transfusion. Some thrombocytopenias are autoimmune induced and may respond to filtration of antibodies via plasmapheresis or immune suppression with corticosteroids. When the spleen is enlarged and tender and these other supportive therapies are unsuccessful, splenectomy can alleviate the autoimmune reaction.

Nursing Interventions

Nursing interventions for the patient with thrombocytopenia are similar to those listed for the bleeding patient. The nurse must recognize and limit complications or interventions that can deplete or shorten the life span of platelets. For example, high fevers and high metabolic activity (e.g., seizures) prematurely destroy platelets.

Desired patient outcomes include adequate tissue perfusion, skin integrity, prompt recognition and treatment of bleeding, and absence of pain.

Disseminated Intravascular Coagulation

Pathophysiology

DIC is a serious disorder of hemostasis characterized by exaggerated microvascular coagulation, depletion of clotting factors, and subsequent bleeding. Because clotting factors are used up in the abnormal coagulation process, this disorder is also termed consumption coagulopathy. The disorder often manifests with acute and severe symptoms, and is associated with a high mortality rate.

The clinical course of DIC ranges from an acute, life-threatening process to a chronic, low-grade condition. Sepsis is the most common cause of acute DIC.[1,15] Acute DIC develops rapidly and is the most serious form of acquired coagulopathy. With chronic DIC, the patient may have more subtle clinical and laboratory findings.

Whatever the initiating event in DIC, procoagulants that cause diffuse, uncontrolled clotting are released. The intrinsic or extrinsic pathways are activated by release of tissue factor, from either endothelial damage (intrinsic) or direct tissue damage (extrinsic). Large amounts of thrombin are produced, resulting in the deposition of fibrin in the microvasculature, the consumption of available clotting factors, and the stimulation of fibrinolysis.

Clotting in the microvasculature of the patient with DIC causes organ ischemia and necrosis. The skin, lungs, and kidneys are most often damaged. Thrombophlebitis, pulmonary embolism, cerebrovascular accident, gastrointestinal bleeding, and renal failure may result from thrombosis. In addition, microvasculature thrombosis may result in cyanosis of the fingers and toes, purpura fulminans, or infarction and gangrene of the digits or tip of the nose.[15]

The fibrinolysis that ensues results in the release of fibrin degradation products, which are potent anticoagulants that interfere with thrombin, fibrin, and platelet activity. RBCs are damaged as they try to pass through the blocked capillary beds; the damage to RBCs causes excess hemolysis. The lack of available clotting factors coupled with the anticoagulant forces results in an inability to form clots when needed and predisposes the patient with DIC to hemorrhage (Figure 16-7).

Assessment and Clinical Manifestations

DIC is always a secondary complication of excessive clotting stimuli and may be triggered by vessel injury caused by disease states, tissue injury, or a foreign

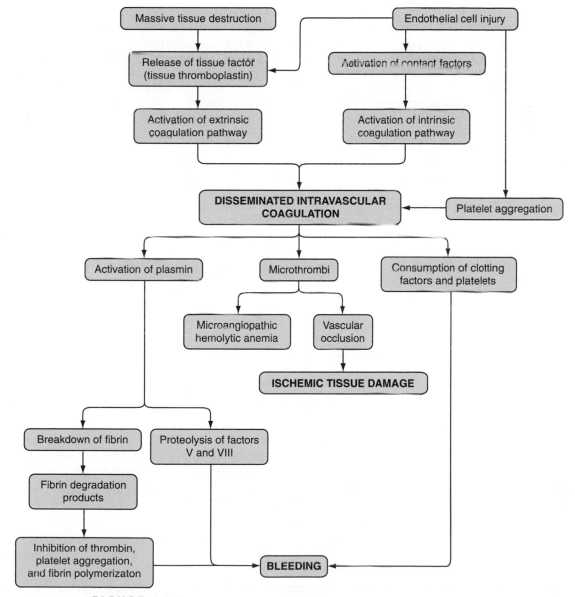

FIGURE 16-7. Pathophysiology of disseminated intravascular coagulopathy.

body in the bloodstream. The greater the clotting stimulus, the higher is the risk of developing the coagulopathy. Sepsis, multisystem trauma, and burns are the main risk factors for DIC and also provide the most significant stimuli for the clotting cascade. Recognition of potential risk factors and conscientious monitoring of the high-risk patient can permit early intervention. A summary of common risk factors for DIC is included in Table 16-12.

Clinically, the patient with DIC first develops microvascular thrombosis. Thrombosis leads to organ ischemia and necrosis that may be manifested as changes in mental status, angina, hypoxemia, oliguria, or nonspecific hepatitis. Cyanosis and infarction of the fingers and toes as well as infarction of the tip of the nose may occur if the DIC is severe. After a thrombotic phase of hours to a few days, depletion of clotting factors and clot lysis cause excessive bleeding. Early signs may include occult blood in the stool, emesis, and urine. Capillary fragility and depleted clotting factors often appear early as mucosal or subcutaneous tissue bleeding seen as gingival bleeding, petechiae, or ecchymoses. Overt bleeding ranges from mild oozing from venipuncture sites to massive hemorrhage from all body orifices. Occult bleeding into body cavities, such as the peritoneal and retroperitoneal spaces, may be detected by vital sign changes or other classic signs of blood loss.[1,15]

Diagnosis of DIC is made based on recognition of pertinent risk factors, clinical symptoms, and the results of laboratory studies. Evidence of factor depletion in the form of thrombocytopenia and hypofibrinogenemia is seen in the early phase; however, definitive diagnosis is made by evidence of excess fibrinolysis detectable by elevated fibrin degradation products, an increased D-dimer level, or a decreased antithrombin III level.[1,15] Altered laboratory values in DIC are noted in Laboratory Findings in Disseminated Intravascular Coagulation.

Nursing Diagnoses

The patient with DIC is likely to have multiple system involvement that encompasses both thrombotic and hemorrhagic manifestations. Nursing diagnoses may include altered tissue perfusion, fluid volume deficit, impaired skin integrity, and pain.

Medical Interventions

Medical treatment of DIC is aimed at identifying and treating the underlying cause, stopping the abnormal coagulation, and controlling the bleeding. Correction of hypotension, hypoxemia, and acidosis is vital, as is treatment of infection if it is the triggering factor. If the cause is obstetrical, evacuation of the uterus for retained fetal tissue or other tissue must be performed. Blood volume expanders and crystalloid intravenous fluids, such as lactated Ringer's solution or normal saline, are given to counteract hypovolemia caused by blood loss.

Blood component therapy is used in DIC to replace deficient platelets and clotting factors and to treat hemorrhage. Platelet infusions are usually necessary because of consumptive thrombocytopenia. They are viewed as the highest priority for transfusion because they will provide the clotting factors needed to establish an initial platelet plug from any bleeding sites. Fresh frozen plasma is administered for fibrinogen replacement. It contains all clotting factors and anti-

---

TABLE 16-12   Causes of Disseminated Intravascular Coagulation

Cause	Examples
Infections	Bacterial (especially gram-negative), fungal, viral, mycobacterial, protozoan, rickettsial
Trauma	Burns; crush or multiple injuries; snakebite
Obstetrical	Abruptio placentae, placenta previa, amniotic fluid embolism, retained dead fetus, missed abortion, eclampsia, hydatidiform mole
Hematological/ immunological disorders	Transfusion reaction, transplant rejections, anaphylaxis, autoimmune disorders, sickle cell crisis
Oncological disorders	Carcinomas, leukemias
Miscellaneous	Extracorporeal circulation, pulmonary or fat embolism, anoxia, acidosis, hyperthermia or hypothermia, hypovolemic shock, ARDS, sustained hypotension

ARDS, Acute respiratory distress syndrome.

GENETICS

FACTOR V LEIDEN: AN INHERITED CLOTTING DISORDER

There are many hereditary blood coagulation disorders. Some inherited disorders cause increased bleeding such as hemophilia. Other inherited disorders result in increased clotting or thrombophilia. The most common thrombophilic disorder with a genetic connection is factor V Leiden. This disorder is named after the city of Leiden, The Netherlands, where it was first identified in 1994.[1] It is an autosomal dominant condition, present in 2% to 15% of the general population.[5]

Factor V is one of the proteins in the clotting cascade. Factor V Leiden is a variation in this protein caused by a single nucleotide polymorphism—a substitution of adenine for guanine in the F5 gene on the long arm of chromosome 1.[6] This single nucleotide polymorphism changes the 506th amino acid of factor V from arginine to glutamine. The substitution of glutamine at this site increases the stability of factor V, resulting in prolonged clotting action. Normally, activated protein C inactivates factor V by cleaving it at three sites. When glutamine is present at the 506th amino acid site, activated protein C cannot inactivate factor V. When factor V remains active, it promotes overproduction of another clotting cascade protein, thrombin, leading to excess fibrin generation and clot formation. Thus, factor V Leiden is resistant to activated protein C. Once the coagulation process begins in someone with the Leiden variant of factor V, coagulation turns "off" more slowly than in someone with normal factor V.

The clinical presentation of factor V Leiden varies. Many individuals with the factor V Leiden allele never develop thrombosis.[2] The most common manifestation is venous thromboembolism (VTE), usually in the deep veins of the legs. The risk for increased thrombosis can also lead to pregnancy loss and placental abruption. When an individual inherits a single variant gene (heterozygous), the risk of venous thrombosis is 3 to 8 times higher than that in the general population. When two copies of the Leiden variant (homozygous) are inherited, the risk of thrombosis increases to 30- to 80-fold over that of the general population; homozygosity may also present with a more catastrophic clotting event.[2,5] About 34% of the individuals homozygous for factor V Leiden experience recurrent clots. The presence of risk factors for VTE, such as immobility, injury, cancer, or other procoagulant conditions coexisting with thrombophilic disorders has synergistic effects in the clotting cascade. Therefore, under many conditions, patients with the Leiden allele are at an even higher risk for thromboses.[1,4]

Treatment of an initial VTE in individuals with factor V Leiden follows the same guidelines for any first episode of VTE. Long-term oral anticoagulation is considered in those with recurrent VTE, multiple thrombophilic disorders, or coexistent risk factors. Heparin or enoxaparin prophylaxis may be used in women to prevent pregnancy loss.[6]

The diagnosis of factor V Leiden is made either by using a coagulation screening test (activated protein C resistance assay) or by DNA analysis of the F5 gene. Factor V Leiden testing should be performed in the following situations: a first VTE before 50 years of age; an unprovoked VTE; a history of recurrent VTE; a VTE at unusual sites such as cerebral, mesenteric, portal, or hepatic veins; VTE during pregnancy or puerperium; VTE with use of estrogen-based therapy; a first VTE in an individual with a first-degree relative with VTE before 50 years of age; or in women with unexplained fetal loss after 10 weeks' gestation.[3]

Although the factor V Leiden allele is fairly common, heterozygosity for the factor V Leiden variant results in only a small increased risk for thrombosis, and therefore routine genetic screening is not recommended. The issues for family testing are unresolved at this time. Clarification of the factor V Leiden genetic status may be indicated for at-risk relatives considering pregnancy, hormonal contraception, or hormone replacement therapy. Education about the signs and symptoms of VTE that require immediate medical attention should be shared with family members of an individual with diagnosed factor V Leiden.

REFERENCES

1. Bertina, R. M., Koeleman, B. P., Kosater, T., Rosendaal, F. R., Dirven, R. J., de Ronde, H., et al. (1994). Mutation in blood coagulation factor V associated with resistance to activated protein C. Nature, 369, 64-67.
2. Gonzalez-Porras, J. R., Garcia-Sanz, R., Alberca, I., López, M. L., Balanzategui, A., Gutierrez, O., et al. (2006). Risk of recurrent venous thrombosis in patients with the G20210A mutation in the prothrombin gene or factor V Leiden mutation. Blood, Coagulation and Fibrinolysis, 17, 23-28.
3. Grody, W. W., Griffin, J. H., Taylor, A. K., Korf, B. R., Heit, J. A., & ACMG Factor V. Leiden Working Group. (2001). American College of Medical Genetics consensus statement on factor V Leiden mutation testing. Genetics in Medicine, 3(2), 139-148.
4. Heit, J. A., Sobell, J. L., Li, H., & Sommer, S. S. (2005). The incidence of venous thromboembolism among factor V Leiden carriers: A community-based cohort study. Journal of Thrombosis and Haemostasis, 3(2), 305-311.
5. Lashley, F. R. (2005). Clinical genetics in nursing practice (3rd ed.). New York: Springer.
6. Ornstein, D. L., & Cushman, M. (2003). Factor V Leiden. Circulation, 107, e94-e97.

LABORATORY FINDINGS
Disseminated Intravascular Coagulation

Test	Normal Value	Alteration
Platelet count	150,000-400,000/microliter	Decreased
Prothrombin time	11-16 seconds	Prolonged
Activated partial thromboplastin time	30-45 seconds	Prolonged
Thrombin time	10-15 seconds	Prolonged
Fibrinogen	150-400 mg/dL	Decreased
Fibrin degradation products	<10 mcg/mL	Increased
Antithrombin III	>50% of control (plasma)	Decreased
D-dimer assay	<100 mcg/L	Increased
Protein C	71%-142% of normal activity	Decreased
Protein S	61%-130% of normal activity	Decreased

thrombin III; however, factor VIII is often inactivated by the freezing process, thus necessitating administration of concentrated factor VIII in the form of cryoprecipitate.[9] Transfusions of packed RBCs are given to replace cells lost in hemorrhage.

Heparin is a potent thrombin inhibitor and may be administered, in low doses, to block the clotting process that initiates DIC. Heparin is given to prevent further clotting and thrombosis that may lead to organ ischemia and necrosis. Although heparin's antithrombin activity prevents further clotting, it may increase the risk of bleeding and may cause further problems. Its use is controversial when it is administered to patients with DIC.[1,15]

Other pharmacological therapy in DIC includes the administration of synthetic antithrombin III, which also inhibits thrombin.[9] Antithrombin III concentrates may shorten the course of the disease and may increase the survival rate. Activated protein C (drotrecogin alfa, [Xigris]) is indicated in patients with severe sepsis and multiorgan failure. Activated protein C decreases inflammation and clotting while increasing fibrinolysis.[1] Administration of aminocaproic acid (Amicar) inhibits fibrinolysis by interfering with plasmin activity. Fibrinolytics should be given only if other treatments have been unsuccessful and hemorrhaging is life-threatening, as there is no clear evidence of the risk versus benefit with their use.[15]

Nursing Interventions

Nursing care of the patient with DIC is aimed at the prevention and recognition of thrombotic and hemorrhagic events. Continuous assessment for complications facilitates prompt and aggressive interventions that may improve outcomes. Psychosocial support of the patient and family is very important. Few patients who survive DIC are without some functional deficit caused by ischemia or hemorrhage. Patients and their family members are assessed for the level of anxiety and coping mechanisms available. Communication is encouraged, and feelings are acknowledged. Maintenance of an open, honest, and supportive environment may lessen stress and anxiety.

Pain relief and promotion of comfort are important nursing priorities. The location, intensity, and quality of the patient's pain are assessed, along with the patient's response to discomfort. The nurse is conscientious not to enhance vasoconstriction, because it contributes to tissue ischemia and its associated discomfort. Relief of discomfort also reduces oxygen consumption, which is important for these patients with limited circulatory flow. Pain medication is offered as ordered and before painful procedures. Positioning, with support and proper body alignment and frequent changes, also enhances the patient's level of comfort.

Coagulation laboratory studies are carefully monitored for evidence of disease resolution. As fewer clots are created, the platelet count and fibrinogen level are among the first laboratory tests to return to normal. The fibrin degradation products and D-dimer levels fall, and antithrombin III levels rise, as fibrinolysis slows. Other coagulation tests are less sensitive and are not usually assessed.

The main desired outcomes for the patient with DIC include adequate oxygenation, adequate tissue perfusion, absence of bleeding, and skin integrity. Absence of pain and effective coping are additional expected outcomes.

CASE STUDY

Mr. F. is a 62-year-old man with acute myelogenous leukemia diagnosed 15 months ago. He received two cycles of induction (high doses) chemotherapy, which resulted in disease remission. He received additional chemotherapy (reduced intensity) over the next 4 months, and underwent an allogeneic peripheral blood stem cell transplant (identical-matched donor; his sister). He was started on standard immunosuppressive drugs to prevent graft-versus-host disease (GVHD). Forty-three days after his transplant, Mr. F. was diagnosed with stage 1 acute GVHD (skin changes on arms and palms of hands). During a routine follow-up visit, Mr. F. complains of mucositis and xerostomia, photosensitivity, dry and irritated eyes, joint pain, a rash on his arms, and an 8-lb weight loss since his last visit 1 month ago.

QUESTIONS
1. What risk factors are associated with developing chronic GVHD?
2. What are possible signs and symptoms of chronic GVHD?
3. What is the priority of care for the patient experiencing chronic GVHD?
4. What are key nursing interventions for the patient with chronic GVHD?

SUMMARY

All critically ill patients have the potential for hematological or immunological dysfunction. A thorough understanding of normal anatomy and physiology provides the critical care nurse with a basis on which a comprehensive assessment and treatment approach can be built. Because nurses play a key role in the outcome of patients with serious alterations in the hematological and immune systems, this knowledge is critical and has great impact on the well-being of patients.

CRITICAL THINKING QUESTIONS

1. What disorders in critical care are associated with anemia?
2. Why is the critical care unit often a dangerous place for the immunosuppressed patient?
3. How can therapeutic choices, such as interventions and medications, worsen the hematological or immunological compromise of critically ill patients?
4. What criteria are to be used for prioritization of nursing and medical interventions for the bleeding patient?

evolve Be sure to check out the bonus material, including free self-assessment exercises, on the Evolve Web site at http://evolve.elsevier.com/Sole.

REFERENCES

1. Armola, R. R. (2007). Monitor patients for disseminated intravascular coagulation. *Nursing 2007 Critical Care, 2*(5), 9-15.
2. Benz, E. J. (2005). Hemoglobinopathies. In D. L. Kasper, E. Braunwald, A. S. Fauci, S. L. Hauser, D. L. Longo, & J. L. Jameson (Eds.), *Harrison's principles of internal medicine* (16th ed., pp. 593-601). New York: McGraw-Hill.

3. Centers for Disease Control and Prevention. (2007). Cases of HIV infection and AIDS in the United States and dependent areas, 2005. *HIV/AIDS Surveillance Report, 2005.* Vol. 17. Rev ed. Retrieved July 6, 2007, from www.cdc.gov/hiv/topics/surveillance/resources/reports.

4. Chernecky, C. C., & Berger, B. J. (2008). *Laboratory tests and diagnostic procedures* (5th ed.). Philadelphia: Saunders.

5. Cosby, C. D. (2007). Hematologic disorders associated with human immunodeficiency virus and AIDS. *Journal of Infusion Nursing, 30*(1), 22-32.

6. DeMille, D., Deming, P., Lupinacci, P., & Jacobs, L. A. (2006). The effect of the neutropenic diet in the outpatient setting: A pilot study. *Oncology Nursing Forum, 33*(2), 337-343.

7. Dzieczkowski, J. S., & Anderson, K. C. (2005). Transfusion biology and therapy. In D. L. Kasper, E. Braunwald, A. S. Fauci, S. L. Hauser, D. L. Longo, & J. L. Jameson (Eds.), *Harrison's principles of internal medicine* (16th ed., pp. 662-667). New York: McGraw-Hill.

8. Galzibo, E., & Williams, L. A. (2006). Chronic graft-versus-host disease. *Oncology Nursing Forum, 33*(5), 881-883.

9. Gulanick, M., & Myers, J. L. (2007). *Nursing care plans: Nursing diagnosis and intervention* (6th ed.). St. Louis: Mosby.

10. Handin, R. I. (2005). Bleeding and thrombosis. In D. L. Kasper, E. Braunwald, A. S. Fauci, S. L. Hauser, D. L. Longo, & J. L. Jameson (Eds.), *Harrison's principles of internal medicine.* (16th ed., pp. 337-343). New York: McGraw-Hill.

11. Handin, R. I. (2005). Disorders of the platelet and vessel wall. In D. L. Kasper, E. Braunwald, A. S. Fauci, S. L. Hauser, D. L. Longo, & J. L. Jameson (Eds.), *Harrison's principles of internal medicine.* (16th ed., pp. 673-680). New York: McGraw-Hill.

12. Holland, S. M., & Gallin, J. I. (2005). Disorders of granulocytes and monocytes. In D. L. Kasper, E. Braunwald, A. S. Fauci, S. L. Hauser, D. L. Longo, & J. L. Jameson (Eds.), *Harrison's principles of internal medicine.* (16th ed., pp. 349-357). New York: McGraw-Hill.

13. Mackman, N., Tilley, R. E., & Key, N. S. (2007). Role of the extrinsic pathway of blood coagulation in hemostasis and thrombosis. *Arteriosclerosis, Thrombosis, and Vascular Biology, 27,* 1687-1693.

14. Mansen, T. J., & McCance, K. L. (2006). Alteration of erythrocyte functions. In K. L. McCance, & S. E. Huether (Eds.), *Pathophysiology: The biologic basis for disease in adults and children* (pp. 927-953). St. Louis: Mosby.

15. Mansen, T. J., & McCance, K. L. (2006). Alteration of leukocytes, lymphoid and hemostatic function. In K. L. McCance, & S. E. Huether (Eds.), *Pathophysiology: The biologic basis for disease in adults and children* (pp. 955-988). St. Louis: Mosby.

16. McCance, K. L. (2006). Structure and function of the hematologic system. In K. L. McCance, & S. E. Huether (Eds.), *Pathophysiology: The biologic basis for disease in adults and children* (pp. 893-926). St. Louis: Mosby.

17. Moody, K., Finlay, J., Mancuso, C., & Charlson, M. (2006). Feasibility and safety of a pilot randomized trial of infection rate: Neutropenic diet versus standard food safety guidelines. *Journal of Pediatric Hematology Oncology, 28*(3), 126-133.

18. Orange, J. S. (2005). Congenital immunodeficiencies and sepsis. *Pediatric Critical Care Medicine, 6*(3), S99-S107.

19. Rote, N. S. (2006). Alterations in immunity and inflammation. In K. L. McCance, & S. E. Huether (Eds.), *Pathophysiology: The biologic basis for disease in adults and children* (pp. 249-292). St. Louis: Mosby.

20. Rote, N. S., & Trask, B. C. (2006). Adaptive immunity. In K. L. McCance, & S. E. Huether (Eds.), *Pathophysiology: The biologic basis for disease in adults and children* (pp. 211-248). St. Louis: Mosby.

21. Trask, B. C., Rote, N. S., & Huether, S. E. (2006). Innate immunity: Inflammation. In K. L. McCance, & S. E. Huether (Eds.), *Pathophysiology: The biologic basis for disease in adults and children* (pp. 175-299). St. Louis: Mosby.

22. Warkentin, T. E. (2007). Heparin-induced thrombocytopenia. *Hematology/Oncology Clinics of North America, 21,* 589-607.

23. Wilkes, G. M., & Barton-Burke, M. (2007). *2007 Oncology Nursing Drug Handbook.* Sudbury, MA: Jones and Bartlett.

CHAPTER 17

Gastrointestinal Alterations

Carl Laffoon, MSN, ARNP, CEN, EMT-P, FACHE
Marthe J. Moseley, PhD, RN, CCRN, CCNS, CNL

INTRODUCTION

Body cells require water, electrolytes, and nutrients (carbohydrates, fats, and proteins) to obtain the energy necessary to fuel body functions. The primary function of the alimentary tract (oropharyngeal cavity, esophagus, stomach, and small and large intestine) and accessory organs (pancreas, liver, and gallbladder) is to provide the body with a continual supply of nutrients. In addition, food must move through the system at a rate slow enough for digestive and absorptive functions to occur, but also fast enough to meet the body's needs. Meeting these goals requires the appropriate and timely movement of nutrients through the gastrointestinal (GI) tract *(motility)*, the presence of specific enzymes to break down nutrients *(digestion)*, and the existence of transport mechanisms to move the nutrients into the bloodstream *(absorption)*. Each part is adapted for specific functions, including food passage, storage, digestion, and absorption. This chapter provides a brief physiological review of each section of the GI system and a general assessment of the GI system. This provides the foundation for the discussion of the GI disorders most commonly encountered in the critical care setting: acute upper GI bleeding, acute pancreatitis, and liver failure. The remainder of the chapter reviews the pathophysiology of each disorder, nursing and medical assessments, nursing diagnoses, nursing and medical interventions, and patient outcomes. Complete nursing plans of care for select nursing diagnoses are provided; these serve as valuable summaries of the most common patient care problems and collaborative interventions.

REVIEW OF ANATOMY AND PHYSIOLOGY

Gastrointestinal Tract

The anatomical structure of the GI system is shown in Figure 17-1. It comprises the alimentary canal (beginning at the oropharynx and ending at the anus) and the accessory organs (pancreas, liver, and gallbladder) that empty their products into the canal at certain points. A review of the anatomy of the gut wall is provided as an introduction to this section because it is the foundation for the understanding of absorption of nutrients and GI protective mechanisms.

Gut Wall

The GI tract begins in the esophagus and extends to the rectum. It is composed of multiple tissue layers.

Mucosa. The innermost layer, the mucosa, is the most important physiologically. This layer is exposed to food substances, and it therefore plays a role in nutrient metabolism. The mucosa is also protective. The cells in this layer are connected by tight junctions that produce an effective barrier against large molecules and bacteria, and protect the GI tract from bacterial colonization. The goblet cells in the mucosa secrete mucus, which provides lubrication for food substances and protects the mucosa from excoriation.

Gastric Mucosal Barrier. In the stomach, the special architecture of cells of the mucosa and the mucus that is secreted are known as the *gastric mucosal barrier*. This physiological barrier is impermeable to hydrochloric acid, which is normally secreted in the

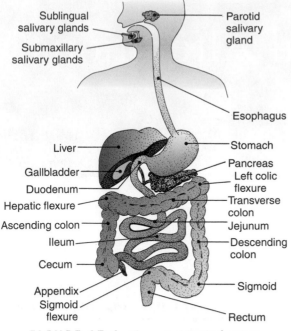

FIGURE 17-1. The gastrointestinal system.

BOX 17-1 Swallowing Stages

Oral: Voluntary
- Initiation of the swallowing process, usually stimulated by a bolus of food in the mouth near the pharynx

Pharyngeal: Involuntary
- Passage of food through the pharynx to the esophagus

Esophageal: Involuntary
- Promotes passage of food from the pharynx to the stomach

stomach, but it is permeable to other substances, such as salicylates, alcohol, steroids, and bile salts. The disruption of this barrier by these types of substances is thought to play a role in ulcer development. In addition, these cells have a special feature—they regenerate rapidly—that explains how disruptions in the mucosa can be quickly healed.

Submucosa. The second layer of the gut wall, the submucosa, is composed of connective tissue, blood vessels, and nerve fibers. The muscular layer is the major layer of the wall. The serosa is the outermost layer.

Beneath the mucosa, submucosa, and muscular layer are various nerve plexuses that are innervated by the autonomic nervous system. Disturbances in these neurons in a given segment of the GI tract cause a lack of motility.

Oropharyngeal Cavity

Mouth. Food substances are ingested into the oral cavity primarily by the intrinsic desire for food called *hunger*. Food in the mouth is initially subject to mechanical breakdown by the act of chewing *(mastication)*. Chewing of food is important for digestion of all foods, but particularly for digestion of fruits and raw vegetables, because they require the cellulose membranes around their nutrients to be broken down. The muscles used for chewing are innervated by the motor branch of the fifth cranial nerve.

Salivary Glands. Saliva is the major secretion of the oropharynx and is produced by three pairs of salivary glands: submaxillary, sublingual, and parotid. Saliva is rich in mucus, which lubricates food. Salivary amylase, a starch-digesting enzyme, is also secreted. Stimuli such as sight, smell, thoughts, and taste of food stimulate salivary gland secretion. Parasympathetic stimulation promotes a copious secretion of watery saliva. Conversely, sympathetic stimulation produces a scant output of thick saliva. The normal daily secretion of saliva is 1200 mL.

Pharynx. Swallowing is a complex mechanism involving oral (voluntary), pharyngeal, and esophageal stages. It is made more complex because the pharynx serves several other functions, the most important of which is respiration. The pharynx participates in the function of swallowing for only a few seconds at a time to aid in the propulsion of food, which is triggered by the presence of fluid or food in the pharynx. Box 17-1 outlines the three broad stages of swallowing.

Esophagus

Once fluid or food enters the esophagus, it is propelled through the lumen by the process of *peristalsis*, which involves the relaxation and contraction of esophageal muscles that are stimulated by the bolus of food. This process occurs repeatedly until the food reaches the lower esophageal sphincter, which is the last centimeter of the esophagus. This area is normally contracted and thus prevents reflux of gastric contents into the esophagus, a phenomenon that would damage the lining by gastric acid and enzymes. Waves of peristalsis cause this sphincter to relax and allow food to enter the stomach. Mucosal layers in the esophagus secrete mucus, which protects the lining from damage by gastric secretions or food and also serves as a lubricant.

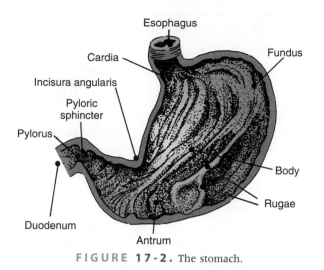

FIGURE 17-2. The stomach.

TABLE 17-1 Gastric Secretions

Gland/Cells	Secretion
Cardiac gland	Mucus
Pyloric gland	Mucus
Fundic (gastric) gland	Mucus
Mucous neck cells	Mucus
Parietal cells	Water
	Hydrochloric acid
	Intrinsic factor
Chief cells	Pepsinogen
	Mucus

Stomach

The stomach is located at the distal end of the esophagus. It is divided into four regions: the *cardia*, the *fundus*, the *body*, and the *antrum* (Figure 17-2). The muscular walls form multiple folds that allow for greater expansion of the stomach. The opening at the distal end of the stomach opens into the small intestine and is surrounded by the pyloric sphincter. The motor functions of the stomach include storage of food until it can be accommodated by the lower GI tract, mixing of food with gastric secretions until it forms a semifluid mixture called *chyme*, and slow emptying of the chyme into the small intestine at a rate that allows for proper digestion and absorption. Motility is accomplished through peristalsis. The pyloric sphincter at the distal end of the stomach prevents duodenal reflux.

Gastric secretions are produced by mucus-secreting cells that line the inner surface of the stomach and by two types of tubular glands: oxyntic (gastric) glands and pyloric glands. Table 17-1 summarizes the major gastric secretions.

An oxyntic gland is composed of three types of cells: mucous neck cells; peptic, or chief, cells; and oxyntic, or parietal cells. *Mucous cells* secrete a viscid and alkaline mucus that coats the stomach mucosa, thereby providing protection and lubrication for food transport. *Parietal cells* secrete hydrochloric acid solution, which begins the digestion of food in the stomach. Hydrochloric acid is very acidic (pH, 0.8). Stimulants of hydrochloric acid secretion include vagal stimulation, gastrin, and the chemical properties of chyme. Histamine, which stimulates the release of gastrin, also stimulates the secretion of hydrochloric acid. Current drug therapies for ulcer disease use H_2-histamine receptor blockers that block the effects of histamine and therefore hydrochloric acid stimulation. The acidic environment of the stomach promotes the conversion of pepsinogen, a proteolytic enzyme secreted by gastric chief cells, to pepsin. Pepsin begins the initial breakdown of proteins. Pepsin is active only in a highly acidic environment (pH < 5); therefore, hydrochloric acid secretion is essential for protein digestion.

An essential protein secreted only by the stomach's parietal cells is *intrinsic factor*. Intrinsic factor is necessary for the absorption of vitamin B_{12} in the ileum. Vitamin B_{12} is critical for the formation of red blood cells (RBCs), and a deficiency in this vitamin causes anemia.

The stomach also secretes fluid that is rich in sodium, potassium, and other electrolytes. Loss of these fluids via vomiting or gastric suction places the patient at risk for fluid and electrolyte imbalances and acid-base disturbances (Table 17-2).

Small Intestine

The segment spanning the first 10 to 12 inches of the small intestine is called the *duodenum*. This anatomical area is physiologically important because pancreatic juices and bile from the liver empty into this structure. The duodenum also contains an extensive network of mucus-secreting glands called *Brunner's glands*. The function of this mucus is to protect the duodenal wall from digestion by gastric juice. Secretion of mucus by Brunner's glands is inhibited by sympathetic stimulation, which leaves the duodenum unprotected from gastric juice. This inhibition is thought to be one of the reasons why this area of the GI tract is the site for more than 50% of peptic ulcers.

The segment spanning the next 7 to 8 feet of the small intestine is called the *jejunum*, and the

TABLE 17-2 Electrolyte and Acid-Base Disturbances Associated with the Gastrointestinal Tract

Fluid Loss	Imbalances
Gastric juice	Metabolic alkalosis Potassium deficit Sodium deficit Fluid volume deficit
Small intestine juice/large intestine juice (recent ileostomy)	Metabolic acidosis Potassium deficit Sodium deficit Fluid volume deficit
Biliary or pancreatic fistula	Metabolic acidosis Sodium deficit Fluid volume deficit

TABLE 17-3 Pancreatic Enzymes and Their Actions

Enzyme	Action
Trypsin*	Digests proteins
Chymotrypsin*	Digests proteins
Carboxypolypeptidase*	Digests proteins
Ribonuclease	Digests proteins
Deoxyribonuclease	Digests proteins
Pancreatic amylase	Digests carbohydrates
Pancreatic lipase	Digests fats
Cholesterol esterase	Digests fats

*Activated only after it is secreted into the intestinal tract.

remaining 10 to 12 feet comprise the *ileum*. The opening into the first part of the large intestine is protected by the *ileocecal valve*, which prevents reflux of colonic contents back into the ileum.

The movements of the small intestine include mixing contractions and propulsive contractions. The chyme in the small intestine takes 3 to 5 hours to move from the pylorus to the ileocecal valve, although this activity is greatly increased after meals. Digestion and absorption of foodstuffs occur primarily in the small intestine. The anatomical arrangement of villi and microvilli in the small intestine greatly increases the surface area in this part of the intestine and accounts for its highly digestive and absorptive capabilities. Located on the entire surface of the small intestine are small pits called *crypts of Lieberkühn*, which produce intestinal secretions at a rate of 2000 mL per day. These secretions are neutral in pH and supply the watery vehicle necessary for absorption.

In the small intestine, digestion of carbohydrates, fats, and proteins begins with degradation by pancreatic enzymes that are secreted into the duodenum. Pancreatic juice contains enzymes necessary for digesting all three major types of food: proteins, carbohydrates, and fats (Table 17-3). It also contains large quantities of bicarbonate ions, which play an important role in neutralizing acidic chyme that is emptied from the stomach into the duodenum. Pancreatic juice is primarily secreted in response to the presence of chyme in the duodenum.

The small intestine also handles water, electrolyte, and vitamin absorption. Up to 10 L of fluid enters the GI tract daily, and fluid composition of stool is only about 200 mL. Sodium is actively reabsorbed in the small intestine. In the ileum, chloride is absorbed and sodium bicarbonate is secreted. Potassium is absorbed and secreted in the GI tract. Vitamins, with the exception of B_{12}, and iron are absorbed in the upper part of the small bowel. Vitamin B_{12} is absorbed in the terminal ileum in the presence of intrinsic factor.

Large Intestine

The large intestine, or colon, is anatomically divided into the ascending colon, transverse colon, descending colon, and rectum (Figure 17-3). The functions of the colon are absorption of the water and electrolytes from the chyme and storage of fecal material until it can be expelled. The proximal half of the colon performs primarily absorptive activities, whereas the distal half performs storage activities. The characteristic contractile activity in the colon is called *haustration*; it propels fecal material through the tract. A mass movement moves feces into the rectal vault, and then the urge to defecate is elicited. The mucosa of the large intestine is lined with crypts of Lieberkühn, but the cells contain very few enzymes. Rather, mucus is secreted, and this protects the colon wall against excoriation and serves as a medium for holding fecal matter together.

Accessory Organs

Pancreas

The pancreas is located in both upper quadrants of the abdomen, with the *head* in the upper right quadrant and the *tail* in the upper left quadrant. The head and tail are separated by a midsection called the *body of the pancreas* (Figure 17-4). Because the pancreas lies retroperitoneally, it cannot be palpated; this characteristic explains why diseases of the pancreas can cause pain that radiates to the back. In addition, a well-developed pancreatic capsule does not exist, and this may explain why inflammatory processes of the pancreas can freely spread and affect the surrounding organs (stomach and duodenum).

The pancreas has both *exocrine* (production of digestive enzymes) and *endocrine* (production of insulin and glucagon) functions. The cells of the pancreas, called *acini*, secrete the major pancreatic enzymes essential for normal digestion (see Table 17-3). Trypsinogen and chymotrypsinogen are secreted in an inactive form so autodigestion of the gland does not occur. Bicarbonate is also secreted by the pancreas and plays an important role in enabling the pancreatic enzymes to work to break down foodstuffs. After breakdown by pancreatic enzymes, food is further digested by enzymes in the small intestine and is absorbed into the bloodstream. The presence of acid in the stomach stimulates the duodenum to produce the hormone secretin, which stimulates pancreatic secretions. Protein substances in the duodenum stimulate the production of cholecystokinin.

The endocrine functions of the pancreas are accomplished by groups of alpha and beta cells that compose the islets of Langerhans. *Beta cells* secrete insulin, and *alpha cells* secrete glucagon. Both are essential to carbohydrate metabolism. When beta cells are affected by disease, blood glucose levels can increase.

The exocrine and endocrine functions of the pancreas are essential to digestion and carbohydrate metabolism, respectively. Therefore, pancreatic dysfunction can predispose the patient to malnutrition and accounts for many clinical problems. (See Chapter 16.)

The pancreatic response to low-flow states (decreased cardiac output), or hypotension, is often ischemia of the pancreatic cells. This ischemia is thought to play a role in the release of cardiotoxic factors (myocardial depressant factor), which decrease cardiac output. Pancreatic ischemia can also result in acute pancreatitis, which is discussed later in the chapter.

Liver

The liver is the largest internal organ of the body; it is located in the right upper abdominal quadrant. The basic functional unit of the liver is the liver lobule (Figure 17-5). Hepatic cells are arranged in

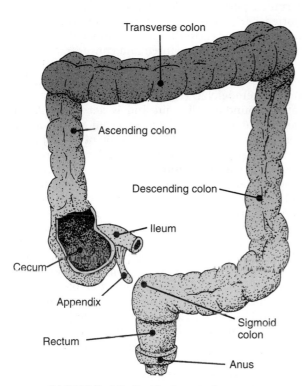

FIGURE 17-3. The intestinal system.

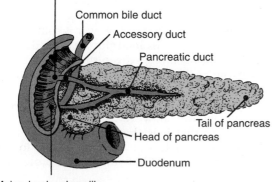

FIGURE 17-4. The pancreas.

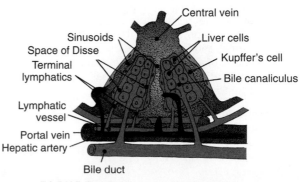

FIGURE 17-5. The normal liver lobule.

cords that radiate from the central vein into the periphery. Blood from portal arterioles and venules empties into channels called *sinusoids*. Lining the walls of the sinusoids are specialized phagocytic cells called *Kupffer's cells*. These cells remove bacteria and other foreign material from the blood.

The liver has a rich blood supply. It receives blood from both the hepatic artery and the portal vein, which drains structures of the GI tract. The blood supplied to the liver by these two vessels accounts for approximately 25% of the cardiac output.

The liver performs more than 400 functions. The following discussion of hepatic functions is based on the classification by Guyton and Hall,[9] and includes vascular, secretory, metabolic, and storage functions. These actions are summarized in Box 17-2.

Vascular Functions

Blood Storage. Resistance to blood flow (hepatic vascular resistance) in the liver is normally low. Any increase in pressure in the veins that drain the liver causes blood to accumulate in the sinusoids, which store up to 400 mL of blood. This blood volume serves as a compensatory mechanism in cases of hypovolemic shock; blood from the liver is shunted into the circulation to increase blood volume.

Blood Filtration. Kupffer's cells that line the sinusoids cleanse the blood of bacteria and foreign material

that have been absorbed through the GI tract. These cells are extremely phagocytic and thus normally prevent almost all bacteria from reaching the systemic circulation.

Secretory Functions

Bile Production. The secretion of bile is a major function of the liver. Bile is composed of water, electrolytes, bile salts, phospholipids, cholesterol, and bilirubin. Approximately 500 to 1000 mL of bile is produced daily. Bile salts emulsify fats and foster their absorption. The bile salts are reabsorbed in the terminal portion of the ileum and are then transported back to the liver, where they can be used again. Bile travels to the gallbladder via the common bile duct, where it is stored and concentrated.

Bilirubin Metabolism. Bilirubin, a physiologically inactive pigment, is a metabolic end product of the degradation of hemoglobin (Hgb). Bilirubin enters the circulation bound to albumin and is *unconjugated*. This portion of the bilirubin is reflected in the *indirect* serum bilirubin level. Accumulation of unconjugated bilirubin is toxic to cells. In the liver, bilirubin is *conjugated* with glucuronic acid. Conjugated bilirubin is soluble and excreted in bile. Some conjugated bilirubin returns to the blood and is reflected in the *direct* serum bilirubin level.

Excess bilirubin accumulation in the blood results in *jaundice*. Jaundice has several categories including hepatocellular, hemolytic, and obstructive. Hemolytic jaundice results from increased RBC destruction, such as that resulting from blood incompatibilities and sickle cell disease. Viral hepatitis is the most common cause of hepatocellular jaundice (jaundice caused by hepatic cell damage). Cirrhosis and liver cancer also decrease the liver's ability to conjugate bilirubin. Obstructive jaundice is usually caused by gallbladder disease such as gallstones.

Metabolic Functions

Carbohydrate Metabolism. The liver plays an important role in the maintenance of normal blood glucose concentration. When the concentration of glucose increases to greater than normal levels, it is stored as glycogen *(glycogenesis)*. When blood glucose levels decrease, glycogen stored in the liver is split to form glucose *(glycogenolysis)*. If blood glucose levels decrease to less than normal and glycogen stores are depleted, the liver can make glucose from proteins and fats *(gluconeogenesis)*.

Fat Metabolism. Almost all cells in the body are capable of lipid metabolism; however, the liver metabolizes fats so rapidly that it is the primary site for these functions. The liver is also the primary site for the conversion of excess carbohydrates and proteins to triglycerides.

Protein Metabolism. All nonessential amino acids are produced in the liver. Amino acids must be

---

BOX 17-2   Functions of the Liver

Vascular Functions
- Blood storage
- Blood filtration

Secretory Functions
- Production of bile
- Secretion of bilirubin
- Conjugation of bilirubin

Metabolic Functions
- Carbohydrate metabolism
- Fat metabolism
- Protein metabolism
- Synthesis of prothrombin (factor I), fibrinogen (factor II), and factors VII, IX, and X
- Removal of activated clotting factors
- Detoxification of drugs, hormones, and other substances

Storage Functions
- Blood
- Glucose
- Vitamins (A, B_{12}, D, E, K)
- Fat

deaminated (cleared of ammonia) to be used for energy by cells, or converted into carbohydrates or fats. Ammonia is released and removed from the blood by conversion to urea in the liver. The urea that is secreted by the liver into the bloodstream is excreted by the kidneys.

With the exception of gamma globulins, the liver also produces all plasma proteins in the blood. The major types of plasma proteins are albumins, globulins, and fibrinogen. *Albumin* maintains blood oncotic pressure and prevents plasma loss from the capillaries. *Globulins* are essential for cellular enzymatic reactions. *Fibrinogen* helps to form blood clots.

Production and Removal of Blood Clotting Factors. The liver synthesizes fibrinogen (factor I); prothrombin (factor II); and factors VII, IX, and X. Vitamin K is essential for the synthesis of other clotting factors. The liver also removes active clotting factors from the circulation and therefore prevents clotting in the macrovasculature and microvasculature.

Detoxification. Drugs, hormones, and other toxic substances are metabolized by the liver into inactive forms for excretion. This process is usually accomplished by conversion of the fat-soluble compounds to water-soluble compounds. They can then be excreted via the bile or the urine.

Storage, Synthesis, and Transport of Vitamins and Minerals. The liver plays a central role in the storage, synthesis, and transport of various vitamins and minerals. It functions as a storage depot principally for vitamins A, D, and B_{12}, where up to 3-, 10-, and 12-month supplies, respectively, of these nutrients are stored to prevent deficiency states.

Gallbladder

The gallbladder is a saclike structure that lies beneath the right lobe of the liver. Its primary function is the storage and concentration of bile. The gallbladder holds approximately 70 mL of bile. Bile salts are secreted into the duodenum when nutrients are ingested. The gallbladder is connected to the duodenum via the common bile duct. Bile flow is controlled by contraction of the gallbladder and relaxation of the sphincter of Oddi, which is located at the junction of the common bile duct and the duodenum. Contraction of the gallbladder is controlled by hormonal *(cholecystokinin)* and central nervous system signals and is initiated by the presence of food in the duodenum. Bile salts emulsify fats and also assist in the absorption of fatty acids.

Neural Innervation of the Gastrointestinal System

Functions of the GI system are influenced by neural and hormonal factors. The autonomic nervous system exerts multiple effects. Parasympathetic cholinergic fibers, or drugs that mimic parasympathetic effects, stimulates to GI secretion and motility. Sympathetic stimulate, or drugs with adrenergic effects, tend to be inhibitory. Parasympathetic and sympathetic fibers also innervate the gallbladder and the pancreas. Other neural regulators of gastric secretions are stimulated by sight, smell, and thoughts of food and by the presence of food in the mouth. In this phase (cephalic), the brain centers reflexively cause parasympathetic stimulation of gastric secretions by chief and parietal cells.

Hormonal Control of the Gastrointestinal System

The GI tract is considered to be the largest endocrine organ in the body. Hormones that influence GI function include those produced by specialized cells in the GI tract and those produced by other endocrine organs (pancreas and gallbladder). GI hormones modulate motility, secretion, absorption, and maturation of GI tissues. Table 17-4 summarizes the common GI hormones and their actions.

Blood Supply of the Gastrointestinal System

Blood supply to organs within the abdomen is referred to as the *splanchnic circulation*. The GI system receives the largest single percentage of the cardiac output. Approximately one third of the cardiac output supplies these tissues. The superior and inferior mesenteric and celiac arteries supply the stomach, small and large intestines, pancreas, and gallbladder. The liver has a dual blood supply and receives part of its blood supply from the hepatic artery. Circulation to the GI system is unique in that venous blood draining the system empties into the portal vein, which then perfuses the liver. The portal vein supplies approximately 70% to 75% of liver blood flow.

Because of the large percentage of cardiac output that perfuses the GI tract, the GI tract is a major source of blood flow during times of increased need, such as during exercise or as a compensatory mechanism in hemorrhage. Conversely, prolonged occlusion or hypoperfusion of a major artery supplying the GI tract can lead to mucosal ischemia and eventually necrosis. Necrosis of intestinal villi can destroy the GI tract's barrier to harmful toxins and bacteria. These bacteria can then enter the blood supply and cause septic shock.

Geriatric Concerns

Several changes occur in the GI system as a result of the aging process. Changes include decreased

TABLE 17-4 Actions of Gastrointestinal Hormones

Action	Gastrin	Cholecystokinin	Secretin	Gastric Inhibitory Peptide
Acid secretion	Stimulates	Stimulates	Inhibits	Inhibits
Gastric motility	Stimulates	Stimulates	Inhibits	—
Gastric emptying	Inhibits	Inhibits	Inhibits	Inhibits
Intestinal motility	Stimulates	Stimulates	Inhibits	—
Mucosal growth	Stimulates	Stimulates	Inhibits	—
Pancreatic HCO_3^- secretion	Stimulates	Stimulates	Stimulates	0
Pancreatic enzyme secretion	Stimulates	Stimulates	Stimulates	0
Pancreatic growth	Stimulates	Stimulates	Stimulates	—
Bile HCO_3^- secretion	Stimulates	Stimulates	Stimulates	0
Gallbladder contraction	Stimulates	Stimulates	Stimulates	—

0, No effect; —, not yet tested; *HCO_3^-*, bicarbonate.

salivation, alterations in taste, delayed esophageal and bowel emptying, decreased gastric secretions, and altered drug metabolism. The Geriatric Considerations feature highlights these changes and related nursing implications.[17]

GENERAL ASSESSMENT OF THE GASTROINTESTINAL SYSTEM

A comprehensive assessment of the abdomen includes a history, inspection, auscultation, percussion, and palpation. Mapping of the abdomen for descriptive purposes is usually performed by use of the four-quadrant method by drawing imaginary lines crossing at the umbilicus: right upper, right lower, left upper, and left lower. Symptoms such as pain may also be described by these landmarks.

History

An assessment of the GI system begins with a history, unless an emergency situation exists that requires immediate physiological assessment and intervention. The patient is questioned about any past problems with indigestion, difficulty swallowing *(dysphagia)*, pain on swallowing, nausea and vomiting, heartburn, belching, abdominal distention or bloating, diarrhea, constipation, or bleeding. Problems such as anorexia, fatigue, and headache also point to specific GI ailments and should be noted. All symptoms should be explored in terms of when the symptoms became apparent, any precipitating factors, what treatment was sought, factors that relieved or made the symptoms worse, and whether the symptom is current. A weight history is also important and includes usual and ideal body weight along with a history of fluctuations, acute weight loss, and interventions or treatments for weight loss.

Careful pain assessment is a challenging aspect of the history. Pain receptors in the abdomen are less likely to be localized and are mediated by common sensory structures projected to the skin. Therefore, distinguishing the pain of a peptic ulcer or cholecystitis from that of a myocardial infarction is often difficult. Abdominal pain is often caused by engorged mucosa, pressure in the mucosa, distention, or spasm. Visceral pain is likely to cause pallor, perspiration, bradycardia, nausea and vomiting, weakness, and hypotension, and should be assessed. Increasing intensity of pain, especially after a therapeutic regimen, is always significant and usually signifies complicating factors, such as increasing inflammation, gastric distention, hemorrhage into tissue or the peritoneal space, or peritonitis from perforation or anastomosis leakage. The nurse obtains a description of the location and the type of pain in the patient's own words.

A history of any GI surgical procedures, including the specific types and dates, should be discussed. A current list of medications is also important, especially because many drugs have GI side effects.

Inspection

General inspection of the abdomen focuses on the following characteristics: skin color and texture, symmetry and contour of the abdomen, masses and pulsations, and peristalsis and movement.

GERIATRIC CONSIDERATIONS

PHYSIOLOGICAL CHANGES	NURSING IMPLICATIONS
Salivation decreased, resulting in dry mouth	Mouth care is essential to keep mucous membranes moist.
Decreased sense of taste	Providing adequate nutrition to those taking oral feedings may be more difficult because food may not be as appealing.
Esophageal emptying delayed	The risk of aspiration is higher; elevate the head of the bed for feedings.
Gastric acid secretion decreased	This may result in anemia; anemia can lead to hypoxemia. Assess complete blood count, arterial blood gases, and pulse oximetry values.
Incidence of gallstones increased	Assess for signs and symptoms of cholecystitis; the patients may be at higher risk for complications of gallbladder disease such as pancreatitis.
Drug metabolism by liver impaired as blood flow decreases by almost half by age 85	Assess for drug toxicity; drug dosages may need to be reduced.
Delayed bowel emptying resulting in higher incidence of constipation	Assess bowel function; patients may need extra fluids, fiber, stool softeners, or laxatives to facilitate bowel function. Provide assistance to facilitate toileting.

Skin Color and Texture

The nurse observes for pigmentation of skin (jaundice), lesions, discolorations, old or new scars, and vascular and hair patterns. General nutrition and hydration status may also be discerned.

Symmetry and Contour of Abdomen

The nurse notes the size and shape of the abdomen and the presence of visible protrusions and adipose distribution. Abdominal distention, particularly in the presence of pain, should always be investigated because it usually indicates trapped air or fluid within the abdominal cavity.

Masses and Pulsations

The nurse looks for any obvious abdominal masses, which are best seen on deep inspiration. Pulsations, if they are seen, usually originate from the aorta.

Peristalsis and Movement

Motility of the stomach may be reflected in movement of the abdomen in lean patients, and is a normal sign. However, strong contractions are abnormal and indicate the presence of disease.

Auscultation

Bowel sounds are high-pitched, gurgling sounds caused by air and fluid as they move through the GI tract. Auscultation of bowel sounds is performed before the abdomen is manipulated so the frequency of bowel sounds is not altered. Optimal positioning of the patient to relax the abdomen is performed before auscultation is begun. A supine position with the patient's arms at the sides or folded at the chest

---

BOX 17-3   Causes of Increased and Decreased Bowel Sounds

Causes of Decreased Bowel Sounds
- Peritonitis
- Gangrene
- Reflux ileus
- Surgical manipulation of bowel
- Late bowel obstruction

Causes of Increased Bowel Sounds
- Early pyloric or intestinal obstruction
- Bleeding ulcers or electrolyte disturbances
- Bleeding esophageal varices
- Diarrhea
- Subsiding ileus

---

is usually the recommended position. Placing a pillow under the patient's knees also helps to relax the abdominal wall.

Bowel sounds are best heard with the diaphragm of the stethoscope and are systematically assessed in all four quadrants of the abdomen. The frequency and character of the sounds are noted. The frequency of bowel sounds has been estimated at 4 to 34 per minute, and the sounds are usually irregular. Therefore, the abdomen must be auscultated for at least 5 minutes before an assessment of absence of bowel sounds can be made. Box 17-3 reviews common causes of increased and decreased bowel sounds as they relate to acute illness.

Vascular sounds such as bruits may also be heard and indicate dilated, tortuous, or constricted vessels.

Venous hums are also normally heard from the inferior vena cava. A hum in the periumbilical region in a patient with cirrhosis indicates obstructed portal circulation. Peritoneal friction rubs may also be heard and may indicate infection, abscess, or tumor.

Percussion

Percussion is aimed at detecting fluid, gaseous distention, or masses. Because of the presence of gas within the GI tract, percussed tympany predominates. Solid masses are dull on percussion. Organ borders of the liver, spleen, and stomach may also be ascertained.

Palpation

Palpation is used to evaluate the major organs with respect to shape, size, position, mobility, consistency, and tension. Palpation is performed last because it often elicits pain or muscle spasm. Deep abdominal tenderness and rebound tenderness must be differentiated. Rebound tenderness occurs when pain is elicited after the examiner's hand is quickly released after deep palpation. Rigidity or guarding of the abdomen is also noted. Masses in the liver, spleen, kidneys, gallbladder, and descending colon can also be palpated.

ACUTE GASTROINTESTINAL BLEEDING

Pathophysiology

GI bleeding results in high patient morbidity and medical care costs. Many causes of acute GI bleeding necessitate admission of a patient to the critical care unit. Box 17-4 reviews the most common causes of this emergency.

Peptic Ulcer Disease
Peptic ulcer disease is characterized by a break in the mucosa that extends through the entire mucosa and into the muscle layers, damaging blood vessels and causing hemorrhage or perforation into the GI wall (Figure 17-6).[13] Duodenal and gastric ulcers are the most common cause of peptic ulcer disease and the most common cause of upper GI bleeding. The ulcer in peptic ulcer disease is a crater surrounded by either acutely or chronically inflamed cells. Over time, the inflamed tissue is replaced by necrotic tissue, then by granulation tissue, and finally by scar tissue.

Acetylcholine (a neurotransmitter), gastrin (a hormone), and *secretin* (a hormone) stimulate the chief cells, which eventually stimulates acid secre-

BOX 17-4   Causes of Gastrointestinal Bleeding

Causes of Upper Gastrointestinal Bleeding
- Duodenal ulcer
- Gastric ulcer
- Esophageal or gastric varices
- Mallory-Weiss tear

Causes of Lower Gastrointestinal Bleeding[8]
- Polyps
- Inflammatory disease
- Diverticulosis
- Cancer
- Vascular ectasias
- Hemorrhoids

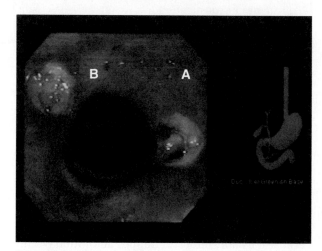

FIGURE 17-6. Duodenal ulcer. *A,* Deep ulceration in the duodenal wall extending as a crater through the entire mucosa and into the muscle layers. *B,* Duodenal ulcer. *(From Huether, S. E. [2006]. Alterations of digestive function. In K. L. McCance, & S. E. Huether [Eds.],* Pathophysiology: The biologic basis for disease in adults and children *[p. 1399]. St. Louis: Mosby.)*

tion. The secretion of acid is important in the pathogenesis of ulcer disease. Parietal cell mass in people with peptic ulcer disease is 1.5 to 2 times greater than in persons with no ulcer disease. Risk factors for the development of peptic ulcer disease are noted in Box 17-5. Contributing factors in ulcer formation are noted in Box 17-6. Infection with *Helicobacter pylori* bacteria is a major cause of duodenal ulcers. Selected studies of GI function are noted in Table 17-5. Characteristics of gastric and duodenal ulcers are presented in Table 17-6.

Stress Ulcers
A stress ulcer is an acute form of peptic ulcer that tends to accompany severe illness, systemic trauma,

BOX 17-5   Risk Factors for Peptic Ulcer Disease

- Smoking: stimulates acid secretion
- *Helicobacter pylori* infection: elevates levels of gastrin and pepsinogen, and releases toxins and enzymes promoting inflammation and ulceration
- Habitual use of nonsteroidal antiinflammatory drugs: inhibits prostaglandins
- Alcohol

BOX 17-6   Contributing Factors to Ulcer Formation[8]

- Increased number of parietal cells in the gastric mucosa
- Gastrin levels remain higher longer after eating
- Gastrin levels continue to stimulate secretion of acid and pepsin
- Feedback mechanism fails
- Rapid gastric emptying overwhelms buffering capacity
- Association of *Helicobacter pylori* with mucosal epithelial cell necrosis
- Decreased muscosal bicarbonate secretion

or neural injury and sometimes mental stress.[13] Stress ulcers are classified as ischemic ulcers or *Cushing's ulcers*.

Ischemic ulcers develop within hours of an event such as hemorrhage, multisystem trauma, severe burns, heart failure, or sepsis.[13] Stress ulcers that develop as a result of burn injury are called *Curling's ulcers*. The shock, anoxia, and sympathetic responses decrease mucosal blood flow leading to ischemia. Stress ulcers associated with severe head trauma or brain surgery are called *Cushing's ulcers*. The decreased mucosal blood flow and hypersecretion of acid caused by overstimulation of the vagal nuclei are associated with Cushing's ulcers.[13]

Administration of antacids and H_2-receptor blockers, and the suppression of vagal stimulation with anticholinergic drugs, are effective forms of therapy. These prophylactic measures are recommended by the Institute of Healthcare Improvement as part of a "bundle" of best practices for care of the critically ill adult. Applying peptic ulcer disease prophylaxis is an appropriate intervention in all patients who are sedentary; however, the higher incidence of stress ulceration in critical illness justifies greater vigilance.[16]

Mallory-Weiss Tear

A Mallory-Weiss tear is an arterial hemorrhage from an acute longitudinal tear in the gastroesophageal mucosa and accounts for 10% to 15% of upper GI

TABLE 17-5   Selected Studies of Gastrointestinal Function[14]

Test	Normal Findings	Clinical Significance
Stool studies	Fat: 2-6 g/24 hr	Steatorrhea can result from intestinal malabsorption or pancreatic insufficiency
	Occult blood: none	Positive tests associated with bleeding
Gastric acid stimulation	11-20 mEq/hr after stimulation	Increased with duodenal ulcers Decreased with gastric atrophy or gastric carcinoma
Breath Tests		
Glucose breath test or D-xylose	Negative for hydrogen or CO_2	May indicate intestinal bacterial overgrowth
Urea breath test	Negative for isotopically labeled CO_2	Presence of *Helicobacter pylori* infection

CO_2, Carbon dioxide.
Adapted from: Huether, S. E. (2006). Structure and function of the digestive system. In K. L. McCance, & S. E. Huether (Eds.), *Pathophysiology: The biologic basis for disease in adults and children.* St. Louis: Mosby.

TABLE 17-6   Characteristics of Gastric and Duodenal Ulcers

Characteristics	Gastric Ulcer	Duodenal Ulcer
Incidence		
Age at onset	50-70 years	20-50 years
Family history	Usually negative	Positive
Gender (prevalence)	Equal in women and men	Equal in women and men
Stress factors	Increased	Average
Ulcerogenic drugs	Normal use	Increased use
Cancer risk	Increased	Not increased
Pathophysiology		
Abnormal mucus	May be present	May be present
Parietal cell mass	Normal or decreased	Increased
Acid production	Normal or decreased	Increased
Serum gastrin	Increased	Normal
Serum pepsinogen	Normal	Increased
Associated gastritis	More common	Usually not present
Helicobacter pylori	May be present (60%-80%)	Often present (95%-100%)
Clinical Manifestations		
Pain	Located in upper abdomen Intermittent Pain-antacid-relief pattern Food-pain pattern	Located in upper abdomen Intermittent Pain-antacid or food-relief pattern Nocturnal pain common
Clinical course	Chronic ulcer without pattern of remission and exacerbation	Pattern of remissions and exacerbations for years

From Huether, S. E. (2006). Alterations of digestive function. In K. L. McCance, & S. E. Huether (Eds.), *Pathophysiology: The biologic basis for disease in adults and children*. St. Louis: Mosby.

bleeding episodes. It is associated with long-term nonsteroidal antiinflammatory drug or aspirin ingestion and with excessive alcohol intake. The upper GI bleeding usually occurs after episodes of forceful retching. Bleeding usually resolves spontaneously; however, lacerations of the esophagogastric junction may cause massive GI bleeding, requiring surgical repair.

Esophageal Varices

In chronic liver failure, liver cell structure and function are impaired, resulting in increased portal venous pressure, called *portal hypertension* (see discussion of hepatic failure). As a result, part of the venous blood in the splanchnic system is diverted from the liver to the systemic circulation by the development of connections to neighboring low-pressure veins. This phenomenon is termed *collateral circulation*. The most common sites for the development of these collateral channels are the submucosa of the esophagus and rectum, the anterior abdominal wall, and the parietal peritoneum. Figure 17-7 shows a liver with collateral circulation. The normal portal venous pressure is 2 to 6 mm Hg. As these veins experience increases in pressure, they become distended with blood, the vessels enlarge, and varices develop. Formation of varices requires that this pressure increase to more than 10 mm Hg. The most common sites for the development of these varices are the esophagus and the upper portion of the stomach. These varices tend to have a low tolerance for pressure and thus tend to bleed. Portal venous pressures of at least 12 mm Hg are needed for varices to bleed.

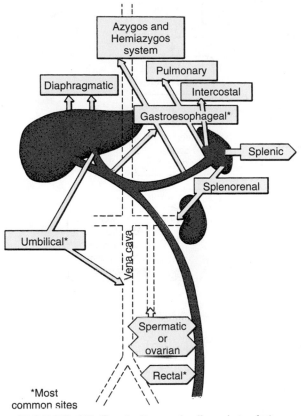

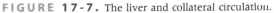

FIGURE 17-7. The liver and collateral circulation.

Assessment

Clinical Presentation

Patients manifest blood loss from the GI tract in several ways. Drainage or lavage from a nasogastric tube that yields blood or coffee-ground–like material confirms upper GI bleeding and can help predict the risk of a high-risk lesion. However, blood or coffee-ground–like contents may not be present if bleeding has ceased, or arises beyond a closed pylorus. Upper GI bleeding commonly presents with *hematemesis*, which is bloody vomitus that is either bright red, indicating fresh blood; or "coffee ground," which is older blood that has been in the stomach long enough for the gastric juices to act on it. Blood may also be passed via the colon. *Melena* is shiny, black, foul-smelling stool and results from the degradation of blood by stomach acids or intestinal bacteria. Bright red or maroon blood (*hematochezia*) can also be passed from the rectum. Hematochezia is usually a sign of a lower GI source of bleeding, but can be seen when upper GI bleeding is massive (>1000 mL). GI blood loss can also be occult, or detected only by testing the stool with a chemical reagent (guaiac). Stool and nasogastric drainage can test guaiac positive for up

to 10 days after a bleeding episode. Hematemesis and melena indicate an episode of acute upper GI bleeding. Upper GI bleeding may also be accompanied by mild epigastric pain or abdominal distress, although it is not very common. Pain is thought to arise from the acid bathing the ulcerated crater.

Finally, patients may manifest clinical signs and symptoms of blood loss. The Clinical Alert summarizes the common presenting manifestations of acute upper GI bleeding. Rapid assessment of the patient is undertaken to determine the seriousness of the bleeding, whether it is acute or chronic, and to determine whether the patient is hemodynamically stable or unstable. Patients with acute upper GI bleeding commonly have signs or symptoms of hypovolemic shock. Figure 17-8 describes the pathophysiology of acute upper GI bleeding.

CLINICAL ALERT
Clinical Signs and Symptoms of Upper Gastrointestinal Bleeding[9]

- Hematemesis
- Melena
- Hematochezia
- Abdominal discomfort
- Signs and symptoms of hypovolemic shock
  - Hypotension
  - Tachycardia
  - Cool, clammy skin
  - Change in level of consciousness
  - Decreased urine output
  - Decreased gastric motility

Special care should be taken to assess comorbid conditions in the older adult. Conditions such as chronic hypertension or cardiovascular disease often mask signs of shock and make resuscitative attempts difficult.

Nursing Assessment

Initial evaluation of the patient with upper GI bleeding involves a rapid assessment of the severity of blood loss, the hemodynamic stability, and the necessity for fluid resuscitation as well as frequent monitoring of vital signs and assessments of body systems for signs of shock. Changes in blood pressure and heart rate depend on the amount of blood loss, the suddenness of the blood loss, and the degree of cardiac and vascular compensation. Vital signs should be monitored at least every 15 minutes. As blood loss

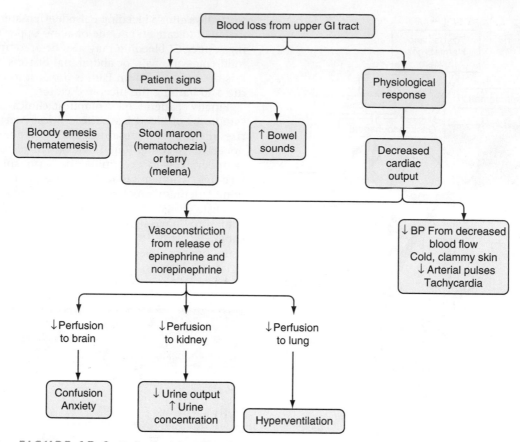

FIGURE 17-8. Pathophysiology flow diagram of acute upper gastrointestinal (GI) bleeding. *BP,* Blood pressure.

exceeds 1000 mL, the shock syndrome progresses, causing decreased blood flow to the skin, lungs, liver, and kidneys.

Hypotension is an advanced sign of shock. As a rule, a systolic pressure of less than 100 mm Hg, a postural decrease in blood pressure of greater than 10 mm Hg, or a heart rate of greater than 120 beats/min reflects a blood loss of at least 1000 mL—25% of the total blood volume.

Hypertension is a common comorbid condition in those at risk of GI bleeding. In the chronically hypertensive patient, normal values for predicting perfusion no longer apply. Emphasis should be placed on other assessment findings, such as level of consciousness and urinary output. As blood pressure decreases, it can be assumed that more blood has been lost.

Rarely, a right atrial or pulmonary artery catheter is inserted to evaluate the patient's hemodynamic response to the blood loss. The electrocardiogram may also show ST-segment depression or flattening of the T waves, both of which indicate decreased coronary blood flow resulting in ischemia.

Abdominal assessment may reveal a soft or distended abdomen. Bowel sounds most often are hyperactive as a result of the sensitivity of the bowel to blood.

In addition to the physical examination, a history is taken to ascertain whether there have been previous episodes of bleeding or surgery for bleeding; a family history of bleeding; or a current illness that may lead to bleeding, such as coagulopathies, cancer, and liver disease. Concurrent diseases also affect the patient's response to the hemorrhage and to the treatment modalities. Patterns of drug or alcohol ingestion and other risk factors need to be assessed and may also help to ascertain the cause.

Medical Assessment

Laboratory Studies. The common laboratory studies ordered for a patient with acute upper GI bleeding are listed in Laboratory Alerts: Upper Gastrointestinal Bleeding. A complete blood count is always ordered. However, the hematocrit (Hct) value does not change substantially during the first few hours after an acute GI bleed. During this time, the severity of the bleeding must not be underestimated. Only when extravascular fluid enters the vascular space to restore volume does the Hct value decrease. This effect is further complicated by fluids and blood that are administered during the resuscitation period. Platelet and white blood cell (WBC) counts may also be increased, reflecting the body's attempt to restore homeostasis. An electrolyte profile is also ordered. Decreases in potassium and sodium levels are common as a result of the accompanying vomiting. Later, serum sodium levels may increase as a result of the loss of vascular volume. The glucose level is often increased related to the stress response. Increases in the blood urea nitrogen (BUN) and creatinine levels reflect decreased perfusion to the liver and kidneys, respectively. Liver function tests, clotting profiles, and serum ammonia levels are ordered to rule out preexisting liver disease. An arterial blood gas analysis is ordered to evaluate the patient's acid-base and oxygenation status. Respiratory alkalosis is common with GI bleeding as a result of the effects of the sympathetic nervous system on the lungs and patient anxiety. As shock progresses, the patient may develop metabolic acidosis as a result of anaerobic metabolism. Hypoxemia may also be present as a result of decreased circulating Hgb levels.

Endoscopy and Barium Study. Endoscopy is the procedure of choice for the diagnosis and treatment of active upper GI bleeding and for the prevention of rebleeding. Endoscopy allows for direct mucosal inspection with the use of a fiberoptic scope. Flexible scopes allow this test to be performed at the patient's bedside, a preferable approach in an unstable, critically ill patient. Endoscopic evaluation of the source of the bleeding is not undertaken until the patient is hemodynamically stable. Barium studies can be performed to help define the presence of peptic ulcers, the sites of bleeding, the presence of tumors, and the presence of inflammatory processes.

Nursing Diagnoses

The nursing diagnoses most commonly seen in patients with acute GI bleeding are found in the Nursing Care Plan for the Patient with Acute Gastrointestinal Bleeding.

Collaborative Management: Nursing and Medical Considerations

The management of acute GI bleeding initially consists of hemodynamically stabilizing the patient and afterward diagnosing the cause of bleeding and initiating specific and supportive therapies (Box 17-7). The nurse's role during the initial management of acute GI bleeding includes assessing the patient, carrying out prescribed medical therapy, monitoring the patient's physiological and psychosocial responses to the interventions, monitoring for complications of the disease process or treatment regimen, and providing supportive care. Patient and family support during the acute phase is a nursing priority. Explanations of the diagnostic tests, the medical therapies, and the critical care environment are extremely

---

LABORATORY ALERTS
Upper Gastrointestinal Bleeding[5]

Complete Blood Count
Hemoglobin: Normal, then ↓
Hematocrit: Normal, then ↓
White blood cell count: ↑
Platelet count: Initially ↑ then ↓

Serum Electrolyte Panel
Potassium: ↓, then ↑
Sodium: ↑
Calcium: Normal or ↓
Blood urea nitrogen, creatinine: ↑
Ammonia: Possibly ↑
Glucose: Hyperglycemia common
Lactate: ↑

Hematology Profile
Prothrombin time, partial thromboplastin time: Usually ↑

Serum Enzyme Levels: ↑

Arterial Blood Gases
Respiratory alkalosis/metabolic acidosis

Gastric Aspirate for pH and Guaiac
Possibly acidotic pH
Guaiac positive

↑ Increased; ↓ decreased.

NURSING CARE PLAN for the Patient with Acute Gastrointestinal Bleeding

NURSING DIAGNOSIS

Fluid volume deficit related to decreased circulating blood volume

PATIENT OUTCOMES
Adequate circulating blood volume

- Hemorrhage controlled or resolved
- Preload indicators WNL
- Hct and Hgb levels stable
- I&O balanced

NURSING INTERVENTIONS	RATIONALES
• Monitor vital signs for hemodynamic instability and orthostatic changes	• Assess volume status
• Measure preload indicators: RAP, PAOP	• Assess volume status
• Monitor ECG, skin, urine output, amount and characteristics of GI secretions	• Monitor volume status and tissue perfusion
• Monitor response to blood and fluid replacement	• Assess response to treatment
• Monitor laboratory values: serial Hct, Hgb, BUN, potassium, sodium	• Assess acute bleeding
• Monitor bowel sounds	• Assess integrity and function of the gut
• Monitor for clinical manifestations of perforation: severe persistent abdominal pain; boardlike abdomen	• Assess for life-threatening complication
• Gastric lavage as ordered until clear	• May help to stop or reduce bleeding
• Administer medications and parenteral fluids	• Control bleeding and maintain fluid volume status
• Prepare for endoscopy, assist as necessary, and monitor for complications	• Assist in diagnosis of clinical problem; patients may not tolerate moderate sedation for GI procedures

NURSING DIAGNOSIS

Altered tissue perfusion related to decreased circulating blood volume

PATIENT OUTCOMES
Adequate tissue perfusion

- Signs and symptoms of decreased perfusion absent: decreased sensorium, chest pain, renal failure
- Hemodynamics stable
- Urine output >30 mL/hr
- Skin warm and dry
- Bowel sounds WNL

NURSING CARE PLAN for the Patient with Acute Gastrointestinal Bleeding—cont'd

NURSING INTERVENTIONS	RATIONALES
• Monitor for hypoperfusion and hemodynamic instability	• Prevent end-organ destruction
• Monitor vital signs every 15 minutes until stable	• Assess for hypovolemia and volume status
• Measure RAP, PAOP, cardiac output every hour until stable	• Assess volume status
• Monitor for tachycardia, chest pain, ST-segment elevation, diaphoresis, and cool/clammy extremities	• Assess for decreased cardiac output and decreased tissue perfusion
• Measure urine output every hour	• Monitor renal tissue perfusion
• Monitor level of consciousness	• Monitor tissue perfusion to the brain
• Assess bowel sounds	• Monitor tissue perfusion to the gut
• Monitor for elevated bilirubin	• Monitor liver dysfunction from hypoperfusion
• Notify the physician of changes and abnormalities	• Promote early intervention and prevent complications

NURSING DIAGNOSIS

Risk for fluid volume excess related to fluid overload from treatment regimen

PATIENT OUTCOMES

• Respiratory pattern normal
• Lung congestion or pulmonary edema absent

NURSING INTERVENTIONS	RATIONALES
• Monitor hemodynamic response to fluid administration	• Monitor for fluid volume excess
• Monitor breath sounds at least every hour during fluid administration	• Monitor for pulmonary interstitial fluid collection, hypoxia, and fluid volume excess
• Monitor for restlessness or anxiety, dyspnea, tachycardia, coughing, crackles, frothy sputum, dysrhythmias, abnormal ABG results, blood pressure, increased RAP, jugular vein distention	• Assess signs and symptoms of fluid volume excess
• Record accurate I&O hourly	• Monitor fluid balance
• Document and report any abnormalities	• Maintain nurse-physician collaboration

ABG, Arterial blood gas; *BUN,* blood urea nitrogen; *ECG,* electrocardiogram; *GI,* gastrointestinal; *Hct,* hematocrit; *Hgb,* hemoglobin; *I&O,* intake and output; *PAOP,* pulmonary artery occlusion pressure; *RAP,* right atrial pressure; *WNL,* within normal limits.

BOX 17-7   Management of Upper Gastrointestinal Bleeding

Hemodynamic Stabilization
- Colloids
- Crystalloids
- Blood or blood products

Definitive and Supportive Therapies
- Gastric lavage
- Pharmacological therapies
  - Antacids
  - H₂-histamine blockers
  - Proton pump inhibitors
  - Mucosal barrier enhancers
- Endoscopic therapies
  - Sclerotherapy
  - Heater probe
  - Laser
- Surgical therapies

important to patients who are often anxious about their diagnosis and the outcome.

Hemodynamic Stabilization

Patients who are hemodynamically unstable need to have immediate venous access (using large-bore intravenous [IV] catheters), and administration of fluid must be started. Refer to Chapter 11 for management of hypovolemic shock. For the restoration of vascular volume, fluids must be infused as rapidly as the patient's cardiovascular status allows and until the patient's vital signs return to baseline.

Patients who continue to bleed, or who have an excessively low Hct value (<25%) and have clinical symptoms, may be resuscitated with blood and blood products. The decision to use blood products is based on laboratory data and clinical examination. Blood is transfused to improve oxygenation (by increasing the number of RBCs) or to improve coagulation (by replacing platelets and plasma). The Hct value may not initially reflect actual blood volume during the first 24 to 72 hours after a hemorrhage and until vascular volume is restored. A reasonable goal for the management of blood transfusions is an Hct value of 30%, but this goal is individually determined for the patient based on clinical assessments. One unit of packed RBCs can be expected to increase the Hgb value by 1 g/dL and the Hct value by 2% to 3%, but this effect is influenced by the patient's intravascular volume status and whether the patient is actively bleeding. Careful monitoring for complications of blood transfusion therapy is also important.

These complications include hypocalcemia, hyperkalemia, infection, increased ammonia levels, hypothermia, and anaphylactic reactions.

Gastric Lavage

Large-volume gastric lavage before endoscopy for acute upper gastrointestinal bleeding is safe and provides better visualization of the gastric fundus.[21] A large-bore nasogastric tube is inserted and is connected to suction. If lavage is ordered, 1000 to 2000 mL of room temperature normal saline is instilled via nasogastric tube and is then gently removed by intermittent suction or gravity until the secretions are clear. Iced lavage is used in some centers, although the evidence for this use is not well documented. After lavage, the nasogastric tube may be left in or removed. Nasogastric tubes left in place may increase hydrochloric acid secretion in the stomach and cause increased bleeding. Of all upper GI hemorrhages, 80% to 90% are self-limiting and stop with lavage therapy alone or on their own. The nurse must carefully document the nature of the nasogastric secretions or vomitus, such as the color, amount, and pH.

Pharmacological Therapy

Pharmacological agents are given to decrease gastric acid secretion or to reduce the effects of acid on the gastric mucosa. The most common agents used include antacids, histamine antagonists (H₂-histamine blockers), proton pump inhibitors, and mucosal barrier enhancers. Antibiotics may also be ordered. Table 17-7 describes the treatments commonly used to decrease gastric acid secretion or reduce the effects of acid on the gastric mucosa.

Antibiotics. *H. pylori* infection is often associated with peptic ulcer disease. Triple-agent therapy with a proton pump inhibitor and two antibiotics for 14 days is the recommended treatment for eradication of *H. pylori*. The regimen consists of omeprazole (the proton pump inhibitor), and amoxicillin and clarithromycin (the two antibiotics).[27,29]

Endoscopic Therapy

Endoscopy is the modality of choice for determining the diagnosis, prognosis, and therapy for upper GI bleeding. Several endoscopic therapies have been developed for the control of peptic ulcer bleeding. Endoscopy is performed only after the patient is stabilized hemodynamically, including volume resuscitation, but within 6 to 12 hours of presentation.[1] The advantage of endoscopic therapies is that they can be applied during the diagnostic procedure. Sclerotherapy involves injecting the bleeding ulcer with a necrotizing agent. The most common agents used are morrhuate sodium, ethanolamine, and tetradecyl

PHARMACOLOGY

TABLE 17-7 Pharmacological Treatments to Decrease Gastric Acid Secretion and/or Reduce Acid Effects on Gastric Mucosa[10]

Classification, Action	Medications	Administration
Histamine Blockers Blocks all factors that stimulate the parietal cells in the stomach to secrete hydrochloric acid	Cimetidine	300-1200 mg/day IV push, administer over not less than 5 minutes Intermittent IV infuse over 15-20 minutes IV infusion 100-1000 mL over 24 hours
	Famotidine	10-20 mg/day IV push, administer over 10 minutes Infuse piggyback over 15-30 minutes
	Nizatidine	150-300 mg/day Not available IV
	Ranitidine	150-300 mg/day IV push, administer over 5 minutes Infuse piggyback over 15-20 minutes IV infusion over 24 hours
Proton Pump Inhibitors Inhibits gastric acid secretion by specific inhibition of the hydrogen potassium–adenosine triphosphatase enzyme system	Esomeprazole	20-40 mg/day IV push administration over not less than 3 minutes For intermittent infusion, infuse over 15-30 minutes
	Lansoprazole	15-30 mg/day IV administration, infuse over 30 minutes
	Omeprazole	20-40 mg/day Not available IV
	Pantoprazole	40 mg/day Infuse 10 mL solution over at least 2 minutes Infuse 100 mL solution over at least 15 minutes
Mucosal Barrier Enhancers Reduces the effects of acid secretion; promotes healing	Sucralfate	1 g four times a day
	Colloidal bismuth	120 mg four times a day
Antacids Direct alkaline buffers to control the pH of the gastric mucosa	Aluminum hydroxide	500-1500 mg 3-6 times a day*
	Calcium carbonate	500-1,500 mg as needed*
	Magnesium hydroxide	Liquid 2.5-7.5 mL up to 4 times a day*
	Magnesium oxide	400-800 mg/day*

* Often given every 1-2 hours to maintain gastric pH >5 *IV*, Intravenous.

sulfate. These agents work by traumatizing the endothelium, causing necrosis and eventual sclerosis of the bleeding vessel. Thermal methods of endoscopic therapy include use of the heater probe, laser photocoagulation, and electrocoagulation. All of these therapies act to tamponade the vessel to stop active bleeding. Because they are performed at the patient's bedside, the nurse assists with the procedures and monitors for untoward effects.

Maintenance of airway and breathing during endoscopic procedures is of major concern. Placement of the patient in a left lateral reverse Trendelenburg position helps to prevent respiratory complications. Other common complications of sclerotherapy include fever and oozing from the bleeding site.

Surgical Therapy
Surgery may be considered in patients who have massive GI bleeding that is immediately life-threatening, in patients who continue to bleed despite medical therapies, and in patients with perforation or unremitting pyloric obstruction. The purpose of emergency surgery in patients with massive upper GI bleeding is the prevention of death

GENETICS
Cytochrome P450 Enzymes and the Patient's Response to Drugs

Variations in the cytochrome P450 (CYP) enzymes found in the gastrointestinal system have important pharmacological implications. The effects and toxicity of drugs vary significantly among individuals because of the way drugs are metabolized. After administration and distribution, drugs are altered usually to make them more water soluble so that they can be excreted by the kidneys.[6] More than half of prescription drugs and many over-the-counter and herbal agents are metabolized by enzymes found in liver and intestinal cells. One group of related enzymes common to both the liver and intestine are the CYP. This name is a result of their red coloration (cytochrome means "colored cell" from a heme molecule in the enzyme structure) and the wavelength of light that these proteins absorb in mass spectrography (450 nanometers).

There are three main cytochrome families involved in drug metabolism in humans: the CYP1, 2, and 3. One isoform of a specific subfamily of CYP3 enzymes, CYP3A4 (A is the subfamily and 4 is the isoform), is abundant in the liver and intestines. Interestingly, CYP3A4 does not have any known polymorphisms, although there may be variations that precede the coding section of this gene that influence its activity. Areas that precede a gene and influence its expression or ability to generate proteins are promoter or inhibitor regions that "turn on" or "turn off" genes, respectively.[3]

The subfamilies in the CYP2 enzymes and their isoforms have polymorphisms that are typically a single nucleotide polymorphism (SNP, pronounced "snip") that leads to altered enzyme activity. For example, the CYP2D4 (D subfamily, 4th isoform) has more than 44 alleles.[7] Some variations result in less metabolic activity, predisposing patients to drug toxicities. Other polymorphisms provide extensive metabolizing effects with a faster metabolism that leads to low drug levels and reduced effects despite administration of a therapeutic dose. The CYP2D6 enzyme affects metabolism of more than 25% of prescription drugs.[5]

Small amounts or ineffective enzymes in the CYP2D4 family affect some beta-blockers, several antidysrhythmics, and drugs used to treat psychiatric disorders including severe depression and schizophrenia. However, because CYP2D6 affects individual drugs but not whole classes of drugs, the prescriber can usually switch prescriptions to an equivalent but alternative drug that is not metabolized by this pathway.[6]

The CYP2D6 enzymes are especially interesting in relationship to patient response to codeine. Poor metabolizers cannot convert codeine to its active form and so codeine provides no pain relief. Increasing the dose or frequency of administration will not change this response.[5] Alternatively, individuals who inherit a genotype that results in extensive metabolism experience a quick conversion of codeine into its active form, causing unanticipated central nervous system effects such as euphoria or hallucinations, which are not generally associated with codeine use.

In addition to metabolizing drugs, CYP enzymes are used to transform procarcinogens, alcohol, fatty acids, prostaglandins, and hormones (both endogenous and exogenous). They also contribute to detoxifying food. Plants develop toxins to limit their consumption, while herbivores develop enzymes to metabolize the plant toxins. It is important to remember that the activity of nearly all the CYP enzymes are affected by foods, temperature (e.g., fever, hypothermia), pH, and other environmental factors.[10]

Clinical observations support the laboratory genotyping for the CYP families as well as other metabolizing enzymes. Reports of "fast" and "slow" metabolizers have appeared for about 50 years in the literature.[9] The potential for clinical genotyping has some advantages over clinical observations. It can limit trial-and-error dosing and avoid adverse complications and undesirable effects from a dose that is too high or inadequate given an individual's ability to metabolize a drug.[9] Results of genotyping can be obtained within 24 hours and are not affected by underlying disease or coadministration of other drugs. Genotype does not change, so it need be done only once. However, since most metabolizing drugs are also affected by other factors such as drug-drug interactions or severity of disease, it is difficult to know whether pharmacological genotype will yield consistently useful data for all patient conditions and responses.[2,4]

This study of genetic variation and its effects on pharmaceuticals is called *pharmacogenetics* or *pharmacogenomics*. Pharmacogenetics specifically refers to the study of individual genetic variability or biochemical and other differences between individuals that influence one person's response to medication. Pharmacogenomics is the study of the whole genome and higher proteins (e.g., RNA, enzymes, and drug receptors) and focuses on how differences within the individual work together to create a response to medications. The terms are used interchangeably as both describe drug-gene interactions that alter patient responses.[8]

Clinicians need to be aware of pharmaco-genetic and—genomic vocabulary and techniques. The study of gene-drug interactions could improve drug testing, clinical trials, and prescriptive approaches. For

GENETICS—cont'd

example, researchers and clinicians recently collaborated to develop a decision tree based on genotyping for two enzymes that affect warfarin metabolism. Patients vary widely in their response to typical doses of warfarin, and its toxic effects can be life-threatening, so developing an approach to dosing that reduces error is highly valued. They tested the algorithm in a small sample and found that it resulted in therapeutic dosing more than 77% of the time; trial-and-error dosing is accurate about 50% of the time.[1] In another example of genotype use, clinicians in oncology routinely test for some types of metabolizing enzymes to avoid toxicities from chemotherapeutic regimens.[9] SNP chips that detail as many as 1000 metabolizing enzymes for individuals may be available in clinical labs in less than 5 years.[4]

REFERENCES

1. Carlquist, J. F., Horne, B. D., Muhlestein, J. B., Lappé, D. L., Whiting, R. M., Kolek, M. J., et al. (2006). Genotypes of the cytochrome P450 isoform, CYP2C9, and the vitamin K epoxide reductase complex subunit 1 conjointly determine stable warfarin dose: A prospective study. *Journal of Thombosis and Thrombolysis, 22*, 191-197.

2. Daly, A. K. (2007). Individualized drug therapy. *Current Opinion in Drug Discovery and Development, 10*, 29-36.

3. FDA/Center for Drug Evaluation and Research. (2006). *Genomics at FDA*. Retrieved April 29, 2008, from www.fda.gov/cder/genomics/.

4. Flockhart, D. A. (2006). *Drug interactions*. Retrieved August 14, 2008, from http://medicine.iupui.edu/flockhart/.

5. Goldstein, D. B., Need, A. C., Singh, R., & Sisodiya, S. M. (2007). Potential genetic causes of heterogeneity of treatment effects. *American Journal of Medicine, 120*, S21-S25.

6. Holford, N. H. G. (2004). *Basic and clinical pharmacology* (9th ed.). New York: McGraw Hill.

7. Ingelman-Sundberg, M. (2005). Genetic polymorphisms of cytochrome P450 2D6 (CYP2D6): Clinical consequences, evolutionary aspects and functional diversity. *Pharmacogenomics Journal, 5*, 6-14.

8. Prows, C. A., & Prows, D. R. (2004). Medication selection by genotype. *American Journal of Nursing, 104*, 59-71.

9. Lashley, F. R. (2005). *Clinical genetics in nursing practice* (3rd ed.). New York: Springer.

10. Testam, B., & Kramer, S. D. (2007). The biochemistry of drug metabolism—An introduction: Part 2: Redox reactions and their enzymes. *Chemical Biodiversity, 4*, 257-405.

from exsanguination. The patient is usually admitted to a critical care unit for initial management and stabilization in preparation for emergency surgery.

The most common reason for emergency surgery is massive rebleeding that occurs within 8 hours of admission. Patients may also become surgical candidates if they continue to bleed despite aggressive medical intervention. Criteria for delayed surgery varies, but it is usually considered in patients who require more than 8 units of blood within a 24-hour period.

Impaired emptying of solids or liquids from the stomach into the small intestine (gastric outlet obstruction) may also necessitate surgical intervention. The major symptoms of obstruction include vomiting and continued ulcer pain that is localized in the epigastrium.

Surgical therapies for peptic ulcer disease include gastric resections (antrectomy, gastrectomy, gastroenterostomy, vagotomy) and combined operations to restore GI continuity (Billroth I, Billroth II) or to prevent GI complications of the surgery (vagotomy and pyloroplasty). An *antrectomy* may be performed for duodenal ulcers to decrease the acidity of the duodenum by removing the antrum, which secretes gastric acid. A *vagotomy* decreases acid secretion in the stomach by dividing the vagus nerve along the

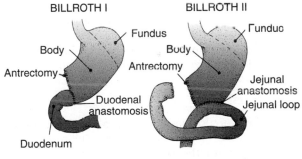

FIGURE 17-9. Billroth I and II procedures.

esophagus. A *pyloroplasty* may be performed in conjunction with a vagotomy to prevent stomach atony, a common complication of the vagotomy procedure. A *Billroth I* procedure involves vagotomy, antrectomy, and anastomosis of the stomach to the duodenum. A *Billroth II* procedure involves vagotomy, resection of the antrum, and anastomosis of the stomach to the jejunum (Figure 17-9). A perforation can be treated by simple closure with the use of a patch to cover the gastric mucosal hole (omental patch) or by excision of the ulcer and suturing of the surrounding tissue.

Postoperative nursing care is focused on prevention and monitoring of potential complications. Fluid and electrolyte imbalances are common from loss of fluids during the surgical procedure and drains that are left in place either to decompress the stomach (nasogastric tube) or to drain the surgical site. In addition, the GI system may not function normally after surgery, with resulting nausea, vomiting, ileus, or diarrhea. Provision of adequate nutrition is essential for proper wound healing. In cases of prolonged ileus after surgery, total parenteral nutrition may be considered. Monitoring for proper wound healing is also a nursing responsibility. Signs and symptoms of wound infection (erythema, swelling, tenderness, drainage, fever, increased WBC count) need to be documented and reported. A systemic infection may result from peritonitis in the case of perforation in which stomach or intestinal contents spill into the peritoneum. Postoperative rupture of the anastomosis may also lead to this complication.

Pain is also an important postoperative nursing concern. Abdominal incisions are associated with postoperative discomfort because of their anatomical location. Postoperative lung infections are also common in patients with abdominal incisions, because incisional pain impairs the ability to cough and breathe deeply.

Nursing Diagnoses

Several nursing diagnoses are associated with the postoperative care of the patient with upper GI bleeding. These diagnoses include risk for infection of wound, peritoneum, or both; altered nutrition; pain; fluid and electrolyte alterations; and impaired gas exchange.

Recognition of Potential Complications

Perforation of the gastric mucosa is the major GI complication of peptic ulcer disease. The nurse must be familiar with the signs and symptoms of acute perforation, which are reviewed in the Clinical Alert. The most common signs of this complication are an abrupt onset of abdominal pain, followed

---

CLINICAL ALERT
Acute Gastric Perforation[9]

- Abrupt onset of severe abdominal pain
- Abdominal tenderness
- Board-like abdomen
- Usually absent bowel sounds
- Leukocytosis
- Presence of free air on x-ray study

---

rapidly by signs of peritonitis. The treatment goal for the patient with acute perforation is preparation for emergent surgery. Fluid and electrolyte resuscitation and treatment of any immediate complications are priorities. These patients almost always have nasogastric tubes placed for gastric decompression. Broad-spectrum antibiotics are also usually prescribed before surgery. Antacids and histamine blockers may or may not be indicated, depending on the cause of the upper GI bleeding. Mortality rates for patients with perforations range from 10% to 40%, depending on the age and condition of the patient at the time of surgery.

Treatment of Variceal Bleeding

Hemorrhaging esophageal or gastric varices are usually a medical emergency because they cause massive upper GI bleeding. The patient typically develops hemodynamic instability and signs and symptoms of shock. Often, the cause of the bleeding is unknown unless the patient has a history of cirrhosis or has previously bled from varices. Initial treatment of patients with esophageal or gastric varices is therefore the same. Top priorities include hemodynamic stabilization and establishment of a patent airway. Gastric lavage may be used to clear the stomach and to document the amount of blood loss. Diagnosis of the cause of the bleeding through endoscopy is the next priority before definitive treatment for the varices can be started.

Somatostatin or Octreotide

Somatostatin or octreotide (a long-acting somatostatin) is commonly ordered to slow or stop bleeding. Early administration provides for stabilization before endoscopy. These drugs decrease splanchnic blood flow and reduce portal pressure, and have minimal adverse effects. Octreotide is given as an IV bolus of 50 to 100 mcg, followed by an infusion of 25 to 50 mcg/hr for up to 3 days. Patients must be monitored for both hypoglycemia and hyperglycemia.[10]

Vasopressin

Vasopressin (Pitressin) (Box 17-8) is a synthetic antidiuretic hormone. Vasopressin lowers portal pressure by vasoconstriction of the splanchnic arteriolar bed. Ultimately, it decreases pressure and flow in liver collateral circulation channels to decrease bleeding. However, vasopressin is not a first-line therapy because of its adverse effects.[11]

Endoscopic Procedures

Sclerotherapy is another option in the treatment of bleeding varices. After the varices are identified, the sclerosing agent is injected into the varix and the

BOX 17-8 Vasopressin (Pitressin) Therapy[10]

Mechanism of Action
- Vasoconstrictor: constricts the splanchnic vascular bed, contracts intestinal smooth muscle, and lowers portal vein pressure

Dose
- Given by intravenous (IV) route, although it may be given intraarterially. IV infusion is started at 0.2-0.4 units/min, increased progressively to 0.9 units/min. The maximum recommended dose is 0.01 unit/kg/min
- Vasopressin should be continued for at least 24 hours after bleeding is controlled. Wean slowly

Side Effects
- *Gastrointestinal:* cramping, nausea, vomiting, diarrhea
- *Cardiovascular:* dizziness, diaphoresis, hypertension, cardiac dysrhythmias, exacerbation of heart failure
- *Neurological:* tremors, headache, vertigo, decreased level of consciousness
- *Integumentary:* pallor, localized gangrene

Nursing Considerations
- Monitor for angina and dysrhythmias
- Infuse through a central line
- Assess serum sodium and neurological status
- Assess neurological status

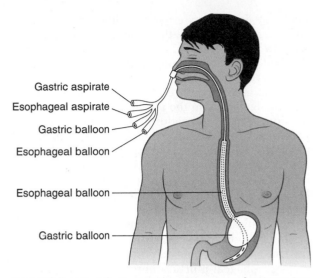

Gastric aspirate
Esophageal aspirate
Gastric balloon
Esophageal balloon

Esophageal balloon

Gastric balloon

FIGURE 17-10. Sengstaken-Blakemore tube. *(From Day, M. W. [2005]. Esophagogastric tamponade tube. In D. J. L. Wiegand, & K. Carlson [Eds.], AACN procedure manual for critical care [5th ed., p. 862]. Philadelphia: Saunders.)*

surrounding tissue. Usually, several applications of the sclerosing agent several days apart are needed to decompress the bleeding varix.

Endoscopic band ligation is another treatment for varices.[28] Under endoscopy, a rubber band is placed over the varix. This treatment results in thrombosis, sloughing, and fibrosis of the varix.

Transjugular Intrahepatic Portosystemic Shunt
Transjugular intrahepatic portosystemic shunting (TIPS) is a nonsurgical treatment for recurrent variceal bleeding after sclerotherapy. Placement of the shunt is performed with the use of fluoroscopy. A stainless steel stent is placed between the hepatic and portal veins to create a portosystemic shunt in the liver and decrease portal pressure.[7] Decreasing portal pressure decreases pressure within the varix, thereby decreasing the risk for acute hemorrhage.

The role of TIPS in treating active hemorrhage uncontrolled by first-line therapy in patients who are good surgical candidates is not well-defined in clinical guidelines, and the choice remains up to the physician.[1] Approximately 10% to 20% of patients

do not stop bleeding with endoscopic treatment combined with somatostatin infusion, while others rebleed in the first couple of days after cessation of the initial bleed. After a second unsuccessful endoscopic attempt, the TIPS procedure is used as a treatment option.

Esophagogastric Tamponade
If bleeding continues despite vasopressin therapy, esophagogastric balloon tamponade therapy may provide temporary control of bleeding. Inflation of the balloon ports applies pressure to the vessels supplying the varices to decrease blood flow, thereby stopping the bleeding. Three types of tubes are used for tamponade: Sengstaken-Blakemore, Minnesota, and Linton tubes. The adult Sengstaken-Blakemore tube has three lumina: one for gastric aspiration, similar to that in a nasogastric tube; one for inflation of the esophageal balloon; and one for inflation of the gastric balloon (Figure 17-10). The Minnesota tube has an additional lumen that allows for aspiration of esophageal secretions. The Minnesota tube is commonly used because it allows for suction of secretions above and below the balloon. The Linton tube has a gastric balloon only, and lumens for gastric and esophageal suction; it is reserved for those with bleeding gastric varices.

Regardless of type, the balloon tip is inserted into the stomach, and the gastric balloon is inflated and clamped. The tube is then withdrawn until resistance is met, so pressure is exerted at the gastroesophageal junction. Correct positioning and traction are maintained by using an external traction source or a nasal cuff around the tube at the mouth or nose. External traction can be attached to a helmet or to the foot of the bed. Proper amounts of traction are essential because too little traction lets the balloon fall away from the gastric wall, resulting in insufficient pressure being placed on the bleeding vessels. Too much traction causes discomfort, gastric ulceration, or vomiting. If bleeding does not stop with inflation of the gastric balloon, the esophageal balloon is inflated and clamped (Sengstaken-Blakemore or Minnesota tube). Normal inflation pressure is 20 to 45 mm Hg. Monitoring inflation pressures is important to prevent tissue damage.

The critical care nurse is responsible for maintaining balloon lumen pressures and patency of the system. The gastric balloon port placement below the gastroesophageal junction must be confirmed by x-ray study. Ideally, the balloons are deflated every 8 to 12 hours to decompress the esophagus and gastric mucosa. The status of the bleeding varices can also be assessed at this time, and the nurse must be prepared for hematemesis during this procedure. It is crucial that the esophageal balloon be deflated before the gastric balloon is deflated, or else the entire tube will be displaced upward and occlude the airway.

Spontaneous rupture of the gastric balloon, upward migration of the tube, and occlusion of the airway are other possible complications that need to be assessed. Esophageal rupture may occur and is characterized by the abrupt onset of severe pain. In the event of either of these two life-threatening emergencies, all three lumina are cut and the entire tube is removed. For this reason, scissors are kept at the patient's beside at all times. Endotracheal intubation is strongly recommended to protect the airway.

Other complications of esophagogastric tamponade include ulcerations of the esophageal or gastric mucosa. In addition, sores can develop around the mouth and nose as a result of the traction devices. Frequent cleansing and lubrication of these areas help to prevent skin breakdown. The nasopharynx requires frequent suctioning because of an increase in secretions and a decreased swallowing reflex. The nasogastric tube should also be irrigated at least every 2 hours to ensure patency and to keep the stomach empty. This measure helps to prevent aspiration and prevents accumulation of blood in the stomach. Ammonia is a byproduct of blood breakdown and cannot be detoxified by the patient with liver failure.

Surgical Interventions

Permanent decompression of portal hypertension can be achieved only through surgical procedures that divert blood around the blocked portal system. These are called *portacaval shunts*. In these operations, a connection is made between the portal vein and the inferior vena cava that diverts blood flow into the vena cava to decrease portal pressure. Several variations of this procedure exist, including the end-to-side shunt and the side-to-side shunt (Figure 17-11). Other surgical techniques for reduction of portal pressure include splenorenal and mesocaval shunting.

Portosystemic shunting reduces portal hypertension and therefore decreases bleeding from esophageal varices. Surgical shunts decrease rebleeding but do not improve survival. The procedure is associated with a higher risk of encephalopathy. The procedure also makes liver transplantation, if needed, more difficult. A temporary increase in ascites occurs after all these procedures, and careful assessments and interventions are required in the care of this patient population (see the later discussion of hepatic failure).

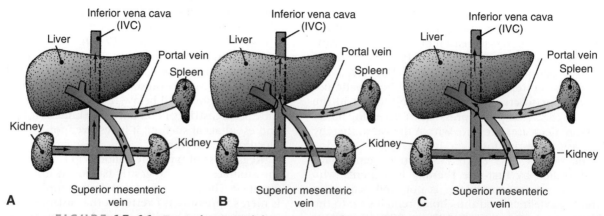

FIGURE 17-11. Types of portacaval shunts. **A,** Normal portal circulation. **B,** End-to-side shunt. **C,** Side-to-side shunt.

Patient Outcomes

Expected patient care outcomes for each nursing diagnosis for the patient with acute GI bleeding are found in the Nursing Care Plan for the Patient with Acute Gastrointestinal Bleeding.

ACUTE PANCREATITIS

Acute pancreatitis is defined as an acute inflammatory disease of the pancreas. The intensity of the disease ranges from mild, in which the patient has abdominal pain and elevated blood amylase and lipase levels, to extremely severe, which results in multiple organ failure. In 85% to 90% of patients, the disease is self-limiting (mild acute pancreatitis), and patients generally recover rapidly. However, the disease can run a fulminant course and is associated with high mortality rates. Severe acute pancreatitis develops in 25% of patients with acute pancreatitis.[2] Management of this more severe form of the disease requires intensive nursing and medical care.

Pathophysiology

Acute pancreatitis is an inflammation of the pancreas with the potential for necrosis of pancreatic cells resulting from premature activation of pancreatic enzymes within the pancreas. It is one of the most common pancreatic diseases, with an incidence rate of 4.9 to 80 cases per 100,000 people per year.[19] Normally, pancreatic juices are secreted into the duodenum, where they are activated. These enzymes are essential to normal carbohydrate, fat, and protein metabolism. The most common theory regarding the development of pancreatitis is that an injury or disruption of pancreatic acinar cells allows leakage of the pancreatic enzymes into pancreatic tissue. The leaked enzymes (trypsin, chymotrypsin, and elastase) become activated in the tissue and start the process of *autodigestion*. The activated enzymes break down tissue and cell membranes, causing edema, vascular damage, hemorrhage, necrosis, and fibrosis.[14] These now toxic enzymes and inflammatory mediators are released into the bloodstream and cause injury to vessel and organ systems, such as the hepatic and renal systems. Box 17-9 reviews the major systemic complications of acute fulminating pancreatitis.

Most patients with mild acute pancreatitis are treatable with a short period of bowel rest, simple IV hydration, and analgesia. Severe acute pancreatitis can be complicated by systemic inflammatory response syndrome. Thus, the current therapy for acute pancreatitis has shifted to intensive hemodynamic and pulmonary management, nutrition support, infection control, and pharmacological treatments.[18]

BOX 17-9 Systemic Complications of Acute Pancreatitis

Pulmonary
- Hypoxemia
- Atelectasis, pneumonia, pleural effusion
- Acute respiratory distress syndrome

Cardiovascular
- Hypovolemic shock
- Myocardial depression
- Cardiac dysrhythmias

Hematological
- Coagulation abnormalities
- Disseminated intravascular coagulation

Gastrointestinal
- Gastrointestinal bleeding
- Pancreatic pseudocyst
- Pancreatic abscess

Renal
- Azotemia
- Oliguria
- Acute renal failure

Metabolic
- Hypocalcemia
- Hyperlipidemia
- Hyperglycemia
- Metabolic acidosis

Acute pancreatitis has numerous causes, but the most common are alcohol ingestion and biliary disease. Box 17-10 lists many causes of this disease. Numerous drugs may initiate acute pancreatitis as a result of either ingestion of toxic doses or a drug reaction. Pancreatitis resulting from blunt or penetrating abdominal trauma, or occurring after endoscopic exploration of the biliary tree, has also been reported.

Metabolic complications of acute pancreatitis include hypocalcemia and hyperlipidemia, which are thought to be related to the areas of fat necrosis. Hypocalcemia is a major complication and almost always indicates a more serious manifestation of acute pancreatitis. Various hormone imbalances, particularly parathyroid hormone imbalance, are also found.

Assessment

History and Physical Examination

A diagnosis of acute pancreatitis is based on clinical examination and the results of laboratory and radiological tests (see Laboratory Alerts: Pancreatitis).

BOX 17-10   Causes of Acute Pancreatitis

- Biliary disease
  - Gallstones
  - Common bile duct obstruction
  - Post ERCP procedure
- Alcohol
- Traumatic injury of the pancreas
- Tumors of pancreatic ductal system or mestastatic
- Medications
  - Estrogen
  - Corticosteroids
  - Thiazide diuretics
  - Azathioprine
  - Sulfonamides
  - Furosemide
  - Pentamidine
  - Octreotide
- Heredity
- Hypercalcemia
- Hypertriglyceridemia
- Infections
- Idiopathic

ERCP, Endoscopic Retrograde Cholangiopancreatography

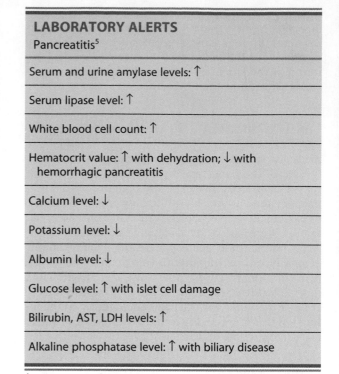

LABORATORY ALERTS
Pancreatitis[5]

Serum and urine amylase levels: ↑
Serum lipase level: ↑
White blood cell count: ↑
Hematocrit value: ↑ with dehydration; ↓ with hemorrhagic pancreatitis
Calcium level: ↓
Potassium level: ↓
Albumin level: ↓
Glucose level: ↑ with islet cell damage
Bilirubin, AST, LDH levels: ↑
Alkaline phosphatase level: ↑ with biliary disease

↑, Increased; ↓, decreased; *AST,* aspartate transaminase; *LDH,* lactate dehydrogenase.

CLINICAL ALERT
Signs and Symptoms of Acute Pancreatitis[9]

- Pain
- Nausea and vomiting
- Fever
- Dehydration
- Abdominal guarding, distention
- Grey Turner's sign
- Cullen's sign

Nurses conduct initial and ongoing clinical assessments; monitor and report physical and laboratory data; and coordinate the multidisciplinary plan of care.

Patients who present with organ failure at admission, or within 72 hours after onset of the disease, have a complicated clinical course with persistence of multisystem dysfunction. Multiorgan dysfunction syndrome triggers additional mechanisms that render translocation of bacteria manifesting as sepsis.[2]

In most cases, patients with acute pancreatitis develop severe abdominal pain.[13] It is most often epigastric or midabdominal pain that radiates to the back. The pain is caused by edema, chemical irritation and inflammation of the peritoneum, and irritation or obstruction of the biliary tract.[14]

Nausea and vomiting are also common symptoms. They are caused by the hypermotility or paralytic ileus secondary to the pancreatitis or peritonitis. Abdominal distention accompanies the hypermotile bowel symptoms along with the accumulation of fluid in the peritoneal cavity.[14] This fluid contains enzymes and kinins that increase vascular permeability and dilate the blood vessels. Hypotension and shock occur from the intravascular volume depletion, which then causes myocardial insufficiency. Fever and leukocytosis are also symptoms of the inflammatory process.

Patients with more severe pancreatic disease may have ascites, jaundice, or palpable abdominal masses. Two rare signs that can be present with any disease associated with retroperitoneal hemorrhage include a bluish discoloration of the flanks *(Grey Turner's sign)* or around the umbilical area *(Cullen's sign),* indicative of blood in these areas.[22] Because of the increase in abdominal size, the abdominal girth is measured at least every 4 hours to detect internal bleeding (see Clinical Alert).

Diagnostic Tests

The clinical diagnosis of acute pancreatitis is based on clinical findings, the presence of associated disorders, and laboratory testing. Because the clinical history, presenting signs and symptoms, and physical findings mimic many other GI and cardiovascular disorders, ultrasound and computed tomography (CT) scans are used in severe cases to determine the extent of involvement and the presence of complications. As an example, the pain associated with acute pancreatitis is similar to that associated with peptic ulcer disease, gallbladder disease, intestinal obstruction, and acute myocardial infarction. This similarity exists because pain receptors in the abdomen are poorly differentiated as they exit the skin surface.

Serum lipase and amylase tests are the most specific indicators of acute pancreatitis because as the pancreatic cells and ducts are destroyed, these enzymes are released. An elevated serum amylase level is a characteristic diagnostic feature. Amylase levels usually rise within 12 hours after the onset of symptoms and return to normal within 3 to 5 days. Serum lipase levels increase within 4 to 8 hours of clinical symptom onset and then decrease within 8 to 14 days. Serum trypsin levels are very specific for pancreatitis but may not be readily available. Urine trypsinogen-2 and urine amylase levels are also elevated. C reactive protein increases within 48 hours and is a marker of severity. The ratio of amylase clearance to creatinine clearance by the kidney can be diagnostic. Other conditions associated with increased serum amylase levels are listed in Box 17-11.

Other common laboratory abnormalities associated with acute pancreatitis include an elevated WBC count resulting from the inflammatory process and an elevated serum glucose level resulting from beta cell damage and pancreatic necrosis. Hypokalemia may be present because of associated vomiting. Hyperkalemia may be a systemic complication in the presence of acute renal failure. Hypocalcemia is common with severe disease and usually indicates pancreatic fat necrosis. Serum albumin and protein levels may be decreased as a result of the movement of fluid into the extracellular space. Increases in serum bilirubin, lactate dehydrogenase, and aspartate transaminase levels, and prothrombin time are common in the presence of concurrent liver disease. Serum triglyceride levels may increase dramatically and may be a causative factor in the development of the acute inflammatory process. Arterial blood gas analysis may show hypoxemia and retained carbon dioxide levels, which indicate respiratory failure.

CT modalities and magnetic resonance imaging are also used to confirm the diagnosis. Contrast-enhanced CT is considered the gold standard for diagnosing pancreatic necrosis and for grading acute pancreatitis.[22] The Balthazar CT index is a scoring system that ranges from 0 to 10 and is obtained by adding the points attributed to the extent of the inflammatory process to the volume of pancreatic necrosis. Endoscopic retrograde cholangiopancreatography (ERCP) combines radiography with endoscopy, and may assist in diagnosis.

Predicting the Severity of Acute Pancreatitis

Patients with acute pancreatitis can develop mild or fulminant disease. As a consequence, research has addressed criteria for predicting the prognosis of patients with acute pancreatitis. The early classification criteria were developed by Ranson[25] (Box 17-12),

---

BOX 17-11 Other Conditions Associated with Increased Serum Amylase Levels

- Salivary gland disease
- Renal insufficiency
- Diabetic ketoacidosis
- Intraabdominal disease (perforations, obstructions, aortic disease, peritonitis, appendicitis)
- Biliary tract disease
- Pregnancy
- Cerebral trauma
- Pneumonia
- Tumors
- Chronic alcoholism
- Burns
- Shock
- Gynecological disorders
- Prostatic disease

BOX 17-12 Ranson Criteria for Predicting Severity of Acute Pancreatitis*

At Admission or on Diagnosis
- Age >55 years (>70)
- Leukocyte count >16,000/microliter (>18,000)
- Serum glucose level >200 mg/dL (>220)
- Serum LDH level >350 IU/L (>400)
- Serum AST level >250 IU/L

During Initial 48 Hours
- Decrease in hematocrit >10%
- Increase in blood urea nitrogen level >5 mg/dL (>2)
- Serum calcium level <8 mg/dL
- Base deficit >4 mEq/L (>5)
- Estimated fluid sequestration >6 L (>4)
- Partial pressure of arterial oxygen <60 mm Hg

*Criteria values for nonalcoholic acute pancreatitis differing from those in alcohol-related disease are in parentheses. LDH, Lactate dehydrogenase; AST, aspartate transaminase. Modified from Ranson, J. C. (1985). Risk factors in acute pancreatitis. *Hospital Practice, 20*(4), 69-73.

where the number of signs present within the first 48 hours of admission directly relates to the patient's chance of significant morbidity and mortality. In Ranson's research, patients with fewer than three signs had a 1% mortality rate, those with three or four signs had a 15% mortality rate, those with five or six signs had a 40% mortality rate, and those with seven or more signs had a 100% mortality rate.

The Atlanta Classification has become accepted worldwide[2] as the first clinically reliable classification system. It defines severe acute pancreatitis as the presence of three or more of Ranson's criteria or a score of 8 or more with APACHE II (Acute Physiologic and Chronic Health Evaluation) criteria.[22] High severity-of-illness scores (APACHE III) and five or more Ranson[25] criteria predict multiple complications or death.

Another scale used to predict multiorgan failure is the Sepsis-Related Organ Failure Assessment.[2]

Nursing Diagnoses

Actual or potential nursing diagnoses associated with acute pancreatitis or with systemic complications of the disease process are found in the Nursing Care Plan for the Patient with Acute Pancreatitis.

Medical and Nursing Interventions

Nursing and medical priorities for the management of acute pancreatitis include several interventions. Managing respiratory dysfunction is a high priority. Fluids and electrolytes are replaced to maintain or replenish vascular volume and electrolyte balance. Analgesics are given for pain control, and supportive therapies are aimed at decreasing gastrin release from the stomach and preventing the gastric contents from entering the duodenum.

Fluid Replacement

In patients with severe acute pancreatitis, some fluid collects in the retroperitoneal space and peritoneal cavity. Patients sequester up to one third of their plasma volume. Initially, most patients develop some degree of dehydration and, in severe cases, hypovolemic shock. Hypovolemia and shock are major causes of death early in the disease process. Fluid replacement is a high priority in the treatment of acute pancreatitis.

The IV solutions ordered for fluid resuscitation are usually colloids or lactated Ringer's solution; however, fresh frozen plasma and albumin may also be used. IV fluid administration with crystalloids at 500 mL/hr is at times required to maintain hemodynamic status.[21] Often, vigorous IV fluid replacement at 240 to 350 mL/hr continues for the first 48 hours.[2]

EVIDENCE-BASED PRACTICE

PROBLEM

For many years patients with acute pancreatitis have been maintained with "nothing by mouth" orders to rest the pancreas. Total parenteral nutrition is often ordered to provide adequate nutrition, yet this therapy increases the risk for complications, including infection and hyperglycemia.

QUESTION

What are the outcomes associated with early enteral feeding in acute pancreatitis?

REFERENCES

Jiang, K., Chen, X. Z., Xia, Q., Tang, W. F., & Wang, L. (2007). Early nasogastric enteral nutrition for severe acute pancreatitis: A systematic review. *World Journal of Gastroenterology, 13*(39), 5253-5260.

Marik, P. E., & Zaloga, G. P. (2004). Meta-analysis of parenteral nutrition versus enteral nutrition in patients with acute pancreatitis. *BMJ, 328,* 1407-1410.

EVIDENCE

Jiang et al reviewed the results of three randomized clinical trials that enrolled a total of 131 patients. The studies were conducted in countries outside the United States and compared enteral nutrition via nasogastric tube with traditional nutritional support, defined as total parenteral nutrition or nasojejunal enteral nutrition. No differences were noted in several outcomes, including mortality (14.9% enteral, 18.8% conventional), length of stay, complications such as sepsis and multisystem organ dysfunction, or pain associated with feeding. Diarrhea was the most common adverse effect of enteral nutrition via nasogastric tube. Although not statistically significant, mortality was lower in the enteral nutrition group, which warrants additional study, since the total number of subjects in these three studies was low.

Marik and Zaloga evaluated the results of six randomized clinical trials (total n = 263) that compared enteral nutrition with total parenteral nutrition in pancreatitis. Enteral nutrition was shown to be statistically better than parenteral nutrition on several outcomes: incidence of infection, surgical interventions to treat pancreatitis, and length of stay. No differences were noted in mortality or noninfectious complications.

IMPLICATIONS FOR NURSING

These meta-analyses show support for early enteral nutritional support in patients with acute pancreatitis. Minimal adverse effects of enteral nutrition were reported. This intervention has the potential of reducing complications.

NURSING CARE PLAN for the Patient with Acute Pancreatitis

NURSING DIAGNOSIS

Fluid volume deficit related to loss of fluid into peritoneal cavity; dehydration from nausea and vomiting; fever; nasogastric suction; and defects in coagulation

PATIENT OUTCOMES
Adequate fluid volume

- Heart rate <100 beats/min
- PAOP WNL
- Urine output >30 mL/hr
- Extremities warm and dry
- Hct and Hgb values stable
- Absence of bleeding

NURSING INTERVENTIONS	RATIONALES
• Monitor hemodynamic status closely: VS, pulmonary artery pressures, urine output, I&O, and peripheral circulation	• Assess fluid volume status
• Administer replacement of fluid, blood, or blood products; monitor response to treatment	• Maintain cardiac output and oxygen-carrying capacity
• Monitor for signs and symptoms of hemorrhage, Hct and Hgb values, Cullen's sign, and Grey Turner's sign	• Assess bleeding in retroperitoneal and abdominal cavities
• Measure abdominal girth every 4 hours	• Assess intraabdominal bleeding

NURSING DIAGNOSIS

Pain related to interruption of blood supply to the pancreas; edema and distention of the pancreas; and peritoneal irritation

PATIENT OUTCOMES

- Relief of pain

NURSING INTERVENTIONS	RATIONALES
• Perform a pain assessment, noting onset, duration, intensity, and location	• Establish baseline assessment
• Control pain with the drug of choice: (morphine) or equivalent analgesic	• Relieve pain, that may be severe
• Schedule pain medication to prevent severe pain episodes	• Provide adequate pain relief
• Differentiate pain from cardiac origin	• Release of myocardial depressant factor and a low cardiac output state increase risk of cardiac events
• Maintain bed rest restriction	• Promote comfort
• Position the patient to optimize comfort	• Relieve pain and promote comfort
• Administer sedation as needed	• Treat anxiety that may be associated with increased pain

Continued

NURSING CARE PLAN for the Patient with Acute Pancreatitis—cont'd

NURSING DIAGNOSIS

Altered nutrition (less than body requirements) related to nausea and vomiting; depressed appetite; alcoholism; and impaired nutrient metabolism and altered production of digestive enzymes

PATIENT OUTCOMES
Adequate nutrition

- Positive nitrogen balance
- Serum albumin level WNL
- Weight stable

NURSING INTERVENTIONS	RATIONALES
• Assess nutritional status through clinical examination and laboratory analysis	• Establish baseline assessment
• Calculate caloric needs and compare intake	• Maintain adequate nutrition
• Consult dietician	• Ensure nutritional support to meet needs
• Provide adequate nutritional intake	• Ensure adequate calories to meet needs
• Administer enteral or TPN as ordered; monitor complications associated with administration	• Promote adequate nutrition (see Chapter 6)

NURSING DIAGNOSIS

Impaired gas exchange related to atelectasis; pleural effusions; acute respiratory distress syndrome; fluid overload; pulmonary embolus; and splinting from pain

PATIENT OUTCOMES
Adequate gas exchange

- PaO_2 >80 mm Hg
- $PaCO_2$ WNL or at baseline
- Pulmonary complications absent or resolved

NURSING INTERVENTIONS	RATIONALES
• Administer oxygen as prescribed	• Optimize oxygenation
• Monitor SpO_2 and ABGs	• Assess adequate gas exchange
• Auscultate breath sounds every 4 hours	• Assess signs of atelectasis or fluid overload
• Monitor the respiratory rate	• Tachypnea is early sign of respiratory compromise
	• Reduce risk for atelectasis
• Administer vigorous pulmonary hygiene, coughing and deep breathing, and humidification therapy	
• Note pulmonary secretions for amount, color, consistency, and presence of an odor	• Assess for pulmonary edema and pneumonia
• Administer analgesia to prevent pain caused by splinting	• Optimize oxygenation
• Reposition the patient frequently	• Maintain normal depth of respiration and avoid atelectasis
	• Maximize ventilation and perfusion and prevent pooling of secretions

NURSING CARE PLAN	for the Patient with Acute Pancreatitis—cont'd

NURSING DIAGNOSIS

Electrolyte imbalance related to prolonged nausea and vomiting; gastric suction; disease process; and therapeutic regimen

PATIENT OUTCOMES

- Electrolyte and glucose values WNL

NURSING INTERVENTIONS	RATIONALES
• Monitor electrolytes and administer replacements according to unit protocol • Monitor blood glucose level according to unit protocol; if using tight glucose control, monitor every hour	• Assess status; ensure normal cellular environment and functions • Monitor response to treatment, prevent complications

ABG, Arterial blood gas; *GI*, gastrointestinal; *Hct*, hematocrit; *Hgb*, hemoglobin; *I&O*, intake and output; *PaCO₂*, partial pressure of carbon dioxide in arterial blood; *PaO₂*, partial pressure of oxygen in arterial blood; *PAOP*, pulmonary artery occlusion pressure; *SpO₂*, oxygen saturation via pulse oximetry; *TPN*, total parenteral nutrition; *VS*, vital signs; *WNL*, within normal limits.

Fluid replacement helps to maintain perfusion to the pancreas and kidneys, reducing the potential for complications.

Critical assessments to evaluate fluid replacement include accurate monitoring of intake and output. A decrease in urine output to less than 50 mL/hr is an early and sensitive measure of hypovolemia and hypoperfusion.[2] Vital signs including blood pressure and heart rate are also sensitive measures of volume status. Expected patient outcomes must be individualized, but reasonable goals are maintenance of systolic blood pressure at greater than 100 mm Hg without an orthostatic decrease, a mean arterial pressure of greater than 60 mm Hg, and a heart rate of less than 100 beats/min. Warm extremities indicate adequate peripheral circulation.

Patients with severe manifestations of the disease may undergo pulmonary artery pressure monitoring to evaluate fluid status and response to treatment. The pulmonary artery occlusion pressure is the most sensitive measure of adequacy of volume status and left ventricular filling pressure. A pulmonary artery occlusion pressure between 11 and 14 mm Hg is a realistic goal for most patients with this disease.

Patients with severe disease who do not respond to fluid therapy alone (i.e., hypotension continues) may need medications to support blood pressure (e.g., vasopressors). Patients with acute hemorrhagic pancreatitis may also need packed RBCs in addition to fluid therapy to restore intravascular volume.

Electrolyte Replacement

Hypocalcemia (serum calcium level <8.5 mg/dL) is a common electrolyte imbalance. It is associated with a high mortality rate. Calcium is essential for catalyzing impulses for nerves and muscles, for maintaining the integrity of cell membranes and vessels, for normal clotting of blood, and for strengthening bones and teeth. Calcium is also essential for increasing contractility in the heart. A sign of hypocalcemia on the electrocardiogram is lengthening of the QT interval. Severe hypocalcemia (serum calcium level <6 mg/dL) may cause tetany, seizures, positive Chvostek's and Trousseau's signs, and respiratory distress. Patients with severe hypocalcemia should be placed on seizure precaution status, and respiratory support equipment should be available (e.g., oral airway, suction). The nurse is responsible for monitoring calcium levels, administering replacement, and monitoring the patient's response to any calcium given. Monitoring serum albumin levels is also important because true serum calcium levels can be evaluated only in comparison with serum albumin levels. The patient is also monitored for calcium toxicity. Symptoms include lethargy, nausea, shortening of the QT interval, and decreased excitability of nerves and muscles. Hypomagnesemia may also be present in hypocalcemia, and magnesium replacement may be required.

Potassium is another electrolyte that may need to be replaced early in the treatment regimen. Hypokalemia is associated with cardiac dysrhythmias, muscle weakness, hypotension, decreased bowel sounds, ileus, and irritability. Potassium must be diluted and administered via an infusion pump per unit protocol.

Hyperglycemia is not a common complication of acute pancreatitis because most of the pancreatic gland must be necrosed before the insulin-secreting islet cells are affected. More commonly, hyperglycemia is a result of the normal body stress response to acute illness.

Nutrition Support

Nasogastric suction and "nothing by mouth" status are classic treatment for patients with acute pancreatitis to suppress pancreatic exocrine secretion by preventing the release of secretin from the duodenum. Normally, secretin, which stimulates pancreatic secretion production, is stimulated when acid is in the duodenum; therefore, nasogastric suction has been a primary treatment. Nausea, vomiting, and abdominal pain may also be decreased with early nasogastric suctioning. A nasogastric tube is also necessary in patients with ileus, severe gastric distention, and a decreased level of consciousness to prevent complications resulting from pulmonary aspiration.

Early nutritional support may be ordered. Enteral nutrition prevents atrophy of gut lymphoid tissue, bacterial overgrowth in the intestine, and increased intestinal permeability.[23] Immediate oral feeding in patients with mild acute pancreatitis is safe and may accelerate recovery.[6] Systematic reviews of early enteral nutrition for severe acute pancreatitis was done to evaluate its effectiveness and safety.[18,23] Early enteral nutrition appears effective and safe (see Evidence Based Practice).

Comfort Management

Pain control is a nursing priority in patients with acute pancreatitis not only because the disorder produces extreme patient discomfort, but also because pain increases the patient's metabolism and thus increases pancreatic secretions. The pain of pancreatitis is caused by edema and distention of the pancreatic capsule, obstruction of the biliary system, and peritoneal inflammation from pancreatic enzymes. Pain is often severe and unrelenting and is related to the degree of pancreatic inflammation.

A baseline pain assessment is performed early after the patient's admission and includes information about the onset, intensity, duration, and location (local or diffuse) of the pain. Analgesic administration is a nursing priority. Adequate pain control requires the use of IV opiates, usually in the form of a patient-controlled analgesia pump (PCA). Opiate analgesics (e.g., morphine) may cause spasm of the sphincter of Oddi and may exacerbate pain; however, some researchers question whether morphine should be avoided. Meperidine (Demerol) may be ordered in place of morphine if pancreatitis occurs secondary to gallbladder disease.[16] In the case in which a PCA pump is not ordered, pain medications are administered on a routine schedule, rather than as needed, to prevent uncontrollable abdominal pain. Insertion of a nasogastric tube connected to low intermittent suction may help ease pain. Patient positioning may also relieve some of the discomfort and should be facilitated by the nurse as the patient's hemodynamic status allows.

Pharmacological Intervention

Various pharmacological therapies have been researched in the treatment of acute pancreatitis. Drugs given to rest the pancreas have been studied, specifically anticholinergics, glucagon, somatostatin, cimetidine, and calcitonin, but these have not been shown to be effective. Prevention of stress ulcers is achieved through the use of histamine blockers and antacids.

Antibiotics have also been studied in the treatment of inflammation of the pancreas with the idea of preventing pancreatic pseudocysts or abscesses. It is not known whether antibiotics improve survival or merely prevent septic complications.[22] The role of prophylactic systemic antibiotics in acute pancreatitis is unsettled since studies evaluating the benefits and harms have produced disparate results.[15]

Treatment of Systemic Complications

Multisystemic complications of acute pancreatitis are related to the ability of the pancreas to produce many vasoactive substances that affect organs throughout the body. These complications are summarized in Box 17-9.

Pulmonary complications are common in patients with both mild and severe manifestations of the disease. Arterial hypoxemia, atelectasis, pleural effusions, and pneumonia have been identified in many patients with acute pancreatitis. Accumulation of fluid in the peritoneum causes restricted movement of the diaphragm. Arterial oxygen saturation is continuously monitored, and arterial blood gases are assessed as needed. Treatment of hypoxemia includes supplemental oxygen and vigorous pulmonary hygiene, such as deep breathing, coughing, and frequent position changes. Some patients may need intubation to ensure adequate ventilation; others can be maintained with noninvasive ventilation modes. Pulmonary emboli have also been documented as a complication of acute pancreatitis. Careful fluid administration is necessary to prevent fluid overload and pulmonary congestion. Patients with severe disease may develop acute respiratory failure.

Close monitoring and management of other systemic complications of acute pancreatitis, such as coagulation abnormalities and hemorrhage, cardiovascular failure and dysrhythmias, and acute renal failure, are also important. Coagulation defects in acute pancreatitis are associated with a high mortality rate, are similar to disseminated intravascular coagulation, and are treated in the same way. The cardiac depression associated with acute pancreatitis may vary, but hypovolemic shock is a grave presentation. Astute cardiovascular monitoring and volume replacement are required to reverse this serious complication. Impaired renal function has been documented in many patients.

GI complications of acute pancreatitis include pancreatic pseudocyst and abdominal abscess. A pseudocyst should be suspected in any patient who has persistent abdominal pain and nausea and vomiting, a prolonged fever, and an elevated serum amylase level. CT can be helpful in diagnosing the location and size of the pseudocyst. Signs and symptoms of an abdominal abscess include an increased WBC count, fever, abdominal pain, and vomiting. CT provides a definitive diagnosis. Early recognition and treatment of a pancreatic pseudocyst are important because this condition is associated with a high mortality rate.

Surgical Therapy

Pancreatic resection for acute necrotizing pancreatitis may be performed to prevent systemic complications of the disease process. In this procedure, dead or infected pancreatic tissue is surgically removed while preserving most of the gland.[22] A variety of surgical treatment modalities are currently in use, with the advantages leaning toward those performed by laparoscopic techniques.[2] The indication for surgical intervention is clinical deterioration of the patient despite the use of conventional treatments, or the presence of peritonitis.

Surgery may also be indicated for pseudocysts; however, surgery is usually delayed because some pseudocysts resolve spontaneously. Surgical treatment of a pseudocyst can be performed through internal or external drainage, or needle aspiration. Acute surgical intervention may be required if the pseudocyst becomes infected or perforated.

Surgery may also be performed when gallstones are thought to be the cause of the acute pancreatitis. A cholecystectomy is usually performed.

Patient Outcomes

Expected outcomes for the patient with acute pancreatitis are found in the Nursing Care Plan for the Patient with Acute Pancreatitis.

HEPATIC FAILURE

Pathophysiology

Hepatic (liver) failure results when the liver is unable to perform its many functions. These functions are reviewed in Box 17-2. Liver failure results from necrosis or a decrease in the blood supply to liver cells. This problem is most often caused by hepatitis or inflammation of the liver. Liver failure also results from chronic liver disease, in which healthy liver tissue is replaced by fibrotic tissue.[24] This form of liver failure is called *cirrhosis*. Finally, liver cells can be replaced by fatty cells or tissue and is known as *fatty liver disease*.

Hepatitis

Hepatitis is an acute inflammation of liver cells *(hepatocytes)*. Other cells in the liver may also be inflamed. This inflammation is accompanied by edema, and early in the course of the disease, no disturbance exists in the architecture of the liver. The normal liver architecture is pictured in Figure 17-5 and is characterized by a basic functional unit of the liver called a lobule. The liver lobule is uniquely made in that it has its own blood supply, which allows the liver cells to be exposed continuously to blood. As the inflammation progresses, the normal pattern of the liver is disturbed by the inflammatory process. This interrupts the normal blood supply to liver cells, causing necrosis and breakdown of healthy cells. Blood backs up in the portal system, causing increased pressure, known as portal hypertension. Liver cells have the capacity to regenerate. Over time, liver cells that become damaged are removed by the body's immune system and are replaced with healthy liver cells. Therefore, most patients with hepatitis recover and regain normal liver function.

Hepatitis is most often caused by a viral disease. Several hepatitis viruses have been identified: hepatitis A, B, C, D, E, and G. Researchers continue to study other viruses that may be associated with acute hepatitis. Modes of transmission are summarized in Box 17-13. Characteristics of hepatitis in terms of type, route of transmission, severity, and prophylaxis are presented in Table 17-8.

Assessment. Patients with hepatitis are often asymptomatic. In many patients, prodromal symptoms of anorexia, nausea, vomiting, abdominal pain, and fatigue may be present. Symptoms then progress to a low-grade fever, an enlarged and tender liver, and jaundice (see Clinical Alert for Signs and Symptoms of Fulminant Hepatic Failure).[4]

Assessment of risk factors often assists in the diagnosis of hepatitis. Laboratory tests show elevated liver function tests. The diagnosis is confirmed by identifying antibodies specific to each type of hepatitis. Recovery from acute hepatitis usually occurs within 9 weeks for hepatitis A, and 16 weeks for hepatitis B. Hepatitis B, C, D, and G may progress to chronic forms.[13]

Nursing Diagnoses. Many nursing diagnoses are associated with viral hepatitis. These include activity intolerance related to fatigue, fever, and flulike symptoms; altered nutrition (less than body requirements) related to loss of appetite, nausea, vomiting, and loss of liver metabolic functions; risk for infection related to loss of liver cell function for phagocytosis of bacteria; and risk for altered thought processes related to medications that require liver metabolism.

Medical and Nursing Interventions. No definitive treatment for acute inflammation of the liver exists. Goals for medical and nursing care include providing rest and assisting the patient in obtaining optimal nutrition. Most patients are cared for at home unless the disease becomes prolonged or fulminant failure develops. Medications to help the patient rest or to decrease agitation must be closely monitored because most of these drugs require clearance by the liver, which is impaired during the acute phase.

Maintenance of the nutritional status of the patient is a nursing priority. Loss of appetite, nausea, and vomiting may persist for weeks. Nursing measures such as administration of antiemetics may be helpful. Small, frequent, palatable meals and supplements should be offered. Evaluation of nutritional status is ongoing and includes assessments of intake and output, daily weights, serum albumin level, and nitrogen balance. Patients must be instructed not to take any over-the-counter drugs that can cause liver damage. Box 17-14 lists common hepatotoxic drugs. Alcohol should be avoided.

BOX 17-13 Modes of Transmission for Hepatitis

- Contact with blood
- Contact with blood products
- Contact with semen
- Contact with saliva
- Percutaneously through mucous membranes
- Direct contact with infected fluids or objects

CLINICAL ALERT

Signs and Symptoms of Fulminant Hepatic Failure[9]

- Hyperexcitability
- Insomnia
- Irritability
- Decreased level of consciousness, coma
- Convulsions
- Sudden onset of high fever
- Nausea and vomiting
- Chills
- Jaundice

TABLE 17-8 Characteristics of Hepatitis

Type	Route of Transmission	Severity	Prophylaxis
Hepatitis A	Fecal-oral, parenteral, sexual	Mild	Hygiene, immune serum globulin, HAV vaccine, Twinrix*
Hepatitis B	Parenteral, sexual	Severe, may be prolonged or chronic	Hygiene, HBV vaccine, Twinrix*
Hepatitis C	Parenteral	Mild to severe	Hygiene, screening blood, interferon-alpha
Hepatitis D	Parenteral, fecal-oral, sexual	Severe	Hygiene, HBV vaccine
Hepatitis E	Fecal-oral	Severe in pregnant women	Hygiene, safe water
Hepatitis G	Parenteral, sexual	Unknown	Unknown

*A bivalent vaccine containing the antigenic components, a sterile suspension of inactivated hepatitis A virus combined with purified surface antigen of the hepatitis B virus.[27]

HAV, Hepatitis A virus; *HBV*, hepatitis B virus.

Adapted from Huether, S. E. (2006). Alterations of digestive function. In K. L. McCance, & S. E. Huether (Eds.), *Pathophysiology: The biologic basis for disease in adults and children* (p. 1420). St. Louis: Mosby.

TRANSPLANTATION Liver

INDICATIONS

Liver transplantation is the standard care of treatment for patients with progressive, irreversible acute or chronic liver disease for which there are no other medical or surgical options. The leading indication for liver transplantation is hepatitis C. As of January 2008, 17,143 patients were waiting for a liver transplant in the United States. Although the number of liver transplants increases each year with 5398 performed in 2007, 1299 patients died while waiting. The survival rate continues to increase, with 85% survival at 1 year, 78% survival at 3 years, and 72% survival at 5 years.[3]

CRITERIA FOR TRANSPLANT RECIPIENTS

Because of the shortage of available organs, selection of appropriate patients is vital and timing of when to list the patient is paramount. Patients must not be so ill that they would not survive the surgery, but must be experiencing deterioration in quality of life. Other contraindications for liver transplantation include metastatic malignancies, active drug or alcohol abuse, advanced cardiopulmonary disease, and acquired immunodeficiency syndrome (AIDS). Once listed, a patient receives a MELD (Model for End-stage Liver Disease) score that prioritizes patients based on the medical urgency of needing a transplantation, with the goal of decreasing the number of deaths of patients awaiting liver transplantation. The MELD score is calculated by using the serum creatinine and serum bilirubin levels and the international normalized ratio. Since the implementation of MELD in 2002, there has been a reduction in waiting time and in waiting list mortality.[2]

CRITERIA FOR DONORS

Donors are carefully screened for blood type, body size, infectious diseases, and metastatic carcinomas, as the latter two disorders can be transmitted to the recipient. Donor liver criteria have expanded to include older donors, livers infected with hepatitis B virus or hepatitis C virus, fatty livers, and livers from donors with a history of cancer. Other efforts to increase the number of liver transplant recipients include reduced-size liver transplants (left lobe of liver transplanted to a recipient), split-liver transplantation (one liver divided between an adult and a child), and living liver donation.

PATIENT MANAGEMENT

The immune system is programmed to recognize a transplanted organ as foreign, and therefore the immune system must be inhibited after organ transplantation (see Chapter 16). Maintenance therapy consists of medications that inhibit T-cell proliferation and differentiation, deplete lymphocytes, and inhibit macrophages. Immunosuppressive medications consist of triple therapy—a calcineurin inhibitor (tacrolimus [Prograf] or cyclosporine [Neoral]), a corticosteroid (prednisone), and mycophenolate mofetil (CellCept) or azathioprine (Imuran). Immunosuppressive regimens are individualized to each patient. Complications associated with immunosuppressive therapy include nephrotoxicity, hypertension, hyperlipidemia, bone loss, new-onset diabetes mellitus, and increased risk of infection.

COMPLICATIONS

Postoperative complications include bleeding, renal failure, infection, pleural effusions, biliary leaks, biliary obstruction, and fluid and electrolyte imbalances. Infection is the leading cause of death in the liver transplant patient. Infections with cytomegalovirus, Epstein-Barr virus, *Pneumocystis carinii*, and *Aspergillus* are often seen 1 to 6 months after transplantation. However, after 6 months, the rate of infection is the same as that for the general population unless the patient requires high doses of immunosuppressive medications.

PREVENTING REJECTION

Rejection after liver transplantation is the result of the patient's immune system response to the donor liver. Compliance with immunosuppressive medication is essential to avoid or decrease the incidence of rejection episodes. Hyperacute rejection occurs within minutes or hours of transplantation and is caused by humoral or antibody-mediated B-cell production against the transplanted organ. Acute rejection occurs days to 3 months after transplantation and involves the activation and proliferation of T cells with destruction of liver tissue. Acute rejection accounts for about 40% of all rejection episodes.[1] Chronic rejection occurs months to years after transplantation and may lead to the need for retransplantation.

Rejection is suspected with a rise in serum levels of aspartate aminotransferase (AST), alanine aminotransferase (ALT), and bilirubin and warrants a liver biopsy. The Banff scale (indeterminate, grade I, grade II, and grade III [severe]) is used for grading acute cellular rejection. Elevated liver AST, ALT, and bilirubin levels are often the first sign of rejection and can be easily monitored with routine blood studies before physical symptoms develop. Most rejection is reversible if diagnosed and treated early, so patient compliance with scheduled laboratory testing is important. Signs and symptoms of rejection include fatigue, fever, tenderness or pain over the liver, dark urine, yellow eyes, yellow skin, ascites, and itching. Management of acute rejection includes increasing the dosages of current immunosuppressive medications.

Continued

TRANSPLANTATION—cont'd

REFERENCES

1. Bufton, S., Emmett, K., & Byerly, A. M. (2008). Liver transplantation. In L. Ohler, & S. Cupples (Eds.), *Core curriculum for transplant nurses*. St. Louis: Mosby.

2. Said, A., Einstein, M., & Lucey, M. R. (2007). Liver transplantation: An update 2007. *Current Opinion in Gastroenterology, 23*(3), 292-298.

3. United Network for Organ Sharing (UNOS). Retrieved August 8, 2008, from www.unos.org.

BOX 17-14   Common Hepatotoxic Drugs

Analgesics
- Acetaminophen (Tylenol)
- Salicylates (aspirin)

Anesthetics
- Enflurane (Ethrane)
- Halothane (Fluothane)
- Methoxyflurane (Penthrane)

Anticonvulsants
- Phenytoin (Dilantin)
- Phenobarbital (Luminal)

Antidepressants
- Monoamine oxidase inhibitors
- Amitriptyline (Elavil)
- Doxepin (Sinequan)

Antimicrobial Agents
- Isoniazid
- Nitrofurantoin (Macrodantin)
- Rifampin
- Sulfonamides (sulfisoxazole acetyl [Gantrisin], silver sulfadiazine [Silvadene])
- Tetracycline

Antipsychotic Drugs
- Haloperidol (Haldol)
- Chlorpromazine (Thorazine)
- Fluphenazine (Prolixin)
- Prochlorperazine (Compazine)
- Promethazine (Phenergan)
- Thioridazine (Mellaril)

Cardiovascular Drugs
- Methyldopa (Aldomet)
- Quinidine sulfate

Hormonal Agents
- Antithyroid drugs
- Oral contraceptives
- Oral hypoglycemics (tolbutamide [Orinase], chlorpropamide [Diabinese])

Sedatives
- Chlordiazepoxide (Librium)
- Diazepam (Valium)

Others
- Cimetidine (Tagamet)

Hepatitis can lead to acute hepatic failure. The clinical manifestations of this disorder are discussed in the sections on impaired metabolic processes and impaired bile formation and flow.

Special precautions must be taken to prevent spread of the virus when caring for the patient with hepatitis. These include the *universal precautions* while handling all items that are contaminated with the patient's body secretions, including patient care items such as thermometers, dishes, and eating utensils.

Several patient outcomes are expected after nursing and medical interventions. These include absence of pain, adequate nutrition, activity tolerance, absence of infection, and resolving/normal laboratory tests.

Cirrhosis

Cirrhosis causes severe alterations in the structure and function of liver cells. It is characterized by inflammation and liver cell necrosis that may be focal or diffuse. Fat deposits may also be present. The enlarged liver cells cause compression of the liver lobule and lead to increased resistance to blood flow and portal hypertension. Necrosis is followed by regeneration of liver tissue, but not in a normal fashion. Fibrous tissue is laid down over time, and this distorts the normal architecture of the liver lobule. These fibrotic changes are usually irreversible, resulting in chronic liver dysfunction. Table 17-9 characterizes the types of cirrhosis.

Fatty Liver

Fatty liver is an accumulation of excessive fats in the liver; it is morphologically distinguishable from cirrhosis. Alcohol abuse is the most common cause of this disorder. Other causes include obesity, diabetes, hepatic resection, starvation, and total parenteral nutrition. Damage caused by the fat deposits may result in liver dysfunction, failure, and death.

Assessment of Hepatic Failure

Presenting Clinical Signs

Initial clinical signs of hepatic failure are vague and include weakness, fatigue, loss of appetite, weight loss, abdominal discomfort, nausea and vomiting, and change in bowel habits. As destruction in the liver progresses, the systemic effects of the disease become apparent. Impaired liver function results in loss of the normal vascular, secretory, and metabolic functions of the liver (see Box 17-2). The functional sequelae of liver disease are divided into three categories: (1) portal hypertension, (2) impaired liver metabolic processes, and (3) impaired bile formation and flow. These derangements and their clinical manifestations are summarized in Box 17-15.

Portal Hypertension. Portal hypertension causes two main clinical problems for the patient: hyperdynamic circulation and development of esophageal or gastric varices. Liver cell destruction causes shunting of blood and increased cardiac output. Vasodilation is also present, which causes decreased perfusion to all body organs, even though the cardiac output is very

TABLE 17-9 Characteristics of Types of Cirrhosis

Type	Cause	Consequences	Sequelae
Alcoholic (Laënnec's)	Long-term alcohol abuse	Fatty liver Fibrotic tissue replaces liver cells	Acetaldehyde, a toxic metabolite of alcohol ingestion, causes liver cell damage and death
Biliary	Long-term obstruction of bile ducts	Decrease in bile flow	Degeneration and fibrosis of the ducts
Cardiac	Severe long-term right-sided heart failure	Decreased oxygenation of liver cells	Cellular death
Postnecrotic	Exposure to hepatotoxins, chemicals, infection, or metabolic disorder	Massive death of liver cells	Development of liver cancer

BOX 17-15 Clinical Signs and Symptoms of Liver Disease

Cardiac
- Hyperdynamic circulation
- Portal hypertension
- Dysrhythmias
- Activity intolerance
- Edema

Dermatological
- Jaundice
- Spider angiomas
- Pruritus

Electrolytes
- Hypokalemia
- Hyponatremia (dilutional)
- Hypernatremia

Endocrine
- Increased aldosterone
- Increased antidiuretic hormone

Fluid Alterations
- Ascites
- Water retention
- Decreased volume in vascular space

Gastrointestinal
- Abdominal discomfort
- Decreased appetite
- Diarrhea
- Varices or gastrointestinal bleeding
- Malnutrition
- Nausea and vomiting

Hematological
- Anemia
- Impaired coagulation
- Disseminated intravascular coagulation

Immune System
- Increased susceptibility to infection

Neurological
- Hepatic encephalopathy

Pulmonary
- Dyspnea
- Hyperventilation
- Hypoxemia
- Ineffective breathing patterns

Renal
- Hepatorenal syndrome

high. This phenomenon is known as *high-output failure* or *hyperdynamic circulation*. Clinical signs and symptoms are those of heart failure and include jugular vein distention, pulmonary crackles, and decreased perfusion to all organs. Initially, the patient may have hypertension, flushed skin, and bounding pulses. Blood pressure decreases and dysrhythmias are common. Increased portal venous pressure causes the formation of varices that shunt blood to decrease pressure. These varices are problematic because they can cause massive upper GI bleeding (see the earlier discussion of upper GI bleeding). The most common sites are in the esophageal and gastric areas. Splenomegaly is also associated with portal hypertension.

Impaired Metabolic Processes. The liver is the most complex organ because of all of its metabolic processes. Liver failure causes the following: altered carbohydrate, fat, and protein metabolism; decreased synthesis of blood clotting factors; decreased removal of activated clotting components; decreased metabolism of vitamins and iron; decreased storage functions; and decreased detoxification functions.

Altered carbohydrate metabolism may result in unstable blood glucose levels. The serum glucose level is usually increased to more than 200 mg/dL. This condition is termed *cirrhotic diabetes*. Altered carbohydrate metabolism may also result in malnutrition and a decreased stress response.

Altered fat metabolism may result in a fatty liver. Fat is used by all cells for energy, and altered metabolism may cause fatigue and decreased activity tolerance in many patients. Alterations in skin integrity, which are common in chronic liver disease, are also thought to be related to this metabolic dysfunction. Bile salts are also not adequately produced, and this leads to an inability of fats to be metabolized by the small intestine. Malnutrition often results.

Protein metabolism, albumin synthesis, and serum albumin levels are decreased. Albumin is necessary for colloid oncotic pressure to hold fluid in the intravascular space and for nutrition. Low albumin levels are also thought to be associated with the development of ascites, a complication of hepatic failure. Globulin is another protein that is essential for the transport of substances in the blood. Fibrinogen is an essential protein that is necessary for normal clotting. A low plasma fibrinogen level, coupled with decreased synthesis of many blood clotting factors, predisposes the patient to bleeding. Clinical signs and symptoms range from bruising and nasal and gingival bleeding to frank hemorrhage. Disseminated intravascular coagulation may also develop.

Kupffer's cells in the liver play an important role in fighting infections throughout the body. Loss of this function predisposes the patient to severe infections, particularly gram-negative sepsis.

The liver also removes activated clotting factors from the general circulation to prevent widespread clotting in the system. Loss of this function predisposes the patient to clot formation, and complications such as pulmonary embolus.

Decreased metabolism and storage of vitamins A, B_{12}, and D, and of iron, glucose, and fat predispose the patient to many nutritional deficiencies. The liver loses a well-known function of detoxifying drugs, ammonia, and hormones. Loss of ammonia conversion to urea in the liver is responsible for many of the altered thought processes seen in liver failure, because ammonia is allowed to enter the central nervous system directly. These alterations range from minor sensory perceptual changes, such as tremors, slurred speech, and impaired decision making, to dramatic confusion or profound coma.

Hormonal imbalances are common in liver disease. The most important physiological imbalance is the activation of aldosterone and antidiuretic hormone, which contribute to some of the fluid and electrolyte disturbances commonly found in liver disease. Sodium and water retention and portal hypertension lead to a third spacing of fluid from the intravascular space into the peritoneal cavity (ascites). The resultant decrease in plasma volume causes activation of compensatory mechanisms in the body to release antidiuretic hormone and aldosterone. This situation causes further water and sodium retention. The renin-angiotensin system is also activated, which causes systemic vasoconstriction. The kidneys are most severely affected, and urine output decreases because of impaired perfusion. Sexual dysfunction is common in patients with liver disease, and this can lead to self-concept alterations. Dermatological lesions that occur in some patients with liver failure, called *spider angiomas*, are thought to be related to an endocrine imbalance. These vascular lesions may be venous or arterial and represent the progression of liver disease.

Impaired Bile Formation and Flow. The liver's inability to metabolize bile is reflected clinically in an increased serum bilirubin level and a staining of tissue by bilirubin, or jaundice. Jaundice is generally present in patients with a serum bilirubin level greater than 3 mg/dL.

Nursing Diagnoses

The nursing diagnoses, actual and potential, can be derived from assessment data in a patient with liver failure. See Nursing Care Plan for the Patient with Hepatic Failure.

NURSING CARE PLAN for the Patient with Hepatic Failure

NURSING DIAGNOSIS

Fluid volume deficit related to variceal hemorrhage; third spacing of peritoneal fluid (ascites); and coagulation abnormalities

PATIENT OUTCOMES
Adequate fluid volume

- Absence or resolution of bleeding
- Hct, Hgb, coagulation factors, protein, albumin values WNL
- Normal VS

NURSING INTERVENTIONS	RATIONALES
- See Nursing Care Plan for the Patient with Acute Gastrointestinal Bleeding - Monitor blood counts and coagulation function test results - Protect the patient from injury - Pad side rails and assist with activities of daily living - Monitor for petechiae and bleeding from the IV site and mucous membranes - Limit punctures for blood draws and IV lines - Guaiac specimens - Administer fluid and blood products as ordered, and monitor patient response - Administer vitamin K and other coagulation products	 - Assess for active bleeding and risk for bleeding from altered liver function - Volume deficits may cause lightheadedness and dizziness from poor perfusion to the brain - Protect from injury - Assess for bleeding - Reduce risk of infection and bleeding from puncture sites - Assess for occult bleeding - Maintain fluid and blood volume - Promote normal coagulation

NURSING DIAGNOSIS

Altered nutrition (less than body requirements) related to altered liver metabolism of food nutrients; insufficient intake; impaired absorption of fat-soluble vitamins; and vitamin B_{12} deficiency

PATIENT OUTCOMES
Adequate nutrition

- Protein intake sufficient for liver regeneration
- BUN level WNL
- Liver function tests results WNL
- Serum albumin level WNL

Continued

NURSING CARE PLAN   for the Patient with Hepatic Failure—cont'd

NURSING INTERVENTIONS	RATIONALES
• Limit protein intake	• Reduce level of ammonia from inadequate protein metabolism
• Monitor serum BUN level	• Determine fluid volume status
• Administer vitamins synthesized by the liver: A, B, D, and K	• Replace essential vitamins
• Monitor nutritional status through serum albumin level and nitrogen balance	• Assess nutritional status
• Consider enteral feeding or TPN if oral intake is insufficient	• Promote normal nutritional status

NURSING DIAGNOSIS

Ineffective breathing pattern and impaired gas exchange related to dyspnea from ascites; and increased risk of pulmonary infections

PATIENT OUTCOMES
Effective breathing

• Effective lung expansion
• Dyspnea absent
• ABGs WNL

NURSING INTERVENTIONS	RATIONALES
• Administer oxygen as ordered according to clinical assessment	• Optimize oxygenation
• Monitor the patient's respiratory status	• Assess deteriorating pulmonary status
• Monitor ABGs for increasing $PaCO_2$ and decreasing PaO_2	• Recognize poor ventilatory efforts; guide treatment
• Encourage the patient to cough and deep breathe	• Mobilize pulmonary secretions, and reduce the risk of pulmonary compromise
• Administer sedatives and analgesics cautiously so as not to impair respiratory effort	• Drugs may not be cleared well when liver function is less than optimal
• Measure abdominal girth every 4 hours	• Assess ascites
• Monitor and restrict fluids and sodium, and administer diuretics as ordered	• Assess and manage ascites
• Assist with paracentesis as needed	• Relieve ascites

NURSING DIAGNOSIS

Altered thought processes related to impaired handling of ammonia; medications that require liver metabolism; and decreased perfusion states

PATIENT OUTCOMES
Normal thought processes

• Hepatic encephalopathy absent or resolved
• BUN level stable

NURSING CARE PLAN for the Patient with Hepatic Failure—cont'd

NURSING INTERVENTIONS	RATIONALES
• Monitor ammonia levels and conduct ongoing neurological assessments	• The neurological assessment slowly returns to normal as ammonia levels return to normal
• Administer lactulose and neomycin, and monitor results	• Reduces ammonia levels
• Restrict protein intake	• Ammonia is a byproduct of protein metabolism
• Reduce the risk of GI bleeding through antacid and H_2-histamine blocker administration	• Prevent bleeding and associated increase in ammonia levels
• Use sedatives and narcotics judiciously	• Drug metabolism is impaired in liver failure
• Prevent and treat infection, dehydration, and electrolyte or acid-base disturbances	• Reduce complications
• Reorient the patient and provide for safety during periods of impaired mentation	• High ammonia levels cause disorientation

ABG, Arterial blood gas; *BUN*, blood urea nitrogen; *GI*, gastrointestinal; *Hct*, hematocrit; *Hgb*, hemoglobin; *I&O*, intake and output; *IV*, intravenous; *PaCO₂*, partial pressure of carbon dioxide in arterial blood; *PaO₂*, partial pressure of oxygen in arterial blood; *TPN*, total parenteral nutrition; *VS*, vital signs; *WNL*, within normal limits.

Medical and Nursing Interventions

Nursing and medical management of the patient with liver failure is aimed at supportive therapies and early recognition and treatment of complications associated with the disease process. Management of acute liver failure challenges the best skills of physicians, intensivists, and nurses.[13]

Diagnostic Tests

Altered laboratory results in patients with liver disease (see Laboratory Alerts: Liver Failure) are a direct result of destruction of hepatic cells (liver enzymes) or of the effects of impaired liver metabolic processes.

Parenchymal tests such as liver biopsy can be performed to study the liver cell architecture directly. The liver is characteristically small and has a marked decrease in functioning hepatic cell structures. This characteristic allows for a definitive diagnosis of the cause of the hepatic failure. An ultrasound study may detect impaired bile flow.

Supportive Therapy

Hemodynamic instability and decreased perfusion to core organs are the end result of portal hypertension and hyperdynamic circulation. Invasive monitoring may be used in the critically ill patient, but it must be weighed in terms of the potential for infection in a patient with an impaired immune response. Administration of vasoactive drugs and fluids may be ordered to support blood pressure and kidney perfusion, which requires close monitoring by the nurse. Portal hypertension also predisposes the patient to esophageal and gastric varices, which have the potential to bleed.

LABORATORY ALERTS

Liver Failure[5]

Serum or Plasma	Alteration
Albumin	↓
Ammonia	↑
Bile Pigments	
Total bilirubin	↑
Direct or conjugated bilirubin	↑
Cholesterol	↑
Coagulation Tests	
Prothrombin time	Prolonged
Partial thromboplastin time	Prolonged
Enzymes	
APT	↑
AST	↑
ALT	↑
Urine	
Bilirubin	↑
Urobilinogen	↑

↑, Increased; ↓, decreased; *ALT*, alanine transaminase; *APT*, alkaline phosphatase; *AST*, aspartate transaminase.
From Chernecky, C. C., & Berger, B. J. (2008). *Laboratory tests and diagnostic procedures* (5th ed.). Philadelphia: Saunders.

Hypoglycemia is common in liver failure. It is caused by depletion of hepatic glycogen stores and loss of ability for gluconeogenesis.[13] Fingerstick glucose measurements are assessed routinely.

The patient with liver failure is at risk for bleeding complications because of decreased synthesis of clotting factors. Patients with a prolonged prothrombin time and partial thromboplastin time and a decreased platelet count should be protected from injury through the use of padded side rails and assistance with all activity. Needle sticks should be kept to a minimum. Blood products may be ordered in severe cases. Antacids, proton pump inhibitors or H_2-blockers are ordered to prevent gastritis and bleeding from stress ulcers.

Administration of all drugs metabolized by the liver must be restricted. The administration of such drugs could cause acute liver failure in a patient with chronic disease.

Support for the Failing Liver

Advances have been made in the development of artificial support of liver function, spurred on by the shortage of donor organs and the high incidence of mortality related to acute or chronic liver failure.[13] Bioartificial liver devices serve as a bridge to liver transplantation or support liver function long enough to allow regeneration of normal liver function.[20] The bioartificial liver circulates the individual's blood around the outside of a system of hollow fibers packed with pig hepatocytes to allow toxins to be removed and nutrients to be replaced.[12]

Another type of support is the Molecular Adsorbents Recirculating System (MARS), an extracorporeal albumin dialysis technique that uses an albumin-impregnated membrane to remove both protein-bound and water-soluble toxins from the blood.[13] Cytokines are believed to play an important role in acute-on-chronic liver failure. Cytokines are cleared from plasma by both MARS and another system, the Fractionated Plasma Separation, Adsorption and Dialysis (Prometheus).[26] However, at present, neither of these treatments is able to change serum cytokine levels.

Treatment of Complications

Ascites. Impaired handling of salt and water by the kidneys and other abnormalities in fluid homeostasis predispose the patient to an accumulation of fluid in the peritoneum, or *ascites*. Ascites is problematic because as more fluid is retained, it pushes up on the diaphragm, thereby impairing the patient's breathing pattern. Nursing assessment of respiratory status through respiratory rate, breath sounds, and arterial blood gas monitoring is critical. Frequent monitoring of abdominal girth alerts the nurse to fluid accumula-

tion. Abdominal girth should be measured at the level of the umbilicus. Positioning the patient in a semi-Fowler's position also allows for free diaphragm movement. Frequent deep-breathing and coughing exercises and changes in position are important to facilitate full/optimal breathing. Some patients may require elective intubation until medical management of the ascites is accomplished. The physiological effects of an increasing abdominal compartment are noted in Box 17-16 and are referred to as *abdominal compartment syndrome*.

Ascites is medically managed through bed rest, a low-sodium diet, fluid restriction, and diuretic therapy. Diuretics must be administered cautiously, however, because if the intravascular volume is depleted too quickly, acute renal failure may be induced. Close monitoring of the serum creatinine level, the BUN level, and urine output is important for the early detection of renal impairment. Careful monitoring of electrolyte balance, particularly serum potassium and sodium levels, is also important when diuretics are administered.

Paracentesis is another medical therapy for ascites, in which ascitic fluid is withdrawn through percutaneous needle aspiration. Close monitoring of vital signs during this procedure is necessary, especially as fluid is withdrawn. Major complications include

---

BOX 17-16   Physiological Effects of Abdominal Compartment Syndrome

Cardiovascular
- Decreased venous return
- Increased systemic vascular resistance and intrathoracic pressure
- Reduction in cardiac output

Respiratory
- Atelectasis
- Pneumonia
- Impaired ventilation
- Respiratory failure

Hepatic and Renal
- Decreased blood flow to liver and kidney
- Functional impairment of both organs

Gastrointestinal
- Impaired lymphatic, venous, and arterial flow
- Poor healing of anastomoses

Neurological
- Simultaneous increased intracranial pressure from both head trauma and intraabdominal hypertension

sudden loss of intravascular pressure (decreased blood pressure) and tachycardia. To prevent these complications, 1 to 2 L of fluid is generally withdrawn at one time. The amount, color, and character of peritoneal fluid obtained is documented. Often, a specimen of the fluid is sent to the laboratory for analysis. The patient's abdominal girth should be measured before and after the procedure. Albumin may be administered to increase colloid osmotic pressure and to decrease loss of fluid into the peritoneal cavity.

Peritoneovenous shunting is a surgical procedure used to relieve ascites that is resistant to other therapies. The LeVeen shunt is inserted by placing the distal end of a tube in the peritoneum and tunneling the other end under the skin into the jugular vein or superior vena cava. A valve that opens and closes according to pressure gradients allows ascitic fluid to flow into the superior vena cava. The patient's breathing normally triggers the valve. During inspiration, pressure increases in the peritoneum and decreases in the vena cava, thereby allowing fluid to flow from the peritoneum into the general circulation. Major complications of this therapy include hemodilution, shunt clotting, wound infection, leakage of ascitic fluid from the incision, and bleeding problems.

A variation of this procedure is use of the Denver shunt, which involves placement of a pump in addition to the peritoneal catheter (Figure 17-12).[3] Fluid is allowed to flow through the pump from the peritoneum into the general circulation at a uniform rate to increase blood volume and renal blood flow, retain nutrients and improve nutritional status, increase diuresis, improve mobility and respiration, and relieve massive, refractory ascites.

Portal Systemic Encephalopathy. *Portal systemic encephalopathy*, commonly known as *hepatic encephalopathy*, is a functional derangement of the central nervous system that causes altered levels of consciousness and cerebral manifestations ranging from confusion to coma. Impaired motor ability is also often present. Asterixis, a flapping tremor of the hand, is an early sign of hepatic encephalopathy that can be assessed by the nurse.

The exact cause of hepatic encephalopathy is unknown, but it is thought to be abnormal ammonia metabolism. Increased serum ammonia levels interfere with normal cerebral metabolism. In acute liver failure, signs and symptoms of this disorder may appear rapidly, whereas in chronic liver failure they often occur over time. Many conditions may precipitate the development of hepatic encephalopathy, including fluid and electrolyte and acid-base disturbances, increased protein intake, portosystemic shunts, blood transfusions, GI bleeding, and many

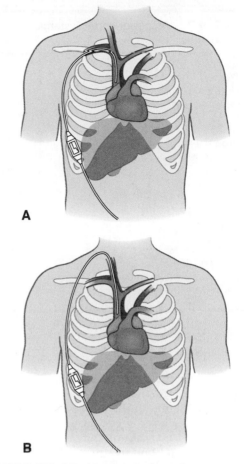

A

B

FIGURE 17-12. The Denver shunt. Percutaneous placement of both the venous and peritoneal catheters of a Denver Ascites Shunt. Venous catheter placement into the **(A)** subclavian and **(B)** internal jugular vein.

drugs such as diuretics, analgesics, narcotics, and sedatives. Progression of hepatic encephalopathy can be divided into stages (Box 17-17).

Measures for decreasing ammonia production are necessary in the treatment of hepatic encephalopathy. Protein intake is limited to 20 to 40 g/day. Neomycin and lactulose are two drugs that can be administered to reduce bacterial breakdown of protein in the bowel.

Neomycin is a broad-spectrum antibiotic that destroys normal bacteria found in the bowel, thereby decreasing protein breakdown and ammonia production. Neomycin is given orally every 4 to 6 hours. This drug is toxic to the kidneys and therefore cannot be given to patients with renal failure. Daily renal function studies are monitored when neomycin is administered.

Lactulose creates an acidic environment in the bowel that causes the ammonia to leave the blood-

BOX 17-17   Stages of Portal Systemic Encephalopathy

Stage 1
- Tremors
- Slurred speech
- Impaired decision making

Stage 2
- Drowsiness
- Loss of sphincter control
- Asterixis

Stage 3
- Dramatic confusion
- Somnolence

Stage 4
- Profound coma
- Unresponsiveness to pain
- Gastrointestinal alterations

stream and enter the colon. Ammonia is trapped in the bowel. Lactulose also has a laxative effect that allows for elimination of the ammonia. Lactulose is given orally or via a rectal enema.

Restriction of medications that are toxic to the liver is another important treatment. All medications that are metabolized by the liver should be reviewed for their therapeutic effect.

Nursing measures for protecting the patient with an altered mental status from harm are a priority.

Many patients with hepatic encephalopathy need to be sedated to prevent them from doing harm to themselves or to others. Oxazepam (Serax), diazepam (Valium), or lorazepam (Ativan) must be used judiciously; however, these drugs are less dependent on liver function for excretion.

Hepatorenal Syndrome. Acute renal failure that occurs with liver failure is called *hepatorenal syndrome*. The pathophysiology of this disorder is not well understood, but it is associated with end-stage cirrhosis and ascites, decreased albumin levels, and portal hypertension. Decreased urine output and an increased serum creatinine level usually occur acutely. The prognosis for the patient with hepatorenal syndrome is generally poor because therapies to improve renal function usually are ineffective. The goals of general medical therapies are to improve liver function while supporting renal function. Fluid administration and diuretic therapy are used to improve urine output. Administration of drugs that are toxic to the kidney is discontinued. Occasionally, hemodialysis is used to support renal function if there is a chance for an improvement in liver function. Because of the poor prognosis, it is appropriate for the critical care nurse to begin to address end-of-life decisions with the patient and family. This is done with consideration of the individual nurse's comfort level, as well as the organizational policy and family dynamics.

Patient Outcomes

Outcomes for the patient with liver failure are included in the Nursing Care Plan for the Patient with Hepatic Failure.

CASE STUDY   *evolve*

You are working evenings in the critical care unit and receive a report from the emergency department of a patient to be admitted to the unit. The patient is a 47-year-old man with a week-long history of severe abdominal pain that worsens with food intake. The pain is associated with nausea and vomiting. The patient is oriented to person and place; however, he is disoriented to day and time and is described as "lethargic." A nasogastric tube and Foley catheter were placed and intravenous access was established in the emergency department.

Vital signs include the following: heart rate, 110 beats/min; respirations, 30 breaths/min; blood pressure, 104/56 mm Hg; and temperature, 38° C.

Laboratory values include the following: white blood cell count, 19,000/microliter; hematocrit, 38%; sodium, 148 mEq/L; potassium, 4.0 mEq/L; chloride, 114 mEq/L; blood urea nitrogen, 25 mg/dL; creatinine, 1.0 mg/dL; glucose, 180 mg/dL; amylase, 500 IU/L; and lipase, 600 IU/L.

QUESTIONS
1. What further data would you like to have from the emergency department?
2. In addition to management of shock in this patient, what is another priority treatment?
3. What further assessment data would be valuable to the long-term management of this patient?

SUMMARY

Acute upper GI bleeding, acute pancreatitis, and liver failure account for potentially life-threatening emergencies that require careful and astute assessment and care by the critical care nurse and medical team. Priorities for care include initial assessments and resuscitation, diagnostic testing for making a definitive diagnosis, and prompt interventions for stabilizing or reversing the pathophysiological process and preventing complications. The nurse's scope of care includes ongoing assessments and monitoring, documentation and reporting of patient responses to diagnostic and treatment regimens, early detection of complications, and supportive care. Patient and family teaching of the ICU routine and all therapies instituted is also a priority. As appropriate, discharge teaching of the underlying pathological process and of the dietary, medication, and activity regimens may also be initiated in the ICU. Successful management of all these patient populations requires a collaborative effort of all disciplines.

CRITICAL THINKING QUESTIONS   *evolve*

1. You are caring for a patient who is admitted with acute abdominal pain and vomiting. His admission vital signs and laboratory values include the following: blood pressure, 94/72 mm Hg; heart rate, 114 beats/min; respiratory rate, 32 breaths/min; potassium level, 3.0 mEq/L; calcium level, 7.0 mg/dL; partial pressure of oxygen in arterial blood (PaO_2), 58 mm Hg; oxygen saturation in arterial blood (SaO_2), 88%; serum amylase level, 280 IU/L; and serum lipase level, 320 IU/L.
   a. What are your priority nursing and medical interventions?
   b. What is the suspected medical diagnosis?

2. A 50-year-old patient is admitted with hematemesis and reports having dark stools for the past 12 hours. Which of the following admission data is the best indicator of the amount of blood lost: blood pressure, 95/60 mm Hg (supine); heart rate, 125 beats/min; respiratory rate, 28 breaths/min; Hct value, 27%; or Hgb level, 14 g/dL?

3. A 45-year-old business executive is admitted to your unit. He tells you that he travels a lot for business and has recently returned from a trip to Mexico. During your initial assessment, he tells you that he is not married, and he relates stories about some of the women he has met and dated on his many trips. His history includes persistent abdominal pain, nausea with occasional vomiting, fatigue, and decreased appetite. Initial vital signs and laboratory results include the following: heart rate, 70 beats/min; urine, clear and dark yellow; liver function test results increased (aspartate transaminase level, 20 IU/L; alanine transaminase level, 70 IU/L); serum albumin level, 3.2 mg/dL, and total serum bilirubin level, 1.5 mg/dL. What is the most likely diagnosis, and what precautions should you take while caring for this patient?

evolve Be sure to check out the bonus material, including free self-assessment exercises, on the Evolve Web site at http://evolve.elsevier.com/Sole.

REFERENCES

1. Bajwa, O., & Marik, P. E. (2005). The management of gastrointestinal bleeding. In M. P. Fink, E. Abraham, J. L. Vincent, & P. M. Kochanek (Eds.), *Textbook of critical care* (5th ed.). Philadelphia: Saunders.
2. Beger, H. G., & Rau, B. M. (2007). Severe acute pancreatitis: Clinical course and management. *World Journal of Gastroenterology, 13*(38), 5043-5051.
3. Cardinal Health. (2007). *Denver Ascites Shunts.* Retrieved November 3, 2007, from www.denverbio.com/physician_ascites_shunts.html.
4. Centers for Disease Control and Prevention (CDC). (2007). *Hepatitis fact sheets.* Retrieved June 1, 2007, from www.cdc.gov/hepatitis.
5. Chernecky, C. C., & Berger, B. J. (2008). *Laboratory tests and diagnostic procedures* (5th ed.). Philadelphia: Saunders.
6. Eckerwall, G. E., Tingstedt, B. B., Bergenzaum, P. E., & Andersson, R. G. (2007). Immediate oral feeding in patients with mild acute pancreatitis is safe and may accelerate recovery: A randomized clinical study. *Clinical Nutrition, 85,* S221-S229.
7. Escorsell, A., & Arroyo, V. (2005). Hepatorenal syndrome. In M. P. Fink, E. Abraham, J. L. Vincent, & P. M. Kochanek (Eds.), *Textbook of critical care* (5th ed.). Philadelphia: Saunders.

8. Gilbert, D., Moellering, R., Eliopoulos, G., & Sande, M. (2007). *The Sandford guide to antimicrobial therapy* (37th ed.). Sperry, VA: Antimicrobial Therapy Inc.

9. Guyton, A. C., & Hall, J. E. (2006). *Textbook of medical physiology* (11th ed.). Philadelphia: Saunders.

10. Hodgson, B. B., & Kizior, R. J. (2007). *Nursing drug handbook*. St. Louis: Mosby.

11. Holzman, N. L., Schirmer, C. M., & Nasraway, S. A. (2005). Gastrointestinal hemorrhage. In M. P. Fink, E. Abraham, J. L. Vencent, & P. M. Kochanek (Eds.), *Textbook of critical care* (5th ed.). Philadelphia: Saunders.

12. Hu, W. S. (2007). *Bioartificial liver*. Retrieved November 2, 2007, from http://hugroup.cems.umn.edu/Research/bal/BAL-howitworks.htm.

13. Huether, S. E. (2006). Alterations of digestive function. In K. L. McCance, & S. E. Huether (Eds.), *Pathophysiology: The biologic basis for disease in adults and children*. St. Louis: Mosby.

14. Huether, S. E. (2006). Structure and function of the digestive system. In K. L. McCance, & S. E. Huether (Eds.), *Pathophysiology: The biologic basis for disease in adults and children*. St. Louis: Mosby.

15. Institute of Healthcare Improvement. (2007). *Critical care*. Retrieved October 31, 2007, from www.ihi.org/IHI/Topics/CriticalCare/.

16. Institute of Healthcare Improvement. (2007). *Implement the ventilator bundle: Peptic ulcer disease prophylaxis*. Retrieved October 31, 2007, from www.ihi.org/IHI/Topics/CriticalCare/IntensiveCare/Changes/IndividualChanges/PepticUlcerDiseaseprophylaxis.htm.

17. Jarvis, C. (2008). *Physical examination and health assessment* (5th ed.). Philadelphia: Saunders.

18. Jiang, K., Chen, X. Z., Xia, Q., Tang, W. F., & Wang, L. (2007). Early nasogastric enteral nutrition for severe acute pancreatitis: A systematic review. *World Journal of Gastroenterology, 13*(39), 5253-5260.

19. Jiang, K., Chen, X. Z., Xia, Q., Tang, W. F., & Wang, L. (2007). Early veno-venous hemofiltration for severe acute pancreatitis: A systematic review. *Chinese Journal of Evidence-Based Medicine, 7*, 121-134.

20. Kramer, D. J. (2005). Liver transplantation. In M. P. Fink, E. Abraham, J. L. Vencent, & P. M. Kochanek (Eds.), *Textbook of critical care* (5th ed.). Philadelphia: Saunders.

21. Lee, S. D., & Kearney, D. J. (2004). A randomized controlled trial of gastric lavage prior to endoscopy for acute upper gastrointestinal bleeding. *Journal of Clinical Gastroenterology, 38*(10), 861-865.

22. Lipsett, P. S. (2005). Acute pancreatitis. In M. P. Fink, E. Abraham, J. L. Vencent, & P. M. Kochanek (Eds.), *Textbook of critical care* (5th ed.). Philadelphia: Saunders.

23. Marik, P. E., & Zaloga, G. P. (2004). Meta-analysis of parenteral nutrition versus enteral nutrition in patients with acute pancreatitis. *British Medical Journal, 328*, 1407-1410.

24. Polson, J., Lee, W. (2005). AASLD guideline: The management of acute liver failure. *Hepatology, 41*, 1179.

25. Ranson, J. C. (1985). Risk factors in acute pancreatitis. *Hospital Practice, 20*(4), 69-73.

26. Stadlbauer, V., Krisper, P., Aigner, R., Haditsch, B., Jung, A., Lackner, C. l., et al. (2006). Effect of extracorporeal liver support by MARS and Prometheus on serum cytokines in acute-on-chronic liver failure. *Critical Care, 10*(6), R169.

27. Twinrix. (2007). *Hepatitis A inactivated & hepatitis B (recombinant) vaccine*. Retrieved November 2, 2007, from www.twinrix.com/.

28. Wendon, J., & Sizer, E. (2005). Portal hypertension. In M. P. Fink, E. Abraham, J. L. Vencent, & P. M. Kochanek (Eds.), *Textbook of critical care* (5th ed.). Philadelphia: Saunders.

29. Zagari, R. M., Bianchi-Porro, G., Fiocca, R., Gasbarrini, G., Roda, E., & Bazzoli, F. (2007). Comparison of 1 and 2 weeks of omeprazole, amoxicillin and clarithromycin treatment for *Helicobacter pylori* eradication: The HYPER Study. *Gut, 56*(4), 475-479.

CHAPTER 18

Endocrine Alterations

Zara R. Brenner, MS, ACNS, BC

Jeanne Powers, MS, RN, CCRN

INTRODUCTION

The endocrine glands form a communication network linking all body systems. Hormones from these glands control and regulate metabolic processes such as energy production, fluid and electrolyte balance, and response to stress. This system is closely linked to and integrated with the nervous system. In particular, the hypothalamus and pituitary gland play a major role in hormonal regulation. The hypothalamus manufactures and secretes several releasing or inhibiting hormones that are conveyed to the pituitary. The pituitary responds to these hormones by increasing or decreasing hormone secretion, thus regulating circulating hormone levels. This system is designed as a feedback control mechanism. Positive feedback stimulates release of a hormone when serum hormone levels are low. Negative feedback inhibits the release of hormones when serum hormone levels are high. Examples of how these feedback systems work to control circulating levels of cortisol are provided in Figure 18-1. This same feedback system also controls the secretion and inhibition of other hormones outside hypothalamic-pituitary control.

Changes in the Endocrine System in Critical Illness

The stress of critical illness provokes a significant response by the endocrine system. Excess glucose in the blood (hyperglycemia) occurs as a result of an increase in gluconeogenesis and decreased peripheral utilization of glucose (increase in insulin resistance). Adrenal insufficiency can occur as a result of insult or damage to the gland itself (primary) or because of dysfunction of the hypothalamus, pituitary, or both (secondary). Relative adrenal insufficiency may occur in critically ill patients whenever elevated cortisol levels are inadequate for the demand. Thyroid hormone balance is disrupted by changes in peripheral metabolism that cause a decrease in triiodothyronine (T_3) levels. Pituitary and hypothalamus dysfunction as a result of brain tumor, trauma, or surgery can cause significant fluid and electrolyte imbalances that complicate critical illness.

Disease States of the Endocrine System

Diseases involving the hypothalamus, the pituitary gland, and the primary endocrine organs (i.e., pancreas, adrenal glands, and thyroid gland) interfere with normal feedback mechanisms and the secretion of hormones. Crisis states occur when these diseases are untreated or undertreated, when the patient is stressed physiologically or psychologically, or as the result of many other factors.

This chapter describes both the endocrine response to critical illness and the crises that occur as a result of imbalances of hormones from the pancreas, adrenal glands, thyroid gland, and posterior pituitary gland. For a summary of endocrine concerns for the older adult, see Geriatric Considerations.

HYPERGLYCEMIA IN THE CRITICALLY ILL PATIENT

Patients in the critical care unit are at high risk for hyperglycemia from a number of different stressors including their disease states, the illness-related hormonal responses to stress, and the critical care environment. See Box 18-1 for risk factors associated with an increase in blood glucose levels.

While stress-induced hyperglycemia is a normal physiological response and is related to the fight-flight mode, it is not beneficial in critical illness.

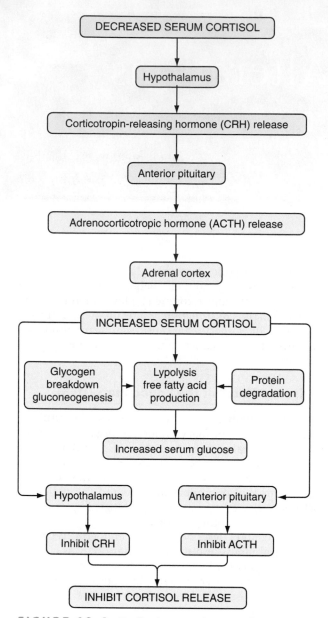

FIGURE 18-1. Feedback system for cortisol regulation.

During hyperglycemic periods, there is decreased white blood cell function, osmotic diuresis, poor wound healing, decreased erythropoiesis, increased hemolysis, endothelial dysfunction, increased thrombosis, vasoconstriction, decreased respiratory muscle function, neuronal damage, and impaired gastric motility. While the adverse effects of hyperglycemia are detrimental, the lack of control of glycemic levels leads to unfavorable outcomes.

In 2001, Van den Berghe et al.[26] published a landmark study which showed that intensive insulin control of hyperglycemia in a surgical population decreased mortality and morbidity, including sepsis, renal failure necessitating dialysis, blood transfusion requirements, and polyneuropathy. Since then, much research has been conducted to examine the role of hyperglycemia on the outcomes in critically ill patients.[25] Hyperglycemia has been shown to contribute to sternal wound infections, to prolong recovery from stroke and acute myocardial infarction, and to increase the risk of morbidity and mortality in patients without a history of diabetes mellitus (DM) who are admitted to critical care units.[19] Control of blood glucose levels is the desired standard of care for critically ill patients.

Achieving Glycemic Control

Control of glycemic levels is an important priority for all patients in a critical care unit, those with DM and those without. The target glucose levels may be somewhat different for medical versus surgical critically ill patients. In critically ill surgical patients, intensive insulin therapy ("tight control") is aimed at maintaining a steady state of euglycemic levels. Target glycemic control for medical patients is in a broader range of serum glucose levels. The American Diabetes Association recommends that glucose levels be controlled as close to 110 mg/dL as possible and that they be kept under 180 mg/dL.[5]

Management of hyperglycemia in the critically ill is attained through the use of protocols.[25] These nurse-implemented protocols include frequent glucose monitoring and insulin dosage adjustments based on those levels. The frequent blood glucose monitoring is intended to ensure the appropriate insulin dosage and to minimize the incidence of hypoglycemia. The key elements of a protocol for glycemic control in the critical care unit are described in Box 18-2. Effective protocols minimize complexity of managing the decision points so there is less chance for error. Computer decision support software as part of the protocol is available and has been shown to be helpful in managing glucose control. Achievement of tight glucose control is time-intensive for the critical care nurse. Concern has been voiced that intensive glucose control contributes to a rise in the cost of caring for patients. However, the significant resultant decreases in morbidity and mortality result in cost-effectiveness for the health care systems.[5]

Hypoglycemia as a Preventable Adverse Effect of Glucose Management

Although the benefits of intensive glycemic control have been established, there is concern about the

GERIATRIC CONSIDERATIONS

Elderly patients present diagnostic and treatment challenges related to endocrine disorders. When critically ill, they are at increased risk for endocrine complications. They have more comorbidities and take more medications that affect fluid and electrolyte balance. The presenting signs and symptoms are frequently atypical and nonspecific, and their responses to dysfunction are blunted. Many of the compensatory mechanisms are lost with advanced age.

PANCREAS

Elderly persons are more prone to develop hyperosmolar hyperglycemic state, type 2 diabetes mellitus, or both. They are also at increased risk of being unaware of hypoglycemia. Elderly patients are more likely to have comorbid conditions, such as cardiac or renal disease, and to take medications that make them more reactive to electrolyte imbalances. They are also slower to respond to treatments.

ADRENAL

Utilization and clearance of cortisol decrease with age, resulting in increased serum cortisol levels. Unfortunately, because the feedback systems are intact, a decrease in cortisol secretion takes place, which tends to exacerbate the situation in the elderly. The absolute level of cortisol needed to maintain homeostasis is unknown. The role of poor nutrition and decreased albumin stores (one of cortisol's binding proteins) remains controversial, especially in the elderly.

THYROID

Thyroid hormone levels can decrease with age, probably as a result of glandular atrophy. Approximately 5% of people older than 60 years are affected by hypothyroidism. Detection of thyroid disease by assessment of signs or symptoms becomes more challenging. In addition, lower amounts of thyroid are needed as replacement, and replacement must be slower to avoid potentially dangerous side effects. Elderly patients are less likely to tolerate urgent treatment with liothyronine sodium.

Older patients may not exhibit the typical signs of thyrotoxicosis. Anorexia, atrial fibrillation, apathy, and weight loss may already be present or misinterpreted. Goiter, hyperactive reflexes, sweating, heat intolerance, tremor, nervousness, and polydipsia are less commonly present. In the elderly, symptoms of thyroid storm may present as increasing angina or worsening congestive heart failure.

PITUITARY

Decreased release of growth hormone and increased sensitivity lead to a decrease in lean body mass and increased blood glucose levels, and they affect the release of thyroid-stimulating hormone (thyrotropin), although usually not significantly. An increase in secretion of antidiuretic hormone occurs with advanced age and places the older person at risk of dilutional hyponatremia. Elderly patients are at greater risk of the syndrome of inappropriate antidiuretic hormone from any cause than are younger patients. Elderly patients can fail to recognize and respond to thirst, and therefore are at an increased risk for hypovolemia.

---

possibility of blood glucose levels falling below the normal range (hypoglycemia). An increased incidence of hypoglycemia in critically ill patients has occurred with a reduction or discontinuation of nutrition without adjustment of insulin therapy, such as the holding of parenteral or enteral feedings during diagnostic exams; a prior diagnosis of DM; sepsis; and the use/change in dosage of inotropic drugs, vasopressor support, and glucocorticoid therapy.

Many episodes of hypoglycemia are preventable. The nurse must ensure that the glucose testing is accurate and consistent. Concurrent and shift-to-shift coordination and adjustment of all medical and nutritional therapies (including increasing, decreasing, or temporarily suspending any of them), is required to prevent hypoglycemia.

The Diabetic Patient in the Critical Care Unit

Stress-induced hyperglycemia affects patients with DM as well as those without. In the critically ill, stress-induced hyperglycemia exacerbates the elevated glucose levels of diabetic patients, predisposes them to an even higher incidence of complications and comorbidities, and impacts treatment for all disease states. Diabetic patients are hospitalized more frequently, are more prone to complications, and have longer hospital stays and higher hospital costs than nondiabetic patients.[24] Therapy aimed at establishing euglycemic levels contributes to improved patient outcomes.[12] Diabetic patients in the critical care unit are managed with insulin therapy regardless of their usual home diabetic regimen. Table 18-1 reviews the variety of insulins.

BOX 18-1 Risk Factors for the Development of Hyperglycemia in the Critically Ill Patient[16,19]

- Preexisting diabetes mellitus, diagnosed or undiagnosed
- Comorbidities such as obesity, pancreatitis, cirrhosis, hypokalemia
- Stress response release of cortisol, growth hormone, catecholamines including epinephrine and norepinephrine, glucagon, glucocorticoids, and the cytokines interleukin-1, interleukin-6, and tumor necrosis factor
- Aging
- Lack of muscular activity
- Relative insulin deficiency/Insulin resistance
- Administration of exogenous catecholamines, glucocorticoids
- Administration of dextrose solutions, nutritional support
- Drug therapy such as thiazides, beta-blockers, highly active antiretroviral therapy, phenytoin, tacrolimus, cyclosporine

BOX 18-2 Key Components of a Glucose Management Protocol

- Frequent plasma blood glucose measurements
- Concentration of insulin infusion (i.e., number of units of insulin mixed in quantity of normal saline)
- Initial intravenous insulin dose if appropriate
- Table with titration for increasing or decreasing insulin infusion based on glucose level
- Interventions for hypoglycemia, should it occur
- Interventions for when feeding is interrupted, either parenteral or enteral
- Interventions for when the patient is transported from the critical care unit for diagnostic testing
- Interventions for discontinuing the intravenous insulin infusion
- Interventions for when the patient is transferred out of the critical care unit

PANCREATIC ENDOCRINE EMERGENCIES

Review of Physiology

Three common critical endocrine disorders associated with the pancreas are diabetic ketoacidosis (DKA), hyperosmolar hyperglycemic state (HHS), and hypoglycemia, which are acute complications of

TABLE 18-1 Types of Insulin

Type	Onset	Peak (hr)	Duration (hr)
Rapid-Acting Insulins			
Aspart (Novolog)	5-10 minutes	1-3	4-6
Lispro (Humalog)	Up to 15 minutes	0.5-1.5	4-6
Glulisine (Apidra)	<30 minutes	0.5-1.5	4-6
Short-Acting Insulin			
Regular (Humulin R, Novolin R)	30-60 minutes	2-3	6-8
Intermediate-Acting Insulins			
NPH (Humulin N, Novolin N)	2-4 hours	4-10	12-18
Long-Acting Insulins			
Glargine (Lantus) Detemir (Levemir)	1 hour	Peakless	≥24

DM. An understanding of the normal physiology of insulin, as well as of the pathophysiology, critical assessments, and collaborative treatment regimens of the aforementioned disorders, is essential to the management and nursing care of these patients.

In response to increased levels of serum glucose, insulin is released from the pancreas by beta cells in the islets of Langerhans. Insulin is essential to normal carbohydrate, protein, and fat metabolism. The physiological activity of insulin is summarized in Box 18-3. Normally, glucose transport into cells occurs as facilitated diffusion using various glucose transport channel proteins.[24] Insulin-mediated glucose transport is necessary for cellular uptake of glucose by most cells in the body, including muscle, fibroblasts, mammary glands, anterior pituitary, lens of the eye, and aorta. Insulin is not required for glucose to enter cells in the liver, kidney tubules, central nervous system, retina, intestinal mucosa, beta islets, or into erythrocytes.

Control of glucose levels and insulin secretion is affected by glucagon and somatostatin, both secreted by the pancreas, as well as circulating catecholamines, cortisol, and growth hormone. These hormones are released in response to decreased glucose levels and in response to stress and are often referred to as counterregulatory or stress hormones.

Without insulin, glucose is unable to enter cells, accumulates in the blood, and triggers a variety of physiological processes as the cells requiring glucose begin to starve. In contrast, levels of circulating insulin that exceed the body's requirement result in decreased serum glucose levels and changes in the level of consciousness, because glucose is the preferred substrate for the central nervous system.

DM is a metabolic disease of glucose imbalance resulting from alterations in insulin secretion, insulin action, or both. The number of people with DM has been increasing, now numbering more than 170 million worldwide.[14] The two most common types of DM are type 1 and type 2. Type 1 DM (autoimmune mediated) is primarily caused by pancreatic islet beta-cell destruction, resulting in an absolute insulin deficiency and a tendency to ketoacidosis. The most prevalent form is type 2 DM, which involves a combination of insulin resistance and an insulin secretory defect, resulting in a relative insulin deficiency. Type 2 DM is commonly accompanied by metabolic syndrome. See Clinical Alert: Metabolic Syndrome for a description. The other types of DM include gestational DM, steroid- or drug-induced DM, and DM associated with genetic disorders such as cystic fibrosis.

There is strong evidence that genetic factors play a role in the development of type 1 DM. Genetic alterations may also contribute to the development of type 2 DM as well as in those conditions, such as obesity and metabolic syndrome, that are more prevalent in patients with type 2 DM (see Genetics feature). Certain populations have a higher incidence of DM, thus leading to an increased awareness of genetic factors and health screening needs for relatives of patients with diagnosed DM. Rates of type 1 DM are especially high in Scandinavia. The incidence of type 2 DM in the United States is higher in Hispanics, African Americans, Native Americans, and Alaskan Native adults.[7]

Effects of Aging

With aging, pancreatic endocrine function declines. Fasting glucose levels trend upwards with age, and glucose tolerance decreases. These changes are due to a combination of both decreased insulin production and increased insulin resistance, independent of any other coexisting disease states. Type 2 DM and postchallenge hyperglycemia (prediabetes) are more common in the older population.

Hyperglycemic Crises

Pathogenesis

The basic underlying mechanism for both DKA and HHS is a reduction in the net effective action of circulating insulin coupled with a concomitant elevation of counterregulatory hormones. Figure 18-2 shows the pathophysiology of DKA and HHS. Together, this hormonal mix leads to increased hepatic and renal glucose production, but it prevents utilization of glucose in the peripheral tissues. DKA and HHS are endocrine emergencies.

BOX 18-3 Physiological Activity of Insulin

Carbohydrate Metabolism
- Increases glucose transport across cell membrane in most cells including muscle and fat
- Within liver and muscle, promotes glycogenesis, the storage form of glucose
- Increases glycolysis in fat and muscle
- Inhibits gluconeogenesis and glycogenolysis in the liver, thus sparing amino acids and glycerol for protein and fatty acid synthesis

Fat Metabolism
- Increases triglyceride synthesis
- Increases fatty acid transport into adipose tissue
- Inhibits lipolysis of triglycerides stored in adipose tissue
- Stimulates fatty acid synthesis from glucose and other substrates

Protein Metabolism
- Increases amino acid transport across cell membrane of muscle and liver
- Augments protein synthesis
- Inhibits proteolysis

CLINICAL ALERT
Metabolic Syndrome

The combination of hypertension, abdominal obesity, high blood glucose levels, and abnormal lipid levels comprise the metabolic syndrome. The generally accepted definitions of the components of the metabolic syndrome are:
- Hypertension = blood pressure >130 mm Hg systolic and >85 mm Hg diastolic
- Abdominal obesity = waist circumference >102 cm (40 inches) for men and >88 cm (35 inches) for women
- High blood glucose levels = fasting blood glucose level >110 mg/dL
- Abnormal lipid levels = triglycerides >150 mg/dL, high-density cholesterol levels <40 mg/dL in men and <50 mg/dL for women

Therapeutic treatment reduces the disease impact of all the components and the severity of complications in hospitalized patients.

GENETICS
Type 2 Diabetes Mellitus: A Complex Disease with Complex Genetics

Type 2 diabetes mellitus (T2DM) is an example of a multifactorial, polygenic disease. *Multifactorial* means that T2DM is a result of an interaction between genes and the environment. *Polygenic* means that more than one gene is implicated in the development of this common, chronic disease. Other multifactorial and polygenic disorders that occur in adults include hypertension, atherosclerosis, many cancers, and manic-depressive psychosis.[5]

Discovering the genetic influences in complex disorders is challenging.[2,5] For example, the age of onset varies, the pathophysiology is incompletely understood, the basic disease lesion may not be known, and differences in the disease within a family may be due to chance. Complex disease genes may have only subtle nucleotide variations, or these variations may be more common than in other diseases. Researchers may need to study large numbers of people with and without the disease to identify the unique genetic contributions. In addition, there may be protective factors that affect susceptibility, and protective factors may differ in populations and in cultures.

Although some subsets of common, complex diseases may be due to single gene polymorphisms, most causation appears to be the result of multiple gene variations and environmental influences.[2] This observation appears to be true for T2DM. For example, there is a single gene variation that is associated with about 5% of people with diagnosed T2DM. The single gene that results in a subset of T2DM is a variation in the coding region of the *HNF4a* gene.[1] Inheriting this gene results in maturity onset diabetes of the young in an autosomal dominant pattern. With this gene, people develop T2DM in their 20s rather than later in life, and do not necessarily have environmental risk factors of obesity or inactivity.[8] Other variations within the *HNF4a* gene result in more traditional signs and symptoms of T2DM with onset of the disease in the fourth or fifth decade and associations with excess weight and a sedentary lifestyle.

Interestingly, many of the variations in genes associated with T2DM are not within the coding section of the gene itself but along the regulatory area preceding the gene. These areas are in close proximity to the actual coding region and regulate the gene by turning it on ("promoter") or off ("inhibitory"), resulting in protein production or cessation. Most of the genes associated with T2DM and their regulatory regions are involved in controlling fuel intake and regulation.[4,6,7] In general, inheriting a single copy of one of these variations increases the risk of developing T2DM; inheriting two copies of the same variation increases the risk for active disease exponentially. Some experts suggest that as much as 50% of the risk for T2DM may be genetic.[7]

People with T2DM may have variations both within a single gene and in different genes. They may also experience greater or reduced environmental effects. The interaction between genes and the environment in patients with diagnosed T2DM has been known for many decades. Specifically, a family history that includes diabetes combined with one's food intake, body weight (specifically, obesity), and low exercise is a strong predictor of T2DM. Environmental and genetic factors combine to influence the onset and progression of diabetes in a number of ways:[2]

1. *Increased or decreased number of pancreatic beta cells that produce insulin.* Inheriting a greater number of beta cells may be protective despite a sedentary lifestyle, whereas few beta cells may result in early-onset or more severe T2DM.
2. *Number of pancreatic beta cells that produce insulin.* The efficiency or effectiveness of the insulin produced by beta cells can be influenced by genes as well as toxic environmental causes, viruses, and other agents.
3. *Secretion of insulin from the beta cells.* Secretion is affected by genetic factors, food intake and exercise.
4. *Insulin-signaling pathways that regulate the uptake of glucose by fat and muscle cells.* Genes influence the response of muscle and fat cells to insulin. The size and number of fat cells and skeletal muscle cells also influence insulin responsiveness.
5. *Control of fat metabolism and storage in the body.* Some genes influence fat absorption from the gastrointestinal tract and fat deposition in the body. Diet and exercise also influence the amount of fat intake and deposition.

The genetics of T2DM are complex and influence an individual's susceptibility to this chronic, complex disease. T2DM is not inherited in a clearly dominant or recessive manner. Genetic polymorphisms appear to increase the risk for developing diabetes, while other genetic variations reduce risk. The American Diabetic Association recommends screening for diabetes onset every 3 years in persons with a positive family history, and in all individuals older than 45 years.[3] Elucidating the genetics of T2DM helps to identify individuals at risk who may benefit from interventions before the disease develops. For the nurse, thinking "genetically" and taking and recording an appropriate family history will help to identify those at higher risk for common diseases influenced by genetic factors.[5]

GENETICS—cont'd

REFERENCES

1. Adams, A. (2000). *Genes can cause type 2 diabetes mellitus.* Retrieved April 22, 2008, from www.GeneticHealth.com.
2. Dean, L., & McEntyre, J. *The genetic landscape of diabetes.* Retrieved April 22, 2008, from www.ncbi.nlm.nih.gov/books/bv.fcgi?rid=diabetes.
3. Fonseca, V., Blonde, L., Gerstein, H. C., Hirsch, I., Kahn, S., Korytkowski, M. T., et al. (2007). Clinical practice recommendations. *Diabetes Care 30,* S1-S60.
4. Freeman, H., & Cox, R. D. (2006). Type-2 diabetes: A cocktail of genetic discovery. *Human Molecular Genetics, 15,* R202-R209.
5. Lashley, F. R. (2005). *Clinical genetics in nursing practice* (3rd ed.). New York: Springer.
6. Malecki, M. T. (2005). Genetics of type 2 diabetes mellitus. *Diabetes in Research and Clinical Practice, 68,* S10-S21.
7. NCBI. (2007). *Online Mendelian inheritance in man (OMIN).* Retrieved April 22, 2008, from www.ncbi.nlm.nih.gov/sites/entrez?db=omim.
8. Olek, K. (2006). Maturity-onset diabetes of the young: An update. *Clinical Laboratory, 52,* 593-598.

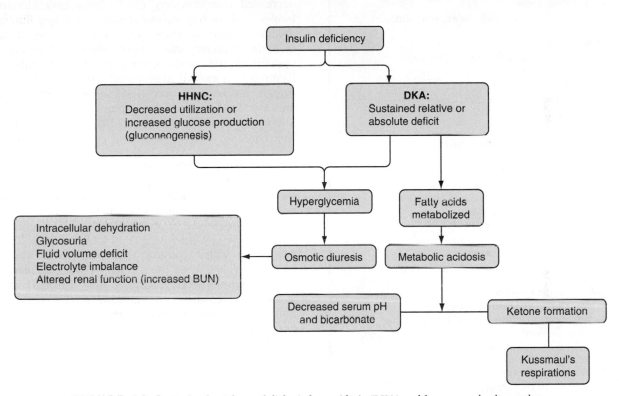

FIGURE 18-2. Pathophysiology of diabetic ketoacidosis (DKA) and hyperosmolar hyperglycemic state (HHS).

Traditionally, DKA had been thought to be the crisis state in type 1 DM, while HHS was thought to be the emergent state in type 2 DM. Increasingly, DKA and HHS are being seen concurrently in the same patient.[3]

Etiology of Diabetic Ketoacidosis. Numerous factors trigger DKA (Box 18-4), the most common being infections, inadequate insulin therapy, and severe stress states (e.g., trauma, surgery, myocardial infarction). Many patients have DKA as the initial indication of previously undiagnosed type 1 DM. Numerous drugs trigger an insulin deficiency, making DKA more likely in these patients. The condition may also occur in patients with known DM who do not administer enough insulin or have increased insulin requirements. In the critically ill, the presence of coexisting autoimmune endocrine disorders must be considered, especially in unstable patients with type 1 DM.[24] In patients using insulin pumps, a malfunctioning pump system can lead to DKA in as little as 12 hours. Lack of knowledge regarding the disease process or insulin administration and/or lack of

BOX 18-4   Factors Leading to Diabetic Ketoacidosis and Hyperosmolar Hyperglycemic State

Common Factors
- Infections: pneumonia, urinary tract infection, sepsis, or abscess
- Omission of diabetic therapy or inadequate treatment
- New-onset diabetes mellitus
- Preexisting illness: cardiac, renal diseases
- Major or acute illness: MI, CVA, pancreatitis, trauma, surgery, renal disease
- Other endocrine disorders: hyperthyroidism, Cushing's disease, pheochromocytoma
- Stress
- Financial issues
- High caloric parenteral or enteral nutrition

Medications
- Steroids (especially glucocorticoids)
- Beta-blockers
- Thiazide diuretics
- Calcium channel blockers
- Phenytoin
- Epinephrine
- Psychotropics, including tricyclic antidepressants
- Sympathomimetics
- Analgesics
- Cimetidine
- Calcium channel blockers
- Immunosuppressants
- Diazoxide
- Chemotherapeutic agents
- "Social drugs" such as cocaine, ecstasy

DKA-Specific Factors
- Malfunction of insulin pump
- Infection at catheter site of insulin pump
- Development of insulin resistance (e.g., during menstruation or pregnancy)

HHS-Specific Factors
- Decreased thirst mechanism
- Difficult access to fluids (e.g., nursing home resident)

DKA, Diabetic ketoacidosis; *HHS*, hyperosmolar hyperglycemic state; *MI*, myocardial infarction; *CVA*, cerebrovascular accident.

The incidence of recurrent DKA is higher in female patients, peaking in the early teenage years. The risk of recurrent DKA is also higher in patients with DM diagnosed at an early age and in those of lower socioeconomic status. The causes of recurrent DKA are unclear but include physiological, psychosomatic, and psychosocial factors. Psychological problems complicated by eating disorders in younger patients with type 1 DM may contribute to 20% of recurrent DKA.[1]

Etiology of Hyperosmolar Hyperglycemic State. HHS is usually precipitated by inadequate insulin secretion or action, and is more commonly seen in patients with newly diagnosed type 2 DM. Some patients may have no history of DM. Most patients are elderly, with decreased compensatory mechanisms to maintain homeostasis in hyperosmolar states. A major illness mediated through glucose overproduction resulting from the stress response may contribute to the development of HHS. High-calorie parenteral and enteral feedings that exceed the patient's ability to metabolize glucose have induced HHS. Several medications are associated with the development of the disorder. The major etiological factors of HHS are included in Box 18-4.

Pathophysiology of Diabetic Ketoacidosis

Figure 18-3 details the intracellular/extracellular shifts that occur in both DKA and HHS. In DKA, high extracellular glucose levels produce an osmotic gradient between the intracellular and extracellular spaces causing fluid to move out of the cells. This process is called osmotic diuresis. When serum glucose levels exceed the renal threshold (approximately 300 mg/dL), glucose is lost through the kidneys (glycosuria). As glycosuria and osmotic diuresis progress, urinary losses of water, sodium, potassium, magnesium, calcium, and phosphorus occur. This cycle of osmotic diuresis causes increases in serum osmolality, further compensatory fluid shifts from the intracellular to the intravascular space, and worsening dehydration.

Typically, body water losses in DKA total 6 L.[1] It is also thought that the hyperosmolarity further impairs insulin secretion and promotes insulin resistance. The glomerular filtration rate in the kidney decreases in response to these severe fluid volume deficits. Decreased glucose excretion (causing increased serum glucose levels) and further hyperosmolarity result. The altered neurological status frequently seen in these patients is partially the result of cellular dehydration and the hyperosmolar state.

Protein stores are depleted through the process of gluconeogenesis in the liver. Amino acids are metabolized into glucose and nitrogen to provide energy. Without insulin, the liberated glucose cannot be

compliance with the therapeutic regimen are also possible causes. DKA characteristically develops over a short period, and patients seek medical help early because of the pathophysiological symptoms they experience.

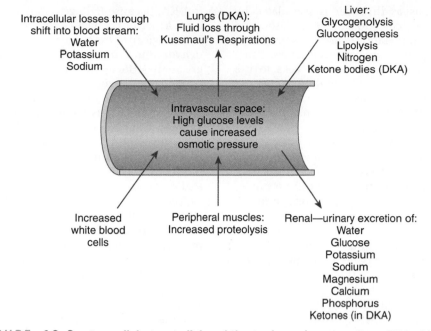

FIGURE 18-3. Intracellular/extracellular shifts in hyperglycemic crises. *DKA*, Diabetic ketoacidosis.

used, further increasing serum blood glucose and urine glucose concentrations and worsening osmotic diuresis. As nitrogen accumulates in the peripheral tissues, blood urea nitrogen (BUN) rises. Breakdown of protein stores also stimulates the shift of intracellular potassium into the extracellular serum (hyperkalemia). This additional circulating potassium may also be lost as a result of osmotic diuresis (hypokalemia). Serum electrolyte levels, particularly potassium, may be falsely elevated in relation to the actual intracellular level. Total body potassium deficits are common and must be considered in the overall management of DKA.

The absence or lack of insulin impairs lipid synthesis as well, with the breakdown of fat cells into free fatty acids. The free fatty acids are released into the blood and are transported to the liver where they are oxidized into ketone bodies (beta-hydroxybutyrate) and acetoacetate. This leads to an increase in circulating ketone concentrations and further increases gluconeogenesis in the liver. Ketonuria accounts for a significant amount of osmotic diuresis. The ketoacids are transported to peripheral tissues where they are oxidized to acetone. Impaired bicarbonate buffering of the excess ketones results in metabolic acidosis from increased carbonic acid concentrations. As ketone and hydrogen ions accumulate and acidosis worsens, the respiratory system attempts to compensate for excess carbonic acid by blowing off another acid, carbon dioxide (CO_2). In

---

BOX 18-5 Calculation for Anion Gap

$(Na^+ + K^+) - (Cl^- + HCO_3^-)$
The normal value is 8 to 16 mEq/L. An elevated value indicates the accumulation of acids, such as is present in diabetic ketoacidosis.

Cl⁻, Chloride; *HCO₃⁻*, bicarbonate; *K⁺*, potassium; *Na⁺*, sodium.

addition to carbonic acid, patients with DKA may have an accumulation of lactic acid (lactic acidosis). The resulting dehydration may cause decreased perfusion to core organs, with consequent hypoxemia and worsening of the lactic acidosis.

Excess lactic acid results in what is called an *increased anion gap* (increased body acids). Sodium, potassium, chloride, and bicarbonate are responsible for maintaining a normal anion gap, which is normally less than 16 mEq/L. Ketone accumulation causes an increase in the anion gap greater than 16 mEq/L. To calculate the anion gap, see Box 18-5.

Many enzymatic reactions within the body function only within a limited range of pH. As the patient becomes more acidotic and enzymes become more ineffective, body metabolism slows. This situation further decreases ketone metabolism, and acidosis worsens. The stress response also contributes to the metabolic alterations as the liver is stimulated by hormones (glucagon, catecholamines, cortisol, and growth hormones) to metabolize protein stores, thus increasing serum glucose and nitrogen levels. Some hormones also decrease the ability of cells to use glucose for ATP production and therefore compound the problem. The alterations in central nervous system function in DKA are thought to be influenced by the acidosis and dehydration.

In summary, cells without glucose starve and begin to use existing stores of fat and protein to provide energy for body processes (gluconeogenesis). Fats are metabolized faster than they can be stored, resulting in an accumulation of ketone acids, a byproduct of fat metabolism in the liver. Ketone acids accumulate in the bloodstream, where hydrogen ions dissociate from the ketones and cause metabolic acidosis. The more acidotic the patient becomes, the less able the body is to metabolize these ketones.

Pathophysiology of Hyperosmotic Hyperglycemic State

The pathophysiology of HHS is similar to that of DKA. However, in HHS, there are significantly lower levels of free fatty acids, resulting in a lack of ketosis, but even higher levels of hyperglycemia, hyperosmolarity, and severe dehydration (see Figure 18-2). HHS is referred to by many different acronyms (Box 18-6).

Hyperglycemia results from decreased utilization of glucose, increased production of glucose, or both. The hyperglycemic state causes an osmotic movement of water from a lesser concentration of solutes to a higher concentration of solutes. This results in expansion of the extracellular fluid volume and intracellular dehydration. The osmotic diuresis and resultant intracellular and extracellular dehydration in HHS are generally more severe than those found

---

BOX 18-6   HHS and Other Synonymous Acronyms

- *HHS:* Hyperosmolar hyperglycemic state
- *HHNC:* Hyperosmolar hyperglycemic nonketotic coma
- *HNS:* Hyperosmolar nonketotic state
- *HHNK:* Hyperosmolar hyperglycemic nonketosis
- *HHNS:* Hyperosmolar hyperglycemic nonketotic state/syndrome
- *HNKDC:* Hyperosmolar nonketotic diabetic coma
- *HONK:* Hyperosmolar nonketosis
- *HNAD:* Hyperglycemic nonacidotic diabetic coma

---

in DKA, because HHS generally develops insidiously over a period of weeks to months. Alterations in neurological status are common because of cellular dehydration. The typical total body water deficit is greater in HHS, approximately 9 L.[1] By the time these patients seek medical attention, they are profoundly dehydrated and hyperosmolar. As a result, the mortality rate of HHS is higher than that of DKA.

Most commonly, patients with type 2 diabetes who develop HHS are older. They are also more likely to have other medical problems that affect morbidity and mortality, such as issues with mobility and access to health care.

Ketoacidosis is usually not seen in patients with HHS. It is believed that insulin levels in these patients are high enough to prevent lipolysis and ketone formation. The levels of glucose counterregulatory hormones that promote lipolysis are lower in patients with HHS than in those with DKA.

Assessment

Clinical Presentation. The presenting symptoms of DKA and HHS are similar (Table 18-2). Signs of DKA and HHS are related to the degree of dehydration present and the electrolyte imbalances. The osmotic diuresis occurring from hyperglycemia results in signs of increased thirst (polydipsia), increased urine output (polyuria), and dehydration. Increased hunger (polyphagia) may also be an early sign. Elderly persons have a decreased sense of thirst, so this sign may not be seen in these patients who develop HHS. Signs of intravascular dehydration are also common as the disease processes continue.

Hyperglycemia and ketosis both contribute to delayed gastric emptying. Vomiting can occur, which worsens total body dehydration. Patients also report symptoms of weakness and anorexia. Abdominal pain and tenderness are common presenting symptoms, particularly in DKA, and are associated with dehydration and underlying pathophysiology, such as pyelonephritis, duodenal ulcer, appendicitis, and metabolic acidosis. Pain associated with DKA most commonly disappears with treatment of dehydration. Weight loss occurs because of the fluid losses and an inability to metabolize glucose.

Altered states of consciousness range from restlessness, confusion, and agitation to somnolence and coma. Visual disturbances, especially blurred vision, are common in hyperglycemia. Generally, altered levels of consciousness are more pronounced in patients with HHS. This is related to the severity of hyperglycemia and serum hyperosmolarity. Seizures and focal neurological signs may also be present and often lead to misdiagnosis in patients with HHS.

TABLE 18-2 Manifestations of Diabetic Ketoacidosis and Hyperosmolar Hyperglycemic State

	Diabetic Ketoacidosis	Hyperosmolar Hyperglycemic State
Pathophysiology	Insulin deficiency resulting in cellular dehydration and volume depletion, acidosis, and protein catabolism	Insulin deficiency resulting in dehydration and hyperosmolality
Health history	History of type 1 diabetes mellitus (DM) or use of insulin Signs and symptoms of hyperglycemia before admission Can also occur in type 2 DM in severe stress	History of type 2 DM (non–insulin-dependent) Signs and symptoms of hyperglycemia before admission Occurs most frequently in elderly, with preexisting renal and cardiovascular disease
Onset	Develops quickly	Develops insidiously
Clinical presentation	Flushed, dry skin Dry mucous membranes ↓ Skin turgor Tachycardia Hypotension Kussmaul's respirations Acetone breath Altered level of consciousness Visual disturbances Polydipsia Nausea and vomiting Anorexia Abdominal pain	Flushed, dry skin Dry mucous membranes ↓ Skin turgor (may not be present in elderly) Tachycardia Hypotension Shallow respirations Altered level of consciousness (generally more profound and may include absent deep tendon reflexes, paresis, and positive Babinski's sign)
Diagnostics	↑ Plasma glucose (average: 675 mg/dL) pH <7.30 ↓ Bicarbonate Ketosis Azotemia Electrolytes vary with state of hydration; often hyperkalemic Plasma hyperosmolality (average: 330 mOsm/kg)	↑ Plasma glucose (usually >1000 mg/dL) pH >7.30 Bicarbonate >15 mEq/L Absence of significant ketosis Azotemia Electrolytes vary with state of hydration; often hypernatremic Plasma hyperosmolality (Average: 350 mOsm/kg) Hypotonic urine

↑, Increased; ↓, decreased.

In DKA, the excessive production and decreased metabolism of ketone bodies result in ketonuria and loss of bicarbonate, with consequent metabolic acidosis. Nausea is an early sign of DKA and is thought to be a result of retained ketones. Increases in the rate and depth of breathing, called Kussmaul's respirations, are common as the patient attempts to compensate for the metabolic acidosis by eliminating CO_2. Acetone ("fruity") breath from fat metabolism may be noted. Later in the disease process, the respiratory status of the patient may be influenced by the neurological status, precipitating impaired breathing patterns and gas exchange. A decreased level of consciousness is also associated with the severe acidotic state (pH <7.15). The flushed face associated with DKA is the result of superficial vasodilation.

Laboratory Evaluation. Numerous diagnostic studies are used to evaluate for DKA and HHS, to rule out other diseases, and to detect complications (see Laboratory Alerts: Pancreatic Endocrine Disorders). In addition, cultures and testing are performed to determine any precipitating factors such as infection or myocardial infarction.

In DKA, an initial arterial blood gas analysis reflects metabolic acidosis (low pH and low bicarbonate). The partial pressure of arterial carbon dioxide

LABORATORY ALERTS
Pancreatic Endocrine Disorders

Laboratory Test*	Critical Value	Significance
Glucose	≥200 mg/dL (2 hours postprandial or random) >140 mg/dL (fasting) >450 mg/dL <50 mg/dL	Combined with symptoms, establishes diagnosis of diabetes mellitus Indicates crisis state; generally higher in HHS Hypoglycemia
Potassium	>6.5 mEq/L <3.0 mEq/L	Potential for heart blocks, bradydysrhythmias, sinus arrest, ventricular fibrillation, or asystole Potential for ventricular dysrhythmias
Sodium	>150 mEq/L	May be a result of stress and dehydration
BUN	>20 mg/dL	Elevated due to protein breakdown and hemoconcentration
Bicarbonate	<20 mEq/L	Decreased in DKA due to compensation for acidosis
pH	<7.3	Decreased in DKA due to accumulation of acids
Osmolality	>330 mOsm/kg H_2O	Elevated in DKA relative to dehydration, higher in HHS
Phosphorus	<2.5 mg/dL	May result in impaired respiratory and cardiac functions
Magnesium	<1.3 mEq/L	Depleted by osmotic diuresis May coincide with decreased potassium and calcium levels; may result in dysrhythmias
Beta-hydroxybutyrate	>3.0 mg/dL	Reflects blood ketosis in DKA

DKA, Diabetic ketoacidosis; *HHS*, hyperosmolar hyperglycemic state.
*Serum tests.

($PaCO_2$) may also be low, reflecting the respiratory system's compensatory mechanism. Acidosis is subsequently monitored by venous pH, which correlates well with arterial pH but is easier to obtain and process. Severe acidosis is associated with cardiovascular collapse, which can result in death.

In HHS, the laboratory results are similar to those in DKA, but with four major differences: (1) the serum glucose concentration in HHS is generally significantly more elevated, (2) plasma osmolality is higher than in DKA and is associated with the degree of dehydration, (3) acidosis is not present or very mild compared with DKA, and (4) ketosis is usually absent or very mild in comparison with DKA. Serum electrolyte concentrations may be low, normal, or elevated and generally are not reliable indicators of total body stores.

Nursing and Medical Interventions
The primary objectives in the treatment of DKA and HHS include respiratory support, fluid replacement, administration of insulin to correct hyperglycemia, replacement of electrolytes, correction of acidosis in DKA, prevention of complications, and patient teaching and support.

Each year, the American Diabetes Association publishes a supplement to *Diabetes Care* that includes its position statement on the treatment of hyperglycemic crises in patients with DM. The reader is referred to the current issue for the most recent recommendations for treating DKA and HHS. In addition, protocols may be in place for the treatment of DKA. These protocols have shown benefits in decreasing the time needed to achieve positive treatment outcomes, as well as decreasing the length of

EVIDENCE-BASED PRACTICE

PROBLEM

Tight glycemic control has been advocated in critically ill patients. Issues and outcomes of achieving glycemic control need to be identified.

QUESTION

What are the outcomes and issues associated with tight glycemic control in critical care?

REFERENCES

Parsons, P., & Watkinson, P. (2007). Blood glucose control in critical care patients—A review of the literature. *Nursing in Critical Care, 12*(4), 202-210.

Pittas, A. G., Siegel, R. D., & Lau, J. (2006). Insulin therapy and in-hospital mortality in critically ill patients: Systematic review and meta-analysis of randomized control trials. *Journal of Parenteral and Enteral Nutrition, 30*, 164-172.

Wilson, M., Wenrch, J., & Soohoo, G. W. (2007). Intensive insulin therapy in critical care. A review of 12 protocols. *Diabetes Care, 30*, 1005-1011.

EVIDENCE

Since the landmark study of Van den Berghe and colleagues in 2001 that demonstrated improved outcomes after initiation of tight glycemic control, most critical care units have implemented various protocols to achieve better glucose levels. Many research studies have been conducted, and the ones cited in this box critically appraise evidence—primarily from randomized controlled trials—on a variety of variables that have been studied. The analysis by Pittas and colleagues noted a significant reduction in hospital mortality when tight glycemic control was implemented in surgical critical care patients, and patients with diabetes. A reduction in mortality, but not a statistically significant one, was also noted in patients with acute myocardial infarction. Numerous protocols are being implemented with little agreement on the best one. Wilson and colleagues' analysis found no consensus on the protocol implementation in the areas of initiation, titration, bolus dosing, and method of adjusting the insulin. They concluded that a standardized protocol may not benefit all patients, primarily because of the variety of patient conditions and responses to treatment. Parsons and Watkinson reviewed 91 articles, including 18 randomized trials and 28 additional research studies. Their analysis identified several issues related to tight glycemic control: mortality (including long-term mortality) has not been shown to be reduced in all patient populations; infections have been shown to be reduced in some studies, but not consistently; hypoglycemia is a negative outcome associated with glycemic protocols; risks may be associated with frequent blood sampling for glucose levels; and the amount of nursing time associated with tight glycemic control is high.

IMPLICATIONS FOR NURSING

Glycemic control has become a standard of practice within critical care settings that reduces complications and mortality in some patient populations. Nurses must be aware of protocols for achieving glycemic control and assist in ensuring that target glucose levels are achieved. Assessing patients for hypoglycemia is an essential nursing implication to prevent complications associated with treatment. Nurses will likely be involved in additional research over the next several years as protocols are refined.

---

stay in the critical care unit and the hospital.[4] (See Evidence-Based Practice feature.)

Respiratory Support. Assessment of the airway, breathing, and circulation is always the first priority in managing life-threatening disorders. Airway and breathing may be supported through the use of oral airways and oxygen therapy. In more severe cases, the patient may be intubated and placed on ventilatory support. Prevention of aspiration is accomplished by elevating the head of the bed. Nasogastric tube suction may be considered in a patient with impaired mentation who is actively vomiting.

Fluid Replacement. Dehydration may have progressed to shock by the time of admission. Immediate intravenous (IV) access and rehydration need to be accomplished. In DKA, the typical water deficit approximates 100 mL/kg, and it may be as high as 200 mL/kg in HHS.[1] Monitoring for signs and symptoms of hypovolemic shock is a priority. Vital signs and neurologic status are recorded at least every hour initially. Unstable patients require constant monitoring and recording of hemodynamic parameters at least every 15 minutes. Right atrial pressure or pulmonary artery pressure monitoring may also be instituted to evaluate fluid requirements and to monitor the patient's response to treatment. This is particularly true of patients with HHS, who tend to be elderly and have concurrent cardiovascular and renal disease. Accurate intake, hourly recording of urine output, and measurement of daily weight are also essential. Changes in mentation may also indicate a change in fluid status. Ongoing assessment of neurological status can alert the nurse to a change in mentation.

Normal saline (0.9% NS) is the fluid of choice for initial fluid replacement because it best replaces extracellular fluid volume deficits. Fluid replacement usually starts with an initial bolus of 1 L of 0.9% NS. This is followed by an infusion of 10 to 20 mL/kg during the first hour.[1] IV fluids are continued at rapid rates until the patient's blood pressure and serum sodium level normalize. The IV fluid is then changed to hypotonic saline (0.45% NS) at slower rates to replace intracellular fluid deficits. The goal is generally to replace half of the estimated fluid deficit over the first 8 hours. The second half of the fluid deficit should be replaced during the next 16 hours of therapy. Serum osmolality should be normalized at a rate of no more than 3 mOsm/hr.

The goal of fluid resuscitation is normovolemia. Hypervolemia must be avoided, especially in patients with ischemic heart disease. Fluid overload from overaggressive fluid replacement can be prevented by monitoring breath sounds and performing cardiovascular assessments. Hemodynamic monitoring may be used to guide fluid resuscitation in some facilities. Signs and symptoms of fluid overload are reviewed in Box 18-7. Rapid fluid administration may also contribute to cerebral edema, a complication associated with DKA. A rapid decrease in the plasma glucose level, combined with rapid fluid administration and concurrent insulin therapy (see next section), may lead to movement of water into brain cells, resulting in brain edema.

Insulin Therapy. Replacement of insulin is definitive therapy for DKA and HHS. Before starting insulin therapy, fluid replacement therapy must be underway and the serum potassium level must be greater than 3 mEq/L. The goal is to restore normal glucose uptake by cells while preventing complications of excess insulin administration, such as hypoglycemia, hypokalemia, and hypophosphatemia. More commonly, hyperglycemic crises are treated with IV insulin infusions because absorption is more predictable. An initial IV bolus of 0.1 to 0.15 units/kg of regular insulin is administered, followed by a continuous infusion of 0.1 units/kg per hour to achieve a steady decrease in serum glucose level of 50 to 75 mg/dL per hour. Some treatment regimens may instead use subcutaneous lispro insulin dosed every hour for patients with mild to moderate DKA.

Serum glucose levels are monitored every 1 to 2 hours. One consistent method of monitoring (e.g., capillary, whole blood) must be used. As the patient's serum glucose level approaches 250 mg/dL, the primary IV solution is changed to 5% dextrose with hypotonic saline (D5 0.45% NS). The addition of dextrose allows for the continued use of insulin and prevents hypoglycemia and cerebral edema. While receiving an insulin drip, patients are generally allowed nothing by mouth. Once serum glucose levels are stabilized in a desirable range, the patient is generally managed with subcutaneous insulin based on a sliding scale, and glucose levels are monitored every 6 to 8 hours.

It is important that serum glucose levels not be lowered too rapidly, not more than 75 to 100 mg/dL per hour, to avoid the potential for cerebral edema, which could result in seizures and coma. Any patient who exhibits an abrupt change in the level of consciousness after initiation of insulin therapy requires frequent blood glucose monitoring and protective steps instituted to prevent harm, such as seizure precautions. Treatment of acute cerebral edema usually involves administration of an osmotic diuretic (e.g., 20% mannitol solution).

Electrolyte Management. Potassium, phosphate, chloride, and magnesium replacement may be required, especially during insulin administration. Osmotic diuresis in DKA and HHS results in total body potassium depletion ranging from 400 to 600 mEq. The potassium deficit may be greater in HHS. Potassium therapy is based on serum laboratory results. In the absence of renal disease, potassium replacement and monitoring should begin after the first liter of IV fluid has been administered, the serum potassium level is greater than 3 mEq/L, and the patient is excreting urine. At that point, 20 to 40 mEq of potassium, based on the serum potassium level, is usually added to each liter of fluid administered. This may be augmented by additional doses of potassium as intermittent infusions. The integrity of the IV site must be maintained to prevent extravasation. Electrocardiographic (ECG) monitoring for cardiac dysrhythmias is also important during potassium administration.

BOX 18-7 Signs and Symptoms of Fluid Overload

- Tachypnea
- Neck vein distention
- Tachycardia
- Crackles
- Increased pulmonary artery occlusion or right atrial pressures
- Declining level of consciousness in cerebral edema

Total body phosphorus levels are also depleted by osmotic diuresis. Phosphate replacement occurs when there is associated respiratory or cardiac dysfunction. Potassium phosphate can be given to treat part of the potassium deficit. Phosphate replacement is used with extreme caution in patients with renal failure because these patients are unable to excrete phosphate and typically have hyperphosphatemia.

Treatment of Acidosis. Acidosis is a hallmark feature of DKA. However, multiple studies have shown that treatment with sodium bicarbonate is not beneficial and may pose some risk to cerebral function. Therefore, sodium bicarbonate is not used to treat acidosis unless the serum pH is 7.0 or less. It is given only to bring the pH up to 7.0, but not to normal levels.[1] Even then, cautious use of sodium bicarbonate is recommended because too rapid correction of acidosis may cause central nervous system acidosis and severe hypoxemia at the cellular level. When administered, the bicarbonate is added to D5W or sterile water and is replaced slowly. Serum blood gas analysis is done frequently to assess for changes in pH, bicarbonate, anion gap, $PaCO_2$, and oxygenation status. Once fluid and electrolyte imbalances are corrected and insulin is administered, the kidneys begin to conserve bicarbonate to restore acid-base homeostasis, and ketone formation will cease.

Patient and Family Education. A primary intervention to prevent DKA is patient education. Managing blood glucose levels with diet, exercise, and medication is a priority. Monitoring of hemoglobin A_{1C} levels, also known as glycosylated or glycated hemoglobin, two to three times a year reflects the patient's long-term control of blood glucose levels. The importance of a regular eating schedule, exercise, rest, sleep, and relaxation needs to be emphasized. Adjustments to the usual diabetic control regimen for illness is known as "sick day management," and all diabetic patients and families need to be instructed in this strategy for prevention of DM complications.

Patient Outcomes

Outcomes for a patient with DKA or HHS are included the nursing care plan. See Nursing Care Plan for the Patient with Hyperglycemic Crisis.

NURSING CARE PLAN for the Patient with Hyperglycemic Crisis

NURSING DIAGNOSIS

Ineffective breathing pattern or impaired gas exchange related to acidosis (DKA), decreased level of consciousness

PATIENT OUTCOMES
Normal respiratory rate and pattern

- RR, 10-25 breaths/min
- Tidal volume >5 mL/kg
- Normal $PaCO_2$ on ABG analysis, pH WNL

NURSING INTERVENTIONS	RATIONALES
• Assess airway and breathing on admission and every 1-2 hours; correlate ABG/venous pH results with clinical examination	• Assess respiratory status; respiratory changes will stabilize as pH improves
• Provide support as needed (e.g., airway, intubation, mechanical ventilation)	• Maintain oxygenation and ventilation
• Assess neurological status every 1-2 hours	• Assess for signs of hypoxemia
• Prevent aspiration: elevate head of bed, NG tube for decompression may be needed	• Prevent aspiration

NURSING DIAGNOSIS

Deficient fluid volume related to osmotic diuresis and total body water loss, ketosis and increased lipolysis, vomiting

Continued

NURSING CARE PLAN for the Patient with Hyperglycemic Crisis—cont'd

PATIENT OUTCOMES
Adequate fluid volume status

- Normal serum glucose
- Hemodynamic stability: BP, HR, RAP, PAOP WNL
- Normal sinus rhythm
- Urine output >0.5 mL/kg/hr
- Balanced I&O
- Stable weight
- Warm, dry extremities
- Normal skin turgor
- Moist mucous membranes
- Serum electrolyte levels WNL: sodium potassium, calcium, phosphorus; osmolality WNL
- pH WNL

NURSING INTERVENTIONS	RATIONALES
• Assess fluid status: Vital signs every hour until stable I&O measurements every 1-2 hours Skin turgor, mucous membranes, thirst Consider insensible fluid losses Daily weight	• Prevent hypovolemic shock and provide data for restoring cellular function
• Initiate fluid replacement therapy: Monitor for signs and symptoms of fluid overload Monitor effects of volume repletion Monitor neurological status closely	• Correct volume deficit and prevent/treat hypovolemic shock; neurological status should improve as electrolytes normalize
• Administer IV insulin infusion per hospital protocol; titrate therapy hourly based on glucose levels	• Provide a steady decrease in serum glucose levels. A decrease of 50 to 75 mg/dL per hour is desired
• Monitor glucose every hour via consistent method (serum or fingerstick capillary) during insulin infusion	• Assess response to therapy
• Monitor for signs and symptoms of hypoglycemia	• Hypoglycemia may occur if the dose is too high
• Add dextrose to maintenance IV solutions once serum glucose level reaches 250-300 mg/dL	• Prevent relative hypoglycemia and a decrease in plasma osmolality that may result in cerebral edema
• Monitor serum electrolyte levels (sodium, potassium, calcium, phosphorus); administer supplements according to protocols; assess causes of continuing electrolyte depletion such as diuresis, vomiting, NG suction	• Prevent complications of electrolyte imbalance. Osmotic diuresis may result in increased excretion of potassium and hyponatremia. Insulin therapy causes potassium to shift to intracellular space
• Monitor pH; administration of bicarbonate may be necessary for severe acidosis	• pH is the best indicator of acidosis and response to treatment

NURSING DIAGNOSIS

Risk for ineffective therapeutic management related to lack of knowledge of disease process, treatment regimen, complications

NURSING CARE PLAN for the Patient with Hyperglycemic Crisis—cont'd

PATIENT OUTCOMES
Effective therapeutic management of diabetes

- Patient/family describe pathophysiology and causes of DKA and HHS, diet, exercise regimen, signs and symptoms of hypoglycemia and hyperglycemia, signs and symptoms of infections that require medical follow-up, sick day management
- Patient/family demonstrate self-glucose monitoring and administration of oral hypoglycemic medications and/or insulin therapy according to glucose values

NURSING INTERVENTIONS	RATIONALES
• Assess patient/family's ability to learn information and psychomotor and sensory skills.	• Identify the type and amount of information and education that is needed
• Implement a teaching program that includes information on pathophysiology and causes of DKA or HHS; diet and exercise restrictions; signs and symptoms of hypoglycemia and hyperglycemia, including interventions; and signs and symptoms of infection, including interventions.	• Provide comprehensive education to prevent complications
• Demonstrate methods for blood glucose monitoring; have the patient repeat the demonstration until proficient. If the patient takes insulin, demonstrate administration. For each skill, have the patient demonstrate abilities with repeat demonstration. Review insulin pump if used for treatment.	• Regular glucose monitoring is essential for patient self-management. Ensure patient/family ability to perform these skills related to at-home monitoring
• Review administration of hypoglycemic medications and/or insulin, including dosage, frequency, action, duration, side effects, and situations when medication may need to be adjusted.	• Facilitate adequate knowledge of medication management
• Consult with dietician regarding diabetic diet needs.	• Assist in identifying the appropriate diet based on the patient's condition and caloric needs
• Encourage patient to wear a form of identification for diabetes.	• Assist in prompt recognition and treatment of complications should they occur
• Provide written materials for all content taught; provide means for the patient to get questions answered after discharge, and schedule follow-up teaching session after discharge.	• Reinforce information taught

ABGs, Arterial blood gases; *BP*, blood pressure; *DKA*, diabetic ketoacidosis; *HHS*, hyperosmolar hyperglycemic state; *HR*, heart rate; *I&O*, intake and output; *IV*, intravenous; *NG*, nasogastric; *PaCO₂*, partial pressure of carbon dioxide in arterial blood; *PAOP*, pulmonary artery occlusion pressure; *RAP*, right atrial pressure; *RR*, respiratory rate; *WNL*, within normal limits.

Hypoglycemia

Pathophysiology

A hypoglycemic episode is defined as a decrease in the plasma glucose level to less than 70 mg/dL and is sometimes referred to as *insulin shock* or *insulin reaction*. Glucose production falls behind glucose utilization, resulting in a change in the level of consciousness. In addition, there is a rise in counter-regulatory hormones (those that work to increase blood glucose levels), including glucagon, epineph-rine, cortisol, and growth hormone. Those at highest risk are diabetic patients taking insulin, children and pregnant women with type 1 DM, and elderly persons with type 1 or type 2 DM.

Hypoglycemia unawareness is a term used to describe those diabetic patients who may not be able to recognize the onset of hypoglycemia. Those at higher risk of hypoglycemia unawareness include the elderly because of their decreased awareness of thirst, and patients with diminished mental function resulting from dementia, concurrent illness, or other factors. Patients taking beta-blockers are at risk of decreased awareness of signs of hypoglycemia because of the drug's impact on the sympathetic nervous system. The pathophysiologic mechanisms associated with acute hypoglycemia are reviewed in Figure 18-4.

Etiology

Patients receiving insulin therapy need to be closely monitored for hypoglycemia or decreased serum glucose levels, especially when the body's requirements are less than the insulin dose or when injection sites are rotated from a hypertrophied area to one with unimpaired absorption. Other causes of hypoglycemia in the hospitalized patient include insufficient caloric consumption because of a missed or delayed meal or snack, decreased intake because of nausea and vomiting, anorexia, and interrupted tube feedings or total parenteral nutrition. Recovery from stress (infections, illness) decreases requirements for exogenous insulin. Other major causes of hypoglycemia are reviewed in Box 18-8.

Patients with renal or liver dysfunction require ongoing assessment when hypoglycemic medications are necessary. Decreased degradation or excretion of hypoglycemic medications prolongs or potentiates the medication effects.

Assessment

Clinical Presentation. The most common signs and symptoms of hypoglycemia are summarized in Table 18-3. Symptoms of hypoglycemia are categorized as (1) mild symptoms from autonomic nervous system stimulation that are characteristic of a rapid decrease in serum glucose levels; and (2) moderate symptoms reflective of an inadequate supply of glucose to neural tissues, associated with a slower, more prolonged decline in serum glucose levels.

With a rapid decrease in serum glucose levels, there is activation of the sympathetic nervous system, mediated by epinephrine release from the adrenal medulla. This compensatory "fight or flight" mechanism may result in symptoms such as tachycardia; palpitations; tremors; cool, clammy skin; diaphoresis; hunger; pallor; and dilated pupils. The patient may also report feelings of apprehension, nervousness, headache, tremulousness, and general weakness.

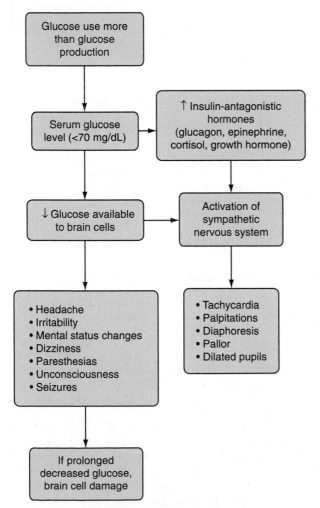

FIGURE 18-4. Pathophysiology of hypoglycemia.

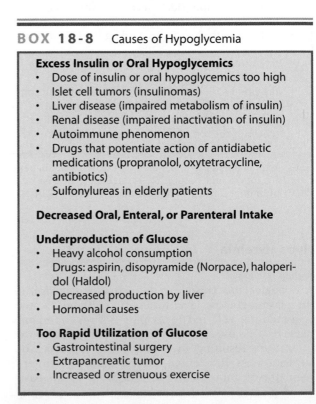

BOX 18-8   Causes of Hypoglycemia

Excess Insulin or Oral Hypoglycemics
- Dose of insulin or oral hypoglycemics too high
- Islet cell tumors (insulinomas)
- Liver disease (impaired metabolism of insulin)
- Renal disease (impaired inactivation of insulin)
- Autoimmune phenomenon
- Drugs that potentiate action of antidiabetic medications (propranolol, oxytetracycline, antibiotics)
- Sulfonylureas in elderly patients

Decreased Oral, Enteral, or Parenteral Intake

Underproduction of Glucose
- Heavy alcohol consumption
- Drugs: aspirin, disopyramide (Norpace), haloperidol (Haldol)
- Decreased production by liver
- Hormonal causes

Too Rapid Utilization of Glucose
- Gastrointestinal surgery
- Extrapancreatic tumor
- Increased or strenuous exercise

TABLE 18-3 Signs and Symptoms of Hypoglycemia

Decrease in Blood Sugar	
Rapid	**Prolonged**
Activation of Sympathetic Nervous System	***Inadequate Glucose Supply to Neural Tissues***
Nervousness	Headache
Apprehension	Restlessness
Tachycardia	Difficulty speaking
Palpitations	Difficulty thinking
Pallor	Visual disturbances
Diaphoresis	Paresthesia
Dilated pupils	Difficulty walking
Tremors	Altered consciousness
Fatigue	Coma
General weakness	Convulsions
Headache	Change in personality
Hunger	Psychiatric reactions
	Maniacal behavior
	Catatonia
	Acute paranoia

BOX 18-9 Treatment of Hypoglycemia

Mild Hypoglycemia
- Patient is completely alert. Symptoms may include pallor, diaphoresis, tachycardia, palpitations, hunger, or shakiness. Blood glucose is less than 70 mg/dL. Patient is able to drink.
- Treatment: 15 g of carbohydrate by mouth

Moderate Hypoglycemia
- Patient is conscious, cooperative, and able to swallow safely. Symptoms may include difficulty concentrating, confusion, slurred speech, or extreme fatigue. Blood glucose is usually less than 55 mg/dL. Patient is able to drink.
- Treatment: 20 to 30 g of carbohydrate by mouth

Severe Hypoglycemia
- Patient is uncooperative or unconscious. Blood glucose is usually less than 40 mg/dL **or** patient is unable to drink
- Treatment with intravenous access: 12.5 g of dextrose as $D_{50}W$
- Treatment without intravenous access: 1 mg of glucagon subcutaneously

$D_{50}W$, 50% dextrose in water.

Slower and more prolonged declines in serum glucose levels result in symptoms related to an inadequate glucose supply to neural tissues (neuroglucopenia). These include restlessness, difficulty in thinking and speaking, visual disturbances and paresthesias. The patient may have profound changes in the level of consciousness, convulsions, or both. Personality changes and psychiatric manifestations have been reported. Prolonged hypoglycemia may lead to irreversible brain damage and coma.

Laboratory Evaluation. The confirming laboratory test for hypoglycemia is a serum or capillary blood glucose level less than 70 mg/dL. The glucose level should be checked in all high-risk patients with the aforementioned clinical signs. In patients with a known history of DM, a thorough history of past experiences of hypoglycemia, including associated signs and symptoms, should be elicited during admission.

Nursing Diagnoses
The nursing diagnoses applicable to a patient with a hypoglycemic episode include the following:
- Imbalanced electrolytes related to excess circulating insulin as compared with glucose
- Disturbed thought processes related to decreased glucose to the brain
- Risk for injury (seizures) related to altered neuronal function associated with hypoglycemia
- Deficient knowledge: prevention, recognition, and treatment of hypoglycemia

Nursing and Medical Interventions
After serum or capillary glucose levels have been confirmed, carbohydrates must be administered. The patient's neurological status and ability to swallow without aspiration determine the route to be used. Box 18-9 details a protocol for treatment of mild, moderate, and severe hypoglycemia. Common food substances that contain at least 15 g of carbohydrate are listed in Box 18-10. Glucose levels should be reassessed 15 to 20 minutes after treatment. If the blood glucose level remains lower than 70 mg/dL, treatment is repeated. Ongoing assessment of vital signs and the ECG during the acute phase is also a priority.

In the event of hypoglycemia, insulin should be stopped temporarily. If the patient has an insulin pump, it should be suspended for moderate or severe hypoglycemia. The patient should determine whether to discontinue the pump for mild hypoglycemia.

Neurological assessments are done to detect any changes in cerebral function related to hypoglycemia. It is important to document baseline neurological status, including mental status, cranial nerve function, sensory and motor function, and deep

BOX 18-10   Sources of 15 Grams
of Carbohydrates

- 4 oz sweetened carbonated beverage
- 4 oz unsweetened fruit juice
- 1 cup skim milk
- Glucose gels or tablets (follow manufacturer's instructions)

tendon reflexes. There is a potential for seizure activity related to altered neuronal cellular metabolism during the hypoglycemic phase, so patients should be assessed for seizure activity. Descriptions of the seizure event and associated symptoms are important to note. Seizure precautions should be instituted, including padded side rails, oxygen, oral airway, and bedside suction, as well as removal of potentially harmful objects from the environment. Neurological status is the best clinical indicator of effective treatment for hypoglycemia.

Patient and family education about hypoglycemic episodes may also be appropriate in the critical care setting. The patient and family members need to be instructed on the causes, symptoms, treatment, and prevention of hypoglycemia. Principles regarding diet, insulin or oral hypoglycemic agents, and exercise may need to be incorporated into the teaching plan, as appropriate. Instruction on the use of home blood glucose monitoring techniques may also be needed.

Patient Outcomes

Outcomes for a patient with a hypoglycemic episode include the following:

- Normal serum or capillary glucose levels
- No signs and symptoms of hypoglycemia
- Mental status returned to baseline
- Absence of seizure activity
- Ability of the patient and family to identify causes of hypoglycemia, state symptoms of hypoglycemia, state type and amount of foods that may be used to treat hypoglycemia, and perform home blood glucose monitoring

ACUTE AND RELATIVE ADRENAL INSUFFICIENCY

Etiology

Hypofunction of the adrenal gland results from either primary or secondary mechanisms that suppress secretion of cortisol, aldosterone, and androgens.

Primary mechanisms, resulting in Addison's disease, are those that cause destruction of the adrenal gland itself. At least 90% of the adrenal cortex must be destroyed before clinical signs and symptoms appear. Primary disorders result in deficiencies of both glucocorticoids and mineralocorticoids. Primary adrenal deficiency has a variety of causes including idiopathic autoimmune destruction of the gland (most common), infection and sepsis, hemorrhagic destruction, and granulomatous infiltration such as neoplasms, amyloidosis, sarcoidosis, and hemochromatosis.

Autoimmune destruction of the adrenal gland may have a genetic component. The disease results in hypofunction and eventual atrophy of the gland. This form of adrenal disease may affect just the adrenal gland or may be part of a constellation of autoimmune problems, such as Hashimoto's thyroiditis or pernicious anemia. Young women with spontaneous premature ovarian failure are at increased risk of developing the autoimmune form of adrenal insufficiency.[11]

Addison's disease, a primary adrenal insufficiency, is a less common cause of adrenal insufficiency. In approximately 50% to 70% of Addison's cases, damage to the adrenal gland is a result of idiopathic autoimmune destruction. Tuberculosis, now a rare cause of adrenal insufficiency in the United States, can play a role in countries where it is endemic.

Secondary mechanisms that can produce adrenal insufficiency are those that decrease adrenocorticotropic hormone (ACTH, also called corticotropin) secretion or simply suppress normal secretion of corticosteroids. These generally result in deficiencies of only glucocorticoids, because stimulation of the mineralocorticoids is not primarily dependent on ACTH secretion. Mechanisms that can produce secondary adrenal insufficiency include long-term steroid use, pituitary and hypothalamic disorders, infection, and sepsis. A more detailed listing of possible causes of primary and secondary adrenal insufficiency is given in Box 18-11.

The most common cause of acute adrenal insufficiency is withdrawal from corticosteroid therapy. Corticosteroids are used in the treatment of various inflammatory, allergic, and immunoreactive disorders (Box 18-12). Long-term corticosteroid use suppresses the normal corticotropin-releasing hormone (CRH)-ACTH-adrenal feedback systems (see Figure 18-1) and can result in adrenal suppression. It is difficult to predict accurately the degree of adrenal suppression in patients receiving exogenous glucocorticoid therapy. Longer-acting agents such as dexamethasone are more likely to produce suppression than are shorter-acting corticosteroids such as hydrocortisone. Once corticosteroid use has been tapered off, it may take several months for these patients to

BOX 18-11   Causes of Adrenal Insufficiency

Primary

- *Autoimmune disease:* idiopathic and polyglandular
- *Granulomatous disease:* tuberculosis, sarcoidosis, histoplasmosis, blastomycosis
- Cancer
- *Hemorrhagic destruction:* anticoagulation, trauma, sepsis
- *Infectious:* meningococcal, staphylococcal, pneumococcal, fungal (candidiasis), cytomegalovirus
- Acquired immunodeficiency syndrome
- *Drugs:* ketoconazole, aminoglutethimide, trimethoprim, etomidate, 5-fluorouracil (suppress adrenals); phenytoin, barbiturates, rifampin (increase steroid degradation)
- Irradiation
- Adrenalectomy
- Developmental or genetic abnormality

Secondary

- Long-term glucocorticoid use
- Pituitary tumors, hemorrhage, radiation, metastatic cancer, lymphoma, leukemia
- Systemic inflammatory states: sepsis, vasculitis, sickle cell anemia
- Infiltrative disorders
- Postpartum hemorrhage (Sheehan's syndrome)
- Trauma, especially head trauma, or surgery
- Hypothalamic disorders

BOX 18-12   Therapeutic Uses of Corticosteroids

Replacement Therapy in Patients with Primary or Secondary Adrenal Cortical Insufficiency

Symptomatic Treatment of Inflammatory, Allergic, or Immunological Disorders, Including the Following:

- *Rheumatic:* rheumatoid arthritis, osteoarthritis, acute gouty arthritis, ankylosing spondylitis, systemic lupus erythematosus
- *Allergic:* allergic rhinitis, bronchial asthma, dermatitis, serum sickness, drug hypersensitivity, anaphylactic shock
- *Ophthalmic:* conjunctivitis, keratitis, iritis, uveitis, acute optic neuritis, chorioretinitis, allergic corneal marginal ulcers
- *Gastrointestinal:* ulcerative colitis, Crohn's disease, chronic active hepatitis
- *Hematological/neoplastic:* thrombocytopenic purpura, hemolytic anemia, leukemia, Hodgkin's disease, multiple myeloma
- *Other:* nephrotic syndrome, gout, hypercalcemia, multiple sclerosis, tuberculosis, meningitis

Supportive Use in Acute Disorders, Including the Following:

- Septic shock
- *Neurological emergencies* (to treat cerebral edema): head trauma, cerebral hypoxia, tumors, hemorrhage, infection
- *Pulmonary disorders:* asthma, chronic bronchitis, adult respiratory distress syndrome

resume normal secretion of corticosteroids. Thus, it is important to be familiar with disorders that may be treated with corticosteroids, because the resulting adrenal suppression may prevent a normal stress response in these patients and may put them at risk of an adrenal crisis.

Infection, sepsis, or both are among the most common causes of adrenal insufficiency in the critical care setting. Sepsis and septic shock can cause thrombotic necrosis of the gland.[9] Hemorrhagic destruction of the adrenal gland has been reported with anticoagulation therapy, after surgical procedures, and during infection. Anticoagulation therapy with heparin can cause selective hypoaldosteronism and, more rarely, cases of hemorrhage resulting in both mineralocorticoid and glucocorticoid deficiencies. A common complication of meningococcal meningitis is massive adrenal hemorrhage, which can result in lethal adrenal insufficiency.

Adrenal crisis can be precipitated in any patient with chronic adrenal insufficiency by providing inadequate hormone replacement during times of acute stress such as infection, trauma, major surgery, or after sudden withdrawal of corticosteroids in a patient receiving long-term therapy. Administration of the drug etomidate to facilitate endotracheal intubation is associated with significant but temporary adrenal dysfunction and increased mortality.[13]

The concept of relative adrenal insufficiency has been debated for several years. It has long been recognized that sepsis and septic shock are hypermetabolic states where cortisol levels normally increase by as much as 10-fold over baseline. Patients with an inadequate physiological response to the demands of this hypermetabolic state have an increased mortality rate. The degree of response and how to best measure the patient's response continue to be investigated.[2]

Review of Physiology

Persons who have suppression or an absolute lack of secretion of corticosteroids are candidates for an adrenal crisis, which represents a life-threatening endocrine emergency. The manifestations of adrenal crisis result from insufficient secretion by the adrenal cortex of glucocorticoids (primarily cortisol), mineralocorticoids (primarily aldosterone), or both. The deficiency of glucocorticoids is especially significant because their influence on the defense mechanisms of the body and its response to stress makes them essential for life. An insufficiency of adrenal androgens may also exist, but the manifestations are not clinically significant.

Cortisol, which is the strongest of the glucocorticoids synthesized by the adrenal cortex, is normally released in response to stimulation by ACTH from the anterior pituitary gland (see Figure 18-1). ACTH is stimulated by CRH from the hypothalamus, which is influenced by circulating cortisol levels, circadian rhythms, and stress. Circadian rhythms affect ACTH, and thus cortisol levels, diurnally, creating peak levels of cortisol in the morning and the lowest levels around midnight. This normal rhythm can be overridden by stress. During stress, plasma cortisol may increase as much as 10 times its normal level. Increased release of cortisol increases the blood glucose concentration by promoting glycogen breakdown and gluconeogenesis in the liver, increases lipolysis and free fatty acid production, increases protein degradation, and inhibits the inflammatory and immune responses. The hemodynamic changes of hypertension, vasoconstriction, and tachycardia also occur. Additional effects are summarized in Box 18-13.

Mineralocorticoids regulate the body's electrolyte and water balance in the renal tubules. Aldosterone is the most important of the mineralocorticoids synthesized by the adrenal cortex. Secretion of aldosterone is regulated primarily by the renin-angiotensin system. Renin is an enzyme stored in the cells of the juxtaglomerular apparatus in the kidneys. Its release occurs in response to sodium levels in the distal tubule, which are influenced by plasma sodium, increased plasma potassium levels, decreased extracellular fluid volume, decreased blood pressure, and decreased sympathetic nerve activity. Once released, renin cleaves with angiotensinogen in the plasma to form angiotensin I. Angiotensin I is then converted to angiotensin II in the lungs under the influence of angiotensin-converting enzyme. Angiotensin II stimulates the secretion of aldosterone by the adrenal cortex while causing vasoconstriction of the arterioles. Aldosterone acts in the kidneys on the ascending loop of Henle, the distal convoluted tubule, and the collecting ducts to increase sodium ion reabsorption and to increase potassium and hydrogen ion excretion. Because reabsorption of sodium creates an osmotic gradient across the renal tubular

---

BOX 18-13   Physiological Effects of Glucocorticoids (Cortisol)

- *Protein metabolism:* promotes gluconeogenesis, stimulates protein breakdown, and inhibits protein synthesis
- *Fat metabolism:* ↑ lipolysis and free fatty acid production, promotes fat deposits in face and cervical area
- *Opposes action of insulin:* ↓ glucose transport and utilization in cells
- *Inhibits inflammatory response:*
  - Suppresses mediator release (kinins, histamine, interleukins, prostaglandins, leukotrienes, serotonin)
  - Stabilizes cell membrane and inhibits capillary dilation
  - ↓ Formation of edema
  - Inhibits leukocyte migration and phagocytic activity
- *Immunosuppression:*
  - ↓ Proliferation of T lymphocytes and killer cell activity
  - ↓ Complement production and immunoglobulins
- ↑ Circulating erythrocytes
- *Gastrointestinal effects:* ↑ appetite; increases rate of acid and pepsin secretion in stomach
- ↑ Uric acid excretion
- ↓ Serum calcium
- Sensitizes arterioles to effects of catecholamines; maintains blood pressure
- ↑ Renal glomerular filtration rate and excretion of water

↑, Increases; ↓, decreases.

---

membrane, antidiuretic hormone (ADH) is activated, causing water to be reabsorbed with sodium. The physiology of aldosterone release is summarized in Figure 18-5.

Pathophysiology

Acute adrenal insufficiency is produced by an absolute or relative lack of cortisol (glucocorticoid) and aldosterone (mineralocorticoid). A deficiency of cortisol results in decreased production of glucose, decreased metabolism of protein and fat, decreased appetite, decreased intestinal motility and digestion, decreased vascular tone, and diminished effects of catecholamines. If a patient with deficient cortisol is stressed, this deficiency can produce profound shock because of significant decreases in vascular tone and the diminished effects of catecholamines.[6]

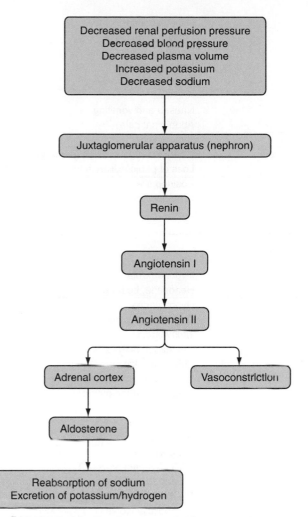

FIGURE 18-5. Physiology of aldosterone release.

BOX 18-14   Risk Factor Analysis
for Adrenal Crisis

Assess carefully for patients who are at risk, have predisposing factors, or have physical findings associated with chronic adrenal insufficiency. Risk factors include:

- *Drug history:* steroids in the past year, phenytoin, barbiturates, rifampin
- *Illness history:* infection, cancer, autoimmune disease, diseases treated with steroids, radiation to head or abdomen, human immunodeficiency virus–positive status
- *Family history:* autoimmune disease, Addison's disease
- *Nutrition:* weight loss, decreased appetite
- *Miscellaneous:* fatigue, dizziness, weakness, darkening of skin, low blood glucose that does not respond to therapy, salt craving (dramatic craving such as drinking pickle juice or eating salt from the shaker)

Deficiency of aldosterone results in decreased retention of sodium and water, decreased circulating volume, and increased potassium and hydrogen ion reabsorption. These effects are seen in patients with underlying primary adrenal insufficiency but not secondary adrenal insufficiency (decreased ACTH), because aldosterone secretion is not primarily dependent on ACTH. A summary of pathophysiological effects of adrenal insufficiency can be found in Figure 18-6.

Assessment

Clinical Presentation

Acute adrenal crisis requires astute and rapid data collection. Box 18-14 gives a risk factor analysis for adrenal crisis. Features of adrenal crisis are nonspecific and may be attributed to other medical

disorders. Signs and symptoms vary, as shown in Figure 18-6. Because this condition is a medical emergency, the diagnosis should be considered in any patient acutely ill with fever, vomiting, hypotension, shock, decreased serum sodium level, increased serum potassium level, or hypoglycemia (see Laboratory Alerts: Adrenal Disorders). Specific system disturbances are widespread.

Cardiovascular System. Cardiovascular signs and symptoms in acute adrenal crisis are related to hypovolemia (decreased water reabsorption), decreased vascular tone (decreased effectiveness of catecholamines), and hyperkalemia. The most common presentation of adrenal insufficiency in the intensive care unit is hypotension refractory to fluids and requiring vasopressors. The patient may also have symptoms of decreased cardiac output; weak, rapid pulse; dysrhythmias; and cold, pale skin. The chest x-ray study may show decreased heart size. Changes in the ECG may result if the degree of hyperkalemia is significant. With mild hyperkalemia, these changes include narrow and taller T waves with a shortened QT interval, whereas with severe hyperkalemia (levels ≥6.0 mEq/L), a depressed ST segment, a prolonged PR interval, and a widened QRS complex may be seen. Hypovolemia and vascular dilation may be severe enough in crisis to cause hemodynamic collapse and shock.

Neurological System. Neurological manifestations in acute adrenal crisis are related to decreases in glucose levels, protein metabolism, volume and perfusion, and sodium concentrations. Patients may complain

			Hypoglycemia
		Decreased production of glucose, metabolism of protein and fat, and appetite	Fatigue, weakness
			Confusion, listlessness
			Lethargy, apathy
			Tachycardia, sweating
Primary and secondary	Lack of cortisol	Decreased intestinal motility/digestion	Anorexia
			Nausea and vomiting
			Abdominal pain
		Decreased vascular tone	Hypotension
		Increased secretion of MSH/decreased androgens	Increased pigmentation (primary)
			Loss of pubic/axillary hair
		Stimulation of lymphoid tissue	Eosinophilia
			Lymphocytosis

			Hyponatremia
		Decreased sodium retention	Headache, Lethargy
		Decreased water retention	Hypovolemia
			Decreased cardiac output
			Tachycardia
			Decreased heart size
Primary only	Lack of aldosterone		Cold, pale skin
			Weak, rapid pulse
			Decreased urine output
			Elevated BUN
			Hypercalcemia
			Hyperuricemia
		Increased potassium reabsorption	Hyperkalemia
			ECG changes: peaked T, long PR, widened QRS
			Dysrhythmias
		Increased hydrogen ion reabsorption	Metabolic acidosis

FIGURE 18-6. Pathophysiological effects of adrenal insufficiency. *BUN,* Blood urea nitrogen; *ECG,* electrocardiogram; *MSH,* melanocyte-stimulating hormone.

of headache, fatigue that worsens as the day progresses, and severe weakness. They may also suffer from mental confusion, listlessness, lethargy, apathy, psychoses, and emotional lability.

Gastrointestinal System. The gastrointestinal signs and symptoms in acute adrenal crisis are related to decreased digestive enzymes and to decreased intestinal motility and digestion. Anorexia, nausea, vomiting, diarrhea, and vague abdominal pain are present in the majority of patients.[7]

Genitourinary System. Decreased circulation to the kidneys from diminished circulating volume and hypotension causes decreases in the glomerular filtration rate and in renal perfusion. Urine output may decline as a result.

Box 18-15 lists the signs associated with progressive onset of chronic adrenal insufficiency.

BOX 18-15   Progressive Signs of Chronic Adrenal Insufficiency

- Weakness
- Fatigue
- Weight loss
- Anorexia, nausea, vomiting
- Abdominal pain
- Hyperpigmentation, especially in the mucous membranes, in scars, and over joints, related to the increased secretion of melanocyte-stimulating hormone that occurs with increases in adrenocorticotropic hormone (corticotropin) secretion
- Loss of pubic and axillary hair related to decreased levels of adrenal androgens

Laboratory Evaluation

Laboratory findings in a patient with acute adrenal crisis include hypoglycemia, hyponatremia, hyperkalemia, eosinophilia, increased BUN level, and metabolic acidosis. Hypercalcemia or hyperuricemia is possible as a result of volume depletion (see Laboratory Alerts: Adrenal Disorders).

The diagnosis of adrenal insufficiency is made by evaluating plasma cortisol levels. These levels vary diurnally in healthy individuals, but this pattern is lost in the critically ill, making the timing of the test unimportant.

Primary and secondary adrenal insufficiency are diagnosed by cortisol levels less than 18 to 20 mg/dL. Differentiating between primary and secondary adrenal insufficiency is accomplished by evaluating serum ACTH levels (elevated in primary insufficiency, normal or decreased in secondary insufficiency).

The diagnosis of relative adrenal insufficiency is less clear. The normal cortisol response to acute illness is a significant increase from baseline. A "normal" cortisol level in a critically ill patient may actually be abnormal and indicate an inadequate response. Because these tests are difficult to interpret, corticosteroid replacement should begin as soon as insufficiency is suspected. Dexamethasone is the only corticosteroid that does interfere with the next test to be done, a cosyntropin (a synthetic ACTH, Cortrosyn) stimulation test. The technique for performing this test is outlined in Box 18-16. The test determines baseline levels as well as response to stimulation. The standard cosyntropin stimulation test uses a dose of 250 mcg, while other regimens use a dose of 1 mcg. Results have been similar with both doses; however, additional research is needed to determine whether the 1-mcg dose should become the standard.[8,22] Regardless of the dose, the expected response is a minimal increase in cortisol level of 7 to 9 mcg/dL. A patient whose cortisol level does not increase by this amount from baseline is deemed a nonresponder and is seen to have an increased risk of mortality.[13]

Nursing Diagnoses

The nursing diagnoses that may apply to a patient with acute adrenal crisis based on the assessment data include the following:
- Deficient fluid volume related to deficiency of aldosterone hormone (mineralocorticoid) and decreased sodium and water retention

LABORATORY ALERTS
Adrenal Disorders

Laboratory Test	Critical Value	Significance
Serum		
Glucose	<50 mg/dL	Hypoglycemia
Cortisol	<10 mcg/dL	In severely ill patient or stressed patient, indicates insufficiency
Potassium	>6.6 mEq/L	Potential for heart blocks, bradydysrhythmias, sinus arrest, ventricular fibrillation, or asystole
	<3.0 mEq/L	Potential for ventricular dysrhythmias
Sodium	>150 mEq/L	May be a result of stress and dehydration
	<130 mEq/L	Resulting from hydration therapy
BUN	>20 mg/dL	↑ From protein breakdown and hemoconcentration
pH	<7.3	↓ From accumulation of acids and dehydration

↑, Increased; ↓, decreased; *BUN*, blood urea nitrogen.

BOX 18-16   Cosyntropin Stimulation Test

Standard Method
- Obtain baseline serum cortisol level
- Administer cosyntropin, 250 mcg IV (synthetic ACTH)
- Obtain serum cortisol level 30 and 60 minutes after cosyntropin

In emergency situations before and during testing, may treat with dexamethasone (Decadron), 2 to 8 mg IV (will not interfere with cortisol levels)

Test Response
An inability to raise cortisol levels to the following indicates adrenal insufficiency (AI):
- Primary/secondary AI: a total level >20 mcg/dL and/or a change from baseline of >7 mcg/dL
- Relative AI: a change from baseline >9 mcg/dL regardless of level

ACTH, Adrenocorticotropic hormone (corticotropin); *IV*, intravenously.

- Ineffective tissue perfusion related to cortisol deficiency, resulting in decreased vascular tone and decreased effectiveness of catecholamines
- Disturbed thought processes related to decreased glucose levels, decreased protein metabolism, decreased perfusion, and decreased sodium levels
- Imbalanced nutrition (less than body requirements) related to cortisol deficiency and resultant decreased metabolism of protein and fats, decreased appetite, and decreased intestinal motility and digestion
- Deficient knowledge: proper long-term corticosteroid management
- Activity intolerance related to use of endogenous protein for energy needs and loss of skeletal muscle mass as evidenced by early fatigue, weakness, and exertional dyspnea

Nursing and Medical Interventions

Adrenal crisis requires immediate recognition and intervention if the patient is to survive. Primary objectives in the treatment of adrenal crisis include identifying and treating the precipitating cause, replacing fluid and electrolytes, replacing hormones, and educating the patient and family.

Fluid and Electrolyte Replacement
Fluid losses should be replaced with an infusion of 5% dextrose and NS until signs and symptoms of hypovolemia stabilize. This not only reverses the volume deficit but also provides glucose to minimize the hypoglycemia. The patient may need as much as 5 L of fluid in the first 12 to 24 hours to maintain an adequate blood pressure and urine output and to replace the fluid deficit.

Hyperkalemia frequently responds to volume expansion and glucocorticoid replacement and may require no further treatment. In fact, the patient may become hypokalemic during therapy and may require potassium replacement. The acidosis also usually corrects itself with volume expansion and glucocorticoid replacement. However, if the pH is less than 7.1 or the bicarbonate level is less than 10 mEq/L, the patient may require sodium bicarbonate.

Hormonal Replacement
If adrenal insufficiency has not been previously diagnosed and the patient's condition is unstable, dexamethasone phosphate (Decadron), 4 mg by IV push, then 4 mg every 8 hours, is given until the cosyntropin test has been done. This drug does not significantly cross-react with cortisol in the assay for cortisol and therefore can be administered to patients pending adrenal testing results.

Initially, glucocorticoid replacement is the most important type of hormonal replacement. Hydrocortisone sodium succinate (Solu-Cortef) is the drug of choice because it has both glucocorticoid and mineralocorticoid activities in high doses. After a bolus dose, IV doses are administered for at least 24 hours or until the patient has stabilized. Cortisone acetate may be given intramuscularly if the IV route is not available.

Once the patient improves, the dose of hydrocortisone is decreased 10% to 20% daily until a maintenance dose is achieved. The patient can be switched to oral replacement once oral intake is resumed. At lower doses (<100 mg/day of hydrocortisone), a patient with primary adrenal insufficiency may also require mineralocorticoid replacement. Fludrocortisone, 0.1 to 0.2 mg daily, is then added. A nutritional consideration if the patient is experiencing excessive sweating or diarrhea would be to increase sodium intake to 15 mEq/day. Table 18-4 describes the drugs used in the treatment of acute adrenal crisis. Box 18-17

BOX 18-17   Treatment of Adrenal Crisis

Identify and Treat Precipitating Event

Replace Fluid and Electrolytes
- Give 5% dextrose in normal saline until hypotension improves
- Acidemia usually corrects with volume expansion; if pH < 7.1, bicarbonate <10 mEq/L, give sodium bicarbonate
- Hyperkalemia responds to volume expansion and glucocorticoids

Hormonal Replacement
- Hydrocortisone (Solu-Cortef), 100 mg IV immediately; then 100 mg every 8 hours
- Cortisone acetate, 50 mg IM every 12 hours (in case IV route is faulty)
- Continue IV replacement at least 24 to 48 hours after recovery from acute phase
- After stabilized, decrease hydrocortisone dose 10% to 20% daily until maintenance dose reached (25.0-37.5 mg/day)
- When dose <100-150 mg/day, add fludrocortisone acetate (oral mineralocorticoid)

Patient Education
- Identification bracelet
- Awareness of signs and symptoms of insufficiency
- Doubling dose with minor stress

Doses are approximate and may vary based on the individual situation.
IM, Intramuscuar; *IV*, intravenous.

PHARMACOLOGY

TABLE 18-4 Medications Used to Treat Adrenal Crisis

Medication	Action/Uses	Dosage/Route	Side Effects	Nursing Implications
Hydrocortisone sodium succinate (Solu-Cortef)	Same as cortisol Antiinflammatory and immunosuppressive effects Salt-retaining (mineralocorticoid) effects in high doses	Individualized: adrenal crisis: 100 mg IV bolus; 50-100 mg every 6-8 hours	Vertigo, headache, insomnia, menstrual abnormalities, fluid and electrolyte imbalance, hypertension, HF, peptic ulcers, nausea and vomiting, immunosuppression, impaired wound healing, increased serum glucose levels, cushingoid state	Institute prophylaxis against GI bleeding Be aware of multiple drug-drug interactions, especially with IV route: oral contraceptives, phenytoin, digoxin, phenobarbital, theophylline, insulin, anticoagulants, salicylates Avoid abrupt discontinuation Monitor serum glucose and electrolyte levels Watch for signs of fluid overload Observe for signs of infection (may mask) Maintain adequate nutrition to avoid catabolic effects Provide meticulous mouth care
Cortisone acetate (Cortone)	Same as hydrocortisone	Individualized: adrenal crisis: 50 mg IM every 12 hours	Same as hydrocortisone	Same as for hydrocortisone
Dexamethasone (Decadron)	Has only glucocorticoid effects	Individualized doses PO, IM, IV	Same as hydrocortisone	Same as for hydrocortisone
Fludrocortisone acetate (Florinef)	Increases sodium reabsorption in renal tubules and increases potassium, water, and hydrogen loss	0.05-0.2 mg/day PO	Increased blood volume, edema, hypertension, HF, headaches, weakness of extremities	Assess for signs of fluid overload, HF Monitor serum sodium and potassium levels Use only in conjunction with glucocorticoids Restrict sodium intake if the patient has edema or fluid overload Not used to treat acute crisis; added as glucocorticoid dose is decreased

GI, Gastrointestinal; *HF,* heart failure; *IM,* intramuscular; *IV,* intravenous; *PO,* orally.

contains a summary of the treatment of adrenal crisis.

Patient and Family Education

In a patient with known adrenal insufficiency and/or receiving corticosteroid therapy, adrenal crisis is preventable. Education of patients, family, and significant others is the key to prevention.

THYROID GLAND IN CRITICAL CARE

Review of Physiology

Thyroid hormones play a role in regulating the function of all body systems. Box 18-18 lists some of the physiological effects of thyroid hormones. The

BOX 18-18   Physiological Effect of Thyroid Hormones

Major Effects
- ↑ Metabolic activities of all tissues
- ↑ Rate of nutrient use/oxygen consumption for ATP production
- ↑ Rate of growth
- ↑ Activities of other endocrine glands

Other Effects
- Regulate protein synthesis and catabolism
- Regulate body heat production and dissipation
- ↑ Gluconeogenesis and utilization of glucose
- Maintain appetite and gastrointestinal motility
- Maintain calcium metabolism
- Stimulate cholesterol synthesis
- Maintain cardiac rate, contractility, and output
- Affect respiratory rate, oxygen utilization, and carbon dioxide formation
- Affect red blood cell production
- Affect central nervous system development and cerebration
- Are necessary for muscle tone and vigor and normal skin constituents

↑, Increase; ↓, decrease.

thyroid hormones thyroxine (T_4) and triiodothyronine (T_3) are secreted by the thyroid gland under the influence of the anterior pituitary gland via secretion of thyroid-stimulating hormone (TSH, also thyrotropin), which in turn is influenced by thyroid-releasing hormone (TRH, also called thyrotropin-releasing hormone) from the hypothalamus. Thyroid hormones are highly bound to globulin, T_4-binding prealbumin, and albumin. Only the unbound (or free) fraction of the circulating hormone is biologically active. Regulation of these hormones occurs via positive and negative feedback mechanisms (Figure 18-7).

T_4 accounts for more than 95% of circulating thyroid hormone, but half of all thyroid activity comes from T_3. T_3 is five times more potent, acts more quickly, and enters cells more easily than T_4. T_3 is derived from conversion of T_4 in nonthyroid tissue by three iodothyronine deiodinases, known as D1, D2, and D3. These iodothyronine deiodinases also convert T_3 into reverse T_3 (rT_3), an inactive metabolite.[17] Certain conditions and drugs can block the conversion of T_4 to T_3, creating a potential thyroid imbalance. Possible causes for blocked conversion are listed in Box 18-19.

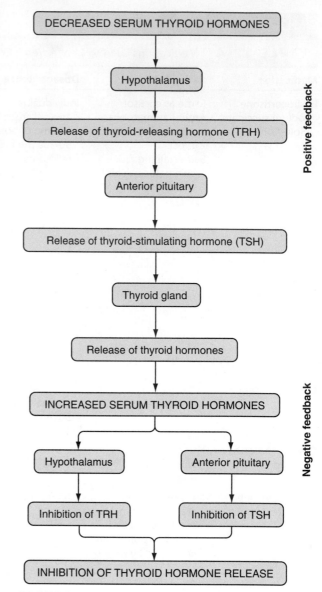

FIGURE 18-7. Feedback systems for thyroid hormone regulation.

BOX 18-19   Causes of Blockage of Conversion from Thyroxine to Triiodothyronine

- *Severe illness:* chronic renal failure, cancer, chronic liver disease
- Trauma
- Malnutrition, fasting
- *Drugs:* glucocorticoids, propranolol (Inderal), propylthiouracil, amiodarone
- Radiopaque dyes
- Acidosis

Effects of Aging

With aging, thyroid function declines. Hypothyroidism occurs in the elderly, frequently with an insidious onset. The decrease in energy level; the feeling of being cold; the dry, flaky skin; and other signs are often mistakenly assumed to be part of aging, whereas they may be signs of decreased thyroid function. Thyroid function should be assessed in any elderly patient with a "sluggish" response to treatments.

Thyroid Function in the Critically Ill

During critical illness, stress-related changes occur in thyroid hormone balance. Initially, there is a decrease in plasma T_3 levels and an increase in rT_3 levels, known as *low T_3 syndrome* or *euthyroid sick syndrome*. These changes are thought to result from alterations in the peripheral metabolism of thyroid hormones and to be an adaptation to severe illness in which the body attempts to reduce energy expenditure.[17] Generally, these changes are considered to be beneficial and do not require intervention. Within approximately 3 days, T_3 levels return to low-normal levels. In severe illness, T_4 levels may also decrease.[15]

In the chronically critically ill, additional thyroid hormone changes occur. Both T_3 and T_4 levels are reduced as is pulsatile TSH secretion. The changes in chronic critical illness are not well understood but are thought to also include central neuroendocrine dysfunction.[6,17,27] Low T_4 levels may serve as a poor prognostic indicator for patient recovery.

THYROID CRISES

Like adrenal insufficiency, thyroid disorders that have been previously diagnosed and adequately treated do not generally result in crisis states. However, if patients with thyroid disorders, especially undiagnosed thyroid disorders, are stressed either physiologically or psychologically, the results can be life-threatening. Hyperthyroidism must be explored as a causative factor in new-onset, otherwise unexplained rapid heart rates.

Etiology

Hyperthyroidism is a common and usually benign illness. The most frequent form of hyperthyroidism is *toxic diffuse goiter*, also known as *Graves' disease*. It occurs most frequently in young (third or fourth decade), previously healthy women. A family history of hyperthyroidism is often present. Graves' disease is an autoimmune disease, and affected patients have abnormal thyroid-stimulating immunoglobulins that cause thyroid inflammation, diffuse enlargement, and hyperplasia of the gland.

Toxic multinodular goiter is the second most common cause of hyperthyroidism. It also occurs more commonly in women, but these patients are generally older (fourth to seventh decades). Crises in patients with toxic multinodular goiter are more commonly associated with heart failure or severe muscle weakness.

Hyperthyroidism can also occur secondary to exposure to radiation, interferon-alpha therapy for viral hepatitis, and other events. Administration of amiodarone, a heavily iodinated compound, can result in either hyperthyroidism or hypothyroidism.[18] These and other possible causes of hyperthyroidism are listed in Box 18-20.

Low levels of thyroid hormones also disrupt the normal physiology of most body systems. Hypothyroidism produces a hypodynamic, hypometabolic state. *Myxedema coma* is a magnification of these disruptions initiated by some type of stressor. This condition takes many months to develop and should be suspected in patients with known hypothyroid-

---

BOX 18-20   Causes of Hyperthyroidism

Most Common
- Toxic diffuse goiter (Graves' disease)
- Toxic multinodular goiter
- Toxic uninodular goiter

Other Causes
- Factitious hyperthyroidism
- Triiodothyronine
- Exogenous iodine in patient with preexisting thyroid disease: exposure to iodine load from radiographic contrast dyes, medications (amiodarone)
- Thyroiditis (transient)
- Postpartum thyroiditis

Rare Causes
- Toxic thyroid adenoma—more common in the elderly
- Metastatic thyroid cancer
- Malignancies with circulating thyroid stimulators
- Pituitary tumors producing thyroid-stimulating hormone (thyrotropin)
- Acromegaly

Associated with Other Disorders*
- Pernicious anemia, idiopathic Addison's disease, myasthenia gravis, sarcoidosis, Albright's syndrome

*The presence of these disorders in a patient in crisis increases the likelihood that the patient has hyperthyroidism.

ism, with a surgical scar on the lower neck, or in those who are unusually sensitive to medications or narcotics.

The underlying causes of myxedema coma are those that produce hypothyroidism. Most cases occur either in patients with long-standing autoimmune disease of the thyroid (Hashimoto's thyroiditis) or in patients who have received surgical or radioactive iodine treatment for Graves' disease and have received inadequate hormone replacement. Only approximately 5% of adults have hypothyroidism as a result of a pituitary (secondary) or hypothalamic (tertiary) disorder. These and other less common causes of hypothyroidism are listed in Box 18-21.

Thyrotoxic Crisis (Thyroid Storm)

Pathophysiology

Thyroid storm occurs in untreated or inadequately treated patients with hyperthyroidism; it is rare in patients with normal thyroid gland function. The crisis is often precipitated by stress related to an underlying illness, general anesthesia, surgery, or infection. As thyroid hormones play a major role in regulating most body systems, uncontrolled hyperthyroidism produces a hyperdynamic, hypermetabolic state that results in disruption of many major body functions. Mortality is more often the

---

BOX 18-21 Causes of Hypothyroidism

Primary Thyroid Disease
- Autoimmune (Hashimoto's thyroiditis)
- Radioactive iodine treatment of Graves' disease
- Thyroidectomy
- Congenital enzymatic defect in thyroid hormone biosynthesis
- Inhibition of thyroid hormone synthesis or release
- Antithyroid drugs
- Iodides
- Amiodarone
- Lithium carbonate
- Oral hypoglycemic agents
- Dopamine
- Idiopathic thyroid atrophy

Secondary (Pituitary) or Tertiary (Hypothalamus) Disease
- Tumors
- Infiltrative disease (sarcoidosis)
- Hypophysectomy
- Pituitary irradiation
- Head injury
- Cerebrovascular accidents
- Pituitary infarction

---

result of the underlying illness rather than the thyrotoxic state.

Thyroid storm is a rare emergency that can result in death within 48 hours without treatment. The specific mechanism that produces thyroid storm is unknown but includes high levels of circulating thyroid hormones, an enhanced cellular response to those hormones, and hyperactivity of the sympathetic nervous system. Certain enzymes may be the key to the dramatic increase in metabolic rate that occurs in thyroid storm. Thyroid hormones normally increase the synthesis of enzymes that stimulate cellular mitochondria and energy production. When excess thyroid hormones are present, the increased activity of these enzymes produces excessive thermal energy and fever. It is believed that the rapidity with which hormone levels rise may be more important than the absolute levels.

Assessment

Clinical Presentation The excess thyroid hormone activity of hyperthyroidism affects the body in many ways. Box 18-22 gives signs associated with hyperthyroidism. Common findings in patients with thyroid storm, their significance, and the actions nurses can take to address each of these findings are listed in Table 18-5.

Thyroid storm has an abrupt onset and is best characterized as a state of unregulated hypermetabolism. The most prominent clinical features of thyroid storm are severe fever, marked tachycardia, heart failure, tremors, delirium, stupor, and coma. Untreated patients die in 1 to 2 days of extreme hyperpyrexia and cardiovascular collapse.

The patient's ability to survive thyroid storm is determined by the severity of the hyperthyroid state and the patient's general health. The severity of the hyperthyroid state is not necessarily indicated by the serum levels of thyroid hormones but rather by tissue and organ responsiveness to the hormones.

Thermoregulation Disturbances. Temperature regulation is lost. The patient's body temperature may be as high as 106°F (41.1°C). The increase in heat production and metabolic end products also causes the blood vessels of the skin to dilate. This enhances oxygen and nutrient delivery to the peripheral tissues and accounts for the patient's warm, moist skin.

Neurological Disturbances. Thyroid hormones normally maintain central nervous system cerebration. Excess thyroid hormones cause hypermetabolism and increased cerebration, resulting in hyperactivity of the nervous system both psychologically and physiologically. Thyroid storm may be heralded by agitation, delirium, psychosis, tremulousness, seizures, extreme lethargy, or coma.

Cardiovascular Disturbances. Thyroid hormones play a role in maintaining cardiac rate, force of contraction, and

BOX 18-22   Progressive Signs
of Hyperthyroidism

- *Cardiovascular:* Increased heart rate and palpitations. Hyperthyroidism may present as sinus tachycardia in a sleeping patient or as atrial fibrillation with a rapid ventricular response.
- *Neurological:* Increased irritability, hyperactivity, decreased attention span, and nervousness. In an elderly patient, these signs may be masked, and depression or apathy may be present.
- *Temperature intolerance:* Increased cold tolerance; heat intolerance; fever; excessive sweating; and warm, moist skin. Older patients may naturally lose their ability to shiver and may be less comfortable in the cold.
- *Respiratory:* Increased respiratory rate, weakened thoracic muscles, and decreased vital capacity are evident.
- *Gastrointestinal:* Increased appetite, decreased absorption (especially of vitamins), weight loss, and increased stools. Diarrhea is not common. Elderly patients may be constipated.
- *Musculoskeletal:* Fine tremors of tongue or eyelids, peripheral tremors with activity, and muscle wasting are noted.
- *Integumentary:* Thin, fine, and fragile hair; soft friable nails; and petechiae. Young women generally have the more classic findings. Young men may notice an increase in acne and sweating. An elderly patient with dry, atrophic skin may not have significant skin changes.
- *Hematopoietic:* Normochromic, normocytic anemia and leukocytosis may occur.
- *Ophthalmic:* Pathological features result from edema and inflammation. Physical findings may include upper lid retraction, lid lag, extraocular muscle palsies, and sight loss. Exophthalmos is found almost exclusively in Graves' disease.

cardiac output. The increase in metabolism and the stimulation of catecholamines produced by thyroid hormones cause a hyperdynamic heart. Contractility, heart rate, and cardiac output increase as peripheral vascular resistance decreases. These effects are magnified by the body's increased demand for oxygen and nutrients. In thyroid storm, the increased demands on the heart produce high-output heart failure and cardiovascular collapse if the crisis is not recognized and treated.

Patients experience palpitations, tachycardia (out of proportion to the fever), and a widened pulse pressure. Atrial fibrillation is common. A prominent third heart sound may be heard as well as a systolic murmur over the pulmonic area, the aortic area, or

both. Occasionally, a pericardial rub may be heard. In the absence of atrial fibrillation, frequent premature atrial contractions or atrial flutter may be present. In an elderly patient with underlying heart disease, worsening of angina or severe heart failure may herald thyroid storm.

Pulmonary Disturbances. Thyroid hormones affect respiratory rate and depth, oxygen utilization, and CO_2 formation. Tissues need more oxygen as a result of hypermetabolism. This increased need for oxygen stimulates the respiratory drive and increases respiratory rate. However, increased protein catabolism reduces protein in respiratory muscles (diaphragm and intercostals). As a result, even with an increased respiratory rate, muscle weakness may prevent the patient from meeting the oxygen demand and may cause hypoventilation, CO_2 retention, and respiratory failure.

Gastrointestinal Disturbances. Excess thyroid hormones increase metabolism and accelerate protein and fat degradation. Thyroid hormones also increase gastrointestinal motility, which may result in abdominal pain, nausea, jaundice, vomiting, and/or diarrhea. The latter two problems contribute to volume depletion during thyrotoxic crises.

Musculoskeletal Disturbances. Muscle weakness and fatigue result from increased protein catabolism. Skeletal muscle changes are manifested as tremors. Thoracic muscles are weak, causing dyspnea. In thyrotoxic crises, patients are placed on bed rest to reduce metabolic demand.

Laboratory Evaluation. The determination of thyroid storm is a clinical diagnosis. Thyroid hormone levels are elevated; however, these levels are generally no higher than those normally found in uncomplicated hyperthyroidism. In any event, the patient must be treated before these results are available. See Laboratory Alerts: Thyroid Disorders for possible laboratory abnormalities that may occur in thyroid storm.

Nursing Diagnoses
The nursing diagnoses that may apply to a patient with thyroid storm are based on assessment data and include the following:

- Hyperthermia related to loss of temperature regulation, increased metabolism, increased heat production
- Disturbed thought processes related to hypermetabolism and increased cerebration, agitation, delirium, psychosis
- Decreased cardiac output related to increased metabolic demands on the heart, extreme tachycardia, dysrhythmias, congestive heart failure
- Ineffective breathing pattern related to muscle weakness and decreased vital capacity resulting in hypoventilation and CO_2 retention, increased oxygen need from hypermetabolism

TABLE 18-5   Thyroid Crises

Clinical Concerns	Significance	Nursing Actions
Thyroid Storm		
Alterations in level of consciousness	Symptoms can be confused with other disorders (e.g., paranoia, psychosis, depression), especially in the elderly	Provide a safe environment. Assess for orientation, agitation, inattention. Control environmental influences. Implement seizure precautions.
↑ Cardiac workload due to hypermetabolic state; ↓ cardiac output	Can lead to heart failure and collapse	Assess for chest pain, palpitations. Monitor for cardiac dysrhythmias (e.g., atrial fibrillation or flutter) and tachycardia. Monitor blood pressure for widening pulse pressure. Auscultate for the development of S_3. Monitor hemodynamic status: CI, SVR, PAOP. Assess urine output. Evaluate response to therapy.
↑ Oxygen demand due to hypermetabolic state; ineffective breathing pattern	↑ Respiratory rate and drive can lead to ↑ fatigue and hypoventilation	Provide supplemental oxygen or mechanical ventilation as needed. Monitor respiratory rate and effort. Monitor oxygen saturation via pulse oximeter. Minimize activity.
Loss of ability to regulate with temperature	Inability to respond to fever exacerbates hypermetabolic demands	Monitor temperature and treat with acetaminophen and/or a cooling blanket as needed.
Myxedema Coma		
↓ Cardiac function	Hypotension and potential to develop pericardial effusion	Perform cardiac monitoring (look for ↓ voltage, indicating effusion). Auscultate for diminished heart sounds. Monitor blood pressure for signs of hypotension.
Muscle weakness, hypoventilation, pleural effusion; ineffective breathing	Potential for respiratory acidosis and hypoxemia	Auscultate the lungs frequently. Monitor respiratory effort (rate and depth) and pattern. Maintain I&O (probable need for fluid restriction). Monitor ABGs/pulse oximetry and CBC (for anemia). Position for optimum respiratory effort.
Alterations in level of consciousness	Ranges from difficulty concentrating to coma Seizures can occur	Assess and maintain patient safety.
Loss of ability to regulate temperature	Inability to respond to cold	Monitor temperature. Control room temperature, provide rewarming measures.

↑, Increased; ↓, decreased; *ABGs*, arterial blood gases; *CBC*, complete blood count; *CI*, cardiac index; *I&O*, intake and output; *PAOP*, pulmonary artery occlusive pressure; *SVR*, systemic vascular resistance.

- Imbalanced nutrition: less than body requirements related to increased requirement, increased peristalsis, decreased absorption
- Activity intolerance related to muscle weakness, tremors, anemia, fatigue, and extreme energy expenditure
- Deficient knowledge: disease process, therapeutic regimen, prevention of complications

Nursing and Medical Interventions

Thyroid storm requires immediate intervention if the patient is to survive. The primary objectives in the treatment of thyroid storm are antagonizing the peripheral effects of thyroid hormone, inhibiting thyroid hormone biosynthesis, blocking thyroid hormone release, providing supportive care, identifying and treating the precipitating cause, and pro-

LABORATORY ALERTS
Thyroid Disorders

Laboratory Test	Critical Value	Significance
Thyroid Storm		
T₃, free (triiodothyronine)	>0.52 ng/dL	Hyperthyroidism
T₃, resin uptake	>35% of total	
T₄ (thyroxine)	>12 mcg/dL	
TSH	<0.01 mU/L	
Glucose	≥200 mg/dL (2 hours postprandial or random) >140 mg/dL (fasting)	↑ Insulin degradation
Sodium	>150 mEq/L	May be a result of stress, dehydration, and/or hypermetabolic state
BUN	>20 mg/dL	↑ Due to protein breakdown and hemoconcentration
CBC	↓ RBCs ↑ WBCs	Normocytic, normochromic anemia
Calcium	>10.2 mg/dL	Excess bone resorption
Myxedema Coma		
T₃, free	<0.2 mg/dL	Hypothyroidism
T₃, resin uptake	<25% of total	
T₄	<5 mcg/dL	
TSH	>25 mU/L	
Sodium	<130 mEq/L	Dilutional from increased total body water
Glucose	<50 mg/dL	Hypoglycemia due to hypermetabolic state
CBC	↓ RBCs	Anemia due to vitamin B₁₂ deficiency, inadequate folate or iron absorption
Platelets	<150,000 cells/microliter	Risk for bleeding
pH	<7.35	Respiratory acidosis from hypoventilation

↑, Increased; ↓, decreased; *BUN*, blood urea nitrogen; *CBC*, complete blood count; *RBCs*, red blood cells; *TSH*, thyroid-stimulating hormone (thyrotropin); *WBCs*, white blood cells.

viding patient and family education. Box 18-23 details the treatment of thyroid storm.

Antagonism of Peripheral Effects of Thyroid Hormones. Because it may take days or longer to impact circulating thyroid hormones, immediate action is necessary to minimize the dramatic effects of thyroid storm on the major organ systems. The mortality rate of thyroid storm has been significantly reduced with the introduction of beta-blockers to block the effects of thyroid hormones. The drug used most frequently

BOX 18-23   Treatment of Thyroid Storm

**Antagonize Peripheral Effects
of Thyroid Hormone**
- Propranolol (Inderal): 1 to 2 IV boluses every 10 to 15 minutes up to 15 to 20 mg IV or 160 to 480 mg daily PO; individualized to response
- If beta-blocker contraindicated, give resperpine or guanethidine

Inhibit Hormone Biosynthesis
- Propylthiouracil: PO loading dose of 400 mg, then 200 mg, then every 4 hours until thyrotoxicosis controlled, or
- Methimazole (Tapazole): 60 to 100 mg PO loading dose; 20 mg PO every 4 hours

Block Thyroid Hormone Release
Give 1-2 Hours after Proplylthiouracil or Methimazole Loading Dose
- Saturated solution of potassium iodide: 5 drops every 6 hours, or
- Lugol's solution: 30 drops daily PO in 3 to 4 doses, or

Secondary Options
- Iopanoic acid: 1 g every 8 hours times 24 hours, 0.5 g PO twice daily
- Ipodate (Oragrafin): 500 to 1000 mg daily
- Lithium carbonate: 300 mg PO or NG every 6 hours

Supportive Therapy
- Hydrocortisone: 100 mg IV drip every 8 hours, or dexamethasone: 0.5 mg PO every 6 hours
- Pharmacotherapy for congestive heart failure or tachydysrhythmia
- Correct fluid and electrolyte imbalance
- Treat hyperthermia (avoid aspirin)
- High-calorie, high-protein diet

Identify and Treat Precipitating Cause

Patient and Family Education

Doses are approximate and may vary based on the individual situation.
IV, Intravenous; *NG,* nasogastric (tube); *PO,* orally.

is propranolol (Inderal). Other beta-blockers such as esmolol hydrochloride (Brevibloc) or atenolol (Tenormin) may also be used. Results should be seen within minutes using the IV route and within 1 hour after the oral route. IV effects should last 3 to 4 hours. In addition, high-dose glucocorticoids are administered to block the conversion of T_4 to T_3 and thereby decreasing the effects of thyroid hormone on peripheral tissues.

Inhibition of Thyroid Hormone Biosynthesis. Two drugs may be used to inhibit thyroid hormone biosynthesis: propylthiouracil and methimazole (Tapazole). Neither of these drugs is available in IV form. Propylthiouracil is used because in large doses it inhibits conversion of T_4 to T_3 in peripheral tissues and results in a more rapid reduction of circulating thyroid hormone levels. Methimazole may be used because of its longer half-life and higher potency.

The disadvantage to both propylthiouracil and methimazole is that they lack immediate effect. They do not block the release of thyroid hormones already stored in the thyroid gland and may take weeks to months to lower thyroid hormone levels to normal.

Blockage of Thyroid Hormone Release. Iodide agents inhibit the release of thyroid hormones from the thyroid gland, inhibit thyroid hormone production, and decrease the vascularity and size of the thyroid gland. Serum T_4 levels decrease approximately 30% to 50% with any of these drugs, with stabilization in 3 to 6 days.

Saturated solution of potassium iodide (SSKI) or Lugol's solution may be given orally or sublingually. All these drugs must be administered 1 to 2 hours after antithyroid drugs (propylthiouracil or methimazole) to prevent the iodide from being used to synthesize more T_4. Ipodate (Oragrafin) and iopanoic acid (Telepaque) are radiographic contrast media that may also be used to block thyroid hormone release. Lithium carbonate also inhibits the release of thyroid hormones but is more toxic, so it is used only in patients with an iodide allergy. Lithium carbonate is given orally or by nasogastric tube and the dose is adjusted to maintain therapeutic serum levels.

Supportive Care. Symptoms are aggressively treated. Acetaminophen is used as an antipyretic. Cooling blankets and ice packs may be used. Cardiac complications are treated with pharmacotherapy. Oxygen is administered to support the respiratory effort. The large fluid losses are replaced. Hemodynamic monitoring may be required. Nutritional support is provided. Precipitating factors are identified and treated and/or removed.

Patient and Family Education. Education of patients, families, and significant others is crucial in identifying and preventing episodes of thyroid storm. Teaching varies depending on the long-term therapy chosen for each patient (e.g., drugs versus radioactive iodine or surgery).

Patient Outcomes

Outcomes for a patient with thyroid storm include the following:
- Temperature within normal range
- Return to baseline mentation and personality
- Stable hemodynamics within normal limits
- Effective breathing pattern

- Nutritional needs met and weight maintained
- Return to baseline activity level
- Verbalization by the patient and significant others of an understanding of the patient's illness, anticipated treatment, and potential complications

Myxedema Coma

Pathophysiology

Myxedema coma is the most extreme form of hypothyroidism and is life-threatening. Myxedema coma in the absence of an associated stress or illness is uncommon, with infection being the most frequent stressor. The addition of stress to an already hypothyroid patient accelerates the metabolism and clearance of whatever thyroid hormone is present in the body. Thus, the patient experiences increased hormone utilization but decreased hormone production, which precipitates a crisis state. Common findings in patients with myxedema coma are contrasted with those of thyroid storm in Table 18-5.

Etiology

Myxedema coma is the end stage of improperly treated, neglected, or undiagnosed hypothyroidism. It is a life-threatening emergency with a mortality rate as high as 50% despite appropriate therapy. Much of this mortality can be attributed to underlying illnesses. Most patients who develop myxedema coma are elderly women. It is rarely seen in young persons. It occurs more frequently in winter as a result of the increased stress of exposure to cold in a person unable to maintain body heat. Known precipitating factors include hypothermia, infection, cerebrovascular accidents, trauma, and critical illness. Medications that may precipitate myxedema coma include those that affect the central nervous system such as analgesics, anesthesia, barbiturates, narcotics, sedatives, tranquilizers, lithium, and amiodarone.

Assessment

Clinical Presentation. Many patients may have had vague signs and symptoms of hypothyroidism for several years. Box 18-24 details signs of hypothyroidism. Many of the manifestations are attributable to the development of mucinous edema. This interstitial edema is the result of water retention and decreased protein. Fluid collects in soft tissue such as the face and in joints and muscles. It can also produce pericardial effusion. The clinical picture of myxedema coma varies with the rate of onset and severity. Diagnosis is based on the clinical signs and symptoms, a high index of suspicion, and a careful history and physical examination.

Cardiovascular Disturbances. Cardiac function is depressed, resulting in decreases from baseline in heart rate,

---

BOX 18-24 Progressive Signs of Hypothyroidism

- *Earliest signs:* Fatigue, weakness, muscle cramps, intolerance to cold, and weight gain.
- *Cardiovascular:* Bradycardia and hypotension.
- *Neurological:* Difficulty concentrating, slowed mentation, depression, lethargy, slow and deliberate speech, coarse and raspy voice, hearing loss, and vertigo.
- *Respiratory:* Dyspnea on exertion.
- *Gastrointestinal:* Decreased appetite, decreased peristalsis, anorexia, decreased bowel sounds, constipation, and paralytic ileus. However, the decreased metabolic rate also leads to weight gain.
- *Musculoskeletal:* Fluid in joints and muscles results in stiffness and muscle cramps.
- *Integumentary:* Dry, flaky, cool, coarse skin; dry, coarse hair; and brittle nails. The face is puffy and pallid, the tongue may be enlarged. The dorsa of the hands and feet are edematous. There may be a yellow tint to the skin from depressed hepatic conversion of carotene to vitamin A. Ecchymoses may develop from increased capillary fragility and decreased platelets.
- *Hematological:* Pernicious anemia and jaundice. Splenomegaly occurs in about 50% of patients. About 10% of patients have a decrease in neutrophils.
- *Ophthalmic:* Generalized mucinous edema in the eyelids and periorbital tissue.
- *Metabolic:* Elevated creatine phosphokinase, aspartate aminotransferase, lactate dehydrogenase, cholesterol, and triglyceride levels. Elevated cholesterol and triglyceride levels predispose persons with hypothyroidism to the development of atherosclerosis.

---

blood pressure, contractility, stroke volume, and cardiac output. The patient may develop a pericardial effusion, making heart tones distant. The ECG has decreased voltage because of the pericardial effusion.

Pulmonary Disturbances. Respiratory system responsiveness is depressed, producing hypoventilation, respiratory muscle weakness, and CO_2 retention. CO_2 narcosis may contribute to decreased mentation. As part of the picture of generalized mucinous edema and fluid retention, these patients may also develop pleural effusions or upper airway edema, further restricting their breathing.

Neurological Disturbances. The low metabolic rate and resulting decreased mentation produce both psychological and physiological changes. The patient in hypothyroid crisis may present with somnolence, delirium, or coma. Grand mal seizures can occur. Personality changes such as paranoia and delusions may be evident.

Patients with hypothyroidism are unable to maintain body heat because of the decreased metabolic rate and decreased production of thermal energy. Because of this, patients may present in crisis after being stressed by exposure to cold. Hypothermia is present in 80% of patients in myxedema coma, with temperatures as low as 80°F (26.7°C). Patients with temperatures less than 88.6°F (32°C) have a grave prognosis. If a patient with myxedema coma has a temperature greater than 98.6°F (37°C), underlying infection should be suspected.

Skeletal Muscle Disturbances. Slowed motor conduction produces decreased tendon reflexes and sluggish, awkward movements.

Laboratory Evaluation. Serum T_4 and T_3 levels and resin T_3 uptake are low in patients with myxedema coma. In primary hypothyroidism, TSH levels are high. If hypothyroidism is the result of disease of the pituitary gland or hypothalamus (secondary and tertiary hypothyroidism), TSH levels are inappropriately normal or low. As in patients with thyroid storm, if myxedema coma is suspected, treatment should not be delayed while awaiting these results to confirm the diagnosis.

Serum sodium levels may be low as a result of impaired water excretion and resultant water retention. Impaired water excretion is the result of the inappropriate ADH secretion and cortisol deficiency that frequently accompany hypothyroidism. The patient should be monitored for signs and symptoms related to hyponatremia such as weakness, muscle twitching, seizures, and coma.

Hypoglycemia is common and may be related to pituitary or hypophyseal disorders and/or adrenal insufficiency. Adrenal insufficiency may also result in serum cortisol levels that are inappropriately low for stress. Laboratory manifestations of myxedema coma are summarized in Laboratory Alerts: Thyroid Disorders.

Nursing Diagnoses

The nursing diagnoses that may apply to a patient in myxedema coma are based on assessment data and include the following:

- Decreased cardiac output related to decreased contractility, decreased heart rate, decreased stroke volume, pericardial effusion, dysrhythmias
- Ineffective breathing pattern related to hypoventilation, muscle weakness, decreased respiratory rate, ascites, pleural effusions
- Disturbed thought processes related to slowed metabolism and cerebration, hyponatremia

- Hypothermia related to inability of body to retain heat
- Excess fluid volume related to impaired water excretion
- Risk for injury related to edema, decreased platelet count
- Activity intolerance related to muscle weakness
- Imbalanced nutrition: less than body requirements related to decreased appetite, decreased carbohydrate metabolism, hypoglycemia
- Deficient knowledge: disease process, therapeutic regimen, prevention of complications

Nursing and Medical Interventions

Myxedema coma requires immediate intervention if the patient is to survive. The primary objectives in the treatment of myxedema coma are identifying and treating the precipitating cause, providing thyroid replacement, restoring fluid and electrolyte balance, providing supportive care, and providing patient and family education. Box 18-25 details the treatment of myxedema coma. It is important to achieve physiological levels of thyroid hormone without incurring the adverse effects of excess thyroid hormones.

BOX 18-25　　Treatment of Myxedema Coma

- Identification and treatment of underlying disorder
- *Thyroid replacement:* levothyroxine sodium, 200 to 500 mcg IV loading dose, then 50 mcg/day IV; or liothyronine sodium, 25 mcg IV every 8 hours for 24 to 48 hours, then 12.5 mcg every 8 hours
- Restoration of fluid and electrolyte balance
- Cautious administration of vasopressors
- *Hyponatremia:* <115 mEq/L, hypertonic saline; <120 mEq/L, fluid restriction
- *Hypoglycemia:* IV glucose
- Supportive care
- Passive warming with blankets (do not actively warm)
- Ventilatory assistance
- Avoidance of narcotics and sedative drugs
- Adrenal hormone replacement: hydrocortisone, 100 mg IV bolus, then 50-100 mg every 6-8 hours for 7-10 days
- Chest x-ray or ultrasound study of the chest possibly needed to assess pleural effusion
- Echocardiogram possibly needed to assess cardiac function and/or pericardial effusion
- Patient and family education

Doses are approximate and may vary based on the individual situation.
IV, Intravenous.

Thyroid Replacement. The best method of thyroid replacement is controversial. Either levothyroxine sodium (Synthroid; T_4) or liothyronine sodium (Cytomel; T_3) can be used. Levothyroxine ultimately provides the patient with both T_4 and, through peripheral conversion, T_3 replacement, whereas liothyronine sodium requires lower doses.

Levothyroxine sodium is the more commonly used drug. It has a smoother effect and a longer activity. The preferred route is IV because absorption of oral or intramuscular levothyroxine is variable. The initial dose may be decreased if the patient has underlying factors such as angina, dysrhythmias, or other heart disease.

Liothyronine sodium has heightened metabolic effects, a more rapid onset (6 hours), and a shorter half-life (1 day) than levothyroxine. Because of liothyronine's potency, its administration may be complicated by angina, myocardial infarction, and cardiac irritability. Thus, it is generally avoided in older populations.

The effects of levothyroxine are not as rapid as those of liothyronine, but its cardiac toxicity is lower. Serum levels of T_4 reach normal in 1 to 2 days. Levels of TSH begin to fall within 24 hours and return to normal in 10 to 14 days.

Fluid and Electrolyte Restoration. If the patient is hypotensive or in shock, thyroid replacement usually corrects this, but cautious volume expansion with saline also helps. Vasopressors should be used with extreme caution because patients in myxedema coma are unable to respond to vasopressors until they have adequate levels of thyroid hormones available. Simultaneous administration of vasopressors and thyroid hormones is associated with myocardial irritability.

Hyponatremia usually responds to thyroid replacement and water restriction; the patient can resume water intake once thyroid hormones are replaced. If hyponatremia is severe (<110 mEq/L) or the patient is having seizures, hypertonic saline with or without furosemide (Lasix) may be administered, but only until symptoms disappear or the sodium level is 120 mEq/L.

Glucose should be added to IV fluids to provide support to a patient with hypoglycemia, concomitant adrenal insufficiency, or both. Hydrocortisone, 100 mg, is given initially, followed by 50 to 100 mg every 6 to 8 hours for 7 to 10 days. The adrenal abnormality may last several weeks after thyroid replacement is begun, so this support should be continued during that time.

Supportive Care. Symptoms are aggressively treated. Hypothermia is treated by keeping the room warm and using warmed blankets. Electric heating blankets are not used because active heat in the presence of

vasodilation may lead to vascular collapse. Drugs that depress respirations, such as narcotics, are avoided. Mechanical ventilation is frequently required. Cardiac function is assessed and treated. Glucocorticoid administration is recommended for all patients in the event that hypoadrenalism coexists with hypothyroidism. IV hydrocortisone is administered every 6 to 8 hours until the patient improves and the pituitary-adrenal axis can be accurately assessed.

Patient and Family Education. The education of patients, family, and significant others is critical in identifying and preventing episodes of myxedema coma.

Patient Outcomes

Outcomes for a patient with myxedema coma include the following:

- Stable hemodynamics within normal limits
- Effective breathing pattern
- Return to baseline mentation and personality
- Maintenance of temperature within normal range
- Normal fluid volume balance and absence of edema
- Intact skin without edema or bleeding
- Return to baseline activity level
- Adequate nutrition and stable body weight
- Verbalization by the patient and significant others of an understanding of the disease, therapeutic regimen, and prevention of complications

ANTIDIURETIC HORMONE DISORDERS

Review of Physiology

The primary function of ADH is regulation of water balance and serum osmolality. ADH (also known as arginine vasopressin, AVP) is produced in the supraoptic nuclei and paraventricular nuclei of the hypothalamus. These nuclei are positioned near the thirst center and osmoreceptors in the hypothalamus (Figure 18-8). Once produced, ADH is stored in neurons in the posterior pituitary. If the supraoptic and paraventricular nuclei are stimulated (via mechanisms described later), their discharge stimulates the nerve endings in the posterior pituitary to release ADH. This stimulation occurs in response to both osmotic and nonosmotic forces. Osmoreceptors in the hypothalamus respond to changes in extracellular osmolality. Stretch receptors in the left atrium and baroreceptors in the carotid sinus and aortic arch respond to changes in circulating volume and blood pressure, respectively. The physiology of ADH release is summarized in Figure 18-9.

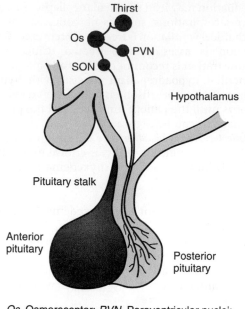

Os, Osmoreceptor; PVN, Paraventricular nuclei;
SON, Supraoptic nuclei

FIGURE 18-8. Hypothalamic–posterior pituitary system.

Once released, ADH acts on the renal distal and collecting tubules to cause water reabsorption. In high concentrations, ADH also acts on smooth muscles of the arterioles to produce vasoconstriction. Normally, ADH is released in response to increased serum osmolality (primary stimulus), elevated serum sodium level, decreased blood volume (by more than 10%), decreased blood pressure (5%-10% drop), stress, trauma, hypoxia, pain, and anxiety. Certain drugs such as narcotics, barbiturates, anesthetics, and chemotherapeutic agents are also known to stimulate ADH release.

Two common disturbances of ADH are diabetes insipidus (DI) and the syndrome of inappropriate ADH (SIADH). A less common disorder is cerebral salt wasting (CSW), which is similar to SIADH but with important differences. CSW is a disorder of sodium and fluid balance that occurs in patients with a neurological insult. Differentiating CSW from SIADH is difficult but crucial because of opposing management strategies. Table 18-6 compares the electrolyte and fluid findings associated with DI, SIADH, and CSW.[21,23]

Diabetes Insipidus

Etiology

Various disorders can produce neurogenic DI (Box 18-26), but the primary cause is traumatic injury to the posterior pituitary or hypothalamus as a result of head injury or surgery. Transient DI may occur after pituitary surgery or trauma resulting from manipula-

---

BOX 18-26   Causes of Diabetes Insipidus

Antidiuretic Hormone Deficiency (Neurogenic Diabetes Insipidus)
- *Idiopathic:* familial, congenital, autoimmune, genetic
- Intracranial surgery, especially in region of pituitary
- *Tumors:* craniopharyngioma, pituitary tumors, metastases to hypothalamus
- *Infections:* meningitis, encephalitis, syphilis, mycoses, toxoplasmosis
- *Granulomatous disease:* tuberculosis, sarcoidosis, histiocytosis
- Severe head trauma, anoxic encephalopathy, or any disorder that causes increased intracranial pressure

Antidiuretic Hormone Insensitivity (Nephrogenic Diabetes Insipidus)
- Hereditary; idiopathic
- *Renal disease:* pyelonephritis, amyloidosis, polycystic kidney disease, obstructive uropathy, transplantation
- *Multisystem disorders affecting kidneys:* multiple myeloma, sickle cell disease, cystic fibrosis
- *Metabolic disturbances:* chronic hypokalemia or hypercalcemia
- *Drugs:* ethanol, phenytoin, lithium carbonate, demeclocycline, amphotericin, methoxyflurane

Secondary Diabetes Insipidus
- Idiopathic
- Psychogenic polydipsia
- Hypothalamic disease: sarcoidosis
- Excessive intravenous fluid administration
- *Drug-induced disease:* anticholinergics, tricyclic antidepressants

---

tion of the pituitary stalk or cerebral edema. Permanent DI occurs when more than 80% to 85% of the supraoptic or paraventricular nuclei or the proximal end of the pituitary stalk is destroyed.

Nephrogenic DI may occur in genetically predisposed persons. It also may be acquired from chronic renal disease, drugs, or other conditions that produce permanent kidney damage or inhibit the generation of cyclic adenosine monophosphate in the tubules.

Pathophysiology

DI results from an ADH deficiency (neurogenic or central DI), ADH insensitivity (nephrogenic DI), or excessive water intake (secondary DI). Regardless of the cause, the effect is impaired renal conservation of water resulting in polyuria (>3 L in 24 hours). As long as the thirst center remains intact and the person

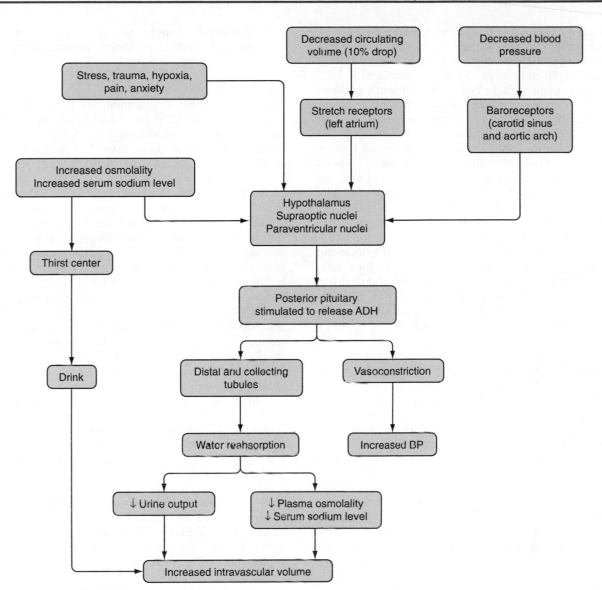

FIGURE 18-9. Physiology of antidiuretic hormone (ADH) release. *BP,* Blood pressure.

TABLE 18-6	Electrolyte and Fluid Findings in ADH Disorders		
Finding	**Diabetes Insipidus**	**Syndrome of Inappropriate ADH**	**Cerebral Salt Wasting**
Plasma volume	Decreased	Increased	Decreased
Serum sodium	Increased	Decreased	Decreased
Serum osmolality	Increased	Decreased	Normal or increased
Urine sodium	Normal	Increased	Increased
Urine osmolality	Decreased	Increased	Normal or increased

ADH, Antidiuretic hormone.

is able to respond to this thirst, fluid volume can be maintained. If the patient is unable to respond, severe dehydration will result if fluid losses are not replaced. DI may be permanent or transient.

Neurogenic DI is the type most frequently encountered in clinical practice. In neurogenic DI, absent or diminished release of circulating levels of ADH from the posterior pituitary produces free water loss and causes serum osmolality and serum sodium to rise. The posterior pituitary is unable to respond by increasing ADH levels; thus, the kidneys are not stimulated to reabsorb water, and excessive water loss results. Neurogenic DI occurs because of disruption of the neural pathways or structures involved in ADH production, synthesis, or release.

In nephrogenic DI, the kidney collecting ducts and distal tubules are unresponsive to ADH; thus, adequate levels of ADH may be synthesized and released, but the kidneys are unable to conserve water in response. In patients with secondary DI, compulsive volume consumption causes polyuria.

Assessment

Clinical Presentation. Neurogenic DI usually occurs suddenly with an abrupt onset of polyuria, as much as 5 to 40 L in 24 hours. The onset of nephrogenic DI is more gradual. The urine is pale and dilute. The thirst mechanism is activated in conscious patients, and polydipsia occurs. If the patient is unable to replace the water lost by responding to thirst, signs of hypovolemia develop: hypotension, decreased skin turgor, dry mucous membranes, tachycardia, weight loss, and low right atrial and pulmonary artery occlusion pressures. Neurological signs and symptoms are seen with hypovolemia and hypernatremia.

Laboratory Evaluation. A classic sign of DI is an inappropriately low urine osmolality in the face of a high serum osmolality. Corresponding with the low urine osmolality is a decreased urine specific gravity. Serum osmolality is greater than 295 mOsm/kg, and the serum sodium level is greater than 145 mEq/L. The presence of hypokalemia or hypercalcemia suggests nephrogenic DI. Other values such as BUN and creatinine may be elevated as a result of hemoconcentration. Further testing to differentiate neurogenic and nephrogenic DI includes water deprivation studies. These tests are inappropriate in the critically ill population and are not performed in this setting. See Laboratory Alerts: Pituitary Disorders.

Nursing Diagnoses

The nursing diagnoses that may apply to a patient with DI include the following:

- Deficient fluid volume related to deficient ADH, renal cells insensitive to ADH, polyuria, and inability to respond to thirst
- Disturbed thought processes related to decreased cerebral perfusion, cerebral dehydration, and hypernatremia

Nursing and Medical Interventions

The primary goals of treatment are to identify and correct the underlying cause and to restore normal fluid volume, osmolality, and electrolyte balance. Identifying the underlying cause is a necessary part of determining appropriate treatment, particularly drug therapy.

Volume Replacement. Monitoring for signs and symptoms of hypovolemia is a priority. Vital signs must be recorded at least every hour, along with urine output. Hemodynamic monitoring may be instituted to evaluate fluid requirements and to monitor the patient's response to treatment. This is particularly important in elderly patients who are likely to have concurrent cardiovascular and renal disease. Accurate intake and output and daily weights are essential. Measurement of urine specific gravity assists in evaluating the patient's response to treatment. Once drug therapy has been instituted, the urine should become more concentrated and the specific gravity should increase.

Patients who are alert and able to respond to thirst generally drink enough water to avoid symptomatic hypovolemia. However, patients in critical care units who develop DI and elderly patients with cognitive impairments are frequently unable to recognize or respond to thirst, so fluid replacement is essential.

If the patient has symptoms of hypovolemia, the volume already lost must be replaced. In addition, fluid is replaced every hour to keep up with current urine losses. Correction of hypernatremia and replacement of free water are achieved by using hypotonic solutions of dextrose in water. If the patient has circulatory failure, isotonic saline may be administered until hemodynamic stability and vascular volume have been restored.

Frequent monitoring of the patient's neurological status is also critical because changes may indicate a change in fluid status, electrolyte status (e.g., sodium), or both. It is important to avoid fluid overload from overaggressive fluid replacement, particularly once drug therapy has been instituted.

Hormone Replacement. Because of the decreased secretion of AVP, neurogenic DI is controlled primarily with exogenous ADH preparations. These drugs replace ADH and enable the kidneys to conserve water. They can be administered intravenously, intramuscularly, subcutaneously, intranasally, or orally. Injectable forms are generally more potent than the intranasal or oral routes. Absorption is more reliable through the IV route.

LABORATORY ALERTS
Pituitary Disorders

Laboratory Test	Critical Value	Significance
	Diabetes Insipidus	
Sodium (serum)	>145 mEq/L	Absent or diminished release of ADH or lack of response by the kidneys leads to free water loss
Osmolality (serum)	>295 mOsm/kg H_2O	Low (neurogenic) ADH High (nephrogenic) Normal (secondary)
Osmolality (urine)	<100 mOsm/kg H_2O	
Specific gravity (urine)	<1.005	
	Syndrome of Inappropriate Antidiuretic Hormone	
Sodium (serum)	<135 mEq/L	Oversecretion of ADH and failure of negative feedback system leading to free water retention
Osmolality (serum)	<280 mOsm/kg H_2O	
ADH	High	
Sodium (urine)	>20 mEq/L	Used as differential for other causes of hypo-osmolality (e.g., HF)

ADH, Antidiuretic hormone; *HF*, heart failure.

The drug most commonly used for management is desmopressin (DDAVP), a synthetic analogue of vasopressin. Unlike aqueous vasopressin and lysine vasopressin, desmopressin is devoid of any vasoconstrictor effects and has a longer antidiuretic action (12 to 24 hours). It also has infrequent and mild side effects: headache, nausea, and mild abdominal cramps.

Overmedication with an ADH preparation can also produce water overload. The patient is monitored for signs of dyspnea, hypertension, weight gain, hyponatremia, headache, or drowsiness.

Nephrogenic Diabetes Insipidus. Treatment of nephrogenic DI depends primarily on solute restriction and the administration of thiazide diuretics such as hydrochlorothiazide. Sodium depletion causes a decrease in the glomerular filtration rate, enhanced reabsorption of fluid, and a reduced capacity to dilute the urine.

Patient and Family Education. Patients who have a permanent ADH deficit require education regarding the following:

- Pathogenesis of DI
- Dose, side effects, and rationale for prescribed medications
- Parameters for notifying the physician
- Importance of adherence to medication regimen
- Importance of recording daily weight measurements to identify weight gain
- Importance of wearing a Medic-Alert identification bracelet
- Importance of drinking according to thirst and avoiding excess drinking

Patient Outcomes

Outcomes for a patient with DI include the following:

- Serum osmolality, 275 to 295 mOsm/kg
- Stable weight and balanced intake and output
- Serum sodium level, 135 to 145 mEq/L
- Return to baseline mentation

Syndrome of Inappropriate Antidiuretic Hormone

Etiology

A common cause of SIADH is ectopic production of ADH by malignant disease, especially small cell carcinoma of the lung. The malignant cells themselves actually synthesize, store, and release ADH and thus place control of ADH outside the normal pituitary-hypothalamus feedback loops. Other types of malignancies known to produce SIADH include pancreatic and duodenal carcinoma, Hodgkin's lymphoma, sarcoma, and squamous cell carcinoma of the tongue.

Nonmalignant pulmonary conditions such as tuberculosis, pneumonia, lung abscess, and chronic obstructive pulmonary disease can also produce SIADH. As with malignant cells, it is believed that benign pulmonary tissue is capable of synthesizing and releasing ADH in certain disease states.

Central nervous system disorders such as head injuries, infections, hemorrhages, surgery, and cerebrovascular accidents can produce SIADH. The problem is caused by stimulation of the hypothalamic or pituitary system, or both.

Many medications are associated with SIADH. (Box 18-27). Of recent concern are reports of the effects of the widely prescribed selective serotonin reuptake inhibitors on ADH levels and function.[20] The mechanisms involved include increasing or potentiating the action of ADH, acting on the renal distal tubule to decrease free water excretion, or causing central release of ADH.

Pathophysiology

SIADH occurs when the body secretes excessive ADH unrelated to plasma osmolality. This occurs when there is a failure in the negative feedback mechanism that regulates the release and inhibition of ADH. The results are an inability to secrete a dilute urine, fluid retention, and dilutional hyponatremia. CSW is similar to SIADH with the primary exception being fluid status. In SIADH, the patient has normal or excessive fluid volume, a decreased serum sodium level, and an increased urinary sodium level. The primary treatment of SIADH is to withhold fluids. In CSW, the patient has volume depletion, a decreased serum sodium level, and an increased urinary sodium level. The treatment of CSW is to replenish fluids.[23]

Assessment

Clinical Presentation. ADH stimulation produces a clinical picture of water intoxication. The clinical manifestations are primarily the result of water retention, hyponatremia, and hypo-osmolality of the serum. The severity of the signs and symptoms is

---

BOX 18-27   Causes of Syndrome of Inappropriate Antidiuretic Hormone

Ectopic Antidiuretic Hormone Production
- Small cell carcinoma of lung
- Cancer of prostate, pancreas, or duodenum
- Hodgkin's disease
- Sarcoma, squamous cell carcinoma of the tongue, thymoma
- *Nonmalignant pulmonary disease:* viral pneumonia, tuberculosis, chronic obstructive pulmonary disease, lung abscess

Central Nervous System Disorders
- Head trauma
- *Infections:* meningitis, encephalitis, brain abscess
- Intracranial surgery, cerebral aneurysm, brain tumor, cerebral atrophy, cerebrovascular accident
- Guillain-Barré syndrome, lupus erythematosus

Drugs
- Angiotensin-converting enzyme inhibitors
- Amiodarone
- Analgesics and narcotics: morphine, fentanyl, acetaminophen
- Antineoplastics: vincristine, cyclophosphamide, vinblastine, cisplatin
- Barbiturates
- Carbamazepine (Tegretol) and oxcarbazepine (Trileptal)
- Chlorpropamide (Diabinese)
- Ciprofloxacin
- General anesthetics
- Haloperidol (Haldol)
- Mizoribine
- Nicotine
- Nonsteroidal antiinflammatory drugs
- Pentamidine
- Serotonergic agents: 3,4-methylenedioxymethamphetamine (MDMA; Ecstasy), selective serotonin reuptake inhibitors
- Thiazide diuretics
- Tricyclic antidepressants

Positive-Pressure Ventilation

---

related to the rate of onset and the severity of the hyponatremia.

Central Nervous System. Manifestations such as weakness, lethargy, mental confusion, difficulty concentrating, restlessness, headache, seizures, and coma may occur in response to hyponatremia and hypo-osmolality. Hypo-osmolality disrupts the intracellular-extracellular osmotic gradient and causes a shift of water into brain cells, cerebral edema, and increased intracranial pressure. If the serum sodium level decreases to less than 120 mEq/L in 48 hours or less, there are usually serious neurological symptoms and a mortality rate as high as 50%. If hyponatremia develops more slowly, the body is able to protect against cerebral edema, and the patient may remain asymptomatic even with a very low serum sodium level.

Gastrointestinal System. Congestion of the gastrointestinal tract and decreased motility because of electrolyte imbalance (hyponatremia) produce nausea and vomiting, anorexia, muscle cramps, and decreased bowel sounds.

Cardiovascular System. In the cardiovascular system, water retention produces weight gain, increased blood pressure, and elevated central venous and pulmonary artery occlusion pressures.

Pulmonary System. Fluid overload in the pulmonary system produces increased respiratory rate; dyspnea; adventitious lung sounds; and frothy, pink sputum.

Laboratory Evaluation. The hallmark of SIADH is hyponatremia and hypo-osmolality in the presence of an inappropriately concentrated urine (a low serum osmolarity should trigger inhibition of ADH secretion, resulting in the loss of water through the kidneys and a dilute urine). Hyponatremia (<135 mEq/L) and hypo-osmolality (<280 mOsm/kg) result from water retention. See Laboratory Alerts: Pituitary Disorders.

High urinary sodium levels (>20 mEq/L) help to differentiate SIADH from other causes of hypoosmolality, hyponatremia, and volume overload (such as congestive heart failure). In SIADH, renal perfusion (a major stimulus for sodium reabsorption) is usually adequate, so sodium is not conserved. In a disorder such as heart failure, renal perfusion is low because of decreased cardiac output, triggering reabsorption of sodium.

Hemodilution may decrease other laboratory values such as BUN, creatinine, and albumin. SIADH should be suspected in a patient with evidence of hemodilution and urine that is hypertonic relative to plasma.

When the cause of the disorder is unclear, additional testing includes water loading. As with the water deprivation test, this test is unsafe in the critically ill population and is not performed in this setting. These tests are best suited to stable patients.

Nursing Diagnoses

The nursing diagnoses that may apply to a patient with SIADH include the following:
- Excess fluid volume related to excess water retention from excess ADH
- Disturbed thought processes related to brain swelling and fluid shift into cerebral cells

Nursing and Medical Interventions

The primary goals of therapy are to treat the underlying cause, to eliminate excess water, and to increase serum osmolality. In many instances, treatment of the underlying disorder (e.g., discontinuation of a responsible drug) is all that is needed to return the patient's condition to normal.

Fluid Balance. In mild to moderate cases (serum sodium level, 125 to 135 mEq/L), fluid intake is restricted to 800 to 1000 mL/day, with liberal dietary salt and protein intake. The patient's response is evaluated by monitoring serum sodium levels, serum osmolality, and weight loss for a gradual return to baseline.

In severe, symptomatic cases (coma, seizures, serum sodium level <110 mEq/L), hypertonic 3% saline may be given following rigorous guidelines and with careful monitoring. Correction of the serum sodium level must be done slowly, no more than 12 mEq within the first 24 hours. Administering hypertonic saline too rapidly, correcting the serum sodium level too rapidly, or both, can result in central pontine myelinolyhhsis, a severe neurological syndrome that can lead to permanent brain damage or death.[10] The risk of heart failure is also significant. A diuretic such as furosemide may be given during hypertonic saline administration to promote diuresis and free water clearance. Treatments for chronic or resistant SIADH are listed in Box 18-28.

BOX 18-28 Treatments for Chronic or Resistant Syndrome of Inappropriate Antidiuretic Hormone

- Water restriction of 800 to 1000 mL/day.
- Administration of loop diuretics in conjunction with increased salt and potassium intake is the safest method for treating chronic hyponatremia. The diuretic prevents urine concentration, and the increased salt and potassium intake increases water output by increasing delivery of solutes to the kidney.
- Demeclocycline is an antibiotic that also decreases renal tubule responsiveness to ADH. Doses of 600 to 1200 mg are given in divided doses twice a day. Its onset is delayed for several days, and it may not be completely effective for 2 weeks, evidenced by a decrease in urine osmolality to therapeutic range. This drug is rarely used. The major side effects are azotemia (nephrotoxicity) and risk of infection.

Doses are approximate and may vary based on the individual situation.
ADH, Antidiuretic hormone.

Nursing. Prevention of SIADH may not be possible, but early detection and treatment may prevent more serious sequelae from occurring. Being aware of the populations at risk and monitoring at-risk populations for clinical signs are key roles for the critical care nurse.

Close monitoring of fluid and electrolyte balance is required. Daily weight, intake and output, and urine specific gravity are measured. Fluid overload may occur from hypervolemia or too rapid administration of hypertonic saline. Cardiovascular symptoms such as tachycardia, increased blood pressure, increased hemodynamic pressures, full bounding pulses, and distended neck veins are all indicators of fluid overload. Respiratory function is monitored for signs of tachypnea, labored respirations, shortness of breath, or fine crackles. Careful monitoring of potassium and magnesium levels is necessary to replace diuresis-induced losses.

Adherence to fluid restrictions is critical but difficult for patients. The nurse should ensure that the patient and the family understand the importance of the restriction and that they are included in planning types and timing of fluids. Patients should be encouraged to choose fluids high in sodium content such as milk, tomato juice, and beef and chicken broth. Measures to relieve some of the discomfort caused by fluid restriction include frequent mouth care, oral rinses without swallowing, chilled beverages, and sucking on hard candy.

Assessment of the patient's neurological status is also critical to monitor the effects of treatment and to watch for complications. The patient is assessed for subtle changes that may indicate water intoxication, such as fatigue, weakness, headache, or changes in level of consciousness. Strict adherence to administration rates of hypertonic (3%) saline solutions and measurement of serial serum sodium levels are essential to prevent neurological sequelae. Seizure precautions should be instituted if the patient's sodium level decreases to less than 120 mEq/L.

Patient and Family Education. In some patients, SIADH may require long-term treatment, ongoing monitoring, or both. These patients and their families require instruction regarding the following:

- Early signs and symptoms to report to the health care provider: weight gain, lethargy, weakness, nausea, mental status changes
- The significance of adherence to fluid restriction
- Dose, side effects, and rationale for prescribed medications
- Importance of daily weights

Patient Outcomes

Outcomes for a patient with SIADH include the following:

- Serum osmolality, 275 to 295 mOsm/kg
- Serum sodium level, 135 to 145 mEq/L
- Hemodynamic measurements within normal limits
- Return of vital signs to patient baseline
- Return of mental status to patient baseline
- Ability of the patient and family to verbalize an understanding of SIADH, the therapeutic regimen, and prevention of complications

CASE STUDY

evolve

Mr. P. F., a 68-year-old man, is admitted to the medical intensive care unit from the emergency department with respiratory failure and hypotension. His history is significant for type 2 diabetes mellitus, steroid-dependent chronic obstructive pulmonary disease, peripheral vascular disease, and cigarette and alcohol abuse. His medications at home include glipizide, prednisone, and Combivent. In the emergency department he received a single dose of ceftriaxone and etomidate for intubation.

On exam he is intubated, on pressure-controlled ventilation, and receiving normal saline at 200 mL/hr and dopamine at 8 mcg/kg/min. His blood pressure is 86/50 mm Hg; heart rate, 126 beats/min; oxygen saturation, 88%; and temperature, 39.6°C. His cardiac rhythm shows sinus tachycardia and nonspecific ST-T wave changes. Arterial blood gas values are as follows: pH, 7.21;

PaO_2, 83 mm Hg; $PaCO_2$, 50 mm Hg; and bicarbonate, 12 mEq/L. Other laboratory values are as follows: serum glucose, 308 mg/dL; serum creatinine, 2.1 mg/dL; and white blood cell count, 19,000/microliter.

QUESTIONS

1. What disease state do you suspect this patient is experiencing and why?
2. What potential endocrine complications do you anticipate?
3. What further laboratory studies would you want? What results do you anticipate?
4. What treatment goals and strategies do you anticipate?
5. In providing patient and family education and support, what issues need to be addressed immediately and which can be delayed?

SUMMARY

The stress of critical illness affects the endocrine system. Control of blood glucose levels is an essential component of critical care because of the adverse outcomes associated with hyperglycemia. Low-dose corticosteroid therapy is a component of managing the inflammatory response seen in many critical illnesses.

Various endocrine disorders are seen in critical care. Patients may be admitted to the critical care unit for treatment of an endocrine disorder (e.g., DKA) or a disorder secondary to another problem (e.g., SIADH after a head injury). Preexisting disorders (e.g., hypothyroidism) may become secondary during treatment of a critical illness.

The critical care nurse must be knowledgeable about the endocrine system, its feedback mechanisms, and its role in maintaining homeostasis. Nursing assessments and interventions can assist in prevention, detection, and early treatment of endocrine imbalance.

CRITICAL THINKING QUESTIONS   *evolve*

1. How does glycemic control impact various body systems?
2. How can the hazards of hypoglycemia be prevented?
3. Insulin therapy is a critical intervention in the treatment of DKA. What crucial parameters must be monitored to ensure optimal patient outcomes?
4. In a patient with neurologic injury, how do lab values help to differentiate DI and SIADH?
5. In which patient population would the nurse expect to administer a cosyntropin stimulation test? What factors affect the interpretation of the test results?

evolve Be sure to check out the bonus material, including free self-assessment exercises, on the Evolve Web site at http://evolve.elsevier.com/Sole.

REFERENCES

1. American Diabetes Association (ADA). (2004). Hyperglycemic crises in diabetes. *Diabetes Care, 27*(Suppl. 1), S94-S102.
2. Arafah, B. (2006). Review: Hypothalamic-pituitary-adrenal function during critical illness: Limitations of current assessment methods. *Journal of Clinical Endocrinology and Metabolism, 91*(10), 3725-3745.
3. Brenner, Z. R. (2006). Management of hyperglycemic emergencies. *AACN Clinical Issues, 17*, 56-65.
4. Bull, S. V., Douglas, I. S., Foster, M., & Albert, R. K. (2007). Mandatory protocol for treating adult patients with diabetic ketoacidosis decreases intensive care unit and hospital lengths of stay: Results of a non-randomized trial. *Critical Care Medicine, 35*, 41-46.
5. Garber, A. J., for the ACE/ADA Task Force on Inpatient Diabetes. (2006). American College of Endocrinology and American Diabetes Association consensus statement on inpatient diabetes and glycemic control: A call to action. *Diabetes Care, 29*(8), 1955-1962.
6. Gonzalez, H., Nardi, O., & Annane, D. (2006). Relative adrenal failure in the ICU: An identifiable problem requiring treatment. *Critical Care Clinics, 22*, 105-118.
7. Guthrie, R. A., & Guthrie, D. W. (2004). Pathophysiology of diabetes mellitus. *Critical Care Nursing Quarterly, 27*(2), 113-125.
8. Hamrahian, A. (2005). Adrenal function in critically ill patients: How to test? When to treat? *Cleveland Clinic Journal of Medicine, 72*(5), 427-432.
9. Jacobi, J. (2006). Corticosteroid replacement in critically ill patients. *Critical Care Clinics, 22*, 245-253.
10. Johnson, A., & Criddle, L. (2004). Pass the salt: Indications for and implications of using hypertonic saline. *Critical Care Nurse, 24*(15), 36-46.
11. Johnson, K. (2006). The hypothalamic-pituitary-adrenal axis in critical illness. *AACN Clinical Issues, 17*(1), 39-49.
12. Langdon, C. D., & Shriver, R. L. (2004). Clinical issues in the care of critically ill diabetic patients. *Critical Care Nurse Quarterly, 27*, 162-171.
13. Lipiner-Friedman, D., Sprung, C. L., Laterre, P. F., Weiss, Y., Goodman, S. V., Vogeser, M., et al. (2007). Adrenal function in sepsis: The retrospective Corticus cohort study. *Critical Care Medicine, 35*(4), 1012-1018.
14. Nugent, B. W. (2005). Hyperosmolar hyperglycemic state. *Emergency Medicine Clinics of North America, 23*, 629-648.
15. Nylen, E. S., & Muller, B. (2004). Endocrine changes in critical illness. *Journal of Intensive Care Medicine, 19*(2), 67-82.
16. Nylen, E. S., Seam, N., & Khosla, R. (2006). Endocrine markers of severity and prognosis in critical illness. *Critical Care Clinics, 22*, 161-179.

17. Peeters, R. P., Debaveye, Y., Fliers, E., & Visser, T. J. (2006). Changes within the thyroid axis during critical illness. *Critical Care Clinics, 22*, 41-55.

18. Porsche, R., & Brenner, Z. R. (2006). Amiodarone-induced thyroid dysfunction. *Critical Care Nurse, 26*(3), 34-42.

19. Raghavan, M., & Marik, P. E. (2006). Stress hyperglycemia and adrenal insufficiency in the critically ill. *Seminars in Respiratory and Critical Care Medicine, 27*(3), 274-285.

20. Rottman, C. (2007). SSRI's and the syndrome of inappropriate antidiuretic hormone secretion. *American Journal of Nursing, 107*(1), 51-58.

21. Singh, S., Bohn, D., Carlotti, A., & Cusimano, M. (2002). Cerebral salt wasting: Truths, fallacies theories and challenges. *Critical Care Medicine, 30*(11), 2575-2579.

22. Siraux, V., De Backer, D., Yalavatti, G., & Melot, C. (2005). Relative adrenal insufficiency in patients with septic shock: Comparison of low-dose and conventional corticotropin tests. *Critical Care Medicine, 33*(11), 2479-2486.

23. Tisdall, M., Crocker, M., Watkiss, J., & Smith, M. (2006). Disturbances of sodium in critically ill adult neurologic patients. *Journal of Neurosurgery and Anesthesiology, 18*(1), 57-63.

24. Turina, M., Christ-Cain, M., & Polk, H. C. (2006). Diabetes and hyperglycemia: Strict glycemic control. *Critical Care Medicine, 34*, S291-S300.

25. Van den Berghe, G., Wilmer, A., Hermans, G., Meersseman, W., Wouters, P., Milants, I., et al. (2006). Intensive insulin therapy in the medical ICU. *New England Journal of Medicine, 354*, 449-461.

26. Van den Berghe, G., Wouters, P., Weekers, F., Verwaest, C., Bruyninckx, F., Schetz, M., et al. (2001). Intensive insulin therapy in critically ill patients. *New England Journal of Medicine, 345*, 1359-1367.

27. Vanhorebeek, I., & Van den Berghe, G. (2006). The neuroendocrine response to critical illness is a dynamic process. *Critical Care Clinics, 22*, 1-15.

CHAPTER 19

Trauma and Surgical Management

Mary Beth Flynn Makic, RN, PhD, CNS, CCNS, CCRN

INTRODUCTION

Trauma is defined as a physical injury caused by external forces or violence.[2] Trauma, or unintentional injury, is the fifth leading cause of death in the United States, claiming the lives of predominately young individuals.[12] Only heart disease, cancer, stroke, and chronic respiratory diseases result in a higher death rate. In 2005, the number of deaths from unintentional injury increased for the seventh consecutive year, and experts expect this trend to continue.[51]

Motor vehicle crashes (MVCs) are the most common cause of traumatic death and often involve the use of alcohol, drugs, or other substance abuse. Trauma is frequently referred to as the disease of the young, because the majority of injured persons range in age from 16 to 44 years. An overarching goal in trauma care is prevention. However, when traumatic injuries occur, the priority is early and aggressive interventions to save life and limb.

This chapter provides a review of trauma systems, the trauma team concept, and phases of trauma care. The nature of traumatic events usually requires surgical interventions; thus the postsurgical management of the trauma patient is discussed. Special populations, frequent traumatic injuries, and mass casualty response are also described.

TRAUMA DEMOGRAPHICS

The incidence of trauma in the United States is a major health care and economic concern because of the loss of life, the societal burden in terms of lost productivity and increased disability of injured persons, as well as the consumption of health care resources.[28] MVCs and firearm incidents are the leading cause of death for persons 16 to 24 years of age.[51] A second peak in trauma-related incidents occurs between the ages of 35 and 44, in which MVCs are the primary mechanism of injury. A third peak in unintentional injuries and deaths occurs between the ages of 72 and 85, consisting of MVCs and fall-related injuries. Males are much more likely to experience traumatic injury (2:1 odds ratio) when compared with the frequency of females experiencing unintentional injury or death.[12,51] In addition, drug and alcohol consumption are leading contributing causes of traumatic events.[25]

MVC-related injuries account for 41% of all unintentional injuries and 44.5% of traumatic deaths, and incidents peak around the age of 19 years.[51] In addition, MVCs are associated with the largest number of hospital and critical care unit days utilized. Falls account for 27% of unintentional injuries, affecting primarily an older population, and are responsible for the second largest number of hospital and critical care unit days utilized. Injuries and deaths from firearms peak around 19 years of age and taper off at 22 years, accounting for 22% of unintentional deaths and 6% of injuries requiring hospital and critical care.[51]

Economic factors to consider with traumatic injury include both direct and indirect costs. Direct costs are related to the actual expense of acute hospitalization and rehabilitative care an individual receives as a result of a traumatic event. Indirect costs are associated with lost work, physical disability (temporary and permanent), psychological disability, and lost productivity. It is estimated that 10% (approximately $120 billion) of total U.S. medical expenditures is attributable to trauma care costs, and more than 400,000 individuals develop permanent disabilities.[28]

Significant advances in trauma prevention during the past 30 years have decreased the frequency and severity of traumatic injuries. Advocates of organized trauma systems identify prevention as an essential component of a structured approach to trauma care. Organized trauma care systems have also decreased patient morbidity and mortality.[11] Nurses play an essential role in the care of the trauma patient, from prevention to resuscitation through rehabilitation.

SYSTEMS APPROACH TO TRAUMA CARE

Trauma System

A model trauma system provides an organized approach to trauma care that includes components of prevention, rapid access, acute hospital care, rehabilitation, and research activities.[2] Regional and state trauma systems provide comprehensive processes to deliver optimal care through an established trauma system network that matches a patient's medical needs to the level of trauma hospital with the resources necessary to provide the best possible care for the type and severity of traumatic injury. A trauma system combines levels of designated trauma centers that coexist with other acute care facilities. Levels of a trauma system are a differentiation of medical care, but are defined by resources available within the specific hospital.[2]

Levels of Trauma Care

Trauma systems are effective in reducing morbidity and mortality of severely injured individuals.[2,11,28,41,61] The development of trauma systems has reduced the preventable death rate from unintentional injuries from 40% 30 years ago to less than 4% today.[25]

Formal categorization of trauma care facilities is considered essential to provide optimal care of the traumatically injured patient. The goal of the trauma system is to match the needs of injured patients to the resources and capabilities of the trauma facility. The first civilian trauma units began in the United States in 1966, and in 1971 the state of Illinois created the first trauma system mandated by state legislation.[2] In 1976, the American College of Surgeons Committee on Trauma (ACS-COT) developed a program of external review and verification of hospitals for trauma care to ensure that certain standards in trauma management were met within hospitals that obtained the trauma verification. In 1992, under the direction of the Health Resources and Services Administration, the Trauma Care Systems Plan was developed, providing a framework for the current trauma system and a verification process in the United States.

The ACS-COT trauma system identifies a trauma center's expected level of care based on categories: Level I, II, III, or IV.[2] *Level I* facilities are regional resource trauma centers that are tertiary care hospitals. Level I centers have maximal resources across the spectrum of trauma care including prevention programs, acute treatment, rehabilitation, and trauma-related research; most are university-based teaching hospitals.[2] Patients who are most severely injured should be cared for in a Level I trauma center to optimize patient outcomes. *Level II* trauma centers are hospitals that provide definitive care to severely injured patients; however, they may not be able to provide the same comprehensive trauma care as a Level I center because of limited resources. A Level II center may care for complex patients, yet may transport patients to a Level I facility if advanced and extended surgical care is required. *Level III* facilities are often in communities where no Level I or II facilities exist. Level III facilities provide prompt assessment, resuscitation, emergency surgery, and stabilization of a patient until transfer of the patient to a higher level of trauma care is arranged. *Level IV* facilities provide advanced trauma life support and prepare for immediate transport of the patient. Level I through IV designated hospitals collaborate to develop transfer agreements and treatment protocols that maximize patients' survival.

All states with an identified trauma system are divided into regions. Each region has an identified lead trauma hospital. The lead hospital is usually the Level I trauma center.[2]

Trauma Continuum

Despite advances in trauma care, the continued high incidence of unintentional death and disability of survivors of traumatic injury remain a health care challenge. Death caused by traumatic injury is described as a trimodal distribution occurring in one of three periods. The first peak of death occurs within seconds to minutes from the time of injury. Death is caused by severe injuries, such as apnea from severe brain or high spinal cord injury, or exsanguinating hemorrhage (e.g., rupture of the heart, aorta, or other large blood vessels). Only trauma prevention will decrease deaths that occur in the first peak. The second peak occurs within minutes to several hours after injury. Death is the result of subdural and epidural hematomas, hemopneumothorax, ruptured spleen, liver lacerations, pelvic fractures, and/or other multiple injuries associated with significant blood loss. This first hour of emergent care, the "golden hour," focuses on rapid assessment, resuscitation, and treatment of life-threatening injuries. The third peak occurs several days to weeks after the initial injury and is most often the result of sepsis, acute respiratory distress syndrome (ARDS), and multiple organ dysfunction syndrome (MODS). Patient outcomes in this time frame are affected by the care provided early in the management of the traumatic injury.[1,61] The trimodal distribution of death supports the central concept of trauma systems matching patients' severity of injury to the available resources for optimal care at an accredited trauma facility. Special resources, including early surgical management of injuries, are needed to decrease the morbidity and mortality of severely injured patients; thus the most critically injured patients should be cared for in higher-level trauma centers to maximize patient outcomes.[11,28,34,41,61]

Injury Prevention

Traumatic injury is considered a preventable public health problem and is the most important aspect of trauma system effectiveness.[34] Injury prevention occurs at three levels. *Primary prevention* involves interventions to prevent the event (e.g., driving safety classes, speed limits, campaigns to not drink and drive). *Secondary prevention* entails strategies to minimize the impact of the traumatic event (e.g., seat belt use, airbags, automobile construction, car seats, helmets). *Tertiary prevention* refers to interventions to maximize patient outcomes after a traumatic event through emergency response systems, medical care, and rehabilitation.

Historically, traumatic events and subsequent injuries were considered accidents or events that resulted from human error, fate, or bad luck. Research that explored antecedents of traumatic events found that traumatic injuries are not random events.[64] An individual's knowledge, risk-taking behaviors, beliefs, and decision to engage in a certain activity influence the outcome of actions. The word *accident* conveys a message of randomness in which an individual cannot prevent the event. Because most traumatic events are considered preventable, the word accident has been removed from discussion of traumatic injury, such as a motor vehicle accident. Current verbiage is a *motor vehicle crash*. Changing the language conveys the message that preventive efforts can be implemented to prevent a MVC, and additional behaviors, such as wearing a seat belt, may minimize the impact of the crash.

Nurses play an important role in the spectrum of trauma prevention. Nurses can role model trauma prevention within their family, community, and through political involvement. Political involvement includes simple efforts such as writing letters to local and national policy makers encouraging changes in laws and/or enforcing public policies favoring injury prevention (e.g., helmet and seat belt laws, driving under the influence of drugs and alcohol laws, limiting access to firearms laws). Involvement in trauma prevention includes supporting community and national coalition networks for trauma prevention (e.g., Mothers Against Drunk Drivers; National Safe Kids Campaign). Nurses provide ongoing injury prevention education to patients and families including fall prevention for older adults, child seat and seat belt safety, helmet safety, and drug and alcohol prevention education. The opportunity to decrease death from unintentional injury lies in preventing the initial traumatic event.

Trauma Team Concept

The term *trauma team*, similar to a code team, refers to health care professionals who respond immediately to and participate in the initial resuscitation and stabilization of the trauma patient. Box 19-1 lists the composition of a typical trauma team. Trauma care begins in the field when the emergency medical response (EMS) team responds to an event. Trauma systems work with EMS teams to create protocols that maximize treatment in the field. Once a patient is transported to a hospital, the acute care trauma team is activated. Essential to the team approach is that each team member is preassigned and understands the specific responsibilities inherent in a particular team role. The *trauma surgeon* is ultimately responsible for the activities of the trauma team and acts as the team leader in establishing rapid assessment, resuscitation, stabilization, and intervention priorities. Other team members, such as emergency department physicians, consulting physicians (e.g., orthopedic surgeons, neurosurgeons, otolaryngologists, thoracic surgeons, ophthalmologists, plastic surgeons), nurses, respiratory therapists, social workers, pastoral care providers, and interventional

---

BOX 19-1   Multidisciplinary Trauma Team

- Emergency medical response (EMS) team
- Trauma surgeon (team leader)
- Emergency physician
- Anesthesiologist
- Trauma nurse team leader (coordinates and directs nursing care)
- Trauma resuscitation nurse (hangs fluids, blood, and medications; assists physicians)
- Trauma scribe (records all interventions on the trauma flowsheet)
- Laboratory phlebotomist
- Radiological technologist
- Respiratory therapist
- Social worker/pastoral services
- Hospital security officer
- Physician specialists (neurosurgeon, orthopedic surgeon, urological surgeon)

radiologists, have specific responsibilities. Each member of the trauma team is vital to meeting the needs of a multitrauma patient.

Prehospital Care and Transport

Reduced morbidity and mortality is achieved with rapid assessment in the field by prehospital personnel and immediate transport of the trauma patient to an appropriate trauma care facility. Once EMS personnel arrive at the scene of a traumatic incident, they direct the situation and prepare the patient for transport. The time from injury to definitive care is a determinant of survival in many critically injured patients, particularly those with major internal hemorrhage.[1,2,11] Treatment of life-threatening problems is provided at the scene, with careful attention given to the *airway* with cervical spine immobilization, *breathing*, and *circulation* (ABCs). Interventions include establishing an airway, providing ventilation, applying pressure to control hemorrhage, immobilizing the complete spine, and stabilizing fractures.[1,2,9] The ultimate goal of any EMS system is to get the patient to the right level of hospital care in the shortest span of time to optimize patients' outcomes.[9] Additional lifesaving prehospital interventions that may be required include occlusive dressings on open chest wounds, endotracheal intubation, and needle thoracotomy to relieve tension pneumothorax.

Large-bore venous access and administration of crystalloid solution to restore blood volume to maintain systemic arterial blood pressure may be initiated. Administration of intravenous (IV) fluids is dependent on the mechanism of injury. Research has shown that patients with isolated penetrating trauma and a short transit time to a hospital are more likely to survive if IV fluids are limited or withheld.[13] It is believed that patients who have isolated penetrating vascular injury form a temporary clot over the injury site, and excessive IV fluid resuscitation may dislodge the clot, increasing bleeding.[9,13,19] The current standard of practice is to infuse a crystalloid solution such as normal saline or lactated Ringer's solution. Both solutions in excess can precipitate complications such as hyperchloremic metabolic acidosis and inflammatory organ injury (e.g., ARDS, MODS). Studies are currently exploring the use of hypertonic IV fluids for resuscitation to effectively restore circulating volume without negative sequelae from excessive fluid administration.[1,9]

Ground or air transport is appropriate for the trauma patient from the scene of the injury to the trauma center. Considerations in the choice of transport include travel time, terrain, availability of air and ground units, capabilities of transport personnel, and weather conditions. Once the decision is made to transport a patient to a trauma center, the trauma team is notified. In most trauma centers, the initial resuscitation and stabilization of the trauma patient occur in a designated resuscitation area, usually within the emergency department. Optimally, the trauma team responds before the patient's arrival and begins preparations based on the report of the patient's injuries and clinical status. Trauma patients in unstable condition may be admitted directly to the operating room for resuscitation and immediate surgical intervention.

Trauma Triage

Triage of an injured patient to the appropriate care facility with the necessary personnel and resources is an essential component of a successful trauma system. *Triage* means sorting the patients to determine which patients need specialized care for actual or potential injuries. Determining the type of patient who requires transport to a trauma center rather than a basic emergency care facility occurs according to the EMS providers' assessment, established protocols, policies, and procedures. Triage decisions are often made by prehospital personnel based on knowledge of the mechanisms of injury and rapid assessment of the patient's clinical status. Medical direction of this process occurs through voice communication and medical review of triage decisions.

Trauma may be classified as minor or major depending on the severity of injury. *Minor trauma* refers to a single-system injury that does not pose a threat to life or limb and can be appropriately treated in a basic emergency facility. *Major trauma* refers to serious multiple system injuries that require immediate intervention to prevent disability, loss of limb, or death. In some regions, an injury scoring system is used to objectively measure and convey the severity of injury an individual has sustained. Several scoring systems are used for this purpose. The Abbreviated Injury Scale (AIS) and the Injury Severity Score (ISS) divide the body into seven regions and use a severity score from 1 to 6 for each injury. The AIS score is calculated from the three most severely injured body regions. The ISS is the sum of scores of the highest AIS score in three body regions. The risk for mortality increases with a higher ISS. A score of 1 indicates minor injury, and a score of 6 is fatal.

Another scoring system that is used to objectively evaluate a patient's severity of neurological injury is the Glasgow Coma Scale. The lower this score, based on three assessment parameters, the more severe the neurological injury, suggesting the need for emergent transport to a trauma center (see Chapter 13).

The Revised Trauma Score (RTS) is another tool. The RTS is a prospective physiological scoring system based on initial assessment of the patient. The variables assessed in determining the RTS are blood pressure, respiratory rate, and Glasgow Coma Scale score. In this scoring system, lower scores are associated with a higher mortality.

The development of and adherence to established triage criteria are essential for maintaining an effective system of optimal care for the trauma patient. Triage decisions are based on abnormal findings in the patient's physiological functions, the mechanism of injury, the severity of injury, the anatomical area of injury, or evidence of risk factors such as age and preexisting disease. Other criteria, such as passenger space intrusion and a 30-inch deformity of an automobile, may be considered in the decision to triage to a trauma center. Prehospital personnel may elect to transport the patient to a trauma center in the absence of accepted triage criteria. This decision is most often based on visualization of the trauma incident and the patient's clinical condition.

Disaster and Mass Casualty Management

A disaster is a sudden event in which local EMS services, hospitals, and community resources are overwhelmed by the demands placed on them. Disasters can be caused by fire, weather (e.g., earthquake, hurricane, floods, tornado), explosions, terrorist activity, radiation or chemical spills, epidemic outbreaks, and human error (e.g., plane crash, multicar crash). Disaster planning and management response have long been considered a primary responsibility of trauma systems. However, each disaster is unique, placing tremendous strain on communities to minimize mortality, injury, and destruction of property.[2]

Disasters are classified by the number of victims involved: mass patient incident refers to fewer than 10 victims; multiple casualty incident refers to 10 to 100 victims; mass casualty incident refers to more than 100 victims.[15] Disasters also vary in resource demand depending on whether any warning was available before the event. For example, with impending bad weather disasters (e.g., hurricane), medical personnel can prepare a tentative plan for response. Unfortunately, some disasters such as plane crashes do not allow for preparation.

Regardless of the event, several principles in disaster management and mass casualty care exist. Initially, the local EMS system notifies the area hospitals of the disaster. Level I trauma centers take the lead in responding and preparing to care for the most severely injured patients. Effective field triage is vital in determining how patients are transported to local hospitals and trauma centers.

Command control centers and communication stations are established at the event site when possible and maintain contact with the lead hospital to facilitate efficient transport of patients.[31] Effective, consistent, and accurate communication of the activities at the disaster site and effective management of the severity and volume of incoming victims at the hospitals are critical to successful disaster and mass casualty management.[2,15,17,32,39]

During disasters, all health care personnel are requested to respond. Hospitals have well-developed disaster plans that outline specific health care provider responses during an event (e.g., disaster plan for weather, bombs, mass casualty). These plans outline the roles and responsibilities of all health care providers including hospital administrators, physicians, nurses, pharmacists, respiratory therapists, and security personnel. All personnel are required to be familiar with the disaster response policy.

Hospitals maintain disaster phone call lists that are activated during a disaster. When a disaster occurs, each area of the hospital activates this phone list and calls all the names on the list. Individuals are informed of when and where to respond within the hospital to help with the disaster management. Both human resources and medical supplies are assessed, and health care personnel are frequently rotated to minimize fatigue. Maximal treatment is provided to the victims; however, supplies are judiciously used to avoid running out of essential items.

Upon arrival at the hospital, victims are further triaged by physicians based on the severity of injury. Many mass casualty triage classification schemes exist. However, the most useful method involves treatment based on three gross category assessments: (1) patients who are dead or have no possibility to survive; (2) patients with survivable injuries needing immediate care; (3) patients who are moderately to minimally injured and can wait several hours for definitive medical care.[1,2,32] Patients receive treatment based on the assessment of greatest chances for survival matched to immediate resources available for medical intervention.

Disasters cause significant psychological stress during the event and after the situation has been stabilized.[17] Too often, the psychological well-being of the health care provider is not acknowledged after a disaster event. Resources to debrief health care professionals involved in disaster and mass casualty response are needed to help process the psychological stress and trauma experienced during the event. Debriefing frequently occurs as a group discussion session involving all health care team members involved in the disaster response; however, individual and ongoing psychological interventions may be necessary.[55] Current standards strongly encourage debriefing of health care providers soon after an event to address the psychological stress of the individual and team.[55]

MECHANISMS OF INJURY

Injury and death result from both unintentional and deliberate (violent aggression and suicide) events. *Mechanism of injury* refers to how a traumatic event occurred, the injuring agent, and information about the type and amount of energy exchanged during the event. Knowledge of the mechanism of injury assists the trauma team in early identification and management of injuries that may not be apparent on initial assessment.[10,29] It guides the assessment and interventions to minimize the chances of missing injuries that are more subtle (e.g., organ contusions). Questions regarding mechanisms of injury are directed to the patient (if applicable), prehospital care providers, law enforcement personnel, or bystanders in an attempt to reenact the scene of the trauma. Questions that may be asked include the following: *Did the victim wear a seat belt? What was the speed of the vehicle on impact? Where was the victim located in the car—driver, passenger? Was the victim in the front seat or rear seat? Did the victim wear a helmet (bike, motorcycle, snow sporting crash)? What type of weapon was used (length of knife, type and caliber of gun)? How far did the patient fall? How long was the patient in the field before EMS arrived?*

Personal and environmental risk factors include patient age, sex, race, alcohol or substance abuse, geography, and temporal variation. Temporal variation describes the pattern and timing of trauma. For example, injury deaths occur most frequently on weekends, unintentional injuries occur during recreational activities, and suicides occur more frequently on Mondays.[65] Injury may also occur when patients are deficient in oxygen, such as drowning or suffocation; or, in response to cold, leading to frostbite.

The transfer of energy causes traumatic injury. Energy may be kinetic (e.g., crashes, falls, blast injuries, penetrating injuries), thermal, electrical, chemical, or from radiation exposure. *Kinetic energy* is defined as mass multiplied by velocity squared, divided by 2. Therefore, the greater the mass and velocity (speed), the more significant the displacement of kinetic energy to the body structures, resulting in severe injury. The effects of the energy released and the resultant injuries depend on the force of impact, the duration of impact, the body part involved, the injuring agent, and the presence of associated risk factors.

Injury patterns from energy exchange are further described as blunt, penetrating, and blast injuries. The incidence of blunt trauma is usually greater in rural and suburban areas, whereas penetrating trauma occurs more frequently in inner-city urban neighborhoods. Blast injuries occur less frequently and include construction site explosions and terrorist attacks.[7]

Blunt Trauma

Blunt trauma is the most common mechanism of injury. It most often results from MVCs, but it also occurs from assaults with blunt objects, falls from heights, sports-related activities, and pedestrians struck by a motor vehicle. The severity of injury depends on the amount of kinetic energy dissipated to the body and its underlying structures. Blunt trauma may be caused by accelerating, decelerating, shearing, crushing, and compressing forces. Vehicular trauma often results from a mechanism of acceleration-deceleration forces. The vehicle and the body accelerate and travel at an identified speed. In normal circumstances, the vehicle and body slow to a motionless state in a timely manner. However, when the vehicle stops abruptly, as in a collision, the body continues to travel forward until it comes into contact with a stationary object such as the dashboard, windshield, or steering column. Bodily injury occurs in the presence of rapid deceleration, when the movement ceases and contents within the body continue to travel within an enclosed space or compartment. An example of this occurs when the patient's head strikes the windshield after impalement of the automobile into a cement barrier. The brain tissue strikes the cranium and is thrown back against the opposite side of the cranial vault, with a resulting coup-contrecoup injury. In addition, shearing forces of the cerebral tissue and the skull cause vessels to stretch and exceed their elasticity, resulting in tears, dissection, or rupture. Figure 19-1 shows potential sites of injury in an unrestrained passenger and driver as a result of blunt trauma.

Body tissues and structures respond to kinetic energy in different ways. Low-density porous tissues and structures, such as the lungs, tolerate energy transference and often experience little damage because of their elasticity. Conversely, organs such as the heart, spleen, and liver are less resilient because of the high-density tissue and the decreased ability to release energy without resultant tissue damage. These types of organs often present with fragmentation or rupture. The severity of injury resulting from a blunt force is contingent on the duration of energy exposure, the body part involved, and the underlying structures.

Blunt trauma requires expert clinical judgment to assess and diagnose actual and potential injury. Organ injury from blunt trauma may not be immediately visible. Knowledge of the mechanism of injury and effects of blunt trauma forces is vital in the care of the blunt trauma patient.

Penetrating Trauma

Penetrating trauma results from the impalement of foreign objects (e.g., knives, bullets, debris) into the

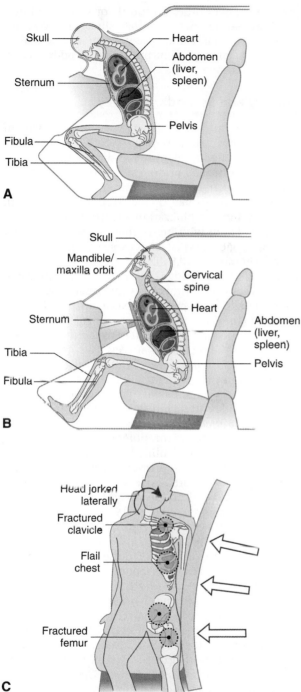

A

B

C

FIGURE 19-1. Potential sites of blunt trauma injury in unrestrained passenger and driver in a motor vehicle crash. **A,** Unrestrained passenger in front seat. **B,** Unrestrained driver. **C,** Lateral impact collision. *(From Herm, R. L. [2003]. Biomechanics and mechanism of injury. In S. S. Cohen [Ed.], Trauma nursing secrets [p. 8]. Philadelphia: Hanley & Belfus.)*

body. Penetrating injuries are more easily diagnosed and treated because of the obvious signs of injury. Stab wounds are low-velocity injuries because the velocity is equal only to the speed with which the object is thrust into the body. The direct path of injury occurs when the impaled object comes into contact with underlying vessels and tissues. Important considerations in a stabbing are the length and width of the impaling object, and the presence of vital organs in the area of the stab wound. Gender differences are seen and may provide information on the trajectory of the injury. Women tend to stab with a downward thrust, whereas male assailants use an upward force.

Ballistic trauma is categorized as either medium- or high-velocity injuries. Medium-velocity weapons are handguns and some rifles. High-velocity weapons are assault weapons and hunting rifles.[10] High-velocity injuries result in greater dissipation of the kinetic energy and more significant bodily injury. The velocity and type of bullet (missile) influence the transfer of energy creating tissue injury. As the missile penetrates the tissues, vessels are stretched and compressed, creating tissue damage referred to as a cavitation. Depending on the range, the distance from the weapon to the point of bodily impact, and the velocity of the missile, the cavitation may be as great as 30 times the diameter of the bullet. As bullets travel through tissues, damage to surrounding tissues and organs may occur. Knowledge of the type of bullet (e.g., size, hollow, shotgun pellet bullets) influences the assessment as to the type of internal tissue damage that may have occurred.

Assessment of penetrating injury from gunshot wounds involves examination of the entrance and exit wound. The entrance wound is usually smaller than the exit wound; however, forensic experts rather than the trauma team determine the direction of the bullet entrance and exit.[10] Penetrating injuries are monitored closely for subsequent complications including organ damage, hemorrhage, and infection.

Blast Injuries

Blast injuries are forms of blunt and penetrating trauma. Energy exchanged from the blast causes tissue and organ damage. Penetrating injury may occur as a result of debris impalement into the body. Blast injuries are classified as primary, secondary, tertiary, and quaternary.[1,7] The primary explosive blast generates shock waves that create changes in air pressure, causing tissue damage. Initially after an explosion, there is a rapid increase in positive pressure for a short period, followed by a longer period of negative pressure. The increase in positive pressure injures gas-containing organs. The tympanic membrane ruptures, and the lungs may show evidence of contusion, acute edema, or rupture. Intraocular hemorrhage and intestinal rupture may occur from the first shock wave after an explosion. Secondary injuries occur from increased negative pressure from the shock wave causing debris to impale the body, creating organ and tissue damage. Tertiary blast injuries are the result of the body being thrown by the force of the explosion, resulting in blunt tissue trauma including closed head injuries, fractures, and visceral organ injury. Quaternary blast injuries occur from chemical, thermal, and biological exposure.

EMERGENCY CARE PHASE

Information obtained during the prehospital phase provides essential data to ensure a coordinated, life-saving approach in the management of trauma patients. Most traumatic events are considered "scoop and run" situations with short transport times, but other patients may come to the hospital by private car. Trauma centers designate rooms or resuscitation areas within the emergency department for the management of trauma patients. These trauma rooms provide a central location for the team to provide a quick initial assessment, stabilization, and determination of the immediate medical needs of the patient.

Procedures exist within hospitals to activate the trauma team, including the operating room team, for emergent surgical interventions. The resuscitation area must always be in a state of readiness for the next trauma patient. Equipment needed for management of the airway with cervical spine immobilization, breathing, circulatory support, and hemorrhage control must be immediately available and easily accessible. The trauma surgeon is the lead health care provider in directing the patient's care throughout the emergent phase as well as the acute hospitalization. The nurse plays an essential role in assisting with assessment, advocating for the patient, and anticipating the needs of the trauma team and patient.

Initial Patient Assessment

Patient survival after a serious traumatic event depends on prompt, rapid, and systematic assessment in conjunction with immediate resuscitative interventions. Priorities of care are based on the patient's clinical presentation, physical assessment, history of the traumatic event (mechanism of injury), and knowledge of preexisting disease. Evaluation of airway patency, ventilation, and venous access with circulatory support are of prime importance and take

precedence over other diagnostic or definitive interventions. Adherence to established protocols for patient assessment and intervention is essential to ensure that management priorities are addressed in a timely manner.

Primary and Secondary Survey

The primary survey is the most crucial assessment tool in trauma care. This rapid, 1- to 2-minute evaluation is designed to identify life-threatening injuries accurately, establish priorities, and provide simultaneous therapeutic interventions. The *primary survey* is a systematic survey of the patient's airway with cervical spine immobilization, breathing and ventilation, circulation with hemorrhage control, disability or neurological status, and exposure/environmental considerations (ABCDEs).[1] During the primary survey, life-threatening conditions are identified and management is instituted simultaneously.[1] Table 19-1 details the critical assessment parameters included in the primary survey. All major life-threatening conditions must be treated before one proceeds to the secondary survey.

The *secondary survey* is a methodical head-to-toe evaluation of the patient using the assessment techniques of inspection, palpation, percussion, and auscultation to identify all injuries. The secondary survey is initiated after the primary survey has been completed and all actual or potential life-threatening injuries have been identified and addressed. Heart rate, auscultated blood pressure, core body temperature, respiratory effort, and level of consciousness are obtained as a baseline for analysis of trends during the resuscitation phase (Table 19-2). A mnemonic (*F through I*) may be used to remember the features of the secondary assessment: F—*full set of vital signs, five interventions* (cardiac monitor, pulse oximetry, urinary catheter, nasogastric tube, laboratory tests), and *facilitate family presence*; G—*give comfort*; H—*history* and *head-to-toe assessment*; and I—*inspect posterior.*[21]

Information about actual and potential injuries are noted and used to establish diagnostic and treatment priorities. Radiological studies are completed according to a standardized trauma protocol or an assessment of suspected injuries. The sequence of diagnostic procedures is influenced by the patient's level of consciousness, the stability of the patient's condition, the mechanism of injury, and the identified injuries. As data are obtained, the team leader determines the need for consultation with specialty physicians such as neurosurgeons, orthopedists, urologists, or others. Supportive interventions such as splinting of extremities, wound care, and administration of tetanus prophylaxis and antibiotics are completed.

TABLE 19-1 Primary Survey: ABCDE	
Assessment	**Observations Indicating Impairment**
A = Airway Open and patent Maintain cervical spine immobilization Patency of artificial airway (if present)	Shallow, noisy breathing Stridor Central cyanosis Nasal flaring Accessory muscle use Inability to speak Drooling Anxiety Decreased level of consciousness Trauma to face, mouth, neck Debris or foreign matter in mouth or pharynx
B = Breathing Presence and effectiveness	Asymmetrical chest movement Absent, decreased, or unequal breath sounds Open chest wounds Blunt chest injury Dyspnea Central cyanosis Respiratory rate <8-10 breaths/ min or >40 breaths/min Accessory muscle use Anxiety Decreased level of consciousness Tracheal shift
C = Circulation Presence of major pulses Presence of external hemorrhage	Weak, thready pulse HR >120 beats/min Pallor Systolic BP <90 mm Hg MAP <65 mm Hg Obvious external hemorrhage Decreased level of consciousness
D = Disability Gross neurological status Pupil size, equality, and reactivity to light Spontaneous/moves to command	Glasgow Coma Scale score ≤11 Agitation Lack of spontaneous movement Posturing Lack of sensation in extremities
E = Expose patient Environmental control Remove patient's clothing Rewarm with blankets, warming lights, fluid-filled or air convection warming blankets	Presence of soft tissue injury, crepitus, deformities, edema

BP, Blood pressure; *HR,* heart rate; *MAP,* mean arterial pressure.

RESUSCITATION PHASE

From the time of initial injury until the patient is stabilized in the emergency department or operating room, the trauma team resuscitates the patient. *Resuscitation* in trauma refers to reestablishing an effective circulatory volume and a stable hemodynamic status in the patient. During the emergency care phase, effective resuscitation is a central component of the primary and secondary survey. The ABCDEs of the emergency care phase are *airway, breathing, circulation, disability* (neurological), and *exposure,* and treating life-threatening injuries (e.g., pneumothorax, cardiac tamponade) emergently. Each of these interventions is discussed in detail.

Establishing Airway Patency

Establishing and maintaining a patent airway is an essential element of trauma management. An effective airway allows for adequate ventilation and optimal oxygenation. Every trauma patient has the potential for an ineffective airway, whether it occurs at the time of injury or develops during resuscitation. The tongue, because of posterior displacement, is the most common cause of airway obstruction. Other causes of obstruction are foreign debris (blood or vomitus) and anatomical obstructions from maxillofacial fractures. Direct injuries to the throat or neck can structurally impair the airway. Patients with an altered sensorium or high spinal cord injuries may not be able to protect their airway.

Opening the airway is easily accomplished by the simple manual technique of a jaw thrust or chin lift. These maneuvers do not hyperextend the neck or compromise the integrity of the cervical spine. These are temporary interventions that move the mandible anteriorly and create a patent airway. The airway must be cleared of any foreign material such as blood, vomitus, bone fragments, or teeth by gentle suction with a tonsillar tip catheter.

Nasopharyngeal and oropharyngeal airways are the simplest artificial airway adjuncts used in patients with spontaneous respirations and adequate ventilatory effort. Both devices help to prevent posterior displacement of the tongue. The oropharyngeal airway is not used in the conscious patient because it may induce gagging, vomiting, and aspiration; if needed, a nasopharyngeal airway is better tolerated.

Endotracheal intubation is the definitive nonsurgical airway management technique and allows for complete control of the airway. Both the oral and nasal routes may be used for intubation. Nasotracheal intubation is indicated for the spontaneously

TABLE 19-2   Secondary Survey

Survey Activities	Actions	Inspection	Palpation	Auscultation
F = Full set of vital signs Five interventions Facilitate family presence	Obtain full set of vital signs (blood pressure, heart rate, respiratory rate, temperature) Insert nasogastric tube, indwelling urinary catheter Obtain oxygen saturation via pulse oximetry Connect to cardiac monitor Obtain blood and urine for laboratory studies Identify family; provide updates; facilitate visitation with patient	Inspect perineal area during insertion of urinary catheter Inspect digits to ensure adequate vascular flow to obtain accurate oxygen saturation	Palpate for radial pulse Palpate for vein to access for blood studies	Auscultate blood pressure
G = Give comfort measures	Provide emotional reassurance Administer narcotics as ordered by trauma surgeon	Inspect patient for relief of pain	Provide touch to facilitate patient comfort and reassurance	
H = History Head-to-toe assessment	Perform head-to-toe assessment Obtain information on allergies, current medications, past illness, pregnancy, last meal	HEAD/FACE: Inspect for wounds, ecchymosis, deformities, drainage, pupillary reaction NECK: Inspect for wounds, ecchymosis, deformities, distended neck veins CHEST: Inspect for breathing rate and depth, wounds, deformities, ecchymosis, use of accessory muscles, paradoxical movement ABDOMEN: Inspect for wounds, distention, ecchymosis, scars PELVIS/PERINEUM: Inspect for wounds, deformities, ecchymosis, priapism, blood at the urinary meatus or in the perineal area EXTREMITIES: Inspect for ecchymosis, movement, wounds, deformities	HEAD/FACE: Palpate for tenderness, crepitus, deformities NECK: Palpate for tenderness, crepitus, deformities, tracheal position CHEST: Palpate for tenderness, crepitus, subcutaneous emphysema, deformities ABDOMEN: Palpate all four quadrants for tenderness, rigidity, guarding, masses, femoral pulses PELVIS/PERINEUM: Palpate the pelvis and anal sphincter tone EXTREMITIES: Palpate for pulses, skin temperature, sensation, tenderness, deformities, crepitus	CHEST: Auscultate breath and heart sounds ABDOMEN: Auscultate bowel sounds; observe for passing flatulence
I = Inspect posterior surfaces	Maintain cervical spine stabilization Log roll using three hospital personnel	Inspect posterior surface for wounds, deformities, and ecchymosis	Palpate posterior surfaces for deformities and pain Assist physician with the rectal examination, if not previously completed	

breathing patient and is used when the urgency of the resuscitation procedure does not allow time to obtain preliminary cervical spine x-ray studies. Nasotracheal intubation is contraindicated for patients with facial, frontal sinus, basilar skull, or cribiform plate fractures.[1] Disadvantages of nasal intubation are that it can cause epistaxis and injury to the nasal turbinates, and can increase the risk for infection. In the presence of documented or suspected cervical spine injury, oral tracheal intubation must be performed carefully to prevent manipulation of the neck. Manual immobilization of the neck must be provided by an assistant during the procedure. Disadvantages of oral tracheal intubation include possible manipulation of the cervical spine, incorrect tube placement in the esophagus or right mainstem bronchus, vocal cord trauma, and injury to the intraoral structures. Before intubation, patients are preoxygenated with 100% oxygen via a bag-valve mask. Rapid sequence intubation (sequential administration of a sedative or anesthetic, and a neuromuscular blocking agent) may be used to facilitate the procedure. Correct position of the tube is verified (see Chapter 9). Mechanical ventilation with 100% oxygen is initiated immediately after intubation. The patient is then attached to a mechanical ventilator to provide ventilation and oxygenation.

In rare circumstances it may be difficult to intubate the trauma patient. In this event, a surgical intervention (cricothyrotomy) is performed to establish an effective airway. Conditions that may require cricothyrotomy are maxillofacial trauma, laryngeal fractures, facial or upper airway burns, airway edema, and severe oropharyngeal hemorrhage. The choice of airway management technique is based on the health care providers' familiarity with the procedures, the clinical condition of the patient, and the degree of hemodynamic stability.

Maintaining Effective Breathing

Interventions to restore normal breathing patterns are directed toward the specific injury or underlying cause of respiratory distress, with the goal of improving ventilation and oxygenation. Basic nursing interventions include application of supplemental oxygen with ventilatory assistance (if applicable), effective positioning, and evaluation of specific interventions. Ineffective breathing patterns are the result of certain traumatic injuries. These injuries and specific interventions are listed in Table 19-3.

The patient is assessed frequently for respiratory rate and effort, heart rate and rhythm, breath sounds, sensorium, skin color, temperature, tracheal position, and jugular venous distention. When spontaneous breathing is present but ineffective, a life-threatening condition must be considered if any of the following are present: altered mental status, central cyanosis, asymmetrical expansion of the chest wall; use of accessory or abdominal muscles, or both; paradoxical movement of the chest wall during inspiration and expiration; diminished or absent breath sounds; tracheal shift from midline position; decreasing oxygen saturation via pulse oximetry; or distended jugular veins. Arterial blood gas analysis and diagnostic studies including chest x-ray and chest computed tomography (CT) imaging may be completed to assist in determining the effectiveness of specific interventions.

Impaired oxygenation follows airway obstruction as the most crucial problem of the trauma patient. Impaired gas exchange can result from ineffective ventilation, an inability to exchange gases at the alveoli, or both. Possible causes include a decrease in inspired air, retained secretions, lung collapse or compression, atelectasis, or accumulation of blood in the thoracic cavity. Any patient presenting with multiple systemic injuries, hemorrhagic shock, chest trauma, and/or central nervous system trauma must be assessed for impaired gas exchange. These conditions have the potential to affect the patient's volume status and oxygen-carrying capacity, interfere with the mechanics of ventilation, or interrupt the autonomic control of respirations. Assessment is ongoing, and the nurse must be prepared to assist with intubation and subsequent mechanical ventilation, needle thoracostomy, chest tube insertion, and restoration of circulating blood volume.

Maintaining Circulation

Maintaining adequate circulation is essential. The most common cause of hypotension and impaired cardiac output in the trauma patient is hypovolemic shock from acute blood loss. Causes may be external (hemorrhage) or internal (hemothorax, hemoperitoneum, solid organ injury, long bone or massive pelvic fractures). Initial interventions include applying pressure to control the bleeding, replacing circulatory volume with crystalloid and blood products, and determining definitive treatment. In the face of hypovolemic shock from hemorrhage, early, rapid surgical intervention is lifesaving and limb saving.[1,2,41]

The management of hypovolemic shock focuses on finding and eliminating the cause of the bleeding and concomitant support of the patient's circulatory system with IV fluids and blood products (see Chapter 11). Frequently, it is difficult to assess a young patient's blood loss, especially with internal hemorrhage from blunt trauma. Sympathetic compensa-

TABLE 19-3 Specific Interventions for Ineffective Breathing Patterns

Etiology	Interventions
Tension pneumothorax	Prepare for decompression by needle thoracostomy with a 14-gauge needle in second intercostal space at the midclavicular line on affected side. Prepare for chest tube insertion on affected side.
Pneumothorax	Prepare for chest tube insertion on affected side.
Open chest wound	Seal the wound with an occlusive dressing and tape on three sides. Prepare for chest tube insertion on affected side.
Massive hemothorax	Establish two 14-gauge or 16-gauge peripheral IV lines for crystalloid infusion. Obtain blood for type and crossmatch. Prepare for chest tube insertion on affected side. Administer blood or blood products as ordered. Anticipate and prepare for emergency open thoracotomy.
Pulmonary contusion	Prepare for early intubation and mechanical ventilation.
Flail chest	Prepare for early intubation and mechanical ventilation. Administer analgesics as ordered.
Spinal cord injury	Avoid hyperextension or rotation of the patient's neck. Observe ventilatory effort and use of accessory muscles. Maintain complete spinal immobilization. Prepare for application of cervical traction tongs or a halo device. Monitor motor and sensory function. Monitor for signs of distributive (neurogenic) shock.
Decreased level of consciousness	Position the patient's head midline with the head of the bed elevated. Anticipate a computed tomography scan. Implement interventions to prevent aspiration. Prepare for intubation and mechanical ventilation.

IV, Intravenous.

tory mechanisms in the body respond to states of hypoperfusion through tachycardia, narrowing pulse pressure, tachypnea, and decreased urine output. These signs and symptoms may not be obvious until the patient is in a later stage of hypovolemic shock.[1] As a result of hypovolemia and hypoxemia, metabolic acidosis occurs secondary to a shift from aerobic to anaerobic metabolism and the production of lactic acid. The serum arterial lactate level and base deficit are markers of effective tissue perfusion. The higher the lactate level and base deficit, the more severe the tissue underperfusion and the higher the morbidity and mortality.[16]

Diagnostic Testing

Determining the cause of bleeding is imperative. Diagnostic testing, including chest and pelvis x-ray studies, abdominal ultrasound, and x-ray studies of suspected extremity fractures, is completed early in the resuscitative phase to determine injuries and potential sources of bleeding. An abdominal CT scan may be completed to assist in identifying a specific source of intraperitoneal bleeding. However, an abdominal CT scan is not the diagnostic test of choice in the presence of hemodynamic instability. In this case, a *focused assessment with sonography for trauma (FAST)* is the method of choice. FAST provides a rapid, noninvasive means to diagnose peritoneal hemorrhage at the patient's bedside. FAST can be used to evaluate accumulation of blood in the pericardium as well as the peritoneum.[37,49] The primary limitation to FAST is related to the skills of the user.[37]

Diagnostic peritoneal lavage may also be used to evaluate intraperitoneal bleeding. This procedure involves the insertion of a lavage catheter into the peritoneum with subsequent gentle syringe aspiration. If frank blood is obtained, the patient is prepared for emergency laparotomy. If frank blood is not found, a sample of the fluid is sent for evaluation of red blood cells, white blood cells, amylase, bile, bacteria, fecal material, or food particles to determine the need for immediate operative intervention.

Occasionally patients with pelvic and long bone fractures and subsequent blood loss are placed in a *pneumatic antishock garment (PASG)*. Compartments in these pants can be inflated to hold pressure on long bones and the pelvis to stabilize a fracture and reduce bleeding during transport. The device may increase intraabdominal and thoracic pressure, compromising effective ventilation, oxygenation, and circulation. Thus, PASGs are infrequently used.

Additional causes of diminished cardiac output are impairment of venous blood return to the heart secondary to tension pneumothorax, and decreased filling and ventricular ejection fraction resulting from pericardial tamponade, cardiac contusions or myocardial infarction. Definitive interventions to relieve the tension of the pneumothorax or pericardial sac are necessary to reestablish effective cardiac output and blood pressure. A chest tube is placed to relieve the pneumothorax. Treatment of the pericardial tamponade requires emergent insertion of a needle into the pericardial sac to remove fluid. If fluid continues to accumulate in the pericardial sac, surgical intervention is necessary.

Adequacy of Resuscitation

Newer technologies are being refined for use during resuscitation to more effectively evaluate the severity of shock before decompensation of vital signs. Two of these technologies are sublingual capnometry and near-infrared spectroscopy (NIRS). Sublingual capnometry is a noninvasive technology that provides information about the degree of hypovolemia and adequacy of fluid resuscitation based on the sublingual partial pressure of carbon dioxide (PCO_2).[27] A probe is placed under the patient's tongue, and PCO_2 levels are derived from the blood flow found in the mucosal bed. During shock, an elevated sublingual PCO_2 indicates poor tissue perfusion. The sublingual PCO_2 is not an exact measure but a derived measure similar to pulse oximetry.

NIRS is a continuous noninvasive technology that uses principles of light transmission to measure skeletal muscle oxygenation as an indicator of shock. The NIRS probe is placed on the thenar muscle, which is located on the palm of the hand by the thumb. The probe measures the oxygen saturation state of tissue by evaluating the amount of infrared light absorption. Low values of tissue oxygenation (<80%) indicate states of shock; the lower the value, the more severe the tissue hypoxemia.[16,18,27]

Fluid Resuscitation

Venous access and infusion of volume are required for optimal fluid resuscitation in the patient with hypovolemic shock. At least two large-bore (14-gauge or 16-gauge) peripheral IV lines are necessary. The forearm or antecubital veins are preferred sites for peripheral lines. A central venous line or a venous cutdown may be necessary because of peripheral vasoconstriction and venous collapse. A central line (single- or multiple-lumen line) may be more beneficial as a resuscitation monitoring tool. A pulmonary artery catheter is not usually helpful in the emergent phase of trauma management, but may be inserted in the critical care unit to evaluate the response to fluid resuscitation. As a general rule, venous access is achieved rapidly with the largest-bore catheter possible to initiate early resuscitation.

Isotonic electrolyte solutions are used for initial fluid resuscitation. Ringer's lactate solution or normal saline are the fluids of choice. A rapid infuser device may be used to facilitate rapid infusion of warm IV fluids. However, alterations in the infusion rate and volume may be necessary for certain trauma populations, such as the patient with cardiac disease. Underresuscitation results in worsening tissue ischemia, and overresuscitation causes life-threatening complications; therefore, assessment of fluid volume status is critical.

Current research is exploring the administration of hypertonic saline for fluid resuscitation. Hypertonic saline provides volume expansion without excessive administration of IV fluids and is associated with fewer adverse effects, such as hyperchloremic metabolic acidosis, abdominal compartment syndrome, ARDS, and MODS.[5,8,16,19,48,60]

The ACS recommends administration of 3 mL of crystalloid solution for each milliliter of blood loss (3 : 1 rule).[1] The patient's response to the initial fluid administration is monitored by assessing urine output (50 mL/hr in the adult), level of consciousness, heart rate, blood pressure, pulse pressure, and laboratory indices (e.g., serum lactate level and base excess).

Three response patterns are used to determine further therapeutic and diagnostic decisions (Table 19-4). These response patterns to initial fluid administration are rapid, transient, or no response.[1] *Rapid responders* react quickly to the initial bolus and remain hemodynamically stable after administration of the initial fluid bolus. Fluids are then slowed to maintenance rates. *Transient responders* improve in response to the initial fluid bolus. However, these patients begin to show deterioration in perfusion when fluids are slowed to maintenance rates. This finding indicates ongoing blood loss or inadequate resuscitation. Continued fluid administration and

TABLE 19-4   Responses to Initial Fluid Resuscitation*

	Rapid Response	Transient Response	No Response
Vital signs	Return to normal	Transient improvement; recurrence of ↓ BP and ↑ HR	Remain abnormal
Estimated blood loss	Minimal (10%-20%)	Moderate (20%-40%)	Severe (>40%)
Need for more crystalloid	Low	High	High
Need for blood	Low	Moderate to high	Immediate
Blood preparation	Type and crossmatch	Type-specific	Emergency blood release
Need for operative intervention	Possibly	Likely	Highly likely
Early presence of a surgeon	Yes	Yes	Yes

*2000 mL Ringer's lactate solution in adults, 20 mL/kg Ringer's lactate bolus in children.
↑, Increased; ↓, decreased; *BP*, blood pressure; *HR*, heart rate; >, greater than.
From the American College of Surgeons, Committee on Trauma. (2004). *Advanced trauma life support for doctors: Instructor's course manual* (7th ed., p. 79). Chicago: American College of Surgeons.

blood transfusion are indicated. If the patient continues to respond in a transient manner, the patient is probably bleeding and requires rapid surgical intervention. *Minimal* or *no responders* fail to respond to crystalloid and blood administration in the emergency department, and surgical intervention is needed immediately to control hemorrhage.

The decision to administer blood is based on the patient's response to initial fluid therapy and the amount of blood lost.[1] If the patient is unresponsive to IV fluid therapy, type-specific blood may be administered. In the event of life-threatening blood loss, the physician may request unmatched, type-specific or type O (universal donor) blood. Crossmatched, type-specific blood should be instituted as soon as it is available. Current practice tolerates lower hemoglobin levels in trauma patients because research has shown that patients receiving massive blood transfusions have poorer outcomes.[33] The decision to give blood is based on the patients' lack of response to only crystalloid resuscitation, the volume of blood lost, the need for hemoglobin to assist with oxygen transport, and the necessity to correct any coagulopathy. If blood loss and coagulopathy are life-threatening, massive blood transfusion may be required. This is defined as administering 10 or more units of packed red blood cells in 24 hours. In this situation, it is necessary to administer platelets and fresh frozen plasma in addition to packed red blood cells to improve patient outcomes. Blood products are given in a 1:1:1 ratio when massive blood transfusions are require—1 unit of packed red blood cells, 1 unit of platelets, and 1 unit of fresh frozen plasma.[31,33,43]

During fluid resuscitation, the patient is monitored for electrolyte imbalances, dilutional coagulopathies, and consequences of excessive third-spacing of IV fluids.[16] Electrolyte imbalances that may develop include hypocalcemia, hypomagnesemia, and hyperkalemia or hypokalemia. These imbalances may lead to changes in myocardial function, laryngeal spasm, and neuromuscular and central nervous system hyperirritability.[16,24]

Dilutional coagulopathy may occur with excessive IV fluid resuscitation and extensive blood loss. Banked blood products have high levels of citrate, which may induce transient hypocalcemia. Decreased serum calcium levels may lead to ineffective coagulation because calcium is a necessary cofactor in the coagulation cascade. Further inhibition of the clotting cascade is observed when platelet dysfunction develops secondary to hypothermia or metabolic acidosis. Management focuses on improving perfusion to the body tissues, increasing the patient's body temperature, and administering clotting factors (fresh frozen plasma, cryoprecipitate, and platelets). Monitoring the hemoglobin level, hematocrit value, plasma fibrinogen level, platelet count, prothrombin time, and partial thromboplastin time is essential.

Third-spacing can pose a significant problem during and within hours of aggressive fluid resuscitation.[16,43,48] During states of hypoperfusion and acidosis, inflammation occurs and vessels become more permeable to fluid and molecules. With aggressive fluid resuscitation, this change in permeability allows the movement of fluid from the intravascular space into the interstitial spaces (third-spacing). Hypovolemia thus occurs in the intravascular space, and patients require a larger volume of fluid replacement. This creates a vicious cycle; as more IV fluids are given to support systemic circulation, fluids continue to migrate into the interstitial space, causing excessive edema and predisposing the patient to additional complications such as abdominal compartment syndrome, ARDS, acute renal failure, and MODS. The goal is to provide adequate fluid resuscitation to prevent tissue hypoxemia. As technological advances continue, specific markers of tissue oxygenation and consumption (sublingual PCO_2 and NIRS) may be used in addition to vital signs, urine output, and level of consciousness to evaluate the effectiveness of fluid resuscitation.

EVIDENCE-BASED PRACTICE

PROBLEM

Aggressive fluid resuscitation of critically ill patients (including those who sustain traumatic injury) with crystalloid solutions can have negative effects of interstitial edema, compromising tissue perfusion and requiring higher volumes of solution for resuscitation. Colloid solutions have also been used in resuscitation. There is ongoing debate about the effectiveness of using colloid solutions compared with crystalloid solutions for effective resuscitation and tissue perfusion.

QUESTION

In critically ill patients, what is the effect on mortality of administering colloids compared with crystalloids for fluid resuscitation?

REFERENCE

Roberts, I., Alderson, P., Bunn, F., et al. (2007). Colloids versus crystalloids for fluid resuscitation in critically ill patients. *Cochrane Database of Systematic Reviews*, issue 3. 1-34.

EVIDENCE

The authors searched the literature from 1994-2007 for all randomized and quasi-randomized trials of administration of colloids compared with crystalloids in critically ill patients requiring volume replacement. Fifty-three studies met the inclusion criteria for review. No evidence from the randomized controlled trials found that resuscitation with colloids reduces the risk of death compared with resuscitation with crystalloids.

IMPLICATIONS FOR NURSING

In critically ill patients, aggressive fluid resuscitation with colloid solutions was not associated with improved survival when compared with aggressive fluid resuscitation with crystalloid solutions. Colloids are expensive, and caution must be exercised when caring for a patient who does not wish to receive blood product components, such as some colloids. Crystalloid resuscitation was found to be effective and may be more cost-effective.

Assessment of Neurological Disabilities

Rapid assessment of patients with neurological injury, along with early intervention, is a vital element of the primary survey. Assessment of neurological disabilities includes evaluation of the patients' level of consciousness, pupillary size and reaction, and spontaneous and reflexive spinal movement, as well as consideration of possible neurological injuries based on the history of the injury (e.g., ejection from motor vehicle, fall, or diving accident).

Hypotension decreases cerebral perfusion; therefore, the patient's response to interventions, and the degree of tissue ischemia are considered in the neurological examination. Recreational drug and/or alcohol use by the patient can mask neurological responsiveness on the neurological examination, leading to misleading findings. If an effective neurological examination cannot be conducted because of the patient's drug use, the health care provider manages the patient based on knowledge of the traumatic event and the patient's neurological response.[1]

Nearly 2 million head injuries occur each year in the United States, and brain injury is the leading single-organ cause of death related to trauma.[6] Close head injury is the cause of 50% of deaths in MVCs involving drivers aged 15 to 24 years.[12,51] Falls are responsible for severe closed head injury in older patients (>65 years). Management priorities focus on the primary injury from the traumatic event and the subsequent secondary injury that occurs as a result of cerebral hypoperfusion, increased intracranial pressure, and/or cerebral edema.

Injuries to the head may result from blunt or penetrating trauma. Primary head injury from blunt trauma typically occurs in the presence of acceleration, deceleration, or rotational forces. Injury may be focal or diffuse. Secondary head injury refers to the systemic (hypotension, hypoxia, anemia, hyperthermia) or intracranial changes (edema, intracranial hypertension, seizures, vasospasm) that result in alterations in the nervous system tissue.[40,53] Patients with secondary injury often have poor outcomes, including death. Nursing interventions focus on ensuring an adequate blood pressure to meet cerebral perfusion needs, maximizing ventilation and oxygenation through effective airway management, maintaining the head in a midline position to enhance cerebral blood flow, administering sedatives to address agitation and increased intracranial pressure, and conducting frequent neurological assessments.[4,40] The key to neurological assessments is recognizing subtle changes and notifying the physician for prompt intervention (see Chapter 13).

Lacerations to the scalp may result in significant bleeding. These wounds are cleansed, debrided, and sutured. Fractures of the skull may be linear, basilar, closed depressed, open depressed, or comminuted. Underlying brain injury may occur with skull fractures. Basilar skull fractures are located at the base of the cranium and potentially involve the five bones that form the skull base. The diagnosis is based on the presence of cerebrospinal fluid in the nose (rhinorrhea), in the ears (otorrhea), or in both; ecchymosis over the mastoid area (Battle's sign); or hemotympanum (blood in the middle ear). Raccoon eyes or periorbital ecchymoses are present after a cribiform plate fracture. Two potential complications that may develop after a basilar skull fracture are infection (meningitis) and cranial nerve injury. Nursing care focuses on assessing the presence and amount of cerebrospinal fluid leak and monitoring for signs and symptoms of possible neurological infection.

Spinal cord injury (SCI) is the second major neurological disability that is assessed early in the emergent phase of traumatic injury. Mechanisms of injuries that may result in SCI include hyperflexion, hyperextension, axial loading, rotation, and penetrating trauma. The initial treatment of a patient with suspected SCI includes the ABCs of resuscitation, spinal immobilization, and prevention of further injury through surgical stabilization of the spine. A complete sensory and motor neurological examination is performed, and x-ray studies of the cervical spine are obtained. A spinal CT scan may be performed to rule out occult injury. It is important to determine the approximate level of SCI because higher cervical spine injuries may result in the loss of phrenic nerve innervations, compromising the patient's ability to breathe spontaneously.

SCI causes a loss of sympathetic output, resulting in distributive shock with hypotension and bradycardia. Blood pressure may respond to IV fluids, but vasopressor therapy is often required to compensate for the loss of sympathetic innervation and resultant vasodilation. Often the patient with an SCI is awake and aware of possible paralysis. Frequently, health care providers discuss care around the patient but do not talk to the patient. The nurse is both an advocate and comforter during the emergent evaluation of the patient. The patient with an SCI presents complex challenges for the trauma team as they attempt to minimize loss of function associated with the injury. Proactive, aggressive, and comprehensive care is necessary to help the patient achieve optimal functional outcomes (see Chapter 13).

Exposure and Environmental Considerations

Standard practice in the management of the patient with trauma is to remove all clothing and expose the patient to allow for full visualization of the body to identify all injuries. Exposure decreases body temperature. Hypothermia, defined as a core body temperature less than 35°C, is caused by a combination of accelerated heat loss and decreased heat production. A person is more susceptible to hypothermia after severe injury (especially older persons), excessive blood loss, alcohol use, and massive fluid resuscitation. Body temperature continues to fall after clothing removal, contact with wet linens, and surgical exposure of body cavities during the patient's initial assessment. Prolonged exposure to hypothermia is associated with the development of myocardial dysfunction, coagulopathies, reduced perfusion, dysrhythmias (bradycardia and atrial or ventricular fibrillation), and decreased metabolic rate. Uncontrolled hypothermia caused by rapid infusion of IV fluids slows the heart rate and eventually decreases cardiac output. Hypothermia inhibits normal clotting mechanisms causing coagulopathies. Optimally, IV fluids are warmed by using a fluid-warming rapid infusion device (Figure 19-2).[31] Crystalloids should not be warmed in a microwave because the temperature cannot be well regulated. Other adjuncts to minimize the negative effects of hypothermia include warming the room, covering the patient's head, applying warm blankets, or using convection air blankets. Suggested techniques for rewarming are listed in Table 19-5.

Other environmental considerations are related to the location of the traumatic event. Environmental

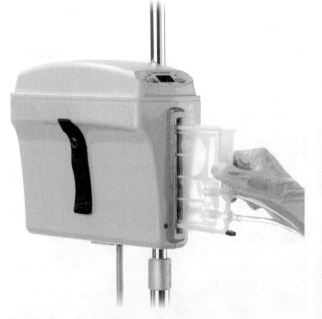

FIGURE 19-2. Medi-Temp Blood and Fluid Warmer. *(Courtesy of Gaymar Industries Inc. Orchard Park, New York.)*

TABLE 19-5	Rewarming Strategies
Type	**Interventions**
Passive external	Removal of wet clothing
	Warm room
	Decrease airflow over patient
	Blankets
	Head coverings
Active external	Radiant lights
	Fluid-filled warming blankets
	Convection air blankets
Active internal	Warmed gases to respiratory tract
	Warmed intravenous fluids, including blood
	Body cavity irrigation (peritoneal, mediastinal, pleural, gastric)
	Continuous arteriovenous rewarming
	Cardiopulmonary bypass

considerations include farming accidents, impalement with machinery or contaminated industrial equipment, exposure to contaminated water, or wound contamination with soil and road dirt.[56] Initial attempts to cleanse the wound are not priorities in the emergent phase of trauma management; however, once the patient is stabilized, the wounds are cleansed and debrided, and appropriate antibiotics are initiated.

ASSESSMENT AND MANAGEMENT OF SPECIFIC ORGAN INJURIES

The following section discusses common, specific traumatic injuries. These injuries may be diagnosed and managed in the emergency care phase or subsequent critical care phase of the traumatically injured patient. Rapid assessment and definitive surgical interventions save lives.[2,11,41] However, not all injuries require surgical intervention. Ongoing assessment, management of specific organ injuries, and an awareness of the response to the stress of the injury are vital during the critical care phase of the traumatically injured patient.

Thoracic Injuries

The thoracic region contains vital organs such as the heart, great vessels, and lungs. It is considered a critical region because injuries to the thoracic organs and structures can quickly become life-threatening.

Cardiac Tamponade

Cardiac tamponade is a life-threatening condition caused by rapid accumulation of fluid (usually blood) in the pericardial sac. As the intrapericardial pressure increases, cardiac output is impaired because of decreased venous return. The development of pulsus paradoxus may occur with a decrease in systolic blood pressure during spontaneous inspiration. Blood, if unable to flow into the right side of the heart, causes increased right atrial pressure and distended neck veins. Classic signs of this injury are hypotension, muffled or distant heart sounds, and elevated venous pressure (Beck's triad). Beck's triad may not be present until late in the development of tamponade.

Cardiac tamponade is generally caused by penetrating trauma to the chest. However, it should also be suspected in any patient with blunt trauma to the chest or multisystem injuries who presents in shock and does not respond to aggressive fluid resuscitation. Pericardial tamponade is often difficult to diagnose in the presence of other injuries that also cause a decreased cardiac output. Cardiac tamponade is diagnosed by using FAST or pericardiocentesis. Pericardiocentesis can also be used to treat the tamponade by decompressing the pericardium. Needle aspiration of the pericardial sac is done by the physician with a 16- to 18-gauge over-the-needle catheter attached to a 35-mL syringe with a three-way stopcock. It is important to differentiate blood from the pericardial sac from other sources. Blood aspirated from the pericardial sac usually does not clot unless the heart itself has been penetrated. Cardiac output may dramatically improve with removal of as little as 15 to 20 mL of blood, as noted by an increase in blood pressure. Nurses should anticipate and obtain equipment for an emergency thoracotomy in the event of cardiac arrest. After pericardiocentesis, immediate operative intervention is required for definitive repair.

Cardiac Contusion

Blunt trauma to the chest is the most frequent cause of cardiac contusion. The force of the traumatic event bruises the heart muscle and can compromise effective heart functioning.[52] Dysrhythmias are the most significant concern with cardiac contusion. Ongoing monitoring for symptomatic cardiac dysrhythmias via continuous monitoring of the electrocardiogram (ECG) is frequently indicated for up to 48 to 72 hours. In the event of significant anterior chest trauma, a 12-lead ECG and serum levels of cardiac isoenzymes and troponin are obtained to rule out ischemia or infarction. With severe cardiac contusion injuries, inotropic agents are occasionally needed to support myocardial function.

Aortic Disruption

Aortic disruption is produced by blunt trauma to the chest, frequently resulting in death at the scene of the traumatic event. Rapid deceleration forces produced by a head-on MVC, ejection, or falls can cause dissection of the aorta in four common sites: (1) just distal to the left subclavian artery at the level of the ligamentum arteriosum, (2) the ascending aorta, (3) the lower thoracic aorta above the diaphragm, and (4) avulsion of the innominate artery at the aortic arch.[35,52] Often the outer two layers of the aorta are torn, leaving the innermost layer intact. Although this is considered a lethal injury, early diagnosis can prevent tearing of the innermost layer, exsanguination, and death.

Signs of aortic disruption include weak femoral pulses, dysphagia, dyspnea, hoarseness, and pain. A chest x-ray study may demonstrate a widened mediastinum, tracheal deviation to the right, depressed left mainstem bronchus, first and second rib fractures, and left hemothorax. The diagnosis is confirmed by an aortogram. Definitive, emergent surgical resection and repair are necessary with this injury.

Tension Pneumothorax

Tension pneumothorax is a rapidly fatal emergency that is easily resolved with early recognition and intervention. It occurs when an injury to the chest allows air to enter the pleural cavity without a route for escape. With each inspiration, additional air accumulates in the pleural space, increasing intrathoracic pressure and leading to lung collapse. The increased pressure causes compression of the heart and great vessels toward the unaffected side, as evidenced by mediastinal shift and distended neck veins. The resulting decreased cardiac output and alterations in gas exchange are manifested by severe respiratory distress, chest pain, hypotension, tachycardia, absence of breath sounds on the affected side, and tracheal deviation. Cyanosis is a late manifestation of this life-threatening clinical situation.

The diagnosis of tension pneumothorax is based on the patient's clinical presentation. Treatment is never delayed to confirm the diagnosis with a chest x-ray study. Immediate decompression of the intrathoracic pressure is accomplished by needle thoracostomy. The physician inserts a 14-gauge needle into the second intercostal space at the midclavicular line on the injured side. This procedure converts a tension pneumothorax to a simple pneumothorax. Subsequent definitive treatment is required with placement of a chest tube.

Hemothorax

Hemothorax is a collection of blood in the pleural space resulting from injuries to the heart, great vessels, or the pulmonary parenchyma. Bleeding can be moderate (from intercostal vessels) or massive (from the aorta or from subclavian or pulmonary vessels). Decreased breath sounds, dullness to percussion on the affected side, hypotension, and respiratory distress may be seen. Placement of a chest tube facilitates removal of blood from the pleural space with resolution of ventilation and gas exchange abnormalities. Nursing interventions include management of the chest tube, close observation of the amount of blood drained from the pleural space, and monitoring the patient's hemodynamic response.

Open Pneumothorax

Open pneumothorax results from penetrating trauma that allows air to pass in and out of the pleural space. The normal pressure gradient between the atmosphere and intrathoracic space no longer exists. Patients present with hypoxia and hemodynamic instability. Management of the open wound is accomplished with a three-sided occlusive dressing. The fourth side is left open to allow for exhalation of air within the pleural cavity. If the dressing becomes completely occlusive on all sides, a tension pneumothorax may occur. A chest tube is inserted on the affected side, and a chest x-ray study is obtained to determine proper placement and to determine whether there is resolution of the pneumothorax.

Pulmonary Contusion

Pulmonary contusion occurs as a result of blunt or penetrating trauma to the chest. Rapid deceleration or blast forces with resulting multiple rib fractures or flail chest injuries can cause a pulmonary contusion. It is one of the most common causes of death after chest trauma, and it predisposes the patient to pneumonia or acute lung injury. A contusion is a parenchymal injury to the lung that often results in some degree of hemorrhage and edema with a subsequent inflammatory process extending beyond the site of injury.[52] It is often difficult to detect because the initial chest x-ray study may be normal. Infiltrates on chest x-ray studies and hypoxemia may not be present until hours or days after injury. The clinical presentation includes chest wall abrasions, ecchymosis, bloody secretions, and a partial pressure of arterial oxygen (PaO_2) of less than 60 mm Hg while breathing room air. The bruised lung tissue becomes edematous, resulting in hypoxia and respiratory distress. Ventilatory support is needed to promote healing of the lungs. Fluids must be administered cautiously to avoid further lung edema. Adequate pain relief with IV narcotics is essential to optimize lung expansion and respiratory effort and to prevent complications including atelectasis and pneumonia.

Rib Fractures and Flail Chest

Rib fractures are the most common injury associated with chest trauma. Rib fractures may lead to significant respiratory dysfunction and may indicate a serious injury to organs and structures below and near the rib cage. The diagnosis of rib fractures is frequently made after a chest x-ray study. However, there are situations in which rib fractures are not visualized on chest x-rays, and the diagnosis is made through clinical assessment. A high-impact force is needed to fracture the clavicle and first rib. Patients with these fractures require careful assessment for hemodynamic instability, which if present may indicate the presence of major vessel injury such as aortic disruption or injury to the subclavian artery. Rib fractures may have associated pneumothoraces or contusions of the heart and lungs. Injury to the liver, spleen, or kidney may accompany fractures of ribs 10 through 12.

The management of rib fractures is dependent on the number of ribs fractured, the degree of underlying injury, and the age of the patient. Interventions focus on assessing the patient's ventilation and oxygenation, and effective pain management. Nurses should provide education on pillow splinting, incentive spirometry, coughing and deep breathing exercises, the benefits of early ambulation, and pain management. Effective pain management enables the patient to maximally participate in pulmonary exercises. Pneumonia is the primary complication associated with rib fractures.

A flail chest occurs when two or more adjacent ribs are broken in two or more places, creating a free-floating segment of the rib cage. The flail segment "floats" freely and results in paradoxical chest movement. The flail segment contracts inward with inhalation and expands outward with exhalation. Normal respiratory mechanics depend on a rigid chest wall to generate negative intrathoracic pressure for effective ventilation. The uncoordinated chest movement with flail chest impairs the ability of the body to generate effective changes in intrathoracic pressure for ventilation. Clinical presentation includes paradoxical chest movement, increased work of breathing, tachypnea, and eventually signs and symptoms of hypoxemia. Management frequently involves endotracheal intubation and mechanical ventilation with adequate pain control, which may include epidural analgesia or a regional block.[35,52] Positioning the patient to enhance ventilation and oxygenation, and frequent pulmonary care, are additional strategies to prevent pneumonia.

Abdominal Injuries

Abdominal injuries are often difficult to diagnose. A normal initial examination does not necessarily rule out intraabdominal injury. The classic sign of abdominal injury is pain. However, pain cannot be used as an assessment tool if the patient has an altered sensorium, drug intoxication, or SCI with impaired sensation.

The liver is the most commonly injured organ after blunt or penetrating trauma.[67] Hemorrhage is the primary cause of death after liver injury. The patient may present with a history of right lower thoracic trauma, fractured lower right ribs, right upper quadrant ecchymosis, right upper quadrant tenderness, and hypotension. The diagnosis is confirmed with the use of FAST, abdominal CT, and/or diagnostic peritoneal lavage. The degree of liver injury is graded on a scale of I to VI, with I representing a nonexpanding subcapsular hematoma and VI signifying hepatic avulsion. Grade I through III injuries are treated with close monitoring (regular abdominal assessment and serial hemoglobin and hematocrit measurements) and bed rest for 5 days. Angiographic embolization or surgical management is indicated for grades IV through VI in which there is expansion of the hemorrhage, a large laceration, or complete avulsion of the liver from its vascular supply.[23,67]

Splenic injury occurs most often as a result of blunt trauma to the abdomen. However, penetrating trauma to the left upper quadrant of the abdomen or fracture of the anterior left lower ribs also contributes to splenic injuries. The patient may present with left upper quadrant tenderness, peritoneal irritation, referred pain to the left shoulder (Kehr's sign), and hypotension or signs of hypovolemic shock. An encapsulated hemorrhage of the spleen produces no immediate signs of bleeding. The diagnosis is confirmed by using the same tests as for liver injuries. The degree of splenic injury is graded on a scale from I to V. Grade I is a subcapsular, nonexpanding hematoma, and a grade V injury results when the spleen is shattered and devascularized. Management of splenic injury is similar to that of liver injuries. Close monitoring of the patient is vital. This includes assessment of the patient's hemodynamic status; the presence of guarding, rebound tenderness, rigidity, or distention of the abdomen; and alterations in the patient's hemoglobin and hematocrit values. Bed rest for 5 days may be appropriate for grade I to III splenic injuries. Operative intervention is often necessary for grade IV and V injuries. Splenic injuries may continue to bleed slowly, and the spleen may ultimately rupture days to weeks after the initial injury. A ruptured spleen is a life-threatening event that requires immediate surgical intervention. Every effort is made to preserve splenic tissue because of its role in immune function. Overwhelming infection has been seen after removal of the spleen.[23,67] Patients undergoing splenectomy are very susceptible to pneumococcal infections, and administration of the pneumococcal vaccine within the first few days postoperatively is recommended.

Gastric and small bowel injuries are most frequently the consequence of penetrating trauma from gunshot wounds. Blast injuries can also cause injury to these hollow organs. The incidence of gastric and bowel injury from blunt trauma is quite low, roughly 1% to 10%.[23] Gastric and bowel injury is suspected based on the mechanism of injury. FAST, diagnostic peritoneal lavage, or both, may also detect trauma to these organs. Surgical intervention is usually required. Postoperative complications include infection and difficulty maintaining nutrition.

Blunt trauma to the abdomen may also injure the kidneys; however, usually only one kidney is affected. Renal trauma is classified as minor, major, or critical (life-threatening). The patient may present with costovertebral tenderness, microscopic or gross hematuria, bruising or ecchymosis over the 11th and 12th ribs, hemorrhage, and/or shock. Diagnostic studies include FAST, CT scan, angiography, IV pyelogram, and cystoscopy.[36] For minor injuries, management focuses on bed rest, hydration, and monitoring of renal function including adequacy of urine output; urinalysis; hematuria; blood urea nitrogen, creatinine, and electrolyte levels; and a complete blood count. Management of major and critical renal injuries focuses on surgical intervention including control of bleeding, repair of the injury, or nephrectomy. Postsurgical complications include refractory hypertension, hemorrhage, fistula formation, and infection.

Blunt trauma causing disruption of the pelvic structure is a challenging clinical problem because of the large vascular supply, nervous system pathways, location of urological structures, and articulation of the hip joint within the pelvic ring. Frequently, treatment of pelvic injuries requires the expertise of many specialties (orthopedics, general surgery, neurosurgery, and urology).[36] The potential for morbidity, loss of function, and death is significant. Pelvic injuries occur most frequently in high-deceleration MVCs, pedestrian-vehicle impacts, and falls. The mortality rate from pelvic injuries is estimated at 50%, primarily related to massive bleeding causing hemodynamic instability and hypovolemic shock.[23] Primary interventions focus on stabilizing the pelvis and aggressive fluid resuscitation to ensure adequate tissue perfusion. Initially, pelvic stabilization can be accomplished by tying a large sheet or pelvic binder around the patient's hips to control the bleeding.[23,36,67] Early definitive treatment is accomplished through interventional radiology techniques that use embolization or coil techniques to stop the bleeding. Surgical repair may be required for internal or external fixation of complex pelvic fractures.

Musculoskeletal Injuries

Musculoskeletal trauma rarely is a priority in the emergent management of the patient unless the injuries result in significant hemodynamic instability

(e.g., pelvic fractures and traumatic amputations). The injuries may be blunt or penetrating, and may involve bone, soft tissue, muscle, nerves, and/or blood vessels. Injuries are classified as fractures, fracture-dislocations, amputations, and tissue trauma (crushing injuries of the soft tissue, nerves, vessels, or tendons). Knowing the mechanism of injury is important in evaluating musculoskeletal injuries because kinetic energy can be distributed from the bony impact to other areas of the body. For example, when a patient falls from a height, ankle fractures are likely, but energy displaced from the impact may have also caused lumbar spine and pelvic fractures.[3]

During the secondary survey, limb swelling, ecchymosis, and deformity are assessed. Extremity assessment is often described by the five Ps: *pain, pallor, pulses, paresthesia*, and *paralysis*. This process of assessment describes the neurovascular status of the injured extremity and is critical in assessing circulation in the extremity. Loss of pulses is considered a late sign of diminished perfusion. Increased pain, pallor, and paresthesia supersede loss of pulses and should be reported immediately to the trauma team.[3,14,30]

Fractures involve a disruption of bony continuity. X-ray studies are taken to diagnose fractures, and the extremity is immobilized. Common types of fractures are shown in Figure 19-3.[30] If the skin is open at the fracture site, it is called an *open fracture*; if the skin is intact, it is called a *closed fracture*. Fractures are further classified into grades based on the degree of bony, soft, and vascular tissue and nerve damage. Early treatment of a fracture involves immobilization with splints or application of traction. Once the patient is hemodynamically stable, surgical management for open fractures (open reduction and internal fixation) is performed to restabilize the bone for effective healing.

Traumatic soft tissue injuries are categorized as contusions, abrasions, lacerations, puncture wounds, crush injuries, amputations, or avulsion injuries. Injury to the skin and soft tissues predisposes the individual to secondary complications including localized and systemic infection, hypoproteinemia, and hypothermia.[42]

Assessment of soft tissue injury is part of the secondary survey unless the loss of tissue (e.g., amputation) is hemodynamically compromising the patient. Traumatic amputation produces a well-defined wound edge with localized injury to soft tissue, nerves, and vessels. These wounds usually require debridement and surgical closure. Avulsion injuries result in stretching and tearing of the soft tissue and may tear nerves and vessels at different levels other than the actual site of bone and tissue trauma.

A crush injury may produce local soft tissue trauma or extensive damage distant from the site of

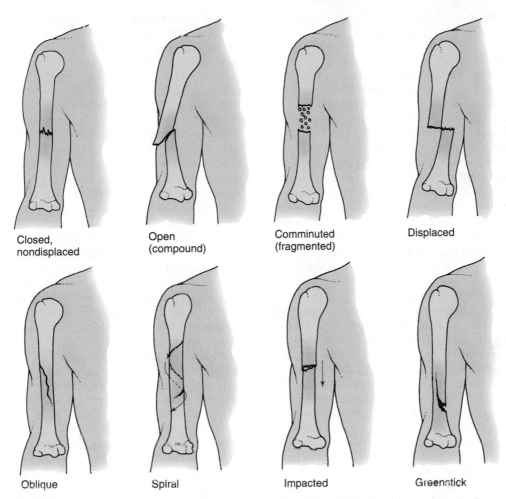

FIGURE 19-3. Common types of fractures. *(From Heron Evans, M. R. [2006]. Interventions for clients with musculoskeletal trauma. In D. Ignatavicius, & M. L. Workman [Eds.], Medical-surgical nursing: Critical thinking for collaborative care [5th ed., p. 1190]. Philadelphia: Saunders.)*

Closed, nondisplaced

Open (compound)

Comminuted (fragmented)

Displaced

Oblique

Spiral

Impacted

Greenstick

injury. Crush injuries of the pelvis and/or both lower extremities or a prolonged entrapment may be life-threatening. Prolonged compression produces ischemia and anoxia of the affected muscle tissue. Third-spacing of fluid, localized edema, and increased compartment pressures cause secondary ischemia. Without aggressive intervention, these injuries can result in irreversible complications.

Contusions do not cause a break in the skin, but localized edema, ecchymosis, and pain occur. Abrasions ("road rash") occur when the skin experiences friction. The abrasion can be superficial or cause deep tissue injury. Traumatic abrasions are frequently contaminated with debris implanted into the skin, resulting in traumatic tattooing. It can take hours to days to effectively remove the debris from the wound. Lacerations are usually caused by sharp objects, and they are treated with cleansing and suturing. Puncture wounds carry a heightened risk of infection. Although they do not cause vast soft tissue destruction or lacerations, puncture wounds can cause an aggressive infection because they deliver bacteria or foreign inoculums deep into the body.[42] Puncture wounds should not be surgically closed until treatment for infection with local and systemic antibiotics has been completed. Animal bites are notorious causes of puncture wounds.

All traumatic wounds are considered contaminated. Wounds must be cleansed and debrided to reduce the risk of infection. Ongoing assessment of the wound includes evaluating healing and investigating any local and systemic signs and symptoms of infection (e.g., increased wound pain, swelling, fever, elevated white blood cell count, increased wound drainage) that arise. Tetanus toxoid administration and antibiotic therapy are also considered.

Complications

Complications of musculoskeletal injury include the systemic effects that may occur after a crush injury, including compartment syndrome, rhabdomyolysis, deep vein thrombosis (DVT), pulmonary embolism, and fat embolism.

Compartment Syndrome. Compartment syndrome occurs when a fascia-enclosed muscle compartment, such as an extremity, experiences increased pressure from internal and external sources. Internal sources include edema, hemorrhage, or both; external forces include splints, immobilizers, or dressings. The closed muscle compartment of an extremity contains neurovascular bundles that are tightly covered by fascia. If the pressure is not relieved, compression of nerves, blood vessels, and muscle occurs, with resulting ischemia and necrosis of muscle and nerve tissue.

Patients with compartment syndrome complain of increasing throbbing pain disproportionate to the injury. Narcotic administration does not relieve the pain. The pain is localized to the involved compartment and increases with passive muscle stretching. The area affected is firm. Paresthesia distal to the compartment, pulselessness, and paralysis are late signs and must be reported immediately to prevent loss of the extremity. The affected limb is elevated to heart level to promote venous outflow and to prevent further swelling. Compartmental pressure monitoring may be performed for definitive diagnosis. Treatment of compartment syndrome is immediate surgical fasciotomy in which the fascial compartment is opened to relieve the pressure.

Rhabdomyolysis. Rhabdomyolysis is a syndrome of hypoperfusion and ischemia, followed by reperfusion, in which injured muscle tissue releases myoglobin into the circulation, compromising renal blood flow.[66] Causes of rhabdomyolysis include crush injuries, compartment syndrome, burns, and injuries from being struck by lightning. Myloglobinuria (the excretion of myoglobin through the urine) is an effective marker of rhabdomyolysis and causes the urine to be a dark tea color. Ultimately, the myloglobin is toxic to the renal tubule, causing acute tubular necrosis, electrolyte and acid-base imbalances, and eventually acute renal failure. Treatment of rhabdomyolysis consists of aggressive fluid resuscitation to flush the myloglobin from the renal tubules. A common protocol includes the titration of IV fluids to achieve a urine output of 100 to 200 mL/hr.[44,66] Administering osmotic diuretics and adding sodium bicarbonate to IV fluids may be used to protect the renal tubules in patients with myoglobinuria.

Deep Vein Thrombosis. DVT is a significant complication of traumatic injury.[50] The risk of DVT in trauma patients is dependent on the severity of injury, the type of injury (e.g., musculoskeletal injuries), the presence of shock, recent surgeries, vascular injury, and immobility. DVT usually occurs in the lower extremities. Thrombus formation is enhanced in the presence of Virchow's triad: vessel damage, venous stasis, and hypercoagulability. If the thrombus dislodges, it becomes an embolus and travels through the body's vasculature until it lodges in either the pulmonary artery or its smaller branches (pulmonary embolism). Once the embolus becomes lodged, blood flow is obstructed distally and the tissues distal to the obstruction become hypoxic. Pulmonary vessels constrict in response to the hypoxia, resulting in ventilation-perfusion mismatches and hypoxemia. Prevention of DVT is essential in the management of trauma patients. If not medically contraindicated, patients should receive pharmacological prophylaxis. Nurses should encourage ambulation, evaluate the patient's overall hydration, and ensure sequential compression devices are in use.

Fat Embolism Syndrome. Fat embolism syndrome is a potential complication that accompanies traumatic injury of the long bones and pelvis that result in multiple skeletal fractures. Typically, the syndrome develops between 24 and 48 hours after injury.[20] Long bone injury may release fat globules into torn vessels and the systemic circulation. The fat particles act as an embolus, traveling through the great vessels and pulmonary system, obstructing flow and causing hypoxia. Hallmark clinical signs that accompany fat embolism syndrome begin with the development of a low-grade fever followed by a new-onset tachycardia, dyspnea, an increased respiratory rate and effort, hypoxemia (PaO_2 <60 mm Hg), sudden thrombocytopenia, and a petechial rash.[20] Late signs and symptoms include ECG changes, lipuria (fat in the urine), and changes in the level of consciousness progressing to coma.

Prevention of fat embolism is the best treatment. Stabilization of extremity fractures to minimize both bone movement and the release of fatty products from the bone marrow must be accomplished as early as possible. Treatment of fat embolism syndrome is directed toward the preservation of pulmonary function and maintenance of cardiovascular stability. Administration of supplemental oxygen and intubation with mechanical ventilation and positive end-expiratory pressure may be required to restore or maintain pulmonary function. Monitoring the patient's cardiovascular stability is continued throughout the critical care phase, with particular attention paid to ECG and hemodynamic changes.

CRITICAL CARE PHASE

The critical care phase for the patient with multisystem traumatic injuries requires the skills and collaboration of a variety of health care professionals.[63] The patient experiences additional physiological stressors from the traumatic injury and subsequent surgeries, psychological stressors, and often disruption of the social or family unit. The nurse is central to the critical care phase, continually assessing the patient's progress, anticipating and evaluating for possible complications, encouraging family-centered care, and acting as the patient's advocate. Interventions that were initiated in the emergent phase to treat and manage the traumatic injuries continue into the critical care phase.

Damage-Control Surgery

Patients with multiple injuries from traumatic events are at greatest risk of death from hemorrhage. Emergent surgical management of traumatically injured patients is the gold standard to stop hemorrhage and stabilize life-threatening injuries.[1] Definitive surgical interventions may require several surgeries to effectively manage traumatic injuries. The initial surgery focuses on cessation of the cause of bleeding; however, long, extensive surgeries can lead to severe complications that contribute to the patient's ultimate death. These complications, now recognized as the leading cause of death in patients who sustain multitraumatic injuries, include the triad of hypothermia, acidosis, and coagulopathy.[46,58]

These complications and resultant mortality have changed the current surgical focus to an approach known as *damage-control surgery* or a *staged surgical repair*. This strategy sacrifices the completeness of immediate repair, yet provides early surgical stabilization and management of active hemorrhage associated with injuries. The first stage includes the operative repair of life-threatening injuries only. Patients are then returned to the critical care unit (second stage) for aggressive rewarming, ongoing resuscitation, and attainment of hemodynamic stability.[46,54] The third stage occurs usually within 24 to 48 hours after the initial operation. This involves the return to the operating room for definitive repair of intraabdominal injuries. This three-stage approach allows for cardiovascular stabilization, correction of metabolic acidosis and coagulopathy, rewarming, and optimization of pulmonary function.[46,54,58] The damage-control concept improves the outcomes of critically ill patients with severe intraabdominal injuries.[58]

Postoperative Management

After surgery, critically ill patients frequently bypass the postanesthesia recovery unit and are admitted directly to the critical care unit. Preparation for admission of the patient provides a smooth transition in care from the operative phase to the critical care phase. The room temperature may be increased to manage anticipated hypothermia, IV infusion pumps are accessed, respiratory therapy is contacted for a ventilator, and the monitoring equipment and room supplies are double-checked to minimize the need to find necessary supplies once the patient is admitted. The bed scale is "zeroed" to obtain a quick admission weight of the patient. The nurse frequently receives a report from the emergency department nurse before the patient goes to surgery; however, a thorough report from the anesthesiologist as part of hand-off communication between health care providers is essential for continuity of care. Elements of the hand-off communication include a review of systems, past medical history, description of the injury, description of the intraoperative procedures, the patient's tolerance of the procedures, vital signs during the surgery and current vital signs, total intake (i.e., crystalloids, colloids, blood products) and output (i.e., urine output, chest tube output, and estimated blood loss), medications administered (i.e., sedation, analgesia, neuromuscular blockade reversal agents, antibiotics, and vasoactive agents), IV access, and location of chest tubes and other drains.

The initial intervention upon admission to the critical care unit is a rapid assessment of airway, breathing, and circulation. The nurse quickly connects the patient to the bedside monitor and ventilator, and completes an assessment of vital signs, cardiac rhythm, pulse oximetry reading, level of consciousness, and pupil reactivity. Hypothermia is a concern postoperatively; thus the nurse keeps the patient covered while assessing the body for surgical incisions, dressings, other injuries, and location and function of drainage devices (e.g., chest tubes, hemovacs). It is important to inspect the posterior surface of the patient, so a quick turn to assess and remove soiled linens is completed early. The nurse reassesses IV access and evaluates the patency of IV catheters, as they may have become dislodged during transport. All IV infusions are traced from the IV fluid, to the infusion pump, and to the IV access in the patient. Calculation of medication dosages and rates is completed as part of the initial assessment. All drainage devices are emptied, such as hemovacs and the urinary drainage bag, and the volume of output is recorded. If a chest tube is in place, the amount of existing drainage is marked on the external collection system. Admission laboratory studies are obtained. The most frequent studies obtained postoperatively include a complete blood count, a complete metabolic panel, coagulation studies, an arterial lactate level, and an arterial blood gas analysis with base deficit. Finally the patient is weighed. The admission weight is important for ongoing assessment of the patient's fluid status and medication administration throughout the critical care unit admission. Once the assessment and initial interventions are completed, the family is contacted to see the patient.

Postoperative management of critically ill patients involves a systematic and thorough assessment, and the monitoring of respiratory and cardiovascular function, neuromuscular abilities, mental status, temperature, pain, drainage and bleeding, urine output, and resuscitation efforts.[19,46] Patients usually have an endotracheal tube in place when they are transferred to the critical care unit for the postoperative recovery period. Patients who do not require extended mechanical ventilation are extubated within minutes to hours of admission, depending on their ability to protect the airway after the reversal of anesthesia and neuromuscular blocking agents. Other critically ill patients are maintained on mechanical ventilation until stable, their injuries are definitively repaired, and/or pulmonary pathological processes have resolved. Monitoring of the patient's oxygenation and ventilation status is part of ongoing critical care management. Modifications in the ventilatory modes, adjuncts, and fraction of inspired oxygen (FiO_2) are made based on assessment.

After ensuring the stability of the patient's airway and adequacy of ventilation, attention is focused on hemodynamic assessment. This includes monitoring heart rate, cardiac rhythm, blood pressure, respiratory rate, pulse oximetry, temperature, drainage (e.g., chest tubes, nasogastric tubes, wound or incisional drains), urinary output, IV fluids, and vasoactive medications. The postoperative standard for monitoring these parameters is every 5 minutes for three measurements, every 15 minutes for three measurements, every 30 minutes for 1 hour, with hourly measurements thereafter. More frequent monitoring is indicated if the patient is hemodynamically unstable. Additional hemodynamic values are obtained if the patient has a pulmonary artery catheter or an intracranial monitor.

Temperature is measured on admission and is monitored at regular intervals. In the event of hypothermia, passive and active strategies are used to rewarm the patient to a normothermic state (see Table 19-5). Shivering is avoided because it increases metabolic rate and results in increased oxygen demands and the potential for hemodynamic insta-

bility. During the rewarming process, vasodilation occurs and the patient is monitored for decreases in blood pressure.

A complete physical assessment is performed on all postoperative patients. All body systems are assessed including the neurological, cardiovascular, pulmonary, gastrointestinal, renal, hematological, immune, musculoskeletal, and integumentary systems. All invasive IV and central lines are also assessed. Continuous collection of assessment data guides therapies aimed at correcting identified problems or injuries, and preventing or minimizing postinjury complications. Elderly patients are at increased risk of complications after traumatic injury because of age-related changes (see Geriatric Considerations).

The patient's mental status is assessed to ensure that a neurological event did not occur intraoperatively. Hand-off communication from the anesthesiologist includes whether anesthesia was reversed pharmacologically and the most recent times of analgesic, amnesic, or sedative medication administration. This provides information on the estimated time of patient wakefulness. Pupils are checked for reactivity. Once the patient is awake, the patient is assessed for alertness and orientation to person, place, and time, as well as the ability to follow commands. In the event that the patient does not awaken, measures must be taken to determine the cause of the unresponsive state. The medical team must determine whether the anesthetic agents, sedation, or analgesic medications are contributing factors. If it is determined that medications are not the contributing cause of the neurological impairment, the patient may require additional diagnostic testing such as a CT scan of the head. Any alterations in the patient's clinical assessment must be analyzed to determine whether intervention is necessary. This may require interdisciplinary collaboration with surgeons, advanced practice nurses, respiratory therapists, and consulting physicians.

Patients must be assessed to determine their level of pain. Multiple pain scales are available to assess the degree of pain (see Chapter 5). Individual institutions determine the most appropriate pain scale for use with their patient population. Postoperative orders include analgesic medication to be administered orally or IV (as needed or as a continuous infusion). If the nurse is unable to assess the patient's pain level postoperatively because of the patient's lack of wakefulness or secondary to a neurological event, the pain level is evaluated by using other parameters including increased heart rate and blood pressure, restlessness, facial grimacing, decreasing oxygen levels, and ventilator dyssynchrony. After administration of analgesia, the patient's pain level is reassessed.

GERIATRIC CONSIDERATIONS

- Falls are the most frequent cause of injury for the elderly population, resulting in fractures of the hips, arms, hands, legs, feet, pelvis, ribs, and vertebrae.
- The elderly patient has three major factors influencing care needs after traumatic injury: known preexisting disease, diminished physiological capacity, and occult disease. The effects of trauma are exacerbated by decreased physiological reserve and host resistance that occur with aging.[59] These patients may present with hemodynamic instability, diminished organ function, and delayed healing.
- The cardiopulmonary effects of aging affect the patient's ability to respond to the pathophysiological effects of trauma. These patients often present with decreased cardiac output, have a risk of volume overload with fluid resuscitation, and have a lack of compensatory response to altered hemodynamics.
- Decreased brain mass, increased neuronal death, decline in sensory nerve function, decreased cerebral perfusion, and decreased autoregulation contribute to the changes seen in neurological assessment. Patients may present with changes in level of consciousness (agitation or coma), more pronounced neurological impairments after intracranial bleeding because of a larger compartment available for blood to accumulate, and an inability to report acute changes in painful stimuli.
- Physiological changes in the elderly include decreased renal blood flow and glomerular filtration rate, increased susceptibility to infection, decreased hematopoiesis, increased insulin resistance, decreased insulin release, diminished bowel motility, delayed wound healing, increased incidence of osteoporosis, decreased inflammatory response, and loss of subcutaneous fat. These changes alter the elderly patient's response to trauma. These patients are monitored closely for the development of decreased urinary output, diminished hemoglobin or hematocrit values, increased blood glucose levels, development of ileus, signs and symptoms of infection, increased number of bony fractures, and alterations in skin integrity.
- Elderly patients often have limitations in mobility and joint flexibility, muscle atrophy, osteoarthritis, and preexisting deformities that complicate their ability to participate in physical and/or occupational therapy and delay their return to pretrauma functional status.
- Knowledge of current medications is important because there may be increased risk of complications. The following drugs may contribute to patient complications:

MEDICATIONS	COMPLICATION
Aspirin	Increase risk of bleeding
Warfarin (Coumadin)	
Antiplatelet medications	
NSAIDs	Gastrointestinal bleeding
Steroids	Delay in healing
Beta-blockers and calcium channel blockers	Inadequate hemodynamic response
Herbal therapies	Severe drug interactions

NSAIDs, Non-steroidal anti-inflammatory drugs.

Resuscitative efforts are evaluated postoperatively to determine the effectiveness of fluid management. Establishing baseline hemodynamic status, laboratory values, and intake and output assists in determining the patient's fluid volume status and the degree of successful resuscitation. Hemoglobin levels, hematocrit values, and coagulation studies provide valuable information on whether the patient is bleeding or has a high probability of bleeding because of unavailable or ineffective clotting factors. A higher arterial lactate level, a more negative base deficit value, or both, indicate inadequate resuscitation resulting in anaerobic metabolism. The presence of abnormal values indicates the need for more aggressive resuscitation.

Ongoing patient care priorities evolve from the patient's diagnosis and the surgical procedure. Careful attention is given to anticipating potential problems and intervening when actual problems are identified. A comprehensive reassessment every 4 hours guides the nurse in identifying changes in the patient's status, preparing for additional diagnostic procedures, and intervening appropriately. It is vital to evaluate the patient continuously for alterations in oxygenation, ventilation, acid-base balance, perfusion, metabolic status, and hemodynamic status, as well as for signs and symptoms of infection.

Effective nutritional support is considered an integral component of care of the critically injured patient. Nutritional needs of the patient are addressed early in the postoperative phase (within 24 to 48 hours) to assist with healing and meeting the body's needs related to an elevated metabolic demand. The route of administration (oral, enteral, or parenteral), type of nutritional replacement, and rate of administration are dependent on the severity of illness or injury and the expected recovery period. A nutritional consult is placed to evaluate the metabolic needs of the patient and determine the optimal feeding formula and rate of administration (see Chapter 6).

Ensuring that the patient has pharmacological prophylaxis for DVT and stress ulceration, as well as an aggressive protocol for mobilization, may prevent untoward complications. Immobility places the patient at increased risk of developing DVT, pneumonia, pressure ulcers, and urostasis. Strategies to prevent complications of immobility include frequent turning, offloading pressure on bony prominences with pillows, frequent skin assessments, application of moisture barriers to skin to prevent maceration from feces or leaking drainage devices, coughing and deep breathing exercises, early extubation, urinary catheter care and early removal of the catheter, and early ambulation.

Variations in hormonal regulation, specifically hyperglycemia and increased gluconeogenesis, are often seen in critically ill patients. Research has demonstrated improved patient outcomes when serum glucose levels are maintained within normal limits.[1] Elevations in serum glucose levels are aggressively treated with IV insulin infusions. Frequent laboratory analysis or monitoring of glucose levels with point-of-care testing is required for these patients.

Patients with multisystem injuries are at high risk of developing a myriad of complications because of the body's compromised condition related to the overwhelming stressors of the injury, prolonged immobility, and consequences of inadequate tissue perfusion. Even with optimal care, the stressors and overwhelming inflammatory responses to injury influence the risk of secondary complications. These include respiratory impairment (abdominal compartment syndrome, acute lung injury, ARDS, pneumonia), infection (catheter infection, sepsis), acute renal failure, high nutritional demands, and MODS. A full discussion of these secondary complications is found in other chapters within this text.

SPECIAL CONSIDERATIONS AND POPULATIONS

Effects of Aging

Elderly patients are at increased risk of complications after traumatic injury because of age-related changes. Trauma in the elderly is primarily from MVCs and falls. The incidence of trauma in geriatric patients is significantly less than that in younger patients;

however, these patients are more likely to require hospitalization and have significantly higher costs for care associated with their injuries.[28,59] Older trauma patients are more likely to have severe morbidity, require longer hospitalization, have more complications, and are less likely to return home after acute hospitalization.[59]

Delirium and pneumonia are the primary complications seen in the elderly after trauma. Delirium is a syndrome with many potential etiologies. Patients with delirium may be withdrawn, agitated and aggressive towards other individuals, or have hallucinations. Their ability to receive, process, store, and recall information is acutely impaired. The development of delirium is associated with a functional decline during hospitalization, a prolonged hospital stay, an increased risk for developing hospital-acquired complications, and a three-fold risk of admission to a long-term–care facility.[38]

Delirium should be investigated if any acute change in an elderly patient's cognition or consciousness is noted. Nursing interventions focus on establishing the cause of the delirium, including electrolyte imbalances, infection, and sleep deprivation. Sedative medications and restraints should be avoided, as these interventions may worsen the delirium and have additional negative consequences related to prolonged immobility and an increased risk for falls.[38] Frequent reorientation of the patient and involvement of the family in the patient's care may be effective in calming the delirious patient.

Pneumonia in the elderly is a life-threatening complication. With aging, the pulmonary system is less able to compensate when stressed, and the immune system is less likely to mount a significant fever, which is one of the main signs that would normally alert the nurse to the possibility that an infection is present.[59] Age-related changes in pulmonary structure and function affect the patient's ability to effectively ventilate and exchange gases. Preexisting pulmonary diseases limit the patient's ability to wean quickly from the ventilator. Pain management is essential for older individuals so that aggressive pulmonary interventions can be effective in preventing pneumonia. Pulmonary exercises (i.e., incentive spirometry, ambulating, coughing and deep breathing exercises) and strategies that prevent aspiration (i.e., evaluate swallowing, head-of-bed elevation to 30 degrees) are imperative in the care of the older trauma patient.

Alcohol and Drug Abuse

The first step in trauma management is effective trauma prevention. Up to 40% of all traumatic events involve alcohol, and an additional 20% include drug intoxicants.[25,26] Overall complications, morbidity, and mortality are higher in traumatically injured patients who tested positive for alcohol, drugs, or both, at the time of admission. Most trauma patients who have high blood alcohol concentration upon admission meet criteria that indicate an alcohol problem.[25,26,47,57] With such a high incidence of traumatic events involving the use of alcohol and drugs, trauma prevention cannot be successful unless these concerns are mutually addressed.

Alcohol problems are treatable, and interventions are effective; however, patients must be involved in alcohol intervention and cessation programs. Research has shown that interventions for problem drinking reduce the incidence of suicide attempts, domestic violence, falls, traumatic injury, and injury-related hospitalizations.[22,25,26,47,57] Trauma centers should develop alcohol and drug intervention programs that can be implemented at the time of admission and maintained throughout the hospitalization to reduce the high correlation of alcohol abuse and serious traumatic injury.[57]

Drug use and abuse impair a patient's cognitive processes and create physiological stress.[21] Multiple categories of drugs may be used by the trauma patient ranging from inhalant intoxicants to hallucinogens, designer drugs (e.g., ecstasy, ketamine), cocaine, and methamphetamine. Injuries frequently are self-inflicted because of the person's altered judgment from the effects of the drug. Mechanisms of injury associated with drug use include jumping from buildings or running through traffic. Drug use, especially drug overdose, causes significant physiological stressors. After addressing the traumatic injury, the physiological consequences of the drug and subsequent drug withdrawal must be addressed.

Nursing care of the trauma patient with an alcohol or drug addiction provides both a challenge and opportunity. Because addiction is associated with physiological dependence, when the patient no longer consumes these agents, serious or life-threatening withdrawal occurs. The nurse must closely monitor the patient's physiological status while a patient is experiencing withdrawal. Common signs and symptoms observed include increased agitation, anxiety, auditory and visual hallucinations, disorientation, headache, nausea and vomiting, paroxysmal diaphoresis, and tremors (Box 19-2).

Discovering the time frame or exact time between the patient's last use of the drug or alcohol, or both, is essential in planning treatment strategies.[22,26,57] As patients experience withdrawal, sedating agents may be ordered to ease the physiological and behavioral symptoms. Haloperidol (Haldol) and lorazepam (Ativan) are commonly ordered. Ongoing and frequent assessments are necessary to ensure patient

---

BOX 19-2 Signs and Symptoms of Alcohol Withdrawal

- Irritability, agitation, confusion, hallucinations, and delusions
- Insomnia
- Anxiety and tremors
- Nausea, vomiting, and diarrhea
- Diaphoresis
- Tachycardia and hypertension
- Fever
- Seizures

---

safety. The patient is observed hourly or more frequently for the presence of worsening anxiety, hallucinations, fall risk, and disorientation. Someone may be designated to sit with the patient at all times to ensure the safety of the individual going through acute drug or alcohol withdrawal. It is important that drug and alcohol prevention interventions begin before discharge from the hospital.

Family and Patient Coping

Traumatic injury is frequently unexpected and is a potentially devastating event, producing physical, psychological, and emotional stress for the patient and family. The event leaves the patient and family feeling overwhelmed, vulnerable, and often ill prepared to cope with ramifications of the injury. The traumatic event often creates a crisis within the family unit of the patient. Critical decisions for the patient frequently must be made by family members in seconds. The trauma team can assist the patient and family in crisis by helping them establish a designated family member as the spokesperson. This allows for consistent communication between the health care team and family. Health care providers need to explore the patient's and family's perception of the event, support systems, and coping mechanisms.[45,62] Early involvement of a social worker assists the patient and family with coping and can diffuse the current crisis, allowing more effective coping and decision-making processes. Family conferences early in the emergent phase and frequently during the critical care phase assist with communication and with understanding the patient's and family's expectations for care, and enhance the decision-making and coping skills of the patient and family.[45]

The traumatic crisis and family dynamics fluctuate throughout the hospitalization. Initially, during the phases of emergent and critical illness, the crisis may focus on whether the individual will survive the injury. As the patient recovers, the patient and the family may experience a crisis as they attempt to adjust to physical or emotional disabilities. During the rehabilitation phase, a crisis may ensue as the patient and family face the difficulties of reintegrating the injured individual into the family and the community.[45] Patient and family responses may fluctuate from anger to remorse, anxiety, denial, and grief. Open communication with the patient is important to assist with effective coping. Clear, calm communication that establishes eye contact reduces anxiety. The nurse may use gentle touch with the patient or family while discussing their fears and concerns. Research has shown that patients with traumatic injury who discussed their perceptions, fears, and emotions soon after sustaining the physical injury have more effective coping and less injury-related distress.[62]

REHABILITATION

The final phase of trauma care encompasses rehabilitation of the patient. The initiation of the rehabilitative process begins the moment the patient is admitted to the trauma center. Prevention of complications that prolong hospitalization and delay rehabilitation is imperative. Early involvement of the physical medicine and rehabilitation personnel is vital to positive functional patient outcomes.

Early in this phase of trauma care, a case manager or discharge planner evaluates the patient for the need for extensive rehabilitation at a specialty center. An individualized plan is developed for each patient based on physical injuries and rehabilitation potential, patient and family preferences, and insurance coverage.

Nursing interventions in the critical care phase influence the patient's rehabilitative needs. For example, the critical care nurse's attention to the position of the immobile patient to prevent foot drop assists with ambulation. Application of splints provides positions of functionality in injured extremities. The nurse also provides much needed emotional support as the patient convalesces through the critical care phase and begins more independent activities, preparing for the rehabilitation phase of trauma recovery.

Transition of the patient into rehabilitation is both an exciting and a frightening time for the patient and family. The patient has relied on the nursing staff for encouragement and support at a critical time in the patient's life. Transferring to another facility brings with it uncertainty in new relationships, as well as excitement, since rehabilitation is the last step before returning to the patient's home.

CASE STUDY

M. L., a 17-year-old male, was involved in a motor vehicle crash. He was wearing a seat belt but was traveling at a high speed when he lost control of the car and crashed into a tree. He was awake at the scene, but his level of consciousness quickly declined during transport to the trauma center by emergency medical services (EMS). The prehospital team was unable to intubate him during transport, and the patient's airway was maintained with bag-valve-mask ventilation using a fraction of inspired oxygen (FiO_2) of 1.00 (100%). Two large-bore intravenous catheters were placed, and normal saline was infused at 250 mL/hr. Three liters of fluid were administered before arrival in the emergency department. M. L. does not have a significant medical history or any drug allergies. Initial vital signs were temperature, 36.6°C; blood pressure, 102/80 mm Hg; heart rate and rhythm, 136 beats/min with sinus tachycardia; respiratory rate, 36 breaths/min with assisted manual ventilation; and oxygen saturation, 97%. He is nonresponsive to verbal commands, and his pupils are 2 mm and reactive to light. He has a 6-cm scalp laceration, a right closed femur fracture, and 4 broken ribs. Initial laboratory results were hemoglobin, 7.2 g/dL; white blood count, 16,000/microliter; platelet count, 200,000/microliter; potassium, 5.5 mEq/L; and other electrolyte levels were unremarkable. Arterial blood gas results were pH, 7.19; partial pressure of arterial oxygen (PaO_2), 160 mm Hg; partial pressure of arterial carbon dioxide ($PaCO_2$), 42 mm Hg; bicarbonate (HCO_3^-), 22 mEq/L; base deficit, −14; and lactate, 9 mEq/L. Aggressive fluid resuscitation continues as he is transported to radiology for computed tomography to evaluate his chest and abdomen for injuries. EMS contacted his parents, who are both in the waiting room of the emergency department.

QUESTIONS

1. What are the possible injuries based on the mechanism of injury?
2. What is the priority intervention at this time based on his vital signs?
3. What is your interpretation of the laboratory results? What interventions do you anticipate based on these results?
4. What are possible reasons for his unresponsiveness?
5. What additional studies or interventions do you anticipate the patient needs after the computed tomography scan?
6. What are the needs of the family?

SUMMARY

Trauma is a leading cause of death in persons between the ages of 14 and 44 years and is considered preventable. Patient survival after traumatic injury depends on prompt, rapid, systematic assessment in conjunction with immediate resuscitative interventions. Evaluation of airway patency, ventilation, and venous access with circulatory support take precedence over other diagnostic interventions. The goal is to ensure the delivery of oxygen to the body tissues, to stop the progression of shock, and to prevent long-term complications. Critical care nurses provide an essential role in the early and ongoing care of the traumatically injured patient.

CRITICAL THINKING QUESTIONS   *evolve*

1. A patient presents to the critical care unit with a gunshot wound to the left lower anterior chest from a 0.45-caliber semiautomatic weapon. What additional prehospital information would be helpful? Considering the mechanism of injury and location of the entrance wound, describe the potential patterns of injury. What are the immediate management priorities?

2. After operative repair, this patient is admitted to the critical care unit. Describe the assessment and intervention priorities during the first postoperative hour.

3. Why is it necessary to administer platelets and fresh frozen plasma along with packed red blood cells in the patient who requires a massive blood transfusion (>10 units)?

4. What are the management priorities for a patient with a traumatic brain injury?

---

evolve Be sure to check out the bonus material, including free self-assessment exercises, on the Evolve Web site at http://evolve.elsevier.com/Sole.

REFERENCES

1. American College of Surgeons, Committee on Trauma. (2004). *Advanced trauma life support for doctors: Instructor's course manual* (7th ed.). Chicago: American College of Surgeons.

2. American College of Surgeons, Committee on Trauma. (2006). *Resources for optimal care of the injured patient 2006.* Chicago: American College of Surgeons.

3. Aresco, C. A. (2005). Trauma. In P. G. Morton, D. K. Fontaine, C. M. Hudak, & B. M. Gallo (Eds.), *Critical care nursing: A holistic approach* (8th ed., pp. 1277-1301). Philadelphia: Lippincott Williams & Wilkins.

4. Bader, M. K., & Arbour, R. (2005). Refractory increased intracranial pressure in severe traumatic brain injury: Barbiturate coma and bispectral index monitoring. *AACN Clinical Issues, 16*(4), 526-541.

5. Boswell, S., & Scalea, T. M. (2009). Initial management of traumatic shock. In K. McQuillan, M. B. Makic, & E. Whalen (Eds.), *Trauma nursing from resuscitation through rehabilitation* (4th ed.). Philadelphia: Saunders.

6. Bourg, P. W. (2007). Head and face trauma. In K. S. Oman, & J. Koziol-McLain (Eds.), *Emergency nursing secrets* (2nd ed., pp. 288-298). St. Louis: Mosby.

7. Bridges, E. J. (2006). Blast injuries: From triage to critical care. *Critical Care Nursing Clinics of North America, 18*(2), 338-348.

8. Brush, K. A. (2007). Abdominal compartment syndrome: The pressure is on. *Nursing, 37*(7), 36-41.

9. Bulger, E. M., & Maier, R. V. (2007). Pre-hospital care of the injured: What's new. *Surgical Clinics of North America, 87*(1), 37-53.

10. Carson, D., & Pickard, K. M. (2007). Mechanism of injury. In K. S. Oman, & J. Koziol-McLain (Eds.), *Emergency nursing secrets* (2nd ed., pp. 269-277). St. Louis: Mosby.

11. Celso, B., Tepas, J., Langland-Orban, B., Pracht, E., Papa, L., Lottenberg, L., et al. (2006). A systematic review and meta-analysis comparing outcome of severely injured patients treated in trauma centers following the establishment of trauma systems. *Journal of Trauma, 60*(2), 371-378.

12. Centers for Disease Control and Prevention. (2006). *Centers for Disease Control: National vital statistic fact book 2004.* Retrieved July 1, 2007, from www.cdc.gov/nchs/fastats/acc-inj.htm.

13. Champion, H. R. (2003). Combat fluid resuscitation: Introduction and overview of conferences. *Journal of Trauma, 54*(Suppl. 5), S7-S12.

14. Cohen, S. S. (2007). Musculoskeletal trauma. In K. S. Oman, & J. Koziol-McLain (Eds.), *Emergency nursing secrets* (2nd ed., pp. 345-356). St. Louis: Mosby.

15. Conners, G. R., & Oman, K. S. (2007). Emergency preparedness. In K. S. Oman, & J. Koziol-McLain (Eds.), *Emergency nursing secrets* (2nd ed., pp. 17-28). St. Louis: Mosby.

16. Cottingham, C. A. (2007). Resuscitation of traumatic shock. *AACN Advanced Critical Care, 17*(3), 317-328.

17. Cox, E., & Briggs, S. (2004). Disaster nursing: New frontiers for critical care. *Critical Care Nurse, 24*(3), 16-22.

18. Crookes, B. A., Cohn, S. M., & Bloch, S. (2005). Can near-infrared spectroscopy identify the severity of shock in trauma patients? *Journal of Trauma, 58*(4), 806-816.

19. Dagi, T. F. (2005). The management of postoperative bleeding. *Surgical Clinics of North America, 85*(4), 1191-1213.

20. DeFeiter, P. W., van Hooft, M. A., Beets-Tan, R. G., & Brink, P. R. (2007). Fat embolism syndrome: Yes or no? *Journal of Trauma, 63*(2), 429-431.

21. Emergency Nurses Association. (2000). *Trauma nursing core course: Provider manual* (5th ed.). Des Plaines, IL: Emergency Nurses Association.

22. Felton, A. M., & Platter, B. K. (2007). Drug and alcohol impaired patients. In K. S. Oman, & J. Koziol-McLain (Eds.), *Emergency nursing secrets* (2nd ed., pp. 468-481). St. Louis: Mosby.

23. Flarity, K. (2007). Abdominal trauma. In K. S. Oman, & J. Koziol-McLain (Eds.), *Emergency nursing secrets* (2nd ed., pp. 315-335). St. Louis: Mosby.

24. Friese, R. S., Dineen, S., Jennings, A., Pruitt, J., McBride, D., Shafi, S., et al. (2007). Serum B-type natriuretic peptide: A maker of fluid resuscitation after injury? *Journal of Trauma, 62*(6), 1346-1351.

25. Gentilello, L. M. (2005). Alcohol interventions in trauma centers: The opportunity and the challenge. *Journal of Trauma, 59*(3), S18-S20.

26. Gentilello, L. M., Samuels, P. N., Henningfield, J. E., & Santora, P. B. (2005). Alcohol screening and intervention in trauma centers. *Journal of Trauma, 59*(11), 1250-1255.

27. Goodrich, C. (2007). Endpoints of resuscitation: What should we be monitoring? *AACN Advanced Critical Care, 17*(3), 306-316.

28. Harrison, J. P., & McLane, C. G. (2005). The importance of level 1 trauma services in U.S. hospitals. *Nursing Economics, 23*(5), 223-232.

29. Herm, R. L. (2003). Biomechanics and mechanisms of injury. In S. S. Cohen (Ed.), *Trauma nursing secrets* (pp. 7-16). Philidelphia: Hanley & Belfus.

30. Heron Evans, M. R. (2006). Interventions for clients with musculoskeletal trauma. In D. Ignatavicius, & M. L. Workman (Eds.), *Medical-surgical nursing: Critical thinking for collaborative care* (5th ed., pp. 1189-1227). Philadelphia: Saunders.

31. Hess, J. R., & Zimrin, A. B. (2006). Massive blood transfusion for trauma. *Current Opinion in Hematology, 12*(4), 488-492.

32. Hoffman, H. (2007). Medical field hospital capability and trauma care. *Journal of Trauma, 62*(6), 97-98.

33. Holcomb, J. B., & Hess, J. R. (2006). Early massive trauma transfusion: State of the art. *Journal of Trauma, 60*(Suppl. 1), S1-S2.

34. Hoyt, D. B., & Coimbra, R. (2007). Trauma systems. *Surgical Clinics of North America, 87*(1), 21-35.

35. Karmy-Jones, R., & Jurkovich, G. J. (2006). Chest trauma. In M. W. Mulholland, K. D. Lillemoe, G. M. Doherty, R. V. Maier, & G. R. Upchurch (Eds.), *Greenfield's surgery: Scientific principles & practice* (4th ed., pp. 406-420). Philadelphia: Lippincott Williams & Wilkins.

36. Kaun, J. K., Routt, M. L., & Wessells, H. (2006). Genitourinary and pelvic trauma. In M. W. Mulholland, K. D. Lillemoe, G. M. Doherty, R. V. Maier, & G. R. Upchurch (Eds.), *Greenfield's surgery: Scientific principles & practice,* (4th ed., pp. 441-449). Philadelphia: Lippincott Williams & Wilkins.

37. Kirkpatrick, A. W. (2007). Clinician-performed focused sonography for the resuscitation of trauma. *Critical Care Medicine, 35*(Suppl. 5), S162-S172.

38. Kress, J., & Hall, J. (2004). Delirium and sedation. *Critical Care Clinics, 20*(3), 419-433.

39. Liebergall, M., Braverman, N., Shapira, S., Rotem, O, Soudry, I, & Mor-Yosef, S. (2007). Role of nurses in a university hospital during mass casualty events. *American Journal of Critical Care, 16*(5), 480-484.

40. Littlejohns, L., & Bader, M. K. (2005). Prevention of secondary brain injury: Targeting technology. *AACN Clinical Issues, 16*(4), 501-514.

41. MacKenzie, E. J., Rivara, F. P., Jurkovich, G. J., Nathens, A. B., Frey, K. P., Egleston, B. L., et al. (2007). A national evaluation of the effect of trauma-center care on mortality. *New England Journal of Medicine, 354*(4), 366-378.

42. Makic, M. B. F., Singh, N., & McQuillan, K. A. (2009). Wound healing and soft tissue trauma. In K. McQuillan, M. B. Makic, & E. Whalen (Eds.), *Trauma nursing from resuscitation through rehabilitation* (4th ed.). Philadelphia: Saunders.

43. Malone, D. L., Hess, J. R., & Fingerhunt, A. (2006). Massive transfusion practices around the globe and a suggestion for a common massive transfusion protocol. *Journal of Trauma, 60*(Suppl. 6), S91-S96.

44. Mann, E., & Makic M. B. F. (2007). Burn injury. In K. S. Oman, & J. Koziol-McLain (Eds.), *Emergency nursing secrets* (2nd ed., pp. 357-372). St. Louis: Mosby.

45. Martinez, R. (2009). Psychosocial impact of trauma. In K. McQuillan, M. B. Makic, & E. Whalen (Eds.), *Trauma nursing from resuscitation through rehabilitation* (4th ed.). Philadelphia: Saunders.

46. McArthur, B. J. (2006). Damage control surgery for the patient who has experienced multiple traumatic injuries. *AORN Journal, 84*(6), 992-1000.

47. McCabe, S. (2006). Substance use and abuse in trauma: Implications for care. *Critical Care Nursing Clinics of North America, 18*(2), 371-382.

48. Moore, F. A., McKinley, B. A., & Moore, E. E. (2004). The next generation in shock resuscitation. *Lancet, 363*(6), 1988-1996.

49. Myers, J. (2007). Focused assessment with sonography for trauma (FAST): The truth about ultrasound in blunt trauma. *Journal of Trauma, 62*(3), S28.

50. Nathens, A. B. (2005). Thrombosis and coagulation: Deep vein thrombosis and pulmonary embolism prophylaxis. *Surgical Clinics of North America, 85*(3), 1163-1177.

51. *National Trauma Data Bank Report 2006, version 6.0.* (2006). American College of Surgeons. Retrieved July 1, 2007, from: www.facs.org/trauma/ntdb.html.

52. Neff, M. J., & Neff, J. A. (2007). Thoracic and neck trauma. In K. S. Oman, & J. Koziol-McLain (Eds.), *Emergency nursing secrets* (2nd ed., pp. 299-314). St. Louis: Mosby.

53. Olson, D. M, & Graffagnino, C. (2005). Consciousness, coma, and caring for the brain injured patient. *AACN Clinical Issues, 16*(4), 441-455.

54. Parr, M. J. (2004). Damage control surgery and intensive care. *Injury, 35*(7), 712-721.

55. Rose, S., Bisson, J, Churchill, R., & Wessely, S. (2007). Psychological debriefing for preventing post traumatic stress disorder (review). *The Cochrane Collaboration, issue 3*, 1-37.

56. Ryan, T. J. (2006). Infection following soft tissue injury: Its role in wound healing. *Current Opinion in Infectious Diseases, 20*(2), 124-128.

57. Schermer, C. R., Moyers, T. B., Miller, W. R., & Bloomfield, L. A. (2006). Trauma center brief interventions for alcohol disorders decrease subsequent driving under the influence arrests. *Journal of Trauma, 60*(1), 29-34.

58. Schreiber, M. A. (2004). Damage control surgery. *Critical Care Clinics, 20*(1), 101-118.

59. Thompson, H. J., & Bourbonniere, M. (2006). Traumatic injury in the older adult from head to toe. *Critical Care Nursing Clinics of North America, 18*(2), 419-431.

60. Tisherman, S., Barie, P., Bokhari, F., Bonadies, J., Daley, B., Diebel, L., et al. (2004). Clinical practice guideline: Endpoints of resuscitation. *Journal of Trauma, 57*(4), 898-912.

61. Utter, G. H., Maier, R. V., Rivara, F. P., Mock, C. N., Jurkovich, G. J., & Nathens, A. B. (2006). Inclusive trauma systems: Do they improve triage or outcomes of the severely injured? *Journal of Trauma, 60*(3), 529-572.

62. Victorson, D., Farmer, L., Burnett, K., Ouellette, A., & Barocase, J. (2005). Maladaptive coping strategies and injury-related distress following traumatic physical injury. *Rehabilitation Psychology, 50*(4), 408-415.

63. VonRueden, K. T. (2009). Cycles of trauma. In K. McQuillan, M. B. Makic, & E. Whalen (Eds), *Trauma nursing from resuscitation through rehabilitation* (4th ed.). Philadelphia: Saunders.

64. Waller, J. A. (1994). Reflections on a half century of injury control. *American Journal of Public Health, 84*(4), 664-670.

65. Weigelt, J. A., Brasel, K. J., & Klein, J. D. (2009). Mechanisms of injury. In K. A. McQuillan, K. M. B. Makic, & E. Whalen (Eds.), *Trauma nursing from resuscitation through rehabilitation* (4th ed.). Philadelphia: Saunders.

66. Wilson, S. (2006). Rhabdomyolysis made easy. *Australian Nursing Journal, 14*(2), 21-23.

67. Wisner, D. H., & Hoyt, D. B. (2006). Abdominal trauma. In M. W. Mulholland, K. D. Lillemoe, G. M. Doherty, R. V. Maier, & G. R. Upchurch (Eds.), *Greenfield's surgery: Scientific principles & practice* (4th ed., pp. 421-440). Philadelphia: Lippincott Williams & Wilkins.

CHAPTER 20

Burns

Karla S. Ahrns-Klas, BSN, RN, CCRP

INTRODUCTION

There is no greater challenge in critical care nursing than caring for a severely burned patient. In a single year, fire departments in the United States responded to an estimated 1,602,000 fires.[29] These fires resulted in an associated civilian death approximately every 2 hours and a civilian burn injury every 29 minutes.[29] Burn injuries result in an estimated 500,000 hospital emergency department (ED) visits and 50,000 acute hospital admissions each year in the United States.[6] Initial management of the seriously injured burn patient dramatically affects the patient's long-term outcome. Many burn patients are treated in hospitals with special capabilities for managing extensive burn injuries. However, even with the expanded network of burn center facilities, most patients are first seen in a community hospital. Consequently, it is crucial that ED and critical care nurses have the skills necessary to provide initial resuscitative care to burn-injured patients. Care of the burned patient requires a multidisciplinary team approach to maximize favorable patient outcomes.

Burn injuries have significant economic and social consequences, as well as marked morbidity and mortality. Historically, burn injuries have been one of the most lethal forms of trauma. However, application of research-based advances in fluid resuscitation, early excision and closure of the wound, metabolic and respiratory support, microbial surveillance, and infection control have dramatically improved survival and recovery from burn injury.[34,38,39] Even with these improvements, morbidity and mortality remain significant in patients with inhalation injuries and burns greater than 50% of total body surface area (TBSA).[5,9,17,18,31,34] Elderly and young patients with a smaller percentage of burned areas involved are also at considerable risk of mortality.[5,12,18,31,38] Knowledge of the physiological changes and the potential complications associated with burn injury prepares the

critical care nurse to care for these complex patients and to optimize their outcome.

REVIEW OF ANATOMY AND PHYSIOLOGY OF THE SKIN

The skin, also called the integumentary system, is the largest organ of the body. It is a vital organ because of its many functions, including a protective barrier against infection and injury, regulation of fluid loss, thermoregulatory (or body heat) control, synthesis of vitamin D, sensory contact with the environment, determination of identity, and presentable cosmetic appearance. The skin is composed of two layers, the *epidermis* and the *dermis*, with an underlying *subcutaneous* fat tissue layer that binds the dermis to organs and tissues of the body (Figure 20-1). The epidermis is the outermost and thinnest skin layer. The dermis is considerably thicker and contains collagen and elastic fibers, blood and lymph vessels, sweat glands, hair follicles, sebaceous glands, and sensory fibers for the detection of pain, pressure, touch, and temperature. The underlying subcutaneous tissue is a layer of connective tissue and fat deposits. When an extensive amount of skin is damaged from burn injury, alterations of these multiple physiological functions place the patient at risk for complications.

Effects of Aging

Elderly skin is much less resilient to mechanical trauma because of a flattened dermal-epidermal junction, loss or atrophy of dermal and subcutaneous mass, and reduced microcirculation. These tissue and turgor changes manifest as skin thinning and predispose this group to deeper burn wounds and to poor or delayed healing. Healing also is impacted by a decline in immune system function that increases susceptibility to infectious complications. Health status before injury greatly affects critical care

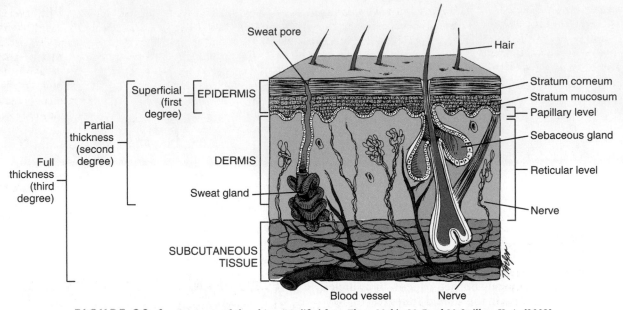

FIGURE 20-1. Anatomy of the skin. *(Modified from Flynn Makic, M. B., & McQuillan, K. A. [2009]. Wound healing and soft tissue injuries. In K. A. McQuillan, M. B. Flynn Makic, & E. Whalen [Eds.],* Trauma nursing: From resuscitation through rehabilitation *[4th ed.]. Philadelphia: Saunders.)*

management and outcome. Older patients have a diminished physiological reserve and capacity to respond to the significant metabolic stress, hemodynamic demand, and inflammatory challenge that occur after a burn injury. The added insult of preexisting disease contributes to difficulties in burn shock fluid resuscitation and increases in morbidity and mortality.

MECHANISMS OF INJURY

Burn injury is classified into three types: thermal, chemical, and electrical. These types of injuries can also occur in conjunction with inhalation injury. Inhalation injury is observed in 20% to 50% of patients admitted to burn centers and significantly increases the risk of death.[4] Approximately 90% of burn injuries are thermally induced. Chemical and electrical burns account for the remaining 10% of the injuries.[4] Although the primary principles of care are the same for all burn injuries regardless of cause, chemical and electrical burns require special initial management and ongoing assessment, as discussed later in this chapter.

Thermal Injury

Thermal injury is caused when the skin comes in contact with a source of sufficient temperature to cause cell injury by coagulation. This can occur from flame (e.g., house fires, ignition of clothing, explosion of gases), scalding liquids (e.g., water, cooking oil, grease), steam (e.g., car radiators, cooking pots, industrial equipment), or direct contact with a heat source (e.g., space heater, metal). The severity of injury is related to heat intensity and duration of contact. For example, a heat source of less than 40°C (111.2°F) does not cause a burn regardless of the length of exposure. However, the extent of damage increases with temperatures greater than this level, in direct proportion to the duration of exposure. Exposure to temperatures of 60°C (140°F) causes full-thickness tissue destruction (third-degree burns) in as little as 3 to 5 seconds. This poses an injury prevention issue, because 140°F is a common setting for home water heaters despite recommendations of maintaining temperature settings of less than 120°F (49°C). Children and the elderly are at greater risk of thermal injury at lower temperatures because of their thinner skin and their decreased agility in moving to avoid harm.

Chemical Injury

Chemical burns are caused by contact, inhalation of fumes, ingestion, or injection. Although chemical injuries account for only a small percentage of admissions to burn centers, they can be severe, and have both local and systemic effects. The severity of injury is related to type, volume, duration of contact, and concentration of the agent. Tissue damage from chemical burns continues until the chemical is completely removed or neutralized. Chemical agents are part of our lifestyle. Thus, the potential for injury from exposure is great. The Occupational Safety and Health Administration's Hazard Communication Standard requires that employees receive educational training regarding hazardous materials in the workplace and that Material Safety Data Sheets (MSDS) be posted in work areas. MSDS list specific information on all chemicals in the workplace including composition, side effects, and potential for systemic toxicity. The Joint Commission also monitors compliance with this mandatory regulation.

Three categories of chemical agents exist: alkalies, acids, and organic compounds. Alkalies are commonly found in cleaning products used in the home and industry, such as oven cleaners, wet cement, and fertilizers. This category of chemical agents produces far more damage than acids because alkalies loosen tissue by protein denaturation and liquefaction necrosis, thereby allowing the chemical to diffuse more deeply into the tissue. Alkalies also bind to tissue proteins and make it more difficult to stop the burning process.

Acids are found in many household and industrial products, such as bathroom cleansers, rust removers, and acidifiers for home swimming pools. Depth of burn injury from acids (except hydrofluoric acid) tends to be limited because acids cause coagulation necrosis of tissue and precipitation of protein. Hydrofluoric acid is a weak acid. However, the fluoride ion is very toxic and is potentially lethal even with small exposures, because it causes hypocalcemia by rapidly binding to free calcium in the blood.

Organic compounds such as phenols and petroleum products (e.g., gasoline, chemical disinfectants) can produce cutaneous burns as well as be absorbed with resulting systemic effects. Phenols cause severe coagulation necrosis of dermal proteins and produce a layer of thick, nonviable tissue called *eschar*.[4] Petroleum products such as gasoline promote cell membrane injury and dissolution of lipids with resulting skin necrosis. Systemic effects such as central nervous system depression, hypothermia, hypotension, pulmonary edema, and intravascular hemolysis may be severe or even fatal. Chemical pneumonitis and bronchitis may occur from inhalation of fumes. Other complications observed with gasoline burns include hepatic and renal failure and sudden death.[4]

Warfare, terrorist attacks, and/or mass casualty incidents can produce burn injuries from chemical or thermal exposure. Approximately 30% of those involved in a disaster event sustain burn injuries, that are on average greater than 50% TBSA.[4] There-fore, every critical care nurse should be aware of the potential impact a mass casualty incident may have on patient admissions to their hospital and critical care units. Disaster management is further discussed in Chapter 19.

An emerging epidemic is burn injury from the manufacturing of methamphetamine in clandestine "laboratories."[12,46] These complex cases involve both thermal and chemical burns, and are highly associated with inhalation injuries.[46] They also pose risk to the clinicians caring for these patients if patients are not properly decontaminated from the chemical exposure. A vague or inconsistent injury history, burns to the face and hands, and signs of agitation or substance withdrawal should alert the nurse to a potential methamphetamine-related injury.[12]

Electrical Injury

Electrical injury is caused by contact with varied electrical sources such as household or industrial current, car batteries, electrosurgical devices, high-tension electrical lines, and lightning. Electrical injuries are frequently work-related and often involve litigation.[30] Electricity flows by either alternating current (AC; e.g., most commercial applications) or direct current (DC; e.g., lightning, car batteries). Although AC and DC are both dangerous, AC has a greater probability of producing cardiopulmonary arrest by ventricular fibrillation. Tetanic muscle contraction occurs that may "lock" the patient to the source of electricity and cause respiratory muscle paralysis. Electrical injuries are arbitrarily classified as high voltage (>1000 V) or low voltage (≤1000 V).[4]

In electrical burns, tissue damage occurs during the process of electrical energy being converted to heat. The resulting dissipation of heat energy is often greatest at the point of contact (entry and exit), which is frequently on the extremities. Many factors affect the extent of injury including the type and pathway of current, the duration of contact, environmental conditions, the body tissue resistance, and the cross-sectional area of the body involved. Therefore, electrical injury wounds are extremely variable in presentation. A small burn may be noted at the point of contact, or there may be a craterlike "blowout" wound. Since electricity follows the path of least resistance, it was historically theorized that the low resistance of nerve tissue placed it at the highest risk of damage or degeneration. More recently it has been proposed that the density of bone tissue and its high resistance generates the most heat.[4,30] The resulting heat energy is dissipated to and damages adjacent deep muscle tissue. Consequently, deep tissue necrosis occurs beneath viable more superficial tissue. On initial presentation, the cutaneous wound

TABLE 20-1   Types of Smoke Inhalation Injury

Type of Injury	Pathology
Carbon monoxide poisoning	Carbon monoxide binds to hemoglobin molecules more rapidly than does oxygen molecules; tissue hypoxia results
Inhalation injury above the glottis	Most often a thermal injury; heat absorption and damage occur mostly in the pharynx and larynx; may cause airway obstruction after resuscitation is initiated
Inhalation injury below the glottis	Usually a chemical injury that produces impaired ciliary activity, erythema, hypersecretion, edema, ulceration of mucosa, increased blood flow, and spasm of bronchi and/or bronchioles

Modified from American Burn Association. (2005). *Advanced burn life support course: Provider's manual.* Chicago: American Burn Association.

may appear minimal or superficial. However, it can manifest as an extensive, deep wound with neurological impairment several days or weeks later.

Lightning injury is caused by a direct strike or a side flash that causes a flow of current between the person and a close object that is struck by lightning.[4] Cutaneous injury is often superficial because the current travels on the surface of the body rather than through it. Lightning injuries frequently result in cardiopulmonary arrest. Approximately 70% of survivors have transient but severe central nervous system deficits.[4]

Inhalation Injury

Lung injury caused by inhalation of smoke and products of incomplete combustion is associated with increased mortality.[4,34] Inhalation injury is classified as (1) injury from carbon monoxide (CO), (2) injury above the glottis, and (3) injury below the glottis.[4] Table 20-1 summarizes characteristics of each type of injury. Inhalation injury often warrants admission to a critical care unit, even when there are no cutaneous surface burn wounds.

Carbon Monoxide Poisoning
Carbon monoxide poisoning is the most frequent cause of death at the burn scene.[4] Carbon monoxide is released when organic compounds, such as wood or coal, are burned, and it has an affinity for hemoglobin that is 200 times greater than that of oxygen.[4] When carbon monoxide is inhaled, it binds to hemoglobin (*carboxyhemoglobin* [COHgb]) and prevents the red blood cell from transporting oxygen to body tissues, leading to hypoxia. Carbon monoxide poisoning is difficult to detect because it may not present with significant clinical findings. Specifically, partial pressure of oxygen in arterial blood (PaO_2) and arte-

TABLE 20-2   Carboxyhemoglobin

Carboxyhemoglobin Level*	Clinical Presentation
<10% to 15%	Headache; impaired visual acuity
15% to 40%	Central nervous system dysfunction: restlessness, confusion, impaired dexterity, dizziness, nausea/vomiting
40% to 60%	Loss of consciousness, tachycardia, tachypnea, cherry red or cyanotic skin
>60%	Coma; death generally ensues

*Percentage of hemoglobin molecules bound with carbon monoxide.

rial oxygen saturation (SaO_2) levels are normal. Therefore, it is essential to measure COHgb levels, which are reported as a percentage of hemoglobin molecules bound with carbon monoxide. Levels lower than 10% to 15% are found in mild carbon monoxide poisoning, and are commonly associated with heavy smokers and people exposed continually to dense traffic pollution (Table 20-2). Central nervous system dysfunction of varying degrees (e.g., restlessness, confusion) manifests at levels of 15% to 40%. Loss of consciousness occurs at COHgb levels of 40% to 60%, and death generally ensues when the COHgb level exceeds 60%.

Injury Above the Glottis
Inhalation injury above the glottis, also referred to as upper airway injury, is caused by breathing in heat or noxious chemicals produced during the burning

- Facial burns
- Presence of soot around mouth and nose and in sputum (carbonaceous sputum)
- Signs of hypoxemia (tachycardia, dysrhythmias, anxiety, lethargy)
- Signs of respiratory difficulty (change in respiratory rate, use of accessory muscles, intercostal or sternal retractions, stridor, hoarseness)
- Abnormal breath sounds
- Abnormal arterial blood gas values
- Singed nasal hairs
- Elevated carboxyhemoglobin levels

- Partial-thickness burns >10% total body surface area
- Full-thickness burns
- Burns involving the face, hands, feet, genitalia, perineum, or major joints
- Chemical and electrical burns
- Inhalation injury
- Preexisting medical disorders
- Associated trauma
- Hospitals without qualified personnel or equipment to care for burn-injured children
- Patients requiring special social, emotional, or rehabilitative intervention

process. The nose, mouth, and throat dissipate the heat and prevent damage to lower airways. However, the resulting upper airway thermal injury causes edema, thereby placing the patient at high risk of airway obstruction. Airway obstruction clinically presents as hoarseness, dry cough, labored or rapid breathing, difficulty swallowing, or stridor.

Injury Below the Glottis

Injury below the glottis is almost always caused by breathing noxious chemical byproducts of burning materials and smoke. Extensive damage to alveoli and impaired pulmonary functioning result from the injury (see Table 20-1 and Clinical Alert: Clinical Indicators of Inhalation Injury). A hallmark sign is *carbonaceous sputum* (soot or carbon particles in secretions). Tracheal and bronchial/bronchiolar constriction and spasms with resulting wheezing can occur within minutes to several hours after injury.[4] Acute respiratory failure and acute respiratory distress syndrome may develop within the first few days. Respiratory tract mucosal sloughing may occur within 4 to 5 days. Admission chest x-rays typically demonstrate normal findings. However, later x-rays may display reduced lung expansion, atelectasis, and diffuse lung edema or infiltrates. Fiberoptic bronchoscopy or xenon ventilation-perfusion lung scanning may be indicated to provide a definitive diagnosis of injury below the glottis.[34,47]

BURN CLASSIFICATION AND SEVERITY

Burn injury severity is determined by the type of burn injury, burn wound characteristics (depth, extent, body part burned), concomitant injuries, patient age, and preexisting health status. Properly classifying and assessing the severity of injury allow appropriate triage and transfer of patients to a burn center. The extent and depth of burn injury are affected by the duration of contact with the injuring agent, the temperature of the agent, the amount of tissue exposed, and the ability of the agent and tissue to dissipate the thermal energy.

Depth of Injury

Burn depth predicts wound care treatment requirements, determines the need for skin grafting, and affects scarring, cosmetic, and functional outcomes. Burn injuries are often classified as first-, second-, or third-degree burns. However, the terms *superficial*, *partial-thickness*, or *full-thickness* burns more closely correlate with the pathophysiology of burn injury and the level of affected skin layer involvement (see Figure 20-1). Accurate depth assessment may be difficult to determine initially, because progressive edema formation and compromised wound blood flow during the first 48 to 72 hours after injury may increase the definitive burn depth.

Superficial burns involve only the first layer of skin or the epidermis (hence termed first-degree injury), and typically heal in 3 to 5 days without treatment. Because superficial burn injuries (e.g., sunburns) only cause erythema and do not involve the dermis, they are not included in the calculation of the size of the burn (extent of injury) used for fluid resuscitation requirements. *Partial-thickness* burns involve injury of the second skin layer or dermal layer (hence a second-degree injury), and are further subdivided into superficial and deep classifications. *Superficial partial-thickness* injuries that involve the epidermis and a limited portion of the dermis heal by growth

TABLE 20-3   Depth of Burn Injury

Degree of Injury	Morphology	Healing Time	Wound Characteristics
Superficial (First degree)	Destruction of epidermis only	3-5 days	Red, dry, painful; blisters rarely present
Superficial partial-thickness (Second degree)	Destruction of epidermis and some dermis	10-21 days	Moist, pink or mottled red; very painful; blisters; blanches with pressure
Deep partial-thickness (Second degree)	Destruction of epidermis and most of dermis; some skin appendages remain	3-6 weeks	Pale, mottled, pearly red/white; moist or somewhat dry; typically less painful; blanching decreased and prolonged; difficult to distinguish from full-thickness injury
Full-thickness (Third degree)	Destruction of epidermis, dermis, and underlying subcutaneous tissue	Does not heal; requires skin grafting	Thick, leathery eschar; dry; white, cherry-red, or brown-black; painless; does not blanch with pressure; thrombosed blood vessels

of undamaged basal cells within 10 to 21 days. *Deep partial-thickness* injuries involve destruction of the epidermis and most of the dermis. Although such wounds may heal spontaneously within 3 to 6 weeks, they are typically excised and grafted to achieve better functional and cosmetic results, to decrease the length of healing time, and decrease hospitalization time.

Destruction of all layers of the skin down to or past the subcutaneous fat, fascia, muscles, or bone is defined as a *full-thickness* injury (third-degree injury). A thick, leathery, nonelastic, coagulated layer of necrotic tissue called *eschar* is created. The nerves are destroyed, resulting in a painless wound. These injuries always require skin grafting for permanent wound closure. Table 20-3 describes the characteristics of superficial, partial-thickness, and full-thickness burn injuries.

Differentiating partial-thickness from full-thickness injuries may initially be difficult because burn wounds mature or progress within the first few days. The three zones of thermal injury explain this phenomenon by illustrating the relationship of depth and extent of injury with damaged tissue viability (Figure 20-2). The outermost area of minimal cell injury is termed the *zone of hyperemia*. It has early spontaneous recovery and is similar to a superficial burn. The greatest area of tissue necrosis is at the core of the wound or the *zone of coagulation*. It is the site of irreversible skin death and is similar to a full-thickness burn. Peripheral to this area is a *zone of stasis*, where vascular damage and reduced blood flow have occurred. Secondary insults, such as inadequate resuscitation or infection, result in conversion of this potentially salvageable area to full-thickness

skin destruction with irreversible tissue *necrosis* or death.

Extent of Injury

The extent of injury or size of a burn is expressed as the percentage of *total body surface area* (%TBSA). The quickest method to initially calculate %TBSA is the *rule of nines*. This technique divides the TBSA into areas representing 9% or multiples of 9% (Figure 20-3). By summing all areas of partial- and full-thickness burns (superficial burns are not included), the %TBSA burned is quickly estimated. For evaluations of injury extent in irregular or scattered small burns, the size of the patient's palm (including fingers) is used for measurement and represents 1% TBSA.[4] The rule of nines varies between adult and pediatric patients because children have a proportionally larger head size compared with adults.

Another surface area assessment method, the *Lund and Browder chart* (Figure 20-4), provides a more accurate determination of the extent of burn injury by correlating body surface area with age-related proportions. This method is used most frequently in a burn center. Accurate calculation of extent of injury is important for assessing burn severity and for estimating fluid resuscitation requirements.

PHYSIOLOGICAL RESPONSES TO BURN INJURY

The body responds to major burn injuries with significant hemodynamic, metabolic, and immunological effects that occur locally and systemically as a

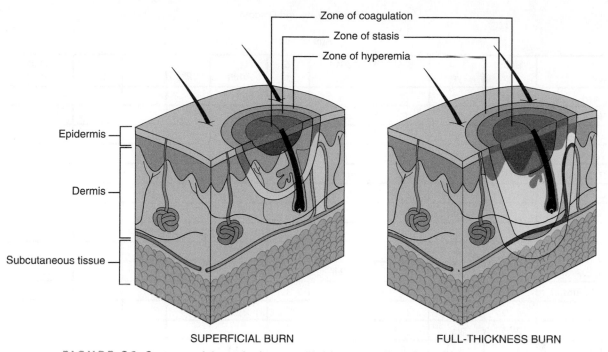

FIGURE 20-2. Zones of thermal injury. *(Modified from Cornwell, P., & Gregory C. [2005]. Management of clients with burn injury. In J. M. Black, & J. H. Hawks [Eds.],* Medical-surgical nursing: Clinical management for positive outcomes *[7th ed.]. Philadelphia: Saunders.)*

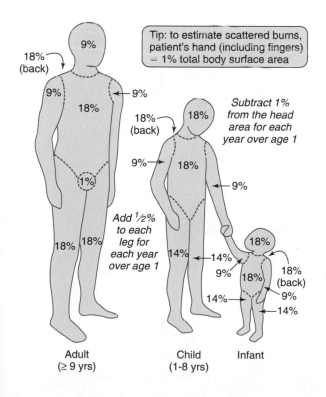

FIGURE 20-3. The rule of nines. *TBSA,* Total body surface area. *(Courtesy of University of Michigan Trauma Burn Center, Ann Arbor, MI.)*

EXAMPLE: An adult with superficial burns to the face and partial-thickness burns to the lower half of the right arm, entire left arm, and chest: 4.5% (lower right arm) + 9% (entire left arm) + 9% (chest or upper anterior trunk) = 22.5% TBSA (the superficial burns to the face are not included in the %TBSA calculation).

result of cellular damage from heat (Figures 20-5 and 20-6). The magnitude and duration of the systemic response and the degree of physiological changes are proportional to the extent of body surface area (%TBSA) injured. Direct thermal damage to blood vessels causes intravascular coagulation, with arterial and venous blood flow ceasing in the wound injury area. The damaged and ischemic cells release *mediators,* endogenously produced substances that the body secretes to initiate a protective inflammatory response. Mediators such as histamine, prostaglandins, bradykinins, catecholamines, and cytokines are stimulated and released, causing myriad vasoactive, cellular, and cardiovascular effects. Gaps between endothelial cells in vessel wall membranes develop, making vessel walls porous or "leaky." This *increased capillary membrane permeability* allows a significant shift of protein molecules, fluid, and electrolytes

Text continued on p. 694

Burn Estimate and Diagram

Age vs. Area

Area	Birth 1 yr	1–4 yr	5–9 yr	10–14 yr	15 yr	Adult	2°	3°	Total	Donor Areas
Head	19	17	13	11	9	7				
Neck	2	2	2	2	2	2				
Ant. Trunk	13	13	13	13	13	13				
Post. Trunk	13	13	13	13	13	13				
R. Buttock	2 ½	2 ½	2 ½	2 ½	2 ½	2 ½				
L. Buttock	2 ½	2 ½	2 ½	2 ½	2 ½	2 ½				
Genitalia	1	1	1	1	1	1				
R. U. Arm	4	4	4	4	4	4				
L. U. Arm	4	4	4	4	4	4				
R. L. Arm	3	3	3	3	3	3				
L. L. Arm	3	3	3	3	3	3				
R. Hand	2 ½	2 ½	2 ½	2 ½	2 ½	2 ½				
L. Hand	2 ½	2 ½	2 ½	2 ½	2 ½	2 ½				
R. Thigh	5 ½	6 ½	8	8 ½	9	9 ½				
L. Thigh	5 ½	6 ½	8	8 ½	9	9 ½				
R. Leg	5	5	5 ½	6	6 ½	7				
L. Leg	5	5	5 ½	6	6 ½	7				
R. Foot	3 ½	3 ½	3 ½	3 ½	3 ½	3 ½				
L. Foot	3 ½	3 ½	3 ½	3 ½	3 ½	3 ½				
						Total				

Burn Diagram

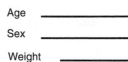

Age _____
Sex _____
Weight _____

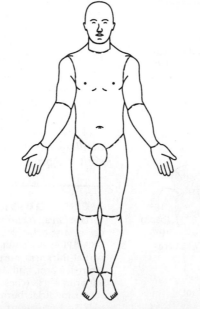
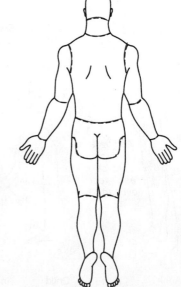

FIGURE 20-4. Burn estimate and diagram. *Ant,* Anterior; *post,* posterior; *L,* left; *R,* right; *R. U.,* right upper; *R. L.,* right lower; *L. U.,* left upper; *L. L.,* left lower.

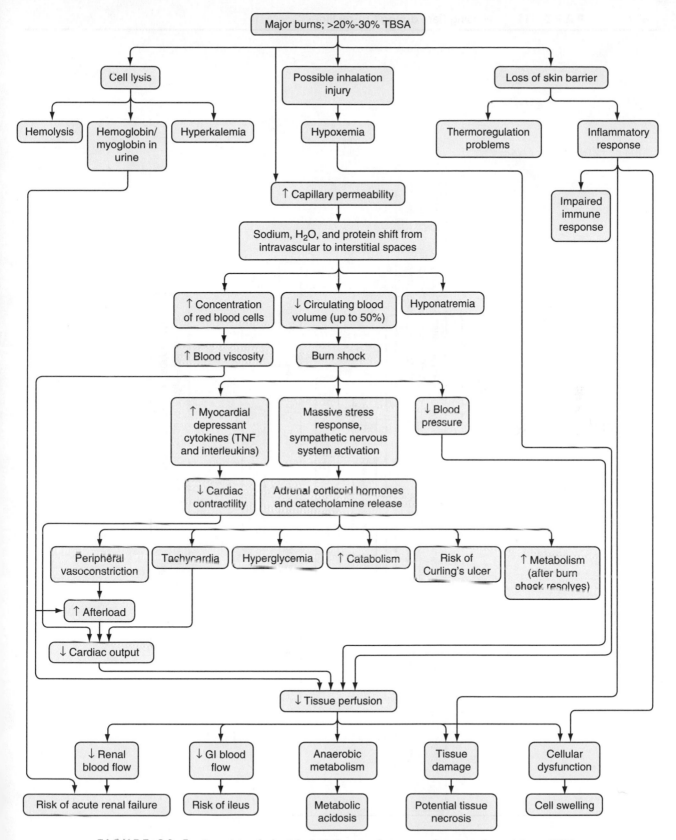

FIGURE 20-5. Overview of physiological changes that occur after acute burn injury. *TBSA,* Total body surface area; *TNF,* tumor necrosis factor. *(Modified from Byers, J. F., & LaBorde, P. J. [2004]. Management of patients with burn injury. In S. C. Smeltzer, & B. G. Bare [Eds.], Brunner & Suddarth's text-book of medical-surgical nursing [10th ed.]. Philadelphia: Lippincott Williams & Wilkins.)*

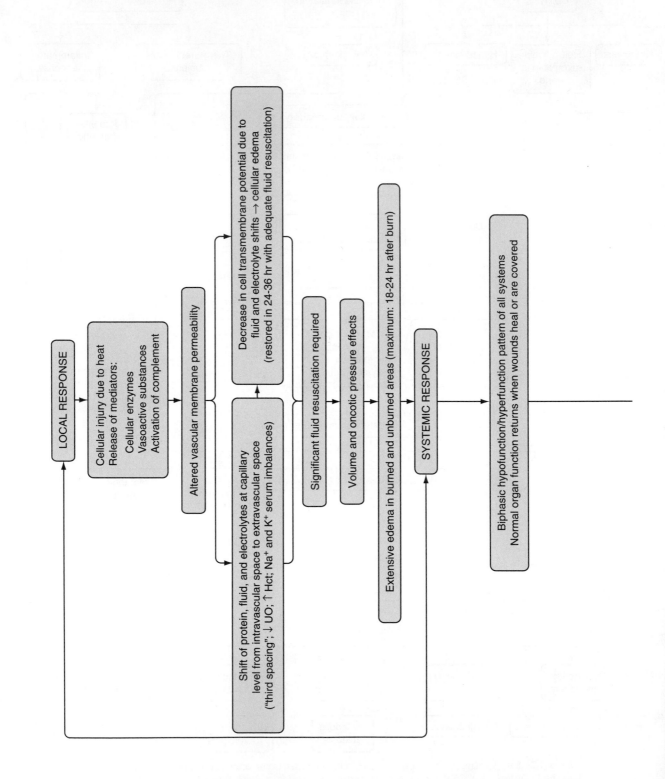

LOCAL RESPONSE

Cellular injury due to heat
Release of mediators:
    Cellular enzymes
    Vasoactive substances
    Activation of complement

Altered vascular membrane permeability

Decrease in cell transmembrane potential due to fluid and electrolyte shifts → cellular edema (restored in 24-36 hr with adequate fluid resuscitation)

Shift of protein, fluid, and electrolytes at capillary level from intravascular space to extravascular space ("third spacing"; ↓ UO; ↑ Hct; Na$^+$ and K$^+$ serum imbalances)

Significant fluid resuscitation required

Volume and oncotic pressure effects

Extensive edema in burned and unburned areas (maximum: 18-24 hr after burn)

SYSTEMIC RESPONSE

Biphasic hypofunction/hyperfunction pattern of all systems
Normal organ function returns when wounds heal or are covered

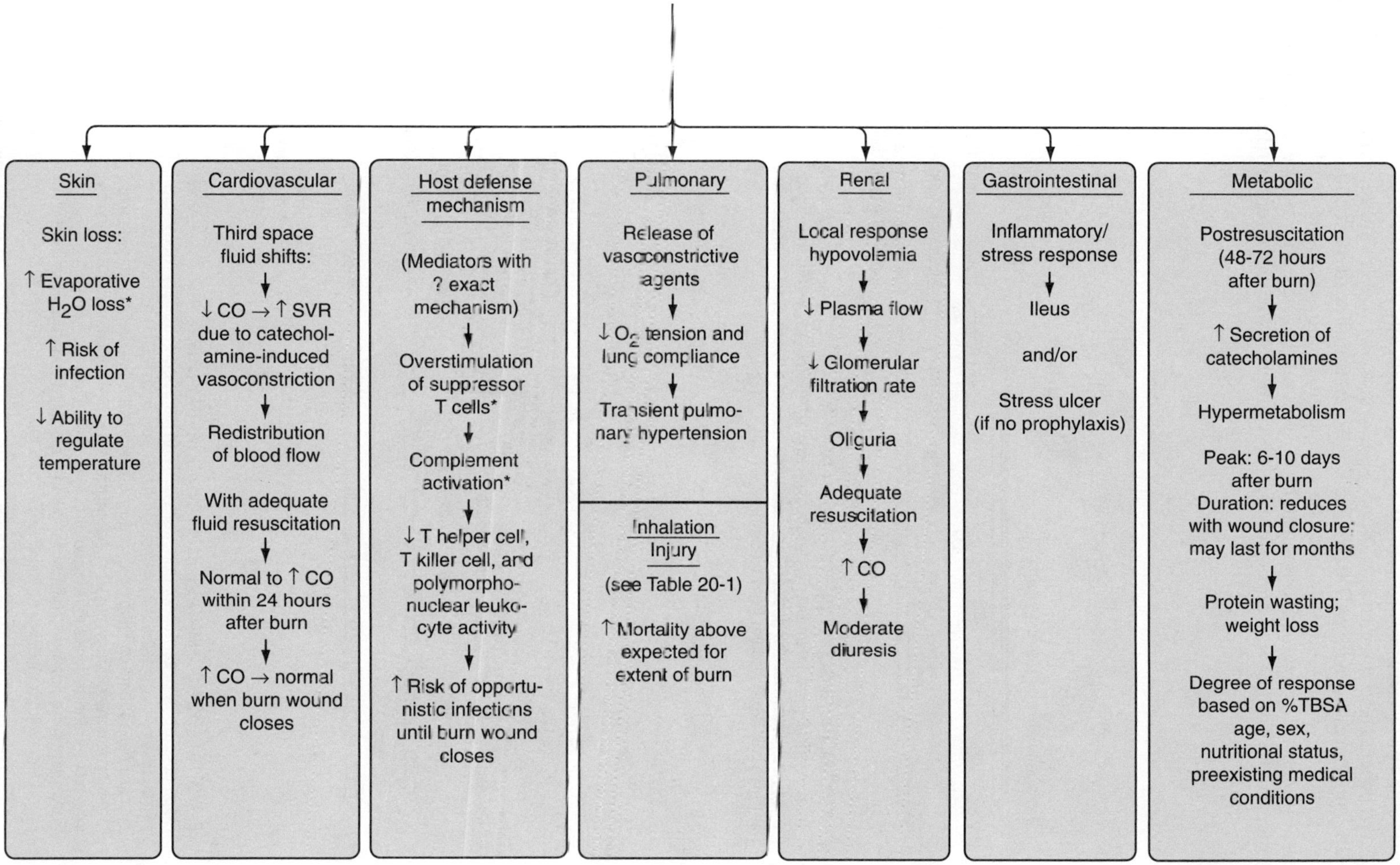

FIGURE 20-6. Pathophysiology of extensive burn injury. *A response associated with burn injury greater than 20% to 25% total body surface area (%TBSA). *CO*, Cardiac output; *H₂O*, water; *Hct*, hematocrit; *SVR*, systemic vascular resistance; *UO*, urinary output.

Skin

Skin loss:

↑ Evaporative H₂O loss*

↑ Risk of infection

↓ Ability to regulate temperature

Cardiovascular

Third space fluid shifts:

↓ CO → ↑ SVR due to catecholamine-induced vasoconstriction

Redistribution of blood flow

With adequate fluid resuscitation

Normal to ↑ CO within 24 hours after burn

↑ CO → normal when burn wound closes

Host defense mechanism

(Mediators with ? exact mechanism)

Overstimulation of suppressor T cells*

Complement activation*

↓ T helper cell, T killer cell, and polymorphonuclear leukocyte activity

↑ Risk of opportunistic infections until burn wound closes

Pulmonary

Release of vasoconstrictive agents

↓ O₂ tension and lung compliance

Transient pulmonary hypertension

Inhalation Injury (see Table 20-1)

↑ Mortality above expected for extent of burn

Renal

Local response hypovolemia

↓ Plasma flow

↓ Glomerular filtration rate

Oliguria

Adequate resuscitation

↑ CO

Moderate diuresis

Gastrointestinal

Inflammatory/stress response

Ileus

and/or

Stress ulcer (if no prophylaxis)

Metabolic

Postresuscitation (48-72 hours after burn)

↑ Secretion of catecholamines

Hypermetabolism

Peak: 6-10 days after burn Duration: reduces with wound closure; may last for months

Protein wasting; weight loss

Degree of response based on %TBSA age, sex, nutritional status, preexisting medical conditions from the *intravascular space* (inside the blood vessels) into the *interstitium* (the space between cells and the vascular system) in a process also referred to as *third-spacing* (Figure 20-7). There is rapid and dramatic edema formation. Cellular swelling also occurs as a result of a decrease in cell transmembrane potential and a shift of extracellular sodium and water into the cell.[13] The leaking of proteins into the interstitium dramatically lowers intravascular *oncotic pressure*, which draws even more intravascular fluid into the interstitium and contributes to the development of edema and *burn shock* (shock from intravascular volume loss, created by the sudden fluid and solute shifts immediately after burn injury). In burns greater

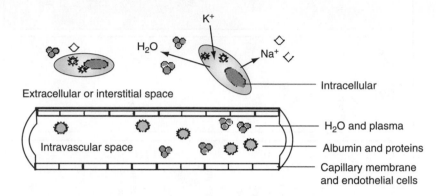

NORMAL PHYSIOLOGY BEFORE BURN INJURY
Intact capillary wall membranes keep large protein molecules within the blood vessels or intravascular space. This maintains normal protein oncotic pressure and retains intravascular fluid volume.

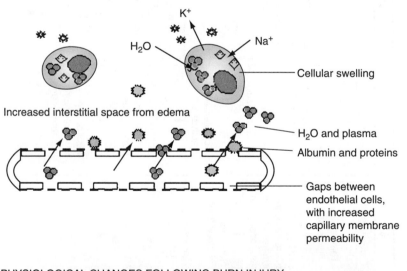

PHYSIOLOGICAL CHANGES FOLLOWING BURN INJURY
Gaps develop between endothelial cells causing increased capillary membrane permeability. Intravascular proteins and fluids flow into the interstitium in a process called third-spacing and produces tissue edema. Loss of intravascular proteins decreases intravascular oncotic pressure, pulls additional fluid into the interstitium, and reduces intravascular fluid volume. Decreased cell transmembrane potential shifts sodium into the cells, drawing in water and producing cellular swelling and further tissue edema.

FIGURE 20-7. Burn edema and shock development. *H_2O*, Water; *K*, potassium; *Na*, sodium.

than 20% TBSA, the increased capillary permeability and edema formation process not only occur locally at the site of burn injury, but also systemically in distant unburned tissues and organs.[4,14] Edema is further exacerbated as lymph drainage flow is obstructed from either direct damage of lymphatic vessels or from blockage by serum proteins that have leaked into the interstitium. Edema is a natural inflammatory response to injury that aids transport of white blood cells to the site of injury for bacterial digestion; however, the extent and rate of edema formation associated with major burn injury far exceed the intended beneficial inflammatory effect.[2] A hallmark study by Demling and colleagues found that edema continues to expand until it reaches a maximum at approximately 24 hours after burn injury.[15] Edema reabsorption and resolution begin 1 to 2 days after a burn injury.

Intravascular fluid volume lost into the interstitium causes the unique phenomenon of burn shock. Burn shock is described as a combination of *distributive* and *hypovolemic shock*. There is a distributive component because third-spacing greatly expands the area in which total body fluid is contained, to include the intravascular space plus intracellular and interstitial spaces. The hypovolemic component is caused by massive loss of intravascular fluid from increased vessel membrane permeability and evaporative losses through the open wound beds. Burn shock ensues when plasma or intravascular volume becomes insufficient to maintain circulatory support and adequate preload, causing cardiac output to decrease and impairing tissue perfusion. Fluid resuscitation is a crucial part of burn management because it directly replaces plasma fluid losses, fills the newly increased body fluid reservoir, and restores preload deficits.

In summary, significant burn injuries trigger local and systemic responses involving a multitude of complex mechanisms and cascades of physiological events that stress all body systems. The magnitude of physiological response is unique to burn injury and is characterized by dramatic shifts in intravascular fluid, mediator activation, hyperexaggerated inflammatory cascade reaction, and extensive edema formation. The specific organ system responses are summarized in the following sections and in Figure 20-6.

Cardiovascular Response

Loss of intravascular volume after major burn injury produces a decrease in cardiac output and oxygen delivery to the body tissues. The sympathetic nervous system is activated as a compensatory mechanism, with the release of catecholamines causing tachycardia and vasoconstriction to maintain arterial blood pressure. Tissue perfusion and multiorgan perfusion are altered when a redistribution of blood flow occurs early in the postburn period to perfuse essential organs such as the heart and brain. Early postburn, myocardial depression is observed and exerts a negative inotropic effect on myocardial tissues. The magnitude of myocardial depression exceeds that which would be explained by intravascular fluid volume loss. Inflammatory cytokine mediators such as tumor necrosis factor and interleukins secreted locally within the myocardium have been implicated as major contributors to this progressive cardiac contractile dysfunction. Extensive activation of the complement system, which produces anaphylatoxins like C5a, has recently been demonstrated to trigger cardiac dysfunction.[23] Cardiac instability in burn patients is further exacerbated by underresuscitation (hypovolemia), overresuscitation (hypervolemia), or increased afterload. Impaired cardiac function improves approximately 24 to 30 hours after injury.[23,24] The purpose of initial postburn fluid resuscitation is to aid in restoring normal cardiac output.

Host Defense Mechanisms

With the loss of skin from burn injury, the primary barrier to microorganisms is destroyed. Tissue damage invokes simultaneous activation of all inflammatory response cascades, including the complement, fibrinolytic, clotting, and kinin systems. The exact mechanism by which postburn immune defects occur remains ambiguous, because inflammatory mediators and cytokines exert numerous, varied, and interrelated effects. However, the end results are overstimulation of suppressor T-cells and depression of other components such as helper T-cell, killer T-cell, and polymorphonuclear leukocyte activity. This immunosuppression interferes with the ability of the patient's host defense mechanisms to fight invading microorganisms and thus places the patient at high risk of developing infection and sepsis.

Pulmonary Response

Release of vasoconstrictive mediator substances causes an initial transient pulmonary hypertension associated with a decrease in oxygen tension and lung compliance. This occurs in the absence of a lung injury and edema.[16,26] The impact of inhalation injury on the pulmonary system is described in Table 20-1.

Renal Response

The renal circulation is sensitive to decreasing cardiac output. Hypoperfusion and a decreased glomerular filtration rate signal the nephrons to initiate the renin-angiotensin-aldosterone cascade. Sodium and water are retained to preserve intravascular fluid in an attempt to increase cardiac preload. Oliguria occurs, and urine becomes more concentrated. If fluid resuscitation is inadequate, acute renal failure can develop. With resuscitation, diuresis occurs approximately 48 hours after injury secondary to an increase in cardiac output.

Gastrointestinal Response

As a consequence of the inflammatory response and hypovolemia after major burn injury, the gastrointestinal (GI) circulation undergoes compensatory vasoconstriction and redistribution of blood flow to preserve perfusion to the brain and heart. The resulting ischemia of the stomach and duodenal mucosa places burn patients at high risk of developing a duodenal ulcer, called a stress ulcer or *Curling's ulcer*. GI motility or peristalsis is also decreased, creating a *paralytic ileus*. The ileus clinically presents as decreased bowel sounds, gastric distention, nausea or vomiting.

Metabolic Response

Two phases of metabolic dysfunction occur after a major burn injury. First, a decreased response in organ function occurs, followed by a second phase of hypermetabolic and hyperfunctional response of all systems. Hypermetabolism begins as resuscitation is completed and is one of the most significant and persistent alterations observed after burn injury. The postburn hypermetabolic response is greater than that seen in any other forms of trauma.[39] Patients with severe burns have metabolic rates that are 100% to 200% above their basal rates, with some degree of elevation continuing for up to 9 to 12 months after injury.[22,39] The rapid metabolic rate is caused by the secretion of inflammatory response mediators or catabolic hormones, such as catecholamines, cortisol, and glucagon, in an effort to support tissue remodeling and repair.[38,39,53] The hypermetabolic state produces a catabolic effect on the body, with skeletal muscle breakdown, decreased protein synthesis, increased glucose utilization, and rapid depletion of glycogen stores.[26,39,42,53] The amount of protein wasting and weight loss that occurs is affected by several factors including %TBSA burned, age, sex, preburn nutritional status, other health problems, and nutrient intake. Wound closure reduces metabolic expenditure.[22,39]

PHASES OF BURN CARE ASSESSMENT AND COLLABORATIVE INTERVENTIONS

Assessment and management of the burn-injured patient is classified into three phases of care: (1) resuscitative, (2) acute, and (3) rehabilitative. The *resuscitative phase* or emergency phase begins at the time of injury and continues for approximately 48 hours until the massive fluid and protein shifts have stabilized. The primary focus of assessment and intervention is on maintenance of the ABCs (airway, breathing, and circulation) and prevention of burn shock. The resuscitative phase spans care in the prehospital setting, in the ED, and transfer to a burn center. With the onset of diuresis approximately 48 to 72 hours after injury, the *acute phase* begins and continues until wound closure occurs. This phase typically occurs in a burn center and may last for weeks or months. Nursing care focuses on the promotion of wound healing, the prevention of infections and complications, and the provision of psychosocial support. Although the critical care nurse is rarely involved in the *rehabilitative phase*, the care given in the first two phases is instrumental in achieving optimal final rehabilitative outcomes. The primary goal in this final phase is to restore the patient's ability to function in society and to return to an established family role and vocation.

Critical care activities usually occur in the resuscitative and acute phases. In both these phases, patient assessment and management are prioritized and guided by following the primary and secondary surveys as described in the Advanced Burn Life Support Course.[4] Pain control, wound management, infection control, special considerations for unique burn injuries, and psychosocial concerns are important issues throughout all the phases of burn care. See the Nursing Care Plan for Resuscitative and Acute Care Phases of Major Burn Injury for more information.

Resuscitative Phase: Prehospital

Primary Survey

Prehospital personnel (e.g., emergency medical technicians, flight nurses) are the first health care providers to arrive at the scene of injury. Care rendered in the first few hours after a significant burn injury greatly affects the patient's likelihood of survival. The priorities of prehospital care and management are to extricate the patient safely, stop the burning process, identify life-threatening injuries, and minimize time on the scene by rapidly transporting the patient to an appropriate care facility. As with any other type of trauma, the primary survey is used to

Text continued on p. 702

NURSING CARE PLAN for Resuscitative and Acute Care Phases of Major Burn Injury

NURSING DIAGNOSIS

Ineffective airway clearance and impaired gas exchange related to tracheal edema or interstitial edema secondary to inhalation injury and/or circumferential torso eschar manifested by hypoxemia and hypercapnia

PATIENT OUTCOMES
Adequate airway clearance and gas exchange

- PaO_2 >90 mm Hg; $PaCO_2$ <45 mm Hg; SaO_2 >95%; COHgb <10%
- Respiration rate 16-20 breaths/min and unlabored; breath sounds present and clear in all lobes; chest wall excursion symmetrical and adequate
- Mentation clear; patient mobilizes secretions, which are clear to white

NURSING INTERVENTIONS	RATIONALES
• Monitor SpO_2 every hour, arterial blood gases and COHgb prn; chest x-ray study as ordered	• Assess oxygenation and ventilation
• Assess respiratory rate, character, and depth every hour; breath sounds every 4 hours; level of consciousness every hour. If not intubated, assess for stridor, hoarseness, and wheezing every hour	• Evaluate respiratory status and response to treatment
• Administer humidified oxygen as ordered	• Expedite elimination of carbon monoxide and prevent/treat hypoxemia
• Evaluate need for chest escharotomy during fluid resuscitation	• Releasing eschar by escharotomy improves ventilation and oxygenation
• Assist patient in coughing and deep breathing every hour while awake. Suction every 1 to 2 hours or as needed. Monitor sputum characteristics and amount	• Promote lung expansion, ventilation, clearing of secretions, and maintaining clear airway
• Turn every 2 hours to mobilize secretions. Out of bed as tolerated	
• Elevate head of bed	• Decrease edema of face, neck, and mouth and facilitate lung expansion
• Schedule activities to avoid fatigue	• Decrease ventilatory effort

NURSING DIAGNOSIS
Adequate fluid volume

Deficient fluid volume secondary to fluid shifts into the interstitium and evaporative loss of fluids from the injured skin

PATIENT OUTCOMES

- Heart rate 80-120 beats/min; BP adequate in relation to pulse and urine output; RAP/CVP/PAOP at upper ends of normal range; sensorium clear; optimal tissue perfusion; nonburn skin warm and pink
- Hourly urine output 30-50 mL/hr; 75-100 mL/hr in electrical injury
- Weight gain based on volume of fluids given in first 48 hours, followed by diuresis over next 3-5 days
- Serum laboratory values WNL; specific gravity normal except during diuresis; urine negative for glucose and ketones

Continued

NURSING CARE PLAN for Resuscitative and Acute Care Phases of Major Burn Injury—cont'd

NURSING INTERVENTIONS

- Monitor: vital signs and urine output q1h until stable; mental status every hour for at least 48 hours
- Titrate calculated fluid requirements in first 48 hours to maintain urinary output and hemodynamic stability
- Record daily weight and hourly intake/output measurements; evaluate trends
- Monitor serum electrolytes, hematocrit, serum glucose, blood urea nitrogen, serum creatinine levels at least twice daily for first 48 hours and then as required by patient status

RATIONALES

- Assess perfusion and oxygenation status
- Restore intravascular volume. Urine output closely reflects renal perfusion and overall tissue perfusion status
- Evaluate fluid loss and replacement
- Evaluate need for electrolyte and fluid replacement associated with large fluid and protein shifts

NURSING DIAGNOSIS

Risk for hypothermia related to loss of skin and/or external cooling

PATIENT OUTCOME
Normothermia

Rectal/core temperature 37°C (98.6°F)-38.3°C (101°F)

NURSING INTERVENTIONS

- Monitor and document rectal/core temperature every 1 to 2 hours; assess for shivering
- Minimize skin exposure; maintain environmental temperatures
- For temperature <37° C (98.6° F), institute rewarming measures

RATIONALES

- Evaluate body temperature status
- Prevent evaporative and conductive losses
- Prevent complications

NURSING DIAGNOSIS

Ineffective tissue perfusion related to compression and impaired vascular circulation in extremities with circumferential burns

PATIENT OUTCOMES
Adequate tissue perfusion

- Peripheral pulses present and strong
- No tissue injury in extremities secondary to inadequate perfusion from edema or eschar

NURSING INTERVENTIONS

- Assess peripheral pulses every hour for 72 hours. Notify physician of changes in pulses, capillary refill, or pain sensation

RATIONALES

- Assess peripheral perfusion and the need for escharotomy

NURSING CARE PLAN for Resuscitative and Acute Care Phases of Major Burn Injury—cont'd

NURSING INTERVENTIONS	RATIONALES
• Elevate upper extremities with IV poles or on pillows; elevate lower extremities with pillows	• Decrease edema formation
• Be prepared to assist with escharotomy or fasciotomy	• Escharotomy or fasciotomy, allows for edema expansion, and permits peripheral perfusion

NURSING DIAGNOSIS

Acute pain related to burn trauma

PATIENT OUTCOMES
Relief of pain

• Identifies factors that contribute to pain. Verbalizes improved comfort level
• Physiological parameters WNL and remain stable after administration of narcotic analgesia

NURSING INTERVENTIONS	RATIONALES
• Monitor physiological responses to pain, such as increased BP, increased heart rate, restlessness, and nonverbal cues. Use validated tools to assess pain and anxiety	• Pain responses are variable and unique to each patient
• Assess response to analgesics or other interventions	• Evaluate effectiveness of interventions
• Administer analgesic and/or anxiolytic medication as ordered; administer IV during critical care phases	• Facilitate pain relief. Intramuscular medications not consistently absorbed
• Medicate patient before bathing, dressing changes, and major procedures as needed	• Assist patient to perform at higher level of function
• Minimize open exposure of wounds	• Exposed nerve endings increase pain
• Use nonpharmacological pain-reducing methods as appropriate	• Reduce need for narcotics

NURSING DIAGNOSIS

Risk for infection related to loss of skin, impaired immune response, and invasive therapies

PATIENT OUTCOMES
Absence of infection

• No inflamed burn wound margins
• No evidence of burn wound, donor site, or invasive catheter site infection
• Autograft or allograft skin is adherent to granulation tissue
• Body temperature WNL
• White blood cell counts WNL
• Sputum, blood, and urine cultures negative
• Glycosuria, vomiting, ileus, and/or change in mentation absent

Continued

NURSING CARE PLAN for Resuscitative and Acute Care Phases of Major Burn Injury—cont'd

NURSING INTERVENTIONS	RATIONALES
• Assess temperature and vital signs and characteristics of urine and sputum every 1 to 4 hours. Monitor WBC, burn wound healing status and invasive catheter sites	• Evaluate effectiveness of treatments and interventions. Facilitate early detection of developing infections
• Use appropriate protective isolation. Provide meticulous wound care with antimicrobial topical agents as ordered. Shave hair (except eyebrows) 1 inch around burn wounds. Adhere to CDC guidelines for invasive catheter care. Instruct visitors in burn unit guidelines	• Prevent infection by decreasing exposure to pathogens. Hair is a medium for microorganism growth. Proper hand washing and use of protective barriers decrease contamination
• Obtain wound, sputum, urine, and blood cultures as ordered	• Determine infection source and specific invading microorganism to guide topical/ systemic antimicrobial therapy

NURSING DIAGNOSES

Risk for Injury: Gastrointestinal Bleeding related to stress response
Imbalanced nutrition: less than body requirements related to ileus and increased metabolic demands secondary to physiological stress and wound healing

PATIENT OUTCOMES
Absence of injury and adequate nutrition

- Decreased gastric motility and ileus resolved
- No evidence of GI hemorrhaging
- Enteral feedings absorbed and tolerated
- Daily requirement of nutrients consumed
- Positive nitrogen balance
- Progressive wound healing
- 90% of preburn weight maintained

NURSING INTERVENTIONS	RATIONALES
• Place NG tube for gastric decompression in >20% TBSA burns	• Prevent nausea, emesis, and aspiration from ileus
• Assess abdomen and bowel sounds every 8 hours	• Evaluate resolution of decreased gastric motility and ileus
• Assess NG aspirate (color, quantity, pH, and guaiac); monitor stool guaiac	• Facilitate early detection of GI bleeding
• Administer stress ulcer prophylaxis	• Prevent stress ulcer development
• Initiate enteral feeding, and evaluate tolerance. Provide high-calorie/protein supplements prn. Record all oral intake and count calories	• Caloric/protein intake must be adequate to maintain positive nitrogen balance and promote healing
• Schedule interventions and activities to avoid interrupting feeding times	• Pain, fatigue, or sedation interferes with desire to eat
• Monitor weight daily or biweekly	• Assess tolerance and response to feeding interventions

NURSING CARE PLAN for Resuscitative and Acute Care Phases of Major Burn Injury—cont'd

NURSING DIAGNOSIS

Impaired physical mobility and self-care deficit related to burn injury, therapeutic splinting, immobilization requirements after skin graft, and/or contractures

PATIENT OUTCOMES

Physical mobility

- Demonstrates ability to care for burn wounds
- No evidence of permanent decreased joint function
- Verbalizes understanding of plan of care
- Vocation resumed without functional limitations, or adjustment to new vocation

NURSING INTERVENTIONS	RATIONALES
• Perform active and passive ROM exercises to extremities every 2 hours while awake. Increase activity as tolerated. Reinforce importance of maintaining proper joint alignment with splints and antideformity positioning	• Prevent contractures and loss of movement/function
• Elevate extremities	• Decrease edema and promote ROM and mobility
• Provide pain relief measures before self-care activities and OT/PT	• Facilitate mobility and assist patient to perform at a higher level of function
• Explain procedures, interventions, and tests in clear, simple, age-appropriate language	• Patient more likely to participate and adhere to treatment plan if the purpose is understood
• Promote use of adaptive devices as needed to assist in self-care and mobility	• Decrease dependency on caregivers

NURSING DIAGNOSIS

Risk for ineffective individual coping and disabled family coping related to acute stress of critical injury and potential life-threatening crisis

PATIENT OUTCOMES

Effective coping

- Verbalizes goals of treatment regimen
- Demonstrates knowledge of support systems
- Able to express concerns and fears
- Patient's and family's coping is functional and realistic for phase of hospitalization; family processes at precrisis level

NURSING INTERVENTIONS	RATIONALES
• Orient patient and family to unit guidelines and support services; provide written information and reinforce frequently; involve in plan of care. Support adaptive and functional coping mechanisms	• Decrease fear and anxiety and enhance feelings of control and self-worth. Reinforce verbal information provided to patient and family
• Use interventions to reduce fatigue and pain	• Adequate pain control and rest facilitate patient coping

Continued

NURSING CARE PLAN for Resuscitative and Acute Care Phases of Major Burn Injury—cont'd

NURSING INTERVENTIONS	RATIONALES
• Use social worker for assistance in discharge planning and psychosocial assessment issues. Consult psychiatric services for inadequate coping skills or substance abuse treatment. Promote use of group support sessions	• Provide expert consultation and intervention. Assist patient and family in understanding experiences and reactions after burn injury and methods of dealing with trauma

BP, Blood pressure; *CDC,* Centers for Disease Control and Prevention; *CO,* carbon monoxide; *COHgb,* carboxyhemoglobin; *CVP,* central venous pressure; *GI,* gastrointestinal; *IV,* intravenous; *NG,* nasogastric; *OT/PT,* occupational therapy/physical therapy; *PaCO₂,* partial pressure of arterial carbon dioxide; *PaO₂,* partial pressure of arterial oxygen; *prn,* as required; *RAP,* right atrial pressure; *ROM,* range of motion; *SpO₂,* arterial oxygen saturation via pulse oximetry; *TBSA,* total body surface area; *WBC,* white blood cell count; *WNL,* within normal limits.

provide a fast systematic assessment that prioritizes evaluation of the patient's airway, breathing, and circulatory status (Figure 20-8).

Stopping the Burning Process. The first priority of patient care is to stop the burning process by removing the patient from the source of burning while preventing further injury.[4] It is crucial that this step be performed safely but quickly, because interventions aimed to stop the burning should not delay the next assessment phases of the primary survey.

Flame burns are extinguished by rolling the patient on the ground, smothering the flames with a blanket or other cover, or dousing the flames with water. Ice is never applied to the wounds because further tissue damage may occur as a result of vasoconstriction and hypothermia. Jewelry is immediately removed because metal retains heat and can cause continued burning. Scald, tar, and asphalt burns are treated by immediate removal of the saturated clothing or immediate cooling with water if available, or both. No attempt is made to remove adherent tar at the scene. Adherent clothing (clothing that is burned into and stuck to the skin) is not removed because increased tissue damage and bleeding may occur; however, water is applied to cool the clothing material. Immediate treatment of electrical injuries involves prompt removal of the patient from the electrical source while protecting the rescuer. The burning process of chemical injuries continues as long as the chemical is in contact with the skin. All clothing is immediately removed, and water lavage is instituted before and during transport. Powdered chemicals are first brushed from the clothing and skin before lavage is performed. Clean water is the lavage solution of choice. If the chemical is in or near the eyes, contact lenses are removed (if present), and the eyes are irrigated with saline or clean water.

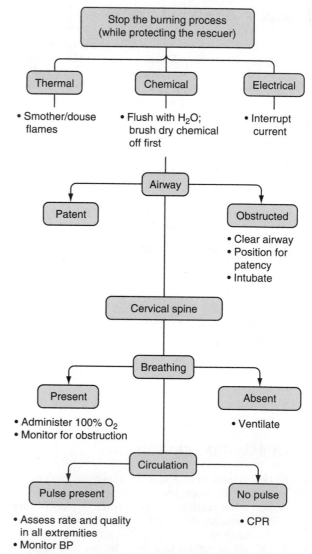

FIGURE 20-8. Major burn injury: primary survey. *BP,* Blood pressure; *CPR,* cardiopulmonary resuscitation.

Cross-contamination of the opposite eye is avoided during lavage by irrigating in the direction from inner to outer canthus. Neutralizing agents are not used on chemical burns. When neutralizing agents come in contact with chemicals, increased heat production occurs and further increases the depth of injury. Health care providers must prevent exposure to themselves during initial treatment and lavage of chemical injuries by wearing protective barrier garments such as plastic gowns, gloves, goggles, and a face shield.

Airway (with Cervical Spine Precautions). A history of the injury event occurring in a closed space alerts the clinician to the high potential for inhalation injury. Any suspicion of inhalation injury requires immediate intervention for airway control while maintaining cervical spine immobilization precautions (if indicated by the injury event). Refer to Clinical Alert: Clinical Indicators of Inhalation Injury for findings indicative of pulmonary injury. Respiratory stridor indicates airway obstruction and mandates immediate endotracheal intubation at the scene. Patients with severe facial burns are prophylactically intubated because delayed or later endotracheal intubation will be difficult or impossible as edema develops.

Breathing. The half-life of carbon monoxide is reduced to 45-60 minutes in the presence of an oxygen concentration of 100% (versus a half-life of 4 hours in the presence of room air). Therefore, all patients with suspected smoke inhalation are treated at the scene with 100% humidified oxygen delivered by nonrebreathing face mask or endotracheal tube. Patients are monitored for clinical signs of decreasing oxygenation such as changes in respiratory rate or neurological status. Pulse oximetry may not be accurate in acute inhalation injuries because the pulse oximeter cannot distinguish between carbon monoxide versus oxygen attached to the hemoglobin.

Circulation. All clothing and jewelry are removed to prevent constriction and ischemia to distal extremities secondary to edema formation during fluid resuscitation. Intravenous (IV) therapy is initiated with insertion of two large-bore (14- or 16-gauge) IV lines, preferably through nonburned tissue, and infusion of lactated Ringer's (LR) solution.[4] The patient is closely monitored for signs of hypovolemia such as changes in level of consciousness, rapid or thready pulses, decreased blood pressure, or narrowing pulse pressure. Burn injury rarely results in hypovolemic shock in the very early prehospital phase. If evidence of shock is present, then associated internal or external injury must be suspected.

Heat loss occurs rapidly in a major burn injury because the protective covering of skin is lost. The burned patient is covered with a clean, dry sheet and blankets to prevent hypothermia and further contamination of the wounds.

Secondary Survey

The secondary survey in the prehospital setting is brief and should not delay transport to a hospital. A rapid head-to-toe assessment to rule out any additional trauma is completed as part of the secondary survey (Figure 20-9). Patients with an injury mechanism suggestive of the potential for spinal injury

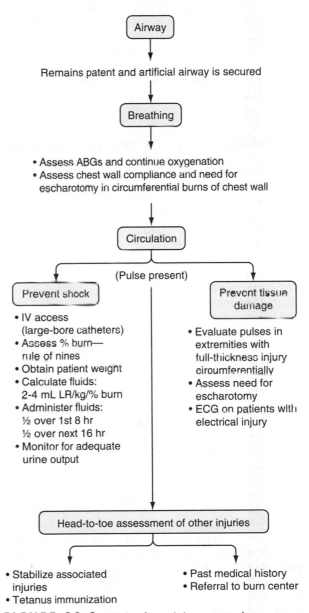

FIGURE 20-9. Major burn injury: secondary survey. *ABG,* Arterial blood gas; *ECG,* electrocardiogram; *IV,* intravenous; *LR,* lactated Ringer's solution.

(e.g., jumping from a burning building, electrical injury) have a cervical collar applied and are placed on a backboard before transport. Often, the patient is the most alert during this initial period after the injury. Therefore, an accurate history of the events that led to the burn injury is obtained, including the date and time of injury, the source of burns, and any events leading to the injury. Acquiring a brief medical history is beneficial, including allergies, current medical problems and medications taken, past surgical procedures and/or trauma, time of last meal, and history of tetanus immunization.[4]

In preparation for transport, a short-acting narcotic such as morphine sulfate may be administered IV for pain relief. No intramuscular medications are given during the resuscitative phase because perfusion of edematous tissues is poor and produces sporadic narcotic absorption. The patient should not receive anything by mouth before and during transport, to prevent vomiting and aspiration.

Resuscitative Phase: Emergency Department and Critical Care Burn Center

The burn patient is transferred from the injury scene to either a community hospital ED or a burn center. Management goals at either facility continue to be restoration and maintenance of the ABCs and the prevention of burn shock.

Transfer to a Burn Center

The care of a patient who has sustained a major burn injury is complex and requires the expertise of a specially trained multidisciplinary health care team. Burn team members include nurses, physicians (general and plastic surgeons), occupational therapists, physical therapists, dietitians, respiratory therapists, infection control specialists, pharmacists, child life specialists, social workers, psychologists, chaplains, injury prevention educators, and physician specialists (e.g., rehabilitation physicians, pediatricians, and neurosurgeons as indicated). A burn center provides the necessary resources to improve burn patient care and outcome, including a dedicated staff delivering specialized clinical care, prehospital and community education, injury prevention, and research. Hospitals without burn units may not have the personnel or medical supplies needed to provide the specialized care these patients require. The American Burn Association has developed guidelines (see Clinical Alert: Guidelines for Burn Center Referral) for determining which patients should be referred to a specialized burn center after initial stabilization.[6]

When transfer to a burn center is considered, the referring physician must make direct contact with the burn center physician. The burn center physician determines the mode of transportation (ground ambulance or air) and the treatment necessary to stabilize the patient for transport.[4] Transport is optimally done early in the postburn period during the resuscitative phase, based on guidelines provided by the receiving burn center. The use of a transfer form to summarize information concerning a burn patient's status promotes good communication between the referring and receiving facilities and ensures continuity of care (Figure 20-10).

Primary Survey

On arrival to either the ED or the burn center, the primary survey is reassessed. Once the patient has arrived in the critical care burn unit, primary and secondary assessments are again performed.

Airway. Ineffective airway clearance related to tracheal edema may occur early, or it may not be apparent until after fluid resuscitation is initiated. Patients with suspected inhalation injuries who are not already intubated must be monitored frequently for hoarseness, stridor, or wheezing. Because massive edema formation is an anticipated response to fluid resuscitation in an extensively burned patient, patients with severe facial burns are intubated as a precaution. The presence of other symptoms suggestive of inhalation injury (see Clinical Alert: Clinical Indicators of Inhalation Injury) necessitates early intubation to maintain adequate oxygenation and perfusion. Fiberoptic bronchoscopy may be performed to confirm the presence of inhalation injury. If the patient is already intubated, accurate tube position is assessed. The endotracheal tube is securely tied (not taped) in place to prevent accidental extubation (Figure 20-11). This measure is especially important with young children, who often require the use of uncuffed endotracheal tubes that can easily dislodge. A dislodged endotracheal tube may be impossible to replace in the presence of massive edema and airway obstruction, thereby necessitating an emergency cricothyroidotomy or tracheostomy. Care must be taken to prevent tube ties from placing pressure on burned ears. The head of the patient's bed is elevated to reduce facial and airway edema.

Breathing. Assessment for impaired gas exchange related to carbon monoxide poisoning or inhalation injury is important. Breath sounds, characteristics of respirations, work of breathing, sputum color and consistency, and symmetry of chest wall excursion are evaluated. Arterial blood gases and COHgb are measured when inhalation injury is suspected. Humidified 100% oxygen is administered via face mask or endotracheal tube until COHgb levels are determined. Once COHgb levels have normalized

MetroHealth Medical Center

Burn Center Transfer Form

Time: _____ Referring Hospital: _____ Physician: _____

Patient name: _____ Age: _____ Sex: _____

Address: _____ Phone: _____

Next of Kin: _____ Phone: _____ Notified: _____

Time of Burn: _____ Cause of Burn: _____ Treatment: _____

Significant Past Medical History: _____

Allergies: _____

Medications: _____

Height: _____ Weight: _____ Last Tetanus: _____

ASSESSMENT	LABS
	ABG
HEENT/NEURO _____	pH _____
PULMONARY _____	PO_2 _____
CARDIAC/CIRC _____	CO_2 _____
	O_2 Sat _____
GI/GU _____	Bicarb _____
MUSCULOSKELETAL _____	CO Level _____
MEDICATIONS GIVEN _____	O_2 Therapy _____

TIME _____

TEMPERATURE _____

PULSE _____

RESPIRATION _____

BLOOD PRESSURE _____

X-RAYS

INTRAVENOUS THERAPY _____

FLUID
SITE GAUGE _____

FLUID
SITE GAUGE _____

FOLEY _____ OUTPUT _____

NG _____

ET _____ SIZE _____

OTHER INFORMATION _____

FLUID RESUSCITATION - PARKLAND FORMULA
4 mL/kg/% Burn

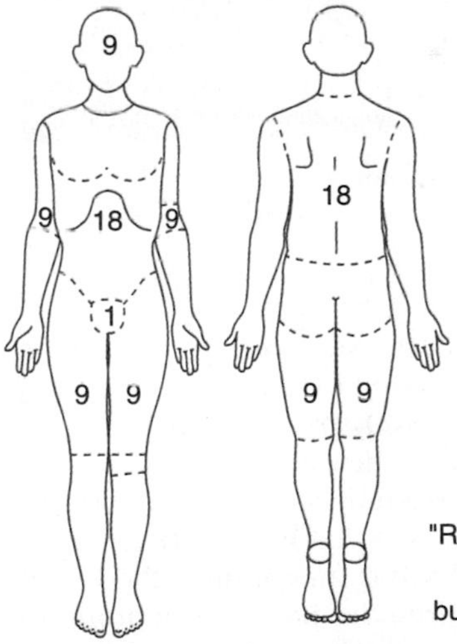

9

9 18 9

18

1

9 9

9 9

"RULES OF NINES"
(Indicate area
burned on diagram)

ESTIMATE % _____

M.D. or NURSE _____

FIGURE 20-10. Burn center transfer form. *ABG*, Arterial blood gas; *CIRC*, circulatory; *CO*, carbon monoxide; *ET*, endotracheal tube; *GI/GU*, gastrointestinal/genitourinary; *HEENT*, head, eyes, ears, nose, throat; *NG*, nasogastric tube; *O_2*, oxygen. *(Courtesy of MetroHealth Medical Center, Cleveland, OII.)*

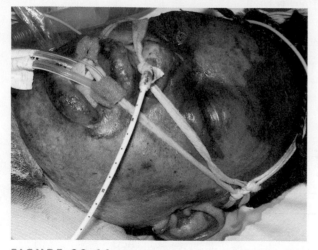

FIGURE 20-11. Facial edema. *(Courtesy of University of Michigan Trauma Burn Center, Ann Arbor, MI.)*

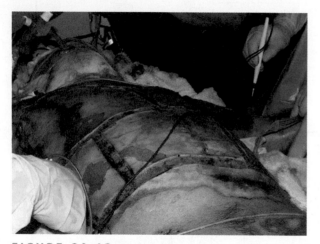

FIGURE 20-12. Escharotomy. *(Courtesy of University of Michigan Trauma Burn Center, Ann Arbor, MI.)*

(lower than 5% to 10%), the 100% oxygen is weaned as tolerated, as demonstrated by maintaining a PaO_2 greater than 90 mm Hg, SaO_2 greater than 95%, and unlabored respirations. If the patient has a circumferential full-thickness burn of the thorax, the nurse assesses for adequate ventilatory effort because edema and restrictive eschar may inhibit chest wall expansion. Young children are particularly prone to this complication because their thoracic walls are more pliable. Therefore, an immediate chest wall *escharotomy* may be indicated to facilitate breathing (Figure 20-12). An escharotomy is an incision performed at the bedside through a full-thickness burn to reduce constriction caused by the tight nonelastic band of eschar. This relieves pressure and restores

ventilation, and blood flow. Local anesthesia is not required because the full-thickness burn eschar is painless. This procedure should be done only in consultation with the burn center. Ongoing assessment of breath sounds, arterial blood gases, and ventilatory status is crucial. All patients with inhalation injuries receive assistance with coughing, deep breathing, suctioning, and repositioning at least every 2 hours. Pulse oximetry and end-tidal carbon dioxide monitoring occur continuously as appropriate.

Circulation

Fluid Resuscitation. Fluid resuscitation is a critical intervention for burn management. To estimate fluid resuscitation requirements, the depth and extent of injury are assessed. Fluid resuscitation requirements are estimated according to body weight in kilograms, the %TBSA burned, and the patient's age. IV fluid resuscitation is instituted in patients with burns greater than 15% to 20% TBSA because these burns are associated with a diffuse capillary leak, large intravascular fluid loss, and ileus. Patients with smaller %TBSA burns may be resuscitated with oral hydration.

One of the most widely used burn resuscitation fluid formulas is the *Parkland formula*. It provides an approximation of fluid replacement requirements by calculating the amount of lactated Ringer's (LR) solution to infuse during the first 24 hours postburn at 4 mL/kg/%TBSA. Half of the calculated amount is given over the first 8 hours after injury, and the remaining half is given over the next 16 hours. A revised version of the Parkland formula, called the *Consensus formula*, is advocated by the Advanced Burn Life Support Course.[4] The Consensus fluid formula outlined in Box 20-1 specifies the fluid requirements for adults and children during the initial 24 hours after the burn.

Two large-bore (14- to 16-gauge) peripheral IV lines are inserted. If an unburned location is not available, the IV lines are placed through burned skin. Central venous catheters are commonly inserted in patients with major burns to facilitate and accommodate large IV fluid infusion requirements. LR solution is the preferred initial IV fluid for burn resuscitation.[4,47] It is a crystalloid that has an osmolality and electrolyte composition most similar to normal body physiological fluids, and it does not contain dextrose, which can cause a misleading high urine output from glycosuria and osmotic diuresis. In addition, LR contains lactate, which helps to buffer the metabolic acidosis associated with hypoperfusion and burn shock. Because LR is a crystalloid, it does not provide any intravascular protein replacement to increase intravascular oncotic pressure. In the presence of increased capillary membrane permeability, the intravascular retention of LR is only about 25% of the infused

BOX 20-1   Burn Fluid Resuscitation Formula

First 24 Hours Administer

ABLS Consensus Formula (Based on the Parkland Formula)

In adults: LR, 2 to 4 mL/kg/%TBSA

In children: LR, 3 to 4 mL/kg/%TBSA

  Half given over the first 8 hours after injury and the remaining half given over the next 16 hours

In infants <12 months and young children: Give fluid with 5% dextrose at a maintenance rate in addition to the resuscitation fluid noted above to prevent hypoglycemia. Maintenance rate is calculated by the following:

  For the first 10 kg of body weight: 100 mL/kg over 24 hours

  For the second 10 kg of body weight: 50 mL/kg over 24 hours

  For each kg of body weight above 20 kg: 20 mL/kg over 24 hours

Titrate fluids to maintain urine output of 30 to 50 mL/hr in adults and 1 mL/kg/hr in children weighing <30 kg

Example: For an adult weighing 75 kg with a 55% TBSA burn and inhalation injury:

  4 mL LR × 75 kg × 55%TBSA = 16,500 mL of LR infused over 24 hours

  First 8 hours after burn injury: 8200 mL of LR infused over 8 hours or 1031.25 mL/hr

  Next 16 hours after burn injury: 8200 mL of LR infused over 16 hours or 515.6 mL/hr

Second 24 Hours Administer

Parkland Formula

Dextrose in water, plus potassium to maintain normal electrolyte balance

Colloid-containing fluid at 20% to 60% of calculated plasma volume, which equals an infusion rate of approximately 0.35 to 0.5 mL/kg/%TBSA

ABLS, Advanced Burn Life Support; *LR,* Lactated Ringer's solution; *TBSA,* total body surface area.

volume, necessitating large fluid volume infusions to maintain circulating blood volume.

Fluid requirements calculated by the Consensus formula serve only as a guide for estimating initial fluid needs. Each patient reacts differently to burn injury and requires varying amounts of IV fluid to support perfusion. The patient's requirements for fluid resuscitation are affected by several factors including age, depth of burn, concurrent inhalation injury, preexisting disease or comorbidities, delay in

burn injury treatment, use of methamphetamine or other polysubstances, and associated injuries. Inhalation injuries increase the extent of %TBSA injury, and these patients typically require more resuscitation fluids. Larger fluid resuscitation volumes are also required in patients with electrical injuries to prevent acute tubular necrosis by clearing the renal tubules from precipitating myoglobin caused by skeletal muscle damage or *rhabdomyolysis.* Children also require relatively more resuscitation fluid because they have a greater ratio of body surface area to mass than that of adults, and higher evaporative losses. Because evaporative fluid losses continue until burn wounds are closed, these losses are calculated as a part of the total daily maintenance fluid replacement formula.

Colloids, such as albumin, contain proteins and are sometimes used in burn resuscitation to increase intravascular oncotic pressure. The increase in intravascular oncotic pressure pulls fluid from the interstitium back into the circulating intravascular volume, thereby reducing edema and combating burn shock. However, during increased permeability, colloids leak into the interstitium and contribute to further intravascular fluid loss. If colloids are used during burn resuscitation, it is generally advocated that they not be administered within 8 to 12 hours of burn injury when capillary permeability is at its highest level.[11,45] Recent reviews suggest colloid use plays an important role in burn resuscitation, as increased crystalloid infusion alone is incapable of restoring cardiac preload in burn shock.[12,24,45]

During the second 24 hours postinjury when capillary permeability has decreased, a fluid formula such as the Parkland (see Box 20-1), which incorporates colloids, dextrose, and electrolyte replacement, may be used. Hypertonic dextrose solutions and colloids increase oncotic pressure, which helps pull third-spaced fluid from the interstitium back into the circulatory system. Potassium is added to IV fluids to replace potassium losses in the urine.

End Point Monitoring. Assessment of fluid volume status related to changes in capillary permeability is essential. The goal of burn resuscitation is to maintain tissue perfusion and organ function while avoiding the complications of inadequate or excessive fluid therapy.[4] Resuscitation fluid infusion rates are titrated to specific measured outcomes of patient response, known as physiological end points.[2] During burn shock resuscitation, IV crystalloids or colloids, or both, are administered according to Consensus formula guidelines, with normalization of urine output and blood pressure used as the hemodynamic end points to titrate fluids. A urinary catheter is inserted to evaluate resuscitation adequacy. IV infusion rates are adjusted to ensure a urinary output of

EVIDENCE-BASED PRACTICE

Compared with other critical care patient populations, the burn-injured population constitutes a relatively small number of patients. Consequently, there are limited numbers of major burn centers in the United States, and they are typically separated by great geographical distances. These facts greatly impact research investigations and the ability to generate rigorous guidelines and standards for evidence-based practice specifically pertinent to burn care. Most burn research studies published to date involve only one center, animal models, small sample sizes, and/or are often retrospective reviews. This limits the strength of any demonstrated findings and study conclusions. There currently is minimal validation of burn clinical care practices by randomized controlled clinical trials, and that which does exist is frequently extrapolated from research performed in other critical care patient populations. Acknowledgment of these issues spurred recent efforts by the American Burn Association to initiate and support collaboration between burn centers to conduct multicenter trials. The resulting research studies should generate evidence-based practice and greatly impact future burn care.

PROBLEM

Burn fluid resuscitation, use of colloids, and end-point monitoring have historically been topics of much discussion and debate. Questions arise regarding whether to administer colloids during resuscitation, and which specific end points to use to guide treatment. National trends in avoiding colloid use and increasing total amounts of fluids administered (deemed "fluid creep") have been criticized as potential contributors to the development of intraabdominal hypertension, abdominal compartment syndrome, and poor patient outcomes.

REFERENCES

American Burn Association, Evidence-Based Guidelines Group. (2001). Practice guidelines for burn care. *Journal of Burn Care & Rehabilitation, 22*(Suppl. 2):S1-S69.

Chung, K. K., Blackbourne, L. H., Wolf, S. E., et al. (2006). Evolution of burn resuscitation in operation Iraqi freedom. *Journal of Burn Care & Research, 27*(5), 606-611.

O'Mara, M. S., Slater, H., Goldfarb, I. W., & Caushaj, P. F. (2005). A prospective, randomized evaluation of intra-abdominal pressures with crystalloid and colloid resuscitation in burn patients. *Journal of Trauma, 58*(5), 1011-1018.

Saffle, J. R. (2007). The phenomenon of "fluid creep" in acute burn resuscitation. *Journal of Burn Care & Research, 28*(3), 382-395.

Silver, G. M., Klein, M. B., Herndon, D. N., et al. (2007). Standard operating procedures for the clinical management of patients enrolled in a prospective study of inflammation and the host response to thermal injury. *Journal of Burn Care & Research, 28*(2), 222-230.

EVIDENCE

Optimal burn resuscitation provides enough fluid to maintain vital organ function without producing iatrogenic negative outcomes. Patients with burns greater than 20% of total body surface area (TBSA) should be closely monitored and given fluid resuscitation with lactated Ringer's solution at an initial estimated rate per Parkland/Consensus formula that is titrated to maintain urine output of 0.3 to 1.0 mL/kg/hr and mean arterial pressure of 60 mm Hg or greater. These recommendations are primarily based on retrospective reviews and expert consensus. A randomized prospective study demonstrated greater fluid volume amounts and an increased incidence of intraabdominal hypertension with crystalloid infusion compared with colloid infusion. Patients requiring fluid volumes exceeding the initial estimate of 4 mL/kg/%TBSA burn to achieve satisfactory urine output and/or who demonstrate hemodynamic instability require intraabdominal pressure and advanced hemodynamic monitoring; use of colloids or vasoactive/inotropic agents, or both, should be considered. Excessive fluid administration has been demonstrated by several retrospective and prospective reviews to produce negative outcomes in burn patients.

IMPLICATIONS FOR NURSING

Patient response to resuscitation should be closely monitored, and fluid infusion aggressively adjusted. Nurses must use skills in hemodynamic monitoring to assess fluid volume status. Bladder pressure monitoring and assessment of ventilation will assist in identifying intraabdominal hypertension. Large burn-specific, randomized controlled trials are needed to generate scientifically validated data and critically evaluate resuscitation therapies, end points, and monitoring strategies.

---

30 to 50 mL/hr in adults and 1 mL/kg of body weight per hour in children weighing less than 30 kg. During the resuscitation phase, steady increases or decreases in IV resuscitation rates are performed, rather than administration of fluid boluses.[2]

Peripheral Circulation. Special attention is given to *circumferential* (completely surrounding a body part) full-thickness burns of the extremities. Pressure from bands of eschar or from edema that develops as resuscitation proceeds may impair blood flow to underlying and distal tissue. Therefore, extremities are elevated to reduce edema. Active or passive range-of-motion (ROM) exercises are performed every hour for 5 minutes to increase venous return and to minimize edema. Peripheral pulses are assessed every hour, especially in circumferential burns of the extremities, to confirm adequate circulation. An ultrasonic flowmeter (Doppler) is used to auscultate radial, palmar, digital, or pedal pulses. Delayed capillary refill, tense skin, progressively decreasing or absent pulse, and other neurovascular changes (e.g., intense pain, paresthesia, paralysis) indicate impaired blood flow and developing *compartment syndrome*. Compartment syndrome occurs when tissue pressure in the fascial compartments of extremities increases, compressing and occluding blood vessels and nerves. If signs and symptoms of compartment syndrome are present on serial examination, preparation is made for an escharotomy to relieve pressure and to restore circulation. If decreased perfusion is not quickly detected, ischemia and necrosis with loss of limb may occur. A *fasciotomy* (incision through fascia) may be indicated for deep electrical burns or severe muscle damage to restore blood flow. Escharotomy and fasciotomy sites are treated with a topical antimicrobial agent and are closely monitored for bleeding. Cautery, silver nitrate sticks, or sutures may be indicated to stop continued bleeding.

Secondary Survey

On admission to the ED or burn center, a chest x-ray is obtained, and other x-ray studies are ordered as indicated by the patient's condition. Spinal immobilization precautions are continued until clinical assessment and radiological studies demonstrate no evidence of vertebral injury. The patient's medical history and the history of the injury event are conveyed to the medical team. The critical care nurse must assess indices or end points of essential organ function to evaluate adequacy of burn shock resuscitation and to prevent complications. Initially, monitoring is performed frequently to detect changes that can rapidly occur during fluid resuscitation. Critical indices monitored at least hourly include blood pressure, heart rate, cardiac rhythm, respiration quality and rate, temperature, peripheral pulse presence and quality, and urinary output. In addition, urine specific gravity, urine glucose and ketones, occult blood tests, and gastric pH levels are typically evaluated every 2 hours. The patient is weighed on admission and daily thereafter until the preburn weight is obtained after diuresis. Pain is closely monitored, and efforts are made to control it adequately. All parameters are documented for analysis of trends. Assessment and intervention in the resuscitative phase focus on early detection and prevention of problems in the systems discussed in the following sections.

Cardiovascular System. Historically, a mean arterial pressure greater than 70 mm Hg and the absence of tachycardia (heart rate <120 beats/min) have been standard assessments of adequate burn shock resuscitation.[2] However, the cardiovascular response of the patient to burn injury warrants special consideration. The burn patient often has an elevated baseline heart rate of 100 to 120 beats/min from postinjury metabolic changes. Compensatory mechanisms do not allow hypotension to develop until significant intravascular volume losses have occurred; therefore, decreasing blood pressure is a late sign of inadequate perfusion. Both arterial and noninvasive cuff pressure readings may be altered by peripheral tissue edema or by catecholamine- and mediator-induced arteriospasm. Changes in heart rate and blood pressure may also be masked or may appear increased from pain, anxiety, or fear rather than from inadequate resuscitation. Therefore, monitoring for a narrowing pulse pressure is helpful, because it provides an earlier indication of shock than assessing systolic blood pressure alone.[33]

The routine insertion of pulmonary artery catheters is not universally supported by the literature. However, patients with significant cardiopulmonary disease, the elderly, or those who have unexplained large resuscitation fluid volume requirements may benefit from insertion of a pulmonary artery catheter to assess cardiac function.[2,11,33,38,47] If a pulmonary artery catheter is used, low right atrial pressure and pulmonary artery occlusion pressure are reflective of hypovolemia and require intervention. Assessing trends in cardiac output variables and oxygen transport variables provide useful information to guide burn shock resuscitation.

Local thermal injury, venous stasis, hypercoagulability, and immobility place the burn patient at risk of developing thromboembolic complications such as deep venous thrombosis (DVT) and pulmonary embolism. However, clinical findings indicative of DVT may not be present, or they may be obscured by extremity burn wound pain, edema, or erythema. Data suggest that the incidence of thromboembolic complications in burn patients is dramatically higher than previously thought.[47,50] Therefore, the investigators recommend that immobile burn patients receive routine DVT prophylaxis with sequential compression devices, low–molecular weight heparin, or another prophylactic modality. The traditional signs of DVT may not be present in the burn patient. Therefore, the nurse must closely monitor for sudden respiratory deterioration, which may indicate pulmonary embolism.

Neurological Status. Severely injured burn patients are initially awake, alert, and oriented. Monitoring of sensorium is crucial. If a burned patient initially presents with a decreased level of consciousness, other injuries or causes should be suspected (e.g., head injury, carbon monoxide poisoning, drug overdose). The patient's sensorium is evaluated hourly because increased agitation or confusion or a continued decreased level of consciousness may be an indication of hypovolemia, hypoxemia, or both. The head of the bed is elevated 30 degrees to prevent cerebral edema during fluid resuscitation.

Renal Status. Urine output closely reflects renal perfusion, which is sensitive to decreasing cardiac output and developing shock. Urinary output is the quickest and most reliable indicator of adequate burn fluid resuscitation. Titration of calculated fluid requirements according to hourly urine output is an essential function of the nurse during resuscitation. Urine output, color, and concentration are also closely monitored. Oliguria occurs if fluid resuscitation is inadequate.

Gastrointestinal System. The GI system is monitored for problems occurring with its initial response to the burn injury (i.e., ileus, Curling's ulcer). It is essential to assess for the presence and quality of bowel sounds, abdominal distention, gastric pH, characteristics of gastric secretions, and the presence of GI bleeding. Because patients with burns greater than 20%TBSA generally develop an ileus, a nasogastric tube is inserted and connected to low suction to prevent vomiting and aspiration. If oral intake is not feasible, enteral feedings by a small bowel feeding tube are started early. Stress ulcer prophylaxis is ordered.

Circumferential torso eschar or bowel edema from fluid resuscitation, the inflammatory response, or both, can cause *intraabdominal hypertension*. There has been increasing awareness and focused research into the incidence of this serious complication, which may likely be related to the change in practice of restrictive colloid use and increased crystalloid infusion in burn resuscitation.[2,11,45] Intraabdominal hypertension causes compression of intraabdominal contents and leads to renal, gut, and hepatic ischemia. If not treated by trunk escharotomies, diuresis, and/or sedation and chemical paralytics, intraabdominal hypertension can progress to abdominal compartment syndrome or death. *Abdominal compartment syndrome* is characterized by the presence of intraabdominal hypertension, decreasing urine output, and difficulty with ventilation (e.g., elevated airway pressure, hypercapnea, or hypoxemia).[36] Abdominal compartment syndrome mandates immediate decompression by laparotomy or percutaneous drainage of peritoneal fluid; otherwise, multiple organ dysfunction and death quickly ensue. Inclusion of bladder pressure monitoring to assess for intraabdominal hypertension during burn resuscitation should be considered in the plan of care.[11,36,45]

Integumentary System. Assessing a burn patient for the first time is frightening and overwhelming to most health care providers. However, other life- or limb-threatening conditions (e.g., airway compromise, burn shock, extremity compartment syndrome) take priority over treating the burn wound during the initial resuscitation phase. The depth and extent of burn injury are assessed to assist with fluid resuscitation predictions. Burn wound management is discussed later in this chapter.

Burn wounds are prone to tetanus, and the patient receives tetanus immunization on ED or burn center admission, if indicated. Tetanus toxoid immunization is administered if more than 5 years have elapsed since the last received dose, or tetanus hyperimmune globulin and tetanus toxoid are given if the patient's immunization history is unknown.[4]

During the resuscitation period, loss of the protective skin layer and administration of large amounts of fluid place the burn patient at risk of developing hypothermia. The patient's temperature is closely monitored. Loss of body heat is minimized by limiting skin exposure and covering the patient with clean, dry sheets and blankets. Fluid/blood warmers are used for IV fluid infusion. The environmental temperature is strictly regulated by increasing the room temperature, closing room doors to prevent air drafts, and using external heat lamps or radiant heat shields.

Blood and Electrolytes. Serum electrolyte levels are determined on admission and as dictated by the patient's status. Serum sodium levels typically approach the concentration of the resuscitation fluid being administered. Serum potassium levels may be increased as a result of release from injured tissue. The blood urea nitrogen level may also be increased when excessive protein catabolism occurs, and hyperglycemia may occur as a result of catecholamine release. Arterial blood gas values and serum lactate levels are evaluated frequently because metabolic acidosis can indicate inadequate tissue perfusion (see Laboratory Alert: Alterations Seen During Acute Care Management of the Burned Patient).

Acute Care Phase: Critical Care Burn Center

With successful resuscitation, burn shock and its dramatic fluid and protein fluctuations stabilize approximately 48 to 72 hours after injury, and the acute phase of burn care begins. Assessments and interventions during the acute phase of burn recovery are

LABORATORY ALERTS

Alterations Seen During Acute Care Management of the Burned Patient

Laboratory Test	Critical Value	Significance
Carboxyhemoglobin	>15%	Present in carbon monoxide poisoning
Hematocrit	<15% >60%	↑ In hypovolemia; ↓ as third-spaced fluid reenters the intravascular compartment or with concomitant traumatic injury
Serum lactate	>2.2 mEq/L	↑ In metabolic acidosis; should ↓ if fluid resuscitation adequate
Potassium	<2.5 mEq/L >6.6 mEq/L	↑ Related to tissue damage; assess for cardiac dysrhythmias. May ↓ as reenters cells
Sodium	<110 mEq/L	Levels approach the concentration of fluids being administered. May ↑ due to inadequate fluid replacement. May ↓ with diuresis
Blood urea nitrogen	>100 mg/dL	May be ↑ secondary to catabolism or falsely ↑ in hypovolemia; monitor nutrition and volume status
White blood cell count	<2000/ microliter >100,000/ microliter	May ↓ due to use of topical silver sulfadiazine ↑ With infection

↑, Increased; ↓, decreased.

implemented to promote wound healing, to prevent complications, and to improve function of the various body systems.

Respiratory System

Assessment continues for signs of respiratory compromise and pneumonia. Tachypnea, abnormal breath sounds, fever, increased white blood cell count, purulent secretions, and infiltrations on chest x-ray films indicate developing pneumonia. Nursing interventions play a key role in preventing ventilator-associated pneumonia, such as regular oral care, maintaining head-of-bed elevation of at least thirty degrees, and eliminating cross-contamination.[51] Aggressive pulmonary hygiene including suctioning, coughing, deep breathing, and early ambulation is essential.

Cardiovascular System

As capillary permeability stabilizes, IV fluid requirements decrease. Patients must receive maintenance IV fluid infusions that match overall fluid output. Monitoring daily weight and intake and output is essential. Increased fluid resuscitation requirements after debridement and grafting operations are often required because the inflammatory response is triggered by the surgical intervention. Frequent monitoring of vital signs continues.

Neurological Status

Changes in neurological status, which may indicate hypoxemia, hypoperfusion, or sepsis are part of ongoing assessment.

Renal Status

Urine output assessment continues. Postburn diuresis starts approximately 48 to 72 hours after injury. Urine output ranging from 100 to 600 mL/hr is commonly observed. Intake and output assessment remains important. After postburn diuresis, urinary output should correlate with intake of IV and oral fluids. In the absence of diabetes, glycosuria may indicate an early sign of sepsis.

Gastrointestinal System

Assessment of GI function continues. The patient is monitored for the development of a stress ulcer. Tolerance of enteral feedings is assessed. Nutritional considerations are a treatment priority and are discussed later in this chapter.

Integumentary System

The burn wound becomes the major focus of the acute phase of burn recovery. Assessment continues to include monitoring for burn wound healing, burn wound depth conversion, and signs of infection.

Blood and Electrolytes

Although fluid and protein shifts stabilize in the acute care phase, blood and electrolyte abnormalities related to other processes may be observed. Hemodilution with an associated decreased hematocrit may result from reentry of fluid into the intravascular compartment and from loss of red blood cells destroyed at the burn injury site. Hyponatremia from diuresis may occur, but it usually resolves within 1 week of onset. Inadequate replacement of evaporative water loss may produce hypernatremia. Hypokalemia may develop as potassium reenters the cells. Electrolyte shifts also affect the ability to maintain a proper acid-base balance and may cause metabolic acidosis. Hypoproteinemia and negative nitrogen balance may occur from an increase in metabolic rate and insufficient nutrition. Leukopenia may develop from administration of the topical antimicrobial agent silver sulfadiazine. Infection and excessive carbohydrate loading contribute to hyperglycemia. In addition, an increase in the white blood cell count, prolonged coagulation times, and a decreased platelet count may result from infection or sepsis.

SPECIAL CONSIDERATIONS AND AREAS OF CONCERN

Burns of the face, ears, eyes, hands, feet, major joints, genitalia, and perineum pose distinct concerns because injuries to these areas contribute to overall burn injury severity and require unique management. Certain types of burns (electrical, chemical, and abuse) also mandate special consideration and intervention.

Burns of the Face

The presence of head or neck burns alerts the clinician to suspect a potential inhalation injury. Associated facial edema may lead to a compromised airway. Close monitoring of the patient's respiratory status is essential. The head of the bed is elevated to facilitate ventilation and edema reabsorption. Special care is taken during cleansing of facial burns to prevent excessive bleeding and damage to new tissue growth. All hair (except for eyebrows) is shaved from the wound each day. Once the wound is cleaned and debrided, a topical antimicrobial agent is applied per unit protocol. Because of the rich blood supply in the face, partial-thickness burns usually heal quickly as long as infection is prevented. Good oral hygiene is essential.

Burns of the Ears

The ears are especially prone to inflammation and infection of the cartilage *(chondritis)*, which leads to complete loss of ear cartilage. Ear burns are treated with a topical antimicrobial agent. Mafenide acetate (Sulfamylon) is the agent of choice because of its ability to penetrate the cartilage. Mechanical pressure on the ears from dressings or other external sources (tube ties, pillows) must be avoided because the pressure impairs blood flow and contributes to the development of chondritis. Cloth ties are used for securing

tubes to the face and are monitored frequently to ensure that pressure is not placed on top of the ears. Pillows are not used for the head. Instead, a foam donut with a hole for the ear to rest in while the patient is in a lateral position is substituted.

Burns of the Eyes

Immediate examination of the eyes is necessary on arrival to the hospital because eyelid edema forms rapidly. Eyelid edema can cause the cornea to become exposed as the eyelid retracts. Contact lenses are removed if present. A thorough examination by an ophthalmologist is mandatory for serious injuries. The eyes are stained with fluorescein to rule out corneal injury, and the eyes are irrigated with copious amounts of physiological saline if injury is confirmed. Nursing care involves the frequent application of ophthalmic ointment or artificial tears to protect the cornea and conjunctiva from drying. Careful observation of eyelashes is also necessary because they may invert and scratch the cornea.

Burns of the Hands, Feet, or Major Joints

Extensive burns of the hands and feet may cause permanent disability, necessitating a long convalescence. An important aspect of critical care nursing care is preservation of function. Burned hands are elevated above the level of the heart on slings or wedges to reduce edema formation. Fingers and toes are wrapped individually during dressing changes with gauze, bandages or biological products to keep digits separated to prevent *webbing* (the skin growing together between burned body parts). Occupational and physical therapists are involved in the patient's plan of care from the day of admission to address and evaluate function and mobility parameters. Although ROM exercises may be painful, they must be initiated as soon as possible after the injury and performed frequently throughout each day. Active ROM exercises prevent muscle atrophy, reduce or prevent the shortening of ligaments, and decrease edema. Passive ROM exercises are indicated if patients are unable to move their extremities actively.

Burn wounds over joints are prone to scar tissue contractures that limit joint ROM. The position of comfort is the position of contracture and deformity development. Therefore, splinting and antideformity positioning (e.g., extension of knees and elbows, extension and supination of wrists, abduction of hips and shoulders) are required to maintain function and prevent deformities of the affected part. When the patient is ambulating or sitting, an elastic bandage is applied over burn wounds of the feet and legs to prevent venous stasis and pooling of blood. Venous pooling delays wound healing and increases the risk of DVT development. The elastic bandage is removed when the feet are elevated. In establishing a nursing plan of care, the nurse must remember that patients with bilateral burned hands are very dependent on nursing personnel for their physical needs.

Burns of the Genitalia and Perineum

Patients with perineal burns often require hospitalization for monitoring of urinary tract obstruction. An indwelling urethral catheter is indicated until the surrounding wounds are healed or grafted. Meticulous wound care is essential because of the high risk of urine or fecal contamination and resulting infection. Perineal hair must be shaved over wound areas. Scrotal edema is common, and the scrotum is elevated on towels or foam.

Electrical Injury

Cardiopulmonary arrest is a common complication of high-voltage electrical injury. Other severe complications related to electrical injury are summarized in Box 20-2. Hypoxemia may occur secondary to tetanic contractions and resulting paralysis of the respiratory muscles. Oxygen and endotracheal intubation with mechanical ventilation are implemented as indicated. Patients are evaluated for spinal fractures from tetanic contractions or from falls during the injury event. Cervical collars and backboards are used to maintain spinal immobilization until radiological tests and clinical examinations have confirmed the absence of injury. All patients with electrical injury are monitored closely for cardiac dysrhythmias. If present, continuous cardiac monitoring or serial electrocardiographic evaluations continue for at least 24 hours after injury. Tea-colored urine indicates the presence of hemochromogens (myoglobin), released as a result of severe deep tissue damage in a process called rhabdomyolysis. Urinary output for these patients is maintained at 100 mL/hr until the urine becomes clear to prevent renal failure.[4] Resuscitation fluid volumes larger than predicted by the Consensus formula are often required to achieve this high urine output. Sodium bicarbonate and mannitol may be administered at the burn center physician's discretion to increase urine pH and output. Affected extremities are closely monitored for the development of compartment syndrome. Often, fasciotomies are required to release compartment pressure.

Chemical Injury

Treatment of chemical injuries focuses on stopping the burning process while maintaining the safety of

> ### BOX 20-2 Manifestations and Complications of Electrical Injury
>
> - Cardiac dysrhythmias or cardiopulmonary arrest
> - Hypoxia secondary to tetanic contractions and paralysis of the respiratory muscles
> - Deep tissue necrosis
> - Compartment syndrome of extremities
> - Long bone or vertebral fractures from tetanic muscle contractions
> - Rhabdomyolysis and acute renal failure
> - Acute cataract formation
> - Neurological deficits such as spinal cord paralysis, traumatic brain injury, peripheral neuropathy, seizures, deafness, motor and sensory deficits

the nurse. Protective gear such as plastic gowns, gloves, masks, and goggles are worn by the burn team during decontamination. If a patient is suspected of having a methamphetamine laboratory–related injury, decontamination is required. During decontamination for all chemical exposures, the patient's clothing is immediately removed. Dry chemicals are brushed off, and the area exposed to chemicals is continuously flushed with water for at least 30 minutes. The nurse questions the patient and significant others to determine the specific chemical agent involved. Some chemicals such as alkalies require even longer lavage, which can be quite uncomfortable for the patient. Nursing interventions include controlling pain and minimizing heat loss caused by continual irrigation. Patients must also be closely monitored for signs of systemic chemical absorption and effects.

Abuse and Neglect

Burns are a prevalent form of abuse and can result from either an active intent to injure or from neglect. Vulnerable populations such as children, the elderly, disabled persons, and mentally impaired persons are at increased risk of abuse and neglect. Critical care nurses play a lead role in recognizing and identifying potential abuse or neglect cases because they spend the most time interfacing with the patient and significant others. Nurses must elicit the history of the story and circumstances surrounding the injury event, meticulously and accurately document the

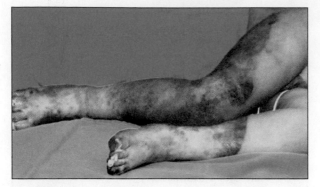

FIGURE 20-13. Child abuse by hot water immersion. The thigh burn wound edges have a clear demarcation line (are in a straight line), and there are no splash marks. The parents delayed seeking medical treatment for the child's burns until 3 days after injury (note the dry, crusty appearance of the wounds). The child also had a forearm fracture and multiple areas of bruising on the body. *(Courtesy of University of Michigan Trauma Burn Center, Ann Arbor, MI.)*

wound appearance and the pattern of injury (including use of photographs), and observe the interactions between the patient and caregivers or family. The injured individual should be questioned separately and privately from the family caregiver. The reported injury history should correlate with physical findings. Discrepancies between reported accounts of the injury event and physical assessment findings indicate a potential abuse/neglect situation. The presence of other injuries (i.e., associated bruising, fractures, abrasions, or other trauma) and the distribution and characteristics of the burn wound also provide key information on the true cause of the burn injury. For example, a scald burn with a clear demarcation and/or symmetrical wound pattern on the extremities without splash mark burns indicates an intentional immersion injury instead of an accidental scald (Figure 20-13). Lack of witnesses to the injury event, blaming of siblings, and delay in seeking care are also indicators of potential abuse situations. All potential or suspected abuse cases must be reported to the appropriate authorities as governed by state laws. The patient is hospitalized until social workers and protective services have investigated the patient's home environment to determine whether the patient will be safe on discharge.

PAIN CONTROL

Pain is a tormenting consequence of burn injury, both immediately after the injury and during the healing of the burn wound.[27] Pain experienced during the acute phase of recovery consists of a constant or *resting pain*, as well as a shorter peak of excruciating pain *(procedural or breakthrough pain)* often associated with therapeutic procedures.[10,38,49] Many aspects of burn treatment produce pain including dressing changes, debridement, surgical intervention, application of topical antimicrobials, and physical and occupational therapy. This situation illustrates the major paradox of burn pain management: the nurse inflicts pain and then must relieve it.

Adequately treating a burn patient's pain is a challenge. Altered pharmacokinetics secondary to changes in volume distribution and hypermetabolism is associated with burn injury. Burn patients commonly have histories of regular alcohol consumption or substance use that further compound pain management and narcotic resistance.[49,52] Therefore, the quantities of analgesics required by burn patients often exceed those of other disease states.[49] Inaccurate assessment of a patient's pain or fears of addiction leads to undermedication. Improved assessment and intervention of severe burn pain are needed.[1,10] A recent study found that burn patients have realistic expectations of their care and do not expect to be completely free of acute pain; however, patients' satisfaction with their care was related to the level of pain experienced.[10] To control a patient's pain successfully and to achieve increased patient satisfaction, accurate serial pain assessments must occur, and the patient must be involved in creating an individualized analgesic treatment plan.[10] Pain levels should be assessed frequently as "the fifth vital sign," with additional assessments before, during, and after all procedures and treatments. The nurse serves as the patient's advocate by ensuring that pain medications are administered by appropriate delivery methods and in adequate dosages to reduce pain intensity.

Opiates are the most common analgesics used to treat burn pain. Subcutaneous or intramuscular injections are ineffective in the resuscitative phase because of impaired circulation in soft tissue. Absorption is sporadic, increasing the risk of undermedication or narcotic overdose. Morphine is the drug of choice, and IV administration is the route of choice. A continuous IV infusion of morphine maintains a consistent level of analgesia, but it is typically used only in critically ill patients requiring mechanical ventilation. Patients have expressed increased satisfaction in being able to have some "control" over their pain.[48] Therefore, patient-controlled analgesia may be beneficial. Analgesic medications can be given safely by the oral route once the patient is hemodynamically stable and any ileus has resolved. Although pain is reduced when wounds are covered with temporary dressings or skin grafts, frequent surgical procedures and wound care procedures produce episodes of pain until permanent wound closure or healing is completed. Itching that occurs during the healing process also contributes to the patient's overall discomfort. Several medications and soothing emollients assist in controlling pruritus.

The entire burn care and treatment experience produces anxiety, which further exacerbates pain.[49] The ideal pain management regimen must incorporate treatment of both pain and anxiety. Fear and a loss of control over their lives and schedules increase patients' anxiety. The critical care nurse must provide frequent and repeated explanations of care plans, interventions, and procedures at an age-appropriate level. Patients are encouraged to participate as much as possible in their wound care, medication administration, feeding, and exercise therapy. Anxiolytics are commonly administered in the acute care phase. Psychological techniques, such as relaxation and guided-imagery techniques, also serve as useful adjuncts for reducing anxiety and enhancing pain relief. Accurate pain and anxiety assessment, close monitoring, and individualized dosing of medications are essential for successful pain control.

INFECTION CONTROL

Burn patients have a high risk of infection related to altered skin integrity and altered immune response. When the skin's natural mechanical barrier protection is lost, the patient's susceptibility to infection increases. In addition, other host defense mechanisms are impaired, and immunosuppression develops. Although great strides in management have been made, the incidence of infection is higher in burn patients than in other patient groups and remains a predominant determinant of outcome.[12,17,23,26] The control of infection is an important nursing intervention in the care of burn patients. Concomitant inhalation injury places the burn patient at particularly high risk of developing pneumonia.[17,26] The added insult of pneumonia doubles mortality rates.[17] Invasive monitoring and the presence of urinary catheters, IV catheters, and endotracheal tubes are also sources of infection.

The goals of infection control in burn care are as follows:

- Preserve existing immune defenses
- Prevent transmission of exogenous organisms
- Control transfer of endogenous organisms (normal flora) to sites at increased risk for infection

Infection control in the burn patient is dependent on the following strategies:

- Aseptic management of the wound and the environment
- Use of topical antibacterial agents
- Aggressive wound management with close monitoring for changes in wound appearance
- Judicious and microbial-guided use of systemic antibiotics based upon patient flora and local unit bacterial resistance patterns[47]
- Provision of adequate nutrition
- Close monitoring of laboratory values and clinical signs of impending sepsis
- Early wound closure to restore the protective barrier of skin
- Continuous observation and implementation of targeted interventions that improve outcomes (e.g., tight glycemic control, prevention of central line infection, head of bed elevated at least 30 degrees, restrictive sedation practice, aggressive ventilator weaning)[51]

Although infection control policies differ among burn units, all policies stress standard precautions, including the use of barrier techniques, strict hand washing, and appropriate garb when caring for a burn-injured patient.

WOUND MANAGEMENT

Patient outcomes from burn injury are optimized by focusing on the goals of prevention and treatment of wound infections, and expedited closure of burn wounds. Interventions performed to obtain these goals are wound cleansing, debridement, topical antimicrobial and/or biological-biosynthetic dressing therapy, and definitive surgical wound closure. Burn wound care protocols and procedures vary among burn centers across the country. However, the underlying goals of wound care are the same: removal of nonviable tissue to promote reepithelialization and prompt coverage via skin grafts when necessary.

Wound Care

To promote prevention of infection and healing of the burn wound, the nurse must focus on performing meticulous wound care. Wound care is typically done once or twice a day, depending on the healing status of the wound, the topical agents or dressing used, and the number of days postoperatively from grafting. Before initiating wound care, the nurse carefully explains the procedure to the patient and significant others and encourages participation as able. Analgesics are administered (and sedatives if indicated) before starting the procedure. All wounds are cleansed with a mild soap or surgical detergent disinfectant and are rinsed with warm tap water. The patient is not immersed in water because immersion has a significant potential for cross-contamination of wounds. Instead, water is allowed to flow over the wounds and immediately drained away. This regimen is best accomplished in a shower or hydrotherapy stretcher, but bed baths may be used for hemodynamically unstable patients. All previously applied topical agents, necrotic tissue, exudate, and fibrous debris are removed from the wound to expose healthy tissue, to control bacterial proliferation, and to promote healing. Loose eschar and wound debris are *debrided* with washcloths or gauze sponges, scissors, and forceps. Mechanical trauma and damage from aggressive cleansing of newly formed epithelial skin buds or healing granulation tissue must be avoided. Hair in and immediately surrounding the wound bed is shaved (except eyebrows) to eliminate a medium for bacterial growth and to facilitate wound assessment. All wounds are inspected closely, with wound location, size, color, texture, and drainage carefully documented so any changes in appearance or developing signs of infection are noted. The patient's core body temperature is closely monitored. During wound care the room temperature must be maintained to prevent chilling and excessive body heat loss.

Topical Agents and Dressings

New prospects for wound treatment using tissue engineering continue to emerge. New topical wound care agents and biosynthetic dressings have been developed. Newer products have broader antimicrobial actions, interact with the wound growth factors and collagen fibers to accelerate healing and to stop the zone of stasis from expanding, help to fill in defects, and may reduce scarring. All these actions positively affect outcomes in patients with burn injury by reducing infection, shortening healing time, preventing wound conversion to full-thickness depth, and improving long-term cosmetic appearance and scarring. After each hydrotherapy session, the unhealed or unexcised burn wound is covered with an antimicrobial topical agent, a dressing, or both. Table 20-4 describes the most commonly used agents and related nursing considerations. The selection of an agent and dressing is determined by burn depth, anatomical location, frequency of wound visualization desired, and presence and type of microorganisms identified. The ideal antimicrobial agent demonstrates broad-spectrum activity against microorganisms with low resistance development, penetrates eschar, and has limited adverse effects. The burn center physician orders the antimicrobial

agent, the frequency of application, and the method of application.

Many advances have been made in the development of wound dressings and skin substitutes to provide coverage for major burns. Temporary wound coverings are classified as either *biological* or *biosynthetic* (a combination of biological and synthetic properties). Table 20-5 describes common types and uses for biological and biosynthetic coverings. Biological or biosynthetic dressings are used as temporary wound coverings for freshly excised (surgically debrided) burn wounds until autograft skin is available. Allograft, Integra, AlloDerm, or xenograft is commonly used for this indication. Biological or biosynthetic products may be used as dressings for partial-thickness burns, meshed autograft skin, or donor sites to promote healing. Allograft, TransCyte, BioBrane, or xenograft is typically used for this type of application. Temporary wound coverings have the added benefits of controlling heat and fluid loss, decreasing infection risk, stimulating healing, and increasing patient comfort.

Enzymatic agents such as collagenase, papain/urea, or sutilains are sometimes used for debridement of smaller necrotic tissue areas on deep partial- and full-thickness burns. Topical enzymatic agents are proteolytic enzyme ointments that act as potent digestants of nonviable protein matter or necrotic tissue, but they are harmless to viable tissue. Enzymatic agents do not have antimicrobial properties; therefore, wounds must be closely monitored for infection.

Burn wounds are treated in one of two ways: open or closed methods. The decision of which method to use depends on the location, size, and depth of the burn, as well as on specific burn unit protocols. Each method has advantages and disadvantages.

With the *open method*, the burn wounds are left open to air after the antimicrobial agent is applied. The open method provides increased wound visualization and more opportunities for observation, eliminates dressing supplies, and improves joint mobility normally limited by the presence of restrictive dressings. However, the open method allows direct contact between the wound and the environment. The topical antimicrobial agent may rub off on clothing, bedding, or equipment. The open method increases wound exposure time and the risk of hypothermia. The open method is commonly used on superficial burns to the face treated with the topical agent bacitracin.

With the *closed method*, a gauze dressing is placed over an agent that was applied directly to the wound, or the wound is covered with gauze dressings that have been saturated with a topical antimicrobial agent. The closed method reduces heat loss and pain or sensitivity from wound exposure, and it assists in

PHARMACOLOGY

TABLE 20-4 Topical Antimicrobial Agents for Burn Wound Management

Agent	Indications	Nursing Considerations
Clotrimazole cream or nystatin (Mycostatin)	Fungal colonization of wounds	Apply once or twice daily. Use in conjunction with an antibacterial topical agent. May cause skin irritation.
Mafenide acetate (Sulfamylon)	Active against most gram-positive, gram-negative, and *Pseudomonas* pathogens; drug of choice for ear burns; penetrates thick eschar and ear cartilage	Apply once or twice daily. Strong carbonic anhydrase inhibitor that can cause metabolic acidosis; monitor respiratory rate, electrolyte values, and ABGs. Hydroscopic (draws water out of tissue) and can be painful/burning for 15-60 minutes after application. Tends to slow eschar separation.
Silver-coated dressings (Acticoat, Aquacel Ag, Silverlon)	Silver-coated, flexible, nonadhesive wound dressings; as long as dressing is moist, provides continuous release of silver ions for 3-14 days (depending on product); effective broad-spectrum coverage for numerous pathogens (gram-negative and gram-positive bacteria, antibiotic-resistant bacteria, yeast, mold); alternative for patients allergic to sulfa drugs	Apply new dressing every 1-7 days by (1) applying to moist open wound, with wound exudate maintaining silver activation until drainage stops or wound healing; or (2) applying to wound, rewetting with sterile water every 4-6 hours to keep dressing moist (not wet). Use sterile water to moisten dressings; saline renders silver ions ineffective. A decrease in number of required dressing changes increases patient comfort and cost-effectiveness. Aquacel Ag does not require wetting; converts to a gel with wound exudate absorption.
Silver nitrate	Effective against wide spectrum of common wound pathogens; acts on surface microorganisms only; poor eschar penetration; used in patients with sulfa allergy or toxic epidermal necrolysis	Apply 0.5% solution wet dressing two or three times daily; rewet dressing every 2 hours to ensure remains moist. Hypotonic solution causes leeching of electrolytes; monitor for hyponatremia, hypochloremia, hypocalcemia, and hypokalemia; replace electrolytes according to protocol. Must be kept in light-resistant container. Stains easily; protect walls, floors, and equipment with plastic.
Silver sulfadiazine (SSD, Silvadene)	Active against wide spectrum of gram-negative, gram-positive, and *Candida albicans* pathogens; acts only on cell wall and membrane; does not penetrate thick eschar	Apply once or twice daily. May wrap wounds or leave as open dressing. Can cause leukopenia; monitor white blood cell count.

ABGs, Arterial blood gases.

protecting wounds from external mechanical trauma. The dressings applied may also assist with debridement. However, the closed method requires a dressing change to assess the wound, and the presence of dressings may impair ROM. The closed method is commonly used on full-thickness burns treated with silver sulfadiazine and new grafts.

A unique dressing system, the vacuum-assisted closure (VAC) system, has been developed for the treatment of grafts, partial-thickness burns, and deep surgical wounds (as seen in the nonburn injury necrotizing fasciitis). The VAC device consists of a sponge and suction tubing placed on the wound bed and covered with an occlusive dressing (Figure 20-14, *A*).

TABLE 20-5   Biological and Biosynthetic Dressings

Type of Dressing	Definition
Biological Dressing	**Temporary Wound Cover from Human or Animal Species Tissue**
Allograft (homograft) skin	Graft of skin transplanted from another human, living or dead
Xenograft (heterograft) skin	Graft of skin (usually pigskin) transplanted between different species
Biosynthetic Dressing	**A Wound Covering Composed of Both Biological and Synthetic Materials**
AlloDerm	Transplantable tissue consisting of human cryopreserved allogeneic dermis from which the epidermal cells, fibroblasts, and endothelial cells targeted for immune response have been removed
Composite cultured skin or cultured dermal substitutes (CCS, CDS, Apligraf, OrCel)	Bilayer *allogeneic* (from another human) skin substitutes typically cultured from neonatal foreskin, consisting of outer *epidermal* layer of cultured epidermal keratinocytes, and bottom *dermal* layer embedded with fibroblasts and collagen
Integra	Dressing system composed of two layers: (1) *dermal* layer made of animal collagen and glycosaminoglycan that interfaces with wound and functions as dermal matrix for cellular growth and collagen synthesis; (2) temporary outer synthetic *epidermal* layer made of Silastic that acts as barrier to water loss and bacteria. Dermal layer biodegrades within months as new wound collagen matrix is synthesized. Silastic epidermal layer removed in 14-21 days and replaced with thin autograft
TransCyte	Temporary skin substitute composed of outer synthetic layer and inner collagen base layer of human neonatal fibroblasts; interacts with wound to amplify tissue regeneration: fibroblasts secrete growth factors, matrix proteins, human fibronectin, and collagen

The device then creates a negative-pressure dressing to decompress edematous interstitial spaces and increase local perfusion, to help draw wound edges closed uniformly, to remove wound fluid, and to provide a closed, moist wound healing environment (Figure 20-14, *B*). VAC also allows the collection and quantification of wound drainage. VAC therapy has been associated with lower wound bacterial counts, earlier reepithelialization, and a reduction in graft loss due to reduced edema and preservation of blood flow.[19,28,32]

Surgical Excision and Grafting

The depth of the injury determines whether a burn will heal or require skin grafting. First- and second-degree burns heal because they are superficial and partial-thickness burns; thus, the necessary elements to generate new skin remain. Full-thickness burns are nonvascular, and all dermal appendages have been destroyed. Full-thickness burns require skin grafting to achieve wound closure. Deep partial-thickness burns are also commonly grafted to decrease the risk of infection by achieving earlier wound closure and to minimize scarring and improve cosmetic appearance. *Excision* is surgical debridement by scalpel or electrocautery to remove *necrotic* (dead)

tissue until a layer of healthy, well-vascularized tissue is exposed. *Skin grafting* is placing skin on the excised burn wound (Figure 20-15, *A*). Several types of skin can be used for skin grafting including *autograft* (skin from oneself that is transferred to a new location on the same individual's body; i.e., the patient's own skin); *allograft*, which is also called *homograft* (skin from another human; e.g., cadaver skin); and *xenograft* (skin from another animal; e.g., pigskin). Autografts are the only permanent type of skin grafting (Table 20-6). Homografts and xenografts are temporary biological dressings (see Table 20-5). With autografts, a partial-thickness wound called a *donor site* is created where the skin was harvested or removed from the patient.

Excision and grafting are performed in the operating room and are typically initiated within the first week after burn injury. Early excision within the first 1 to 3 days is advocated because it has been associated with decreased mortality and morbidity.[9,26,47] Advantages reported include modulation of the hypermetabolic response, reduced infection and wound colonization rates, increased graft take, and decreased length of hospitalization.[8,9,26] Depending on the size of the burn and the presence of infection, sequential or repeated surgical debridements and grafting may be required. In major burns, it is often

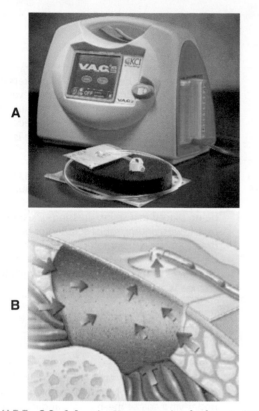

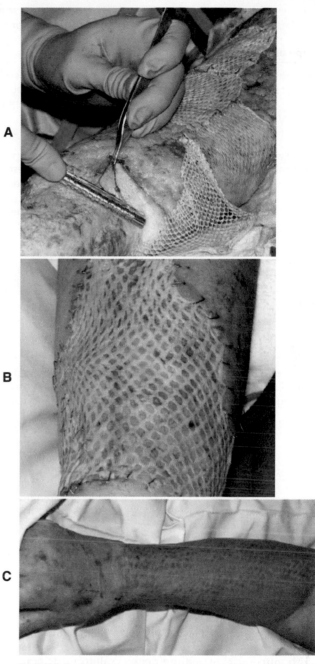

FIGURE 20-14. A, Vacuum-assisted closure (VAC) device. **B,** The device creates a negative-pressure dressing to decompress edematous interstitial spaces and to increase local perfusion, help draw wound edges closed uniformly, remove wound fluid, and provide a closed, moist healing environment. *(Courtesy of Kinetic Concepts, Inc., San Antonio, TX.)*

FIGURE 20-15. Excision and autografting. **A,** Surgical debridement (excision) with meshed autograft placement in the operating room. **B,** Meshed autograft postoperative day 2. **C,** Comparison of sheet autograft (on hand) versus meshed autograft (on forearm) 3 weeks postoperatively. Use of meshed autograft allows larger body surface area coverage, but it also typically leads to more scarring and a less cosmetically pleasing appearance. *(Courtesy of University of Michigan Trauma Burn Center, Ann Arbor, MI.)*

not possible to graft all full-thickness wound areas initially either because of the patient's instability from the size and severity of burned areas or because of a lack of donor sites to provide adequate coverage. Priority areas for autograft skin application include the face, the hands, the feet, and over joints. In addition, other temporary and permanent synthetic products have been developed to substitute for a person's own skin (see Table 20-5). These products allow early burn wound coverage, while delaying autografting until previously used donor sites have healed and can be reharvested.

Autograft skin can be applied as meshed grafts or as sheet grafts. *Sheet* (nonmeshed) grafts are often used on the face and hands for better cosmetic results. Meshed grafts are commonly used elsewhere on the body (Figure 20-15, *B*). A meshed graft is created by using a tool *(dermatome)* that places multiple tiny slits or holes in the piece of skin that was harvested from the donor site. The wider the mesh of the graft is, the larger the area that can be covered with the autograft skin. However, wider mesh grafts also

TABLE 20-6   Autograft Skin: Nursing Implications

Type of Autograft	Definition	Nursing Implications
Split-thickness *sheet* skin graft	Sheet of skin composed of epidermis and a variable portion of dermis harvested at a predetermined thickness. Sheet kept intact (not meshed) to improve cosmetic appearance; often used on face and hands.	Grafted area must be immobilized; pockets of serous/serosanguinous fluid must be evacuated by needle aspiration or rolling of the fluid with cotton tip applicator toward the skin edges; if fluid is not evacuated, graft adherence is compromised.
Split-thickness *meshed* skin graft	Split-thickness sheet graft that is mesh-cut by a dermatome, to expand the graft from 1.5 to 9 times its original size before being placed on a recipient bed of granulation tissue; used to cover large surface areas.	Grafted area is immobilized; skin graft is covered with layers of fine and coarse mesh gauze and wrapped with absorbent gauze roll before being placed in a splint; dressings must be kept moist (with antimicrobial solution or biological dressing) but not saturated to prevent desiccation and to promote epithelialization of interstices of the meshed skin; first dressing change is in 3-5 days.
Full-thickness skin graft	Skin graft that contains the full thickness of skin down to the subcutaneous tissue, typically used for eyelids or later reconstructive procedures.	Requires same care as a sheet skin graft.
Cultured epidermal autograft (CEA)	Layered sheets of autologous human epidermal cells grown in a laboratory with tissue culture techniques to expand keratinocytes; derived from small skin biopsy specimen from the patient. Provides potential to cover extensive wound areas more quickly without having to wait for healing of limited donor site skin surfaces. Epidermal layer replacement only. Epicel is trade name of commercially manufactured CEA as opposed to on-site burn center production.	During first 7-10 days after surgery, daily dressing changes involve only outer layer of fluffy gauze; underlying coarse mesh gauze and petroleum jelly gauze, which are sutured over the graft, are not disturbed. Outer dressing must remain dry; many topical antimicrobial agents are toxic to CEA skin and should not come in contact with graft dressings. Once petroleum jelly gauze is loose (7-10 days) it is removed, and wet saline dressings are used until approximately 21 days after surgery when the skin graft is usually well adherent. Gentle passive range-of-motion exercises can begin once petroleum jelly gauze is removed.

contribute to more scarring and a less cosmetically pleasing appearance (Figure 20-15, *C*). Table 20-6 summarizes the types of skin autografts used, along with nursing care requirements. Splinting of graft sites is indicated to prevent movement and shearing of the grafts until healing is complete. Extremities are elevated to prevent pooling of blood and edema, which can lead to increased pressure and graft loss.

Many types of dressings can be used on donor sites (Table 20-7), but the product chosen must promote healing of the donor site within 8 to 14 days. Donor sites can be reused or reharvested once healed. When patient donor sites are limited because of the severity of the burn injury, cultured epithelium autograft (CEA) can be used to provide coverage for a major

burn injury. With CEA, a biopsy specimen is obtained from the patient's skin and is sent to a laboratory where keratinocytes are cultured and grown. The process usually takes 2 to 3 weeks and results in small pieces of skin. These fragile pieces of skin are surgically applied to a clean, excised burn wound. The disadvantage of CEA is its extreme fragility, partly the result of the lack of a durable dermis. Researchers have been investigating the development of different types of cultured skin substitutes that incorporate CEA with a dermal layer to increase durability.[8]

Burn units vary in their protocols to treat grafted areas and donor sites. Basic wound care principles are applied, and prevention of infection is always the primary goal. Although the critical care nurse may not actually develop the wound care plan, involvement by the entire burn team to promote compliance with the plan is essential for positive patient outcomes. A method of documenting wound treatment that facilitates day-to-day team communication of care requirements should be used.

Inherent in all wound care management is the necessity to improve and maintain function. Occupational and physical therapists are essential members of the burn team and are consulted on the day of admission. Often, the position of comfort for the patient is one that leads to dysfunction or deformity. Specialized splints and exercises are required for the prevention of future complications.

NUTRITIONAL CONSIDERATIONS

Adequate nutrition plays an important role in the survival of extensively burned patients. A major burn injury produces a stress-induced hypermetabolic-catabolic response that is greater than that of any other disease process or injury. Skeletal muscle is the major protein store in the body. Postburn hypermetabolism leads to deleterious consequences including significant skeletal muscle breakdown with protein degradation, weight loss, marked delays in wound healing, skin graft loss, impaired immunological responsiveness, sepsis, or even death if adequate nutrition is not provided and an anabolic or positive nitrogen balance is not achieved.[26,42,51] Muscle weakness and atrophy also contribute to prolonged mechanical ventilation and delayed ambulation.[54]

Nutritional therapy must be instituted immediately after the burn injury to meet energy demands, to maintain host defense mechanisms, to replenish body protein stores, and to curtail progressive loss of lean body mass. The nurse collaborates with the patient, the registered dietitian, and the physician to coordinate a nutritional plan. If the patient is able to tolerate an oral diet, a high-calorie, high-protein diet with supplements is instituted with daily calorie counts performed to monitor dietary intake. If oral intake is not tolerated or caloric intake is insufficient, enteral tube feeding is begun. Early enteral feeding within the first 24 hours after burn injury decreases the production of catabolic hormones, improves nitrogen balance, maintains gut integrity, lowers the incidence of diarrhea, and decreases hospital stay.[26,42,44,47,53]

Recent research efforts have focused on using beta-blockade, anabolic hormones, and other pharmacological interventions to ameliorate the hypermetabolic-catabolic response to burn injury.[7,26,39,53] Fatal outcome and wound healing time are reduced with administration of beta blockers.[7,26]

TABLE 20-7 Types of Donor Site Dressings

Dressing	Description
BioBrane	Bilaminate wound dressing composed of nylon mesh embedded with a collagen derivative with an outer silicone rubber membrane; permeable to wound drainage and topical antimicrobial agents; peels away as wound heals
DuoDerm	Hydrocolloid dressing that interacts with moisture on skin, creating a bond that makes it adhere
Fine mesh gauze	Cotton gauze placed directly on donor site; a crust or "scab" is formed as gauze dries and epithelialization of wound occurs under the dressing; gauze peels away easily as wound heals
Kaltostat	Hydrophilic, nonwoven fiber that converts to a firm gel when it is activated by wound exudates; creates warm, moist environment that is nonadherent to the wound
N-terface	Translucent, nonabsorbent, and nonreactive surface material used between the burn wound and outer dressing
Op-Site	Thin elastic film that is occlusive, waterproof, and permeable to moisture, vapor, and air; fluid under dressing may need to be evacuated
Vigilon	Colloidal suspension on a polyethylene mesh support that provides a moist environment and is permeable to gases and water vapor
Scarlet Red	Cotton gauze is impregnated with a blend of lanolin, olive oil, petrolatum, and red dye "scarlet red"; healing occurs as with fine mesh gauze dressing
Silver-coated dressings	Acticoat, Aquacel Ag, and Silverlon. Silver-coated, flexible dressings that provide continuous release of silver ions for 3-14 days while dressing is moist
Xeroform	Fine mesh gauze containing 3% bismuth tribromophenate in a petrolatum blend; promotes healing as with other mesh gauze dressings

A hallmark prospective, randomized, blinded, multicenter trial demonstrated that treatment with the anabolic hormone oxandrolone in burn patients significantly decreased the hospital length of stay.[53] While further analysis is required to determine the exact cause of this reduction, proposed contributing factors are normalization of metabolism, decreased inflammation, improved organ function, increased strength, and/or improved wound healing.[53] It is advocated that all patients with greater than 20%TBSA burns be treated with oxandrolone while monitoring levels of hepatic transaminases.[53] Refer to Chapter 6 for additional nutrition information.

PSYCHOSOCIAL CONSIDERATIONS

Burn injury is one of the most psychologically devastating injuries to patients and their families. Not only is there a very real threat to survival, but also psychological and physical pain, fear of disfigurement, and uncertainty of long-term effects of the injury on the future can precipitate a crisis for the patient and family. Before appropriate functioning returns, the patient may exhibit stages of psychological adaptation (Box 20-3). A patient may not manifest every stage, but support and therapy are necessary for any patient and family experiencing major burn injury.

To facilitate a person's emotional adjustment to burn trauma, it is necessary to consider the complex interaction of preinjury personality, extent of injury, social support systems, and home environment. For example, many burn injuries are the result of suicide attempts, abuse, assaults, or arson. The patient may be dealing with loss of loved ones in the fire, injury event flashbacks, loss of home and belongings, job or financial concerns, or fear of assailants. The patient may also be facing legal consequences. Preinjury psychiatric disorders such as depression, mood disorders, psychoses, and alcohol and drug abuse frequently exist in the burn patient population.[12,52] Therefore, the critical care nurse must assess the patient's and family's support systems, coping mechanisms, and potential for developing posttraumatic stress disorder. Inadequate coping is demonstrated by changes in behavior, manipulation, regression, sleep deprivation, or depression. Interventions based on individual assessments are the most beneficial and may require assistance from support personnel such as chaplains, clinical nurse specialists, child life specialists, psychiatrists, psychologists, and social workers. As the patient is transferred from the critical care unit, support mechanisms and continuity of care must be maintained because psychosocial recovery can take months, years, or a lifetime.

GERIATRIC CONCERNS

As a group, older patients are more prone to and more adversely affected by burns.[3,18,31,41] Diminished

---

BOX 20-3   Stages of Postburn Psychological Adaptation

Survival Anxiety
Manifested by lack of concentration, easy startle response, tearfulness, social withdrawal, and inappropriate behavior. Instructions must be repeated, and the patient has to be allowed time to verbalize concerns and fears. Increased reports of pain are frequently associated with high levels of anxiety.

Search for Meaning
Patient repeatedly recounts events leading to the injury and tries to determine a logical explanation that is emotionally acceptable. It is important to avoid judging the patient's reasoning and to listen actively and to participate in the discussions with the patient.

Investment in Recuperation
Patient is cooperative with the treatment regimen, motivated to be independent, and takes pride in small accomplishments. The nurse should educate the patient concerning discharge goals and involve both patient and family in planning for a program of increased self-care. Patient requires much praise and verbal encouragement.

Investment in Rehabilitation
As self-confidence increases, patient is focused on achieving as much preburn function as possible. Depression may occur as new losses in function are realized. Staff support is limited in this phase, which usually occurs after patient is discharged from the hospital and is undergoing outpatient rehabilitation. Praise, support, and continued information are beneficial.

Reintegration of Identity
Patient accepts losses and recognizes that changes have occurred. Adaptation is completed, and staff involvement is terminated.

Modified from Watkins, P., Cook, E., May, S., & Ehleben, C. (1988). Psychological stages in adaptation following burn injury: A method for facilitating psychological recovery of burn victims. *Journal of Burn Care & Rehabilitation,* 9(4), 376-384.

---

manual dexterity, reaction time, vision, hearing, and judgment render the elderly vulnerable to burn injuries. Many older people live alone and are often physically or mentally unable to respond appropriately to an emergency. In addition, elderly skin is much less resilient to mechanical trauma. A growing concern is the incidence of elder abuse or neglect. It may be more difficult to identify potential elderly abuse cases since older individuals often live alone and predominantly interact with the abusing caregiver.[20] The physiological and psychosocial trauma of a burn injury in the elderly patient provides a tremendous challenge for the burn team.

Many variables influence outcome of the elderly burn patient and increase mortality including the size and extent of the burn, the number and severity of coexisting diseases, and the development of postinjury complications (see Geriatric Considerations).[3,38,43] Preinjury hydration status, nutritional deficiencies, and diseases may contribute to a higher mortality or difficulties in fluid resuscitation and combating burn shock. Older patients with heart failure may require administration of positive inotropic medications to increase cardiac contractility. Elderly patients with inhalation injury frequently require mechanical ventilation support and are more prone to episodes of pneumonia and sepsis. Wound care presents a challenge. Skin changes associated with aging, such as a flattened dermal-epidermal junction and a loss of dermal and subcutaneous mass, manifest as skin thinning and predispose this group to deeper burn wounds and to poor or delayed healing. This situation affects not only the healing of the original burn wounds, but also the skin graft recipient beds and donor sites. A decline in immune system function increases susceptibility to infectious complications in this group as well. Older patients also have a diminished physiological reserve and capacity to respond to the metabolic stress and bacterial challenge after a burn injury.

Advances in technology and treatment have improved survival after burn injury.[9,34,38,39] However, data suggest that advanced age, especially in combination with inhalation injury, continues to be a major determinant of mortality after thermal injury.[18,31] The decision to proceed with resuscitation in elderly patients with large burns and concomitant inhalation injury should be carefully considered, with advanced directives, health care surrogate, or next of kin.[18,38,41] Preexisting dementia exacerbated by injury and medications has major implications for elderly patients being able to participate in rehabilitation to regain function and independence. It may be more prudent to target interventions to reduce pain, maintain independence and sustain quality of life, rather than increase life span.[38] Poor outcomes after injury highlight that prevention of burn injuries in the elderly is of utmost importance. Avoidance of high-risk activities by the elderly and their caregivers should occur. Cooking, yard work, smoking, hot bathing water, and home heating devices are often reported as sources of burn injuries in this group.[3,31]

GERIATRIC CONSIDERATIONS

- Determine as early as possible whether the patient has an advanced directive.
- Elderly patients have reduced physiological reserves and capacity to respond to the metabolic stress of burn injury.
- Preexisting cardiovascular, renal, and pulmonary diseases lead to challenges in fluid resuscitation.
- Fluid administration may be guided by hemodynamic monitoring.
- Physiological changes in the skin from aging predispose elderly patients to deeper burn wounds and poor or delayed wound healing. Burn wounds, grafts, and donor sites must be monitored carefully.
- Decline in immune system functioning contributes to increased susceptibility to infection.
- Mechanical ventilation contributes to a higher risk of pneumonia, sepsis, and complications of immobility. Ventilator weaning may be prolonged because of muscular weakness.
- Reduced renal and hepatic functioning predisposes elderly patients to delayed clearance of medications (antibiotics, analgesics) and increased potential for toxicity or overdose.
- Elderly patients have greater morbidity and mortality compared with younger patients with similar percentages of total body surface area burn.[18,31,38]

NONBURN INJURY

The experience of the burn team in providing excellent wound and critical care leads to burn unit admissions of patients with a variety of other severe exfoliative and necrotizing skin disorders such as toxic epidermal necrolysis (TEN), staphylococcal scalded skin syndrome, and necrotizing fasciitis. These conditions create a clinical wound picture similar to that of a burn wound and require similar patient management and wound care. Management of these patients in a burn center has been associated with a marked increase in survival.[4,19,21,40]

Severe Exfoliative Disorders

Toxic Epidermal Necrolysis, Stevens-Johnson Syndrome, Erythema Multiforme

TEN, Stevens-Johnson syndrome, and erythema multiforme are similar conditions in which the body sloughs its epidermal layer in response to some causative agent. The skin separation occurs at the epidermal-dermal junction, with varying degrees of dermal involvement. Clinically, it is difficult to diagnose these similar disorders. Assessment of the extent of cutaneous involvement and skin biopsy for histopathology are required for differential diagnosis. However, nursing diagnoses and interventions are the same for all severe exfoliative disorders.

TEN is the most extensive form of severe exfoliative disorder and is the focus of discussion. It is associated with a mortality rate of 32%.[35] The most common cause of TEN is drug reaction, particularly from sulfa drugs, phenobarbital, and phenytoin. However, up to 26% of cases have no identified etiology.[4] Patients initially have fever and flulike symptoms, with erythema and blisters developing within 24 to 96 hours. As large bullae develop, the skin and mucous membranes slough, resulting in a significant and painful partial-thickness injury. TEN is also associated with mucosal wound involvement of conjunctival, oral, GI tract, and/or urogenital areas.[4,21,35,40] Immune suppression occurs and contributes to life-threatening complications such as sepsis and pneumonia. Primary treatment includes discontinuation of the offending drug. Optimal wound treatment consists of early coverage of cutaneous wounds with biological dressings. Severe exfoliative disorders typically require intensive critical care management to provide fluid resuscitation and nutritional support. Corticosteroids should not be given.[4,40] IV immune globulin administration may be beneficial.[40] Care is primarily supportive, with prevention of infection being crucial to stop progression of wounds to full-thickness depth. Long-term follow-up with the burn team is important to monitor for the development of commonly reported ophthalmic, skin, nail, and vulvovaginal complications and to address continued issues in health-related quality of life.[21]

Staphylococcal Scalded Skin Syndrome

Staphylococcal scalded skin (SSS) syndrome occurs primarily in children and often presents with a clinical picture similar to that of TEN. SSS syndrome is caused by a reaction to a staphylococcal toxin, with intraepidermal splitting (unlike epidermal-dermal separation in TEN) resulting in skin sloughing. The differential diagnosis is made by microscopic examination of the denuded skin to determine the level of skin separation.[4,40] SSS syndrome is limited to epidermal involvement and does not affect the mucous membranes. A low mortality rate (5%) exists with this condition in children, although the mortality rate may be as high as 60% in adults.[37] SSS syndrome is best treated with antibiotic therapy and wound care management.

Necrotizing Soft Tissue Infections

Names for necrotizing soft tissue infections include necrotizing fasciitis, gas gangrene, hemolytic strep-tococcal gangrene, and necrotizing cellulitis. When a necrotizing infection involves the perineum and scrotum, it is referred to as Fournier's gangrene.[19] Necrotizing fasciitis occurs more frequently in adults and is associated with a 17% mortality rate.[19] It is caused by toxin-producing organisms, often introduced from minor skin disruptions such as insect bites or cuts, that lead to widespread fascial and muscle necrosis. Diabetes, obesity, and hypertension are risk factors for the development of necrotizing fasciitis.[19] Necrotizing fasciitis has a subtle initial presentation of a localized, painful edematous area with increasing erythema and crepitus. The pain is severe and out of proportion to cutaneous findings. Early diagnosis, aggressive surgical excision and wound care, and antibiotic therapy are essential for a positive outcome.

DISCHARGE PLANNING

Discharge planning for critically ill burned patients or those who have sustained a nonburn injury must begin on the day of admission. Assessments are made regarding patient survival, the potential or actual short-term or long-term functional disabilities secondary to the burn or nonburn injury, the financial resources available, the family roles and expectations, and the psychological support systems. Patient and family education is essential to prepare for transfer from the critical care unit and eventual discharge from the hospital. Patients and families who are returning home must understand how to manage their physical requirements, as well as care for their psychological and social needs. Nurses play an important role in multidisciplinary discharge planning by providing patient and family education and by evaluating the need for additional resources to meet the patient's long-term rehabilitative and home care requirements.

BURN PREVENTION

The overwhelming majority of burns and fire-related injuries are preventable. Typically, injuries do not occur from random events or "accidents," but rather predominately from predictable incidents. If people are not aware of potential risks, they do not take appropriate precautions to prevent an injury from occurring. Successful prevention efforts consider the targeted population and focus on interventions involving education, engineering/environment (i.e., modifications in safety designs), or enforcement (i.e., laws or safety regulations). Critical care nurses play an active and vital role in teaching prevention concepts and in promoting fire safety legislation that assists in preventing fires and burn injuries. The incidence of burn injuries has been successfully decreased with government-mandated regulations on industrial environments, products, and home safety (e.g., hot water heater temperature, self-extinguishing cigarettes, and mandatory smoke detectors).[25] Box 20-4 lists strategies for preventing burn injuries.

BOX 20-4   Strategies for Preventing Burn Injuries

Cook with Care
- Turn pot handles toward back of the stove.
- Keep appliances with long cords toward back of the counter.
- Always use cooking mitts, and never carry more than you can safely handle.
- Never wear loose sleeves or other loose clothing while cooking.
- Always set a kitchen timer as reminder to turn off burners and oven.
- If a pan of food catches fire, carefully slide a lid over the pan and turn off burner.
- Never throw water on a grease or electrical fire. Turn off heat source and, if necessary, use a smothering substance such as salt or baking soda.
- Many injuries occur when hot liquids are pulled from the microwave.
- Stir microwave foods to distribute heat, and test all heated foods before giving to a child.
- Create a safety zone for children by using gates, playpens, and highchairs to keep them at a safe distance from all hot items.

Hot Liquids Cause Scalds
- Never hold an infant or child while pouring or drinking hot liquids.
- Bath water is a potentially dangerous hot liquid; keep water heater at 120° F; use a thermometer to check water temperature before touching bath water.

Home Precautions
- Teach children to use the stop, drop, and roll technique when they or their clothes are on fire.
- Small children often use their teeth to pull apart plugs; keep electrical cords out of reach, and teach safety.
- Keep all matches and lighters out of the reach of children.
- Teach children to stay away from high-voltage utilities.
- Teach older children how to use appliances safely and about the danger of electricity near water.
- Do not overload outlets.
- Use only Underwriters Laboratory UL-approved portable space heaters, and keep space heaters 3 feet away from everything, including yourself; do not use them with extension cords.

- Be safe when smoking: use large, deep ashtrays, and dispose of ashes in toilet; do not smoke while lying down or in bed (quitting smoking is the best safety precaution of all).
- There is only one acceptable use of gasoline: fueling an engine.
- Put sunscreen on you and your children.
- Be prepared for a fire emergency: practice escape routes with children and babysitters; small children could become frightened and hide when faced with an unfamiliar emergency situation.
- Keep all flame sources away from home oxygen.
- Acknowledge that alcohol, drugs, and some medications impair balance, judgment, and reaction time; use caution around fire sources.
- Closely supervise burning candles; keep them out of reach of children and pets who may knock them over; never leave candles burning while sleeping.
- Never store flammable liquids (gasoline, propane, cleaners, paint solvents) near fire sources such as a furnace or pilot light.

Fire Extinguishers and Smoke Detectors
- Fire extinguishers must be easily accessible (near exits).
- Learn how to use your fire extinguisher.
- Properly working smoke detectors are burn prevention tools; they prevent injury and save lives.
- Install several smoke detectors; check batteries and sensors regularly.

Occupation-Related Precautions
- Always wear safety equipment and personal protection gear.
- Fatigue contributes to carelessness and accidents; take breaks to prevent accidents.
- Know the location of emergency exits, fire extinguishers, safety showers and eye washers, and main electrical and/or gas shutoff valves.
- Be familiar with potential chemical hazards in the workplace; review Material Safety Data Sheets.

CASE STUDY

evolve

Mrs. J. is a 70-year-old woman who sustained a thermal burn injury in a house fire. An electric heater ignited her bedspread while she was asleep. She was trapped in the room for approximately 15 minutes before being rescued by firefighters.

QUESTIONS

1. Once Mrs. J. is removed from the fire, what priorities are essential in her initial management?
2. She has singed nose hair and is coughing up sooty sputum. The emergency department is 15 minutes away. Based on this assessment, what should the paramedics do?
3. What diagnostic tests and assessments do you anticipate once Mrs. J. reaches the emergency department?
4. Mrs. J. weighs 65 kg. She has burned an estimated 30% of her body. What is her estimated fluid requirement during the first 24 hours?
5. How much fluid will be given in the first 8 hours after the injury?
6. Given Mrs. J.'s age, what are important assessments during aggressive fluid resuscitation?
7. Mrs. J. has circumferential, white, leathery burn wounds on both arms. What type of burn wound does she have? What assessments should be performed? What type of surgical treatment and wound care should be expected during the resuscitative phase, and later in the acute care phase?
8. What type and route of pain medication should be administered to Mrs. J.?

SUMMARY

The physiological response to a major burn injury is one of a biphasic pattern of multiorgan system hypofunction followed by hyperfunction. A major goal of resuscitative care is the prevention of burn shock. The critical care nurse's observations of patient responses are crucial for the prevention of complications related to increased capillary permeability and massive resuscitation fluid therapy. In the acute phase, therapeutic goals include prevention of further tissue loss, maintenance of function, prevention of infection, and wound closure. As the patient progresses through various stages of wound care management, the nurse must not only provide skilled care but also monitor the patient's and family's responses to the treatment regimen. Psychosocial support is integral to the entire process. Although providing care to the burned patient is a team effort, it is the critical care nurse who is with the patient 24 hours a day. The skill and support of the nurse make the critical difference in the patient's outcome.

CRITICAL THINKING QUESTIONS

evolve

1. Explain why patients with burns need extensive fluid resuscitation even though they are extremely edematous.
2. What strategies might you use to meet the high caloric needs of burn patients who can take foods by mouth?
3. What interventions can be used in the critical care unit to promote early rehabilitation of a burned patient?
4. Many burned patients must be treated at institutions far away from home. What approaches can be used to meet the psychosocial needs of these patients and their families?

evolve Be sure to check out the bonus material, including free self-assessment exercises, on the Evolve Web site at http://evolve.elsevier.com/Sole.

REFERENCES

1. Agency for Health Care Policy and Research. (1992). *Clinical practice guideline. Acute pain management: Operative or medical procedures and trauma* (No. 92-0032). Rockville, MD: U.S. Department of Health and Human Services.

2. Ahrns, K. S. (2004). Trends in burn resuscitation: Shifting the focus from fluids to adequate endpoint monitoring, edema control, and adjuvant therapies. *Critical Care Nursing Clinics of North America, 16*(1), 75-98.

3. Alden, N. E., Bessey, P. Q., Rabbitts, A., Hyden, P. J., & Yurt, R. W. (2007). Tap water scalds among seniors and the elderly: Socio-economics and implications for prevention. *Burns, 33*(5), 666-669.

4. American Burn Association. (2005). *Advanced burn life support course: Provider's manual.* Chicago: American Burn Association.

5. American Burn Association (ABA). (2007). *National burn repository: 2006 report.* Chicago: American Burn Association.

6. American Burn Association/American College of Surgeons. (2007). Guidelines for the operation of burn centers. *Journal of Burn Care & Research, 28*(1), 134-141.

7. Arbabi, S., Ahrns, K. S., Wahl, W. L., Hemmila, M. R., Wang, S. C., Brandt, M. M., et al. (2004). Beta-blocker use is associated with improved outcomes in adult burn patients. *Journal of Trauma, 56*(2), 265-271.

8. Atiyeh, B. S., & Costagliola, M. (2007). Cultured epithelial autograft (CEA) in burn treatment: Three decades later. *Burns, 33*(4), 405-413.

9. Barret, J. P., & Herndon, D. N. (2003). Effects of burn wound excision on bacterial colonization and invasion. *Plastic and Reconstructive Surgery, 111*(2), 744-752.

10. Carrougher, G. J., Ptacek, J. T., Sharar, S. R., Wiechmans, S., Honari, S., Patterson, O. R., et al. (2003). Comparison of patient satisfaction and self-reports of pain in adult burn-injured patients. *Journal of Burn Care & Rehabilitation, 24*(1), 1-8.

11. Chung, K. K., Blackbourne, L. H., Wolf, S. E., White, C. E., Renz, E. M., Cancio, L. C., et al. (2006). Evolution of burn resuscitation in operation Iraqi freedom. *Journal of Burn Care & Research, 27*(5), 606-611.

12. Cone, J. B. (2005). What's new in general surgery: Burns and metabolism. *Journal of the American College of Surgeons, 200*(4), 607-615.

13. Cope, O., & Moore, F. D. (1947). The redistribution of body water in the fluid therapy of the burn patient. *Annals of Surgery, 126*, 1010-1018.

14. Demling, R. H. (2005). The burn edema process: Current concepts. *Journal of Burn Care & Rehabilitation, 26*(3), 207-227.

15. Demling, R. H., Mazess, R. B., Witt, R. M., & Wolberg, W. H. (1978). The study of burn wound edema using dichromatic absorptiometry. *Journal of Trauma, 18*(2), 124-128.

16. Demling, R. H., Wong, C., Jin, L. J., Hechtman, H., Lalonde, C., & West, K. (1985). Early lung dysfunction after major burns: Role of edema and vasoactive mediators. *Journal of Trauma, 25*(10), 959-966.

17. Edelman, D. A., Khan, N., Kempf, K., & White, M. T. (2007). Pneumonia after inhalation injury. *Journal of Burn Care & Research, 28*(2), 241-246.

18. Edelman, D. A., White, M. T., Tyburski, J. G., & Wilson, R. F. (2006). Factors affecting prognosis of inhalation injury. *Journal of Burn Care & Research, 27*(6), 848-853.

19. Endorf, F. W., Supple, K. G., & Gamelli, R. L. (2005). The evolving characteristics and care of necrotizing soft-tissue infections. *Burns, 31*(3), 269-273.

20. Greenbaum, A. R., Horton, J. B., Williams, C. J., Shah, M., & Dunn, K. W. (2006). Burn injuries inflicted on children or the elderly: A framework for clinical and forensic assessment. *Plastic and Reconstructive Surgery, 118*(2), 46e-58e.

21. Haber, J., Hopman, W., Gomez, M., & Cartotto, R. (2005). Late outcomes in adult survivors of toxic epidermal necrolysis after treatment in a burn center. *Journal of Burn Care & Rehabilitation, 26*(1), 33-41.

22. Hart, D. W., Wolf, S. E., Mlcak, R., Chinkes, D. L., Ranzy, P. I., Obeng, M. K., et al. (2000). Persistence of muscle catabolism after severe burn. *Surgery, 128*(2), 312-319.

23. Hoesel, L. M., Niederbichler, A. D., Schaefer, J., Ipakchi, K. R., Gao, H., Rittirsch, D., et al. (2007). C5a-blockade improves burn-induced cardiac dysfunction. *Journal of Immunology, 178*(12), 7902-7910.

24. Holm, C., Mayr, M., Tegeler, J., Hürbrand, F., Henckel von Donnersmarck, G., et al. (2004). A clinical randomized study on the effects of invasive monitoring on burn shock resuscitation. *Burns, 30*(8), 798-807.

25. Hunt, J. L., & Purdue, G. F. (2002). Prevention of burn injuries. In D. N. Herndon (Ed.), *Total burn care* (2nd ed.). London: Harcourt Publishers.

26. Ipaktchi, K., & Arbabi, S. (2006). Advances in burn critical care. *Critical Care Medicine, 34*(Suppl. 9), S239-S244.

27. Jonsson, C. E., Holmsten, A., Dahlstrom, L., & Jonsson, K. (1998). Background pain in burn patients: Routine measurement and recording of pain intensity in a burn unit. *Burns, 24*(5), 448-454.

28. Kamolz, L. P., Andel, H., Haslik, W., Winter, W., Meissl, G., Frey, M. (2004). Use of subatmospheric pressure therapy to prevent burn wound progression in human: First experiences. *Burns, 30*(3), 253-258.

29. Karter, M. J. (2006). *Fire loss in the United States during 2005—Full report.* Quincy, MA: National Fire Protection Association, Fire Analysis and Research Division.

30. Kidd, M., Hultman, C. S., Van Aalst, J., Calvert, C., Peck, M. D., & Cairns, B. A. (2007). The contemporary management of electrical injuries: Resuscitation, reconstruction, rehabilitation. *Annals of Plastic Surgery, 58*(3), 273-278.

31. Lionelli, G. T., Pickus, E. J., Beckum, O. K., Decoursey, R. L., & Korentager, R. A. (2005). A three decade analysis of factors affecting burn mortality in the elderly. *Burns, 31*(8), 958-963.

32. Llanos, S., Danilla, S., Barraza, C., Armijo, E., Piñeros, J. L., Quintas, M., et al. (2006). Effectiveness of negative pressure closure in the integration of split thickness skin grafts: A randomized, double-masked, controlled trial. *Annals of Surgery, 244*(5), 700-705.

33. Mikhail, J. (1999). Resuscitation end points in trauma. *AACN Clinical Issues, 10*(1), 10-21.

34. Mlcak, R. P., Suman, O. E., Herndon, D. N. (2007). Respiratory management of inhalation injury. *Burns, 33*(1), 2-13.

35. Palmieri, T. L., Greenhalgh, D. G., Saffle, J. R., Spence, R. J., Peck, M. D., Jeng, J. C., et al. (2002). A multicenter review of toxic epidermal necrolysis treated in U.S. burn centers at the end of the twentieth century. *Journal of Burn Care & Rehabilitation, 23*(2), 87-96.

36. Parra, M. W., Al-Khayat, H., Smith, H. G., & Cheatham, M. L. (2006). Paracentesis for resuscitation-induced abdominal compartment syndrome: An alternative to decompressive laparotomy in the burn patient. *Journal of Trauma, 60*(5), 1119-1121.

37. Patel, G. K., & Finlay, A. Y. (2003). Staphylococcal scalded skin syndrome: Diagnosis and management. *American Journal of Clinical Dermatology, 4*(3), 165-175.

38. Pereira, C. T., Barrow, R. E., Sterns, A. M., Hawkins, H. K., Kimbrough, C. W., Jeschke, M. G., et al. (2006). Age-dependent differences in survival after severe burns: A unicentric review of 1674 patients and 179 autopsies over 15 years. *Journal of the American College of Surgeons, 202*(3), 536-548.

39. Pereira, C. T., Murphy, K. D., & Herndon, D. N. (2005). Altering metabolism. *Journal of Burn Care & Rehabilitation, 26*(3), 194-199.

40. Pereira, F. A., Mudgil, A. V., & Rosmarin, D. M. (2007). Toxic epidermal necrolysis. *Journal of the American Academy of Dermatology, 56*(2), 181-200.

41. Pomahac, B., Matros, E., Semel, M., Chan, R. K., Rogers, S. O., Demling, R., et al. (2006). Predictors of survival and length of stay in burn patients older than 80 years of age: Does age really matter? *Journal of Burn Care & Research, 27*(3), 265-269.

42. Prelack, K., Dylewski, M., & Sheridan, R. L. (2007). Practical guidelines for nutritional management of burn injury and recovery. *Burns, 33*(1), 14-24.

43. Rao, K., Ali, S. N., & Moiemen, N. S. (2006). Aetiology and outcome of burns in the elderly. *Burns, 32*(7), 802-805.

44. Rose, J. K., & Herndon, D. N. (1997). Advances in the treatment of burn patients. *Burns, 23*(Suppl. 1), S19-S26.

45. Saffle, J. R. (2007). The phenomenon of "fluid creep" in acute burn resuscitation. *Journal of Burn Care & Research, 28*(3), 382-395.

46. Santos, A. P., Wilson, A. K., Hornung, C. A., Polk, H. C., Rodriguez, J. L., & Franklin, G. A. (2005). Methamphetamine laboratory explosions: A new and emerging burn injury. *Journal of Burn Care & Rehabilitation, 26*(3), 228-232.

47. Silver, G. M., Klein, M. B., Herndon, D. N., Gamelli, R. L., Gibran, N. S., Alstein, L., et al. (2007). The Inflammation and the Host Response to Trauma, Collaborative Research Program. Standard operating procedures for the clinical management of patients enrolled in a prospective study of Inflammation and the host response to thermal injury. *Journal of Burn Care & Research, 28*(2), 222-230.

48. Sim, K. M., Hwang, C., Chan, Y. W., & Seah, C. S. (1996). Use of patient-controlled analgesia with alfentanil for burn dressing procedures: A preliminary report of five patients. *Burns, 22*(3), 238-241.

49. Summer, G. J., Puntillo, K. A., Miaskowski, C., Green, P. G., & Levine, J. D. (2007). Burn injury pain: The continuing challenge. *Journal of Pain, 8*(7), 533-548.

50. Wahl, W. L., Brandt, M. M., Ahrns, K. S., Zajkowski, P. J., Proctor, M. C., Wakefield, T. W., et al. (2002). Venous thrombosis incidence in burn patients: Preliminary results of a prospective study. *Journal of Burn Care & Rehabilitation, 23*(2), 97-102.

51. Wahl, W. L., Dawson, C., Pennington, K., et al. (2007). ICU core measures for burn patients. *Journal of Burn Care & Research, 28*(2), S95.

52. Wisely, J. A., Hoyle, E., Tarrier, N., & Edwards J. (2007). Where to start? Attempting to meet the psychological needs of burned patients. *Burns 33*(6), 736-746.

53. Wolf, S. E., Edelman, L. S., Kemalyan, N., Donison, L., Cross, J., Underwood, M., et al. (2006). Effects of oxandrolone on outcome measures in the severely burned: A multicenter prospective randomized double-blind trial. *Journal of Burn Care & Research, 27*(2), 131-139.

54. Wray, C. J., Mammen, J. M. V., & Hasselgren, P. (2002). Catabolic response to stress and potential benefits of nutrition support. *Nutrition, 18*(11/12), 971-977.

Index

Page numbers followed by f indicate figures; t, tables; b, boxes.